Neurologic Disease in Women

Second Edition

Neurologic Disease in Women

Second Edition

EDITED BY

PETER W. KAPLAN, MB, FRCP

Professor of Neurology
Johns Hopkins University School of Medicine
and
Chairman, Department of Neurology
Johns Hopkins Bayview Medical Center
Baltimore, Maryland

2006

Demos

New York

Demos Medical Publishing, Inc.

386 Park Avenue South, New York, New York 10016

Visit our website at www.demosmedpub.com

Library of Congress Cataloging-in-Publication Data

Neurologic disease in women / edited by Peter W. Kaplan.
     p. ; cm.
   Includes bibliographical references and index.
   ISBN 1-888799-85-4 (hardcover : alk. paper)
   1. Nervous system—Diseases.   2. Women—Diseases.   3. Sex factors in disease.
I. Kaplan, Peter W., 1951–   .
   [DNLM: 1. Nervous System Diseases.   2. Sex Factors.   3. Women's Health.
WL 140 N49157 2006]
   RC361.N465   2006
   616.8'082—dc22

                                                            2005016608

Made in the United States of America

Copyeditor: Joann Woy, Freelance Editorial Services
Production/Typesetter: Patricia Wallenburg, TypeWriting
Printer: The Maple-Vail Book Manufacturing Group
Indexer: Joann Woy, Freelance Editorial Services

Dedication

To Nora, Emma, and Alexander,
    Lenna and Martin,
    Alexa and Jeffrey,
    who have been a limitless source of support and inspiration

Contents

II LIFE STAGES AND NEUROLOGIC DISEASE EXPRESSION IN WOMEN

III NEUROLOGIC DISORDERS IN WOMEN

Preface

Although a general understanding persists that the human brain functions similarly in women and in men, an increasing body of knowledge indicates that neuronal connectivity, recruitment, and disease patterns exhibit gender differences. Imaging techniques such as positron emission computerized tomography (PET) and single photon emission computerized tomography (SPECT) have highlighted some gender-based differences in human brain function.

Clear gender differences are present in genetic expression, physiologic function, metabolism, hormonal makeup, and psychosocial profile, which often modify the clinical expression of neurologic and other diseases. In addition, ethnic, cultural, and economic factors are frequently overlooked in dealing with the health problems of women, even though they undoubtedly have a strong influence on the clinical course of the illness. The World Health Organization (WHO) has highlighted a number of relevant factors, including women's lower social and economic status that adversely affect health in early childhood; in many countries girls receive less food, education, and health care than do boys. Each year, half a million women die from causes related to pregnancy and childbirth; 90% of them are in poorer countries. Women carry the burden of care within the family, and their health has a strong generational impact on the children they bear and rear, and hence on society.

We now have many clinical studies demonstrating gender differences in disease prevalence, clinical features, and response to treatment, yet many studies propose similar management and medication guidelines for both sexes. Furthermore, for various reasons, drug trials have often avoided including women and children and, in so doing, have generated data that fail to enlighten us on important medical issues relating to these populations. Of particular concern is the situation of the pregnant woman, for whom the treating physician is often uncertain about how to proceed and is in need of information regarding conditions, diseases, and their treatment—as, for example, in migraine, epilepsy, depression, autoimmune disease, and other neurologic disorders. Finally, there is the elderly woman, whose longer life expectancy now renders her more vulnerable to dementia and many other medical problems that may give rise to a condition of physical and/or mental "frailty." The need for special attention is intensified by the aging of this population and the attendant problems such as increasing instability of gait, multiple falls, and reliance on supportive care. Much new data have appeared on the risks and benefits of hormone replacement therapy (HRT) in postmenopausal women.

This second edition of *Neurologic Disease in Women* was designed to help physicians and other medical personnel seeking information relevant to patient care, and to this end is divided into three sections. The first addresses general anatomic, hormonal, epidemiologic, and drug aspects of women's health. The second relates to neurologic conditions that arise during childhood, pregnancy, adulthood, and old age. The third covers specific neurologic conditions that present differently or predominantly in females. Because this book is organized by subject, with the authors' particular viewpoints, some overlap occurs in areas common to several chapters. For example, each chapter may discuss medications useful in particular disorders, but will also address these issues in chapters on pregnancy and drug treatment trials in women. Similarly, particular diseases or gender issues may arise in several chapters, but are further focused in the chapter on genetics. I believe that this cross-referencing of subject and chapter will permit the reader to pursue the breadth and depth of neurologic issues in women.

Important advances in several areas led to the inclusion of new chapters, new approaches, and additional information provided in the chapters on hormonal effects in women and the use of HRT; the adverse effects of antiepileptic drugs on hormonal homeostasis, weight, and bone health; and cardiovascular diseases in women. New chapters include reproductive and metabolic disorders with antiepileptic drug use and movement disorders. Other chapters remain relatively unchanged, for example, regarding women, law, and neurologic disease, and the effects of menstruation and pregnancy on neurologic disease.

The authors and I hope that this reference text will help in a more directed approach to understanding and treating neurologic diseases in women.

Acknowledgments

This is a multiauthored and multidisciplinary work. I am grateful to all the contributors for their efforts and patience throughout the rather prolonged revisions of the manuscripts. I would especially like to thank Joyce Caplan, who performed expert secretarial assistance and editing functions on the draft manuscript.

Contributors

Joan C. Amatniek, MD
Visiting Research Associate
Columbia University
G. H. Sergievsky Center and Department of Neurology
College of Physicians and Surgeons
New York, New York
and
Director, Clinical Development
Alzheimer's Disease
Ortho-McNeil Neurologics, Inc.
Titusville, New Jersey

J. Thomas Benson, MD
Clinical Professor, Obstetrics and Gynecology
Indiana University School of Medicine
Director, Female Pelvic Medicine and Reconstructive
    Surgery Fellowship
Indianapolis, Indiana

H. Richard Beresford, MD
Adjunct Professor of Law
Cornell Law School
Myron Taylor Hall
Ithaca, New York
and
Professor of Neurology
University of Rochester School of Medicine
Rochester, New York

Gretchen L. Birbeck, MD, MPH
Associate Professor
Departments of Neurology and Epidemiology
Michigan State University
African Studies Center Core Faculty
East Lansing, Michigan

Yvette M. Bordelon, MD, PhD
Assistant Professor
Department of Neurology
UCLA Medical Center
Los Angeles, California

Linda Brubaker, MD
Professor and Fellowship Director
Department of Obstetrics and Gynecology
Female Pelvic Medicine and Reconstructive Surgery
Loyola University Medical Center
Maywood, Illinois

P. K. Coyle, MD
Professor of Neurology and Acting Chair
Department of Neurology
SUNY at Stony Brook
    and
Director of Stony Brook MS Comprehensive Care Center
SUNY at Stony Brook
Stony Brook, New York

James O. Donaldson III, MD
Professor of Neurology
University of Connecticut Health Center
Farmington, Connecticut

Stanley Fahn, MD
H. Houston Merritt Professor of Neurology
Director, Center for Parkinson's Disease and Other
    Movement Disorders
Columbia University Medical Center
Neurological Institute
New York, New York

Lauren C. Frey, MD
Instructor
Department of Neurology
Anschutz Outpatient Pavilion
University of Colorado Health Sciences Center
Denver, Colorado

James M. Gilchrist, MD
Professor of Neurology
Department of Clinical Neuroscience
Brown Medical School
Rhode Island Hospital
Providence, Rhode Island

Angela S. Guarda, MD
Assistant Professor of Psychiatry
Johns Hopkins University School of Medicine
and
Director, Eating Disorders Program
The Johns Hopkins Hospital
Baltimore, Maryland

Mustafa Hammad, MD
Attending Physician
The Brain and Spine Center
Panama City, Florida

W. Allen Hauser, MD
Professor of Neurology and Public Health–
Epidemiology
Columbia University
G. H. Sergievsky Center and
Department of Neurology
College of Physicians and Surgeons
Mailman School of Public Health
New York, New York

David B. Hellmann, MD, MACP
Mary Betty Stevens Professor of Medicine
Department of Medicine
Johns Hopkins University School of Medicine
and
Chairman, Department of Medicine
Johns Hopkins Bayview Medical Center
Baltimore, Maryland

Orest Hurko, MD
Assistant Vice President
AVP Discovery Medicine
Wyeth Research
Collegeville, Pennyslvania

David N. Irani, MD
Assistant Professor of Neurology
Department of Neurology
Johns Hopkins University School of Medicine
and
Assistant Professor of Molecular Microbiology and
Immunology
Johns Hopkins University Bloomberg School of Public
Health
Johns Hopkins Hospital
Baltimore, Maryland

Julene K. Johnson, PhD
Assistant Professor of Medicine
Department of Neurology
Memory and Aging Center
University of California San Francisco
San Francisco, California

Peter W. Kaplan, MB, FRCP
Professor of Neurology
Johns Hopkins University School of Medicine
and
Chairman, Department of Neurology
Johns Hopkins Bayview Medical Center
Baltimore, Maryland

Ramesh Khurana, MD
Assistant Professor of Neurology
Johns Hopkins University School of Medicine
Clinical Associate Professor of Neurology
University of Maryland
and
Chief, Division of Neurology
Union Memorial Hospital
Baltimore, Maryland

Pavel Klein, MB, BChir
Mid-Atlantic Epilepsy and Sleep Center
Champlain Building
Bethesda, Maryland

Allan Krumholz, MD
Professor of Neurology
Department of Neurology
University of Maryland
Baltimore, Maryland

John J. Laterra, MD, PhD
Professor of Neurology, Oncology & Neuroscience
Johns Hopkins University School of Medicine
and
The Kennedy Krieger Research Institute
Baltimore, Maryland

Rafael H. Llinas, MD
Assistant Professor
Department of Neurology
Johns Hopkins University School of Medicine
and
Johns Hopkins Bayview Medical Center
Baltimore, Maryland

Aileen MacLaren Loranger, CNM, PhD
Clinical Assistant Professor, Family & Child Nursing
University of Washington School of Nursing
Seattle, Washington

E. Wayne Massey, MD
Clinical Associate Professor of Neurology
and
Clinical Director, MDA Clinics
Duke University Medical Center
Durham, North Carolina

Janice M. Massey, MD
Professor of Medicine
Division of Neurology
Duke University Medical Center
and
Director, EMG Laboratory
Durham, North Carolina

E. Jeffrey Metter, MD
Medical Officer
National Institutes on Aging
Clinical Research Branch
NIA-ASTRA
Harbor Hospital
and
Associate Professor
Department of Neurology
Johns Hopkins University School of Medicine
Baltimore, Maryland

Neil R. Miller, MD
Professor Neuro-Ophthalmology and Orbital Disease
Johns Hopkins University School of Medicine
and
Johns Hopkins Hospital
Baltimore, Maryland

Alan R. Moore, MD
Clinical Assistant Professor
Department of Neurology
University of Mississippi Medical Center
Jackson, Mississippi

Martha Morrell, MD
Clinical Professor of Neurology
Stanford University
and
Chief Medical Officer
NeuroPace, Inc.
Mountain View, CA

Holly Mussell, MD
Birmingham, Alabama

Errol R. Norwitz, MD, PhD
Associate Professor
Yale University School of Medicine
and
Director of Perinatal Research
Co-Director, Division of Maternal-Fetal Medicine
Department of Obstetrics, Gynecology and Reproductive Sciences
Yale–New Haven Hospital
New Haven, Connecticut

Alessandro Olivi, MD
Professor and Vice Chairman
Department of Neurosurgery
Johns Hopkins University School of Medicine
Chairman, Department of Neurosurgery
Johns Hopkins Bayview Medical Center
and
Director of Neurosurgical Oncology
Johns Hopkins Hospital
Baltimore, Maryland

Michelle Petri, MD, MPH
Professor of Medicine
Department of Medicine
Johns Hopkins University School of Medicine
Baltimore, Maryland

John T. Repke, MD
Professor and Chairman
Department of Obstetrics and Gynecology
Penn State University, College of Medicine
and
Obstetrician-Gynecologist-in-Chief
Milton S. Hershey Medical Center
Hershey, Pennsylvania

Susan M. Resnick, PhD
Senior Investigator
Laboratory of Personality and Cognition
National Institute on Aging
Gerontology Research Center
Baltimore, Maryland

S. Lane Rutledge, MD
Associate Professor of Pediatrics, Neurology, and
    Genetics
University of Alabama at Birmingham
    and
The Children's Hospital
Birmingham, Alabama

Donald L. Schomer, MD
Professor of Neurology
Harvard University
Director
Laboratory of Clinical Neurophysiology
Chief, Comprehensive Epilepsy Program
Beth Israel Deaconess Medical Center
Boston, Massachusetts

Stephen D. Silberstein, MD
Professor of Neurology
Thomas Jefferson University
School of Medicine
Director, Jefferson Headache Center
Thomas Jefferson University Hospital
Philadelphia, Pennsylvania

Karen L. Swartz, MD
Assistant Professor of Psychiatry
Johns Hopkins University School of Medicine
    and
Co-director, Mood Disorders Program
Johns Hopkins Hospital
Baltimore, Maryland

Tricia Ting, MD
Assistant Professor
Department of Neurology
University of Maryland School of Medicine
Baltimore, Maryland

Carla J. Weisman, MD
Faculty Practice Attending
Department of Obstetrics and Gynecology
Sinai Hospital
Baltimore, Maryland

Nancy Fugate Woods, PhD, RN, FAAN
Dean and Professor
University of Washington School of Nursing
Seattle, Washington

Kristine Yaffe, MD
Associate Professor of Psychiatry, Neurology, and
    Epidemiology
University of California San Francisco
    and
Chief, Geriatric Psychiatry
University of California San Francisco and San
    Francisco Veterans Association Medical Center
San Francisco, California

I

GENERAL ISSUES
IN WOMEN

1 Gender Differences in Disease of the Nervous System

Joan Amatniek, Lauren Frey, and W. Allen Hauser

The emphasis on women's issues in neurology and other health fields represents a trend that reflects the awareness that a particular disease may affect women in a way different from men and that diseases predominantly affecting women have been understudied. Although the management of conditions may vary by gender for biologic and sociologic reasons, more basic questions of epidemiologic interest arise. Are there conditions that are differentially distributed in populations by gender, and how do we interpret the differences in distribution to develop meaningful interventions that might be gender-specific?

CLUES TO OVERALL ETIOLOGY

Despite the difficulties in interpretation, basic descriptive epidemiologic data are important in hypothesis development, both to understand disease processes and develop interventions. Conditions that universally affect one gender with greater or lesser frequency suggest that some universal biologic factor associated with gender functions as a modifier of disease susceptibility or expression. A variation in frequency by gender across studies suggests that gender-specific environmental factors are important in the underlying disease mechanisms.

SPECIFICITY FOR WOMEN'S ISSUES

The identification of conditions that differentially affect one gender can alert the provider to altered risk and thus earlier intervention or therapy. This identification not only allows for the development of gender-specific preventive strategies, but also the development of gender-specific therapeutic interventions. Although recent emphasis in this area has been on the uniqueness of the female gender, the better understanding of factors such as hormonal influences on the disease process will be of universal benefit.

A number of strategies have been used to identify differential disease frequency by gender. None is perfect, and all are open to some criticism. Various levels of certainty of difference are based upon data source.

CLINICAL IMPRESSION

We all have impressions of the differential frequency of disease based upon our clinical perceptions. This may be driven by the most recent cases that have been evaluated, or, for specialists, may be driven by referral patterns. Although such data are important for hypothesis generation, such data must be considered anecdotal unless confirmed by other strategies.

CLINICAL SERIES

Collections of cases from individual clinicians, referral centers, or hospitals may provide somewhat better information regarding gender specificity. Despite substantial numbers, conclusions regarding the ratio of male to female cases from such collections of cases can be considerably flawed. One seldom is aware of the general referral base, much less its distribution by gender. Other important considerations may bias the impressions derived from such series.

Problems of Referral Bias in the Interpretation of Clinical Series

Several examples exist of neurologic conditions for which specific patterns of referral are influenced by gender. Table 1.1 lists the studies reviewed in this chapter.

Referral Bias: Parkinson Disease or Epilepsy in the Elderly

A difference clearly exists in health-seeking behavior in terms of referral between the elderly and the young. Younger individuals are much more likely to be referred for medical care than the elderly. For example, the age distribution of patients with Parkinson disease reported from clinical series from referral centers underenumerates the proportion in the oldest age groups. This is related to referral patterns and the tendency in the elderly not to seek specialized medical care (1). In this same situation, in many societies, elderly men are more likely to be referred than women.

Many studies of people with epilepsy depend upon the identification of cases through clinical neurophysiology laboratories. The elderly are much less frequently referred for such testing (2). Failure to take these referral patterns into account may in part explain differences in the frequency and gender distribution of epilepsy cases in some studies within the same region (3,4). Thus, an inappropriate perception of both age and gender distribution may occur in clinical series or epidemiologic studies if incomplete methods of ascertainment are used.

Self-Selection for Medical Care: The Young with Headache

Studies of headache identifying differences in health-seeking behavior between men and women. Women are more likely to seek medical care for this condition than men (5).

TABLE 1.1
Age/Gender Adjusted Incidence (per 100,000 Population)
Age Adjusted to the 1990 U.S. Population Unless Otherwise States

LOCATION	DURATION	MALE	FEMALE	AGE	COMMENTS	
STROKE: TOTAL						
Shiga, Japan (15)	1989–93	189.9	94.1	35 to 85+	*1980 Japanese population	
Southern Greece (16)	1994–95	362.4	276.1	18 to 85+	*European population	
Lund–Orup, Sweden (17)	1993–95	194.2	126.2	15 to 85+	*European population	
Melbourne, Australia (18)	1996–97	153	117	0 to 85+	*"World" population of Segi	
Hisayama, Japan (19)	1961–93	640	340	40+	*Unidentified "standard" population	
Bavaria, Germany (20)	1994–98	129.6	101.4	0 to 85+	*WHO standard European population	
Vittoria, Italy (21)	1991	200.9	194.7	0 to 85+		
No. Manhattan, N.Y. (22)	1993–96	204.5	143.8	20 to 85+		
No. Manhattan, N.Y. (22)	1993–96	259	222	20 to 85+	Black	*1990 US census for No. Manhattan
No. Manhattan, N.Y. (22)	1993–96	118	80	20 to 85+	White	*1990 US census for No. Manhattan
No. Manhattan, N.Y. (22)	1993–96	232	172	20 to 85+	Hispanic	*1990 US census for No. Manhattan
Belluno, Italy (23)	1992–93	208.2	166.2	<35 to 85+		
Shibata, Japan (24)	1977–92	849.3	680.3	40 to 70+		
Warsaw, Poland (25)	1991–92	169.2	125.1	<30 to 85+		
Malmo, Sweden (26)	1989	165.3	110.8	<45 to 85+		
Valle d'Asota (27)	1989	228.6	180.2	<55 to 85+		
Fredericksburg, Denmark (28)	1989–90	224.5	132.2	<55 to 85+		
Fredericksburg, Denmark (28)	1972–74	164.5	121.4	<55 to 85+		

(continued on next page)

TABLE 1.1

Age/Gender Adjusted Incidence (per 100,000 Population)
Age Adjusted to the 1990 U.S. Population Unless Otherwise States (continued)

LOCATION	DURATION	MALE	FEMALE	AGE	COMMENTS	
Umbria, Italy (29)	1986–89	193.2	147.8	<55 to 85+		
Dijon, France (30)	1985–86	188.5	101.7	<15 to 85+		
Perth, Australia (31)	1986	349.8	164.4	30 to 85+		
Soderham, Sweden (32)	1983–86	429.7	395.3	25 to 85+		
Soderham, Sweden (32)	1975–78	392.8	285.9	25 to 85+		
Auckland, New Zealand (33)	1981–82	204.3	178.7	15 to 85+		
Oxfordshire, England (34)	1981–82	177	162	<55 to 75+		
STROKE: SUBARACHNOID HEMORRHAGE						
Shiga, Japan (15)	1989–93	18.0	22.6	35 to 85+		*1980 Japanese population
Sweden (35)	1996	6.4	13.5	0 to 85+	ICH and SAH	*Swedish population
No. Manhattan, N.Y. (22)	1993–96	26.2	3.2	20 to 85+	Black	*1990 US census for No. Manhattan
No. Manhattan, N.Y. (22)	1993–96	4.9	11.9	20 to 85+	White	*1990 US census for No. Manhattan
No. Manhattan, N.Y. (22)	1993–96	6.3	15.6	20 to 85+	Hispanic	*1990 US census for No. Manhattan
Belluno, Italy (23)	1992–93	5.5	4.7	<35 to 85+		
Shibata, Japan (24)	1977–92	34.7	42.7	40 to 70+		
Valle d'Asota (27)	1989	5.0	5.0	<55 to 85+		*1988 Italian working population
STROKE: INTRACEREBRAL HEMORRHAGE						
Shiga, Japan (15)	1989–93	58.0	47.5	35 to 85+		*1980 Japanese population
No. Manhattan, N.Y. (22)	1993–96	37.2	34.9	20 to 85+	Black	*1990 US census for No. Manhattan
No. Manhattan, N.Y. (22)	1993–96	15.3	10.8	20 to 85+	White	*1990 US census for No. Manhattan
No. Manhattan, N.Y. (22)	1993–96	44.2	22.0	20 to 85+	Hispanic	*1990 US census for No. Manhattan
Belluno, Italy (23)	1992–93	33.9	34.8	<35 to 85+		
Shibata, Japan (24)	1977–92	94.1	15.9	40 to 70+		
Valle d'Asota (27)	1989	22.0	36.0	<55 to 85+		*1988 Italian working population
EPILEPSY AND SEIZURES						
Martinique (36)	1994–95	109.2	57.6	0 to 70+	Provoked and unprovoked seizures	
Houston, Texas (37)	1988–1994	30.0	30.3	0 to 75+	Epilepsy	
Umea, Sweden (4)	1992–94	54.1	51.3	17 to 80+	Unprovoked seizures	
Umea, Sweden (38)	1985–87	67.7	89.7	0 to 15	Unprovoked seizures	
Rural Iceland (39)	1993	55.2	35	0 to 85+	Epilepsy	
Geneva, Switzerland (40)	1990–91	90.2	51.9	0 to 80+	Provoked and unprovoked seizures	
Rural central Ethiopia (41)	1986–90	54.5	41	0 to 70+	Epilepsy	
El Salvador, Chile (42)	1984–88	101.4	89.7	0 to 60+	Epilepsy	
Rochester, Minn. (43)	1935–84	49.6	41.5	0 to 85+	Eepilepsy	
Rochester, Minn. (43)	1975–84	53.3	45.2	0 to 85+	Epilepsy	
Rochester, Minn. (43)	1935–44	46.9	40.3	0 to 85+	Epilepsy	
Rochester, Minn. (43)	1935–84	30.4	26.5	0 to 85+	Epilepsy of unknown cause	
Rochester, Minn. (43)	1935–84	68.6	56.2	0 to 85+	All unprovoked seizures	
Rochester, Minn. (44)	1935–84	45	27	0 to 75+	Acute Symptomatic seizures	*1970 US population
Rochester, Minn. (43)	1955–84	53.8	30	0 to 75+		

(continued on next page)

TABLE 1.1

Age/Gender Adjusted Incidence (per 100,000 Population)
Age Adjusted to the 1990 U.S. Population Unless Otherwise States (continued)

Location	Duration	Male	Female	Age	Comments
STATUS EPILEPTICUS					
Rochester, Minn. (45)	1965–84	23.2	13.1	0 to 80+	*1980 US population
Western Switzerland (46)	1997–98	12.1	7.8	0 to 75+	*1980 US population
Hessen, Germany (47)	1997–99	26.1	13.7	18 to 60+	* German census data
SUDEP					
Midwestern US (48)	1991–96	79.5	108	0 to 80+	* Compared to full cohort population
VASCULAR DEMENTIA					
Canada (49)	1991–96	331.6	111.7		*Compared to undemented cohort population
Rochester, Minn. (50)	1985–89	21.7	34.1	50 to 85+	
EURODEM (51)	1992–97	31.0	37.4	65–85+	
ALZHEIMER DISEASE					
EURODEM (51)	1992–97	60.7	189.7	65–85+	
Rochester, Minn. (52)	1985–89	77.1	155.1	50–85+	
Seattle, WA (53)	1994–2002	89.6	193.8	65–85+	
Baltimore, MD (54)	1985–98	1000	2200	55–85+	
Rural India (55)	1991–99	41.0	86.4	55 to 85+	
Stockholm, Sweden (56)	1990–92	912	1943.2	75 to 84	
Rochester, Minn. (57)	1980–84	95.7	103.5	0 to 85+	
Rochester, Minn. (57)	1975–79	85.3	96.6	0 to 85+	
Rochester, Minn. (57)	1970–74	60.6	91.2	0 to 85+	
Rochester, Minn. (57)	1965–69	66.8	60	0 to 85+	
Rochester, Minn. (57)	1960–64	76.7	78.5	0 to 85+	
Cambridge, England (58)	Unspecified	1483	3134.9	75 to 85+	Mild + Alzheimer disease
Cambridge, England (58)	Unspecified	6139	9039.1	75 to 85+	Minimal + Alzheimer disease
MILD COGNITIVE IMPAIRMENT					
Southwest France (59)	1988–98	57.9	37.4	70–85+	
MULTIPLE SCLEROSIS					
Bagheria City, Sicily (60)	1985–94	3.55	5.85	0 to 45+	
Catania, Sicily (61)	1975–94	2.31	2.73	0 to 75+	
Enna, Italy (62)	1986–95	5.46	6.25	0 to 45+	
Sassari, Sardinia, Italy (63)	1965–85	3.6	7.3	10 to 54	
Olmsted County, Minn (13)	1905–84	2.8	6.8	0 to 65+	*1950 US white population
Rochester, Minn (13)	1905–84	3.4	7.7	0 to 65+	*1950 US white population
Perth, Australia (64)	1961–81	0.6	2.2	0 to 85+	
New Castle, Australia (64)	1961–81	2.2	2.6	0 to 85+	
Hobart, Australia (64)	1961–81	3.5	4.1	0 to 85+	
Barbagia, Sardinia, Italy (65)	1961–80	5.4	6.6	10 to 49	
PARKINSON DISEASE					
Ilan County, Taiwan (66)	1993–95	11.1	9.8	40 to 80+	*1970 US census population
Washington Heights, N.Y. (67)	1989–91	31.9	10.3	45 to 85+	Black	*1990 US census for Washington Heights
Washington Heights, N.Y. (67)	1989–91	13.3	11.8	45 to 85+	White	*1990 US census for Washington Heights
Washington Heights, N.Y. (67)	1989–91	12.2	11.3	45 to 85+	Other	*1990 US census for Washington Heights

(continued on next page)

TABLE 1.1

Age/Gender Adjusted Incidence (per 100,000 Population)
Age Adjusted to the 1990 U.S. Population Unless Otherwise States (continued)

LOCATION	DURATION	MALE	FEMALE	AGE	COMMENTS
Ferrara, Italy (68)	1962–87	9.3	10.7		*Italian standard working population
Pozan, Poland (69,70)	1985–86	13	10	0 to 85+	*1970 US population
Rochester, Minn. (68,71)	1967–79	25	16	0 to 85+	*1970 US population
Turku, Finland (68,72)	1968–70	13	12	0 to 895+	*1970 US population
Yonago, Japan (73)	1975–79	159.1	181.3	30 to 80+	
MIGRAINE					
Olmsted County, Minn. (74)	1989–90	192.1	466.9	0 to 85+	
Washington County, Md. (75)	1986–87	285.9	1047.6	10 to 21	Migraine with aura
Washington County, Md. (75)	1986–87	782.4	1659.5	10 to 21	Migraine without aura
Olmsted County, Minn. (76)	1979–81	137.3	284.6	0 to 60+	Migraine
PRIMARY INTRACRANIAL TUMORS					
New York state (77)	1976–1995	0.28	0.18	AA	*1970 US census population
New York state (77)	1976–1995	1.48	1.05	ANOS	*1970 US census population
New York state (77)	1976–1995	3.49	2.27	GBM	*1970 US census population
Valle d'Aosta, Italy (78)	1992–99	17.3	18.5	0 to 85+	
Valle d'Aosta, Italy (79)	1986–91	21.62	28.09	0 to 75+	*1988 Italian population
AMYOTROPHIC LATERAL SCLEROSIS					
Western Washington state (80)	1990–95	2.1	1.9	0 to 85+	
Parma, Italy (81)	1960–90	0.9	0.6	0 to 70+	
Sardinnia, Italy (82)	1971–80	0.6	0.4	0 to 80 +	
Sardinnia, Italy (82)	1981–90	0.9	0.5	0 to 80+	
Harris County, Texas (10)	1985–88	1.8	1.5	15 to 75+	
Messina, Italy (10,83)	1976–85	0.9	0.22	0 to 85+	*1970 US population
Palermo, Italy (84)	1973–84	0.7	0.4	20 to 79	
Minnesota (10,85)	1925–84	2.9	1.9	0 to 85+	*1970 US population
Ferrara (110,86)	1964–82	0.6	0.3	0 to 85+	*1970 US population
Middle Finland (87)	1976–81	5.7	6.4	40 to 79	
Florence, Italy (10,88)	1967–76	0.7	0.5	0 to 85+	*1970 US population
Israel (10,89)	1959–74	0.9	0.6	0 to 85+	*1970 US population
Mexico (10,90)	1962–69	0.3	0.5	0 to 85+	*1970 US population
GUILLAIN–BARRE SYNDROME					
Harbin, China (91)	1997–98	0.74	0.57	0 to 60+	
Emilia–Romagna, Italy (92)	1992–93	1.4	0.7	0 to 70+	
Ferrara, Italy (93)	1981–93	2	1.3	0 to 70+	
Stockholm County, Sweden (94)	1973–91	1.6	1.4	0 to 80+	
Benghazi, Libya (95)	1983–85	2.2	2.5	0 to 60+	
PSEUDOTUMOR CEREBRI					
Rochester, Minn. (96)	1976–90	0.2	1.6	0 to 45+	
Benghazi, Libya (97)	1982–89	0.2	6.3	0 to 60+	
BELL PALSY					
Laredo, Texas (98)	1974–82	31.5	37.7	0 to 70+	
Rochester, Minn. (99)	1968–82	26.3	28.1	0 to 70+	
Rochester, Minn. (100)	1955–67	25	27.6	0 to 70+	

Supported in part by NINDS grants.

Thus, if one bases perceptions on data based upon medical contact alone, an erroneous perception of frequency and conceivably age distribution may occur.

EPIDEMIOLOGIC CONSIDERATIONS

All the potential biases associated with clinical series can also influence epidemiologic studies. Hopefully, some of these factors are considered in the study design by the epidemiologic investigator. The availability of a denominator based upon population surveys may provide some reassurance of the validity of gender-specific comparisons, but this may not be the case for all comparisons.

Gender and Prevalence

Prevalence studies exist for most neurologic conditions, but for several reasons, these studies may provide inappropriate conclusions if one wishes to compare gender-specific disease frequency. Despite the obvious problems of need for age adjustment (seldom performed even in the most sophisticated studies), many other problems arise in the interpretation of gender-specific prevalence.

Differential Mortality

Prevalence is a complex measure driven by the influence of incidence and duration of illness. If there is differential survivorship by gender [as may exist for amyotrophic lateral sclerosis (6) or for epilepsy (7,8), for example], one may come to erroneous conclusions about gender-specific frequency.

Differential Remission

Not all diseases are life-long. An example of this is epilepsy, in which 65% to 70% of all cases go into remission (9). Differential remission by gender could again provide misleading perceptions of the true frequency of the condition in the sexes.

Incidence

A much better perception of gender-specific frequency is provided through the study of newly identified (or incidence) cases. These cases eliminate the potential biases associated with differential mortality or disease duration, although they are subject to the same problems of patient identification that can cause difficulty in the interpretation of clinical series. For conditions that would invariably require medical attention (amyotrophic lateral sclerosis, for example), identification through hospital or medical referrals may be adequate (10). For conditions for which medical care may not be sought, such as

headache or movement disorders, population surveys may be necessary. The use of these strategies must be taken into account when interpreting studies. Unfortunately, because of considerations of the expense and time required, few incidence studies of neurologic conditions exist. Those that do exist have been done predominately in developed countries. This may lead to some bias in interpretation if the age or gender distributions underlying developed populations in some way differ systematically from those underlying other populations.

Several design strategies are used in those incidence studies providing gender-specific data. Each has advantages and disadvantages.

Historical Cohort Studies

The determination of incidence through the retrospective review of medical records for a defined community has represented a successful strategy for the determination of incidence. This strategy has been used successfully in studies of neurologic disease from Rochester, Minnesota. These studies require medical records from the entire population at risk, preferably both inpatient and outpatient. They provide reliable data for conditions likely to require medical attention. Thus, conditions such as stroke or epilepsy can be successfully studied in such populations, whereas data may be unreliable for conditions such as migraine. The advantage of these studies is the ability to document occurrence and associated factors. The disadvantage is the lack of ability to ask contemporary questions. The influence of these studies on changes in diagnostic criteria and in disease perception may need to be taken into account if the data cover a long interval. The possibility of time trends in disease frequency unrelated to technology advancement is also important. This could be gender specific.

Reconstructed Cohorts

A variation on the historical cohort study is the reconstruction of incidence through interview of prevalence cases. For nonfatal conditions, this could be a successful strategy, although one is also at the mercy of recall bias and inability to verify the condition. These strategies have been used in the study of migraine incidence.

Cross-Sectional Surveys that Provide Incidence

Incidence has been determined in cross-sectional studies associated with community-based prevalence surveys. Incident cases are those with "recent" onset of symptoms. These surveys offer the advantage of case verification and can be successful in conditions not rapidly fatal, but most neurologic conditions require huge populations to provide useful information, thus making these studies expensive.

Prospective Studies

Prospectively followed cohorts can provide detailed information not only on incidence but also on factors associated with onset, which may modify interpretation of incidence, because targeted data can be collected at the time of onset or of diagnosis of the disease in question. Examples of these studies include the Framingham studies, limited by a small population, and studies by health maintenance organizations. The latter studies may cause difficulties in interpretation because of the selection of those included. Data are, in all likelihood, reliable for conditions affecting healthy young individuals, but unreliable for disease associated with poverty or with highest frequency in the elderly.

Need for Age Adjustment

Regardless of the method of incidence determination, the need for age adjustment should be obvious, but it is seldom done. If wide variation occurs in the age distribution by gender, crude incidence may be misleading. An example is the frequency of Parkinson disease in Rochester, Minnesota (11). Crude incidence was equal for males and females, but age-adjusted incidence was 60% higher in males compared with females. Age adjustment is also needed to compare disease frequency across populations, although this is not the objective of this chapter.

Cumulative Incidence

Cumulative incidence may also be used to compare gender differences. This may offer some statistical advantages, but may also be more difficult to interpret, and may be misleading if applied to restricted age groups.

Gender as a Risk Factor in Case Control and Cohort Studies

Gender may be assessed as a variable in either case control studies or in cohort studies. The advantage of using gender in this fashion is the ability to control for other factors to establish an idea about the independent contribution of gender, if any. For example, the age-adjusted incidence of stroke was 10% higher for men compared with women in the Cardiovascular Health Study (12). In proportional hazards analysis, the adjusted risk for male sex was 0.97, suggesting that other factors measured were responsible for differences in incidence.

GENDER-SPECIFIC FREQUENCY OF SELECTED NEUROLOGIC DISEASES

For reasons discussed above, we limit our discussion to data provided by incidence studies. Further, age- and gen-der-specific incidence must be provided to allow age adjustment to a standard population, or the authors must have done such an adjustment. If not specified, age adjustment to the 1990 U.S. population has been performed by us using only the age groups presented by the author. For studies that have provided an age-adjusted incidence, we have tried to designate the standard population and the age groups used for adjustment. All comparisons should be made across gender *within* studies. Comparisons across studies may be made, but the varying age groups included in different studies make such comparisons difficult, and these are not the purpose of this paper. Further, definitions of the disease of interest may vary across studies and require more interpolation. We do not include conditions that are determined through modification of the X or Y chromosomes.

Stroke

The age-adjusted incidence of all cerebrovascular disease is substantially higher in men compared with women across all studies. This finding holds true across racial lines in the one study that examined age, sex, and race together. A review of gender-specific incidence within age strata, however, suggests a substantially higher incidence in women in the oldest age group (85+). This is true for many but not all studies. The comparatively small population of that age makes the contribution to the overall age-adjusted figure low.

For stroke subtypes other than ischemic, the case for gender specificity is less clear. For both intracerebral and subarachnoid hemorrhage, studies vary in regard to gender predominance. For the Northern Manhattan study, which examined age, race, and sex, a male excess of intracerebral hemorrhage existed for each racial group, while a female excess of subarachnoid hemorrhage existed for whites and Hispanics only.

Convulsive Disorders and Epilepsy

Regardless of the definitions used, seizures occur more frequently in men than women. This is true for epilepsy, status epilepticus, all unprovoked seizures, and symptomatic seizures. The higher incidence of acute symptomatic seizures in men is not surprising, since most of the conditions associated with this class of seizure are more frequent in men. The male predominance persists after an exclusion of cases of epilepsy of presumed cause.

A single study has been done to determine the gender-specific incidence of sudden unexplained death in epilepsy patients (SUDEP). This study showed a female predominance, a finding that should be confirmed with additional studies.

The cumulative incidence of epilepsy through age 85 in Rochester, Minnesota was 5% in men compared to 4%

in women. A reversal in epilepsy risk by gender may occur in the oldest age groups (over age 75).

Alzheimer Disease

The age-adjusted incidence of Alzheimer disease is substantially higher in women compared with men across all studies. A review of gender-specific incidence within age strata in some studies suggests a slightly higher incidence in men in the younger age groups (65 to 70). The overall differences are, therefore, likely driven by a dramatically higher female incidence with advancing age.

Other Dementias

Increasing clinical attention has been focused on two other subtypes of cognitive dysfunction: vascular dementia and mild cognitive impairment. Two studies have now suggested that the incidence of vascular dementia may be higher in women, an unexpected finding given the male predominance of cerebrovascular disease. One additional study from Canada showed a clear male excess in the incidence of vascular dementia, although, in multivariate analysis, gender was not a significant predictor of disease. The one study that has been done on mild cognitive impairment suggests a male predominance, although, clearly, additional studies are needed to confirm this finding.

Multiple Sclerosis

Data on the gender-specific incidence of multiple sclerosis (MS) are consistent with clinical series and with prevalence studies. A consistently higher incidence of MS occurs in women than men. This is consistent across age groups.

Migraine

Migraine is a condition that is universally believed to have a female excess. The incidence studies seem to confirm this perception. In addition to the studies cited, an incidence study in an HMO reported the cumulative incidence between the third and fourth decades of life to be 10% in women and 3% in men. When age-specific incidence is evaluated however, incidence is higher in men than women in the youngest age groups. The female excess is not evident until the teenage years.

Amyotrophic Lateral Sclerosis

Studies are consistent in showing a male excess; this is true for age-adjusted incidence and for incidence within age groups. The sole exception is a study from Mexico, performed some 30 years ago, in which incidence was substantially lower in men than in the other studies.

Parkinson Disease

Incidence studies of Parkinson disease generally suggest a slight male excess, but this is by no means consistent across all studies. In Italy, a slight female excess occurs, and in Japan, the female preponderance is substantial. Differences in Washington Heights are mainly attributable to the substantially greater incidence in black men. The substantial male excess for "parkinsonism" noted in Rochester, Minnesota may be misleading, because it includes cases with "arteriosclerotic" and "postencephalitic" features.

Pseudotumor Cerebri

Studies of the incidence of pseudotumor cerebri are few but show a consistent female excess.

Guillain-Barré Syndrome

Several studies of Guillain-Barré syndrome provide gender-specific incidence. There seems to be a slight male excess in these studies.

Bell Palsy

Few incidence studies of peripheral nerve dysfunction exist. Bell palsy is the only condition for which incidence has been systematically studied and for which gender-specific incidence is available. A slight but consistent female excess is noted. The difference may be greater in younger age groups.

Brain Tumor

A number of studies of brain tumor incidence using national registries have suggested that brain tumor incidence may be increasing, although this may be a reflection of the greater use of imaging procedures. Detailed statistical evaluation fails to confirm this observation—at least in the United States (13). In studies in Rochester, Minnesota, almost 35% of brain tumors are noted incidentally at autopsy. The majority of these incidental tumors were meningiomas (14). No statistically significant increase in total incidence over time has occurred in Rochester, Minnesota. The gender-specific differences in incidence of primary brain tumors varies by tumor type, with a slightly higher incidence of gliomas and astrocytomas in men. The incidence of mengiomas is consistently higher in women. The age-adjusted incidence of symptomatic brain tumors was higher in women in this community.

Other Conditions

Other conditions seem to have a definite gender preponderance, such as myasthenia gravis (female excess), although there are no studies that allow age adjustment. There may be an increased risk for females in the younger age groups and a male excess in older age groups.

SUMMARY

Women clearly are more frequently affected by MS, migraine, meningioma, Alzheimer disease, pseudotumor cerebri, and possibly some conditions of the peripheral nervous system (such as Bell palsy). For cerebrovascular disease, generally a male excess exists, although this is not consistent for subarachnoid or intracerebral hemorrhage. For Parkinson disease, there is a slight but consistent male excess. For epilepsy, amyotrophic lateral sclerosis, and Guillain-Barré syndrome, a definite male excess occurs. These gender-specific differences must be further explored to better understand the underlying pathophysiologic mechanisms associated with gender and its effect on disease susceptibility or expression.

*R*eferences

1. Kurland LT, Hauser WA, Okazaki H, Nobrega FT. Epidemiologic studies of Parkinsonism with special reference to the cohort hypothesis. *Proc Sympos Parkinson's Dis*. E&S Livingstone, 1970.
2. Ólafsson E, Hauser WA, Luovigsson P, Gudmundsson G. Incidence of epilepsy in rural Iceland. *Epilepsia* 1996:37(10):951–955.
3. Forsgren L. Prospective incidence study and clinical characterization of seizures in newly referred adults. *Epilepsia* 1990;31:292–301.
4. Forsgren L, Bucht G, Eriksson S, Bergmark L. Incidence and clinical characterization of unprovoked seizures in adults: a prospective population-based study. *Epilepsia* 1996;37:224–229.
5. Lipton RB, Stewart WF, Celentano DD, Reed ML. Undiagnosed migraine headaches. A comparison of symptom-based and reported physician diagnosis. *Arch Intern Med* 1992;152:1273–1278.
6. Grundman M, Donnenfeld H, Masdeu JC, Hauser WA. Do women with ALS present with more severe disease? *Neurology* 1992;42:3–16.
7. Hauser WA, Annegers JF, Elveback LR. Mortality in patients with epilepsy. *Epilepsia* 1980;21:399–412.
8. Ólafsson E, Hauser WA, Luovigsson P, Gudmundsson G. Incidence of epilepsy in rural Iceland. *Epilepsia* 1996;37(10):951–955.
9. Annegers JF, Hauser WA, Elveback LR. Remission of seizures and relapse in patients with epilepsy. *Epilepsia* 1979;20:729–737.
10. Annegers JF, Appel S, Lee RJ, Perkins P. Incidence and prevalence of amyotrophic lateral sclerosis in Harris County, Texas, 1985–1988. *Arch Neurol* 1991;48:590–594.
11. Rajput AH, Offord KP, Beard CM, Kurland LT. Epidemiology of Parkinsonism: incidence, classification, and mortality. *Ann Neurol* 1984;16:278–282.
12. Manolio TA, Kronmal RA, Burke GL, et al. Short term predictors of incident stroke in older adults. The Cardiovascular Health Study. *Stroke* 1996;27:1479–1486.
13. Ahsan H, Neugut AI, Bruce JN. Trends in incidence of primary malignant brain tumors in USA, 1981–1990. *Int J Epidemiol* 1995;24:1078–1085.
14. Radhakrishnan K, Mokri B, Parisi JE, O'Fallon WM, Sunku J, Kurland LT. The trends in incidence of primary brain tumors in the population of Rochester, Minnesota. *Ann Neurology* 1995;37:67–73.
15. Kita Y, Okayama A, Ueshima H, Wada M, Nozaki A, Choudhury SR, Bonita R, Inamoto Y, Kasamatsu T. Stroke incidence and case fatality in Shiga, Japan 1989–1993. *Int J Epidemiol* 1999;28:1059–1065.
16. Vemmos KN, Bots ML, Tsibouris PK, Zis VP, Grobbee DE, Stranjalis GS, Stamatelopoulos S. Stroke incidence and case fatality in southern Greece: the Arcadia stroke registry. *Stroke* 1999;30:363–370.
17. Johansson B, Norrving B, Lindgren A. Increased stroke incidence in Kund-Orup, Sweden, between 1983 to 1985 and 1993 to 1995. *Stroke* 2000;31:481–486.
18. Thrift AG, Dewey HM, Macdonell RA, McNeil JJ, Donnan GA. Stroke incidence on the east coast of Australia: the North East Melbourne Stroke Incidence Study (NEMESIS). *Stroke* 2000;31:2087–2092.
19. Tanizaki Y, Kiyohara Y, Kato I, et al. Incidence and risk factors for subtypes of cerebral infarction in a general population: the Hisayama study. *Stroke* 2000;31:2616–2622.
20. Kolominsky-Rabas PL, Weber M, Gefeller O, Neundoerfer B, Heuschmann PU. Epidemiology of ischemic stroke subtypes according to TOAST criteria: incidence, recurrence, and long-term survival in ischemic stroke subtypes: a population-based study. *Stroke* 2001;32:2735–2740.
21. Lemolo F, Beghi E, Cavestro C, Micheli A, Giordano A, Caggia E. Incidence, risk factors and short-term mortality of stroke in Vittoria, southern Italy. *Neurol Sci* 2002;23:15–21.
22. Sacco RL, Boden-Albala B, Gan R, Chen X, Kargman DE, Shea S, Myunghee CP, Hauser WA and the Northern Manhattan Stroke Study Collaborators. Stroke incidence among white, black and hispanic residents of an urban community. *Am J Epidemiology* 1998;147:1–10.
23. Lauria G, Gentile M, Fassetta G, et al. Incidence and prognosis of stroke in the Belluno province, Italy. First-year results of a community-based study. *Stroke* 1995;6:1787–1793.
24. Nakayama T, Date C, Yokoyama T, Yoshiike N, Yamaguchi M, Tanaka H. A 15.5-year follow-up study of stroke in a Japanese provincial city. The Shibata Study. *Stroke* 1997;28:45–52.
25. Czlonkowska A, Ryglewicz D, Weissbein T, Baranska-Gieruszak M, Hier DB. A prospective community based study of stroke in Warsaw, Poland. *Stroke* 1994;25:547–551.
26. Jerntorp P, Berglund Goran. Stroke registry in Malmo, Sweden. *Stroke* 1992; 23:356–361.
27. D'Alessandro G, Di Giovanni M, Roveyaz L, Ianizzi L, Compagnoni MP, Blanc S, Bottacchi E. Incidence and prognosis of stroke in the Valle d'Aosta, Italy: first year results of a community-based study. *Stroke* 1992;23:1712–1715.
28. Jorgensen HS, Plesner AM, Hubbe P, Larsen K. Marked increase of stroke incidence in men between 1972 and 1990 in Frederiksberg, Denmark. *Stroke* 1992;23:1701–1704.

29. Ricci S, Celani MG, La Rosa F, et al. SEPIVAC: a community-based study of stroke incidence in Umbria, Italy. *J Neurol Neurosurg Psychiatry* 1991;54:695–698.

30. Giroud M, Gras P, Chadan N, Beuriat P, Milan C, Arveux P, Dumas R. Cerebral haemorrhage in a French prospective population study. *J Neurol Neurosurg Psychiatry.* 1991;54:595–598.

31. Ward G, Jamrozik K, Stewart-Wynne E. Incidence and outcome of cerebrovascular disease in Perth, Western Australia. *Stroke* 1988;19:1501–1506.

32. Terent A. Increasing incidence of stroke among Swedish women. *Stroke* 1988;19:598–603.

33. Bonita R, Beaglehole R, North JDK. Event, incidence and case fatality rates of cerebrovascular disease in Aukland, New Zealand. *Am J Epidemiol* 1984;120:236–243.

34. Oxfordshire Community Stroke Project. Incidence of stroke in Oxfordshire: first years experience of a community stroke register. *British Med J* 1983;287:713–717.

35. Nilsson OG, Lindgren A, Stahl N, Brandt L, Saveland H. Incidence of intracerebral and subarachnoid hemorrhage in southern Sweden. *J Neurol Neurosurg Psychiatry* 2000;69:601–607.

36. Jallon P, Smadja D, Cabre P, Le Mab G, Bazin M. EPI-MART: prospective incidence study of epileptic seizures in newly-referred patients in a French Carribean island (Martinique). *Epilepsia* 1999;40:1103–1109.

37. Annegers JF, Dubinsky S, Coan SP, Newmark ME, Roht L. The incidence of epilepsy and unprovoked seizures in multiethnic, urban health maintenance organizations. *Epilepsia* 1999;40:502–506.

38. Sidenvall R, Forsgren L, Blomquist HK, Heijbel J. A community-based prospective incidence study of epileptic seizures in children. *Acta Paediatrica* 1993;82:60–65.

39. Ólafsson E, Hauser WA, Luovigsson P, Gudmundsson G. Incidence of epilepsy in rural Iceland. *Epilepsia* 1996; 37(10):951–955.

40. Jallon P, Goumaz M, Haenggeli C, Morabia A. Incidence of first epilepstic seizures in the canton of Geneva, Switzerland. *Epilepsia* 1997;38:547–552.

41. Tekle-Haimamot R, Forsgren L, Ekstedt J. Incidence of epilepsy in rural central Ethiopia. *Epilepsia* 1997;38: 541–546.

42. Lavados J, Germain L, Morales A, Campero M, Lavados P. A descriptive study of epilepsy in the district of El Salvador, Chile, 1984–1988. *Acta Neurologica Scand* 1992;85:249–256.

43. Hauser WA, Annegers John F, Kurland LT. Incidence of epilepsy and unprovoked seizures in Rochester, Minnesota: 1935–1984. *Epilepsia* 1993;34(3):453–468.

44. Annegers JF, Hauser WA, Lee JR-J, Rocca WA. Incidence of acute symptomatic seizures in Rochester, Minnesota: 1935–1984. *Epilepsia* 1995;36(4):327–333.

45. Hesdorffer DC, Logroscino G, Cascino G, Annegers JF, Hauser WA. Incidence of status epilepticus in Rochester, Minnesota: 1965–1984. *Neurology* 1998;50:735–741.

46. Coeytaux A, Jallon P, Galobardes B, Morabia A. Incidence of status epilepticus in French-speaking Switzerland: (EPISTAR). *Neurology* 2000;55:693–697.

47. Knake S, Rosenow F, Vescovi M, et al. Incidence of status epilepticus in adults in Germany: a prospective, population-based study. *Epilepsia* 2001;42:714–718.

48. Walczak TS, Leppik IE, D'Amelio M, et al. Incidence and risk factors in sudden unexpected death in epilepsy: a prospective cohort study. *Neurology* 2001;56:519–525.

49. Hebert R, Lindsay J, Verreault R, Rockwood K, Hill G, Dubois M-F. Vascular dementia: incidence and risk factors in the Canadian Study of Health and Aging. *Stroke* 2000;31:1487–1493.

50. Knopman DS, Rocca WA, Cha RH, Edland SD, Kokmen E. Incidence of vascular dementia in Rochester, Minnesota: 1985–1989. *Arch Neurol* 2002;59:1605–1610.

51. Andersen K, Launer LJ, Dewey ME, et al. Gender differences in the incidence of AD and vascular dementia: The EURODEM studies. EURODEM Incidence Research Group. *Neurology* 1999;53:1992–1997.

52. Edland SD, Rocca WA, Petersen RC, Cha RH, Kokmen E. Dementia and Alzheimer disease rates do not vary by sex in Rochester, Minnesota. *Arch Neurol* 2002;59: 1589–1593.

53. Kukull WA, Higdon R, Bowen JD, et al. Dementia and Alzheimer disease incidence: a prospective cohort study. *Arch Neurol* 2002;59:1737–1746.

54. Kawas C, Gray S, Brookmeyer R, Fozard J, Zonderman A. Age-specific incidence rates of Alzheimer's disease: the Baltimore Longitudinal Study of Aging. *Neurology* 2000;54:2072–2077.

55. Chandra V, Pandav R, Dodge HH, et al. Incidence of Alzheimer's disease in a rural community in India: the Indo-US study. *Neurology* 2001;57:985–989.

56. Lavados J, Germain L, Morales A, Campero M, Lavados P. A descriptive study of epilepsy in the district of El Salvador, Chile, 1984–1988. *Acta Neurologica Scand* 1992;85:249–256.

57. Kokmen E, Beard CM, O'Brien PC, Offord KP, Kurland LT. Is the incidence of dementing illness changing? A 25-year time trend study in Rochester, Minnesota: (1960-1984). *Neurology* 1993;43:1887–1892.

58. Brayne C, Gill C, Huppert FA, et al. Incidence of clinically diagnosed subtypes of dementia in an elderly population. Cambridge Project for Later Life. *Brit J Psychiat* 1995;167:255–262.

59. Larrieu S, Letenneur L, Orgogozo JM, et al. Incidence and outcome of mild cognitive impairment in a population-based prospective cohort. *Neurology* 2002;59: 1594–1599.

60. Salemi G, Ragonese P, Aridon P, et al. Incidence of multiple sclerosis in Bagheria City, Sicily, Italy. *Neurol Sci* 2000;21:361–365.

61. Nicoletti A, Lo Bartolo ML, Lo Fermo S, et al. Prevalence and incidence of multiple sclerosis in Catania, Sicily. *Neurology* 2001;56:62–66.

62. Grimaldi LM, Salemi G, Grimaldi G, et al. High incidence and increasing prevalence of MS in Enna (Sicily), southern Italy. *Neurology* 2001;57:1891–1893.

63. Rosati G, Aieloo I, Mannu L, et al. Incidence of multiple sclerosis in the town of Sassari, Sardinia, 1965 to 1985: evidence for increasing occurrence of the disease. *Neurology* 1988;38:384–388.

64. Hammond SR, McLeod JG, Millingen KS, et al. The epidemiology of multiple sclerosis in three Australian cities: Perth, Newcastle and Hobart. *Brain* 1988;111:1–25.

65. Granieri E, Rosati G, Tola R, et al. The frequency of multiple sclerosis in Mediterranean Europe. An incidence and prevalence study in Barbagia, Sardinia, insular Italy. *Acta Neurologica Scand* 1983;28:84–89.

66. Chen RC, Chang SF, Su CL, et al. Prevalence, incidence, and mortality of PD: a door-to-door survey in Ilan county, Taiwan. *Neurology* 2001;57:1679–1686.

67. Mayeux R, Marder K, Cote LJ, et al. The frequency of idiopathic Parkinson's disease among middle-aged and elderly Black, Hispanic and White men and women in New York City. *Am J Epidemiol* 1995;142:820–827.

68. Granieri E, Carreras M, Casetta I, et al. Parkinson's disease in Ferrera, Italy 1967 through 1987. *Arch Neurol* 1991;48:854–857.
69. Zhang Z-X, Roman GC. Worldwide occurrence of Parkinson's disease: An updated review. *Neuroepidemiology* 1993;12:195–208.
70. Wender M, Pruchink D, Kowal P, Florezak J, Zalejski T. The epidemiology of parkinsonism in the Poznan region. *Przegal Epidemiol* 1989;43:150–155. (As cited in Zhang Z-X.)
71. Rajput AH, Offorf KP, Beard CM, Kurland LT. Epidemiology of parkinsonism: incidence, classification, and mortality. *Ann Neurol* 1984;16:278–282. (As cited in Zhang Z-X.)
72. Marttila RJ, Rinne UK. Epidemiology of Parkinson's disease in Finland. *Acta Neurol Scand* 1976;53:81–102. (As cited in Zhang Z-X.)
73. Harada H, Nishikawa S, Takahashi K. Epidemiology of Parkinson's disease in a Japanese city. *Arch Neurol* 1983;40:151–154.
74. Rozen TD, Swanson JW, Stang PE, McDonnell SK, Rocca WA. Incidence of medically recognized migraine: a 1989-1990 study in Olmsted County, Minnesota. *Headache* 2000;40:216–223.
75. Stewart WF, Linet MS, Celentano DD, Van Natta M, Ziegler D. Age and sex-specific incidence rates of migaine with and without visual aura. *Amer J Epidemiol* 1991;134:1111–1120.
76. Stang PE, Yanagihara PA, Swanson JW, et al. Incidence of migraine headache, a population based study in Olmsted County, Minnesota. *Neurology* 1992;42:1657–1662.
77. McKinley BP, Michalek AM, Fenstermaker RA, Plunkett RJ. The impact of age and sex on the incidence of glial tumors in New York state from 1976 to 1995. *J Neurosurg* 2000;93:932–939.
78. Cordera S, Bottacchi E, D'Alessandro G, Machado D, De Gonda F, Corso G. Epidemiology of primary intracranial tumours in NW Italy, a population based study: stable incidence in the last two decades. *J Neurol* 2002;249:281–284.
79. D'Alessandro G, Di Giovanni M, Iannizzi L, Guidetti E, Bottachi E. Epidemiology of primary intracranial tumors in the Valle d'Aosta (Italy) during the 6-year period 1986–1991. *Neuroepidemiology* 1995;14:139–146.
80. McGuire V, Longstreth WT Jr, Koepsell TD, van Belle G. Incidence of amyotrophic lateral sclerosis in three counties in western Washington state. *Neurology* 1996;47:571–573.
81. Bettoni L, Bazzani M, Bortone E, Dascola I, Pisani E, Mancia D. Steadiness of amytrophic lateral sclerosis in the province of Parma, Italy, 1960–1990. *Acta Neurol Scand* 1994;90:276–280.
82. Giagheddu M, Mascia V, Cannas A, et al. Stroke in a French prospective populaton study. *Neuroepidemiology* 1989;8:97–104.
83. DeDomenico P, Malara CE, Marabello L, Puglisi RM, et al. Amyotrophic lateral sclerosis: an epidemiological study in the province of Messina, Italy 1976–1985. *Neuroepidemiology* 1988;7:152–158.
84. Salemi G, Fierro B, Arcara A, Cassata M, Castiglione MG, Savettieri G. Amyotrophic lateral sclerosis in Palermo, Italy: an epidemiological study. *Ital J Neurolog Sci* 1989;10:505–509.
85. Yoshida S, Mulder DW, Kurland LT, Chu CP, Okazaki H. Follow-up study on amyotrophic lateral sclerosis in Rochester, Minnesota: 1925 through 1984. *Neuroepidemiology* 1986;5:61–70. (As cited in Annegers JF, 1990.)
86. Granieri E, Carreras M, Tola R, et al. Motor neuron disease in the province of Ferrara, Italy, in 1964–1982. *Neurology* 1988;38:1604–1608. (As cited in Annegers JF, 1990.)
87. Murros R, Fogelholm R. Amyotrophic lateral sclerosis in middle Finland: an epidemiological study. *Acta Neurol Scand* 1983;67:41–47. (As cited in Annegers JF, 1990.)
88. Bracco L, Antuono P, Amaducci L. Study of epidemiological and etiological factors of amyotrophic lateral sclerosis in the province of Florence, Italy. *Acta Neurol Scand* 1979;60:112–124. (As cited in Annegers JF, 1990.)
89. Kahana E, Zilber N. Changes in the incidence of amyotrophic lateral sclerosis in Israel. *Arch Neurol* 1984;41:157–160. (As cited in Annegers JF, 1990.)
90. Olivares L, San Estaban E, Alter M. Mexican 'resistance' to amyotrophic lateral sclerosis. *Arch Neurol* 1972;27:397–402. (As cited in Annegers JF, 1990.)
91. Cheng Q, Wang DS, Jiang GX, et al. Distinct pattern of age-specific incidence of Guillain-Barre syndrome in Harbin, China. *J Neurol* 2002;249:25–32.
92. Emilia-Romagna Study Group on Clinical and Epidemiological Problems in Neurology. A prospective study in the incidence and prognosis of Guillain-Barré syndrome in Emilia-Romagna region, Italy 1992–1993. *Neurology* 1997;48:214–221.
93. Govoni V, Granieri E, Casetta I, et al. The incidence of Guillain-Barré syndrome in Ferrara, Italy: is the disease really increasing? *J Neurol Sci* 1996;137(1):62–68.
94. Jiang GX, de Pedro-Cuesta J, Fredrikson S. Guillain-Barré syndrome in south-west Stockholm, 1973–1991. Quality of registered hospital diagnoses and incidence. *Acta Neurologica Scand* 1995;91:109–117.
95. Radhakrishnan K, El-Manghoush A, Gerryo SE. Descriptive epidemiology of selected neuromuscular disorders in Benghazi, Libya. *Acta Neurol Scand* 1987; 75:95–100.
96. Radhakrishnan K, Ahlskog E, Shelley A, Kurland LT, O'Fallon WM. Idiopathic intracranial hypertension (pseudotumor cerebri). Descriptive epidemiology in Rochester, Minnesota: 1976–1990. *Arch Neurol* 1993; 50:78–80.
97. Radhakrishnan K, Thacker AK, Bohlaga NH, Maloo JC, Gerryo SE. Epidemiology of idiopathic intracranial hypertension: a prospective and case-control study. *J Neurol Sci* 1993;116:18–28.
98. Brandenberg N, Annegers JF. Incidence and risk factors for Bell's palsy in Laredo, Texas. 1974–1982. *Neuroepidemiology* 1993;12:313–325.
99. Katusic SK, Beard M, Wiederholt WC, Bergstralh EJ, Kurland LT. Incidence, clinical features and prognosis in Bell's palsy, Rochester, Minnesota: 1968–1982. *Annals of Neurology* 1986;20:622–627.
100. Hauser WA, Karnes WE, Annis J, Kurland LT. Incidence and prognosis of Bell's palsy in the population of Rochester, Minnesota: *Mayo Clinic Proc* 1971;46: 258–264.

2 Sex Differences in Regional Brain Structure and Function

Susan M. Resnick, PhD

S ex differences in human behavior have led to the hypothesis that sex differences in brain anatomy and physiology contribute to these behavioral differences. Behavioral measures for which sex differences have been reported include some aspects of cognition and memory (1). For example, men, on average, achieve higher scores on some tests of mathematical reasoning ability (2,3) and spatial ability, particularly spatial rotation, the ability to mentally rotate an object in two- or three-dimensional space (4). Conversely, average scores for women are higher on some language tests, such as verbal fluency (1), on some measures of verbal memory (5,6), on tests of verbal articulation (1), and on tests that assess attention to detail or perceptual speed and accuracy (1,7). Sex differences in hemispheric specialization have also been reported, with men showing greater asymmetry for both verbal and nonverbal material (8–10). Early studies suggest that sex differences in brain lateralization become manifest in certain neurologic disorders, particularly stroke, with men exhibiting more frequent and severe aphasias following left hemisphere stroke (8,11). However, more recent studies using these indirect approaches to examine brain sex differences offer no consistent evidence of sex differences in the incidence, severity, or type of language disturbance following stroke (12–14).

By offering a direct approach to the study of sex differences in the brain, neuroimaging technology holds the promise of elucidating the neuroanatomic and neurophysiologic correlates of behavioral differences. A greater understanding of sex differences in brain structure and function is important in defining brain–behavior associations and how they are affected by normal aging and disease. In this chapter, we examine the evidence for morphologic and physiologic sex differences in animal models and in the brains of neurologically normal individuals to provide a foundation for understanding the impact of neurologic disease on brain and behavior in women.

NEUROANATOMIC SEX DIFFERENCES

Songbirds and Rodents

From songbirds to humans, morphologic sex differences exist in the brain. In songbirds, the sex difference in the brain is lateralized and has been linked to a specific behavior: the capacity of males to learn a species-specific song (15). The anatomic sex difference and the singing behavior are influenced by both hormonal factors, as shown by experimental studies in which hormones are manipulated (16), and by seasonal factors, as indicated by cyclical seasonal variation in brain morphology and singing behavior (17). Interestingly, recent studies have demonstrated that testosterone implants in the brain can actually induce the seasonal-like growth in the neural circuitry underlying singing behavior (18).

Similarly, a number of sex differences have been documented in rodent brains, most often in regions thought to be directly involved in rodent sexual behavior and neuroendocrine regulation, such as the preoptic area of the hypothalamus. Morphologic and behavioral sex differences in rats, mice, guinea pigs, and other rodents are highly influenced by neonatal hormones (19–21). The neonatal administration of testosterone to female rats masculinizes brain morphology and increases the probability that females will display male-typical sexual behavior as adults (19). Gonadal steroids also influence a number of nonsexual behaviors, including maternal behavior, activity levels, aggression, juvenile play, and learning and memory. For example, early androgen treatment increases aggression and activity levels in female rodents. Conversely, neonatal castration of male rats demasculinizes behavior (21).

In addition to morphologic sex differences in brain regions mediating sexual behavior, rodent studies of the corpus callosum indicate differences between male and female rats that are influenced by early hormonal manipulation (22,23). Subtle sex differences in the hippocampus have also been reported that may influence spatial learning and memory [see McEwen and Alves for more detailed review (24)]. Male rats have a larger dentate gyrus than females and a greater number of mossy fiber synapses from granule neurons in the dentate gyrus. Sex differences are apparent also in the density and branching of dendrites of CA3 pyramidal neurons, with male rats having more excrescences for CA3 mossy fiber contacts and females having greater branching of CA3 apical dendrites. Some of these anatomic differences can be modulated by neonatal hormonal manipulation or changes in the rearing environment. In addition, hormonal manipulations influence sex differences in spatial learning ability using a Morris water maze. Neonatal testosterone administration to female rats improved spatial learning performance, whereas neonatal castration of male rats produced female typical spatial learning. Because testosterone is aromatized to estradiol in the brain, testosterone's effects on behavior may reflect either androgen or estrogen effects on spatial learning.

Nonhuman Primates

Sex differences have been demonstrated in the brains of nonhuman primates. Sex differences exist in the dendritic structure of the preoptic area of juvenile macaque monkeys (25) and in the maturation of the orbital frontal cortex (26) and temporal lobe of rhesus monkeys (27). At 75 days of age, males, but not females, with orbital frontal lesions showed deficits on an object discrimination reversal task, sensitive to damage in this region. These sex differences were dependent on perinatal androgen exposure (26) and were not evident in monkeys tested after 18

months of age (28,29). Developmental sex differences in learning abilities (30) and in the effects of selective temporal lobe lesions on visual discrimination tasks have also been reported in the rhesus monkey (27). Three-month-old female monkeys with neonatal lesions show greater deficits on these tasks than males. This sex difference in 3-month-old monkeys is influenced by neonatal androgen exposure (31). The same lesions in adult monkeys produce severe deficits in both males and females (27). These results are consistent with sex differences in the rate of maturation and vulnerability to damage of cortical regions associated with specific behaviors. In addition to sex differences in cortical regions, one MRI-based study of rhesus monkeys showed a larger splenial area in female compared to male animals (32), but another postmortem study found no consistent evidence of sex differences for the corpus callosum in New and Old World monkeys (33).

Humans

Given the frequency with which morphologic sex differences are observed in the brains of many species, it is not surprising that morphologic sex differences in the human brain have also been reported. Early studies of neuroanatomic sex differences in humans were based on postmortem examination of gross anatomic differences. Men were reported to have a larger preoptic area of the hypothalamus (34,35). Men were also more likely to be missing the massa intermedia, a midline structure between the right and left thalamus that is not present in all individuals (36). Table 2.1 lists general sex-related differences between men and women, in brain structure and function.

More recently, advances in neuroimaging techniques have allowed the noninvasive study of the human brain in vivo, initially using computed tomography (CT) and later magnetic resonance imaging (MRI). MRI provides excellent resolution and high contrast among gray matter, white matter, and cerebrospinal fluid (CSF), thus permitting the quantification of increasing numbers of brain regions as both image acquisition and processing techniques advance. In fact, current advances in automated image analysis provide the capability for quantitative MRI studies in large epidemiologic investigations.

To date, a number of sex differences in brain structure have been reported through the quantification of a limited number of brain areas, although several recent studies have examined differences throughout the brain. In this section, we focus primarily on sex differences in the adult brain [see Durston (37) for a comprehensive review of sex differences earlier in development]. Earlier studies of structural differences between the male and female brain focused on more global regions or specific brain structures through the manual or semiautomated

TABLE 2.1
Sex Differences in Brain Structure and Function: Selected Findings in Humans*

Brain structure:

Cerebrum	Larger in males
Cerebellum	Larger in males*
Preoptic area of hypothalamus	Larger in males
Massa intermedia	More likely to be missing in males
Corpus callosum	Splenium larger in females*
Corpus callosum	Isthmus larger in females*
Planum temporale	Greater asymmetry in males*
Ventricular volume	Relative size larger in men, particularly in elderly*
Sulcal volume	Relative size larger in men, particularly in elderly

Brain Function:

EEG:

Beta and theta activity	Higher in females
Alpha activity	Higher in males

ERP:

P300	Shorter latency and greater amplitude in females

PET, SPECT, and ^{133}Xenon techniques:

Global cerebral blood flow	Higher in females
Global cerebral glucose metabolism	Higher in females*
Regional distribution of glucose metabolism and CBF	Higher relative activity in males in lateral and ventro-medial temporal lobe, hippocampus, inferior frontal regions, and cerebellum
	Higher relative activity in females in posterior and middle cingulate and parietal regions
	Higher absolute glucose metabolic rates in males in hippocampus but lower absolute rates in thalamus#

Functional MRI (most based on single study):

Phonological processing	Greater left hemisphere lateralization in males and more symmetric activation in females
Passive listening	Greater asymmetric activation of anterior and posterior temporal regions in men
Lexical visual field task	Greater left-lateralized activation in inferior frontal and fusiform gyrus in men and more symmetric activation in language areas in women
Working memory	Women show greater left lateralization and men more bilateral or right-lateralized
Odor identification	Greater activation of frontal and perisylvian regions in women
Mood induction negative affect	Right-lateralized amygdala activation in men but not women

Neuroreceptor systems (most findings based on single study):

Dopamine	Greater decline of striatal D2-dopamine receptors with age in women
	Greater striatal uptake of $_{18}$F-fluorodopa in women
	Greater striatal dopamine transporter availability in women
	Higher binding potentials for D2-like receptors in the frontal cortex for women
Serotonin	Greater 5HT2 receptor binding in men than women, most pronounced for frontal and cingulate cortex
	Greater binding in women for the 5HT$_{1A}$ receptor in the dorsal raphe, amygdala, cingulate gyrus and prefrontal cortex
	Higher rates of serotonin synthesis in men than women
Mu opioid system	Men had greater activation in anterior thalamus, ventral striatum, and amygdala in response to sustained pain

*Findings are often inconsistent, but summary statement reflects the direction of effect in studies reporting sex differences
#Results of a single study

definition of specific regions of interest (ROIs). Evidence exists that both younger (38) and older men (39) have larger brains than women of comparable ages, even after adjusting for variability in height. Although Nopoulous and colleagues reported similar sex differences for frontal, parietal, temporal, and occipital lobes in younger individuals, Resnick and colleagues found that sex differences in older adults were greater for frontal and temporal than parietal and occipital regions. Sex differences in brain volume are apparent for the cerebrum, but are inconsistent for the cerebellum (38,40).

Sex differences have also been reported for more specific regions. Gur and colleagues (41) found larger volumes of orbital frontal regions in young women compared with men, but similar volumes of hippocampus, amygdala, and dorsal frontal prefrontal cortex. Pujol and colleagues (42) reported that young men had a larger anterior but not posterior cingulate cortex on the right.

Several recent studies have used voxel-based analysis to investigate sex differences throughout the brain. In this approach, each individual MRI is elastically deformed (through expansion and contraction) to a standard template MRI or average MRI, transforming all brains to a standard stereotaxic coordinate space. Using software, such as Statistical Parametric Mapping (43), differences between groups of subjects can be investigated for each voxel in the standardized space. In a large study of 465 normal adults, ranging from 18 to 79 years of age, Good and colleagues (44) used voxel-based morphometry (VBM) to examine sex differences throughout the brain. Adjusting for global volumes, they found greater gray matter volumes for women compared with men in the regions adjacent to the banks of the central sulci, in the right Heschl's gyrus and planum temporale, in right inferior frontal and frontomarginal gyrus and in the cingulate gyrus, and greater white matter volumes bilaterally in the posterior frontal regions and in the right temporal stem. Conversely, men had increased gray matter volumes bilaterally in the mesial temporal lobes, entorhinal and perirhinal regions, and in the anterior lobes of the cerebellum, and greater white matter volumes bilaterally in the anterior temporal white matter extending into the internal capsules.

One region that has received much attention in investigations of morphologic sex differences in the human brain is the corpus callosum, perhaps due to implications of callosal size for interhemispheric transfer of information and hemispheric specialization. In 1982, DeLacoste-Utamsing and Holloway (45) reported that adult women had a more bulbous splenium—the posterior portion of the corpus callosum—in a study based on post-mortem samples of 14 brains. While the finding of a larger splenial area in females was replicated (46) and extended to the fetal corpus callosum (47) by the same research group, other investigators have been unable to replicate these results in post-mortem investigations of adults (48,49) and children (50).

The capacity for detailed in vivo visualization of the corpus callosum has led to many more recent studies of sex differences in size of the corpus callosum, with inconsistent findings across studies (46,51). For example, a larger callosal isthmus in females but no sex difference in splenial area was reported in autopsy (52) and MRI (53) studies. Similarly, findings from studies of the effects of sex on the association between age and callosal size are inconsistent. In an autopsy sample, Witelson (54) reported significant negative correlations between age and total callosal area in 23 men aged between 26 and 69 years old but no significant association in 39 women aged 35 to 68 years. In contrast, other investigators have not found sex differences in the association between age and MRI-assessed callosal size in adults (51,55–57). In an MRI study of children aged 4 to 18 years, callosal size increased with age, but there were no differences between males and females (58).

It has been suggested that the varied findings across studies may reflect the way in which sections of the callosum are divided for measurement (36,59) and that there may be sex differences in the shape but not size of the corpus callosum (36). Another issue is that some authors examine sex differences in callosal regions, adjusted for brain volume. Because males have larger brains than females, it is important to investigate whether sex differences occur in the relative size of callosal subunits after adjusting for variability in total brain or callosal volume.

Davatzikos and colleagues (60) applied an earlier version of voxel-based morphometry to the analysis of sex differences in corpus callosum morphology. This deformation-based method avoids many of the drawbacks of previous methods and allows the examination of size and shape differences, separately. Using an elastic deformation, each point on an individual's corpus callosum is mapped with reference to a standard atlas of the callosum, and a coefficient—the deformation function—is calculated for each point. The deformation function for each point describes the relative shrinkage or expansion of the structure for that point; that is, how much each individual's corpus callosum must be warped to move into spatial registration with the corpus callosum of the atlas. The deformation functions can then be averaged for groups of subjects, and differences between groups can be calculated to reflect average differences in the shrinkage or expansion at each point of the structure. Illustrating this technique on MRIs from eight men and eight women, who are participants aged 60 to 85 years in the Baltimore Longitudinal Study of Aging (BLSA), we found significantly larger splenial size in women as well as sex differences in average callosal shape. This finding was extended and confirmed in a larger sample of 114 right-handed participants in the longitudinal neuroimaging study of the BLSA (61). In the larger sample, we also found significant positive associations between cognitive performance and splenial size in women, but no such associations for men (Figure 2.1). Greater interhemispheric connectivity may be more essential to performance in women than men due to their greater reliance on the bilateral processing of information.

Sex differences have also been reported in other types of MRI-based measures. A greater percentage of gray matter compared with white matter was found in one study of young women compared with men (using proton density/T2-weighted images) (62), but higher contrast volumetric images did not support this finding in other samples (39,63). Sex differences have also been found in tissue contrast and signal intensities on MRI (64), thus reflecting qualitative differences in tissue composition. In two large samples of older adults, women had more extensive evidence of white matter signal abnormalities (65) and nonsignificant trends toward more frequent subcortical and periventricular white matter lesions (66). A study of chemical shift imaging in a large sample of elderly individuals revealed sex differences in levels of creatine, N-acetylaspartate, and choline in some brain regions (67).

CT and MRI have also allowed the investigation of sex differences in age-associated brain changes (68). The majority of studies of the influence of sex on brain aging have been cross-sectional, although as noted above, our group at the National Institute on Aging is conducting a longitudinal investigation of brain changes in the BLSA. Sex differences in brain aging have been reported throughout the lifespan. In an MRI study of children and adolescents aged 4 to 18 years, Giedd and colleagues (69) reported larger cerebral and cerebellar volumes, even after adjusting for height and weight, in males compared with females. In addition, after adjusting for cerebral volume, the putamen and globus pallidus were larger in males than females, whereas the volume of the caudate nucleus was larger in females. In males only, the regression of brain volumes on age revealed a significant positive slope for the lateral ventricles, suggesting increases with age, and negative slopes for the caudate and putamen, suggesting decreases with age.

Early cross-sectional CT (70) and MRI (71,72) studies of adults aged 20 to 80 years indicated greater brain atrophy, as indexed by increased CSF volumes, in older compared with younger individuals. Although these early studies suggested the possibility of greater and earlier increases in atrophy in men compared with women, sex differences in age-associated increases in ventricular and/or sulcal volumes were not significant. More recent MRI and CT studies have shown significant sex differences in the effects of age on brain atrophy. Gur and colleagues (73) reported a significant influence of sex on age differences in MRI-assessed CSF volumes. Older individuals (aged 55–80 years) had more CSF than younger individuals (aged 18–54 years), and this difference was greater for men, particularly for sulcal CSF. In a CT study

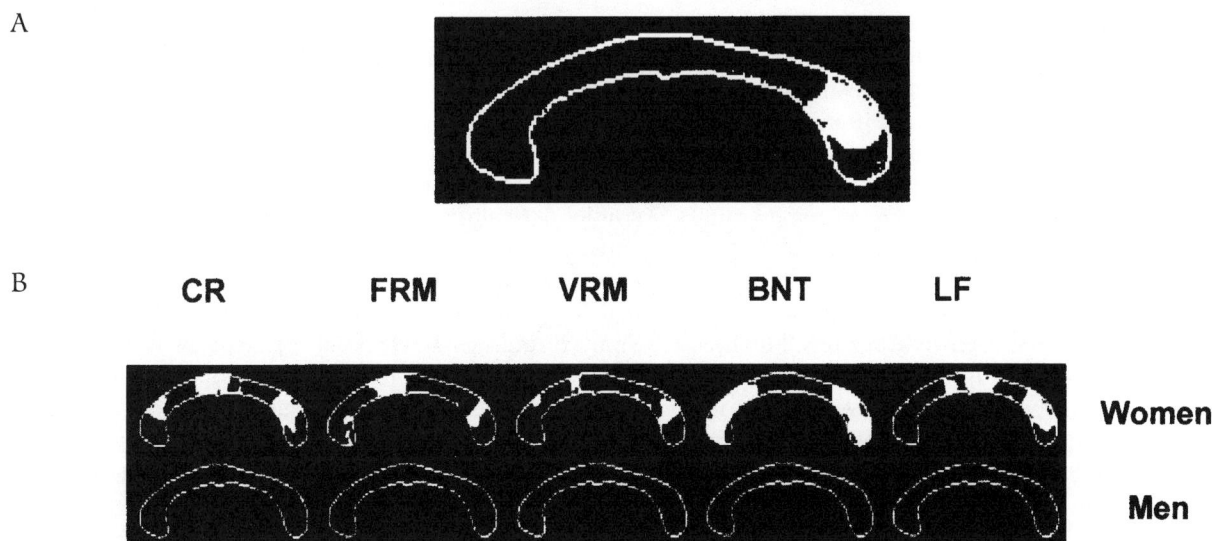

A

B

FIGURE 2.1

A. Sex differences in corpus callosum morphology. Regions in white depict areas of the corpus callosum that are larger in women than men, p<0.0001. **B.** Correlations between the deformation functions and five neuropsychologic tests for women (top row) and men (bottom row). White regions show points of significant positive correlations, p<0.05. The five tests are: Card Rotations (CR), Figural Recognition Memory (FRM), Verbal Recognition Memory (VRM), Boston Naming Test (BNT), and Letter Fluency (LF). Greater callosal size, particularly in the splenial region, is associated with better cognitive performance in women only. Effects are adjusted for sex differences in total callosal size. Adapted from Davatzikos and Resnick (61).

of ventricular volumes, sex differences in lateral ventricular volume, adjusted for cranial volume, were demonstrated for each decade from the 20s to the 80s (74). MRI-based ratings of ventricular and sulcal atrophy on 3,660 community-dwelling individuals aged 65 years and older (65) in the Cardiovascular Health Study are consistent with greater atrophy in older men compared with women. Greater age differences for men compared with women were also reported for quantitative volumes of sulcal and Sylvian fissure CSF in a subgroup of this elderly sample (68). In summary, most CT and MRI studies examining CSF as an index of brain atrophy have found greater age effects on CSF volumes in men than women.

Sex differences in the effects of age on other brain regions have also been explored. Cowell and colleagues (75) quantified frontal and temporal volumes from MRI images of 96 younger (aged 18–40 years) and 34 older (aged 41–80 years) adults. These investigators reported greater differences between age groups for men than women, with older individuals having lower volumes in both regions. Murphy and colleagues (76) reported sex effects on age differences in frontal, parietal, temporal, and hippocampal volumes. Consistent with the findings of Cowell and colleagues, decreases in frontal and temporal volumes in older, compared with younger, subjects were greater in men than women. Conversely, decreases in parietal and hippocampal volumes in older subjects were greater in women. However, it is important to note that hippocampal volumes were actually greater in younger women than younger men and were not significantly different among older men and women. In a large sample of Japanese subjects, men showed greater age-related decreases in tissue volume than women in the posterior right frontal lobe, right temporal lobe, left basal ganglia, and bilaterally in the parietal lobe and the cerebellum (77). More recently, Gur and colleagues (78) showed that sex differences in age effects on some brain regions may emerge early in adulthood. In a sample ranging in age from 18 to 49 years, they found greater age effects in men than women for cortical gray matter, most pronounced for dorsolateral prefrontal regions. Further delineation of sex differences in age effects on specific regional brain volumes awaits further investigation in larger samples with more sophisticated image processing methods.

In addition to the investigation of morphologic sex differences in specific brain volumes, sex differences in neural asymmetry have also been reported in animals and humans (79,80). For example, the planum temporale, a superior temporal brain region involved in language function, is thought to be greater on the left than right side of the human brain in right-handed individuals (81,82). It has been reported that this asymmetry may depend on sex (83,84). In one MRI study of 24 adults (12 men, 12 women), men typically had greater left than right areas

for the planum temporale, whereas women showed a more symmetric and less consistent pattern (85). This finding was not replicated in one study of 40 post-mortem brains (20 men, 20 women) (86), which reported sex differences in the bifurcation patterns of the sylvian fissure. The availability of high-resolution MRI and new image processing techniques has facilitated the investigation of larger samples to clarify sex differences in brain asymmetries. Applying voxel-based analysis to a large sample of subjects (described above), Good and colleagues (44) replicated the greater leftward asymmetry of tissue volume in the region of Heschl's gyrus and the planum temporale for men versus women.

SEX DIFFERENCES IN REGIONAL BRAIN PHYSIOLOGY

A number of physiologic techniques have been employed to assess sex differences in brain function. These include electroencephalography (EEG) and evoked potentials, ^{133}Xenon inhalation and single photon emission computed tomography (SPECT) measures of regional cerebral blood flow (rCBF), and positron emission tomography (PET) to measure regional cerebral glucose metabolism, rCBF, and neuroreceptor distribution, and functional MRI (fMRI) to measure blood volume and oxygenation changes.

EEG

Sex differences in some EEG parameters have been described in young (87) and elderly (88) individuals. The most consistent findings in the literature are greater spectral power and increased beta and theta activity in women, and increased alpha activity in men (88,89). In studies of healthy elderly adults, these sex differences are consistent across different age groups (88). Sex differences are commonly found in sensory evoked potentials (ERPs), with women showing shorter latencies (90–92). Similar findings have been reported in event-related potential studies involving simple attentional activation tasks. Although sex effects are not commonly analyzed, a number of studies reported sex differences in the amplitude and latency of the P300, with women showing greater amplitude and shorter latency than men (93,94). It has been argued that sex differences in skull thickness or myogenic activity (95), head size or core body temperature (91), and limb and trunk size could account for these sex-related effects in evoked potentials.

Sex differences in EEG activity elicited by more complex activational tasks have also been reported. In a study of continuous recognition performance, Erwin and colleagues found that women showed greater hemispheric asymmetry of activation than men did, in both verbal and spatial tasks (95). Interestingly, these results paralleled findings of sex differences in rCBF in a study involving a similar activation task (96). Others, however, have failed to find hemispheric differences in similar activation tasks, and instead have found sex differences in the effects of test material (i.e., figural or spatial) on the spatial topography of brain activity (94). Overall, sex differences in EEG during the performance of complex cognitive tasks are less consistent than those focusing on baseline sex differences.

Global Cerebral Blood Flow and Glucose Metabolism

Higher CBF throughout the gray matter in females compared with males has been a consistent finding in [133]Xenon topographic studies (96,97) and SPECT (98,99) studies of rCBF. Findings of increased levels of global brain activity in females also received support from two studies examining gender differences in regional cerebral glucose metabolism, using ^{18}F-fluorodeoxyglucose (FDG) and PET. Baxter et al. (100) and Yoshii et al. (101) found higher cerebral metabolic rates for glucose in females compared with males, although the latter authors argued that differences in brain volume accounted for the sex differences in metabolism. Other investigators have reported no significant sex differences in global cerebral glucose metabolism (76,102–104) or nonsignificant trends to higher metabolism in women (105).

PET/SPECT Studies of Regional Distribution of Brain Activity during a Resting Condition

Gur and colleagues (103) reported sex differences in the regional distribution of cerebral metabolic activity during a resting state in a sample of 61 younger individuals (mean ages: 27.3 ± 6.5 and 27.7 ± 7.4 years for 37 men and 24 women, respectively). Relative metabolism (regional radioactivity count rates divided by counts for the whole brain) did not differ between men and women for nonlimbic frontal, parietal, and occipital regions. In contrast, men had higher relative metabolism in temporal cortex, hippocampus, parahippocampal gyrus, insula, inferior frontal regions, the putamen, and the cerebellum, whereas women had higher relative metabolism in the middle and posterior cingulate gyrus. Conversely, in a sample of 55 men and 65 women over a broader age range (mean 54 ± 22 years for men and 52 ± 23 years for women), Murphy and colleagues (76) found greater hippocampal metabolism in old but not young men compared with women, suggesting sex differences in the effect of age on hippocampal glucose metabolism.

Studies using SPECT and ^{99m}Tc-ECD or ^{99m}Tc-HMPAO to measure regional perfusion have also demonstrated sex differences in the regional pattern of cerebral perfusion. In a sample of adults ranging in age from 20 to 81 years, voxel-based analysis demonstrated significantly greater perfusion for women in the right parietal lobe and for men in anterior temporal, inferior frontal, and cerebellar regions (106). Using a different approach to image analysis in a study of individuals between the ages of 50 and 92 years, women were found to have higher regional perfusion in the mid-cingulate/corpus callosum, inferior temporal, and inferior parietal areas (107).

In addition to sex differences in regional metabolism, sex differences in interregional correlations have also been reported (104), suggesting different patterns of neural connectivity during a resting state for men and women.

Brain Activation in Response to Cognitive Challenge

The examination of sex differences in regional brain activity during the performance of specific cognitive tasks has been facilitated by PET studies using oxygen-15-labeled water to measure rCBF and developments in fMRI imaging, which allow the measurement of changes in blood oxygenation as an index of changes in brain activity. In an early study using the [133]Xenon clearance technique to measure cortical blood flow, Gur and colleagues found sex differences in hemispheric activation patterns during the performance of verbal analogies and spatial judgment of line orientation tasks (96). Applying an adapted version of these tasks for use in an fMRI paradigm, this group reported sex differences in hemispheric lateralization in response to the spatial but not verbal task (108). The expected left hemispheric lateralization for the verbal task was found in the inferior parietal and planum temporale regions in both men and women, but only men showed the right lateralized increase for these regions during the spatial task. These findings contrasted somewhat with an earlier fMRI study demonstrating greater hemispheric specialization for language in a group of young men compared with women (109). Although men showed highly lateralized increases in activity in the left inferior frontal gyrus during phonologic processing, women showed bilateral activation of this region during task performance. The phonologic processing and verbal analogies tasks employed in the two studies, however, involved different task demands and brain regions responsive to these tasks.

Other sex differences in the aspects of language processing include more asymmetric activation of the anterior and posterior temporal region (110,111) in men versus women during passive listening tasks, greater left-lateralized activation in inferior frontal and fusiform gyrus in men, and more symmetric patterns in language-related areas in women during a lexical visual field task

(112). Sex differences have also been reported in the functional organization of the brain for working memory (women show left lateralization across a number of tasks and men show more bilateral or right-sided activation) (113); spatial navigation (activation of the left hippocampus in males and right parietal and prefrontal cortex in females) (114); odor identification (greater spatial extent of activation of frontal and perisylvian regions in women) (115), and primary visual cortex response to red and blue light (116).

The use of neuroimaging techniques to investigate sex differences in brain activation patterns has yielded a variety of often conflicting findings. The results of these studies must be interpreted within the context of the specific samples studied (e.g., young versus older) and the particular task demands of the activation *and* control tasks employed in each paradigm. Because the statistical analysis of these studies is typically based on image subtraction or another form of direct comparison between activation and control tasks, the demands of the latter are as critical in determining the result as the particular activation task.

Brain Activation in Response to Emotional Stimuli

Sex differences have also been reported in neural activity during receptive and expressive emotion. Using a mood induction paradigm and fMRI, Schneider and colleagues (117) found increased right amygdala activity in men but not women during negative affect. Different patterns of brain activation for men and women have also been reported for tasks tapping receptive emotions, with sex differences in activation during the discrimination of happy, sad, and neutral faces (118,119). Sex differences in activation patterns have also been observed during the retrieval of emotional words (120) and during the encoding of emotional pictures (121).

Neurotransmission

Few in vivo studies have been done of sex differences in brain neurotransmitter levels and receptor binding distributions. In an early study using PET and ^{11}CN-methylspiperone (^{11}C-NMSP) as a radiotracer, Wong and colleagues (122) reported sex differences in the rate of decline with age in D2-dopamine receptor binding. Males had a steeper slope or decline with age than females for D2 dopamine receptor binding, but no sex differences occurred in association with age for serotonin binding using this tracer. Preliminary PET ^{11}C-NMSP studies of D2 dopamine receptor binding in women over the menstrual cycle suggested cyclic variation in dopamine binding (123). In a small sample of six women, dopamine receptor binding tended to increase from the follicular to the luteal phase. Nordstrom and colleagues, however, found no differences in raclopride binding to striatal D2-dopamine receptors across the menstrual cycle (124). Menstrual cycle variation in neurotransmitter receptor binding characteristics, an area that has received little attention, has important implications for the efficacy of pharmacotherapies in women.

More recently, additional sex differences in the dopamine system have been described. In a PET study using ^{18}F-fluorodopa as a radiotracer, women had significantly higher striatal uptake of fluorodopa than men, with the difference more pronounced in the caudate than putamen (125). Using SPECT and a technetium^{99m} labeled analog of cocaine (TRODAT-1) to measure the availability of the dopamine transporter, women had higher availability than men in the caudate nucleus (126). Furthermore, dopamine transporter availability was associated with executive and motor functioning in women but not men. In another study of the dopamine transporter (using ^{123}IB-CIT and SPECT), women had higher uptake than men in the striatum, diencephalon, and brainstem (127). New radiotracers also allow the investigation of extrastriatal dopamine receptor activity. Using ^{11}C-FLB475, women had higher D2-like receptor binding potentials than men in the frontal cortex, most pronounced in bilateral anterior cingulate cortex (128). Thus, a number of studies support greater dopaminergic activity in both striatal and extrastriatal cortical regions in women, and these sex differences in neurotransmitter activity in healthy individuals may have important implications for the pathophysiology and treatment of neuropsychiatric diseases involving the dopamine system.

Although sex differences in dopaminergic activity have been the most widely studied in humans, several recent studies suggest that there may also be sex differences in other neurotransmitter systems. Using PET and ^{18}F-altanserin, Biver and colleagues found greater 5HT2 receptor binding in men than women in a number of cortical regions, most pronounced in frontal and cingulate cortex. However, using PET and ^{11}C-WAY-100635 to measure serotonin 5-HT1A binding potential, Parsey and colleagues reported greater binding in women compared with men in the dorsal raphe, amygdala, cingulate gyrus, and prefrontal cortex (129). The rates of serotonin synthesis, measured with PET and alpha-^{11}C-methyl-tryptophan, were higher in men than women (130). Sex differences in the regional activation of the mu opioid system in response to sustained pain have also been observed (131). Men had greater activation than women (during follicular phase) in the anterior thalamus, ventral basal ganglia, and amygdala, whereas women showed reduced activation in the nucleus accumbens in a basal state during pain. For comparable levels of pain intensity, men and women differed in the response of the mu opioid system in specific brain regions. The majority of in vivo studies of neurotransmission have been performed in younger individuals and do not address sex differences in neurotransmitter systems in older adults or differential aging for men and women.

CONCLUSION

The present overview of sex differences in brain neuroanatomy and neurophysiology highlights recent findings from the nascent field of neuroimaging. Although we have only begun to appreciate the effects of sex, age, and individual differences on brain structure, this direct approach to the investigation of brain sex differences provides a useful method for testing those hypotheses generated from more indirect approaches and from studies on animals. Advances in image acquisition and processing now allow a more detailed investigation of morphometric and functional differences in the human brain. It is critical to consider potential sex effects on brain and cognitive aging throughout the lifespan, because different maturational rates for men and women may lead to age-specific findings of sex differences in brain structure and function. As we advance our understanding of sex differences in the human brain across the lifespan, the potential contributions of organizational hormones early in development and activational hormones throughout maturation should also be investigated.

It is important to emphasize that sex differences in brain and behavior refer to average differences between men and women and that differences between individuals within each sex are much greater than the average differences between sexes. Given that scores for men and women largely overlap, one cannot predict an individual's score on a cognitive test or the volume of a particular brain structure on the basis of her sex any more than one can predict a particular blood assay level from group averages. Nonetheless, just as normative values for laboratory tests provide useful clinical guidelines for evaluating patients, sex- and age-specific normative values for brain imaging measures may be indicated. As neurophysiologic techniques assume an increasingly important role in neuroscience and clinical investigations, it is critical to understand the effects of sex on these measures as they relate to the correct interpretation and application to clinical practice.

Acknowledgments

Wendy Elkins, BA provided assistance in updating this chapter, and Pauline Maki, PhD provided helpful input into the original chapter. Their contributions are gratefully acknowledged.

References

1. Maccoby EE, Jacklin CN. *The Psychology of Sex Differences*. Stanford: Stanford University Press, 1974.
2. Benbow CP, Stanley JC. Sex differences in mathematical reasoning ability: more facts. *Science* 1983; 222(4627):1029–1031.
3. Benbow CP, et al. Sex differences in mathematical reasoning ability at age 13: their status 20 years later. *Psychol Sci* 2000;11(6):474–480.
4. Voyer D, Voyer S, Bryden MP. Magnitude of sex differences in spatial abilities: a meta-analysis and consideration of critical variables. *Psychol Bull* 1995;117: 250–270.
5. Bleecker ML, et al. Age-related sex differences in verbal memory. *J Clin Psychol* 1988;44:403–411.
6. Kramer JH, et al. Age and gender interactions on verbal memory performance. *J Int Neuropsychol Soc* 2003; 9(1):97–102.
7. Wilson JR, Vandenberg SG. Sex differences in cognition: evidence from the Hawaii Family Study. In: McGill TE, Dewsbury DA, Sachs BD, (eds.) *Sex and Behavior*. New York, NY: Plenum, 1978;317–335.
8. McGlone J. Sex differences in human brain asymmetry: a critical survey. *Behavioral Brain Sci* 1980;3:215–263.
9. Kimura D, Harshman RA. Sex differences in brain organization for verbal and non-verbal functions. In: DeVries GJ, (eds.) *Sex Differences in Primates*. New York, NY: Elsevier 1984;423–441.
10. Harshman RA, Hampson E, Berenbaum SA. Individual differences in cognitive abilities and brain organization, part I: sex and handedness differences in ability. *Can J Psychol* 1983; 37(1):144–192.
11. Lansdell H. A sex difference in effect of temporal lobe neurosurgery on design preference. *Nature* 1962;194: 842–854.
12. Hier B, et al. Gender and aphasia in the Stroke Data Bank. *Brain Language* 1994;47(1):155–167.
13. Kertesz A, Benke T. Sex equality in intrahemispheric language organization. *Brain Language* 1989;37:401–408.
14. Kimura D. Sex differences in cerebral organization for speech and praxic functions. *Can J Psychol* 1983;37: 19–35.
15. Nottebohm F, Arnold AP. Sexual dimorphism in vocal control areas of the songbird brain. *Science* 1976;194: 211–213.
16. Gurney ME, Konishi M. Homone-induced sexual differentiation of brain and behavior in zebra finches. *Science* 1980;208:1380–1383.
17. Nottebohm F. A brain for all seasons: cyclical anatomical changes in song control nuclei of the canary brain. *Science* 1981;214:1368–1370.
18. Brenowitz EA, Lent K. Act locally and think globally: intracerebral testosterone implants induce seasonal-like growth of adult avian song control circuits. *Proc Natl Acad Sci USA*, 2002;99(19):12421–12426.
19. Beatty WW. Gonadal hormones and sex differences in non-reproductive behaviors in rodents: organizational and activational influences. *Hormones Behavior* 1979; 12:112–163.
20. Reinisch JM. Fetal hormones, the brain and human sex differences: a heuristic, integrative, review of the recent literature. *Arch Sexual Behavior* 1974;3:51–90.
21. Goy RW, McEwen BS. *Sexual Differentiation of the Brain*. Cambridge, Mass: MIT Press, 1980.

22. Fitch RH, et al. Corpus callosum: effects of neonatal hormones on sexual dimorphism in the rat. *Brain Res* 1990;515:111–116.

23. Mack CM, et al. Ovarian estrogen acts to feminize the female rat's corpus callosum. *Develop Brain Res* 1993;71:115–119.

24. McEwen BS, Alves SE. Estrogen actions in the central nervous system. *Endocr Rev* 1999;20(3):279–307.

25. Ayoub DM, Greenough WT, Juraska JM. Sex differences in dendritic structure in the preoptic area of the juvenile macaque monkey brain. *Science* 1983;219:197–198.

26. Clark AS, Goldman-Rakic PS. Gonadal hormones influence the emergence of cortical function in nonhuman primates. *Behavioral Neuroscience* 1989;103(6):1287–1295.

27. Bachevalier J, et al. Age and sex differences in the effects of selective temporal lobe lesion on the formation of visual discrimination habits in rhesus monkeys (Macaca mulatta). *Behavioral Neuroscience* 1990;104(6):885–899.

28. Goldman PS, et al. Sex-dependent behavioral effects of cerebral cortical lesions in the developing rhesus monkey. *Science* 1974;186:540–542.

29. Goldman PS. Age, sex, and experience as related to the neural basis of cognitive development. In: Buchwald NA, Brazier MAB, (eds.) *Brain Mechanisms in Mental Retardation*. New York, NY: Academic Press, 1975;379–392.

30. Bachevalier J, Hagger C. Sex differences in the development of learning abilities in primates. *Psychoneuroendocrinology* 1991;16(1-3):177–188.

31. Hagger C, Bachevalier J. Visual habit formation in 3-month-old monkeys (Macaca mulatta): reversal of sex difference following neonatal manipulations of androgens. *Behav Brain Res* 1991;45(1):57–63.

32. Franklin MS, et al. Gender differences in brain volume and size of corpus callosum and amygdala of rhesus monkey measured from MRI images. *Brain Res* 2000;852(2):263–267.

33. Holloway RL, Heilbroner P. Corpus callosum in sexually dimorphic and nondimorphic primates. *Am J Phys Anthropol* 1992;87(3):349–357.

34. Swaab DF, Fliers E. A sexually dimorphic nucleus in the human brain. *Science* 1985;228:1112–1115.

35. Allen LS, et al. Two sexually dimorphic cell groups in the human brain. *J Neurosci* 1989;9(2):497–506.

36. Allen LS, et al. Sex differences in the corpus callosum of the living human being. *J Neurosci* 1991;11(4):933–942.

37. Durston S, et al. Anatomical MRI of the developing human brain: what have we learned? *J Am Acad Child Adolesc Psychiatry* 2001;40(9):1012–1020.

38. Nopoulos P, et al. Sexual dimorphism in the human brain: evaluation of tissue volume, tissue composition and surface anatomy using magnetic resonance imaging. *Psychiatry Res* 2000;98(1):1–13.

39. Resnick SM, et al. One-year age changes in MRI brain volumes in older adults. *Cereb Cortex* 2000;10(5):464–472.

40. Raz N, et al. Age and sex differences in the cerebellum and the ventral pons: a prospective MR study of healthy adults. *AJNR Am J Neuroradiol* 2001;22(6):1161–1167.

41. Gur RC, et al. Sex differences in temporo-limbic and frontal brain volumes of healthy adults. *Cereb Cortex* 2002;12(9):998–1003.

42. Pujol J, et al. Anatomical variability of the anterior cingulate gyrus and basic dimensions of human personality. *Neuroimage* 2002;15(4):847–855.

43. Frackowiak RSJ, et al. *Human Brain Function*. San Diego, Calif: Academic Press, 1997.

44. Good CD, et al. Cerebral asymmetry and the effects of sex and handedness on brain structure: a voxel-based morphometric analysis of 465 normal adult human brains. *Neuroimage* 2001;14(3):685–700.

45. DeLacoste-Utamsing C, Holloway RL. Sexual dimorphism in the human corpus callosum. *Science* 1982;216:1431–1432.

46. Holloway RL, et al. Sexual dimorphism of the human corpus callosum from three independent samples: relative size of the corpus callosum. *Amer J Physical Anthropology* 1993;92:481–498.

47. DeLacoste MC, Holloway RL, Woodward D. Sex differences in the fetal corpus callosum. *Human Neurobiology* 1986;5:93–96.

48. Witelson SF, The brain connection: the corpus callosum is larger in left-handers. *Science* 1985;229:665–668.

49. Demeter S, Ringo JL, Doty RW. Morphometric analysis of the human corpus callosum and anterior commissure. *Human Neurobiology* 1988;6:219–226.

50. Bell AD, Variend S. Failure to demonstrate sexual dimorphism of the corpus callosum in childhood. *J Anatomy* 1985;143:143–147.

51. Parashos IA, Wilkinson WE, Coffey CE. Magnetic resonance imaging of the corpus callosum: predictors of size in normal adults. *J Neuropsychiatry* 1995;7:35–41.

52. Witelson SF. Hand and sex differences in the isthmus and genu of the human corpus callosum: a postmortem morphological study. *Brain* 1989;112:799–835.

53. Steinmetz H, et al. Sex but no hand difference in the isthmus of the corpus callosum. *Neurology* 1992;42:749–752.

54. Witelson SF. Sex differences in neuroanatomical changes with aging. *N Engl J Med* 1991;325:211–212.

55. Johnson SC, et al. Corpus callosum surface area across the human adult life span: effect of age and gender. *Brain Res Bull* 1994;35(4):373–377.

56. Pozilli C, et al. No differences in corpus callosum size by sex and aging. *J Neuroimaging* 1994;4:218–221.

57. Sullivan EV, et al. Sex differences in corpus callosum size: relationship to age and intracranial size. *Neurobiol Aging* 2001;22(4):603–611.

58. Giedd J, et al. A quantitative MRI study of the corpus callosum in children and adolescents. *Brain Res Dev Brain Res* 1996;91(2):274–280.

59. Constant D, Ruther H. Sexual dimorphism in the human corpus callosum? A comparison of methodologies. *Brain Res* 1996;727:99–106.

60. Davatzikos C, et al. A computerized approach for morphological analysis of the corpus callosum. *J Comput Assist Tomog* 1996;20(1):88–97.

61. Davatzikos C, Resnick SM. Sex differences in anatomic measures of interhemispheric connectivity: correlations with cognition in women but not men. *Cereb Cortex* 1998;8(7):635–640.

62. Gur RC, et al. Sex differences in brain gray and white matter in healthy young adults: correlations with cognitive performance. *J Neurosci* 1999;19(10):4065–4072.

63. Nopoulos PC, et al. Sex differences in the absence of massa intermedia in patients with schizophrenia versus healthy controls. *Schizophr Res* 2001;48(2-3):177–185.

64. Kim DM, et al. MR signal intensity of gray matter/white matter contrast and intracranial fat: effects of age and sex. *Psychiatry Res* 2002;114(3):149–161.

65. Yue NC, et al. Sulcal, ventricular, and white matter changes at MR imaging in the aging brain: data from the Cardiovascular Health Study. *Radiology* 1997;202: 33–39.

66. de Leeuw FE, et al. Prevalence of cerebral white matter lesions in elderly people: a population based magnetic resonance imaging study. The Rotterdam Scan Study. *J Neurol Neurosurg Psychiatry* 2001;70(1):9–14.

67. Sijens PE, et al. Human brain chemical shift imaging at age 60 to 90: analysis of the causes of the observed sex differences in brain metabolites. *Invest Radiol* 2001; 36(10):597–603.

68. Coffey CE, et al. Sex differences in brain aging: a quantitative magnetic resonance imaging study. *Arch Neurol* 1998;55:169–179.

69. Giedd JN, et al. Quantitative magnetic resonance imaging of human brain development: ages 4–18. *Cereb Cortex* 1996;6:551–560.

70. Takeda S, Matsuzawa T. Age-related brain atrophy: a study with computed tomography. *J Gerontol* 1985;40: 159–163.

71. Grant R, et al. Human cranial CSF volumes measured by MRI: sex and age influences. *Magn Res Imag* 1987;5:465–468.

72. Condon B, et al. Brain and intracranial cavity volumes: in vivo determination by MRI. *Acta Neurol Scand* 1988;78:387–393.

73. Gur RC, et al. Gender differences in age effect on brain atrophy measured by magnetic resonance imaging. *Proc Nat Acad Sci USA* 1991;88:2845–2849.

74. Kaye JA, et al. The significance of age-related enlargement of the cerebral ventricles in healthy men and women measured by quantitative computed x-ray tomography. *J Amer Geriatr Soc* 1992;40:225–231.

75. Cowell PE, et al. Sex differences in aging of the human frontal and temporal lobes. *J Neurosci* 1994;14(8): 4748–4755.

76. Murphy DGM, et al. Sex differences in human brain morphometry and metabolism: an in vivo quantitative magnetic resonance imaging and positron emission tomography study on the effect of aging. *Arch Gen Psychiatry* 1996;53:585–594.

77. Xu J, et al. Gender effects on age-related changes in brain structure. *AJNR Am J Neuroradiol* 2000;21(1): 112–118.

78. Gur RC, et al. Brain region and sex differences in age association with brain volume: a quantitative MRI study of healthy young adults. *Am J Geriatr Psychiatry* 2002;10(1):72–80.

79. Hines M, Gorski RA. Hormonal influences on the development of neural asymmetries. In: Benson DF, Zaidel E, (eds.) *The Dual Brain.* New York, NY: The Guilford Press, 1985;75–96.

80. Hines M, Green R. Human hormonal and neural correlates of sex-typed behaviors, in *Review of Psychiatry.* Washington, D.C.: American Psychiatry Press, 1991; 536–555.

81. Geschwind N, Levitsky W. Human brain: left-right asymmetries in the temporal speech region. *Science* 1968;161:186–187.

82. Galaburda AM, et al. Right-left asymmetries in the brain. *Science* 1978;199:852–856.

83. Wada JA, Clarke R, Hamm A. Cerebral hemispheric asymmetry in humans. Cortical speech zones in 100 adult and 100 infant brains. *Arch Neurol* 1976;32: 239–246.

84. Shapleske J, et al. The planum temporale: a systematic, quantitative review of its structural, functional and clinical significance. *Brain Res Brain Res Rev* 1999;29(1): 26–49.

85. Kulynych JJ, et al. Gender differences in the normal lateralization of the supratemporal cortex: MRI surface-rendering morphometry of Heschl's gyrus and the planum temporale. *Cerebr Cortex* 1994;4:107–118.

86. Ide A, et al. Bifurcation patterns in the human sylvian fissure: hemispheric and sex differences. *Cerebr Cortex* 1996;6:717–725.

87. Matsura M, et al. Age development and sex differences of various EEG elements in healthy children and adults —quantification by a computerized wave form recognition method. *Electroencephalo Clin Neurophysiol* 1985; 60:394–406.

88. Brenner RP, Ulrich RF, Reynolds CFI. EEG spectral findings in healthy, elderly men and women—sex differences. *Electroencephalo Clin Neurophysiol* 1995;94:1–5.

89. Veldhuizen RJ, Jonkman EJ, Poortvliet DCJ. Sex differences in age regression parameters of healthy adults— normative data and practical implications. *Electroencephalo Clin Neurophysiol* 1993;86:377–384.

90. Allison T, Wood CC, Brainstem GWR. Auditory, pattern-reversal visual, and short-latency somatosensory evoked potentials: latencies in relation to age, sex and brain and body size. *Electroencephalo Clin Neurophysiol* 1983;55: 619–636.

91. Stockard JJ, Hughes JF, Sharbrough FW. Visually evoked potentials to electronic pattern reversal: latency variations with gender, age and technical factors. *Am J EEG Technol* 1979;19:171–204.

92. Emerson RG, et al. Effects of click polarity on brainstem auditory evoked potentials in normal subjects and patients: unexpected sensitivity of wave V. *Ann NY Acad Sci* 1982;388:710–721.

93. Polich J, Martin S. P300, cognitive capability, and personality: a correlational study of university undergraduates. *Personality and Individual Differences* 1992;13: 533–543.

94. Taylor MJ, Smith ML, Iron KS. Event-related potential evidence of sex differences in verbal and nonverbal memory tasks. *Neuropsychologia* 1990;28:691–705.

95. Erwin RJ, et al. Effects of task and gender on EEG indices of hemispheric activation: Similarities to previous rCBF findings. *Neuropsychi, Neuropsychol, Behav Neurol* 1989;2:248–260.

96. Gur RC, et al. Sex and handedness differences in cerebral blood flow during rest and cognitive activity. *Science* 1982;217:659–661.

97. Mathew RJ, et al. Abnormal resting regional cerebral blood flow patterns and their correlates in schizophrenia. *Arch Gen Psychiatry* 1988;45(6):542–549.

98. DeVoogd T, Nottebohm F. Gonadal hormones induce dendritic growth in the adult avian brain. *Science* 1981;214:202–204.

99. Jones K, et al. Use of singular value decomposition to characterize age and gender differences in SPECT cerebral perfusion. *J Nucl Med* 1998;39(6):965–973.

100. Baxter LR, et al. Cerebral glucose metabolic rates in normal human females versus normal males. *Psychiatry Res* 1987;21:237–245.

101. Yoshii F, et al. Sensitivity of cerebral glucose metabolism to age, gender, brain volume, brain atrophy, and cerebrovascular risk factors. *J Cerebr Blood Flow Metabolism* 1988;8:654–661.

102. Miura SA, et al. Effect of gender on glucose utilization rates in healthy humans: a positron emission tomography study. *J Neurosci Res* 1990;27:500–504.

103. Gur RC, et al. Sex differences in regional cerebral glucose metabolism during a resting state. *Science* 1995; 267:528–531.

104. Azari NP, et al. Gender differences in correlations of cerebral glucose metabolism rates in young normal adults. *Brain Res* 1992;574:198–208.

105. Andreason PJ, et al. Gender-related differences in regional cerebral glucose metabolism in normal volunteers. *Psychiatry Res* 1994;51:175–183.

106. Van Laere K, et al. 99mTc-ECD brain perfusion SPECT: variability, asymmetry and effects of age and gender in healthy adults. *Eur J Nucl Med* 2001;28(7):873–887.

107. Pagani M, et al. Regional cerebral blood flow as assessed by principal component analysis and (99m)Tc-HMPAO SPET in healthy subjects at rest: normal distribution and effect of age and gender. *Eur J Nucl Med Mol Imaging* 2002;29(1):67–75.

108. Gur RC, et al. An fMRI study of sex differences in regional activation to a verbal and a spatial task. *Brain Lang* 2000;74(2):157–170.

109. Shaywitz BA, et al. Sex differences in the functional organization of the brain for language. *Nature* 1995;373:607–609.

110. Phillips MD, et al. Temporal lobe activation demonstrates sex-based differences during passive listening. *Radiology* 2001;220(1):202–207.

111. Kansaku K, Yamaura A, Kitazawa S. Sex differences in lateralization revealed in the posterior language areas. *Cereb Cortex* 2000;10(9):866–872.

112. Rossell SL, et al. Sex differences in functional brain activation during a lexical visual field task. *Brain Lang* 2002;80(1):97–105.

113. Speck O, et al. Gender differences in the functional organization of the brain for working memory. *Neuroreport* 2000;11(11):2581–2585.

114. Gron G, et al. Brain activation during human navigation: gender-different neural networks as substrate of performance. *Nat Neurosci* 2000;3(4):404–408.

115. Yousem DM, et al. Gender effects on odor-stimulated functional magnetic resonance imaging. *Brain Res* 1999;818(2):480–487.

116. Cowan RL, et al. Sex differences in response to red and blue light in human primary visual cortex: a bold fMRI study. *Psychiatry Res* 2000;100(3):129–138.

117. Schneider F, et al. Gender differences in regional cerebral activity during sadness. *Hum Brain Mapp* 2000;9(4):226–238.

118. George MS, et al. Gender differences in regional cerebral blood flow during transient self-induced sadness or happiness. *Biol Psychiatry* 1996;40(9):859–871.

119. Lee TM, et al. Gender differences in neural correlates of recognition of happy and sad faces in humans assessed by functional magnetic resonance imaging. *Neurosci Lett* 2002;333(1):13–16.

120. Bremner JD, et al. Gender differences in cognitive and neural correlates of remembrance of emotional words. *Psychopharmacol Bull* 2001;35(3):55–78.

121. Canli T, et al. Sex differences in the neural basis of emotional memories. *Proc Natl Acad Sci USA* 2002;99(16):10789–10794.

122. Wong DF, et al. Effects of age on dopamine and serotonin receptors measured by positron emission tomography in the living human brain. *Science* 1984;226:1393–1396.

123. Wong DF, et al. D2 dopamine receptor density measured in human brain in vivo by positron emission tomography: age and sex differences. *Ann NY Acad Sci* 1988;203–214.

124. Nordstrom AL, Olsson H, Halldin C. A PET study of D2 dopamine receptor density at different phases of the menstrual cycle. *Psychiatry Res* 1998;83(1):1–6.

125. Laakso A, et al. Sex differences in striatal presynaptic dopamine synthesis capacity in healthy subjects. *Biol Psychiatry* 2002;52(7):759–763.

126. Mozley LH, et al. Striatal dopamine transporters and cognitive functioning in healthy men and women. *Am J Psychiatry* 2001;158(9):1492–1499.

127. Staley JK, et al. Sex differences in [123I]beta-CIT SPECT measures of dopamine and serotonin transporter availability in healthy smokers and nonsmokers. *Synapse* 2001;41(4):275–284.

128. Kaasinen V, et al. Sex differences in extrastriatal dopamine d(2)-like receptors in the human brain. *Am J Psychiatry* 2001;158(2):308–311.

129. Parsey RV, et al. Effects of sex, age, and aggressive traits in man on brain serotonin 5-HT1A receptor binding potential measured by PET using [C-11]WAY-100635. *Brain Res* 2002;954(2):173–182.

130. Nishizawa S, et al. Differences between males and females in rates of serotonin synthesis in human brain. *Proc Natl Acad Sci USA* 1997; 94(10):5308–5313.

131. Zubieta JK, et al. Mu-opioid receptor-mediated antinociceptive responses differ in men and women. *J Neurosci* 2002;22(12):5100–5107.

3 Women's Lives and Their Experiences with Health Care

Aileen MacLaren Loranger, CNM, PhD and Nancy Fugate Woods, PhD, RN

Women's health is inextricably related to women's lives. What women do in everyday life, the resources available to them, and notions of what a woman "should be" converge to create the social context in which women experience health and illness. A woman's own personal development is shaped not only by that social context, but also by her personal development, which contributes to the context in which she lives her life. "Social causation" is an important determinant of how biology interacts with sociocultural factors to produce differences in women's health (1). It is unlikely that a health care clinician can understand fully how women experience health or illness without understanding the context of their lives. This chapter examines how the context of women's lives and their personal development influence their health and their experiences with health care.

GENDER

Gender influences people's lives in multiple, complex ways. Gender refers to the social experience and self-expression of being a woman or man, whereas sex refers to the biological dimensions of being female or male, based on chromosomal assignment. Gender, as a social category, organizes people's lives and ultimately influences health and disease through social structures that encompass socially assigned life roles, access to resources such as money and power, and the society's image of what it is to be female or male (2,3). Indeed, gender and sex differences have been increasingly incorporated into research design, public policy, and clinical practice as the impetus to improve the health of and health care services for women has gained momentum over the past 15 years. Understanding gender influences attributed to economic, social, cultural, geographic, and behavioral factors, as well as unique sex-based biologic differences, will better shape health care and health care services in the future (4).

Economically, a gender-based division of labor is reflected in the allocation of work both outside and inside the home. Segregation within the labor market is prevalent in the United States despite laws to the contrary, resulting in inequality of wages for men and women. In 2002, the median income for women was 75 percent of the median income of men (5). Women are over-represented in the lower paying occupations, such as clerical or service workers. In addition, subtle (and not so subtle) discrimination remains in skills training that influences who gets trained for better paying jobs and who experiences discrimination in promotions—the so-called "glass ceiling" for women. The appropriation of gender-based work is further reflected in the design of work and tools to perform work. For example, household appliances are sized to women's hands, whereas most tools used in certain types of manufacturing have been sized to fit men's hands.

Women disproportionately assume the allocation of childrearing responsibilities, with few men undertaking primary parental responsibility. Approximately 40% of women in the U.S. workforce have children younger than 18 years of age (6). In addition, some working women also have caregiving responsibilities for mentally or physically disabled or aging family members (7). In 1998, 9% of women were caring for a sick or disabled relative. Of those women, 43% provided more than 20 hours of care per week, and a majority (53%) had annual household incomes of $35,000 or less (8). Caregivers also report that they are in poorer health than noncaregivers.

As a result of the allocation of labor market opportunities and women's disproportionate responsibility for childrearing and/or caregiving in the United States, women are more frequently poor than men. Not surprisingly, poverty is one of the major social issues affecting women's lives and their health. In 2000, 11.9 million women aged 18 and older were living with incomes below the federal poverty level, when compared with 7.6 million men of similar age (9). Single women with young children or who are elderly are most likely to live in poverty, and they remain poor for longer periods than do men. Indeed, 29% more women than men live in poverty (10). Women heads of households are five times more likely to be poor than men; teen mothers and residents of rural areas are especially at risk of being poor (11,12).Recently, 26.4% of all female-headed families were poor compared to 4.9% of families in which males were present (13). Poverty is particularly acute among older women, and health care costs are often responsible for older women's poverty.

Acute care health services are supported through entitlement programs such as Medicare, but the services women need as they age without a spouse or children to care for them, such as home care services and nursing home care, have limited coverage through Medicare. Thus, women must spend down their savings and apply for Medicaid to finance caregiving for themselves.

A substantial decrease in health insurance coverage for American women occurred during the last decade of the twentieth century. The proportion of uninsured women increased by 16.8%, whereas the total uninsured population rose by 11.5%, and the proportion of men who were uninsured rose by 7.1%. Approximately one in five working-age women (17.7%) is uninsured. Between 1990 and 1999, the number of uninsured Americans reached 43 million, including over 20 million uninsured women, despite a national focus on the uninsured and the unparalled economic prosperity over the previous nine years (14).

As a result of this inequity, uninsured women are more likely to be disenfranchised from the health care system; women are up to five times more likely to report no usual source of care and twice as likely to report no recent physician visit. A lack of coverage limits access to essential preventive care, reproductive health care, and both acute and chronic care needs. Without adequate insurance, women are five times more likely to report unmet health needs and nearly six times more likely to use the emergency room as their only source of health care. Uninsured women experience higher mortality and nearly twice the risk of avoidable hospitalizations for conditions that could have been treated as outpatient care or prevented altogether (14).

Power is also allocated according to gender. This gender-related disparity is reflected in the dynamics of domestic relationships, including the control of money and other resources and the tacit approval of violence against women, in particular, domestic violence. In the United States, one woman is beaten in her home by someone she knows every 14 seconds (15). Nearly 45% of women aged 18 to 64 years report having experienced one or more forms of violence, including child abuse (17.8%), physical assault (19.1%), rape (20.4%), and intimate partner violence (34.6%) during the course of their lifetime (16). Hierarchies of state and business reflect the gender order of the society; therefore, the subordination of women to men is assured through rules that make change difficult.

Cathexis refers to ideas about gender, including the ideology governing the social patterning of relationships or links to one another. The image of a woman as a reproductive or sexual object constrains what women can aspire to be in a society. Sexism pervades Western societies in subtle as well as overt ways (17). Sexual harassment of women in the workplace, sexual discrimination in hiring and promotion practices, and differential access to education persist despite changes in the law. Incest, sexual abuse, unwanted sex or "date rape," homicide, and violent acts against women such as rape and battery, are increasingly recognized and reflect both the image of women as objects and gender differences in power. Taken together, the division of labor, power, and imagery about women shape contemporary women's lives.

CONTEMPORARY WOMEN'S LIVES

The lives of women from different birth cohorts vary considerably. The unique experiences of different birth cohorts are exemplified by comparing the lives of women born in the two decades following World War II (1946 to 1964), referred to as the Baby Boomers, with their mothers. The large postwar population surge that produced the Baby Boomers has had a dramatic impact on U.S. society as a whole. The mothers of the Baby Boomers were unusual in that they had larger families, less formal education, and married at younger ages than their own mothers. The Baby Boomer generation of women has differentiated itself from women of previous generations in that many have fashioned their lives as individuals. Whereas past generations of women organized their life roles and goals around their family's objectives, women now spend more of their lives as single, independent adults, organizing their lives to meet their personal and work objectives. The Baby Boomer woman is better educated, lives alone longer than her mother's generation, and participates in the labor force throughout her life regardless of her marital status and the ages of her children. She experiences greater financial independence and fertility control than her mother. Marriage and family are no longer the single controlling institutions around which the Baby Boomer generation of women organized their lives. Moreover, it is likely that daughters of the Baby Boomers will be profoundly influenced by these changing norms and that their lives will be more similar to their mothers' lives than those of their grandmothers (18).

Employment

Since the late 1960s a profound shift has occurred in the relationship of women to the family and economic system, most evident in the integration of work and family roles. The next generation of women is a product of the transition made by Baby Boomer women who entered adulthood with work and family attitudes similar to those of their mothers, but who underwent dramatic transitions. These changes have been reflected in women's roles, particularly those of educational attainment and paid employment, along with parenting, partnerships, and caregiving, which remain significant components of women's work.

Data from the U.S. Bureau of Labor (19) reveal that 58% of all women aged 16 and older are employed outside of their homes for pay. Motherhood is an important component of many—but not all—women's work lives. Nearly three-quarters (71%) of married women with children under age 18 were employed in 1997, whereas the rate of labor participation of single mothers was 68% (20). In 1998, among women with infants under the age of one year, 36% were working full-time, 17% were working part-time, and 6% were actively seeking employment—representing a record high of almost 60% of new mothers participating in the labor force (21). An estimated two-thirds of preschool children in the United States have mothers who are employed. Only 20% of mothers of preschoolers in the United States are full-time homemakers. Most women are employed because their incomes are essential to their family's well-being. This is so for over 70% of black married women and 50% of white married women in the United States (22).

Women have worked throughout U.S. history, but much of women's work has been unpaid work performed in the home and invisible to the larger society. Contemporary women have experienced an increase in their paid work without a compensatory decrease in the responsibilities for the unpaid work benefiting their families. As a result, many experience conflicts among their complex multiple roles and report feeling overloaded.

Adult Partnerships

Although over 51% of U.S. women are married (21), the proportion of women who are single heads of households, assuming responsibility for their children, has grown dramatically since the 1950s. This change is largely attributable to U.S. divorce rates escalating, but to some extent women choosing not to marry but live with a male partner or a series of partners. As women have been able to provide financial support for themselves, the financial necessity to marry has been reduced. Estimates are that 12% of 25- to 29-year-old women may never marry. Median age at first marriage is now approximately 25 years (23) and duration of marriages is about 23 years. About half of all divorces occur within the first seven years of marriage (18).

Parenting

As women's labor market participation has increased dramatically, their childbearing and childrearing activities have slowed somewhat. Currently, women have an average of 1.9 children, but estimates are that now one of five women will have no children during her lifetime. Median age at first birth is 23 years, but 11% of women have their first birth after age 30. Both education and employment opportunities for women have slowed the birth rate in the United States. Indeed, only 30% of college educated women have had their first child by age 25 years (18).

Estimates are that employed women work another 11 or more hours more each week at home than employed men. Employed women with young children are among the most overloaded. In the United States, on-site child care for employed women has begun to be available, but it is not the norm. When child care is available, child care workers (most of whom are women) are not well remunerated. Indeed, most child care workers (94%) in the United States earn wages below the poverty level (24).

Some women with children have pursued employment by working at home. Over 11.2 million women in the United States are self-employed, working in their homes (8). Although it would seem that women with young children might welcome some assistance by cutting back on employment, the concept of a "mommy track," a slower career progression than that typifying men, has met with criticism from women in the United States. Perhaps more assistance with work at home and with child care would be the preferable solution for many women.

Caregiving

In addition to caring for their children, women in the United States contribute disproportionately to caring for their elderly parents and other family members during times of sickness. Informal or unpaid family care is often an overlooked yet essential component of the U.S. health care system for the nation's sick, disabled, frail, and terminally ill (25). The fastest growing portion of the population in the United States is the group between 75 and 85 years of age. U.S. estimates are that women constitute 72% of the 2.2 million people caring for 1.2 million elderly living at home (26). Often these women are elderly themselves, but many are midlife women who also have children at home. This situation is so common in the United States that women with responsibilities to multiple generations are described as the "sandwich generation." Women are sandwiched into caregiving roles by their children and adolescents on one hand and by caregiving responsibilities for their elderly parents and spouses' parents. These responsibilities add about 20 to 28 hours to women's work weeks, in some cases causing then to leave employed positions, reduce hours in the workplace, and lose benefits such as health insurance and pensions. A growing body of scientific evidence exists about these financial, emotional, physical, or familial threats that face caregivers (both women and men) (25).

U.S. women have an estimated average lifespan of nearly 80 years. This fact should alert us to an increasing number of elderly in our society who will need care. As the lifespan increases, so does the necessity for family caregiving by future generations. Indeed, Baby Boomer women will soon require the supportive caregiving of their children, who will also be involved in paid labor, childrearing, and their own life partnerships.

Multiple Roles

The challenges of balancing multiple roles have become commonplace for the Baby Boomer generation of women. Although work generally has been shown to have positive effects on women's health, and studies of women performing multiple roles reveal health benefits (27), other situations may be health-damaging for women. In the United States, an estimated 55% of women return to work within 1 year of the birth of their children (28). This fact may reflect women's satisfaction with their work as well as concern about continuing their employment due to economic necessity, because health care benefits are linked to employment in the United States. Work that is physically demanding, coupled with heavy responsibilities for child care and home maintenance, may have negative health effects. Moreover, the combination of long stressful hours at poorly paid, unrewarding, physically exhausting work that includes exposure to toxic substances or illnesses may combine to produce health problems.

The Framingham Heart study (29) revealed some interesting findings about women who did not seem to benefit from employment. Data from a birth cohort a generation older than the Baby Boomers indicated that women who worked at home had the lowest incidence of heart disease, whereas women who were currently employed and those who had been employed previously had higher rates of disease. The incidence of heart disease was highest among women who were clerical workers, who were married to blue collar (working class) husbands, and who had three or more children. Clerical workers with blue collar husbands were likely to be working due to economic necessity and were likely to receive little spousal support for their employment. Moreover, aspects of their work situation also influenced women's health. Clerical workers who had remained in jobs with a nonsupportive boss and who were unable to express their anger experience a higher incidence of heart disease than do other women (29).

Later studies show that employment has the most beneficial health effects for women without an alternative source of social integration and self-esteem. Women who were not married, did not have children, and were not well educated, benefited the most from being employed (30).

More recent research has focused on the consequences of combining work and family responsibilities. Workplace exposure to stressors was studied among women employed as managers in a Swedish manufacturing industry using norepinephrine levels as an indicator of stress. During the day, women's norepinephrine levels resembled those of male managers. When women went home from work, however, their norepinephrine levels rose. Their male counterparts' norepinephrine levels fell; suggesting that going home was a relaxing part of their daily experiences, unlike women's experiences of going home (31). A study of U.S. partnered women and men who were both employed documented that women work a second shift when they come home from their paid employment (32). Women, more than men, continue to participate in unpaid work as well as their paid labor.

U.S. studies show that young adult women who were employed and had children and who received both emotional support and help with the work from their husbands had better mental health than those who did not receive this type of support. Moreover, when women juggling multiple responsibilities were convinced that it was appropriate for women to be involved in nontraditional roles, their mental health was better than for those with more traditional norms (33). When women had partners who did not assume an equitable load of the work at home, they became depressed. This was most pronounced when the women felt overloaded (34). For women who were working at home, emotional support and positive affirmation from their spouses were most important (33).

The profile of a woman's life course is shaped in large part by the constellation of her roles. The shape of the Baby Boomer's life course differs from that of her mother's in two significant ways: the continuity of employment throughout her reproductive years and the discontinuities in adult life partnerships due to divorce and remarriage. What remains similar in the life course of Baby Boomers and their mothers is parenting. Those women who become parents remain parents—usually developing adult relationships with their children that persist throughout the life course (35). As the nature of work is changing in U.S. society, another dimension of women's lives is also changing—education. Women once completed their formal education before entering the labor force, but now increasingly punctuate their lives with educational episodes geared toward re-training, as the labor market requires it.

WOMEN'S ADULT DEVELOPMENT

The current concepts of women's adult development emphasize women's relational nexus and interdependence in contrast to accounts of men's lives that emphasize individuation and independence. The use of the concept "self-in-relation" has revolutionized the concepts of women's adult development. Seeking an identity as being in a relationship with others implies developing all aspects of oneself in increasingly complex ways, in the context of increasingly intricate relationships. When the nature of those relationships is suppressive or oppressive, women's development is thwarted (36). Instead of emphasizing separation-individuation, the self-in-relation theorists proposed that relationship-differentiation is central to women's development.

The basic elements of women's core self, then, are: i) interest in and attention to the other person, forming the basis for emotional connection and empathy; ii) the expectation of a mutual empathic process in which the sharing of experience enhances development of oneself and another; and iii) the expectation of interaction and relationships as a process of mutual sensitivity and responsibility that stimulates the growth of empowerment and self knowledge (37).

In the context of self-in-relation theory, relationship has a specific meaning. Relationship means the "experience of emotional and cognitive intersubjectivity: the ongoing, intrinsic inner awareness and responsiveness to the continuous existence of the other or others and the

expectation of mutuality in this regard" (37, p. 59). One comes to know oneself and others in the context of mutual relational interaction and in the continuity of emotional-cognitive dialog. Communication is interaction rather than debate.

Power, in the context of self-in-relation theory, is the capacity to move or produce changes. This definition is in contrast to power as dominion, control, or mastery. Power is not seen as "power over" but "power with" (37). The contrast to empowerment is disempowerment, which makes it difficult to create or sustain a healthy relational context. As one develops "power with," one has a sense of being part of the growth and empowerment of others. One develops while seeing another become more of who she is as one does the same. The "power over" model limits growth because it limits the relational context (37).

Female Friendships

Women have overlapping relational networks that span many domains of life, including their personal, educational, work, and political involvements (38). Although women's networks provide a great deal of support, particularly in times of crisis, little is known about these structures and their development across a woman's lifespan. Female friendship provides a unique context in which women can experience happiness in relation to women's lives, not defined in relation to men's lives. Importantly, female friendship makes women visible to one another. The dual vision of what is and what can be includes making women visible to themselves and to one another in a world that frequently keeps women and women's doings invisible by design (39).

Cognitive Development and Moral Reasoning

The new accounts of women's development have also examined women's cognitive development and women's moral reasoning. Relational experiences may contribute to a special style of knowing for women. Belenky and colleagues (40) have proposed that connected learning, taking the views of others and connecting them to one's own knowledge, contributes to a larger understanding of human experience. This approach discourages a split between thinking and feeling. In addition, their work illustrates how differential access to social resources and definitions of self have kept some women silent rather than promoted their ability to construct knowledge.

Carol Gilligan's works (41) illustrate how women's ethical development differs from men's by evolving around an ethic of caring versus an orientation of entitlement. Gilligan found that women live in networks or webs of attraction, a fact that influences the development of an ethic of caring. Women make decisions about moral acts using the criterion of caring or responsibility versus an orientation of rights or privilege.

One important caveat in considering adult development and research on women's roles and their health is that most work has involved white women who have above-average economic resources. Studies often do not reflect the reality of poor women's lives, and women of color are disproportionately poor.

WOMEN'S EXPERIENCES OF HEALTH CARE

Women have well established themselves as expert consumers of health care services in the United States and as a primary resource for their family's health care decisions (1,42). Recent innovations in the field of information technology are greatly increasing the access to knowledge of health maintenance and health care, including the expanding interactive capacities of the Internet, electronic mail (e-mail), handheld computers, and cellular telephones. The Science Panel on Interactive Communication and Health (43) defines these tools of communication technology or interactive health communications (IHC) as "the interaction of individuals—consumer, patient, caregiver, or professionals—with or through an electronic device or communication technology to access or transmit health information or to receive guidance and support on a health related issue" (43, p. 1264). The convergence of rapidly developing scientific advances and IHC is changing the nature of contemporary health care experiences and health care communications. The accessibility of up-to-date medical information through the Internet adds another dimension to the consumer power held by women, one which potentially fosters more active participation in health, health care decisions, and confidence in obtaining appropriate health care for themselves and their families (44).

Equally important to an understanding of women's experiences of health care are the effects that sociocultural influences have. Acknowledging and sensitively addressing the cultural characteristics and needs of diverse groups during the provision of health care will reduce existing socioeconomic, ethnic, and racial disparities, stereotyping, and gender bias.

Women as Health Care Consumers

Women represent the largest proportion of health services consumers at all ages in the United States (even after adjusting for childbearing) (45). American women make three-fourths of the health care decisions in their households and spend nearly two of every three health care dollars. More than 61% of physician visits are made by women, 59% of prescription drugs are purchased by women, and 75% of nursing home residents over 75 years of age are women (46). Increasingly savvy regarding their health and well-being, women want to be taken seriously during visits with their health care clinicians and yet, frequently find themselves frustrated and dissatisfied when they feel they are not being listened to (47–49).

Women regularly express a longing to be more comfortable asking questions and getting clearer answers from their physicians, despite the pressures of today's managed care environment, in which time efficiency is at a premium during the medical encounter (47). The advent of IHC holds great promise for enhancing women's focused interactions with their clinicians, and results in better informed decision-making and greater patient satisfaction.

The Influence of Telecommunications on Health Care

In 2002, the adoption of Internet use in the United States was at a rate of 2 million new Internet users per month. Over half the nation is now online, and overall Internet use is steadily increasing, regardless of income, education, age, race, ethnicity, or gender. Low family incomes, low levels of overall education, and English as a second language are still the strongest predictors of those within the "unconnected" population (50). Yet, the exponential growth rate in the Internet's user base, with the greatest increase occurring among younger, school-aged user groups, is rapidly narrowing the "digital divide" (44,51).

Women and men demonstrate equal rates of computer utilization. Not surprising, women go online to find information on health services or practices more frequently than men (39.8% of female computer users contrasted with 29.6% of male computer users). Regular e-mail use was reported by 85.1% of female users versus 82.8% of male users. Routine computer use and Internet access at work, school, or libraries is substantially narrowing the "unconnected population" in computer applications nationwide, which subsequently influences increased household usage (50).

As the Internet becomes a more conventional information tool, expectations have increased about the reliability of health or medical information found online. According to the Pew Internet & American Life Project (52), 67% of Americans believe that health care information found online is reliable, which explains why such information plays an increasing role in people's interactions with their health care providers and in their more active participation in decision-making.

Most Internet "health seekers" are women, who say that they are still careful to consult with a medical professional before acting on online medical advice. Fifty-eight percent of Internet health seekers predict that they will first go online when next they need reliable health care information versus 35% who say that their first move will be to contact a health care professional (52).

In an exploratory study to determine the motivations of women who use the Internet to obtain health information, health consciousness as well as health needs and cost-effectiveness were each significant (44). In particular, the efficiency of Internet searching was premium for women whose full daily schedules included managing child care, elder care, and/or personal health issues.

Advances in telecommunications and interactive media offer both advantages and potential risks in health communication. The Science Panel on Interactive Communication and Health (43) found that the benefits of IHC include enhanced opportunities for the provision of information "tailored" to the specific needs or characteristics of those searching the Web; increased access to information and support at the user's convenience; greater opportunities for interaction with clinical experts as well as obtaining support from others with similar conditions through e-mail or chat rooms; and enhanced abilities for the widespread dissemination and currency of content.

Potential problems with direct Internet access also exist, including the lack of regulation on the quality of the health information presented, which potentially compromises the accuracy and appropriateness of the material online. This can result in patients obtaining inappropriate treatment or delay in seeking necessary medical care. Further, greater reliance on IHC can erode people's trust in their health care professionals and prescribed therapies if there are substantial differences of opinion. Privacy and confidentiality may be violated (43).

E-mail is also becoming a useful adjunct to patient–clinician communications, replacing the telephone in efficiency and provider accessibility. Typically, important aspects of health care take place via telephone—patients call to ask advice, get prescription refills, and give feedback on previously prescribed therapies, whereas providers call to discuss lab results or follow a patient's progress. Problems encountered with this technology include missed telephone calls in either direction, lines that are often busy, or interruptions to the recipient's activity. Misunderstanding or misinterpretation is common over the phone and can lead to poor compliance with medical advice. The documentation of these calls is often incomplete, which makes the subsequent decision-making process challenging and increases the clinician's legal liability (53).

For nonemergent medical issues, e-mail has the potential to improve patient–clinician communications. For the patient, e-mail can reduce the inconvenience of waiting for call-backs; questions can be formulated more purposefully; the clinician's instructions can be read, saved, and later reread; sensitive questions may be easier to ask electronically; and the ability to ask quick questions between visits gives a sense of greater access to med-

ical care. For the professional, unsuccessful calls are minimized, messages can be read and responded to at more convenient times, medical advice can be carefully worded before it is provided, communications can be saved in print form for the patient's record, and easy references to other sources of information can be provided either in hand-outs or web-links (53,54).

As with any new technology, potential problems exist with "digital doctoring" through electronic communications, including concerns over privacy issues; uncertainty as to the reception of the message; nonuniversal access, especially for those more vulnerable and already underserved populations (55,56); the potential for managing staggering e-mail volume; or an inability to respond in an efficient manner, which could create increasing patient dissatisfaction or enhance the impersonal nature of medical encounters (56,53). Specific recommendations for clinical e-mail and medicolegal and administrative e-mail guidelines have been developed to enhance the use of this technology in positive and productive ways (54).

These technologies can have a democratizing effect on access to and control of information between health care professionals and laypersons. These types of interactions have the potential for increased availability, a better understanding of various aspects of the diagnosis or management of a health condition, and better preparation for health care visits (44).

Despite all its potential, it is equally important to recognize that these newest information technologies continue to emphasize the gaps between the privileged and the less fortunate of our society (55). Whether the issues are access to obtaining health care, health insurance, or health information, the largest barrier for a substantial portion of women remains the acquisition of adequate education and income to afford these essentials. A major challenge of the future will include finding solutions to bridge the "digital divide" to improve health care services for all.

Traditional Communication within Health Care

A fundamental component of effective health care is the dialog that occurs between patients and their clinicians. The communication that is exchanged between women and their physicians is central to the quality of the therapeutic alliance that they establish. It is through talk that unique interpersonal relationships are shaped, essential medical information is exchanged, health problems or risks are identified, health education and counseling is discussed, and decisions about treatment options or prevention measures are negotiated and carried out.

Widely studied, the significant benefits of proficient communication between patients and clinicians include reduced patient anxiety, enhanced patient understanding and recall, increased perceptions of personal control over one's health, satisfaction with medical care, adherence to medical therapeutics, and subsequent improved health status (57–65).

Yet, women's experiences of the health care system often reflect a less than courteous climate. Women patients may encounter a physician's inappropriate use of familiar forms of address (i.e., using the patient's first name), disparagement of their abilities to use medical information rationally, a condescending manner, or withholding technical information, such as the benefits and risks of informed consent. These kinds of exchanges have been described and interpreted as ways in which the physician controls the medical visit and the patient's behavior (66–68).

The consequences of communication problems, based on a review of studies on physician and patient relations by Stewart (69), include inaccurate medical diagnoses, lack of patient participation in medical care discussions, or inadequate provision of information to the patient.

Ineffective communication most commonly results in patient dissatisfaction with a physician's care and consequently, the patient's termination of their professional relationship (57). From the Commonwealth Fund women's health survey data, women were approximately twice as likely as men to have changed physicians due to dissatisfaction. Women were also more likely to report communication problems with their physicians, and this issue was cited as the most important contributing factor for switching health care providers for both men and women (70). Ineffective communication is also a major source of stress and anxiety for the patient during the medical encounter (71).

Social Context

The social context of the medical encounter also influences patient–provider interaction. The dialog between women and their physicians occurs in a variety of clinical settings, between individuals of unequal power, involving issues of vital importance that are both culturally and emotionally laden and thus, necessitate joint cooperation. The ideal patient–provider relationship in which mutual trust exists, communication is reciprocal, and therapeutic goals and decisions are agreed upon, is not easily achieved (64).

Communication Styles

Communication style differences between genders account for the distinct ways in which men and women use questions, volume and pitch, indirectness, interruptions, silence, or polite refusals. From birth, women and men are treated differently, related to differently, and they talk differently as a result. Girls and boys grow up in different worlds, even when they grow up in the same households. These differences continue into adulthood and reinforce communication patterns established in childhood (72, p. 133). Recognizing these gender differences, which include differing expectations about the role of talk in relationships, is essential to the provision of quality health care to women.

In studies of patient–provider communication, women are more likely to recognize and report symptoms as well as be more articulate and knowledgeable when talking with their physicians during annual medical visits (73). Perhaps because they are more familiar and comfortable with health system utilization, women talk more and offer more complaints during medical visits (74,61,62); ask more questions (756–77); receive more information and a greater number of explanations from both male and female physicians (78–80), and generally have longer medical visits than men (61,77,62) (as reviewed in 70,81). Among patients with chronic disease, women are more likely to prefer an active role in decision-making that males (82).

Hooper and colleagues (78) determined that female patients got more information and empathy from their doctors as well as fewer physician-initiated disruptions during their visits. Findings by Stewart (83) revealed that physicians demonstrated more tension release (e.g., laughter) with female patients and were more likely to solicit their feelings and opinions (81).

Power

Studies of interactions between physicians and patients, however, have also described the constrained structure of typical medical encounters and the use of power or domination to limit and control medical dialog. The use of interruption and the amount of talk or words, question-asking, information-giving, and adversativeness are examples of methods that physicians employ to control the course of the medical interview (84–88). One study (89) revealed that physicians interrupt patients an average of 18 seconds into the patient's opening remarks. The patient was only able to complete her primary complaint or concern 23% of the time. But, as Allen and colleagues (90) suggest, perhaps it is not the interruption, but the missed opportunity to disclose information about themselves and their situation that leaves patients feeling that they have not been taken seriously.

Meaning

Patients must be able to tell their stories, but may be confronted with their clinicians' incompatible frame of reference as to what information should be shared during medical visits (91). Physicians may not be aware of or understand women's "explanatory models" of their health concerns or their attitudes, values, and beliefs as related to illness and health care (92,93). These models are the patient's underlying assumptions about their medical condition and its related therapies, which often explain the types of questions that the patient asks about their condition's etiology, symptoms, the degree of severity, the type of sick role (chronic or acute) they assume, and various treatment options (94). These beliefs are directly influenced by one's cultural groups and social class (93,95).

In analyzing medical discourse, Mischler (96) identifies two opposing voices: the voice of medicine (reflecting a scientific, detached attitude) and the voice of the "lifeworld" (patient's meaning of illness and how this disrupts the achievement of personal goals). He sees the medical encounter as a situation of conflict between two distinct efforts to construct meaning (97, p. 81). As Kleinman (92) suggests, the effectiveness of professional communication and health care outcomes is a function of the agreement between the patient's and clinician's explanatory models.

Understanding the patient's perspective of her condition is a prerequisite for successful clinician–patient dialogue. It is also important to recognize how frequently this perspective differs (93). Studies that have explored issues of potential patient–provider conflict include the degree to which physicians meet patient expectations (98), how often physicians are aware of patients' concerns (99,100), the rate of agreement between patients and physicians about those problems that require follow-up visits (101), and levels of agreement between patients and their physicians regarding the patient's health status (102).

Implications of Cultural Diversity

Racial, ethnic and social disparities exist in U.S. health care and have become the focus of a recent Institute of Medicine report uncovering "unequal treatment" (103). Even after controlling for age, insurance status, income, comorbid conditions, and symptom expression, racial and ethnic groups are more likely to experience a substandard quality of health care. Explanations for this disparity in health care, embedded in historic and contemporary socioeconomic inequalities, are complex. Accountabilities exist on many levels: health systems, administrative and bureaucratic policies, utilization managers, and clinicians and patients (103).

As the growth of ethnic populations currently referred to as minorities continues, they will comprise 40% of the U.S. population by 2035, and 47% by 2050 (104). The health care needs of an increasingly diverse U.S. population are now established as a goal of public health, thus cultural, linguistic, and literacy differences must addressed (105,106).

Clinicians are challenged to examine the part they play in creating these disparities: their expressions of bias (or discrimination), greater clinical uncertainty when interacting with minority patients, and the beliefs (or stereotypes) held by professionals about the behavior or health of minorities. In response, patients may contribute to these dynamics through mistrust, treatment refusal, or poor compliance with prescribed therapies. Additional barriers to health care access for minorities can include language, geography, and cultural familiarity. Health systems may also contribute to these inequities because of heavy time pressures, cognitive complexities within the clinical encounter, and the push for cost containment (103).

As one example, a study by Rivadeneyra and colleagues (107) revealed that Spanish-speaking patients experience a double disadvantage when receiving medical care from English-speaking physicians. Primary care patients who spoke through an interpreter made markedly fewer comments than did patients speaking directly with clinicians. Due to time consumed by the interpretation process, these patients had fewer opportunities to explain their symptoms or raise concerns. Further, when they did offer comments, they were more likely to be ignored than the English-speaking patients. These findings illustrate that non-English speaking patients have communication barriers beyond just difficulties with translation. Rivadeneyra and associates suggest that both physician and patient may change their behavior in subtle ways that may compromise the development of mutual trust, increase the likelihood of physician misunderstanding of the complexity associated with the patient's symptoms, and decrease the possibility of patient compliance with medical advice (107).

Other studies have also found that clinicians deliver less information, less supportive remarks, and less proficient clinical performance to black and Hispanic patients and patients from lower economic status than they do to more advantaged patients, even in the same setting (78,80,108).

The ability to establish effective interpersonal and working relationships that transcend cultural differences defines "cultural competence." Within health care, cultural competence describes the process by which a clinician continuously attempts to be effective within the cultural context of a patient, who may be an individual, family, or community (109,106).

Strategies to bridge the sociocultural inequities in health care include providing interpreters as well as linguistic competency to health education materials, the incorporation of clinical staff who share similar cultural backgrounds in addition to the inclusion of family or community health workers, and clinic accommodations that adjust hours of operation and physical environment, and increasing the ability of professionals to interact effectively within the culture of the patient population through regular continuing education (110,106).

Gender Bias

Research has also investigated gender bias in the delivery of health care—that is, if and how female patients are treated and perceived in a way different from male patients by physicians. Twenty years ago, McCranie, Horowitz, and Martin (111) reported no evidence that physicians attribute psychogenic illness more frequently to women than men or recommend psychological treatments more to women. Verbrugge and Steiner (112) also failed to identify any significant gender differences in tests and procedures in their analyses of National Ambulatory Medical Care Survey data.

More recent research in coronary artery disease, kidney dialysis and transplantation, and the diagnosis of lung cancer (113–115) provides convincing evidence that differences in the quality of the technical care received by women cannot be explained by other factors, such as poorer health status (116).

Bernstein and Kane (117) investigated the relative impact of patient gender and expressivity on attitudes of primary care physicians toward patients. Their research determined that physicians believed that women were more likely to make excessive demands as compared to men, women's health complaints were assessed as more likely to be influenced by emotional factors, and women were identified more frequently with psychosomatic complaints than men. Their results supported their hypotheses that physicians have preconceptions about female patients. They also argue, however, that differences in physicians' responses are not simply due to bias against women, but may be a complex response to the open and expressive behavioral style more frequently identified in women. They suggest that their findings underline the necessity for physicians to rise above stereotypes and treat each patient as an individual, instead of a member of a group (118, p. 607).

Collaboration

Increasing evidence exists for the value of a collaborative model of communication that promotes mutual interaction between patients and providers. Roter and Hall (87) offer a framework for understanding patient–provider communication as a partnership, each having certain responsibilities to contribute to the quality of their exchange. This model suggests associations between the patient's question-asking (and the information that is subsequently offered by the provider) with the patient's overall comprehension, agreement with treatment, and continuance with prescribed therapies.

The value of patient involvement during the medical encounter is revealed through enhanced patient satisfaction and loyalty to the clinician (70); among patients with chronic diseases, active patient participation is associated with better health outcomes (116). Patients are also most satisfied by interactions with physicians who encourage them to talk about psychosocial issues in an atmosphere that is characterized by the absence of domination by the physician (118).

In summary, women's experiences of health care services and physician interactions are different from those of their male patient counterparts. The role of communication is paramount to ensuring maximal health outcomes. As information technology becomes more accessible and more widely utilized, the nature of this communication will change. Yet, interpersonal interactions are essential to health care provision. A mutual appreciation and respect for the expertise that each individual (patient or clinician) brings to the medical encounter will facilitate more substantive dialog. Assimilating the principles of cultural competence enhances the interactions and significantly influences the outcomes of care. Just as physicians are technical experts in medical science and therapeutic options, so women are experts in how they feel, both physically and emotionally. Women can usually talk about how their health or illness affects the complexity of their lives, their careers, and families or relationships. Women must be listened to without interruption and believed by their care providers. Physicians must attempt to integrate the complex, contextual aspects of women's health or illness and not focus solely on the pathology of their medical condition and its treatment.

References

1. Weisman CS. *Women's health care: activist traditions and institutional change.* Baltimore, Md: The Johns Hopkins University Press, 1998;10–36.
2. Wizemann TM, Pardue M-L (eds). *Exploring the Biological contributions to human health: does sex matter?* Washington, DC: National Academy Press, 2001.
3. Connell R. *Gender and power.* Stanford, Calif: Stanford University Press, 1987.
4. Pinn VW. Sex and gender factors in medical studies: implications for health and clinical practice. *JAMA* 2003;289(4):397–399.
5. U.S. Department of Labor, Bureau of Labor Statistics, August 2001. *Highlights of women's earnings in 2000* (Report 952). http://www.bls.gov/cps/cpswom2000.pdf. Accessed 1/12/03.
6. U.S. Department of Health and Human Services. *Women, work and health.* DHHS Pub No. (PHS) 98-1791. Washington, DC: USDHHS, 1997.
7. Messing K. Multiple roles and complex exposures: hard-to-pin down risks for working women. In: Goldman MB, Hatch MC, (eds.) *Women & Health.* San Diego, Calif: Academic Press, 2000;455–462.
8. Collins KS, Schoen C, Joseph S, et al. *Health concerns across the lifespan: 1998 Survey of Women's Health.* New York, NY: The Commonwealth Fund, 1999.
9. U.S. Census Bureau and Bureau of Labor Statistics, Current Population Survey, Annual Demographic Survey, March 2000 (Table 1). http://ferret.bls.census.gov/macro/032001/pov/toc.htm. Accessed 1/12/03.

10. U.S. Bureau of the Census. *Poverty in the United States 1998: current population reports.* Washington, DC: U.S. Bureau of the Census.

11. Wilson J. Women and poverty: a demographic overview. *Women's Health* 1987;12(3/4):21–40.

12. Richardson H. The health plight of rural women. *Women's Health* 1987;12(3/4):41–54.

13. Institute for Research on Poverty (IRP). *Who was poor in 2001?* http://www.ssc.wisc.edu/irp/faqx/faq3.htm. Accessed 1/13/03.

14. American College of Physicians-American Society of Internal Medicine. White paper: *No health insurance? It's enough to make you sick.* Philadelphia, Pa: American College of Physicians-American Society of Internal Medicine, 2000.

15. Campbell J, Landenberger K. Violence against women. In: Fogel C, Woods N, (eds.) *Women's health care: A comprehensive handbook.* Thousand Oaks, Calif: Sage, 1995.

16. Plichta SB, Falik M. Prevalence of violence and its implications for women's health. *Women's Health Issues* 2001;11(3):244–258.

17. Faludi S. *Backlash.* New York, NY: Crown Books, 1991.

18. McLaughlin S, Melber B. The changing lifecourse of American women: Life-style and attitude changes, draft. Seattle, Wash: Battelle Human Affairs Research Centers, 1986.

19. U.S. Department of Commerce News. *US Census Bureau releases profile of nation's women, 2001.* Washington, DC: http://www.census.gov/Press-Release/www/2001/cb01-49.html.

20. Bernstein AB. Motherhood, health status, and health care. *Women's Health Issues* 2001;11(3):173–184.

21. U.S. Department of Commerce News. *U.S. Census Bureau releases record share of new mothers in labor force, Census Bureau Reports.* Washington, DC: 2000. http://www.census.gov/Press-Release/www/2000/cb00-175.html. Accessed 1/12/03.

22. Collins K, Rowland D, Salganicoff A, Chait E. Assessing and improving women's health. In: Costello C, Stone A, (eds.) *The American woman: 1994–: Where We Stand.* New York, NY: Norton, 1994;154–196.

23. U.S. Census Bureau Public Affairs Information Office. *U.S. Census Bureau facts for features: women's history month: March 1-31.* Washington, DC: 2001. http://www.census.gov/Press-Release/www/2001/cb01ff03.html. Accessed 1/12/03.

24. McGovern P, Gjerdingen D, Froberg D. The parental leave debate: implications for policy relevant research. *Women's Health* 1992;18:97–118.

25. Donelan K, Falik M, DesRoches CM. Caregiving: challenges and implications for women's health. *Women's Health Issues* 2001;11(5):185.

26. Russo N. Overview: forging research priorities for women's mental health. *Am Psych* 1990;45(3):368–373.

27. Verbrugge L. Role burdens and physical health of women and men. *Women's Health* 1986;11(1):47–77.

28. U.S. Census Bureau Public Affairs Information Office. *U.S. Census Bureau facts for features: mother's day 1999: May 9.* Washington, DC: 1999. http://www.census.gov/Press-Release/www/1999/cb99ff07.html. Accessed 1/12/03.

29. Haynes S, Feinleib M. Women, work, and coronary heart disease: prospective findings from the Framingham Heart Study. *Am J Public Health* 1980;70(2):133–141.

30. Nathanson C. Social roles and health status among women: the significance of employment. *Soc Sci Med* 1980;14a:463–471.

31. Frankenhauser M. The psychophysiology of sex differences as related to occupation. In: Frankenhauser M, Lundberg U, Chesney M, (eds.) *Women, work and health: stress and opportunities.* New York, NY: Plenum, 1991;35–64.

32. Hochschild A, Machung A. *The second shift.* New York, NY: Avon Books, 1990.

33. Woods N. Employment, family roles, and mental ill health in young adult married women. *Nursing Research* 1985;34(1):4–9.

34. Van Fossen B. Sex differences in the mental health effects of spouse support and equity. *J Health Soc Behav* 1981;22:130–143.

35. McBride A. Multiple roles. *Am Psych* 1990;45:381–384.

36. Miller J. The development of a woman's sense of self. In: Jordan J, Kaplan A, Miler J, Stiver I, Surrey J, (eds.) *Women's growth in connection: writings from the Stone Center.* New York, NY: Guilford, 1991;11–26.

37. Surrey J. The "self-in-relation": A theory of women's development. In: Jordan, op cit. 1991;51–66.

38. Jordan J. *Empathy and self boundaries.* In Jordan, op cit. 1991;67–80.

39. Raymond J. *A Passion for friends: toward a philosophy of female affection.* Boston, Mass: Beacon, 1986.

40. Belenky M, et al. *Women's ways of knowing: the development of self, voice, and mind.* New York, NY: Basic Books, 1986.

41. Gilligan C. *In a different voice: psychological theory and women's development.* Cambridge, Mass: Harvard University Press, 1982.

42. Nussbaum R. Studies of women's health care: selected results. *Permanente Journal* 2000;4(3):62–67.

43. Robinson TN, Patrick K, Eng TR, Gustafson D, for the Science Panel on Interactive Communication and Health. An evidence-based approach to interactive health communication: a challenge to medicine in the information age. *JAMA* 1998;280(14):1264–1269.

44. Pandey SK, Hart JJ, Tiwary S. Women's health and the Internet: understanding emerging trends and implications. *Soc Sci Med* 2003;56:179–191.

45. Weisman CS. Women's use of health care. In: Falik MM, Collins KS, (eds.) *Women's Health: the Commonwealth Fund survey.* Baltimore, Md: Johns Hopkins University Press, 1996;19–48.

46. Society for Women's Health Research. Women's Healthlinks. http://www.womens-health-org/healthfactsheet2.html. Accessed 5/18/01.

47. Healy BP. Editorial: listening to America's women. *J Wom Health* 1995;4(6):589–590.

48. Rothert M, Padonu G, Holmes-Rovner M, et al. Menopausal women as decision makers in health care. *Exp Gerontol* 1994;29:(3/4):463–468.

49. Rothert M, Rovner D, Holmes M, et al. Women's use of information regarding hormone replacement therapy. *Res Nurs Health* 1990;13(6):355–366.

50. U.S. Department of Commerce. A nation online: how Americans are expanding their use of the Internet. Washington, DC: 2/2002. http://www.nti.doc.gov/ntiahome/dn/html. Accessed 12/15/02.

51. Hoffman D, Novak T. Bridging the racial divide on the Internet. *Science* 1998;390–391.

52. Pew Internet & American Life Project http://pewinternet.org/reports/reports.asp. Accessed 12/2/02.

53. Leber S, Mack K. The Internet and clinical practice of child neurology. *Curr Op Neurol* 2000;13:147–153.

54. Kane B, Sands DZ and the American Medical Informatics Association Task Force on Guidelines for the Use of Clinic-Patient Electronic Mail. Guidelines for the clinical use of electronic mail with patients. *J American Inform Assoc* 1998;5:104–111.

55. Eng TR, Maxfield A, Patrick K, Deering MJ, Ratzan SC, Gustafson DH. Access to health information and support: a public highway or a private road? *JAMA* 1998;280:1371–1375.

56. Mandl DK, Kohane IS, Brandt AM. Electronic patient-physician communication: problems and promises. *Ann Intern Med* 1998;129:495–500.

57. Hall J, Roter D, Katz NR. Correlates of provider behavior: a meta-analysis. *Med Care* 1988;26(7):657–675.

58. Kaplan SH, Greenfield S, Ware JE Jr. Assessing the effects of physician-patient interactions: the outcomes of chronic disease. *Med Care* 1989;27(suppl 3):S110–S127.

59. Brody DS, Miller SM, Lerman CE, Smith DG, Caputo GC. Patient perception of involvement in medical care: relationship to illness attitudes and outcomes. *J Gen Intern Med* 1989;4(Nov/Dec):506–511.

60. Anderson LA, Sharpe PA. Improving patient and provider communication: a synthesis and review of communication interventions. *Patient Education Counseling* 1991;17:99–134.

61. Meeuwesen L, Schaap C, Van der Staak C. Verbal analysis of doctor-patient communication. *Soc Sci Med* 1991;32(10):1143–1150.

62. Bensing J, van der Brink-Muinen A, de Bakker D. Gender differences in practice style: a Dutch study of general practitioners. *Medical Care* 1993;31(3):219–229.

63. Hodne CJ, Reiter RC. Decision-making in women's health care. *Clin Obstet Gynecol* 1994;37(1):162–178.

64. Ong LML, DeHaes JCJM, Hoos AM, Lammes FB. Doctor-patient communication: a review of the literature. *Socl Sci Med* 1995;40(7):903–918.

65. Lin CT, Albertson GA, Schilling LM, et al. Is patients' perception of time spent with the physician a determinant of ambulatory patient satisfaction? *Arch Intern Med* 2001;161:1437–1442.

66. Fisher S. *In the patient's best interest: women and the politics of medical decisions.* New Brunswick, NJ: Rutgers University Press, 1986.

67. Ruzek S. *The women's health movement.* New York, NY: Praeger, 1979.

68. Weisman C, Teitelbaum M. Women and health care communication. *Patient Ed Counse* 1989;13:183–189.

69. Stewart MA. Effective physician-patient communication and health outcomes: a review. *Canadian Med Assoc J* 1995;152(9):1423–1433.

70. Kaplan SH, Sullivan LM, Spetter D, Dukes KA, Khan A, Greenfield S. Gender and patterns of physician-patient communication. In: Falik MM, Collins KS, (eds.) *Women's health: The commonwealth fund survey.* Baltimore, Md: Johns Hopkins University Press, 1996; 76–95.

71. Roter DL. Patient question asking in physician-patient interaction. *Health Psych* 1984;3(5):395–409.

72. Tannen D. *Gender and discourse.* New York, NY: Oxford University Press, 1994.

73. Weisman C, Teitelbaum M. Women and health care communication. *Patient Ed Counse* 1989;13:183–189.

74. Verbrugge L. Sex differences in complaints and diagnoses. *J Behav Med* 1980;3:327–355.

75. Wallen J, Waitzkin H, Stoeckle J. Physician stereotypes about female health and illness: a study of patient's sex and the informative process during medical interviews. *Wom Health* 1979;4:135.

76. Kaplan SH, Greenfield S. Gender differences in physician-patient communication for patients seeing the same and opposite gender physicians [Abstract]. *Soc Gen Intern Med* 1991.

77. Roter DL, Lipkin M, Korsgaard A. Sex differences in patients' and physicians' communication during primary care visits. *Med Care* 1991;29(11):1083–1093.

78. Hooper EM, Comstock LM, Goodwin JM, Goodwin JS. Patient characteristics that influence physician behavior. *Med Care* 1982;20(6):630–638.

79. Pendleton DA, Bochner S. The communication of medical information in general practice consultations as a function of patients' social class. *Soc Sci Med* 1980;14A(6):669–673.

80. Waitzkin H. Information giving in medical care. *J Health Soc Behav* 1985;26(2):81–101.

81. Hall JA, Irish JT, Roter DL, Ehrlich CM, Miller LH. Gender in medical encounters: an analysis of physician and patient communication in a primary care setting. *Health Psych* 1994;13(5):384–392.

82. Arora NK, McHorney CA. Patient preferences for medical decision making: who really wants to participate? *Med Care* 2000;38(3):335–341.

83. Stewart M. Patient characteristics which are related to the doctor-patient interaction. *Fam Prac* 1983;1:30–36.

84. Svarstad BL. *The doctor-patient encounter: an observational study of communication and outcome.* Doctoral dissertation, University of Wisconsin, Madison, 1974.

85. West C, Zimmerman DH. Small insults: a study of interruptions in cross-sex conversations between unacquainted persons. In: Thorne B, Kramarer C, Henley N (eds.) *Language, gender and society.* Rowley, Mass: Newbury House, 1983;103–117.

86. West C, Zimmerman DH. Doing gender. *Gender in Society* 1987;1:125–151.

87. Roter DL, Hall JA. Health education theory: an application to the process of patient-provider communication. *Health Ed* 1991;6:1301–1306.

88. Tannen D. *You just don't understand: women and men in conversation.* New York, NY: William Morris, 1990.

89. Beckman HB, Frankel RM. The effect of physician behavior on the collection of data. *Ann Intern Med* 1984;101(5):692–696.

90. Allen D, Gilchrist V, Levinson W, Roter D. Caring for women: is it different? Schroeder H, ed. *Patient Care* Nov 1993;183–196.

91. Mathews JJ. The communication process in clinical settings. *Soc Sci Med* 1983;17(18):1371–1378.

92. Kleinman AM. *Patients and healers in the context of culture.* Los Angeles, Calif: University of California Press, 1987.

93. Helman CG. Communication in primary care: the role of patient and practitioner explanatory models. *Soc Sci Med* 1985;20(9):923–931.

94. Joos SK, Hickam DH. How health professionals influence health behavior: Patient-provider interaction and health care outcomes. In: Glanz K, Lewis FM, Rimer BK, (eds.) *Health behavior and health education.* San Francisco, Calif: Jossey-Bass, 1990;216–241.

95. Kleinman A, Eisenberg L, Good B. Culture, illness, and care: clinical lessons from anthropologic and cross-cultural research. *Ann Intern Med* 1978;88(2):251–258.

96. Mischler EG. *The discourse of medicine: dialectics of medical interviews.* Norwood, NY: Ablex, 1984.

97. Weston WW, Brown JB. The importance of patients' beliefs. In: Stewart M, Roter D, (eds.) *Communicating with medical patients.* Newbury Park, Calif: Sage Publications, 1989;77–85.

98. Bell RA, Kravitz RL, Thorn D, Krupat E, Azari R. Unmet expectations for care and the patient-physician relationship. *J Gen Intern Med* 2002;17:817–824.

99. Krupat E, Rosenkranz SL, Yeager CM, Barnard K, Putnam SM, Inui TS. The practice orientations of physicians and patients: the effect of doctor-patient congruence on satisfaction. *Patient Ed Counsel* 2000;39:49–59.

100. Levinson W, Gorawar-Bhat, Lamb J. A study of patient clues and physician responses in primary care and surgical settings. *JAMA* 2000;284:1021–1027.

101. Starfield B, Steinwachs D, Morris I, Bause G, Siebert S, Westin C. Patient-doctor agreement about problems needing follow-up visit. *JAMA* 1979;242(4):344–346.

102. Rakowski W, Hickey T, Dengiz A. Congruence of health and treatment perceptions among older patients and providers of primary care. *Int J Aging Hum Devel* 1987;25:67–81.

103. Smedley BD, Stith AY, Nelson AR, (eds.) *Unequal treatment: confronting racial and ethnic disparities in health care.* Washington, DC: The National Academies Press, 2002.

104. U.S. Bureau of the Census. *Current population reports, series P25-1130: population projections for the U.S. by sex, race and Hispanic origin, 1995-2050.* Washington, DC: U.S. Bureau of the Census, 1996.

105. Agency for Health Care Policy and Research. *Understanding and eliminating minority health disparities* (RFA: HS-00-003). Rockville, Md: Agency for Health Care Policy and Research, 1999.

106. Cooper LA, Roter DL. Patient-provider communication: the effect of race and ethnicity on process and outcomes of health care. In: Smedley BD, Stith AY, Nelson AR, (eds.) *Unequal treatment: confronting racial and ethnic disparities in health care.* Washington, DC: The National Academies Press, 2002;330–354.

107. Rivadeneyra R, Elderkin-Thompson V, Cohen Silver R, Waitzkin H. Patient centeredness in medical encounters requiring an interpreter. *Am J Med* 2000;108:470–474.

108. Wasserman RC, Inui TS, Barriatua RD, Carter WB, Lippincott P. Pediatric clinicians' support for parents makes a difference: an outcome-based analysis of clinician-parent interaction. *Pediatrics* 1984;74:1047–1053.

109. Camphina-Bacote J. A model and instrument for addressing cultural competence in health care. *J Nurs Ed* 1999;38:203–220.

110. Brach C, Fraser I. Can cultural competency reduce racial and ethnic disparities? A review and conceptual model. *Med Care Res Rev* 2000;57(suppl 1):181–210.

111. McCranie EW, Horowitz AJ, Martin RM. Alleged sex-role stereotyping in the assessment of women's physical complaints: a study of general practitioners. *Soc Sci Med* 1978;12(2A):111–116.

112. Verbrugge LM, Steiner RP. Physician treatment of men and women patients: sex bias or appropriate care? *Med Care* 1981;19(6):609–632.

113. Wenger NK, Speroff L, Packard B. Cardiovascular health and disease in women. *N Engl J Med* 1993;329(4): 247–256.

114. Ayanian JZ, Epstein AM. Differences in the use of procedures between men and women hospitalized for coronary artery disease. *N Engl J Med* 1991;325:221–225.

115. Council on Ethical and Judicial Affairs, American Medical Association. Gender disparities in clinical decision-making. *JAMA* 1991;266(4):559–562.

116. Kaplan SH, Gandek B, Greenfield S, Rogers WH, Ware JE Jr. Patient and visit characteristics related to physicians' participatory decision-making style: results from the medical outcomes study. *Med Care* 1995;33(12): 1176–1187.

117. Bernstein B, Kane R. Physicians' attitudes toward female patients. *Med Care* 1981;19(6):600–608.

118. Bertakis KD, Helms LJ, Callahan EJ, Azari R, Robbins JA. The influence of gender of physician practice style. *Med Care* 1995;33(4):407–416.

4 Drug Treatments and Trials in Women

Stephen D. Silberstein

D rugs are usually developed and tested in young to middle-aged adults despite the fact that age and gender differences exist in pharmacokinetics (how individuals handle drugs) and pharmacodynamics (how individuals respond to drugs) (1). Drugs are not usually developed for or specifically evaluated in children, and the adult drug dose cannot always be safely converted to its pediatric equivalent (1). Pharmacodynamic differences can lead to unexpected outcomes and adverse effects. For example, antihistamines and barbiturates, which generally sedate adults, often cause children to become hyperactive. Chronic phenobarbital therapy can affect learning and behavior in children (1). In infants, pharmacokinetic differences may affect drug bioavailability. Low gastric acidity, slower absorption rates, and a difference in gastric emptying time may influence the absorption of orally administered drugs in the neonate.

Pregnant women are often excluded from drug trials, despite the fact that they may metabolize drugs in a way different from nonpregnant women. Differences between breast-feeding mothers and other women of the same age could cause changes in drug distribution. Fat accumulated during pregnancy is still present in the nursing mother and may affect the distribution of fat-soluble drugs. Sex bias may result in the perception that women have a higher biologic vulnerability than do men. For example, the belief that reproduction and fetal health are exclusively women's health issues has resulted in a lack of investigation of male-mediated reproductive toxicity (2).

GENDER DIFFERENCES

Gender can lead to differences in pharmacokinetics. Women often have higher plasma drug concentrations than men receiving the same dose; for example, lidocaine and chlordiazepoxide levels are higher in women because of longer elimination half-life (3). Oral contraceptive (OC) use, sex differences in basal metabolism, and hormone and enzyme levels all influence drug metabolism. OCs can prolong the elimination half-life of drugs that are metabolized by hepatic oxidation. Differences in vascular resistance, muscle mass, and muscle composition may cause a variation in absorption from intramuscular injections. Differences in gastric motility and secretion and metabolic rate may influence plasma levels of orally administered drugs (3).

Gender differences may be present in psychotropic drugs. In one study, male schizophrenic patients required less medication and had a more favorable outcome than female patients (3). Findings from a more recent study by Yonkers and coworkers (4), however, indicate that antipsychotic agents have greater efficacy in women as well as greater likelihood of adverse reactions.

41

Gender differences depend in part on which sex hormone milestone a woman has passed. Menarche marks the onset of the cyclic ovarian function that spans the time between puberty and menopause, which themselves are transitional periods of increasing or decreasing ovarian activity. Menses are a peripheral marker of steroid hormone withdrawal that bridges smooth changes in hormone levels: Follicular growth with rising estrogen levels is followed by ovulation and rising progesterone levels. Other sex hormone milestones include pregnancy, OC use, and estrogen replacement therapy. Differences in sex hormone levels can influence drug metabolism, and drugs can influence sex hormone levels (5).

The phase of the menstrual cycle can affect alcohol metabolism. Decreased elimination times, reduced area under the curves (AUCs; a measure of bioavailability), and faster disappearance rates occur during the midluteal phase compared with the early follicular and ovulatory phases. The midluteal phase is associated with higher progesterone levels, elevated progesterone-estradiol ratios, and lower follicle-stimulating hormone (FSH) levels (6).

When postmenopausal women take oral replacement estrogen, alcohol ingestion can lead to a threefold increase in circulating estradiol levels, similar to the changes that occur when women use transdermal estrogen. Estrone levels decrease after alcohol ingestion, perhaps due to decreased conversion from estradiol. Increased oxidation of sulfated estrogen precursor androgens to estradiol occurs in rats in response to alcohol and may account in part for higher estradiol levels (7).

Gender differences can also be caused by nonhormonal factors, such as (i) poverty and socioeconomic status; (ii) nutritional deficits related to poverty or to eating behavior, such as cyclical dieting; and (iii) occupational selection biases that favor women, as in nursing or housecleaning. Each of these factors can affect a woman's metabolism, and some can increase her exposure to toxins (2).

Gender, disease state, and drugs can interact. Polycystic ovarian syndrome (PCOS), characterized clinically by hirsutism and menstrual irregularities, is frequently (30 to 50%) associated with obesity. Multiple follicular cysts and increased stroma in the ovaries may be found on ultrasonography. Hyperandrogenism is caused by elevated serum levels of testosterone, androstenedione, or dehydroepiandrosterone sulfate. Elevated luteinizing hormone (LH), FSH, and prolactin levels are common.

Menstrual disorders, altered pulsatile secretion of LH, and PCOS are common among women with epilepsy. Herzog and colleagues found a 60% frequency of menstrual disorders and a 30% frequency of PCOS among 20 women with untreated complex partial seizures (8), whereas another group (9) found higher LH pulse frequency in untreated epileptics compared with controls (increased LH pulse frequency promotes the development of PCOS).

Valproate use in women with epilepsy is associated with a higher incidence of PCOS (10,11) than other antiepileptic drugs (AEDs). Isojärvi and coworkers (11) have suggested that this is due to valproate-induced weight gain and induced insulin resistance. PCOS, however, is more common in valproate-treated obese women with epilepsy than in obese normal control subjects. Herzog (12) has speculated that the fundamental problem is epilepsy itself, which is associated with PCOS, and that the other AEDS induce cytochrome P450 and accelerate the biotransformation of testosterone, whereas valproate does not. This association occurs only in women with epilepsy treated with valproate and has not been shown to occur with increased frequency in women with other disorders, such as mania or migraine. Women with epilepsy can be treated with valproate, but they should be followed up for menstrual irregularities. If irregularities occur, ultrasound may be indicated.

RISK OF DRUG TREATMENT

A teratogen is usually defined as any agent, physical force, or other factor that can induce a congenital anomaly through the alteration of normal development during any stage of embryogenesis (8).

The recognition of the teratogenicity of aminopterin and thalidomide and the rubella epidemic of 1963–1964, resulted in extremely conservative drug use during pregnancy. In 1977, the Food and Drug Administration (FDA) developed a policy against phase I and early phase II testing for pregnant women or women of childbearing potential, and many practitioners now avoid drug treatment in pregnancy even when it is indicated. More than 2,500 agents are listed in Shepard's catalog of teratogenic agents. About 1,200 can produce congenital anomalies in experimental animals, but only about 40 of these are known to cause defects in the human (8). Insufficient knowledge exists about the birth defect risks from drug exposure, despite the fact that 67% of women take drugs during pregnancy, and 50% take them during the first trimester (9).

Most drugs cross the placenta and have the potential to adversely affect the fetus, and although studies have not absolutely established the safety of any medication during pregnancy, some drugs are believed to be relatively safe (see Tables 4.7 through 4.21) (10–13).

In 1966, the FDA replaced the Multigeneration Continuous Feeding Reproductive Study with a three-segment design, identified as Segment I (Fertility and General Reproductive Performance), Segment II (Teratology), and Segment III (Perinatal and Postnatal Evaluations), for testing drugs. These studies were designed to detect agents that specifically interrupt reproduction. More than 3,300 chemicals have been tested; of these, 37% are teratogenic. These studies frequently used very high doses of drugs, which then produced maternal toxicity, not fetal teratogenicity. Currently 19 drugs, or drug groups, and two chemicals have been established as human teratogens. Negative results in other species cannot predict a lack of teratogenicity in humans, and drugs that are teratogenic at high doses in these species may not be teratogenic in humans at lower doses (14). Thalidomide, which has no teratogenic effect in mice and rats, has profound teratogenic effects in humans (10,15).

WOMEN AND DRUG TRIALS

A negative pregnancy test is often a condition of enrollment in a study, and postenrollment pregnancy can lead to the termination of participation. This poses a problem for pregnant women who are sick and in need of treatment. If the drug has not been tested in pregnant women during the research phase, information is lacking about the safety and efficacy of the drug for the woman as well as for the fetus (16). The Institute of Medicine Committee on Research in Women made the controversial recommendation that pregnant and lactating women should be considered eligible for enrollment in clinical studies on a routine basis (16). This report reversed the existing exclusion of pregnant women and the severely restricted enrollment of women of "childbearing potential" in most clinical studies. With regard to enrollment, the Committee recommended that women who are or may become pregnant during the course of a study should be viewed as any other potential research subject.

With more women of childbearing age participating in clinical trials, more information will be gained about the risks of birth defects, but uncertainty will still persist. If the medication is associated with a very high level of birth defects (e.g., thalidomide), however, very few exposures need to be followed to detect this risk; if the medication is associated with a slight increase in the overall occurrence of birth defects, approximately 300 exposed pregnancies need to be followed up to detect a doubling of risk; and if the medication is associated with a rare increase of a specific defect (e.g., 1 in 1,000), approximately 10,000 exposed pregnancies need to be followed up to detect a doubling of risk (17).

DRUG USE DURING PREGNANCY

The World Health Organization (WHO) completed an international survey of 14,778 pregnant women on prescription drug utilization during pregnancy. Eighty-six percent of the subjects took medication, each receiving an average of 2.9 prescriptions. Of a total of 37,309 prescriptions, 73% were given by obstetricians, 12% by general practitioners, and 5% by midwives (11). In a survey of pregnant women at Parkland Memorial Hospital in Dallas, 40% took some type of medication other than iron or vitamin supplements, and up to 20% used an illicit drug or alcohol (18). In contrast, in England only 35% of pregnant women took drugs or medications during pregnancy, and only 6% used medications other than vitamin or iron supplements during the first trimester. Among 18,886 Medicaid patients in Michigan, women received an average of 3.1 prescriptions for medications other than vitamins or iron during their pregnancies (19). Approximately 70% of pregnant women in the United States took prescribed drugs, according to two surveys (20,21). The National Hospital Discharge Survey found a 576% increase in discharges of drug-using parturient women and a 456% increase in discharges of drug-affected newborns in the United States between 1979 and 1990.

Adverse Effects

Adverse drug effects depend on the dose and route of administration, concomitant exposures, and timing of the exposure relative to the period of development, which consist of the preimplantation period, embryogenesis, and fetal development. The preimplantation period lasts from conception to 1 week postconception, during which time the conceptus is relatively protected from drugs (18). Embryogenesis is the time of organogenesis, which occurs from the time of implantation to 58 to 60 days postconception (18). Most congenital malformations arise during this time. Placental transport is not well established until the fifth week after conception. This may protect the embryo from maternal drugs. The final phase, fetal development, follows embryogenesis. The fetus grows mainly in size, although structural changes such as neuronal arrangement also occur. Malformations can develop at this time in normally formed organs due to their necrosis and reabsorption (18).

Death to the conceptus, teratogenicity, fetal growth abnormalities, perinatal effects, postnatal developmental abnormalities, delayed oncogenesis, and functional and behavioral changes can result from drugs or other agents (Table 4.1) (10). According to the Perinatal Collaborative Project, a prospective and concurrent epidemiologic study of more than 50,000 pregnancies, many drugs have little or no human teratogenic risk (10,22).

Spontaneous Abortion

Nearly one-half of early pregnancies (0 to 58 days) spontaneously abort, most due to chromosomal abnormalities.

TABLE 4.1
Definitions and Drug Effects (10)

Spontaneous abortion:	Death of the conceptus. Most due to chromosomal abnormality.
Embryotoxicity: anomalies:	The ability of drugs to kill the developing embryo.
Congenital	Deviation from normal morphology or function.
Teratogenicity:	The ability of an exogenous agent to produce a permanent abnormality of structure or function in an organism exposed during embryogenesis or fetal life.
Fetal effects:	Growth retardation, abnormal histogenesis (also congenital abnormalities and fetal death). The main outcome of fetal drug toxicity during the second and third trimesters of pregnancy.
Perinatal effects:	Effects on uterine contraction, neonatal withdrawal, or hemostasis.
Postnatal effects:	Drugs may have delayed long-term effects: delayed oncogenesis, and functional and behavioral abnormalities.

Before the time of organogenesis, exposure to a potential teratogen or toxic drug has an all-or-none effect. An exposure around the time of conception or implantation may kill the conceptus, but if the pregnancy continues, there is no increased risk of congenital anomalies (10).

Developmental Defects

Developmental defects may result from genetic or environmental causes, or from interactions between them. Teratogenic drug effects are generally visible anatomic malformations; they are defined as the production of a permanent alteration of an organ's structure or function due to intrauterine exposure. These effects are dose- and time-related, with the fetus at greatest risk during the first trimester of pregnancy. Drug exposure accounts for only 2 to 3% of birth defects; approximately 25% are genetic, and the causes of the remainder are unknown (10). The incidence of major malformations either incompatible with survival (e.g., anencephaly) or requiring major surgery (e.g., cleft palate or congenital heart disease) is approximately 2 to 3% in the general population. If all minor malformations are included (ear tags or extra digits), the rate may be as high as 7 to 10%. The risk of malformation after drug exposure must be compared with

this background rate.

Birth defects are more common in the children of epileptics, even those who are not taking drugs. The risk is further increased if AEDs are used. Treatment with multiple AEDs increases the teratogenic risk; therefore, monotherapy is advocated (23,24). Overlapping drugs during AED change may expose the fetus to higher concentrations of toxic metabolites and is relatively contraindicated.

The classic teratogenic period in the human is a critical 6 weeks, lasting from approximately 31 days through 10 weeks from the last menstrual period. A teratogenic effect depends on the timing of the exposure as well as on the nature of the teratogen. Exposure early in the pregnancy, when the heart and central nervous system are forming, may result in an anomaly such as congenital heart disease or neural tube defect, whereas later exposure may result in malformation of the palate or ear (10). After the teratogenic period has passed, the major risk of congenital anomaly is gone, but other abnormalities can occur. These include fetal effects, neonatal effects, and postnatal effects.

Fetal Effects

Fetal effects include damage to normally formed organs, damage to systems undergoing histogenesis, growth retardation, or fetal death. Growth retardation is the most common of these.

Neonatal and Postnatal Effects

Certain drugs are associated with adverse neonatal effects, such as drug withdrawal and neonatal hypoglycemia, or adverse maternal effects, such as hemostasis and uterine contracture disorders. Chronic exposure to psychoactive medications, such as alcohol, during the second and third trimesters may cause mental retardation, which may not be recognized until later in life (10). Developmental delay and long-term cognitive dysfunction have been reported in children born to mothers who took AEDs during pregnancy.

Delayed Oncogenesis

Exposure to diethylstilbestrol as late as 20 weeks' gestation may cause reproductive organ anomalies that are not recognized until after puberty.

Drug Risk Categories

The FDA lists five categories of labeling for drug use in pregnancy (Table 4.2) (11,25). These categories are intended to provide therapeutic guidance, weighing the risks as well as the benefits of the drug. Although this sys-

TABLE 4.2
FDA Risk Categories

Category A:	Controlled human studies show no risk
Category B:	No evidence of risk in humans, but there are no controlled human studies
Category C:	Risk to humans has not been ruled out
Category D:	Positive evidence of risk to humans from human and/or animal studies
Category X:	Contraindicated in pregnancy

tem is an improvement over previous labeling, it is not ideal. An alternate system is TERIS, an automated teratogen information resource wherein the rating for each drug or agent is based on a consensus of expert opinion and on the literature (Table 4.3) (26). It was designed to assess the teratogenic risk to the fetus from a drug exposure. The FDA categories have little if any correlation to the TERIS teratogenic risk. This discrepancy results in part from the fact that the FDA categories were designed to provide therapeutic guidance, and the TERIS ratings are useful for estimating the teratogenic risks of a drug and not vice versa (27).

TABLE 4.3
TERIS Risk Rating

N	—	None (A)
UN	—	Unlikely
N-Min	—	None, minimal (A)
Min	—	Minimal (B)
Min-S	—	Minimal-small (D)
S	—	Small
S-Mod	—	Small-Moderate
Mod	—	Moderate
H	—	High (X)
U	—	Undetermined (C)

Equivalent FDA ratings in parentheses.

Prevention

A woman's risk of having a child with a neural tube defect is associated with early pregnancy red cell folate levels in a continuous dose–response relationship (28). Low serum and red blood cell folate levels are associated with spontaneous abortion and fetal malformations in animals and in humans (29–32). Treatment with some drugs, including phenytoin, carbamazepine, and barbiturates, can impair folate absorption. Valproic acid does not produce folate deficiency, but it may interfere with the production of folinic acid by inhibiting glutamate formyl transferase (33). In a small study, women with epilepsy who were taking phenytoin needed 1 mg of folate supplementation a day to maintain a normal serum level (34). Some suggest increasing folic acid intake by 4 mg, which might result in a 48% reduction in neural tube defects (28). Supplementing this by fortifying food with folate benefits all women.

Drug Exposure

During pregnancy, the patient's neurologist and obstetrician should work together. If a woman inadvertently takes a drug when she is pregnant or becomes pregnant while taking a drug, determine the dosage, timing, and duration of the exposure(s). Ascertain the patient's past and present state of health and the presence of mental retardation or chromosomal abnormalities in the family. Using a reliable source of information (such as TERIS), determine whether the drug is a known teratogen (although for many drugs, this is not possible) (8,10,11,18,26).

If the drug is teratogenic or the risk is unknown, have the obstetrician confirm the gestational age by ultrasound. If the exposure occurred during embryogenesis, then high-resolution ultrasound can be performed to determine whether damage to specific organ systems or structures has occurred. If the high-resolution ultrasound is normal, it is reasonable to reassure the patient that the gross fetal structure is normal (within the 90% sensitivity of the study) (18). Fetal ultrasound, however, cannot exclude minor anomalies or guarantee the birth of a normal child. Delay in achieving developmental milestones, including cognitive development, are potential risks, especially for children born to epileptics, that cannot be predicted or diagnosed prenatally (35). Maternal serum alpha-fetoprotein (MSAFP) can be used to screen pregnancies for open neural tube defects. Amniocentesis can also be used to assess an abnormal alpha-fetoprotein level (18). Have the obstetrician discuss the results of these studies with the mother and the significant other; formal prenatal counseling may be helpful in uncertain cases (18).

Maternal Physiology

Profound structural and physiologic changes occur during pregnancy (Table 4.4) (36). The uterus rapidly increases in size, transformed from an almost solid structure weighing 70 g into a relatively thin-walled, muscular organ large enough to accommodate the fetus, placenta, and amniotic fluid (37). Uterine growth depends on estrogen and, to a lesser extent, on progesterone during the first few months of pregnancy. After 12 weeks, growth results from the pressure exerted by the expanding products of conception. Cell and tissue growth is dependent on the increased synthesis of polyamines (including spermidine and spermine and their immediate precursor, putrescine) (37).

TABLE 4.4
Physiologic Changes during Pregnancy

PARAMETER	CHANGE	POTENTIAL IMPLICATIONS FOR TOXICOLOGY
Extracellular volume	4–6 L	Dilution of substances in circulation
Plasma volume	by 40%	Same
Plasma renin/aldosterone		Renal retention/excretion
Renal blood flow	30–50%	Same
Glomerular filtration rate	30–50%	Same
Sodium and calcium retention		Retention of other divalent cations
Cardiac output	by 40%	Increased sensitivity to cardiotoxins (?)
Increased blood flow to skin		Dermal uptake
Food intake	70 kcal/day (average)	Increased
Energy demand*	~300 kcal/day	Increased dose and metabolic shift
Lipid stores*	~3–4 kg over pregnancy	Same
Oxygen consumption*	51 mL O$_2$/min	Metabolic shift (?)
Basal metabolic rate	13%	Metabolic shifts
Hepatic triglyceride synthesis		Redistribution

*Depends on nutrition, activity levels, and gestational state.
Adapted from Metcalfe et al. (36).

Metabolic changes occur in response to the rapidly growing fetus and placenta. Weight gain, due to the increase in the uterus and its contents, the breasts, the blood volume, and the extravascular extracellular fluid, averages approximately 11 kg, with approximately 1 kg occurring during the first trimester (37). Water retention (approximately 6.5 L by term) is a normal occurrence, mediated in part by a fall in plasma osmolality of 10 mOsm/kg, due to a resetting of the osmoreceptor. The fetus, placenta, and amniotic fluid contain approximately 3.5 L of water. Another 3.0 L of water results from increased maternal blood volume and the increase in uterine and breast size. Near term, blood volume is approximately 45% above baseline. Weight loss during the first 10 days postpartum averages approximately 2 kg (37).

Although pregnancy is potentially diabetogenic, in healthy pregnant women, the fasting plasma glucose concentration may fall due to increased plasma insulin levels. Progesterone, when administered to a nonpregnant adult in an amount similar to that which is produced during pregnancy, results in an increased basal insulin concentration and response to an oral glucose challenge similar to that of a normal pregnant woman. Additionally, estradiol induces hyperinsulinism in both control and ovariectomized rats (37).

Lipid, lipoprotein, and apolipoprotein plasma concentrations increase during pregnancy. A positive correlation exists between lipid concentrations and levels of estradiol, progesterone, and human placental lactogen.

The kidneys barely increase in size during pregnancy (38). Early in pregnancy, at the beginning of the second trimester, the glomerular filtration rate and renal plasma flow increase by approximately 50% (39,40). The elevated glomerular filtration rate persists to term, whereas the renal plasma flow decreases during late pregnancy (40). The human liver does not increase in size during pregnancy, and we are not certain whether hepatic blood flow increases.

The profound physiologic changes that occur during pregnancy can alter drug pharmacokinetics: Plasma volume increases by half, cardiac output increases by 30 to 50%, and renal plasma flow and glomerular filtration rate increase by 40 to 50%. Serum albumin decreases by 20 to 30%, resulting in decreased drug binding and increased drug clearance. Increased extracellular fluid and adipose tissue increases the volume of drug distribution. Drug metabolism may also be increased, modulated in part by the high concentration of sex hormones (41).

Seizure frequency can increase during pregnancy due to changes in AED concentration. Total concentrations of carbamazepine, phenytoin, phenobarbital, and valproic acid fall due to decreased plasma protein binding, whereas free or unbound drug concentrations of only phenobarbital fall significantly. Valproate free concentrations actually increase by 25% by the time of delivery (42).

The placenta is a lipid membrane barrier that separates the maternal and fetal circulation. Most drugs cross this barrier by simple diffusion. The rate of transfer is dependent on the drug's molecular size, lipid solubility, and protein binding. Drugs with a very high molecular weight, such as heparin, do not cross the placenta easily, whereas drugs with a low molecular weight (<6,000 daltons) cross it easily. Most drugs have steady-state levels at or near maternal levels, although some drugs may be trapped with fetal levels two to three times maternal levels (43,44).

Breast-Feeding

Milk is a suspension of fat and protein in a carbohydrate-mineral solution. A nursing mother secretes 600 mL of milk a day that contains sufficient protein, fat, and carbohydrate to meet the nutritional demands of the growing and developing infant (11). The transport of a drug into breast milk depends on its lipid solubility, molecular weight, degree of ionization, protein binding (inversely proportional), and the presence or absence of active secretion (12). Species differences in the composition of milk can result in differences in drug transfer. Because human milk (pH usually >7.0) has a much higher pH than cow's milk (pH usually <6.8), bovine drug transfer data may not be accurate in humans (11).

Many drugs can be detected in breast milk at levels that are not clinically significant to the infant. The concentration of a drug in breast milk is a variable fraction of the maternal blood level. The infant dose is usually 1 to 2% of the maternal dose, which is usually trivial. However, any exposure to a toxic drug or potential allergen may be inappropriate (12).

Drug concentration in breast milk depends on drug characteristics (pKa, lipid solubility, molecular weight, protein binding) and breast milk characteristics (composition and volume). Breast milk is given its unique physicochemical properties by the active transport of electrolytes and the formation and excretion of lactose and proteins by glandular epithelial cells in the breast through the passive diffusion of water. The volume produced depends on nutritional factors, the amount of milk removed by the suckling infant, and the increase in mammary blood flow that occurs with breast-feeding. Volume production slowly increases from an average of 600 mL a day to 800 mL a day by the time the infant is 6 months old, and undergoes a diurnal variation, with the greatest quantity occurring in the morning. For the first 10 days of production, milk composition is characterized by a gradual increase in fat and lactose from a milk that is higher in protein content (colostrum).

Because most drugs are either weak acids or bases, the transfer across a biologic membrane is greatly influenced by the ionization characteristics (pKa) and pH differences across the membrane. Because the pH of breast milk (7.0) is slightly lower than that of plasma (7.4), there is a tendency toward ion trapping of basic compounds.

Classification of Drugs Used during Lactation

The American Academy of Pediatrics Committee on Drugs has reviewed and categorized drugs for use in lactating women (Table 4.5) (12,45). The following prescribing guidelines should be followed (45):

- Is the drug necessary? If so:
- Use the safest drug (e.g., acetaminophen instead of aspirin).
- If there is a possibility that a drug may present a risk to the infant (e.g., phenytoin, phenobarbital), consider measuring the blood level in the nursing infant.
- Minimize the nursing infant's drug exposure by having the mother take the medication just after completing a breast-feeding.

CONTRACEPTION

Women of reproductive potential who have neurologic disease, especially if they are taking medications, require contraceptive counseling. Hormonal contraceptive failure can occur with drug use, especially with AEDs. More than one-fourth of the neurologists (27%) and 21% of the obstetricians among 307 responders to a Johns Hopkins survey reported contraceptive failure (46). The AEDs

---

TABLE 4.5
Drug Use during Lactation

(1) — Contraindicated
(2) — Requires temporary cessation of breast-feeding
(3) — Effects unknown but may be of concern
(4) — Use with caution
(5) — Usually compatible

TABLE 4.6
Relationship between Antiepileptic Drugs and Liver Microsomal Cytochrome P450

INDUCERS	NONINDUCERS
Carbamazepine	Benzodiazepines
Phenobarbital	Gabapentin
Phenytoin	Lamotrigine
Felbamate	Levetiracetam
Primidone	

PARTIAL INDUCERS	INHIBITORS
Oxcarbazepine	Valproic acid
Tiagabine	
Topiramate	

phenobarbital, primidone, phenytoin, and carbamazepine induce the hepatic cytochrome P450 system of mixed function oxidases, resulting in a reduction of exogenous estradiol and progesterone levels (Table 4.6). Steroid hormone binding globulins may also be increased, resulting in a decrease in free hormone levels.

The failure rate of OCs is 0.7 per 100 women years. This rate is increased to 3.1 per 100 women years in women who use high-dose estrogen-containing OCs (50 μg or more) and enzyme-inducing anticonvulsants (47). Because the failure rate is higher when more commonly used, lower estrogen-dose OCs are used, an OC containing 50 μg or more of ethinyl estradiol or mestranol is recommended (48). In contrast, valproic acid inhibits the hepatic microsomal enzyme system, and gabapentin, vigabatrin, levetiracetam, and lamotrigine have no effect. Because these AEDs have not been reported to result in hormonal contraceptive failure, they could be used if oral contraception is desired (49). Topiramate, in high (>200 mg/day) but not in low doses, may compromise the efficacy of OCs by decreasing estrogen exposure (25).

Intramuscular medroxyprogesterone (Depo-Provera®) and levonorgestrel implants (Norplant®) are not viable alternatives. Both are progestins whose efficacy is reduced by AEDs (50).

DRUGS AND THE ELDERLY

Many elderly patients fail to take their medicine as prescribed. More than half make at least one drug error, and more than 25% make potentially serious medication errors (51), perhaps because they cannot afford their medicines, their treatment schedules are too complicated (52), or they do not understand the need for and uses of the drug (53). Changes in drug pharmacokinetics and pharmacodynamics that occur with age may result in variable drug plasma levels.

Pharmacokinetics

The rate of gastric emptying is delayed, gastrointestinal motility is decreased, gastric pH levels rise, and active drug transport is reduced in the elderly (54). Most drugs are absorbed by passive diffusion, and xylose absorption, which reflects the passive transport ability, is reduced by 40 to 50%. When transport is not rate-limiting, absorption is not affected. The rate and extent of acetaminophen, phenylbutazone, and sulfamethizole absorption are similar in elderly and young patients (53), whereas galactose, thiamine, calcium, and dextrose absorption, which depends on active transport, is reduced (54).

Pharmacokinetic changes result from changes in body composition and drug-eliminating organ function.

The reduction in lean body mass, serum albumin, and total body water, and the increase in body fat percentage that occur in the elderly produce changes in drug distribution. Cardiac output and kidney blood flow decrease, whereas cerebral, coronary, and skeletal muscle blood flow are unchanged. Hepatic blood flow is reduced. Altered blood flow has a major impact on drug elimination by the liver and kidney and may alter tissue distribution. Renal function declines to approximately half that of the young adult. Hepatic cytochrome P450 enzymes are reduced, whereas conjugation mechanisms are relatively well preserved. Other factors that affect metabolic activity include (i) enzyme-inducing drugs; (ii) disease states, such as hyperthyroidism and osteomalacia; and (iii) exogenous factors, such as bed rest, cigarette smoking, and certain diets. The clearance of drugs that undergo hepatic metabolism is often reduced in the elderly.

The elderly have a decrease in both lean body mass and total body water. The total body fat percentage increases with age in both sexes, increasing from 18 to 36% in men and from 33 to 48% in women between 18 and 85 years of age (55). Drugs that distribute through the total body weight, such as ethanol, have a decreased volume of distribution. Drugs that are primarily distributed through the extracellular fluid show little change in their volume of distribution. In contrast, lipid-soluble drugs (e.g., the benzodiazepines) have larger volumes of distribution due to the greater percentage of fat in elderly persons.

The elimination half-life of lipid-soluble drugs is increased because of a larger volume of distribution. Elimination half-life may decrease because of decreased renal or metabolic clearance. A low plasma albumin level often results in decreased drug binding. The increased free drug fraction results in (i) an enhanced pharmacologic effect; (ii) an increase in the volume of distribution; and (iii) an alteration in the elimination rate.

Pharmacodynamics

The effect of a drug depends on the interaction between it and its receptors. Although pharmacokinetic changes may result in an increased or decreased quantity of drug reaching the receptor, the drug's action depends on how it interacts with its receptors. Central nervous system (CNS) depressant drugs are more potent in the elderly. This is important because psychotherapeutic drugs are the second most commonly prescribed category of drugs for elderly persons. In one study, 32% of all people aged 60 to 70 had used a psychotropic drug within the previous year (56,57). Increased sensitivity to adverse effects, such as hypotension from psychotropic medications and hemorrhage from anticoagulants, can occur even if the dosage is appropriately adjusted (1).

INDIVIDUAL CLASSES OF DRUGS

The use of various medications is reviewed in pregnancy, during lactation, and in the elderly (11).

Acute Specific Antimigraine Drugs

Ergotamine

The use of ergot alkaloids during pregnancy is contraindicated (58,59) (Table 4.7). The abortifacient action of uterotonic ergots in humans has been known for years, but the teratogenic effects of ergotamine and DHE are uncertain. Attempted (but failed) abortion has rarely been associated with certain congenital defects. The Collaborative Perinatal Project (22) reported on 25 exposures to ergotamine and 32 exposures to other ergot derivatives, with the relative risk of malformation being 1 in 24 and 1 in 45, respectively.

Wainscott (60) believed that it was unlikely that ergotamine tartrate posed any teratogenic hazard, but Hughes (61) thought that, because the actual number of exposed women and the severity of exposure were unknown, no definite conclusion could be drawn. Ergot alkaloids, which are frequently present in medication for migraine headaches, enter breast milk and have been reported to cause vomiting, diarrhea, and convulsions in nursing infants.

SUMATRIPTAN. This is a selective serotonin agonist that is safe and effective in the treatment of the nonpregnant migraineur. Sumatriptan at very high doses (three times higher than human plasma concentration after a recommended 6 mg subcutaneous dose) caused embryo lethality in rabbits but not in rats, even when given at higher doses. There is no evidence that sumatriptan is a human teratogen, but no adequate, well-controlled studies have been done in pregnant women.

Sumatriptan is excreted in breast milk in animals. No data exist in humans. Use with caution in nursing women.

NARATRIPTAN. Naratriptan is used for the acute treatment of migraine headaches. It is not an animal teratogen, but it does produce dose-related embryo and fetal developmental toxicity. Human pregnancy experience is too limited to assess the safety of the drug or its teratogenic potential. It is excreted in the milk of nursing rats but there are no reports describing the use of naratriptan during human lactation. The molecular weight of the hydrochloride salt (about 372) is low enough, however, that passage into the milk should be expected. The effects of this exposure, if any, on a nursing infant are unknown (11).

RIZATRIPTAN. Rizatriptan is indicated for the treatment of acute migraine attacks with or without aura in adults. The Merck Pregnancy Registry program has data on 24 pregnancies exposed to rizatriptan. No adverse outcomes were observed in liveborn offspring, but the limited number of exposures studied are not sufficient to detect a risk of rare disorders such as birth defects. No reports describe the use of rizatriptan in

TABLE 4.7
Ergots and Serotonin Agonists

	FETA FDA	L RISK TERIS	BREAST-FEEDING
Ergotamine	X	Min	Contraindicated
Dihydroergotamine	X	U	Contraindicated
Methylergonovine	C	U	Caution
Methysergide	D	U	Caution
Almotriptan	C	U	Caution
Eletriptan	C	U	Caution
Frovatriptan	C	U	Caution
Naratriptan	C	U	Caution
Rizatriptan	C	U	Caution
Sumatriptan	C	U	Caution
Zolmitriptan	C	U	Caution

TABLE 4.8
Analgesics

	FETA FDA	L RISK TERIS	BREAST-FEEDING
Simple Analgesics			
Aspirin	C*	N-Min	Caution
Acetaminophen	B	N	Compatible
Caffeine	B	N-Min	Compatible
NSAIDs			
Fenoprofen	B*	U	Compatible
Ibuprofen	B*	N-Min	Compatible
Indomethacin	B*	N	Compatible
Ketorolac	B*	U	Caution
Meclofenamate	B*	U	Compatible
Naproxen	B*	U	Compatible
Sulindac	B*	U	Compatible
Tolmetin	B*	U	Compatible
COX-2			
Celecoxib	C*	U	Concern
Rofecoxib	C*	U	Concern

*D if third trimester

human lactation. The relatively low molecular weight of free base (about 269) suggests that the drug will be excreted into breast milk. The effects of this exposure on a nursing infant are unknown (11).

ASPIRIN (11,62). Concerns about the safety of aspirin in pregnancy came from earlier data (63,64), when aspirin was used in therapeutic doses for analgesic or antipyretic purposes. There is no evidence that aspirin has any teratogenic effect. Although three retrospective epidemiologic trials looking at aspirin consumption among mothers of children with malformations have found higher consumption in patients than in controls, these studies suffer from memory bias or a possible coincident teratogen for which the aspirin was taken. A large prospective study of 50,282 pregnancies found no evidence of aspirin teratogenicity in humans (22,62). Aspirin in analgesic doses does have perinatal effects. It can inhibit uterine contraction and result in narrowing of the ductus arteriosus and increased maternal and newborn bleeding. Aspirin users have longer gestations and labors than control patients (11).

Increased teratogenic risks, as well as disturbances of platelet function with the risk of hemorrhage in the mother and infant, have been reported. Based on extensive clinical experience, none of these side effects has been seen at low dose; however, it is generally recommended not to start treatment before 15 weeks of pregnancy and to stop it 7 to 10 days before delivery. Aspirin has a clear-cut effect on the hemostasis of the newborn and should not be used in late pregnancy. It can also cause hyperbilirubinemia. Low-dose aspirin, however, may help prevent preeclampsia or the fetal wastage associated with autoimmune diseases.

BREAST-FEEDING. Aspirin is excreted in moderate amounts in breast milk. Occasional aspirin use during lactation appears to be safe, but studies have not been performed on infants of nursing mothers who ingest high doses of aspirin over long periods of time. It should be used cautiously during breast-feeding.

ELDERLY. Aspirin may produce serious problems in the elderly. Even in small doses, aspirin may prolong bleeding time and cause gastric erosions with bleeding.

ACETAMINOPHEN. Acetaminophen is the drug most commonly taken during pregnancy. Its mean half-life (3.7 hours) is not significantly different from the nonpregnant value. Its absorption, metabolism, and renal clearance are unchanged. The decrease in the mean AUC during pregnancy may be due to its increased volume of distribution. Potentially hepatotoxic metabolites were not found in maternal serum. The absorption and disposition of a standard oral dose is not affected by

pregnancy (65). There is no evidence of any teratogenic effect. Its use is compatible with breast-feeding (11).

ELDERLY. Acetaminophen metabolism is not affected by age (66).

CAFFEINE (11,62). In moderate amounts (<300 mg a day), caffeine consumption in pregnancy does not pose a measurable risk to the fetus. High doses may be associated with spontaneous abortion, infertility, or low birth weight. Moderate caffeine use is compatible with breast-feeding. Accumulation may occur in infants whose mothers use excessive amounts of caffeine, however.

Nonsteroidal Antiinflammatory Drugs (11,62)

PREGNANCY. None of the NSAIDs in Table 4.8 has been shown to have a teratogenic effect. Their use should be limited during the third trimester because they inhibit labor, prolong the length of pregnancy, and decrease amniotic fluid volume. A combined 2001 population-based observational cohort study and a case-control study estimated the risk of adverse pregnancy outcome from the use of NSAIDs. The use of NSAIDs during pregnancy was not associated with congenital malformations, preterm delivery, or low birth weight, but a positive association was discovered with spontaneous abortions. NSAID use is compatible with breast-feeding.

The use of indomethacin, which successfully suppresses uterine contractions even after the failure of other tocolytics, has been extensively reviewed (67). Indomethacin crosses the human placenta and has multiple effects on the fetus, including constriction of the ductus arteriosus and reduction of urine production. The risk of ductus arteriosus constriction depends on the gestational age, with a dramatic increase at 32 weeks, when almost 50% of cases show a significantly increased blood flow through the ductus. Because of this high incidence, indomethacin should not be used beyond 32 weeks.

ELDERLY. Adverse reactions in the elderly are similar to those of salicylates, but some are unique to this group of drugs. Gastrointestinal side effects with dyspepsia, nausea, diarrhea, ulcers, and hemorrhage may occur. CNS symptoms of somnolence, dizziness, tinnitus, tremor, and confusion may occur, but these are usually mild. Cognitive dysfunction, manifested by memory loss, inability to concentrate, confusion, and personality change, has been reported in patients over age 65 who have received either naproxen or ibuprofen (68).

Second-Generation NSAIDs

Rofecoxib and celecoxib are second-generation NSAIDs that inhibit prostaglandin synthesis via the inhibition of cyclooxygenase-2 (COX-2). In animal reproduction studies with rats and rabbits, rofecoxib caused peri- and postimplantation losses and reduced embryo and fetal survival at doses approximately nine and two times, respectively. No teratogenicity was observed in rats. In rabbits, a slight, nonstatistically significant increase in the incidence of vertebral malformations was seen. Data from the Merck Pregnancy Registry for Vioxx® (rofecoxib), as of July 31, 2000, include eleven exposed pregnancies. The outcomes in these cases were two normal live-born infants, one lost to follow-up, and three ongoing pregnancies. Constriction of the ductus arteriosus in utero is a pharmacologic consequence arising from the use of prostaglandin synthesis inhibitors during pregnancy. Although animal studies with rofecoxib did not show this effect, it is not known if humans would be similarly unaffected. There are no reports describing the use of rofecoxib during human lactation. The drug is excreted in the milk of lactating rats at concentrations similar to those in the plasma. The relatively long adult serum half-life of rofecoxib (about 17 hours) and the absence of clinical pharmacologic data in infants suggest that this agent should be avoided during nursing (11).

Celecoxib is in the same NSAID subclass (COX-2 inhibitors) as rofecoxib. Teratogenicity studies have been conducted in rats and rabbits. In pregnant rats, a dose-related increase in diaphragmatic hernias was observed in one of two studies at doses of 30 mg/kg/day (about six times the MRHD). No teratogenic effects occurred in pregnant rabbits. The use of first-generation NSAIDs during the latter half of pregnancy has been associated with oligohydramnios and premature closure of the ductus arteriosus. Similar effects should be expected if celecoxib is used during the third trimester or close to delivery. No reports describing the use of celecoxib during human lactation have been located. The drug is excreted in the milk of lactating rats in concentrations similar to those mea-

sured in plasma. The relatively long adult serum half-life of celecoxib (11.2 hours) and the absence of clinical pharmacologic data in infants suggest that this agent should be avoided during nursing (11).

All opioids can produce maternal and neonatal addiction. Their use for prolonged periods and in high doses at term is contraindicated. The amount of morphine and meperidine excreted in breast milk is small, and these medications may be used safely in therapeutic doses. Addicts, however, may excrete significant amounts of morphine and heroin, and symptoms of withdrawal can be prevented by allowing their infants to breast-feed. Narcotic use is compatible with breast-feeding (11,12,62).

CODEINE (11,62). Indiscriminate codeine use may present a risk to the fetus during the first or second trimester. Cleft lip, cleft palate, dislocated hips, inguinal hernia, and cardiac and respiratory system defects have been reported. Codeine passes into breast milk in very small amounts.

PROPOXYPHENE (11,62). Three case reports have linked propoxyphene use to congenital abnormalities, but because other drugs were also used, the association may be coincidental. The Collaborative Perinatal Project found no evidence of increased malformations among 2,914 exposures (22).

OTHER DRUGS. Butorphanol, hydromorphone, meperidine, methadone, and morphine are probably not teratogenic (11,62).

ELDERLY. The acute analgesic effect of narcotics is enhanced in the elderly (66).

Anticoagulants

Heparin is a relatively large molecule with a molecular weight of approximately 20,000. It is highly charged and fails to cross the placenta in any detectable amount.

TABLE 4.9
Opioids

| | FETAL RISK | | |
	FDA	TERIS	BREAST-FEEDING
Butorphanol	B**	N-Min	Compatible
Codeine	C**	N-Min	Compatible
Hydromorphone	B**	N-Min	Compatible
Meperidine	B**	N-Min	Compatible
Methadone	B**	N-Min	Compatible
Morphine	B**	N-Min	Compatible
Propoxyphene	C**	N-Min	Compatible

**D if prolonged or at term

TABLE 4.10
Anticoagulant and Antiplatelet Drugs

| | FETAL RISK | | |
	FDA	TERIS	BREAST-FEEDING
Heparin	C	N-M	Safe
Low molecular weight heparin	C	N-M	Safe
Warfarin	X	S-M	Compatible
Pentoxifylline	C	U	Not recommended

Although the protracted use of heparin may result in osteoporosis and thrombocytopenia in the mother, there has been no evidence that heparin is teratogenic, because it does not cross the placenta. Heparin is not excreted in breast milk, and mothers who use heparin may breast-feed safely (69). Low-molecular-weight heparin has a molecular weight of approximately 4,000 to 6,000 and does not cross the placenta. Omri and associates (70) reported on the use of low-molecular-weight heparin in 17 women without adverse effects, and Gillis and associates (71) reported on its use in six pregnant women without apparent adverse effects. Dulitzki and associates (72) recently reported their experience with low-molecular-weight heparin in 41 pregnancies from 34 women and found it to be both safe and efficacious (69).

Pentoxifylline is a synthetic xanthine derivative used as a vasodilator and to lower blood viscosity in peripheral vascular and cerebrovascular disease. No epidemiologic studies of pentoxifylline use during either the first trimester or the later stages of pregnancy are available (69).

Warfarin is a coumarin derivative that produces its anticoagulant effect by interfering with clotting factors II, VII, IX, and X. This anticoagulant and its derivatives are relatively low in molecular weight and cross the placenta readily, thus resulting in significant fetal levels. The pattern of anomalies called the *warfarin embryopathy* or *fetal warfarin syndrome*, includes nasal hypoplasia, stippled epiphyses on radiographs, and growth retardation, and occurs in approximately 10% of exposed infants. The period of greatest susceptibility is between the sixth and ninth postmenstrual weeks of gestation. Adverse outcomes, such as fetal effects, neonatal deaths, stillbirths, spontaneous abortions, and premature births, occur in 31% of treated pregnancies. Warfarin therapy during the second and third trimesters can produce CNS and eye anomalies in approximately 3% of children. Warfarin use in late pregnancy causes fetal, placental, or neonatal hemorrhage (69).

BREAST-FEEDING. Although many review articles state that oral anticoagulants are contraindicated in nursing mothers, recent evidence indicates that warfarin and dicumarol may be used safely. LeOrme and coworkers (73) measured warfarin levels in the breast milk of 13 mothers who were receiving therapeutic doses of warfarin. They found a concentration of less than 25 mg/ml.

ELDERLY. Patients over 70 years of age are more sensitive to the anticoagulation effect of warfarin and frequently require lower doses. Older persons who are receiving several drugs are at greater risk for drug interactions that may lead to enhanced or diminished effects of warfarin (Table 4.11).

Thrombolytics

The major thrombolytics include streptokinase, urokinase, and tissue plasminogen activator. There are no large randomized studies regarding their use during pregnancy. Turrentine and colleagues (74) recently reviewed 36 reports involving 172 pregnant women treated with thrombolytics for a variety of thromboembolic conditions. A summary of the results revealed maternal mortality in 1.2%, hemorrhagic complications in 8.1%, and pregnancy loss in 5.8%. Pregnancy is considered to be a relative contraindication to thrombolytic therapy, but it would appear that it may be of benefit in some cases and is relatively safe (69,74).

TABLE 4.11
Oral Anticoagulant Drug Interactions

INCREASED EFFECT		DECREASED EFFECT	
DRUG	MECHANISM	DRUG	MECHANISM
Nortriptyline	Absorption	Cholestyramine	Absorption
Allopurinol	Metabolism	Barbiturates	Metabolism
Cimetidine			
Disulfiram			
Alcohol			
Sulfonamides	Protein-binding	Alcohol (chronic)	Metabolism
Phenylbutazone			
Salicylates >3g/day			
Antibiotics	Protein-binding, vitamin K synthesis by bacteria		

Anticonvulsants (11,75,76)

Most AEDs (Table 4.12) have teratogenic potential; mechanisms include induced folate deficiency, interference with folate metabolism, and the production of teratogenic intermediary metabolites such as free radicals. One biologically active metabolite, epoxide, is metabolized by the enzyme epoxide hydrolase. Reduced amniocyte activity correlates with the occurrence of congenital anomalies (77).

TABLE 4.12 *Antiepileptic Drug Classification*			
	FETAL RISK FDA	TERIS	BREAST-FEEDING
Carbamazepine	C	S	Compatible
Gabapentin	C	U	Uncertain
Lamotrigine	C	U	Not recommended
Levetiracetam	C	U	Caution
Oxcarbazepine	C	U	Caution
Phenobarbital	D	M-S	Compatible
Phenytoin	D	S-Mod	Compatible
Primidone	D	S-Mod	Caution
Tiagabine	C	U	Caution
Topiramate	C	U	Uncertain
Valproic Acid	D	S-Mod	Compatible
Vigabatrin	—	U	Uncertain

BREAST-FEEDING. The major AEDs currently in use are usually compatible with breast-feeding. In women with epilepsy who are taking sedating AEDs, close monitoring of the newborn for sedation is necessary. Levels of phenytoin, carbamazepine, and valproic acid in breast milk represent a small fraction of the dose that would produce therapeutic levels in the infant. Sedating AEDs, such as benzodiazepines, primidone, and phenobarbital, should not preclude a trial of breast-feeding, although close monitoring of the newborn is necessary. If the infant becomes sedated, it is advisable to discontinue breast-feeding (78).

CARBAMAZEPINE (13,78). Carbamazepine is probably a human teratogen, having a pattern of congenital malformation whose principal features consist of minor craniofacial defects, fingernail hypoplasia, and developmental delay (similar to the fetal hydantoin syndrome). There may also be a ninefold risk of neural tube defects (0.6% incidence).

GABAPENTIN. It is not known whether gabapentin crosses the human placenta. Because of its lack of protein binding and low molecular weight (about 171), however, transfer to the fetus should be expected. A 1996 review reported 16 pregnancies exposed to gabapentin from preclinical trials and postmarketing surveillance. The outcomes of these pregnancies included five elective abortions, one ongoing pregnancy, seven normal infants, and three infants with birth defects. No specific information was provided on the defects other than the fact that there was no pattern of malformation, and all were receiving polytherapy for epilepsy. The limited human data do not allow an assessment of gabapentin's safety in pregnancy. No reports describing the use of gabapentin during human lactation have been located. Because of its low molecular weight (about 171), transfer into milk should be expected. The effects of this exposure on a nursing infant are unknown (11).

LAMOTRIGINE. Lamotrigine was not teratogenic in animal reproductive studies involving mice, rats, and rabbits using oral doses that were 1.2, 0.5, and 1.1 times, respectively, the highest usual human maintenance dose. Lamotrigine crosses the human placenta. An interim report of the Lamotrigine Pregnancy Registry, an ongoing project conducted by the manufacturer, was issued in 2000. A total of 362 prospective pregnancies (reported before the pregnancy outcome was known) have been enrolled in the Registry. Of these, 66 outcomes are pending and 52 have been lost to follow-up. Outcomes are known for 244 pregnancies. The earliest exposure to lamotrigine occurred in the first trimester in 235 pregnancies, three in the second trimester, two in the third trimester, and four with an unspecified time of earliest exposure. Lamotrigine monotherapy was used in 98 outcomes with earliest exposure in the first trimester, two outcomes with earliest exposure in the second trimester, and five outcomes (one set of triplets) with unspecified exposure timing. For first trimester exposures, the outcomes were nine spontaneous pregnancy losses (<20 weeks gestation), 27 elective abortions (two with birth defects), one fetal death (≤20 weeks), 14 live infants with birth defects, and 186 live infants without birth defects (includes two sets of twins). When the earliest exposure was in the second or third trimesters, or the exposure timing was unspecified, the outcomes were three, two, and six live-born infants, respectively, without birth defects. Lamotrigine monotherapy during the first trimester is associated with esophageal malformation, cleft soft palate, and right club foot. The animal and human data do not appear to indicate a major risk for congenital malformations or fetal loss following first trimester exposure to lamotrigine. At least two reviews have concluded that this anticonvulsant may be associated with a lower risk of teratogenicity. Lamotrigine is excreted into breast milk. No adverse effects have been seen in nursing infants of mothers taking lamotrigine, but the number of known cases is too small to adequately assess the safety of this drug during lactation. Monitoring infant serum levels of lamotrigine may be required (11).

PHENOBARBITAL (11,12,76). Phenobarbital has been in use since 1912, and phenytoin has been used since 1938. It was not until the early 1960s that case reports began to appear suggesting that phenytoin was associated with the development of birth defects. In the late 1960s, phenytoin was demonstrated to be a teratogen in rodents, with the subsequent recognition of a pattern of abnormalities in infants exposed to the drug in utero.

Phenobarbital therapy in the pregnant woman with epilepsy presents to the fetus a risk of minor congenital abnormalities, hemorrhage at birth, and withdrawal. The pregnant woman with epilepsy who is taking phenobarbital in combination with other AEDs has a two- to three-fold increased risk of having a child with a congenital malformation. It is not known if this is due to the drug, the disease, or a combination of these factors. Barbiturates have been demonstrated in breast milk, but therapeutic doses appear to have little or no effect on the infant. A greater amount of phenobarbital was transmitted when a single dose of 1.5 g was administered than when the same amount was given in divided doses throughout the day (76). Phenobarbital may cause sedation in nursing infants, and it should be used with caution in nursing mothers.

PHENYTOIN (11,76). The use of phenytoin during pregnancy involves significant risk (10%) to the fetus in terms of major and minor congenital anomalies and hemorrhage at birth.

TOPIRAMATE (25). There are no studies of topiramate use in pregnant women. Topiramate should be used during pregnancy only if the potential benefit outweighs the potential risk to the fetus. Topiramate is excreted in the milk of lactating rats. It is not known whether topiramate is excreted in human milk. Because many drugs are excreted in human milk, the potential for serious adverse reactions in nursing infants is unknown.

VALPROIC ACID (11,76). Valproic acid is a human teratogen. The absolute risk of producing a child with a neural tube defect when used between day 17 and day 30 after fertilization is 1 to 2%. A characteristic pattern of facial defects is apparently also associated with valproic acid (79–81). Valproic acid may also result in impaired cognition in children born to mothers with epilepsy (35).

The teratogenic potential of the new AEDs (vigabatrin, felbamate, tiagabine, and topiramate) is uncertain.

Antidepressants

In utero exposure to either tricyclic antidepressant drugs or fluoxetine does not affect global intelligence quota, language development, or behavioral development in preschool children (82). Antidepressant use may be a concern during breast-feeding. The exception is fluoxetine, which should be used with caution. Its specific use during pregnancy is described subsequently. The American Academy of Pediatrics classifies all antidepressants as drugs whose effect on the nursing infant may be of concern (11) (Table 4.13).

TABLE 4.13 *Antidepressants*			
	FETAL RISK		
	FDA	**TERIS**	**BREAST-FEEDING**
Tricyclics			
Amitriptyline	D	N-Min	Concern
Amoxapine	C	U	Concern
Desipramine	C	U	Concern
Doxepin	C	U	Concern
Imipramine	D	N-Min	Concern
Nortriptyline	D	U	Concern
Protriptyline	C	U	Concern
SSRIs			
Citalopram	C	N	Concern
Fluoxetine	B	N	Concern
Paroxetine	C	U	Concern
Sertraline	B	U	Concern
MAOIs			
Phenelzine	C	U	Concern
Others			
Bupropion	B	U	Concern
Venlafaxine	C	U	Concern

Tricyclics

- *Amitriptyline* (11). Limb reduction anomalies have been reported but not confirmed. Other malformations have been reported.
- *Amoxapine* (11). No case reports of teratogenicity.
- *Desipramine* (11). No case reports of teratogenicity. Neonatal withdrawal symptoms reported.
- *Doxepin* (11). No case reports of teratogenicity. One serious adverse reaction has been reported in a nursing infant.
- *Imipramine* (11). Malformations have been reported but are rare. Neonatal withdrawal symptoms have been reported.

- *Nortriptyline* (11). See amitriptyline.
- *Phenelzine* (11). Increased risk found.
- *Protriptyline* (11). No data available.

ELDERLY. All tricyclic antidepressants exert both central and peripheral anticholinergic activities and block the histamine H-1 and H-2 receptors (which may be responsible for weight gain) (83). Elderly persons are especially sensitive to these side effects. The patient's tolerance of a tricyclic is often determined by a patient's ability to tolerate these effects.

Selective Serotonin Reuptake Inhibitors (SSRIs)

CITALOPRAM. Citalopram does not appear to be a major human teratogen, although the data are still limited. Citalopram is excreted into human milk. In their product information, the manufacturer describes two infants whose mothers were receiving citalopram and who had excessive somnolence, decreased feeding, and weight loss associated with nursing.

FLUOXETINE (25). There is no evidence of teratogenicity in animals. Chambers and colleagues (84) concluded that women who take fluoxetine during pregnancy do not have an increased risk of spontaneous pregnancy loss or major fetal anomalies, but that they are at increased risk for minor anomalies, indicating a teratogenic effect. Women who are exposed during the third trimester are at increased risk for premature delivery, poor neonatal adaptation, cyanosis on feeding, and jitteriness (84). In contrast to these results, five cohort studies, which included approximately 450 pregnancies and focused on the relationship between fluoxetine and developmental effects, suggested that children exposed in utero, whether early or late in gestation, do not have an increased risk of birth defects, poor perinatal condition, or neurodevelopmental delay (85). Maternal age was higher in the fluoxetine group in the study of Chambers and coworkers (84), which may partly explain the observed excess of poor perinatal outcomes. Prematurity, admission to a special-care nursery, and poor neonatal adaptation are also associated with maternal psychiatric disorders. The comparison between the early-exposure and late-exposure groups led the authors to conclude that exposure to fluoxetine in late pregnancy increases the risk of perinatal problems. This finding might also be explained by the fact that patients with severe depressive illness need treatment throughout pregnancy, whereas those with mild forms of the illness do not.

PAROXETINE. The animal reproductive data and limited human pregnancy experience does not appear to indicate that paroxetine poses a major teratogenic risk.

However, the available human studies lack the sensitivity to identify minor anomalies because of the absence of standardized examinations. Late-appearing major defects may also have been missed in at least two of the studies because of the short time frame. Withdrawal symptoms were reported in four infants exposed to paroxetine during gestation, but other drug exposures may have contributed to the conditions. Paroxetine is excreted into human breast milk. Its effect on the infant is unknown, thus the mother should be given this information so that she can actively participate in any decision (11).

SERTRALINE. Sertraline is an SSRI. The limited animal and human data do not support a major teratogenic risk from sertraline use during pregnancy. In a 1998 study, the mean milk:plasma ratios of sertraline and the metabolite in eight lactating women (mean dose 1.05 mg/kg/day) were 1.93 and 1.64, respectively. The estimated infant doses were 0.2% and 0.3%, respectively, of the weight-adjusted maternal dose. No adverse effects from the drug exposure were noted in the infants. All had achieved normal development milestones.

Other Antidepressants

BUPROPION. Bupropion is a unique antidepressant of the aminoketone class. After reviewing the 90 prospectively reported pregnancy outcomes, the Bupropion Pregnancy Registry Advisory Committee concludes that this sample is insufficient to reliably compute a birth defect risk, and no conclusions can be made regarding the possible teratogenic risk of bupropion. Bupropion is excreted into human breast milk.

VENLAFAXINE. Reproduction studies in rats and rabbits at doses up to 2.5 and 4 times the maximum recommended human daily dose based on body surface area (MRHD), respectively, did not reveal teratogenicity. A 1994 review of venlafaxine included citations of data from the clinical trials of this drug involving its use during gestation in 10 women for periods ranging from 10 to 60 days, apparently during the first trimester. No adverse effects of the exposure were observed in four of the infants (information was not provided for the other six exposed pregnancies). The FDA has not received any reports of adverse pregnancy outcomes involving the use of the drug during gestation. Venlafaxine is excreted into human breast milk. The American Academy of Pediatrics considers the effects of other antidepressants on the nursing infant to be unknown, although they may be of concern.

Antihypertensives

BETA-BLOCKERS (11,12,86–88). There is no evidence of human teratogenicity of the beta-blockers, but fetal and neonatal toxicity may occur. A 1988 review of beta-blocker use during pregnancy concluded that these drugs are relatively safe. Newborn infants, however, should be observed for bradycardia, hypoglycemia, and other symptoms of beta-blockage (87).

BREAST-FEEDING. Beta-blocker use is compatible with breast-feeding.

- *Atenolol* (11). No fetal malformations have been reported. Reduced birth weight and perinatal beta-blockade in the newborn have been reported.
- *Metoprolol* (11). No fetal malformations reported.

TABLE 4.14 *Antihypertensives*			
	FETAL RISK		
	FDA	**TERIS**	**BREAST-FEEDING**
Beta-Blockers			
Atenolol	C	U	Compatible
Metoprolol	B	U	Compatible
Nadolol	C	U	Compatible
Propranolol	C	U	Compatible
Timolol	C	U	Compatible
Adrenergic Blockers			
Clonidine	C	U	Compatible
Calcium Channel Blockers			
Diltiazem	C	U	Compatible
Nifedipine	C	U	Compatible
Nimodipine	C	U	Uncertain
Verapamil	C	U	Compatible
Ace Inhibitors			
Enalapril	D	Mod	Compatible

- *Nadolol* (11). One case report of growth retardation and beta-blockade.
- *Propranolol* (11,12,86) (Table 4.15).

A number of fetal and/or neonatal adverse effects have been reported (61,87,88). Whether these are due to propranolol, maternal disease, or other drugs is not clear. Daily doses of 160 mg or higher seem to produce more serious complications. Most case reports show intrauterine growth retardation, hypoglycemia, bradycardia, and respiratory depression. Propranolol is probably not a teratogen, but fetal and neonatal toxicity may occur.

ELDERLY. Propranolol is cleared by the liver; its half-life in plasma lengthens with age, from approximately 3 hours in young adults to 6 to 8 hours in elderly persons (89). The tissue distribution slows, while an increase in bioavailability secondary to decreased metabolism occurs. Metoprolol's first-pass metabolism decreases with age, which leads to increased bioavailability (90), but this produces no change in its half-life or metabolite accumulation (91). There is decreased beta-adrenoceptor sensitivity to both agonists (isoproterenol) and antagonists (propranolol) (92).

Adrenergic Blockers

- *Clonidine* (11). There are no reports of teratogenicity, but experience is limited.

Calcium Channel Blockers (Table 4.14)

- *Cardizem* (11). No studies or reports in pregnant women.
- *Nifedipine* (11). Experience is limited. Adverse reactions have occurred when the drug is combined with magnesium sulfate.

TABLE 4.15 *Beta-Blockers in the Elderly*					
DRUG	**HALF-LIFE**	**CARDIO-SELECTIVE**	**ACTIVE METABOLITES**	**ROUTE OF EXCRETION**	**STARTING DOSE**
Propranolol	3 hours (young adults) 6 to 8 hours (elderly)	No	Yes	Hepatic and renal	10 mg bid qid
Metoprolol	3 to 6 hours	Yes	No	Hepatic	25 mg bid
Timolol	3 to 4 hours	No	No	Hepatic	5 mg bid
Nadolol	24 hours (young adults) 30 to 72 hours (elderly)	No	No	Renal	20 mg qd
Atenolol	6 to 9 hours (young adults) 16 to 27 hours (elderly)	Yes	No	Renal	25 mg qd

- *Verapamil* (11). There is no evidence of teratogenicity in animals. There are no adequate, well-controlled studies in women.

ELDERLY. The side effects of calcium channel blockers may be particularly troublesome in the elderly. Verapamil may cause headaches, hypotension, flushing, dizziness, constipation, and nausea. High-grade heart block and congestive heart failure occur, but these complications are rare. Noncardiogenic pedal edema occurs in approximately 25% of all patients.

Antiparkinsonian Drugs

TABLE 4.16
Antiparkinsonian Drugs

| | FETAL RISK | | |
	FDA	TERIS	BREAST-FEEDING
Dopaminergic			
Bromocriptine	C	U	Contraindicated
Pergolide	B	U	Unknown
Levodopa	C	U	Unknown
Carbidopa	C	U	Unknown
Amantadine	C	U	Not recommended

BROMOCRIPTINE (11). Bromocriptine does not pose a significant risk to the fetus. The pattern and incidence of anomalies is similar to those expected in a nonexposed population. Because bromocriptine suppresses lactation, its use is contraindicated during breast-feeding.

ELDERLY. Levodopa clearance is reduced, and side effects such as postural hypotension and confusion are aggravated. Bromocriptine and pergolide are not better tolerated in patients who become confused. Anticholinergic agents should be avoided.

Antiviral Drugs

Most pediatric HIV cases result from vertical transmission of the virus from the mother to the infant during pregnancy or at the time of labor and delivery. Anti-HIV nucleoside drugs (Table 4.17) are used in pregnancy and have two objectives: (i) to reduce progression of the disease in the mother, and (ii) to reduce transmission of the virus from the mother to the infant or modify the severity of the transmitted infection.

ACYCLOVIR. Acyclovir is the most commonly used antiviral drug for the treatment of herpes simplex virus

TABLE 4.17
Antiviral Drugs

| | FETAL RISK | | |
	FDA	TERIS	BREAST-FEEDING
Amantadine	C	U	Not recommended
Acyclovir	C	U	Caution
Zidovudine	C	U	Unknown
Famciclovir	B	U	Not recommended

and varicella zoster virus infections. No placental tissue metabolism can be shown (93). Cord blood levels are close to maternal blood levels, whereas amniotic fluid levels are three to six times the corresponding cord plasma levels.

ZIDOVUDINE. When zidovudine was given during the third trimester of pregnancy to HIV-infected asymptomatic pregnant women, it was well tolerated and appeared safe for both mother and infant (94).

Corticosteroids (11)

Cortisone

Reports of congenital defects reflect greater cortisone use and do not necessarily suggest that it is a more potent teratogen than other glucocorticoids. The Collaborative Perinatal Project found no relationship between cortisone and congenital malformations (22). Some concern regarding neonatal adrenal hyperplasia or insufficiency from maternal corticosteroid administration has been raised.

Dexamethasone

No reports link the use of dexamethasone to congenital defects. Leukocytosis has been observed in mothers and in newborn infants. Animal studies have been associated

TABLE 4.18
Corticosteroids

| | FETAL RISK | | |
	FDA	TERIS	BREAST-FEEDING
Cortisone	D	N-Min	Compatible
Dexamethasone	C	N-Min	Compatible
Prednisone	B	N-Min	Compatible

with toxic effects, including increased fetal liver weight, reduced fetal head circumference, and reduced adrenal, thymus, and placental weight. These effects have not been observed in humans.

Prednisone

Along with prednisolone, prednisone poses a very small risk to the developing fetus. The drugs do not cross the placenta easily, except in large doses. Their use is compatible with breast-feeding.

Neuroleptics and Antiemetics

Neuroleptics

CHLORPROMAZINE (11,95). One survey found an increased incidence of defects, and there is one report of ectromelia (gross hypoplasia or aplasia of one or more long bones or limbs). Most studies, however, have found chlorpromazine to be safe for both mother and fetus if used occasionally in low doses. Its effect on the nursing

infant is unknown, but it may cause drowsiness or galactorrhea in the infant.

HALOPERIDOL (11,95). Haloperidol has been associated with two case reports of limb malformation. Other investigators have not found these defects. Its effect on the nursing infant is unknown, but may be of concern.

METOCLOPRAMIDE (11). No congenital malformations have been reported. Normal infant development for up to 4 years following the use of metoclopramide has been reported. Despite theoretic concerns, there is no evidence that metoclopramide in moderate doses of 45 mg or less presents a risk to the nursing infant.

PROCHLORPERAZINE (11,95). Despite occasional reports of congenital defects in children exposed to prochlorperazine, the majority of evidence indicates that the drug and the general class of phenothiazines (promethazine, promazine) are safe for mother and fetus if used occasionally and in low doses.

Antiemetics

DOXYLAMINE (95). Doxylamine alone, or in combination with vitamin B6 (Bendectin®), is not associated with an increased risk of congenital malformations.

EMETROL (95). Emetrol is a phosphorylated carbohydrate solution that acts locally on the wall of the gastrointestinal tract.

TRIMETHOBENZAMIDE (95). Trimethobenzamide has been associated with a low risk of congenital malformations.

Sedatives, Hypnotics, and Antihistamines

Barbiturates

BUTALBITAL (11). Butalbital is a short-acting barbiturate that has not been found to be associated with malformations. Severe neonatal withdrawal can occur from prolonged overuse. Data relating to breast-feeding are not available.

Benzodiazepines (11,62)

CHLORDIAZEPOXIDE (11). Chlordiazepoxide has been associated with an increased risk of congenital malformation in some, but not all, studies. Neonatal withdrawal can occur when chlordiazepoxide is given at term.

TABLE 4.19 *Neuroleptics/Antiemetics*			
	FETAL RISK		
	FDA	**TERIS**	**BREAST-FEEDING**
Other			
Emetrol	B	U	Compatible
Doxylamine and Vitamin B6	B	N	NA
Trimethobenzamide	C	N-Min	NA
Neuroleptics			
Phenothiazines			
Chlorpromazine	C	N-Min	Concern
Prochlorperazine	C	N	Compatible
Promethazine	C	N	NA
Promazine	C	U	NA
Butyrophenones			
Haloperidol	C	N-Min	Concern
Thioxanthenes			
Thiothixene	C	U	NA
Other			
Metoclopramide	B	N-Min	Concern
Olanzapine	C	U	Not recommended
Risperdal	C	U	Not recommended
Quetiapine	C	U	Not recommended

TABLE 4.20
Sedatives, Hypnotics, and Antihistamines

| | FETAL RISK | | |
	FDA	TERIS	BREAST-FEEDING
Antihistamines			
Cyclizine	B	U	NA
Cyproheptadine	B	U	Contraindicated
Dimenhydrinate	B	U	NA
Meclizine	B	N-Min	NA
Barbiturates			
Butalbital	C	N-Min	Caution
Phenobarbital	D	N-Min	Caution
Benzodiazepam			
Chlordiazepoxide	D	N-Min	Concern
Clonazepam	D	U	Concern
Diazepam	D	N-Min	Concern
Lorazepam	D	U	Concern
OTHER			
Zolpidem	B	U	Not recommended

DIAZEPAM (11). Diazepam has been associated with congenital abnormalities, including inguinal hernia, cardiac defects, and pyloric stenosis. Small doses during labor are not harmful to the mother or her infant. Diazepam and its active metabolite, desmethyldiazepam, are excreted in breast milk in measurable quantities, even though the drug is highly protein bound. Therefore, there is a risk of accumulation if this drug is used in lactating women. The effect of diazepam on the nursing infant is unknown, but it may be of concern because of its potential for sedation.

Recently it has been suggested that the high rate of teratogenicity after heavy maternal benzodiazepine use may be a result of coincident alcohol and substance abuse and not due solely to benzodiazepine exposure.

LORAZEPAM (11). No reports linking lorazepam with congenital defects have been located. It is excreted in breast milk and may be of concern because of its potential for sedation.

ELDERLY. Toxic effects arise from both an increased sensitivity to central nervous system effects and alterations in pharmacokinetics. The benzodiazepines that rely on hepatic oxidative metabolism (diazepam, flurazepam, nitrazepam, and chlordiazepoxide) have an increased elimination half-life, with higher plasma levels of both the drug and its active metabolites. This may produce lethargy, excessive sedation, confusion, orthostatic hypotension, and ataxia. Benzodiazepines

that are metabolized by conjugation with glucuronic acid (temazepam, oxazepam, and lorazepam) do not have significant metabolic changes in the elderly (96).

Antihistamines (11,12,95)

Meclizine, cyclizine, and dimenhydrinate are probably not associated with an increased risk of malformations.

CYPROHEPTADINE (11). There is no evidence of fetal abnormalities. Contraindicated for nursing mothers because of sedation of the infant.

ZOLPIDEM (25). No teratogenic effects have been reported in animals. No studies in humans. Risk for withdrawal in neonates exists. Not recommended in nursing mothers because of sedation of the infant.

Other Drugs

Diphenoxylate (11) (in combination with atropine)

One case of an infant with multiple defects, including Ebstein's anomaly, has been reported.

Lidocaine (11)

There is no evidence of an association with large categories of major or minor malformations or individual defects.

Lithium (11)

Lithium should be avoided during pregnancy if possible, especially during the first trimester. Infants with cardiovascular defects, including the rare Ebstein's anomaly, have been reported, but this association may be less frequent than previously thought (97). Lithium use near term may produce severe, usually reversible, toxicity in

TABLE 4.21
Other Drugs

| | FETAL RISK | | |
	FDA	TERIS	BREAST-FEEDING
Diphenoxylate	C	U	Compatible
Lidocaine	C	None*	NA
Lithium	C	Small	Contraindicated
Paregoric	B	U	Compatible

*As local anesthetic

the newborn. Lithium is excreted in breast milk and results in serum levels in nursing infants of approximately one-third to one-half the maternal serum levels. Several authors (98) have reported toxic effects of lithium in neonates born to women who received lithium during pregnancy. Lithium is contraindicated during breast-feeding.

Paregoric (11)

Paregoric is a mixture of opium powder, anise oil, benzoic acid, campho, glycerin, and ethanol. No evidence has been found to suggest a relationship to any major or minor malformation or to individual defects.

References

1. Nies AS. Principles of therapeutics. In: Hardman JG, Limbird LC, (eds.) *The pharmacological basis of therapeutics*. New York, NY: McGraw-Hill, 2001;45–66.
2. Roberts JS, Silbergeld EK. Pregnancy, lactation, and menopause: how physiology and gender affect the toxicity of chemicals. *Mt Sinai J Med* 1995;343–355.
3. Matthews HW. Racial, ethnic and gender differences in response to medicines. In: Matthews HW, (ed.) *Drug metabolism and drug interactions*. Freund Publishing House, 1995:77–91.
4. Yonkers KA, Kando JC, Cole JO, Blumenthal S. Gender differences in pharmacokinetics and pharmacodynamics of psychotropic medication. *Am J Psychiatry* 1992;149: 587–595.
5. Silberstein SD, Merriam GR. Sex hormones and headache. In: Goadsby PJ, Silberstein SD, (eds.) *Headache*. Newton: Butterworth-Heinemann, 1997:143–173.
6. Sutker PB, Goist KC, King AR. Acute alcohol intoxication in women: relationship to dose and menstrual cycle phase. *Alcohol Clin Exp Res* 1987;2(1):74–79.
7. Ginsburg ES, Mello NK, Mendelson JH, et al. Effects of alcohol ingestion on estrogens in postmenopausal women. *JAMA* 1996;276(21):1747–1751.
8. Shepard TH. *Catalog of teratogenic agents*, 8th ed. Baltimore, Md: The Johns Hopkins University Press, 1995.
9. Drug treatment of the pregnant woman: the state of the art. Proceedings from the Food and Drug Administration conference on regulated products and pregnant women. Virginia, November 1995.
10. Yankowitz J. Use of medications in pregnancy: general principles, teratology, and current developments. In: Yankowitz J, Niebyl JR, (eds.) *Drug therapy in pregnancy*. Philadelphia, Pa: Lippincott, 2001:1–4.
11. Briggs GG, Freeman RK, Yaffe SJ. *Drugs in pregnancy and lactation*, 6th ed. Philadelphia, Pa: Lippincott, 2002.
12. Niebyl JR. Teratology and drugs in pregnancy and lactation. In: Winters R, (ed.) *Danforth's obstetrics and gynecology*. New York, NY: Lippincott, 1990.
13. Rayburn WF, Lavin JP. Drug prescribing for chronic medical disorders during pregnancy: An overview. *Am J Obstet Gynecol* 1986;155(3):565–569.
14. Traditional reproductive toxicology studies and their predictive value. FDA conference on regulated products and pregnant women. Virginia, 1994.
15. Silberstein SD. Headaches, pregnancy, and lactation. In:
16. Ethical conflicts and practical realities. Proceedings from the Food and Drug Administration conference on regulated products and pregnant women. 1994.
17. Use of observational methods to monitor the safety of marketed medications for risks of birth defects. Proceedings form the Food and Drug Administration conference on regulated products and pregnant women. 1994.
18. Little BB, Gilstrap LC. Human teratology principles. In: Gilstrap LC, Little BB, (eds.) *Drugs and pregnancy*. New York, NY: Chapman & Hall, 1998:7–24.
19. Piper JM, Baum C, Kennedy DL. Prescription drug use before and during pregnancy in a Medicaid population. *Am J Obstet Gynecol* 1987;157:148.
20. Fitzgerald M. Prescription and over-the-counter drug use during pregnancy. *J Am Acad Nurse Practitioners* 1995; 7(2):87.
21. Rubin JD, Ferencz C, Loffredo C. Use of prescription and nonprescription durgs in pregnancy. The Baltimore-Washington Infant Study Group. *J Clin Epidemiol* 1993; 46(6):581.
22. Heinonen OP, Sloan S, Shapiro S. *Birth defects and drugs in pregnancy*. Littleton: Publishing Sciences Group, 1977.
23. Martin PJ, Millac PA. Pregnancy, epilepsy, management and outcome: a ten-year perspective. *Seizure* 1993; 2(suppl 4):277–280.
24. Oguni M, Dansky L, Andermann E, Sherwin A, Andermann F. Improved pregnancy outcome in epileptic women in the last decade: relationship to maternal anticonvulsant therapy. *Brain Dev* 1993;14(suppl 6): 371–380.
25. Thomson Healthcare. *Physicians' Desk Reference*, 57th ed. Montvale, NJ: Thomson PDR, 2003.
26. Friedman JM, Polifka JE. *Teratogenic effects of drugs: a resource for clinicians (TERIS)*, 2nd ed. Baltimore, Md: Johns Hopkins University Press, 2000.
27. Friedman JM, Little BB, Brent RL, Cordero JF, Hanson JW, Shepard TH. Potential human teratogenicity of frequently prescribed drugs. *Obstet Gynecol* 1990;75: 594–599.
28. Daly LE, Kirke PN, Molloy A, Weir Dg, Scott JM. Folate levels and neural tube defects: implications for prevention. *JAMA* 1995;274:1698–1702.
29. Ogawa Y, Kaneko S, Otani K, Fukushima Y. Serum folic acid levels in epileptic mothers and their relationship to congenital malformations. *Epilepsy Res* 1991;8(suppl 1):75–78.
30. Jordan RL, Wilson JG, Shumacher HJ. Embryotoxicity of the folate antagonist methotrexate in rats and rabbits. *Teratology* 1977;15:73–80.
31. Dansky LV, Andermann E, Rosenblatt D, Sherwin AL, Andermann F. Anticonvulsants, folate levels, and pregnancy outcome: a prospective study. *Ann Neurol* 1987;21(suppl 2):176–182.
32. Reynolds EH. Anticonvulsants, folic acid and epilepsy. *Lancet* 1973;1:1376–1378.
33. Wegner C, Nau H. Alteration of embryonic folate metabolism by valproic acid during organogenesis: implications for mechanism of teratogenesis. *Neurology* 1992; 42(suppl 5):17–24.
34. Berg MG, Stumbo PJ, Chenard CA, Fincham RW, Schneider PJ, Schottelius DD. Folic acid improves phenytoin pharmacokinetics. *J Am Diet Assoc* 1995;95(3): 352–356.

Yankowitz J, Niebyl JR, (eds.) *Drug therapy in pregnancy*. Philadelphia, Pa: Lippincott, 2001:231–254.

35. Adab N, Jacoby A, Smith D, Chadwick D. Additional educational needs in children born to mothers with epilepsy. *J Neurol Neurosurg Psychiatr* 2001;70:15–21.

36. Metcalfe J, Stock MK, Barron DH. Maternal physiology during gestation. In: Knobel E, Neill J, (eds.) *The physiology of reproduction*. New York, NY: Raven Press, 1988:2145–2174.

37. Cunningham FG, MacDonald PC, Leveno KJ, Gant NF, Gilstrap LC. Maternal adaptations to pregnancy. In: Cunningham FG, MacDonald PC, Leveno KJ, Gant NF, Gilstrap LC, (eds.) *Williams obstetrics*. Stamford, CT: Appleton and Lange, 1993:209–246.

38. Bailey RR, Rolleston GL. Kidney length and ureteric dilatation in the puerperium. *Br J Obstet Gynecol* 1971;78:55.

39. Chesley LC. Renal function during pregnancy. In: Carey HM, (ed.) *Modern trends in human reproductive physiology*. London: Butterworth, 1963.

40. Dunlop W. Serial changes in renal hemodynamics during normal human pregnancy. *Br J Obstet Gynecol* 1981;88:1.

41. Chaudhuri G. *Pharmocokinetics in pregnancy*. VA, 11-7-8. 1994 (Abstract).

42. Yerby MS, Friel PN, McCormick K. Antiepileptic drug disposition during pregnancy. *Neurology* 1992;42(suppl 5):12–16.

43. Murray L, Seger D. Drug therapy during pregnancy and lactation. *Emerg Med Clin N Amer* 1994;12:129–149.

44. Szeto HH. Kinetics of drug transfer to the fetus. *Clin Obstet Gynecol* 1993;36:246–254.

45. American Academy of Pediatrics Committee on Drugs. The transfer of drugs and other chemicals into human milk. *Pediatrics* 2001;108(3).

46. Krauss GL, Brandt J, Campbell M, Plate C. Reproductive issues in epilepsy are poorly understood by U.S. neurologists and obstetricians. *Epilepsia* 1995 36(suppl 3),12.

47. Mattson RH, Cramer JA, Darney PD, Naftolin F. Use of oral contraceptives by women with epilepsy. *JAMA* 1986;256(2):238–240.

48. So EL. Update on epilepsy. *Med Clin N Amer* 1993;77(1):203–214.

49. Shuster EA. Epilepsy in women. *Mayo Clin Proc* 1996;71:991–999.

50. Haukkamaa M. Contraception by Norplant subdermal capsules is not reliable in epileptic patients on anticonvulsant therapy. *Contraception* 1986;33:559–565.

51. Schwartz D, Wang M, Geitz L. Medication errors made by elderly chronically ill patients. *Am J Public Health* 1962;52:2018–2029.

52. Brand FN, Smith RT, Brand PA. Effect of economic barriers to medical area on patients' noncompliance. *Pub Health Rep* 1977;92:72–78.

53. Triggs EJ, Nation RL, Long A, et al. Pharmacokinetics in the elderly. *Eur J Clin Pharmacol* 1975;8:55–62.

54. Bender AD. Effect of age on intestinal absorption: implications for drug absorption in the elderly. *J Am Geriatr Soc* 1968;16:1331–1339.

55. Novak LP. Aging, total body potassium, fat free mass and cell mass in males and females between the ages 18 and 85 years. *J Gerontol* 1972;27:438–443.

56. Stilwell JE. Psychotherapeutic drugs. In: Cassel CK, Walsh JR, (eds.) *Geriatric medicine*. New York, NY: Springer-Verlag, 1984:637–647.

57. Parry JH, Balter MB, Mellinger GD, et al. National patterns of psychotherapeutic drug use. *Arch Gen Psychiatry* 1973;28:269–283.

58. Dalessio DJ. Classification and treatment of headache during pregnancy. *Clin Neuropharmacol* 1986;9:121–131.

59. Saameli K. Effects on the uterus. In: Berde B, Schild HO, (eds.) *Ergot alkaloids and related compounds*. Berlin: Springer-Verlag, 1978:231–319.

60. Wainscott G, Volans GN. The outcome of pregnancy in women suffering from migraine. *Postgrad Med J* 1978;54:98–102.

61. Hughes HE, Goldstein DA. Birth defects following maternal exposure to ergotamine, beta-blockers, and caffeine. *J Med Genet* 1988;25:396–399.

62. Norton ME. Analgesic use in pregnancy. In: Yankowitz J, Niebyl JR, (eds.) *Drug therapy in pregnancy*. Philadelphia, Pa: Lippincott, 2001:119–126.

63. Stuart MJ, Gross SJ, Elrad H, Graeber JE. Effects of acetylsalicylic acid ingestion on maternal and neonatal hemostasis. *N Eng J Med* 1982;307:909–912.

64. Hertz-Pigiotto C, Hopenhay-Rich C, Golub M, Hooper K. The risks and benefits of taking aspirin during pregnancy. *Epidemiology Rev* 1990;12:108–148.

65. Rayburn W, Shukla U, Stetson P, Piehl E. Acetaminophen pharmacokinetics: comparison between pregnant and nonpregnant women. *Am J Obstet Gynecol* 1986;155:1353–1356.

66. Merck. *Clinical pharmacology*. 1995:255–276.

67. VandenVeyver JB, Moise KJ. Prostaglandin synthetase inhibitors in pregnancy. *Obstet Gynecolog Survey* 1993;48:493–502.

68. Goodwin JS, Regan M. Cognitive dysfunction associated with naproxen and ibuprofen in the elderly. *Arthritis Rheum* 1982;25:1013–1014.

69. Gilstrapp LC, Little BB. Anticoagulants, thrombolytics and hemostatics during pregnancy. In: Gilstrap LC, Little BB, (eds.) *Drugs and pregnancy*. New York, NY: Chapman & Hall, 1998:149–160.

70. Omri A, Delaloye JF, Anderson H, Bachmann F. LMW heparin Novo (LHN-1) does not cross the placenta during the second trimester of pregnancy. *Thromb Haemost* 1989;61:55.

71. Gillis S, Shushan A, Eldor A. Use of low molecular weight heparin for prophylaxis and treatment of thromboembolism in pregnancy. *Int J Gynecol Obstet* 1992;39:297.

72. Dulitzki M, Pauzner R, Langevitz P, Pras M, Many A, Schiff E. Low molecular weight heparin during pregnancy and delivery: preliminary experience with 41 pregnancies. *Obstet Gynecol* 1996;87:380.

73. LeOrme M, Lewis PJ, Deswiet M, et al. May mothers given Warfarin breast feed their infants? *Br Med J* 1977;1:564.

74. Turrentine MA, Braems G, Ramirez MM. Use of thrombolytics for the treatment of thromboembolic disease during pregnancy. *Obstet Gynecol* 1995;50:534.

75. Uknis A, Silberstein SD. Review article: migraine and pregnancy. *Headache* 1991;31:372–374.

76. Wylen M, Yankowitz J. Anticonvulsants in pregnancy. In: Yankowitz J, Niebyl JR, (eds.) *Drug therapy in pregnancy*. Philadelphia, Pa: Lippincott, 2001:221–230.

77. Buehler BA, Delimont D, VanWaes M, Finnell RH. Prenatal prediction of risk of the fetal hydantoin syndrome. *N Engl J Med* 1990;322:1567–1572.

78. Practice parameter: a guideline for discontinuing antiepileptic drugs in seizure-free patients (summary statement). 1994.

79. Robert E, Biubaud P. Maternal valproic acid and congenital neural tube defects. *Lancet* 1982;2:937.

80. Lindhout D, Schmidt D. In utero exposure to valproate and neural tube defects. *Lancet* 1986;1:1392–1393.

81. Omtzigt JG, Los FJ, Grobee DE, et al. The risk of spina bifida aperta after first trimester exposure to valproate in a prenatal cohort. *Neurology* 1992;42(S5):119–125.

82. Nulman I, Rovet J, Stewart DE, et al. Neurodevelopment of children exposed in utero to antidepressant drugs. *N Engl J Med* 1997;336:258–262.

83. Hollister LE. Treatment of depression with drugs. *Ann Intern Med* 1978;89:78–84.

84. Chambers CD, Johnson KA, Dick LM, Felix RJ, Jones KL. Birth outcomes in pregnant women taking fluoxetine. *N Engl J Med* 1996;335:1010–1015.

85. Robert E. Treating depression in pregnancy. *N Engl J Med* 1996;1056–1058.

86. Robinson JN, Norwitz ER, Repke JT. Antihypertensive use during pregnancy. In: Yankowitz J, Niebyl JR, (eds.) *Drug therapy in pregnancy*. Philadelphia, Pa: Lippincott, 2001:101–118.

87. Pruyn SC, Phelan JP, Buchanan GC. Long-term propranolol therapy in pregnancy: maternal and fetal outcome. *Am J Obstet Gynecol* 1979;135:485–489.

88. Featherstone HJ. Fetal demise in a migraine patient on propranolol. *Headache* 1983;23:213–214.

89. Shand DG. Propranolol. *N Engl J Med* 1975;293:280–285.

90. Koch-Weser J. Metoprolol. *N Engl J Med* 1979;301:698–703.

91. Fishman WH. Beta-adrenoceptor antagonists: new drugs and new indications. *N Engl J Med* 1982;306:1456–1462.

92. Vestal RE, Wood AJ, Shand DG. Reduced beta-adrenoceptor sensitivity in the elderly. *Clin Pharmacol Ther* 1979;26:181–186.

93. Henderson GI, Hu ZQ, Johnson RF, Perez AB, Yang Y, Schenker S. Acyclovir transport by the human placenta. *J Lab Clin Med* 1992;120:885–892.

94. O'Sullivan MJ, Boyer PJ, Scott GB, et al. The pharmacokinetics and safety of zidovudine in the third trimester of pregnancy for women infected with human immunodeficiency virus and their infants: Phase I acquired immunodeficiency syndrome clinical trials group study (Protocol #082). The Zidovudine Collaborative Working Group. *Am J Obstet Gynecol* 1993;168:1510–1516.

95. McMahon MJ. Drug therapy for the treatment of gastrointestinal disorders in pregnancy and lactation. In: Yankowitz J, Niebyl JR, (eds.) *Drug therapy in pregnancy*. Philadelphia, Pa: Lippincott, 2001:77–100.

96. Conrad KA. Antianxiety agents and hypnotics. In: Conrad KA, Bressler R, (eds.) *Drug therapy for the elderly*. Saint Louis: Mosby, 1982:262–276.

97. Jacobson SJ, Jones K, Johnson K, et al. Prospective multicenter study of pregnancy outcome after lithium exposure during first trimester. *Lancet* 1992;339:530–533.

98. Wilbanks GC, Bressler B, Peete CH, et al. Toxic effects of lithium carbonate in a mother and newborn infant. *JAMA* 1970;213:865.

5 Reproductive and Metabolic Disorders with AED Use

Martha J. Morrell, MD

A

ntiepileptic drugs (AEDs) represent a rapidly growing pharmaceutical class with efficacy in a number of neurological and psychiatric disorders, including epilepsy, pain, migraine, depression, bipolar disorder, and social anxiety disorders. Maintaining familiarity with the efficacy and tolerability profiles of individual agents, as well as the pharmacokinetics profiles, is challenging. In addition, the long-term health consequences of taking AEDs must be considered for the many patients who must take these agents for years or even a lifetime. This chapter focuses on AED use in women. Relevant information is also contained in Chapter 15, *Seizures and Epilepsy in Women*, including information about the dosing and pharmacokinetics characteristics of each AED.

CONTRACEPTION IN WOMEN WITH EPILEPSY

Women taking cytochrome P450 (CYP450) enzyme–inducing AEDs have perhaps a fivefold increase in the failure rate of oral contraceptive agents (1,2) because the metabolism of the contraceptive steroid is increased. The hormone dosage, particularly with low-dose hormone pills (the minipill), may not be sufficient to be effective. Phenytoin, carbamazepine, and the barbitu-

rates phenobarbital and primidone, induce CYP450 enzymes, increase steroid hormone metabolism, and bind to sex hormone binding globulin (SHBG) (Table 5.1). Both mechanisms reduce the bioavailable concentration of steroid hormone. Oxcarbazepine at doses in excess of 1,200 mg per day also induces cytochrome P450 enzymes, as does topiramate at dosages in excess of 200 mg per day. Valproate effectively inhibits this enzyme system, thereby slowing the metabolism of contraceptive hormones. Gabapentin, lamotrigine, levetiracetam, and zonisamide do not alter steroid hormone metabolism and thus do not interfere with hormonal contraceptives.

Women taking CYP450 enzyme–inducing AEDs who wish to use oral hormonal contraception should consider using a product containing at least 50 µg of the estrogen product (3) to regulate menstrual bleeding, rather than the commonly used minipill, which contains 35 µg of estrogen or less. Other forms of hormonal contraception, such as subdermal levonorgestrel (Norplant®), a slow-release contraceptive containing only progesterone, also carry a higher risk for failure (4,5).

EFFECTS OF AEDs ON PHYSIOLOGICAL SEX STEROID HORMONES

Just as the AEDs alter concentrations of sex steroid hormones used for contraception, so they alter concentrations

TABLE 5.1
*Antiepileptic Drug Effects on Oral
Hormonal Contraception*

AEDs that induce liver enzymes and may compromise
OC efficacy
    Carbamazepine (Tegretol®, Carbatrol®)
    Phenytoin (Dilantin®)
    Phenobarbital®
    Mysoline (Primidone®)
    Oxcarbazepine (Trileptal®)[1]
    Topiramate (Topamax®)[2]

AEDs that do not compromise OC efficacy
    Gabapentin (Neurontin®)
    Levetiracetam (Keppra®)
    Lamotrigine (Lamictal®)
    Valproate (Depakote®, Depakene®)
    Zonisamide (Zonegran®)

[1]At dosages above 1,200 mg/day
[2]At dosages above 200 mg/day

of endogenous ovarian and adrenal steroid hormones. This subject is reviewed in more detail in Chapter 6. In brief, CYP450 enzyme–inducing AEDs reduce the concentrations of ovarian estradiol and testosterone, as well as adrenal androgens such as androstenedione and DHEAS. Some authors have associated these reductions in androgens with sexual dysfunction in women using AEDs. Valproate, as a CYP450 enzyme inhibitor, is associated with elevations in ovarian and adrenal androgens. The clinical implications of this are discussed in the sections on polycystic ovary syndrome and carbohydrate metabolism. AEDs that have no effect of CYP450 enzymes probably do not change steroid hormone concentrations. This has been studied directly for gabapentin and lamotrigine. Women receiving either of these AEDs in monotherapy for epilepsy had no difference from nonepileptic untreated controls in concentrations of any steroid hormone (6).

EFFECTS OF AEDs ON BONE HEALTH

Some AEDs alter bone mineral metabolism and compromise bone health, especially in women who have smaller bone mass. Women using phenytoin, phenobarbital, and perhaps carbamazepine and valproate, are at higher risk for bone disorders such as osteopenia, osteoporosis, osteomalacia, and fractures (7–9). A prospective study evaluating the risk of hip fractures in women older than 65 years found that women taking AEDs were twice as likely to have a hip fracture (10).

AED associated bone disease is the consequence of a number of biochemical abnormalities of bone metabo-

lism (11). AEDs may alter bone mineral metabolism by decreasing calcium and increasing bone turnover. AEDs that interfere with intestinal calcium absorption could directly affect bone cell function, possibly through the inhibition of cellular responses to phenytoin (8,12), but this cannot be the only mechanism. Whereas reproductive-age women taking carbamazepine, phenytoin, and valproate had significantly reduced calcium levels compared with women receiving lamotrigine, only phenytoin was associated with increased bone turnover (13), as measured by metabolic markers indicating enhanced osteoblast and osteoclast activity. Valproate was associated with impaired osteoblastic differentiation but not with a change in osteoclast activity. Women receiving lamotrigine showed no abnormalities in any marker of bone metabolism.

Given the available data, women with epilepsy receiving AEDs should engage in good bone health practices, including adequate daily calcium (1,200 mg/day) and vitamin D, and gravity-resisting exercise. Bone density scans should be obtained after treatment with phenytoin, carbamazepine, or valproate for 5 or more years, although it seems reasonable to consider this after 3 years. Treatment with bisphosphonates, calcitonin, estrogen, or testosterone may be recommended for women with bone loss. Individuals with bone loss by density scan should be monitored with density scans yearly, or until bone loss begins to reverse.

AEDs AND POLYCYSTIC OVARY SYNDROME

The neurology community has been concerned about the increased prevalence of polycystic appearing ovaries and anovulatory menstrual cycles in women with epilepsy receiving AEDs (see Chapter 15 for detail). One question has been whether these observations imply that women with epilepsy are at greater risk for polycystic ovary syndrome and if such risk applies to women using AEDs for other indications.

Polycystic ovary syndrome is a gynecological syndrome affecting 7% of reproductive-aged women. Polycystic ovaries are found in 15% to 20% of reproductive-aged women and are not a component of the diagnostic criteria for polycystic ovary syndrome. The syndrome diagnosis requires frequent anovulatory cycles and phenotypic or serologic evidence for hyperandrogenism. This may present as centripetal obesity, hirsuitism with increased facial and body hair and loss of scalp hair over the crown and temporal recession, and acne. Serum androgens may be elevated, and there is often an elevation in the ratio of luteinizing hormone (LH) to follicle stimulating hormone (FSH). The metabolic defect underlying the syndrome is believed to be related to insulin insensitivity, perhaps because of a genetically determined abnormality in the insulin receptor. The importance of diagnosis comes from concerns about the long-term health risks associated with the syndrome. These risks include infertility, carbohydrate intolerance and diabetes, dyslipedemia with accelerated atherosclerosis, and endometrial carcinoma. Therefore, treatment is advocated, even for women not actively trying to conceive. Treatment includes dietary alterations, regulation of pituitary and gonadal hormones with oral contraceptives, and even hypoglycemic and lipid-lowering agents (14).

Women with epilepsy and women with bipolar disease have a high frequency of menstrual cycles that are abnormally long and thus suggestive of anovulatory cycles (see Chapter 15). In studies of women with epilepsy, 25% to 50% of cycles are anovulatory, depending on the epilepsy syndrome. A similar prevalence of anovulatory cycles is believed to affect women with bipolar disorder. Although epilepsy and bipolar disorder appear to be one variable associated with this polycystic-ovary-like syndrome, valproate—an AED that is an effective treatment for both disorders—seems to promote weight gain, carbohydrate intolerance, and elevated androgens in some women. Therefore, some women with these disorders who are receiving valproate present with a physical appearance, endocrinopathy, and cycle disturbance that very much resembles polycystic ovary syndrome. It is not known, however, whether this phenomenon has long-term health consequences similar to polycystic ovary syndrome.

Given present knowledge, the strategy is to watch closely for weight gain, cycle lengths shorter than 23 days or longer than 35 days (which is suggestive of anovulation), and query regarding changes in body or facial hair, as well as acne. This topic is discussed in detail with relevant references in Chapter 15.

AEDs AND LIPID, INSULIN, AND CARBOHYDRATE METABOLISM

Changes in lipid metabolism and body weight are associated with use of some AEDs and may cause long-term adverse health effects. Carbamazepine, phenytoin, and phenobarbital increase high-density lipoproteins (HDLs) and may have cholesterol-lowering effects (15–18). Carbamazepine does not alter trigycerides (19). Counteracting these favorable lipid trends, carbamazepine and phenytoin elevate low-density lipoproteins (LDLs). Valproate increases triglycerides, LDLs as well as HDLs, leading to an unfavorable lipid profile (20). Valproate-associated dyslipidemia may be a consequence of valproate-associated obesity and hyperinsulinemia (21). Until the nature and mechanisms of AED-associated alterations in lipid metabolism are better understood, clinicians should monitor cholesterol and lipid profiles in persons receiving AEDs.

Changes in carbohydrate metabolism induced by some AEDs are associated with a change in body mass index. Carbamazepine, gabapentin, and valproate are associated with weight gain in some patients, whereas felbamate, topiramate, and zonisamide are associated with weight loss. Levetiracetam, lamotrigine, and oxcarbazepine are weight neutral and do not change fasting or postprandial insulin levels (21,22). Lamotrigine is not associated with changes in weight in adults (21) or adolescents (23).

Approximately 50% of persons taking valproate for epilepsy experience significant weight gain, defined as more than 4 kg (24–26). Significant weight gain affects children and adolescents, as well as adults (23,27–29), and is usually evident early in therapy (within 3 to 6 months).

The mechanism for weight gain with valproate appears related to changes in lipid and carbohydrate metabolism, so may be relatively resistant to dietary manipulations. Valproate inhibits mitochondrial beta-oxidation and impairs the utilization of free fatty acids, which are then stored as fat (26). Increased free fatty acids increase insulin production and appetite. Valproate also increases GABA, an inhibitory neurotransmitter that increases appetite. Leptin, which also mediates appetite, is elevated in persons gaining weight on valproate (23,30).

Individuals gaining weight on valproate may have some degree of underlying insulin resistance. This hypothesis is supported by observations that fasting and postprandial insulin and proinsulin levels are elevated in obese adolescents and in adults taking valproate (19,20,22). Persons who gain weight on valproate have higher insulin levels than those who do not gain weight (30).

Topiramate is associated with weight loss in persons with epilepsy and in nonepileptic patients. Persons with weight gain associated with use of serotonin reuptake inhibitors lose weight when treated with topiramate (31,32). Glycemic control is improved in persons with type II diabetes taking topiramate (33). Topiramate is also associated with a reduction in the number of binge eating episodes and weight loss in persons with eating disorders (34).

The mechanism of topiramate associated weight loss is not known. In rodents, topiramate decreases lipoprotein lipase and inhibits fat deposition, reduces food intake, and enhances thermogenesis. Weight loss may be mediated through first- and second-messenger systems and augmentation of serotonin receptors, or through the antagonism of glutamate (35). Topiramate may also increase insulin sensitivity, thus reducing insulin levels.

AED USE IN PREGNANCY

Women taking AEDs are understandably concerned that these agents will compromise pregnancy and harm the fetus. Accumulating data allow health care providers to

TABLE 5.2
FDA Use-in-Pregnancy Risk Categories

Category C
Animal studies have shown no adverse effect on the fetus (teratogenic, embryocidal, or other) but there are no adequate studies in humans. The benefit from the use of the drug in pregnant women may be acceptable despite its potential risks.

Gabapentin
Felbamate
Lamotrigine
Levetiracetam
Oxcarbazepine
Tiagabine
Zonisamide

Category D
Positive evidence of human fetal risk exists, but the potential benefits of the drug in pregnant women may be acceptable despite its potential risks (e.g., for a life-threatening condition or a serious disease for which safer drugs cannot be used or are ineffective).

Carbamazepine
Phenobarbital
Phenytoin
Valproate (valproic acid, divalproex sodium)

TABLE 5.3
Maternal and Fetal AED Concentrations

AED	FETAL-TO-MATERNAL TOTAL CONCENTRATION	FETAL-TO-MATERNAL FREE CONCENTRATION
Phenobarbital	0.86	1.13
Phenytoin	0.91	1.10
Carbamazepine	0.73	1.42
Valproate	1.59	0.50
Lamotrigine	1.02 to 1.55	—

Reproduced with permission from Myllyne, et al.

better counsel women receiving AEDs about pregnancy and fetal risks.

AEDs taken by the mother pass the placenta and enter the fetal circulation. Significant concentrations of the total and nonprotein-bound (free) AEDs are detected in the newborn (36). As shown in Table 5.2, the individual fetal-to-maternal total AED concentration is inversely correlated with the fetal to maternal free fraction ratios for carbamazepine, phenobarbital, and phenytoin. The maternal free fraction of valproate is much higher in the mother than the fetus because the increase in free fatty acids during later pregnancy increases the free fraction of valproate. Data are not available for all the newer AEDs.

AED concentrations may change during pregnancy. Changes in total AED concentrations are related to an increase in plasma volume of 40% to 50%, and an increase in renal clearance and hepatic metabolism. The pharmacokinetics of some AEDs are more profoundly affected than that of others, probably because of pregnancy-related differential effects on CYP450 enzymes (Table 5.3). Although the total concentration falls for many AEDs, there tends to be an increase in the percentage of the nonprotein bound fraction of drug because of a reduction in albumin and, thus, in protein binding (37). Therefore, it is necessary to follow the non–protein-bound drug concentration, especially for AEDs that are highly protein bound, such as carbamazepine, phenytoin, and valproate. Dose adjustments should aim to maintain a stable nonprotein-bound fraction. Significant pregnancy-related reductions can be anticipated in concentrations of carbamazepine, phenytoin, phenobarbital, lamotrigine, and sometimes valproate (see Chapter 15 for more information).

AED-ASSOCIATED BIRTH DEFECTS

The older AEDs (benzodiazepines, phenytoin, carbamazepine, phenobarbital, and valproate) are associated with a higher risk of fetal major malformations, including cleft lip and palate and cardiac defects (atrial septal defect, tetralogy of Fallot, ventricular septal defect, coarctation of the aorta, patent ductus arteriosus, and pulmonary stenosis) (38–40). Cleft lip and palate are increased by a factor of 4.7 in children of AED treated mothers with epilepsy compared to the background rate (40). Carbamazepine and valproate are also associated with neural tube defects (NTDs) such as spina bifida (41,42). Exposure to AEDs, rather than the maternal trait of epilepsy, appears to be the cause of malformations. This suggests that women taking AEDs during pregnancy for indications other than epilepsy will have similar risks for birth defects.

The incidence of major malformations in infants born to mothers with epilepsy taking carbamazepine or phenytoin is believed to be 4% to 6%, compared with 2% to 4% for the general population. Neural tube defects (spina bifida and anencephaly) occur in 0.5% to 1% of infants exposed to carbamazepine (42) and 1% to 2% of infants exposed to valproate during the first month of gestation (41). Minor congenital anomalies associated with AED exposure include facial dysmorphism and digital anomalies, which arise in 6% to 20% of infants exposed in utero to the older AEDs (43). This represents a twofold increase over the general population. Minor anomalies in infants of epileptic mothers taking carbamazepine, phenobarbital, phenytoin, or valproate include ocular hypertelorism, epicanthal folds, nasal growth deficiency, abnormal ears, low hairline, distal digital hypoplasia, nail hypoplasia, and low arched fingertip dermotoglyphic patterns (44).These dysmorphisms are essentially identical to those seen with fetal alcohol syndrome and may be outgrown in the first several years of life (38).

The risk of teratogenicity is partly related to the extent of fetal exposure to the AED (45). The risk of birth defects increases significantly with AED polytherapy (38,45) and with higher daily doses (41,46). In one study in Japan (45), the risk of malformation after exposure to a single AED was 2% to 4%, whereas the risk had increased to more than 20% after exposure to four or more AEDs. Some investigators have suggested that it is the peak dose to which the fetus is exposed rather than the cumulative dose exposure that determines teratogenic risk (Morrell, 1997). This concern has led some clinicians to divide the total AED dose into more frequent intervals, particularly for women who require a higher daily dose. Please see Chapter 4 for further review of drug safety.

Children born to women with a history of seizures on and off AEDs, delivering at one of five maternity hospitals in the Boston area, were examined for birth defects (47). Identified mother–infant pairs were compared with control pairs of nonepileptic mothers and infants. Considering major malformations alone, 4.5% of women with epilepsy taking a single AED gave birth to a child with a major malformation, whereas 8.6% of women taking two or more AEDs had a child with a major malformation. No women with a history of seizures not taking an AED gave birth to a child with a major malformation. Major malformations were detected in 1.8% of infants born to controls. When major malformations, growth retardation, microcephaly, and hypoplasia of the midface and fingers were considered, 20.6% of the infants born to mothers with epilepsy taking AEDs had one or more of these birth defects, in contrast to 28% of the infants born to mothers taking two or more AEDs, 6.1% of the infants born to mothers with a history of seizures but not taking AEDs, and 8.5% of controls.

Prospective registries have been established to learn more about pregnancy and fetal outcome in women using AEDs. The North American Antiepileptic Drug Pregnancy Registry was established in 1997 to ascertain the fetal effects of AEDs taken during the first trimester of pregnancy. This is a purely prospective registry with women identified in the first trimester, before pregnancy outcome is known. Although most pregnancies represent women with epilepsy, the registry is open to pregnant women using AEDs for any indication. At the time that this chapter was written, the registry had released data on only two AEDs. The registry reports that malformations were present in only 1.62% of pregnancies with no AED exposure. There was evidence of increased risk of birth defects in offspring of women exposed to phenobarbital. Major malformations were seen in 7.8% of 65 pregnancies exposed to phenobarbital in monotherapy and enrolled in the first trimester (48). Major malformations were heart defects in four and cleft lip and palate in one. There were 123 completed pregnancies in which the fetus was exposed during the first trimester to valproate in monotherapy. Major birth defects were seen in 8.9% of these pregnancies (49). Anomalies included heart defects in four, NTDs in two, and one each of hypospadias, polydactyly, bilateral inguinal hernia, dysplastic kidneys, and clubfoot.

Since 1993, a number of new AEDs have been introduced. Little information exists regarding the effects of some of these drugs on the developing human fetus. Animal reproductive toxicology studies for AEDs provide some useful information, but may not be specifically predictive of the human experience. Data from the U.S. Food and Drug Association (FDA) on fetal outcome in animals exposed to the newer AEDs are favorable.

Data are available for lamotrigine through a drug-specific prospective pregnancy registry established by the manufacturer, GlaxoSmithKline (50). As of March 2003, the registry accumulated prospective data on 302 pregnancies resulting in a live birth, in which the fetus was exposed to lamotrigine during the first trimester in monotherapy. Nine pregnancies resulted in a child with a major malformation (3.0%; 95% confidence interval 1.5–5.8%). The 95% confidence interval indicates that the incidence of major malformations is no more than a twofold increase over the background population, and this may be similar to the background malformation rate.

Data are also available for outcomes after first-trimester exposure to lamotrigine in polytherapy. Twelve of 215 pregnancies with known outcomes resulted in a child with a major defect (5.6%). There were 67 prospectively identified pregnancies in which the polytherapy included valproate. Malformations occurred in seven children (10.4%; 95% confidence interval 4.7–20.9%). AED polytherapy that did not include valproate resulted in major malformations in 5 of 148 outcomes (3.4%; 95% CI 1.3–1.8%). No specific patterns of malformation were seen in the registry as a whole or in any subgroup.

Although the sample sizes for the individual regimens are too small for small frequencies of major malformations or large frequencies of very rare malformation to be ruled out, this experience is thus far reassuring. Confirmation of these findings comes from experience in a registry maintained in the United Kingdom (51).

Pregnancy experience with oxcarbazepine has been reported in several single-center studies. A report from Argentina on 42 pregnancy exposures to oxcarbazepine (25 in monotherapy and 17 in combination with other

AEDs) found no malformations in the monotherapy group and one ventricular septal defect in an infant also exposed to phenobarbital (52). A Finnish series that included 740 pregnancies exposed to AEDs during the first trimester found that the occurrence of major malformations was independently associated with use of oxcarbazepine [odds ratio (OR) 10.8%; 95% CI 1.1–106], as well as with caramazepine [OR 2.5; 95% CI 1–6], and valproate (4.1; 95% CI 1.6–11] (53). The wide confidence intervals indicate that these data should not be considered conclusive.

Presently, the European Registry (EURAP) is enrolling actively across the globe, while the North American Antiepileptic Drug Registry and pharmaceutical company registries continue to gather data. A registry should be contacted regarding any woman who becomes pregnant while taking AEDs.

Mechanisms for AED-Mediated Teratogenesis

Several biochemical and molecular mechanisms are likely for AED mediated teratogenicity, including interference with the folate and methionine metabolic pathways (54), alteration of gene expression (55), generation of reactive metabolites via epoxidation or the prostaglandin co-oxidation pathway (56), and interference with endogenous retinoid metabolism (57). The embryotoxicity associated with folate deficiency and exposure to epoxide intermediates can be minimized through simple treatment strategies.

The teratogenicity of some AEDs (carbamazepine, phenobarbital, phenytoin) may be mediated in part by oxidative (free radical) metabolites generated by the bioactivation of the parent compound by the hepatic CYP450 enzymes. These intermediates may be inactivated by one of several biochemical pathways. Free radical scavenging enzymes, such as glutathione, bind with and disable these reactive intermediates and may be cytoprotective. When glutathione is inhibited, phenytoin embryotoxicity is enhanced (56). These intermediates are also metabolized by the enzyme epoxide hydrolase to a nonreactive dihydrodiol. The activity of this enzyme is genetically mediated, and fetuses with low levels of enzyme activity appear to be at the highest risk for birth defects (55,58,59). The CYP450 enzyme-inducing AEDs accelerate the formation of epoxide derivatives, and valproate inhibits epoxide metabolism by inhibiting the enzyme epoxide hydrolase. Polytherapy with an enzyme inducer and valporate may promote epoxide production and inhibit epoxide metabolism.

Vitamin A (retinol) and its oxidative metabolite, all-trans-retinoic acid, mediate embryonic growth, differentiation, and morphological development. Vitamin excess and deficiency, and low doses of retinoic acid, are associated with birth defects in animals (57). In a study of 75 patients with epilepsy and 29 healthy untreated controls, patients with epilepsy receiving valproate alone or in combination had increased levels of retinol (vitamin A) and decreased levels of retinoic acid (57).

Folic acid deficiency has been identified as a contributing factor to the development of NTDs and other nongenetic malformations, and folate supplementation has been conclusively shown to have a beneficial effect in reducing this risk. Women with epilepsy appear to be at especially high risk for folate deficiency (60). Serum folate is reduced in up to 90% of patients receiving phenytoin, carbamazepine, or barbiturates (61). Valproate does not cause a reduction in folate levels but does interfere with folate and methionine metabolism (62). In mice, valproate reduces levels of 5-formyl- and 10-formyl-tetrahydrofolates and increases the level of tetrahydrofolate, apparently by inhibiting the transfer of the formyl group via glutamate formyltransferase (63). Lamotrigine, an AED that has weak folate properties in vitro, had no effects on serum or red blood cell folate in a small number of patients (64).

Low serum and red blood cell folate levels are associated with an increased incidence of spontaneous abortions and malformations in animals and in women with epilepsy (61,65). Folate supplementation significantly reduces the risk of occurrent and recurrent NTDs in nonepileptic women (66–71). The presumption has been that folic acid supplementation will also reduce the risk of major malformations after fetal exposure to AEDs. There is, however, no proof that this is so. In fact, at least one report exists of a child born with a NTD after in utero exposure to valproate despite folic acid supplementation (72).

The best method to determine folate status has not been established, because serum folate appears to be a relatively insensitive indicator of functional folate status. Red blood cell folate levels more accurately reflect chronic folate status than do serum levels. In one study, women who had given birth to two or more children with NTDs had lower red cell folate levels than did controls (178 ng/mL versus 268 ng/mL). Serum folate, however, was equivalent between the two groups (73). A vulnerability to develop malformations may be associated with defective folate metabolism rather than folate deficiency (74). Results from one recent study suggest that the neurotoxic effects of valproate are mediated by disruption of folate-mediated biochemical processes rather than by causing a folate deficiency (63).

In addition, vitamin B12 deficiency, either related to insufficient dietary intake or abnormalities of the B12 binding proteins (apotranscobalamins), could contribute to AED-mediated teratogenesis by impairing folate metabolism. Mills et al. (75) found higher homocysteine values in mothers of children born with NTDs than in controls. Elevated homocysteine levels are also found in persons taking AEDs, particularly valproate (76,77). This could be explained by reduced activity of the enzyme methionine synthetase, which requires both folate and B12 as cofactors. One assessment of women who had previously given birth to a child with a NTD found evidence of intolerance to methionine loading that was consistent with pathologic homocysteinemia. This response is usually a consequence of heterozygosity for homocysteinemia (78). Carriers for inborn errors of homocysteine metabolism might be identified antenatally, and when possible, exposure to AEDs associated with neural tube abnormalities could be avoided. In women receiving drugs associated with elevated risk for neural tube abnormalities, pathological homocysteinemia could be corrected with high doses of pyridoxine or folic acid.

PRENATAL CARE AND DIAGNOSTIC TESTING

The American Academy of Neurology recommends that, in order to reduce pregnancy risks, treatment consist of a single AED at the lowest effective dose (79). Of course, this is not always possible, but it remains a worthwhile goal.

The malformations associated with AED exposure are readily detected by modern diagnostic testing (80). Neural tube defects can be detected by week 16 of fetal gestation with more than 95% sensitivity by obtaining a maternal serum alpha-fetoprotein (elevated with neural tube abnormalities) and a level II ultrasound to detect neural tube or cardiac malformations. In women who have independent risk factors for malformation, such as advanced maternal age, amniocentesis may be indicated. Amniocentesis to obtain fetal alpha feto-protein (elevated with NTDs) is also recommended if maternal serum alpha-fetoprotein is elevated or if the spinal cord cannot be adequately visualized by ultrasound. Women with fetuses having significant neural tube abnormalities or other major malformations may be given the option of a first-trimester termination.

The optimal concentration of folate to prevent NTDs has not been established for women with epilepsy on AEDs. Data regarding folate dosage comes entirely from populations of medically well women. In nonepileptic women, red blood cell folate levels higher than 906 nmol/l (400 ng/mL) may be optimal for the prevention of folate-responsive NTDs (81). In nonepileptic women who are users of folic acid supplements, dietary folate intakes of greater than or equal to 450 μg/day achieved levels of red blood cell folate in excess of 906 nmol/l. In nonepileptic women who did not use folate supplements, dietary intake of folate needed to exceed 500 μg/day to attain desirable red blood cell folate levels (82). In one evaluation of nonepileptic, healthy, well-educated, middle-income women, one in eight had folate levels indicative of a negative balance and 44% had red blood cell

folate levels that were lower than optimal (less than 680 nmol/l). Only one in four had red blood cell folate levels that exceeded the optimal 906 nmol/l.

The United States Public Health Service recommends that all women of childbearing age in the United States who are capable of becoming pregnant consume 0.4 mg/day of folic acid for the purpose of reducing their risk of having a child affected with a NTD (83). Women who have already had a child with a NTD are referred to a 1991 CDC guideline suggesting a dosage of 4 mg/day, based on the Medical Research Council recurrent risk study (68). The Canadian College of Medical Geneticists recommend that 0.8 to 5.0 mg/day of folic acid be given to women who are at increased risk of having offspring with NTDs and who are planning a pregnancy (84). Whether women with epilepsy require a dosage higher than 0.4 mg/day is not known.

To protect against NTDs, folate supplementation must be provided during the first 28 days of fetal gestation. In the United States, 40% of pregnancies are not planned, and of planned pregnancies, 50% do not consult a health care provider during the first trimester (85). The wide availability of reliable home pregnancy testing kits may further reduce preconceptional and first-trimester physician contacts. Therefore, folate supplementation should be considered in anticipation of conception.

Neonatal Hemorrhage

Neonates of mothers with epilepsy are at risk for early hemorrhage, which is believed to be a consequence of a coagulopathy caused by AED interference with vitamin K metabolism. Vitamin K–dependent proteins include the clotting factors II, VII, IX, and X and the anticoagulant proteins, protein C and protein S. Two forms of vitamin K occur naturally—vitamin K1 (phylloquinone), which is found in green plants and is the major dietary form of vitamin K, and vitamin K2 (menaquinone), which is synthesized by intestinal bacteria. Although vitamin K nutritional deficiency is rare in otherwise healthy populations, vitamin K levels in the cord blood of unsupplemented neonates exposed in utero to AEDs are reported to be below detection (86,87). In addition, assays for protein induced by vitamin K absence (PIVKAs), nonfunctional procoagulants that appear in blood when vitamin K is deficient, are elevated in neonates exposed to AEDs. The assay for PIVKAII is the most sensitive assay for vitamin K deficiency. How AEDs cause vitamin K deficiency in the fetus is not known, but may be a consequence of maternal and fetal induction of CYP450 liver enzymes by AEDs, which increases the rate of oxidative degradation of vitamin K. Therapeutically, this deficiency can be corrected by supplying vitamin K1 at a dose of 10 mg/day to the mother during the last month of gestation. Placental transfer of vitamin K to the fetus occurs, although slowly. Supplying the neonate with vitamin K at birth is safe and has been shown to be efficacious in preventing neonatal hemorrhage. The neonate receives vitamin K at a dose of 1 mg, intramuscular. Cord-blood specimens can be submitted for immediate clotting studies. If a reduction in vitamin K-dependent clotting factors is detected, then fresh frozen plasma can be administered at 20 mL/kg over 1 to 2 hours (88).

BREAST-FEEDING

Breast-feeding is strongly recommended by most health organizations to promote mother–child bonding and reduce the risk of infection and later-life immunologic disorders (89). AEDs cross into breast milk to variable extents. Passage is usually through simple diffusion, and the ratio is determined by the drug's molecular weight, pKa, lipophilicity, and, most important, the extent of protein binding (36,90,91). For phenytoin, carbamazepine, valproate, and tiggabine, the concentration in breast milk is negligible because of their high protein binding. Ethosuximide, phenobarbital, and PRM result in measurable concentrations. Lamotrigine reaches approximately 30% of the maternal serum concentration (92). Topiramate, oxcarbazepine, and oxcarbazepine metabolite levels are similar in maternal serum, cord blood, and placental tissue (93,94), indicating extensive transplacental passage. However, this does not necessarily indicate the ultimate exposure for breastfed infants. For topiramate, the milk-to-maternal-plasma ratio is 0.69 at 3 months, and breast-fed infants have concentrations below the limit of quantification (93).

For most women, the best advice is to seriously consider breast-feeding. Once started, the infant can be observed for proper weight gain and sleep cycles. The mother must also be advised that AED metabolism and clearance will remain elevated as long as breast-feeding continues. When breast-feeding stops, the mother may experience an increase in serum AED concentrations that requires a dosage adjustment.

CONCLUSION

Clinicians selecting an AED should consider its potential impact on reproductive and metabolic health. CYP450 enzyme–inducing AEDs reduce concentrations of bioavailable sex steroid hormones, thus affecting oral contraceptive regulation of the menstrual cycle and contraceptive efficacy. These agents also reduce endogenous sex steroid hormones, which may contribute to sexual dysfunction.

AED-related reproductive endocrine disorders and ovarian dysfunction may present as an alteration in the length or regularity of the menstrual cycle. Development of male pattern hair growth, obesity, or acne is a sign of elevated androgens and/or androgen hypersensitivity. Lipid abnormalities and glucose intolerance may accompany hyperandrogenism and confer significant long-term health risks.

AEDs may also affect bone health. Although mechanisms of bone loss and resultant osteopenia and osteoporosis are not elucidated, compelling data implicate the enzyme–inducing AEDs, particularly phenytoin and phenobarbital. Bone density should be monitored, and all women receiving AEDs should be strongly encouraged to observe good bone health practices, including gravity-resisting exercise, calcium (at least 1,200 mg/day) and vitamin D supplementation, and periodic bone density scans.

The rates of major morphologic abnormalities after fetal exposure to the older AEDs are presently believed to be 4% to 6% for carbamazepine and phenytoin respectively, 8.9% for valproate, and 7.8% for phenobarbital. Information regarding lamotrigine suggests a low risk for major malformations after monotherapy exposure. Data regarding risks for the other new-generation AEDs are pending. In the meantime, limiting exposure to high AED dosages and AED polytherapy, supplementing with periconceptional folic acid, and ensuring rigorous prenatal diagnostic testing with an anatomic ultrasound can enhance the odds for a normal pregnancy outcome.

Health care providers for women receiving AEDs for epilepsy and other indications can benefit from the mass of new information coming from the work of a number of investigators, including those involved in the prospective pregnancy registries. The detection of AED-associated reproductive and metabolic health disturbances can be accomplished easily, and reasonably simple and effective interventions can be readily incorporated into clinical practice. The sophisticated treatment of the woman receiving AEDs provides treatment for the disease state and also optimizes overall health.

References

1. Mattson RH, Cramer JA, Darney PD, Naftolin F. Use of oral contraceptives by women with epilepsy. *JAMA* 1986;256:238–240.
2. Coulam CB, Annegers JF. Do oral anticonvulsants reduce the efficacy of oral contraceptives? *Epilepsia* 1979;20:519–526.
3. Zahn CA, Morrell MJ, Collins SD, Labiner DM, Yerby MS. Management issues for women with epilepsy: a review of the literature. American Academy of Neurology Practice Guidelines. *Neurology* 1998;51:949–956.
4. Haukkamaa M. Contraception by Norplant subdermal capsule is not reliable in epileptic patients on anticonvulsant treatment. *Contraception* 1986;33(6):559–565.
5. Odlind V, Olsson SE. Enhanced metabolism of levonorgestrel during phenytoin treatment in a woman with Norplant implants. *Contraception* 1986;33:257–261.

6. Morrell MJ, Flynn KL, Seale CG, et al. Reproductive dysfunction in women with epilepsy: antiepileptic drug effects on sex-steroid hormones. *CNS Spectrums* 2001;6:771–786.

7. Sheth R, Wesolowski C, Jacob J, et al. Effect of carbamazepine and valproate on bone mineral density. *J Pediatr* 1996;127:256–262.

8. Valimaki M, Tiihonen M, Laitinen K, et al. Bone mineral density measured by dual-energy x-ray absorptiometry and novel markers of bone formation and resorption in patients on antiepileptic drugs. *J Bone Miner Res* 1994;9:631–637.

9. Chang S, Ahn C. Effects of antiepileptic drug therapy on bone mineral density in ambulatory epileptic children. *Brain Dev* 1994;16:382–385.

10. Bogliun G, Beghi E, Crespi V, Delodovick L, d'Amico P. Anticonvulsant drugs and bone metabolism. *Acta Neurol Scand* 1986;74:284–288.

11. Pack AM, Morrell MJ. Adverse effects of antiepileptic drugs on bone structure. Epidemiology, mechanisms and therapeutic implications. *CNS Drugs* 2001;15(8):633–642.

12. Gough H, Goggin T, Bissessar A, Baker M, Crowley M, Callaghan N. A comparative study of the relative influence of different anticonvulsant drugs, UV exposure and diet on vitamin D and calcium metabolism in outpatients with epilepsy. *QJM, New Series 59*. 1986;230:569–577.

13. Pack AM, Olarte LS, Morrell MJ, Flaster E, Resor SR, Shane E. Bone mineral density in an outpatient population receiving enzyme-inducing antiepileptic drugs. *Epilepsy Behav* 2003 Apr;4(2):169–174.

14. American College of Obstetric and Gynecologic Physicians Practice Bulletin #41. *Polycystic ovary syndrome*. 2002;100(6):1389–1402.

15. Calandre EP, Rodriguez-Lopez C, Blazquez A, et al. Serum lipids, lipoproteins and apolipoproteins A and B in epileptic treated with valproic acid, carbamazepine or phenobarbital. *Acta Neurol Scand* 1991;83:250–253.

16. Louma PV, Sotaniemi EA, Peklonen RO, et al. Plasma high density lipoprotein cholesterol and hepatic cytochrome P450 concentrations in epileptics undergoing anticonvulsant treatment. *Scand J Clin Lab Invest* 1980;40:163–167.

17. Eiris JM, Lojo S, Del Rio MC, et al. Effects of long-term treatment with antiepileptic drugs on serum lipid levels in children treated with anticonvulsants. *Neurology* 1995;45:1155–1157.

18. Verrotti A, Domizio S, Angelozzi B, et al. Changes in serum lipids and lipoproteins in epileptic children treated with anticonvulsants. *J Paediatr Child Health* 1997;33:242–245.

19. Pylvanen V, Knip M, Pakarinen AJ, et al. Fasting serum insulin levels and lipid levels in men with epilepsy. *Neurology* 2003;60(4):571–574.

20. Luef G, Abraham I, Hoppichler F, Trinka E, Unterberger I, Bauer G, Lechleitner M. Increase in postprandial serum insulin levels in epileptic patients with valproic acid therapy. *Metabolism* 2002;51(10):1274–1278.

21. Isojarvi JI, Rattya J, Myllyla VV, et al. Valproate, lamotrigine, and insulin-mediated risks in women with epilepsy. *Ann Neurol* 1998;43(4):446–451.

22. Stephen LJ, Kwan P, Shapiro D, Dominiczak M, Brodie MJ. Hormone profiles in young adults with epilepsy treated with sodium valproate or lamotrigine monotherapy. *Epilepsia* 2001;42(8):1002–1006.

23. Biton V, Levisohn P, Hoyler S, Vuong A, Hammer AE. Lamotrigine versus valproate monotherapy-associated weight change in adolescents with epilepsy: results from a post hoc analysis of a randomized, double-blind clinical trial. *J Child Neurol* 2003;18(2):133–139.

24. Corman CL, Leung NM, Guberman AH. Weight gain in epileptic patients during treatment with valproic acid: a retrospective study. *Can J Neurol Sci* 1997;24(3):240–244.

25. Dinesen H, Gram L, Andersen T, Dam M. Weight gain during treatment with valproate. *Arch Neurol Scand* 1984;70(2):65–69.

26. Gidal BE, Anderson GD, Spencer NW, Maly MM, et al. Valproate associated weight gain in persons with epilepsy: potential relationships to energy expensiture and metabolism. *J Epilepsy* 1996;9:234–241.

27. Morrell MJ, Isojarvi J, Taylor A, et al. Higher androgens and weight gain with valproate compared with lamotrigine for epilepsy. *Epilepsy Res* 2003;54:189–199.

28. Rattya J, Vainionpaa L, Knip M, Lanning P, Isojarvi JI. The effects of valproate, carbamazepine and oxcarbazepine on growth and sexual maturation in girls with epilepsy. *Pediatrics* 1999;103(3):588–593.

29. Novak, GP, Maytal J, Alshansky A, Eviatar L, Sy-Sho R, Siddique Q. Risk of excessive weight gain in epileptic children treated with valproate. *J Child Neurol* 1999;14(8):490–495.

30. Verrotti A, Basciani F, Morresi S, de Martino M, Morgese G, Chiarelli F. Serum leptin changes in epileptic patients who gain weight after therapy with valproic acid. *Neurology* 1999;53(1):230–232.

31. Van Amerigen M, Mancini C, Pipe B, et al. Topiramate treatment for SSRI-induced weight gain in anxiety disorders. *J Clin Psychiatry* 2002;63:981–984.

32. Van Ameringen M, Mancini C, Pipe B, Campbell M, Oakman J. Topiramate treatment for SSRI-induced weight gain in anxiety disorders. *J Clin Psychiatr* 2002;63(11):981–984.

33. Chengappa R, Levine J, Rathore D, Parepally H, Atzert R. Long-term effects of topiramate on bipolar mood instability, weight change and glycemic control: a case-series. *Eur Psychiatry* 2001;16(3):186–190.

34. McElroy S, Arnold L, Shapira N, et al. Topiramate in the treatment of binge eating disorder associated with obesity: a randomized, placebo-controlled trial. *Am J Psychiatry* 2003;160:255–261.

35. Richard D, Ferland J, Lalonde J, Samson P, Deshaies Y. Influence of topiramate in the regulation of energy balance. *Nutrition* 2000;16(10):961–966.

36. Takeda A, Okada H, Tanaka H, Izumi M, Ishikawa S, Noro T. Protein binding of four antiepileptic drugs in maternal and umbilical cord serum. *Epilepsy Res* 1992;13:147–151.

37. Yerby MS, Friel PN, McCormick K. Pharmacokinetics of anticonvulsants in pregnancy: alterations in plasma protein binding. *Epilepsy Res* 1990;5:223–228.

38. Koch S, Loesche G, Jager-Roman E, et al. Major birth malformations and antiepileptic drugs. Neurology 1992;42(suppl 5):83–88.

39. Annegers JF, Hauser WA, Elveback LR, Anderson VE, Kurland LT. Congenital malformations and seizure disorders in the offspring of parents with epilepsy. *Int J Epidemiol* 1978;7:241–247.

40. Friis ML. Facial clefts and congenital heart defects in children of parents with epilepsy: genetic and environmental etiologic factors. *Acta Neurol Scand* 1989:79:433–459.

41. Omtzigt JGC, Los FJ, Grobee DE, et al. The risk of spina bifida aperta after first-trimester exposure to valproate

in a prenatal cohort. *Neurology* 1992;42(suppl 5): 119–125.

42. Rosa FW. Spina bifida in infants of women treated with carbamazepine during pregnancy. *N Engl J Med* 1991; 324:674–677.

43. Gaily E, Granstrom ML. Minor anomalies in children of mothers with epilepsy. *Neurology* 1992;42(S5):128–131.

44. Gaily E, Kantola-Sorsa E, Granstrom ML. Intelligence of children of epileptic mothers. *J Pediatr* 1988;113: 677–684.

45. Kaneko S, Otani K, Fukushima Y, et al. Teratogenecity of antiepilepsy drugs: analysis of possible risk factors. *Epilepsia* 1988;29:459–467.

46. Oguni M, Dansky L, Andermann E, Sherwin A, Andermann F. Improved pregnancy outcome in epileptic women in the last decade: relationship to maternal anticonvulsant therapy. *Brain Dev* 1992;14:371–380.

47. Holmes, et al. Evidence of increased risk of birth defects in offspring of women exposed to phenobarbital as a monotherapy. *Teratology* 2001;63:250.

48. Holmes LB, Harvey EA, Coull BA, et al. The teratogenicity of anticonvulsant drugs. *N Engl J Med* 2001; 344:1132–1138.

49. Holmes, et al. Evidence of increased risk of birth defects in offspring of women exposed to valproate (Depakote, Depakene, Epival). *Am J Obstet Gynecol* 2002;187(S):S137.

50. Tennis P, Eldridge RR, and the International Lamotrigine Pregnancy Registry Scientific Advisory Committee. Preliminary results on pregnancy outcomes in women using lamotrigine. *Epilepsia* 2002;43:1161–1167.

51. Morrow JI, Russell A, Craig JJ, et al. Major malformations in the offspring of women with epilepsy: a comprehensive prospective study. *Epilepsia* 2001;42(suppl 2):125.

52. Rabinowicz AL, Meischenguiser R, D'Giano CH, Ferraro SM, Carrazanna EJ. Report of a single centre pregnancy registry of AEDS: focus on outcomes with oxcarbazepine. *Epilepsia* 2002;43(suppl 8):159.

53. Kaaja E, Kaaja R, Hiilesmaa V. Major malformations in offspring of women with epilepsy. *Neurology* 2003;60: 575–579.

54. Wegner C, Nau H. Alteration of embryonic folate metabolism by valproic acid during organogenesis: implications for mechanism of teratogenesis. *Neurology* 1992;42 (suppl 5):17–24.

55. Finnell RH, Buehler BA, Kerr BM, Ager PL, Levy RH. Clinical and experimental studies linking oxidative metabolism to phenytoin-induced teratogenesis. *Neurology* 1992;42:25–31.

56. Miranda AF, Wiley MJ, Wells PG. Evidence for embryonic peroxidase-catalyzed bioactivation and glutathione-dependent cytoprotection in phenytoin teratogenicity: modulation by eicosatetraynoic acid and buthione sulfoximine in murine embryo culture. *Toxicol Appl Pharmacol* 1994;124:230–241.

57. Nau H, Tzimas G, Mondry M, Plum C, Spohr HL. Antiepileptic drugs alter endogenous retinoid concentration: a possible mechanism of teratogenesis of anticonvulsant therapy. *Life Sci* 1995;57:53–60.

58. Buehler BA, Delimont D, Van Waes M, Finnell RH. Prenatal prediction of risk of the fetal hydantoin syndrome. *N Engl J Med* 1990;322:1567–1572.

59. Strickler SM, Dansky LV, Miller MA, Seni MH, Andermann E, Spielberg SP. Genetic predisposition to phenytoin-induced birth defects. *Lancet* 1985;2:746–749.

60. Tomson T, Lindborn U, Sundqvist A, Berg A. Red cell folate levels in pregnant epileptic women. *Eur J Clin Pharmacol* 1995;48:305–308.

61. Ogawa Y, Kaneko S, Otani K, Fukushima Y. Serum folic acid levels in epileptic mothers and their relationship to congenital malformations. *Epilepsy Res* 1991;8:75–78.

62. Alonso-Aperte E, Ubeda N, Achon M, Perez-Miguelsanz J, Varela-Moreiras G. Impaired methionine synthesis and hypomethylation in rats exposed to valproate during gestation. *Neurology* 1999;52(4):750–756.

63. Elmazar MM, Nau N. Trimethoprim potentiates valproic acid-induced neural tube defects (NTDs) in mice. *Reprod Toxicol* 1993 May-June;7(3):249–254.

64. Sander JW, Patsalos PN. An assessment of serum and red blood cell folate concentrations in patients with epilepsy on lamotrigine therapy. *Epilepsy Res* 1992;13(1): 89–92.

65. Dansky L, Andermann E, Roseblatt D, Sherwin AL, Andermann F. Anticonvulsants, folate levels and and pregnancy outcome. *Ann Neurol* 1987;21:176–182.

66. Werler MM, Shapiro S, Mitchell AA. Periconceptional folic acid exposure and risk of occurrent neural tube defects. *JAMA* 1993;269:1257–1261.

67. Czeizel AE, Dudas I. Prevention of the first occurrence of neural tube defects by periconceptional vitamin suplementation. *N Engl J Med* 1992;327:1832–1835.

68. Medical Research Council Vitamin Research Group. Prevention of neural tube defects: results of the Medical Research Council Vitamin Study. *Lancet* 1991;338: 131–137.

69. Mulinare J, Corder JF, Erickson JD, et al. Periconceptional use of multivitamins and the occurrence of neural tube defects. *JAMA* 1988;260:3141–3145.

70. Milunsky A, Jick H, Jick SS, et al. Multivitamin/folic acid supplementation in early pregnancy reduces the prevalence of neural tube defects. *JAMA* 1988;262:2847–2852.

71. Laurence KM, James N, Miller MH, Tennant GB, Campbell H. Double-blind, randomized controlled trial of folate treatment before conception to prevent the recurrence of neural-tube defects. *BMJ* 1981;282:1509–1511.

72. Craig J, Morrison P, Morrow J, et al. Failure of periconceptional folic acid to prevent a neural tube defect in the offspring of a mother taking sodium valproate. *Seizure* 1999;8:253–254.

73. Yates JRW, Ferguson-Smith MA, Shenkin A, Guzman-Rodriguez R, White M, Clark BJ. Is disordered folate metabolism the basis for the genetic predisposition to neural tube defects? *Clin Genet* 1987;31:279–287.

74. Gordon N. Folate metabolism and neural tube defects. *Brain Dev* 1995;17:307–311.

75. Mills JL, McPartlin JM, Kirke PN, et al. Homocysteine metabolism in pregnancies complicated by neural tube defects. *Lancet* 1995;345:149–151.

76. Apeland T, Mansoor MA, Strandjord RE. Antiepileptic drugs as independent predictors of plasma total homocysteine levels. Epilepsy Res 2001;47(1-2):27–35.

77. Apeland T, Mansoor MA, Strandjord RE, Kristensen O. Homocysteine concentrations and methionine loading in patients on antiepileptic drugs. *Acta Neurol Scand* 2000;101(4):217–223.

78. Steegers-Theunissen RPM, Boers GHJ, Trijbels FJM, Eskes TKAB. Neural-tube defects and derangement of homocysteine metabolism. *N Engl J Med* 1991;324: 199–200.

79. American Academy of Neurology. Quality Standards Subcommittee. Practice parameter: management issues

for women with epilepsy (summary statement). *Neurology* 1998;51:944–948.

80. American College of Obstetric and Gynecologic Physicians Educational Bulletin. *Seizure disorders in pregnancy.* 1996;231:1–13.

81. Daly LE, Kirke PN, Molloy A, Weir DG, Scott JM. Folate levels and neural tube defects: implications for treatment. *JAMA* 1995;274:1698–1702.

82. Brown JE, Jacobs DR Jr, Hartman TJ, et al. Predictors of red cell folate level in women attempting pregnancy. *JAMA* 1997;277(7):548–552.

83. MMWR. Recommendations for the use of folic acid to reduce the number of cases of spina bifida and other neural tube defects. *MMWR* 1992;41:1–7.

84. Van Allen M, Fraser FC, Dallaire L, et al. Recommendations on the use of folic acid supplementation to prevent the recurrence of neural tube defects. *CMAJ* 1993;149:1239–1243.

85. Grimes DA. Unplanned pregnancies in the U.S. *Obstet Gynecol* 1986;67:438–442.

86. Cornelissen M, Steegers-Theunissen R, Kollee L, Eskes T, Motohara K, Monnens L. Supplementation of vitamin K in pregnant women receiving anticonvulsant therapy prevents neonatal vitamin K deficiency. *Am J Obstet Gynecol* 1993;168:884–888.

87. Cornelissen M, Steegers-Theunissen R, Kollee L, et al. Increased incidence of neonatal vitamin K deficiency resulting from maternal anticonvulsant therapy. *Am J Obstet Gynecol* 1993;168:923–928.

88. Thorp JA, Gaston L, Caspers DR, Pal ML. Current concepts and controversies in the use of vitamin K. *Drugs* 1995;49:376–387.

89. American Academy of Pediatrics. The transfer of drugs and other chemicals into human milk. *Pediatrics* 1994;93:137–150.

90. Hagg S, Spigset O. Anticonvulsant use during lactation. *Drug Saf* 2000;22:425–440.

91. Bar-Oz B, Nulman I, Koren G, et al. Anticonvulsants and breast-feeding: a critical review. *Pediatr Drugs* 2000;2:113–126.

92. Ohman I, Vitols S, Tomson T. Lamotrigine in pregnancy: pharmacokinetics during delivery, in the neonate and during lactation. *Epilepsia* 2000;41:709–713.

93. Ohman I, Viols S, Luef G, Soderfeldt B, Tomson T. Topiramate pharmacokinetics during delivery, lactation, and in the neonate: preliminary observations. *Epilepsia* 2002;43:1157–1160.

94. Myllynen P, Pienimaki P, Jouppila P, Vahakangas K. Transplacental passage of oxcarbazepine and its metabolites in vivo. *Epilepsia* 2001;42:1482–1485.

6 Effect of Ovarian Hormones on the Nervous System

Pavel Klein, MB, BChir and Donald L. Schomer, MD

Hormones play an important role in the expression of many neurologic conditions. In some of these disorders, endocrine abnormalities are an integral part of the disease process, for example, the abnormal insulin response to a glucose load seen in myotonic dystrophy. In other disorders, the endocrinologic abnormality produces the neurologic disorder, such as the peripheral neuropathy of chronic diabetes mellitus. In other endocrinologic disorders such as primary hypothyroidism, Cushing, or Addison disease, neurologic dysfunction can be more subtle and manifest itself as an alteration in cognition or a change in personality. In all these conditions, men and women can be similarly affected. In women, the cyclical alterations of the ovarian hormones and related endocrine factors can have very particular effects. These effects are the subjects of this chapter.

To best approach this subject, the development, anatomic substrates, and physiologic function of the female endocrine reproductive axis are reviewed. We outline how steroid hormones affect nervous system function, with brief examples of how ovarian and other steroid hormones affect neurologic diseases. In the last section, we illustrate how ovarian and other steroid hormones affect neurologic functioning and diseases. Many of the neurologic disorders are dealt with in far greater detail in other chapters in this book; here we discuss a couple of well-known genetically based diseases. We also discuss in detail how partial epilepsy, an intermittent physiologically based disorder, may be influenced by and, in turn, influence normal cycling behavior. This will serve as a model for how a disease process can interact in a complex way with neuroendocrinologic control mechanisms.

ANATOMICAL, DEVELOPMENTAL, AND PHYSIOLOGICAL CONSIDERATIONS

The cells of the ventromedial and arcuate nuclei and of the preoptic area of the hypothalamus are responsible for the production of the decapeptide hormone gonadotrophin releasing hormone (GnRH), also known as luteinizing hormone releasing hormone (LHRH) (1,2). This hormone controls the release of the anterior pituitary–derived hormones follicle stimulating hormone (FSH) and luteinizing hormone (LH), collectively referred to as gonadotrophins. The cyclical changes in FSH and LH regulate the ovarian cycle, which includes follicular development, ovulation, and corpus luteum maturation. These stages are associated with the variable production of estrogen, progesterone, and testosterone which, in turn, have pleuripotent effects on numerous organs and feedback to hypothalamic and cortical areas related to their own regulation.

The GnRH-containing neurons, estimated at 1,000 to 3,000 total, project their axons to the median eminence at the base of the hypothalamus (2). They release GnRH into the hypothalamic-portal circulation, which delivers it to the LH- and FSH-containing cells (gonadotrophs) in the anterior pituitary. There, GnRH induces the secretion and release of LH and FSH. The GnRH neurons release GnRH in rhythmic synchronized bursts, or pulses, which, in turn, cause pulsatile secretion of LH and FSH. The pulsatile nature of LH and FSH release by the pituitary gland is an essential feature of the gonadotropic control of ovarian function.

LH and FSH are glycoproteins composed of two different carbohydrate-containing protein subunits called *a* and *b*. The *a* subunit is identical in LH and FSH. The *b* subunit differs in its protein sequence in the two hormones and confers specific activity on each hormone. A higher frequency of GnRH pulses induces the preferential formation of LH and high LH pulse frequency, which leads to ovarian hypersecretion of androgens and polycystic ovarian syndrome. Slower frequency (e.g., every 2 to 3 hours) increases FSH production, lowers LH/FSH pulse frequency, and causes anovulation or amenorrhea.

GnRH secretion begins at 20 to 30 weeks of gestation, following the migration of GnRH neurons from the olfactory placode to the hypothalamus. Fetal FSH and LH secretion is high: Fetal FSH and LH levels reach menopausal concentrations. Their secretion subsides after the first postnatal year and stays low until puberty. The reason for this is not well understood, but is likely due to the active suppression of GnRH neurons by the central nervous system (CNS). Puberty is initiated by a resumption of the pulsatile release of GnRH (Figure 6.1). At first, this occurs only at night and causes predominantly FSH secretion. Later, daytime GnRH secretion and LH responsiveness occur coincident with the onset of menarche.

During the menstrual cycle, the pulsatile secretion of LH and FSH changes through the cycle (2). During the first (follicular) half of the menstrual cycle, FSH and LH pulses occur every 1 to 1.5 hours. During the second (luteal) half of the cycle, LH/FSH pulses occur every 3 to 6 hours, as a result of the inhibitory effect of progesterone and inhibin A. During perimenopause and menopause, a decline in the ovarian secretion of inhibin, progesterone, and, eventually, estrogen leads to the disinhibition of pituitary production of FSH and LH, resulting in an elevation of the gonadotropins.

The intrinsic rhythmicity of the GnRH neurons is modulated by gonadal steroids and by the hypothalamic and extrahypothalamic nervous system, including the limbic system (2,3). GnRH neurons receive inhibitory GABA-ergic input from the estrogen and progesterone receptor–containing neurons in the preoptic area and the ventromedial nucleus of the hypothalamus. The steroids thus exert a negative feedback

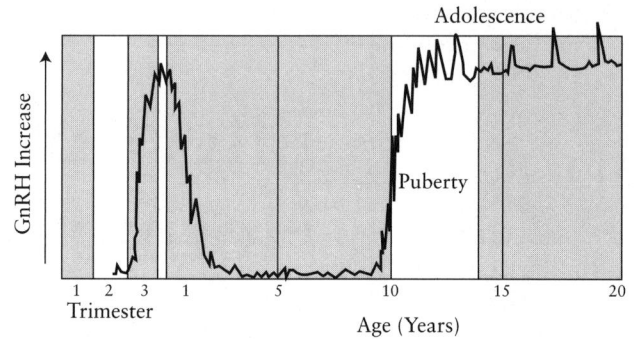

FIGURE 6.1

Ontogeny of GnRH secretion from fetal life to adolescence.

onto the GnRH neurons as well as, more potently, on the gonadotrophs. GnRH neurons are also inhibited by opioidergic neurons from the central gray matter of the pons and by the corticotrophin releasing hormone (CRH)–containing neurons in the paraventricular hypothalamic nucleus. Glutamate stimulates GnRH neurons. The onset of this stimulation occurs at the beginning of puberty, for which it is critical. GnRH release is further stimulated by input from noradrenergic (b1-receptor mediated) and dopaminergic (DA 1-receptor mediated) brain stem nuclei and from the NPY-containing neurons in the arcuate nucleus. Through these inputs, neural factors mediating stress, pain, energy balance, reward, and other functions modulate reproductive endocrine function.

The GnRH neurons receive both direct and multisynaptic modulatory input from limbic structures, most notably from the corticomedial amygdaloid nuclei, from the bed nucleus of the stria terminalis, and from the hippocampus (4,5). The input from the amygdala is particularly important for reproductive endocrine function. The amygdala has reciprocal relationships with the hypothalamus. The amygdala has two distinctive subnuclear regions that are, at least partially, distinguished by their outflow pathway (4). The corticomedial region has as its output—the stria terminalis—and the basolateral region has output through the ventral amygdalofugal pathway. Both of these projections are reciprocal to and from the hypothalamus, particularly to those regions high in GnRH-containing cells. Stimulation and ablation studies in the amygdala and in the output pathways have produced consistent but often species-specific changes in the output of LH and FSH. The effects produced have included the following observations:

- Simulation of the corticomedial nuclei induces ovulation and uterine contractions.
- Stimulation of the basolateral nuclei inhibits sexually orienting behavior in an ovulating female.

- Sectioning of the stria terminalis (cortico-medial outflow tract) blocks ovulation.
- Sectioning of the ventral amygdalofugal pathway (basolateral nuclei outflow tract) has no effect, but lesions bilaterally in the basolateral nuclei blocks ovulation (4,6).

The pulsatile secretion of LH and FSH from pituicytes controls follicular development, ovulation, luteal development, and the associated hormonal production. The menstrual cycle can be divided into four phases: follicular (early, mid-, and late), ovulatory, luteal (early, mid-, and late), and menstrual (2). The ovarian life cycle is schematically illustrated in Figure 6.2. The associated pattern of hormonal changes is shown in Figure 6.3.

About 2 days before menstruation, the falling ovarian production of progesterone, estradiol, and a glycoprotein secreted by the corpus luteum, inhibin A, disinhibit FSH secretion and FSH levels rise. This leads to follicular recruitment for the next cycle, which continues during the first 4 to 5 days of the follicular phase. It is followed by the selection of a single dominant follicle from a cohort of follicles (menstrual cycle days 5 to 7), maturation of the follicle (days 8 to 12), ovulation (days 13 to 15), and formation of the corpus luteum. FSH secretion is suppressed during the luteal phase by progesterone, estradiol, and inhibin A. The demise of corpus luteum at the end of the cycle (days 26–30) results in a decline in levels of progesterone, estradiol, and inhibin A, and in initiation of a new cycle.

All ovarian steroids are synthesized from serum-derived cholesterol. Cholesterol is converted to pregnenolone, then to progesterone or dehydroepiandrosterone (DHEA). These are made into the respective androgens—testosterone or androstenedione—which are aromatized to the estrogens, estradiol, and estrone (Figure 6.4).

The steroidogenic enzymes are regulated by LH and FSH. The two rate-limiting enzymes are cholesterol side chain cleavage enzyme, or CYP450-scc, which catalyzes the conversion of cholesterol to pregnenolone, and the other, aromatase, which catalyzes the conversion (aromatization) of androgens to estrogens.

The follicle is composed of three parts: The oocyte in the center is surrounded by granulosa cells which, in turn, are separated by a basement membrane from the interstitial or thecal cells. The theca cells have LH receptors that, when activated by LH, induce the synthesis and release of androgens. Androgens diffuse into the neighboring granulosa cells. Granulosa cells have FSH (as well as LH) receptors. The activation of FSH receptors by FSH induces aromatase, the enzyme that converts androgens

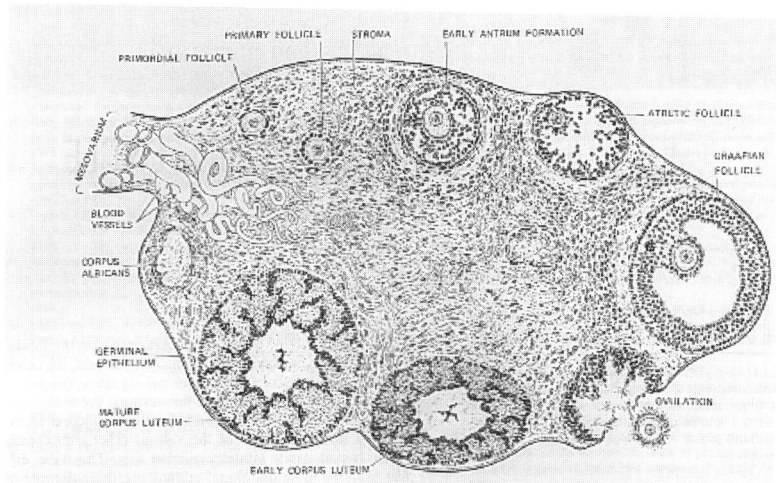

FIGURE 6.2

The life cycle of the human ovary.

Reproduced with permission from Yen SC, Jaffe RB, Barbieri RL (eds.) *Reproductive Endocrinology*, 4th ed. Philadelphia, Pa: WB Saunders, 1999.

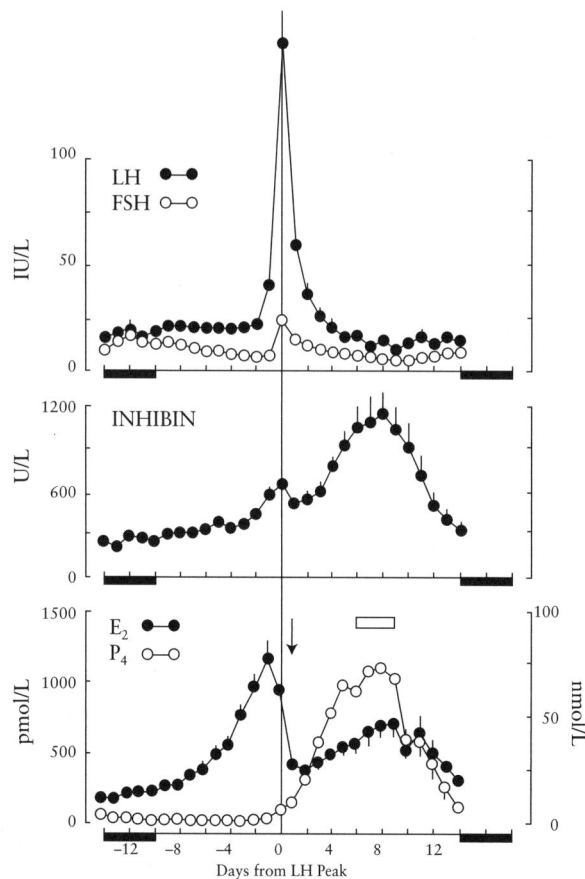

FIGURE 6.3

The hormonal pattern in the human menstrual cycle.

E_2 = estradiol, P_4 = progesterone

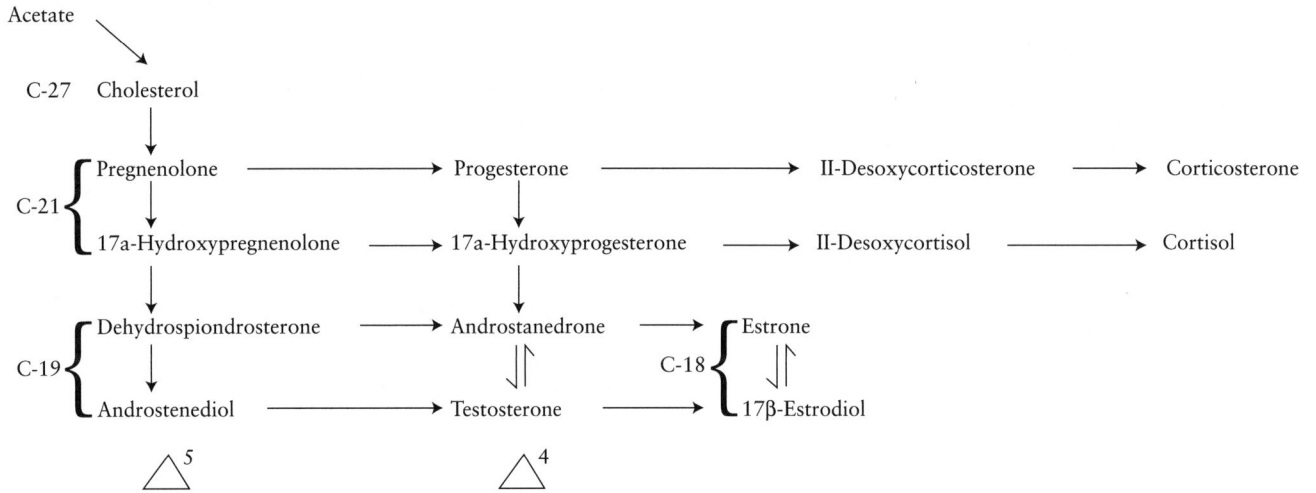

Acetate

C-27 Cholesterol

C-21 { Pregnenolone ⟶ Progesterone ⟶ II-Desoxycorticosterone ⟶ Corticosterone

17a-Hydroxypregnenolone ⟶ 17a-Hydroxyprogesterone ⟶ II-Desoxycortisol ⟶ Cortisol

C-19 { Dehydrospiondrosterone ⟶ Androstanedrone ⟶ { Estrone

Androstenediol ⟶ Testosterone ⟶ 17β-Estrodiol   C-18

△⁵   △⁴

FIGURE 6.4

Biosynthetic pathways of steroid hormone production. Steroids with a double bond between the carbon 5 and 6 positions are shown on the left; those with a double bond between the 4 and 5 positions are shown on the right.

to estrogens. Thus, activation of the granulosa cells in response to FSH results in estrogen secretion. The follicle thus consists of two functionally distinct compartments, the theca cells, which secrete androgens in response to LH, and the granulosa cells, which secrete estrogens in response to FSH (the two compartment hypothesis, Figure 6.5).

Steroid synthesis differs during different cycle phases. During the early follicular phase, pituitary FSH secretion drives the production of estrogen, which grad-

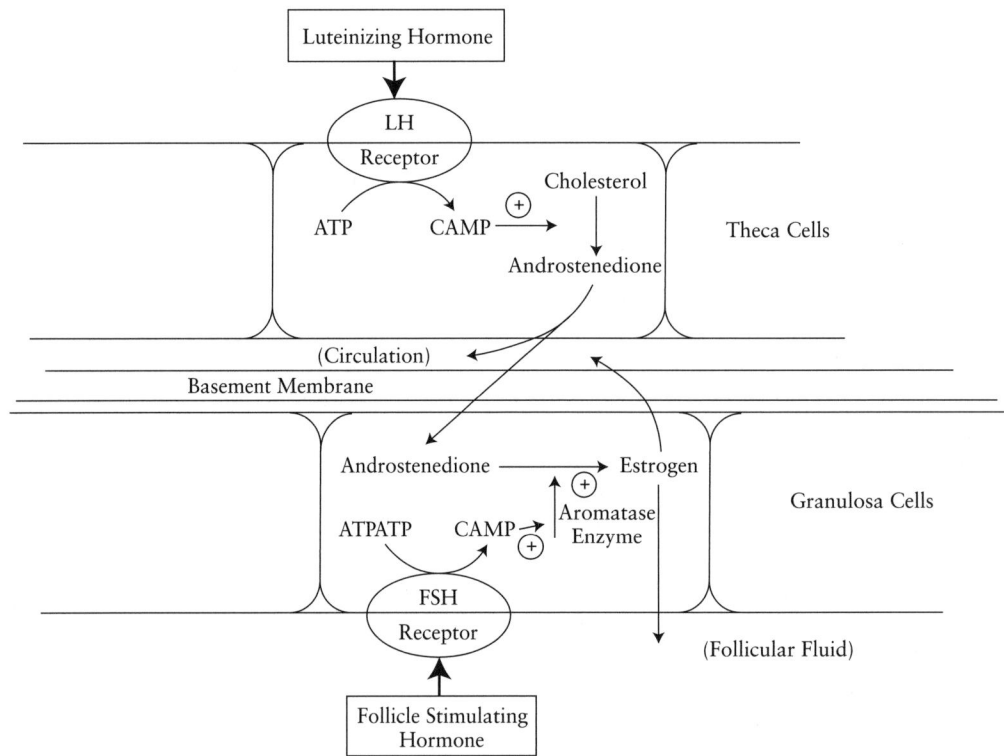

Luteinizing Hormone

LH Receptor

ATP   CAMP ⟶ ⊕   Cholesterol   Theca Cells

Androstenedione

(Circulation)

Basement Membrane

Androstenedione ⟶ ⊕ Estrogen   Granulosa Cells

ATPATP   CAMP ⟶ ⊕   Aromatase Enzyme

FSH Receptor

(Follicular Fluid)

Follicle Stimulating Hormone

FIGURE 6.5

The two cell-two gonadotropin hypothesis of follicular androgen and estrogen production.

ually increases throughout the follicular phase. Just before ovulation, a negative feedback of estrogen on pituitary LH/FSH changes to a positive feedback, with a resulting LH surge, a surge of estradiol secretion, and a release of the oocyte from the follicle in the ovary into the fallopian tubes (ovulation). The granulosa cell remnants of the follicle form the corpus luteum, which secretes progesterone in large quantities in response to LH stimulation (Figure 6.3). Estrogen secretion initially falls after ovulation, but then rises again. The high mid-luteal concentrations of progesterone and estradiol prepare the endometrium for the implantation of the fertilized egg. The secretion of progesterone, estradiol, and inhibin A inhibits pituitary FSH and LH production during the luteal phase of the menstrual cycle. Towards the end of the luteal phase, luteolysis occurs and ovarian secretion of progesterone fails, followed shortly by failure of estrogen secretion. Pituitary FSH production is disinhibited, new follicles begin to grow again, and the cycle repeats itself.

During an anovulatory cycle, the periovulatory estradiol surge does not occur. Otherwise, estrogen secretion occurs the same as during an ovulatory cycle. Because no follicle is released and corpus luteum is not formed, there is little production of progesterone. The absence of progesterone secretion is the endocrine difference between ovulatory and anovulatory cycles. It may contribute to differences in neurologic symptoms in ovulating versus nonovulating women in diseases such as epilepsy or affective disorders.

EFFECTS OF OVARIAN STEROIDS ON THE NERVOUS SYSTEM

Ovarian steroids have a wide-ranging influence upon neuronal activity, neuronal survival, and neuronal differentiation and growth. During embryogenesis, they regulate the formation of parts of the nervous system. Later during life, they alter neuronal response to injury, including trauma and stroke. They affect neuronal excitability by modulating the synthesis, release, and catabolism of neurotransmitters and the sensitivity of neurotransmitter receptors. They affect neuronal plasticity throughout life by affecting synaptogenesis and neurite growth. These actions affect reproductive endocrine function, but also behavior, mood, memory and cognition, and a number of major neurologic and psychiatric diseases.

Ovarian steroid effects on the CNS occur by both receptor-mediated (genomic) and membrane-related (nongenomic) mechanisms (7). In the classic steroid hormone action, the hormone diffuses into the cell, binds to an intracellular receptor, travels in the receptor-bound complex to the nucleus, binds to a specific DNA recognition sequence (the hormone-response element), and initiates a particular mRNA transcription and protein synthesis. The latency of this action is in hours to days. It affects processes related to neuronal survival and growth, and to neurotransmitter synthesis and receptor function.

In addition, certain steroids, including progesterone and estrogen, have a direct, nongenomic effect on neuronal membrane (7). Latency of this action is within seconds to minutes. The main effects are the modulation of transmission of the two main CNS neurotransmitters, glutamate and γ-aminobutyric acid (GABA), and of neuronal membrane excitability.

The effects of the ovarian hormones on the structure of the CNS are sometimes thought of as "organizational"; that is, affecting the hard wiring of the CNS during its formation. The effects on the CNS that occur after completion of the network hard wiring are thought of as "activational."

Organizational and Structural Effects

In most vertebrate species, structural differences are present in certain parts of the brains of males and females. Structures that show such differences are termed *sexually dimorphic* (8,9). In rodents, parts of the hypothalamus and the limbic system are sexually dimorphic. For instance, the medial preoptic nucleus of the hypothalamus has a sexually dimorphic part (SD-MPN) that is four times larger in males than in females. SD-MPN mediates sexual behavior, including mounting and intromission, a male reproductive behavior. Conversely, another hypothalamic area, the anteroventral preoptic nucleus (AVPNv), is several times larger in the female compared to the male. The AVPNv regulates the reproductive endocrine events related to ovulation, a female-specific activity. Examples of other sexually dimorphic areas include the corticomedial amygdala and the bed nucleus of the stria terminalis in the limbic system, structures that modulate reproductive and aggressive behaviors, among others (8,9). (See also Chapter 2 for further information on gender-based brain anatomic differences.)

This difference is determined by pre- and perinatal exposure to sex steroids. Nature's default blueprint for the development of both genitalia and the brain appears to be female. In the absence of perinatal androgens, a female pattern of sexually dimorphic brain structures and a female pattern of GnRH secretion and sexual behavior occur. Pre- and perinatal exposure of the brain to androgens induces the development of a male pattern of CNS structure and function. For instance, even a single androgen injection to a genetic female rat during the first week after birth inhibits the development of the ovulatory trigger mechanism in the preoptic area of the hypothalamus (POA) and the loss of female reproductive behavior, lordosis. This is due to the perinatal induction by androgens of an inhibitory neural circuit between the POA and the septum. If this connection is severed in an adult genetic *male*, female sexual behavior, lordosis, occurs (8,9).

The size differences of the sexually dimorphic structures are due to differences in the number of neurons and of dendritic branches. During the second half of gestation, the testis secrete large amounts of androgens (while the ovary is inactive). Androgens are taken up by the developing neurons and the supporting glia. Paradoxically, the masculinizing effects of pre- and perinatal androgens are in many instances due to their conversion to estrogens in the CNS. Androgen and estrogen receptors are expressed in neurons, astrocytes, and oligodendrocytes in different regions of both the developing and adult CNS (Figure 6.6) (10). Aromatase is present in neurons in some areas such as the preoptic-hypothalamic and the limbic areas, particularly in the developing brain, and particularly in the male (11). Those neurons convert androgens to estrogens, such as testosterone to estradiol.

Estrogens inhibit apoptosis perinatally in the SD-MPN via estrogen receptor–mediated mechanisms (8,9). Estradiol also causes neuronal differentiation and neurite growth. Perinatal exposure to androgens or estradiol therefore increases the number of neurons and the density of dendritic branching in the SD-MPN, thus accounting for the greater size of this nucleus in the males compared to the females. The apoptotic effect is region-specific. In the AVPN, by contrast, estradiol (or testosterone) promotes apoptosis.

In humans, the homologous structure of SD-MPN is the interstitial nucleus of the anterior hypothalamus (INAH). Two subdivisions of this nucleus, INAH-2 and INAH-3, are two to three times larger in men than in women. Furthermore, INAH-3 is larger in heterosexual men than in homosexual men (8,9,12,13). Similarly, in the limbic structure, bed nucleus of the stria terminalis (BNST), which is an outflow relay station from the amygdala and regulates both sexual and aggressive behavior, is also bigger in men than in women, and in heterosexual than in homosexual men. Thus, it is possible that pre- or perinatal sex steroid–induced changes in CNS structures underlie gender-specific differences in reproductive behavior and aggression in humans as well as in nonhuman mammals (8).

Sexual dimorphism of brain structures may also underlie gender differences in nonreproductive behavior. For instance, women are better than men in verbal fluency and other language-related tasks (Chapter X). The language areas, Broca's and Wernicke's areas and the planum temporale, are 20% to 30% larger in women than in men (14), and neuronal and dendritic density in Wernicke's area is greater in women than in men (14,15). It is not known, however, at what time of development the morphologic differences in the language areas become established.

These effects on the CNS are referred to as *organizational* because they determine the organization or the hard wiring of the CNS. Steroids also have an *activational* effect—they modulate which parts of the formed CNS structure will be used, or activated, and how. The administration of testosterone to adult women, for instance, can induce aggression. More subtly, male- and female-specific cognitive patterns can be induced in adults by the administration of androgens and estrogens, respectively. In transsexual men receiving estrogens prior to sex-change surgery, estrogens enhance verbal skills. In transsexual women, treatment with testosterone before sex change surgery enhances visuospatial ability.

It is well known that certain psychiatric and neurologic diseases have different prevalence in men and women. Depression, for instance, is two times more common in women than in men, anxiety four times, anorexia nervosa nine times, migraine four times, and benign intracranial hypertension between four and eight times more common. Aggression and Tourette disease, by contrast, are eight to ten times more common in males (16). What is striking is that the incidence and prevalence of many of these diseases is the same in men and women until puberty, when the difference emerges. The possible activational effects of gonadal steroids on the CNS at the time of puberty that might underlie these clinical phenomena are unknown.

Effects on Neurotransmitter Systems: Genomic Effects

The genomic mechanisms of ovarian steroids are mediated by cytosolic neuronal estrogen, progesterone, and androgen receptors (ER, PR, AR). Estrogen receptors (α,β) and progesterone receptors are distributed in different parts of the brain, including outside of the hypothalamic areas involved in the regulation of endocrine and behavioral aspects of reproduction (10,17).

These receptors are found in great density in the cortical and medial amygdaloid nuclei, and in lesser numbers in the hippocampus and neocortex (10,17). Estrogen and progesterone receptors are present in similar areas. ER-containing neurons colocalize with other neurotransmitters, including GABA, acetylcholine (Ach), 5-hydroxytryptamine (5HT), and dopamine (DA) (1,7,18,19). By regulating the expression of genes affecting the activity, release, and postsynaptic action of different neurotransmitters and neuromodulators, estrogens and progesterone may affect the function of the neurons that take them up. For instance, E2 reduces GABA synthesis in the corticomedial amygdala and in the hippocampus by decreasing the activity of glutamic acid decarboxylase (19). This affects the excitability of hippocampal and amygdaloid neurons.

As another instance, ER and PR colocalize with tryptophan hydroxylase (TH) in the dorsal raphe nucleus, the source of the ascending serotonergic innervation of the limbic and neocortical structures (20). TH is the rate-limiting enzyme in the synthesis of 5-hydroxytryptamine. Estrogen induces tryptophan hydroxylase activity and 5HT synthesis, whereas progesterone counters that effect. In this way, estrogen contributes to upregulation of mood, while progesterone mitigates that effect. This may relate to mood changes during the menstrual cycle, such as late luteal dysphoria (premenstrual syndrome), or to depression during the menopause. Estrogen also inhibits noradrenaline catabolism by inhibiting monoamine oxidase, which catabolizes noradrenaline, and by initiating the competition of estrogen metabolites (catecholestrogens) for the other noradrenergic catabolic enzyme, catechol-O-methyltransferase. These actions result in fluctuations of noradrenaline levels through the menstrual cycle that occur inversely with estrogen levels (21,22) and may similarly contribute to a fluctuation in the levels of arousal and mood during the menstrual cycle and during menopause.

Estradiol also promotes the synthesis of cholineacetyl transferase (ChAT), the rate limiting enzyme of acetylcholine synthesis (23). Levels of ChAT and acetylcholine synthesis and release from cholinergic nerve terminals in the forebrain and in the hippocampus fluctuate across the estrous cycle in rats, being highest during proestrus when estrogen secretion is high (24). Ovariectomy decreases and estrogen replacement increases by 20% to 80% ChAT activity in the basal forebrain neurons and acetylcholine release in target areas of the basal forebrain's cholinergic projections, such as the hippocampus and the frontal cortex (23,25). This effect is magnified when estradiol administration is followed by progesterone. This may explain the clinical findings of cognitive fluctuation during the menstrual cycle, when verbal memory and creativity are highest during the ovulatory and midluteal menstrual cycle phases, when estradiol levels are correspondingly highest. It may also explain the decline in verbal memory seen in postmenopausal women and the observation that in surgical menopause, such decline is seen in untreated but not in estrogen-treated women (26).

Effect of Ovarian Steroids on Neuronal Excitability

Gonadal steroid hormones have a profound influence upon neuronal excitability. Generally, estrogens increase neuronal excitability and facilitate seizure occurrence and epileptogenesis. Progesterone has the opposite effect: It inhibits neuronal excitability, seizures, and epileptogenesis.

Estrogens

In adult female rats, the seizure threshold fluctuates during the estrous cycle. Susceptibility to seizures is highest during proestrus, when serum estrogen levels are highest (27). Estrogens activate spike discharges, lower seizure threshold, and promote epileptogenesis in different animal models (28,29). Ovariectomy in adult rats, however, does not alter the seizure threshold (30). Thus, a lack of estrogen may not protect against seizures, whereas an excess of estrogen promotes them.

Estrogens affect neuronal excitability by genomically dependent mechanisms, by nongenomic, direct effect on neuronal membrane, and by affecting neuronal plasticity and the number of excitatory synapses. As noted earlier, the genomic mechanisms include a reduction of GABA synthesis through the inhibition of the GABA-synthesizing enzyme glutamic acid decarboxylase in the estrogen-containing inhibitory interneurons of the hippocampus and in the amygdala, structures critical in the generation and propagation of temporolimbic seizures (7,18,19,28).

Estrogens also exert a direct excitatory effect at the neuronal membrane, where estradiol (E2) augments both the n-methyl-d-aspartate (NMDA) and non-NMDA glutamate receptor activity (31,32). This increases neuronal excitability, for example of the hippocampal CA1 pyramidal neurons, thus facilitating seizure generation and spread.

Finally, estrogens potentiate neuronal excitability by regulating neuronal plasticity and synaptogenesis. E2 increases the density of the dendritic spines carrying excitatory, NMDA-receptor–containing synapses on hippocampal CA1 pyramidal neurons (33,34). In rats, the density of the excitatory synapses fluctuates during the estrous cycle. It is highest by about one-third during the proestrus—the equivalent to human ovulatory phase—when estrogen levels are highest, compared to diestrus, when they are low. It decreases markedly following oophorectomy (33). This estrogen-driven increase in excitatory synapses results in an enhanced excitatory input to the CA1 neurons and in the synchronization of neuronal outflow that promotes seizure genesis and propagation (34). The increase in excitatory synapses may also enhance memory and learning.

Progestins

Progesterone depresses neuronal firing, lessens epileptiform discharges, and inhibits seizures and epileptogenesis in animal models of epilepsy (28–30,35). The seizure threshold during the rat estrous cycle is high during diestrus, when the serum progesterone level is high. The same occurs in women with epilepsy, in whom seizures are least likely to occur during the lutal phase, when serum progesterone levels are high (36), thus suggesting a protective effect of progesterone against seizures.

Like estrogens, progesterone affects neuronal excitability by genomic and nongenomic mechanisms.

Progesterone genomically influences the enzymatic activity controlling the synthesis and release of various neurotransmitters and neuromodulators (7). Progesterone decreases the number of dendritic spines and synapses on hippocampal CA1 pyramidal neurons, thus counteracting the stimulatory effects of E2 (33). It has inhibitory direct membrane effects, described in the next section.

Neuroactive Steroids

The anticonvulsant effect of progesterone is largely mediated by its 3α-hydroxylated metabolite, 3-α-hydroxy-5-α-pregnan-20-one or allopregnanolone (AP) (37,38). Allopregnanolone and the 3α,5α-hydroxylated natural metabolite of the mineralocorticoid deoxycorticosterone, allotetrahydro-deoxycorticosterone (allo-THDOC), are the two most potent of a number of endogenous neuroactive steroids with a direct membrane effect on neuronal excitability (37,39). Allopregnanolone is devoid of hormonal effects. It may be thought of as an endogenous regulator of brain excitability with anxiolytic, anticonvulsant, and sedative-hypnotic properties (37). Allopregnanolone and allo-THDOC hyperpolarize hippocampal and other neurons by potentiating GABA-mediated synaptic inhibition. They act as positive allosteric modulators of the GABA-A receptor, interacting with a steroid-specific site near the receptor to facilitate chloride (Cl) channel opening and prolong the inhibitory action of GABA on neurons (7,37,39). Allopregnanolone is one of the most potent ligands of GABA-A receptors in the CNS, with affinities similar to the potent benzodiazepines and approximately a thousand times higher than pentobarbital (37,39). Progesterone by itself enhances GABA-induced Cl- currents only weakly and only in high concentrations (37). Plasma and brain levels of allopregnanolone parallel those of progesterone, and plasma levels of AP correlate with progesterone levels during the menstrual cycle and pregnancy (37). Brain activity of progesterone and AP, however, is not dependent solely on ovarian and adrenal production, because they are both synthesized de novo in the brain (40). Their synthesis is region-specific and includes the cortex and the hippocampus.

Allopregnanolone and allo-THDOC have potent anticonvulsant effects in animal seizure models and in status epilepticus (37,38,41). Allopregnanolone's anticonvulsant properties resemble those of clonazepam, but with lower relative toxicity and with little habituation to its anticonvulsant effect (42). The abrupt withdrawal of allopregnanolone induces seizures, possibly by a modulation of the α-4 GABA-A receptor subunit that confers GABA-insensitivity on the GABA-A receptor. This may be a mechanism of the perimenstrual seizure exacerbation seen in some women with epilepsy (43).

Although the 3- and 5-α-reduced steroids potentiate GABA-A receptor activity and enhance neuronal inhibition, some of the sulfated neuroactive steroids have neuroexcitatory effects. These include pregnenolone sulfate and DHEAS, the naturally occurring sulfated esters of the progesterone precursor pregnenolone and of the progesterone metabolite DHEA (Figure 6.4; 37,44). These steroids increase neuronal firing when directly applied to neurons by antagonizing GABA action at the GABA-A receptor and by facilitating glutamate-induced excitation at the NMDA receptor (45). In animals, pregnenolone sulfate and DHEAS have a proconvulsant effect that is prevented by chronic pretreatment with progesterone (37,45).

These neurosteroids may also affect cognition and memory (46). Pregnenolone sulfate stimulates ACh release as well as glutamatergic activity in adult rat hippocampus. DHEAS and PS improve memory and learning in aging mice. In humans, DHEA has been reported to have mood elevating and memory-enhancing effects in middle-aged healthy men and women and in patients with depression (47,48).

Trophic Effects

In addition to their neuromodulatory effect on neuronal excitability, gonadal steroids also exert a trophic effect on neurons and glial cells. Estrogen is an important neural trophic factor throughout life, with influences on neuronal differentiation, survival, and plasticity (49–51). The trophic effects of estrogen may ameliorate the degeneration of neurons in diseases such as Alzheimer disease (see also Chapter 30), reduce apoptotic neuronal death in ischemic and traumatic brain injury, and promote neuronal regeneration and growth following such injuries.

Trophic Effects and Cholinergic Function in Basal Forebrain and Cortex

Estrogen plays an important role in the function of the basal forebrain cholinergic system involved in memory and cognition. In ovariectomized rats, estradiol replacement improves spatial memory and maze learning (52). The basal forebrain cholinergic neurons of the nucleus basalis myenert (NBM) and of the diagonal band of Broca (DBB) innervate the forebrain and the hippocampus, areas important in cognition, learning, and memory. Their degeneration is a key feature of Alzheimer disease.

Estradiol protects cholinergic neurons against excitotoxic neuronal damage (53). It does so by potentiating the endogenous trophic effects of the neurotrophins, nerve growth factor (NGF), and brain-derived neurotrophic factor (BDNF). These trophins are produced in the target areas of basal forebrain cholinergic projections and exert a trophic effect on cholinergic neurons by binding with specific tyrosine kinase receptors, tyrosine kinases A and B (trkA and trkB). TrkA and BDNF mRNA levels in the cholinergic neurons fluctuate across the estrous cycle in parallel with estrogen levels (54). Estradiol and estradiol with progesterone increase trkA and trkB levels in the basal forebrain cholinergic neurons and BDNF in the hippocampus (55). The protective effects of estrogen on cholinergic neurons may underlie the observed protective effect of postmenopausal estrogen replacement therapy against the development of Alzheimer disease (26,56,57).

Role in Neuronal Injury and Neuroprotection

Estradiol protects neurons against a wide variety of neurotoxic stimuli, including ischemic CNS injury, oxidative stress, excitotoxic insults, and b-amyloid-induced toxicity (49,50,58).

In the middle cerebral artery (MCA) occlusion animal model of cerebrovascular accident (CVA), low levels of estradiol replacement reduce infarct size by 50%. The treatment must precede ischemia by several days (59). Low-dose estradiol pretreatment has a similar neuroprotective effect on the pyramidal CA1 neurons of the hippocampus in status epilepticus in rats (60) and protects explant cultures of both neurons and astrocytes against cell death.

The mechanism of this neuroprotection may include the estrogen receptor–mediated inhibition of the apoptotic signaling pathways (58), regulation of growth factor genes and their receptors, and modulation of neurite outgrowth and plasticity (51). In the neocortex, estrogen α receptor (ER-α) is expressed at high levels only during development, when neocortical differentiation occurs, thus suggesting a developmental role (10). Neocortical estrogen β receptor (ER-β), by contrast, is expressed throughout life. In adulthood, ER-α is expressed in the cortex only after neuronal injury such as CVA. In ER-α knockout rats, estradiol has no protective effect against CVA (58). Thus, ischemia or injury induces the expression of ER-α, the activation of which by estradiol protects against ensuing neuronal injury. Recently, another membrane-associated estrogen receptor (ER-X) has been identified; ER-X is also expressed perinatally and is only expressed in adulthood following neuronal injury such as stroke. Its activation may also be involved in injury-related neuroprotection (49–51).

Pregnenolone also may be important in neuroprotection. It reduces the degree of the histopathological injury and increases the recovery of motor function in rats after traumatic spinal cord injury (61). The mechanism is unclear.

Other poorly understood, potentially neuroprotective effects include a reduction of cerebral edema by progesterone following cortical contusion, first suggested by the observations that males have more edema after similar degrees of cortical contusion than females (61).

Myelination

Finally, gonadal steroids may play a hitherto little appreciated role in myelination.

Oligodendrocytes and Schwann cells express estrogen and progesterone receptors. Estradiol increases the proliferation of Schwann cells. This finding may relate to the exacerbation of neurofibromatosis during perimenarche (62).

Schwann cell synthesize progesterone from pregnenolone. Progesterone synthesis may be important in myelin formation. Expression of the synthesizing enzyme, 3-β-hydroxysteroid dehydrogenase (3βHSD) and progesterone synthesis increase in Schwann cells during myelin formation. Progesterone, in turn, promotes myelin formation by Schwann cells. Following cryolesion of the sciatic nerve, progesterone concentrations in the regenerating nerve are about sixfold higher than in plasma. Blocking progesterone synthesis or receptor inhibits the formation of new myelin. Conversely, local application of progesterone or pregnenolone accelerates remyelination (61,63).

Oligodendrocytes also express progesterone receptors and 3βHSD, and progesterone may also promote myelination in the CNS.

CLINICAL IMPLICATIONS

Genetically Based Disorders

Disorders that have a genetic basis may encompass an altered ovarian hormonal production, which may affect neurologic function and may affect those neurologic disorders that have a recognized relationship to fluctuations in cyclical hormones. Most of these disorders are dealt with in a more detailed fashion in other chapters of this book, but a few of these conditions deserve additional comments here.

Turner syndrome is an example of a chromosomal deletion. About 1 in every 5,000 live-born females has 45 chromosomes plus a single X chromosome; that is, there is a deletion of one X chromosome. Girls have ovarian dysgenesis, absence of ovarian hormonal secretion, high FSH levels, and delayed adolescence as well as a number of associated somatic developmental anomalies. When sexual maturation is desired, patients must be treated with exogenous hormone replacement. Women with Turner syndrome exhibit male cognitive patterns—they perform better on visuospatial tasks than on verbal tasks. When untreated with estrogen, patients with Turner syndrome have memory, attention, and spatial performance impairment and hippocampal volume loss on magnetic resonance imaging (MRI) (64).

Another genetically based disorder is *congenital adrenal hyperplasia* (CAH). This autosomal recessive disorder can be caused by a defect in one of six recognized steroid synthesizing enzymes. It affects both men and women. In three forms, only the adrenal gland is affected. In the other three, both the adrenal gland and the ovary are affected. The enzymatic deficiency (e.g., of the CYP450-c21 hydroxylase) results in impaired adrenal synthesis of cortisol, reduced inhibitory feedback of ACTH, and increased adrenal synthesis of the cortisol precursors that can be converted to androgens. Clinically, women with this condition have mild to moderate virilization that manifests itself early in life, and that is occasionally associated with a delay in the onset of sexual development. Two clinical forms of the disease present neonatally, one in late childhood, adolescence, or adulthood. In the neonatal forms, there is an increased prenatal production of androgens. The classic form of CAH due to 21-hydroxylase deficiency is a rare disorder of adrenal steroid synthesis that affects approximately 1 in 15,000 live births as a result of a gene mutation on the short arm of chromosome 6. Males or females with CAH are exposed to high levels of androgens during gestation, beginning in the third month of fetal life. As the disease is now readily diagnosable and treatable at birth, the hormonal abnormalities are confined to prenatal and early neonatal exposure. CAH has been associated with some behavioral changes that have been attributed to intrauterine exposure to increased androgen levels. Women with CAH have an increased risk of gender identity disorder (e.g., of adopting male sexual identity), increased incidence (33%–45%) of homosexual tendencies, and show masculine play behavior in childhood and male-typical cognitive performance in adulthood (65). In addition, women with CAH have a higher incidence of polycystic ovarian syndrome, which may have neurologic consequence (2).

Physiologic Disorders

Changes in the secretion of ovarian hormones associated with menarche, menstrual cycles, pregnancy, and menopause may all affect the clinical manifestation of a number of disorders such as epilepsy, migraines, multiple sclerosis, movement disorders, and pseudotumor cerebri during a woman's life.

Partial Epilepsy

Several researchers have noted that epilepsy commonly starts around the time of menarche (66,67). In one study, seizures began at menarche in 19% of all adult women with epilepsy. In another study, 35% of epilepsy that began between the ages of 0.5 and 18 years began within 2 years of menarche. Epilepsy was much more likely to start within 2 years of menarche (perimenarche) and during the year of menarche than during any other postnatal childhood period (66). In girls with pre-existing epilepsy, approximately one-third experience seizure exacerbation during puberty (66–68). This is more likely to occur in girls with focal epilepsies, refractory seizures, evidence of CNS damage, and delayed menarche.

Changes in reproductive hormones may be responsible for these observations. Sexual maturation begins with adrenarche, which starts between the age of 8 and 10 with a marked increase in the secretion of DHEAS and DHEA (69). This is followed by gonadarche, which starts around the age of 10 with the secretion of estrogen, but without the secretion of progesterone. The ovarian secretion of estrogens gradually rises through menarche (median age 12.8 years) until the onset of ovulation. In the majority of girls, menstrual cycles are initially anovulatory. Ovulation only starts 12 to 18 months after menarche. It is only at this point that the ovarian secretion of progesterone begins, with a parallel increase in serum allopregnanolone levels in late puberty (70). Thus, the secretion of the neuroexcitatory steroids, DHEAS and estrogen, precedes the secretion of progesterone, the neuroinhibitory steroid, by several years. Continued exposure of the brain during this time to the proconvulsant effects of estrogen and DHEAS without the anticonvulsant effect of progesterone may facilitate the development of epilepsy (epileptogenesis) in susceptible girls.

The cyclical pattern of estradiol and progesterone secretion may influence the likelihood of seizures (36). Catamenial seizures broadly refer to an identifiable and predictable occurrence of seizures in relationship to the menstrual cycle (28,71–73). Herzog et al. described three patterns of catamenial seizure exacerbation (74). The two more easily recognized patterns are (i) worsening of seizures during the mid-cycle and (ii) perimenstrually in women with normal ovulation. In the first case, the occurrences of seizures coincide with ovulation, whereas in the second form, the occurrences happen 1 to 2 days before the onset and 1 to 2 days after the onset of menstruation. The third pattern occurs in women who fail to ovulate, when seizures occur throughout the entire late stage of the cycle, which may vary considerably in duration. It is sometimes easier to note that seizures decrease in occurrence from day 2 through days 8 to 10, and then increase until menstruation.

As mentioned earlier, estradiol has proconvulsant effects on the brain, whereas progesterone has anticonvulsant effects. In women with ovulatory cycles, the surge of ovarian secretion of estrogen before and during ovulation may be responsible for the periovulatory seizure exacerbation. During the luteal phase, the anticonvulsant effect of progesterone secreted by the corpus luteum may protect against seizures, resulting in lower seizure frequency (71,72,74). Perimenstrual seizure exacerbation may be due to the withdrawal of progesterone and its GABA-mediated anticonvulsant effect, similar to the withdrawal seizures seen with a discontinuation of barbiturates, benzodiazepines, or alcohol (42,43). In women with anovulatory cycles, the ovary secretes essentially normal quantities of estrogen during the late follicular and luteal phases (not the periovulatory phase) but does not secrete progesterone. Thus, an elevated estrogen:progesterone ratio occurs from late follicular phase until menstruation. This may explain the unusual pattern of seizure exacerbation, when seizures occur from about menstrual cycle day 8 to 10 until menstruation. In essence, such women are only protected against seizure exacerbation when the ovary secretes very little estrogen during the early and mid-follicular phase of the cycle.

Menopause may also affect epilepsy. The term *menopause* refers to a complex process that encompasses both menopause, cessation of all menstruation, and perimenopause, the preceding decline in reproductive endocrine function. Perimenopause often extends for several years. Early in perimenopause ovulatory cycles change to anovulatory, and progesterone secretion declines (75). By contrast, estrogen secretion remains normal through most of perimenopause and may even increase episodically when, as a result of erratic follicular development, multiple follicles develop during some menstrual cycles. Estrogen levels only drop consistently late in the perimenopause, during the last few months before cessation of menses, as the follicle pool becomes exhausted. Thus, for a period of time that may last for several years, there may be a relative excess ratio of estrogen to progesterone. Based on the pattern of hormonal change, an evolving seizure pattern with seizure exacerbation during the perimenopause might be expected: initial seizure exacerbation when progesterone secretion declines but estrogen secretion continues, followed by stabilization or improvement after menopause, as estrogen secretion ceases. This pattern did, in fact, occur in a recent study (76). Sixty-four percent of women experienced seizure exacerbation, and only 13% of women experienced seizure improvement during the perimenopause. By contrast, 43% of women had seizure improvement during the menopause, with only 31% experiencing seizure exacerbation. Partial epilepsy may also begin during the climacteric, sometime without an apparent cause (77). It is possible that the chronic exposure of the brain to estrogen without progesterone during the perimenopausal years could "kindle" an occult nonepileptic CNS lesion into an epileptic one, in a way similar to the suggested epileptogenic effect of perimenarche. Estrogen replacement therapy may also be associated with seizure exacerbation during the perimenopause and menopause (76). We believe that if there is a clinically significant increase in seizure frequency, hormonal replacement should include both estrogen together with natural progesterone.

In addition, epilepsy, particularly temporal lobe epilepsy, can influence the menstrual cycle. As mentioned, the amygdala, a mesial temporal lobe structure, has reciprocal relationships with hypothalamic structures that influence gonadotrophin secretion. In our study of 50 women with clinical and electroencephalographic evidence of temporal lobe onset partial epilepsy, 38% had significant reproductive abnormality (78). Approximately 20% had polycystic ovarian syndrome (PCOS), and 12% had hypogonadotrophic hypogonadism (HH). Two of the women had premature menopause, and one had hyperprolactinemia. An increased risk of premature menopause among women with epilepsy was also observed in another study (79). In humans, it appears that a significant right temporal lobe versus left temporal lobe differential effect occurs in the hypothalamic gonadotrophin response to temporal lobe seizure activity. We first observed that the LH levels in women with temporal lobe epilepsy varied considerably compared to age-matched controls (80). Women with left temporal seizures had more LH surges during an 8-hour period than controls. These women all had PCOS. In women with hypothalamic hypogonadism (HH), there was a marked decrease in the number of LH surges during an 8-hour period compared to controls, and the seizure focus was more often right-sided. A possible explanation for these findings may include a differential effect of altered input from the right and left amygdala on the hypothalamic GnRH neuronal pulsatile activity (80).

In addition to the above observations regarding the complex interactions of seizure type and seizure location on hormonal cyclicity and the hormonal effect on seizure frequency, medications play an important and often confounding role. Similarly, pregnancy may have a major effect on seizures through its effect on endogenous hormone production and its effect on the metabolism of the antiseizure medication. These effects are discussed in more detail in a later chapter.

Migraine

Migraine is equally prevalent in boys and girls until adolescence, when the ratio changes to 3:1 in favor of women: 17.6% of women suffer from migraines compared with 5.7% of males (81). In approximately 60% of women, migraine attacks are linked to the menses, and in approximately 15% of women with migraines, attacks occur exclusively perimenstrually. The catamenial exacerbation of migraines begins at menarche in approximately 33% of women with menstrual migraines. During pregnancy, migraines may worsen during the first trimester and remit during the last two trimesters, although the pattern of improvement or exacerbation is highly variable and individual; approximately 25% of women with migraines experience no change in their headaches during pregnancy (82). Migraines may worsen transiently, but at times markedly and for a prolonged time, during perimenopause; migraines may improve after completion of menopause when the female:male ratio drops to 2:1 (83).

The pathophysiologic underpinnings of these clinical phenomena remain essentially obscure. A popular hypothesis is that estrogen withdrawal perimenstrually alters vascular tone, leading to vascular instability and a greater susceptibility to cerebrovascular dilatation and headache. Estrogen receptors are found on the media of medium-size cerebral vessels. Estrogen stimulates the production of nitric oxide and causes cerebrovascular dilatation (84). Blood flow in the internal carotid artery increases by 15% during the ovulatory phase of the menstrual cycle in normal women (85). However, no difference has been found in the systemic levels of estrogens, progesterone, androgens, LH, or FSH between women with catamenial migraines and controls (86). No blood hormone–blood flow correlation studies have been performed in women with migraines. Progesterone has not been thought to be a significant factor in migraine, but it is noteworthy that in an animal model of migraine, pretreatment with both progesterone and the 3,5-a reduced metabolites allopregnanolone and tetrahydrodeoxycorticosterone ameliorated plasma extravasation within the meninges (87). This would suggest that progesterone—via allopregnanolone—may play an anti-inflammatory role in the CNS. Perimenstrual withdrawal of progesterone could thus theoretically contribute to an increase in the vasogenic inflammation that may be part of the pathophysiology of migraine.

Other possible mechanisms that have been suggested include a perimenstrual reduction of hypothalamic opioid secretion, increased prostacyclin activity, and prostacyclin-related vasodilation and modulation of prolactin secretion (83). Of particular interest is the influence of estrogen on opioids. Estradiol colocalizes with the opioids endorphins, encephalin, and dynorphin in rat neurons of a number of brain regions, including the hypothalamus and the dorsal spinal cord sensory neurons. It induces the expression and release of the endogenous opioid peptides and activate μ-pioid receptor activation in the hypothalamus and in the amygdala (88). Expression of endorphin in hypothalamic neurons and the release of opioids into the hypothalamic-portal circulation fluctuates during the menstrual cycle. It is highest at the time of ovulation (estrus) and falls as serum estrogen levels fall (89). Thus, estradiol potentiates the analgesic effects of endogenous opioids. It may, possibly, by its effect in the amygdala, even alter the subjective perception or "emotional content" of painful stimuli. Its withdrawal perimenstrually may contribute to the menstrually related migraine. Conversely, its large rise during the last two trimesters is associated with an elevation of the pain threshold during gestation (90). Thus, it may contribute to the alleviation of migraine during this part of pregnancy.

These theories have led to limited therapeutic trials with estrogen and, paradoxically, antiestrogen therapy, for example, with tamoxifen, with androgens such as danazol, and with dopamine agonists such as bromocriptine and pergolide to suppress prolactin secretion (91). These studies have been limited in scope and therapeutic success, although anecdotal reports of success using all these agents abound.

Multiple Sclerosis

Multiple sclerosis (MS) is also more common in women than men, with approximately a 2.5:1 ratio. The onset of the disease is also most common during the second and third decades of life, although the incidence rises after puberty, during the second half of the second decade. Anecdotal reports of MS show perimenstrual exacerbation (92), but also improvement with estrogen contraceptive treatment (93). One of the most notable features of MS, however, is the reduction of relapsing attacks in remitting and relapsing MS during the last trimester of pregnancy, with a subsequent rebound of attacks during the postpartum period (94).

The relapse decrease of the last trimester may be mediated by a shift in immune responses from the inflammatory response promoting T helper 1 lymphocytes (Th1 cells) to the inflammatory response dampening T helper 2 lymphocytes (Th 2 cells). A number of hormones rise dramatically during the second half of pregnancy. The serum levels of estradiol, estriol, progesterone, cortisol, and 1,25-vitamin D, among others, rise tenfold during this time, compared with their preconception levels. All these hormones affect the immune system. Estradiol, estriol, cortisol, and 1,25-vitamin D have been shown to have an immunosupressant effect and a suppressant effect on experimental allergic encephalomyelitis (EAE), the animal model of MS (95). Estrogens affect CD4+ T lymphocytes, with differential effects at low versus high dose. High levels of estrogen favor T-2 anti-inflammatory cytokine and humoral immune response (96). Progesterone also facilitates the T-2 profile, with the induction of the messenger RNA of the anti-inflammatory interleukin-4 (97).

Clinically, the number and volume of gadolinium-enhancing MRI lesions in women with MS do not fluctuate between the follicular and the luteal phases of the menstrual cycle. A positive relationship, however, has been demonstrated between MRI lesion number and volume and the serum progesterone:estradiol ratio (98).

Attempts at the therapeutic manipulation of reproductive hormones other than in MS have not been systematic and have been largely unsuccessful. Bromocriptine, which suppresses the secretion of prolactin, was found to be very effective in suppressing EAE in animals when administered both before and after the EAE-inducing agent

(95). Attempts at human studies, however, were not promising and have been abandoned (99). 1,25-vitamin D was similarly promising in EAE models and disappointing in limited human studies (100). Recently, the weak estrogen estriol, a major estrogen product of the second half of human pregnancy, was found to suppress EAE and to decrease delayed-type hypersensitivity responses in peripheral blood mononuclear cells and gadolinium-enhancing MRI lesion number and volumes in nonpregnant women with MS compared with pretreatment baseline. The beneficial MRI effects receded when the treatment was stopped and re-emerged when it was reinstituted (101). A placebo-controlled study is being planned.

Neuropsychiatric Diseases

As already mentioned, most neuropsychiatric diseases are "sexually dimorphic," with a greater predilection for women (depression, anxiety disorders, anorexia-bulimia) or for men (aggression, schizophrenia) (16). The differences in incidence and prevalence of these disorders between men and women emerges during puberty. Menarche has been aptly named "the forgotten milestone" of female psychiatric diseases (16). Affective and anxiety disorders are commonly affected by the menstrual cycle, and commonly exacerbate or present de novo during the postpartum period or during the perimenopause (22).

Both estrogens and progesterone have psychoactive properties. Estrogens, via diverse mechanisms that may include augmentation of NMDA and non-NMDA glutamatergic activity, serotonergic, noradrenergic, and opiate activity, have an arousing, antidepressant, and potentially anxiogenic effect (102). Progesterone and allopregnanolone, by contrast, have anxiolytic, sedating and, in higher doses, depressive and anesthetic effects similar to those of the benzodiazepines, due to their potentiation of GABA-ergic activity. Progesterone withdrawal may therefore be pathophysiologically important in the perimenstrual exacerbation of anxiety disorders, and of rapid cycling in bipolar affective disorders, and in premenstrual dysphoric dysfunction (PMDD) or premenstrual syndrome (PMS). PMDD women with greater levels of premenstrual anxiety and irritability have significantly reduced allopregnanolone levels in the luteal phase relative to less symptomatic PMDD women (103). This suggests that a dysfunction of metabolism of progesterone to allopregnanolone may be one factor in the causation of PMDD. The withdrawal of progesterone and low serum allopregnanolone levels may also be implicated in postpartum depression. Serum allopregnanolone levels were similarly decreased after delivery in women with postpartum dysthymia compared to euhymic women (104), with a negative correlation between Hamilton Depression Rating score and serum allopregnanolone level. A significant negative correlation was observed between the Hamilton score and levels of serum allopregnanolone.

Movement Disorders

Parkinsonian symptoms can worsen perimenstrually in women with Parkinson disease. In one large survey, 75% of women with natural menstrual cycles noted a worsening of symptoms before or during the period (105). The pathophysiologic mechanisms have not been investigated.

In chorea gravidarum, chorea occurs during pregnancy, sometimes in patients with previous postrheumatic fever chorea (Sydenham chorea). Its pathogenesis is unclear, but may be related to a pregnancy-associated rise in gonadal hormones, particularly estrogens. This hypothesis is supported by the observation that estrogen-containing oral contraceptive may be a trigger for chorea, sometimes in a patient who also suffers from chorea gravidarum (106). (See also Chapter 24.)

CONCLUSION

The study of the effects of hormones on the nervous system, mood, memory, cognition, and behavior in health and in disease is beginning to receive the attention that it deserves. Hopefully, over the next few years, the complex interrelationships between hormonal fluctuations and the various neurotransmitter systems and metabolic pathways, as well as neuronal survival, brain plasticity, neuronal remodeling, and synaptogenesis will be more fully understood so that we might predict and treat the normal and pathologic conditions that arise from the cyclical behavior of ovarian hormones.

On a final note, a word of caution. Although a good deal is known about the effects of ovarian hormones on the nervous system, very little is known about two aspects that may be important. The first is the adaptive response of the nervous system to the fluctuation levels of the steroids. Serum steroid levels may change dramatically without clinical effects. During the last trimester of the pregnancy, for instance, serum levels of progesterone and estradiol rise to approximately 10 times the level of the luteal phase of the menstrual cycle and approximately 40 to 200 times the level of the early follicular phase. Within 24 to 48 hours after delivery, the secretion returns to the follicular phase level. Yet in the majority of women, no neurologic complications occur during the last trimester of the pregnancy or the puerperium (2). Thus, adaptive changes must mitigate the effects of such large fluctuations in serum levels on the nervous system.

Second, we know very little about the functional significance of in situ synthesis of neurosteroids in the CNS. This synthesis is larger than peripheral steroid synthesis for several major gonadal and adrenal steroids such

DHEA, DHEAS, and pregnenolone (brain levels of which are up to 10 times higher than serum levels), as well as for neuroactive progesterone metabolites such as allopregnanolone and TH-DOC (105). Such knowledge will be important in determining the overall role of steroids, including ovarian steroids, in the healthy and diseased functioning of the nervous system.

References

1. Greenspan FS, Strewler GJ, (eds.) *Basic and clinical endocrinology*, 5th ed. Stamford, Conn: Appleton and Lange, 1997.
2. Yen SSC, Jaffe RB, Barbieri RL, (eds.) *Reproductive endocrinology*, 4th ed. Philadelphia, Pa: WB Saunders, 1999.
3. Funabashi R, Shinohara K, Kimura F. Neuronal control circuit for the gonadotropin-releasing hormone surge in rats. In: Handa RJ, Hayashi S, Terasawa E, Kawata M, (eds.) *Neuroplasticity, development and steroid hormone action.* Boca Raton, Fla: CRC Press, 2002;169–177.
4. Dreifuss JJ, Murphy JT, Gloor P. Contrasting effects of two identified amygdaloid efferent pathways on single hypothalamic neurons. *J Neurophysiol* 1986;31:37–248.
5. Canteras NS, Simerly RB, Swanson LW. Organization of projections from the medial nucleus of the amygdala: a PHAL study in the rat. *J Comp Neurol* 1995;360:213–245.
6. Herzog AG, Russell V, Vaitukaitis J. Neuroendocrine dysfunction in temporal lobe epilepsy. *Arch Neurol* 1982;39:133.
7. McEwen BS. How do sex and stress hormones affect nerve cells? *Ann NY Acad Sci* 1994;743:1–16.
8. Matsumoto A, (ed.) *Sexual differentiation of the brain.* Boca Raton, Fla: CRC Press, 1999.
9. Breedlove SM. Sexual dimorphism in the vertebrate nervous system. *J Neurosci* 1992;12:4133–4142.
10. Shughrue PJ, Lane MV, Merchenthaler I. Comparative distribution of estrogen receptor-alpha and -beta mRNA in the rat central nervous system. *J Comp Neurol* 1997; 388:507–525.
11. Roselli CE, Resko JA. Cytochrome P450 aromatase (CYP19) in the non-human primate brain: distribution, regulation, and functional significance. *J Steroid Biochem Mol Biol* 2001;79:247–253.
12. LeVay SA. A difference in hypothalamic structure between heterosexual and homosexual me. *Science* 1991;253:1034–1037.
13. Zhou JN, Hofman MA, Gooren LJG, et al. A sex difference in the human brain and its relation to transsexuality. *Nature* 1995;378:68–70.
14. Harasty J, Double KL, Holliday GM, et al. Language-associated cortical regions are proportionally larger in the female brain. *Arch Neurol* 1997;54:171–176.
15. Rabinowicz T, MavDonald-Comber Petetot J, Gartside PS, et al. Structure of the cerebral cortex in men and women. *J Neuropathol and Exp Neurol* 2002;61:46– 57.
16. Angold A, Worthman CW. Puberty onset of gender differences in rates of depression: a developmental, epidemiologic and neuroendocrine perspective. *J Affect Disord* 1993;29:145–158.
17. Simerly RB, Chang M, Muramatsu, et al. Distribution of androgen and estrogen receptor mRNA-containing cells in the rat brain: an in situ hybridization study. *J Comp Neuro* 1990;294:76–95.

18. Wallis GJ, Luttge W. Influence of estrogen and progesterone on glutamic acid decarboxylase activity in discrete regions of rat brain. *J Neurochem* 1980;34:609–613.
19. Murphy DD, Cole NB, Greenberger V, Segal M. Estradiol increases dendritic spine density by reducing GABA neurotransmission in hippocampal neurons. *J Neurosci* 1998;18:2550–2559.
20. Pecins-Thompson M, Brown NA, Kohama SG, et al. Ovarian steroid regulation of tryptophan hydroxylase mRNA expression in rhesus macaques. *J Neurosc* 1996;16:7021–7029.
21. Briggs M. The relationship between monoamine oxidase activity and sex hormone concentrations in human blood plasma. *J Reprod Fertil* 1972;29:447–450.
22. Klein P, Versi E, Herzog AG. Mood and the menopause. *Br J Obstet Gynaecol* 1999;106:1–4.
23. Gibbs RB. Fluctuations of relative levels of choline acetyl transferase mRNA in different regions of the rat basal forebrain across the estrous cycle: effects of estrogen and progesterone. *J Neurosci* 1996;16:1049.
24. Luine VN. Estradiol increases choline acetyltransferase activity in specific basal forebrain nuclei and projection areas of female rat. *Exp Neurol* 1985;89:484.
25. Gibbs RB. Effects of estrogen on potassium-stimulated acetylcholine release in the hippocampus and overlying cortex of adult rats. *Brain Res* 1997;749:143–146.
26. Sherwin BB. Estrogen and cognitive aging in women. *Trends Pharmacol Sci* 2002;23:527–534.
27. Teresawa E, Timiras P. Electrical activity during the estrous cycle of the rat: cyclic changes in limbic structures. *Endocrinology* 1968;83:207.
28. Klein P, Herzog AG. Hormonal effects on epilepsy in women. *Epilepsia* 1998;39(suppl 8):S9–S16.
29. Edwards HE, Burnham WM, Mendonca A, et al. Steroid hormones affect limbic afterdischarge thresholds and kindling rates in adult female rats. *Brain Res* 1999;838: 136–150.
30. Woolley DE, Timiras PS. The gonad-brain relationship: effects of female sex hormones on electroshock convulsions in the rat. *Endocrinol* 1962;70:196–209.
31. Wong M, Moss R. Long-term and short-term electrophysiological effects of estrogen on the synaptic properties of hippocampal CA1 neurons. *J Neurosci* 1992;12: 3217–3225.
32. Foy MR, Xu J, Xie X, et al. 17beta-estradiol enhances NMDA receptor-mediated EPSPs and long-term potentiation. *J Neurophysiol* 1999;81:925–929.
33. Woolley CS, McEwen BS. Role of estradiol and progesterone in regulation of hippocampal dendritic spine density during the estrous cycle in the rat. *J Comp Neurol* 1993;336:293–306.
34. Yankova M, Hart SA, Woolley CS. Estrogen increases synaptic connectivity between single presynaptic inputs and multiple postsynaptic CA1 pyramidal cells: a serial electron-microscopic study. *Proc Natl Acad Sci USA* 2001;98:3525–3530.
35. Landgren S, Aasly J, Backstrom T, et al. The effect of progesterone and its metabolites on the interictal epileptiform discharge in the cat's cerebral cortex. *Acta Physiol Scand* 1987;131:33–42.
36. Backstrom T, Zetterlund B, Blom S, et al. Effects of intravenous progesterone infusions on the epileptic discharge frequency in women with partial epilepsy. *Acta Neurol Scand* 1984;69:240–248.
37. Paul SM, Purdy RH. Neuroactive steroids. *FASEB* 1992;6:2311–2322.

38. Kokate TG, Banks, MK, Magee T, et al. Finasteride, a 5a-reductase inhibitor, blocks the anticonvulsant activity of progesterone in mice. *J Pharmacol Exp Ther* 1999;288:679–684.

39. Majewska MD, Harrison NL, Schwartz RD, et al. Steroid hormone metabolites are barbiturate-like modulators of the GABA receptor. *Science* 1986;232:1004–1007.

40. Cheney DL, Uzunov D, Vosta E, et al. Gas chromatographic-mass fragmentographic quantitation of 3a-hydroxy-5a-pragnan-20-0ne (allopregnanolone) and its precursors in blood and brain of adrenalectomized and castrated rats. *J Neurosci* 1995;15:4641–4650.

41. Reddy DS, Kim HY, Rogawski MA. Neurosteroids withdrawal model of perimenstrual catamenial epilepsy. *Epilepsia* 2001;42:328–337.

42. Reddy DS, Rogawski MA. Enhanced anticonvulsant activity of neuroactive steroids in a rat model of catamenial epilepsy. *Epilepsia* 2001;42:337–344.

43. Smith SS, Gong OH, Hsu FC, et al. GABA(A) receptor alpha-4 subunit suppression prevents withdrawal properties of an endogenous steroid. *Nature* 1998;30:392:926–930.

44. Reddy DS, Kulkami SK. Proconvulsant effects of neurosteroids pregnenolone sulfate and dehydroepiandrosterone sulfate in mice. *Eur J Pharmacol* 1998;345:55–59.

45. Kokate TG, Juhng KN, Krkby RD, et al. Convulsant actions of the neurosteroid pregnenolone sulfate in mice. *Br Res* 1999;831:119–124.

46. Flood JF, Morle JE, Roberts E. Pregnenolone sulfate enhances posttraining memory processes when injected in very low doses into limbic system structures. *Proc Natl Acad Sci USA* 1995;92:10806.

47. Morales AJ, Nolan J, Nelson G, et al. Effects of replacement dose of dehydroepiandrosterone (DHEA) in men and women of advancing age. *J Clin Endocrinol Metab* 1994;78:1360.

48. Wolfowitz OM, Reus VI, Roberts E, et al. Dehyepiandrosterone (DHEA) treatment of depression. *Biol Psychiatry* 1997;41:311.

49. Green PS, Simpkins JW. Neuroprotective effects of estrogens: potential mechanisms of action. *Int J Dev Neurosci* 2000;18:347–358.

50. Garcia-Seguera LLM, Azcoitia I, Don Carlos LL. Neuroprotection by estradiol. *Prog Neurobiol* 2001;63:29–60.

51. Toran-Allerand CD, Guan X, MacLusky NJ, et al. ER-X: a novel, plasma membrane-associated, putative estrogen receptor that is regulated during development and after ischemic brain injury. *J Neurosci* 2002;22:8391–8401.

52. Gibbs RB. Estrogen replacement enhances acquisition of a spatial memory task and reduces deficits associated with hippocampal muscarinic receptor inhibition. *Horm Behav* 1999;36:222–233.

53. Horvath KM, Hartig W, Van der Veen R, et al. 17beta-estradiol enhances cortical cholinergic innervation and preserves synaptic density following excitotoxic lesions to the rat nucleus basalis magnocellularis. *Neuroscience* 2002;110:489–504.

54. Gibbs RB. Levels of trkA and BDNF mRNA, but not NGF mRNA, fluctuate across the estrous cycle and increase in response to acute hormone replacement. *Brain Res* 1998;810:294.

55. Gibbs RB. Treatment with estrogen and progesterone affects relative levels of brain-derived neurotrophic factor mRNA and protein in different regions of the adult rat brain. *Brain Res* 1999;844:20–27.

56. Paganini-Hill A, Henderson VW. Estrogen replacement therapy and risk of Alzheimer disease. *Arch Intern Med* 1996;156:2213–2217.

57. Lerner AJ. Commentary:women and Alzheimer's disease. *J Clin Endocrinol Metab* 1999;84:1830.

58. Wise PM, Wilson M, Dubal DB, Rau SW. In Vitro and in vivo approaches to the study of the neuroprotective actions of estradiol. In: Handa RJ, Hayashi S, Terasawa E, Kawata M, (eds.) *Neuroplasticity, development and steroid hormone action*. Boca Raton, Fla: CRC Press 2002;81–91.

59. Wise PM, Dubal DB, Wilson ME, et al. Estradiol is a protective factor in the adult and aging brain: understanding of mechanisms derived from in vivo and in vitro studies. *Brain Res Brain Res Rev* 2001;37:313–319.

60. Veliskova J, Velisek L, Galanopoulou AS, Sperber EF. Neuroprotective effects of estrogens on hippocampal cells in adult female rats after status epilepticus. *Epilepsia* 2000;41(suppl 6):S30–35.

61. Beaulieu E, Schumacher M. Progesterone as a neuroactive neurosteroid, with special reference to the effect of progesterone on myelination. *Steroids* 2000;65:605–612.

62. Jay JR, MacLaughlin DT, Badger TM, et al. Hormonal modulation of Schwann cell tumors. I. The effects of estradiol and tamoxifen on methylnitrosourea-induced rat Schwann cell tumors. *Ann NY Acad Sci* 1986;486:371–382.

63. Koenig HL, Ferzaz B, et al. Progesterone synthesis and myelin formation by Schwann cells. *Science* 1995;268:1500–1503.

64. Murphy DG, DeCarli C, Daly E, et al. X-chromosome effects on female brain: a magnetic resonance imaging study of Turner's syndrome. *Lancet* 1993;342:1197–1200.

65. Hines M. Gonadal hormones and sexual differentiation of human behavior: effects on psychosexual and cognitive development. In: Matsumoto A, (ed.) *Sexual Differentiation of the Brain*. Boca Raton, Fla: CRC Press, 1999;257–278.

66. Klein P, Van Passell-Clark LM, Pezzullo JC. Onset of epilepsy at the time of menarche. *Neurology* 2003;60:495–497.

67. Morrell MJ, Hamdy SF, Seale CG, Springer A. Self-reported reproductive history in women with epilepsy: puberty onset and effects of menarche and menstrual cycle on seizures. *Neurology* 1998;50(suppl 4):A448.

68. Rosciszewska D, The course of epilepsy in girls at the age of puberty. *Neurol Neurochir Pol* 1975;9:597–602.

69. Speroff L, Glass RH, Kase NG, (ed.) *Clinical gynecologic endocrinology and infertility*, 5th ed. Baltimore, Md: Williams & Wilkins, 1994.

70. Genazzani AR, Bernardi F, Monteleone P, et al. Neuropeptides, neurotransmitters, neurosteroids, and the onset of puberty. *Ann NY Acad Sci* 2000;900:1–9.

71. Laidlaw J. Catamenial epilepsy. *Lancet* 1956;217:1235–1237.

72. Backstrom T. Epileptic seizures in women related to plasma estrogen and progesterone during the menstrual cycle. *Acta Neurol Scand* 1976;54:321–347.

73. Mattson RH, Cramer JA, Caldwell BV. Seizure frequency and the menstrual cycle: a clinical study. *Epilepsia* 1981;22:242.

74. Herzog AG, Klein P, Ransill BJ.Three patterns of catamenial epilepsy. *Epilepsia* 1997;38:1082–1088.

75. Burger HC. The endocrinology of the menopause. *Maturitas* 1996;23:129–136.

76. Harden CL, Pulver MC, Ravdin L, Jacobs AR. The effect of menopause and perimenopause on the course of epilepsy. *Epilepsia* 1999;40:1402–1407.

77. Abbasi F, Krumholz A, Kittner SJ, Langenberg P. Effects of menopause on seizures in women with epilepsy. *Epilepsia* 1999;40:205–210.

78. Herzog A, Seibel M, Schomer DL, Vaitukaitis JL, Geschwind N. Reproductive endocrine disorders in women with partial seizures of temporal lobe origin. *Arch Neurol* 1986;43:341–346.

79. Klein P, Serje A, Pezzullo JC. Premature ovarian failure in women with epilepsy. *Epilepsia* 2001;42:1584–1589.

80. Drislane FW, Coleman AE, Schomer DL, et al. Altered pulsatile secretion of luteinizing hormone in women with epilepsy. *Neurology* 1994;44:306–310.

81. Stewart WF, Lipton RB, Celentano DD, et al. Prevalence of migraine headache in the United States. Relation to age, income, race, and other sociodemographic factors. *JAMA* 1992;267:64–69.

82. Ratinahirana H, Darbois Y, Bousser MG. Migraine and pregnancy: a prospective study in 703 women after delivery. *Neurology* 1990;40(suppl 1):437.

83. Silberstein SD. Hormone-related headache. *Med Clin North Am* 2001;85:1017–1035.

84. Geary GG, Krause DN, Duckles SP. Estrogen reduces mouse cerebral artery tone through endothelial NOS- and cyclooxygenase-dependent mechanisms. *Am J Physiol Heart Circ Physiol* 2000;279:H511–519.

85. Krejza J, Mariak Z, et al. ICA flow correlates with serum estradiol levels during the menstrual cycle. *Stroke* 2001;32:30–36.

86. Epstein MT, Hockaday JM, Hockaday TD. Migraine and reproductive hormones throughout the menstrual cycle. *Lancet* 1975;1:543–548.

87. Limmroth V, Lee WS, Koskowitz MA. GABAA-receptor-mediated effects of progesterone, its ring-A-reduced metabolites and synthetic neuroactive steroids on neurogenic oedema in the rat meninges. *Br J Pharmacol* 1996;117:99–104.

88. Eckersell CB, Popper P, Micevych PE. Estrogen-induced alteration of mu-opioid receptor immunoreactivity in the medial [preoptic nucleus and medial amygdala. *J Neurosci* 1998;q8:3967–3976.

89. Cheung S, Salinas J, Hammer RP Jr. Gonadal steroid hormone-dependence of beta-endorphin-like immunoreactivity in the medial preoptic area of the rat. *Brain Res* 1995;675:83–88.

90. Dawson-Basoa M, Gintzer AR. Gestational and ovarian sex steroid antinociception: synergy between spinal kappa and delta opioid systems. *Brain Res* 1998;794:61–67.

91. Herzog AG. Continuous bromocriptine therapy in menstrual migraine. *Neurology* 1997;48:101–102.

92. Zorgdrager A, DeKeyser J. Menstrually related worsening of symptoms in multiple sclerosis. *J Neurol Sci* 1997;149:95–97.

93. McFarland HR. The management of multiple sclerosis. 3. Apparent suppression of symptoms by an estrogen-progestin compound. *Mo Med* 1969;66:209–211.

94. Confavreux C, Hutchinsoon M, Hours MM, et al. Rate of pregnancy-related relapse in multiple sclerosis. *N Engl J Med* 1998;339:285–291.

95. Riskind PN, Massacesi L, Doolittle TH, Hauser SL. The role of prolactin in autoimmune demyelination: suppression of experimental allergic encephalomyelitis by bromocriptine. *Ann Neurol* 1991;29:542–547.

96. Gilmore W, Weiner LP, Correale J. Effects of estradiol on cytokine secretion by proteolipid protein-specific T cell clones isolated from multiple sclerosis patients and normal control subjects. *J Immunol* 1997;158:446–451.

97. Piccinni MP, Giudizi MG, Biagiotti R, et al. Progesterone favors the development of human T helper cells producing Th2-type cytokines and promotes both IL-4 production and membrane CD 30 expression in established Th1 cell clones. *J Immunol* 1995;155:128–133.

98. Pozzilli C, Falaschi P, Mainero C, et al. MRI in multiple sclerosis during the menstrual cycle: relationship with sex hormone patterns. *Neurology* 1999;53:622–624.

99. Bissay V, De Klippel N, Herroelen L, et al. Bromocriptine therapy in multiple sclerosis: an open label pilot study. *Clin Neuropharmacol* 1994;17:473–476.

100. Fleming JO, Hummel AL, Beinlich BR, et al. Vitamin D treatment of relapsing-remitting multiple sclerosis: a MRI-based pilot study. *Neurology* 2000;50(suppl 3)A:338.

101. Sicotte NL, Liva SM, Klutch R, et al. Treatment of multiple sclerosis with the pregnancy hormone estriol. *Ann Neurol* 2002;52:421–428.

102. Bernardi M, Vergoni AV, Sandrini M, et al. Influence of ovariectomy, estradiol and progesterone on the behavior of mice in an experminetal model of depression. *Physiol Behav* 1989;45:1067–1068.

103. Girdler SS, Straneva PA, Light KC, Pedersen CA, Morrow AL. Allopregnanolone levels and reactivity to mental stress in premenstrual dysphoric disorder. *Biol Psychiatry* 2001;49:788–797.

104. Nappi RE, Petraglia F, Luisi S, Polatti F, Farina C, Genazzani AR. Serum allopregnanolone in women with postpartum "blues." *Obstet Gynecol* 2001;97:77–80.

105. Thulin PC, Carter JH, Nichols MD, et al. Menstrual-cycle related changed in Parkinson's Disease. *Neurology* 1996;46(suppl)A:376.

106. Omdal R, Roalso S. Chorea gravidarum and chorea associated with oral contraceptives—diseases due to antiphospholipid antibodies? *Acta Neurol Scand* 1992; 86:219–220.

107. Baulieu EE. Neurosteroids: of the nervous system, by the nervous system, for the nervous system. *Recent Prog Horm Res* 1997;52:1–32.

7 Genetic Disorders in Women

Orest Hurko, MD

Orest Hurko, MD

F or the most part, genetic diseases do not discriminate between the sexes, affecting both men and women with equal severity and in a similar manner. In a small number of heritable disorders, however, special considerations arise in the clinical management of women that differ considerably from those in men.

Uniquely, in genetics, the clinician is concerned about manifestations not only in the patient but also in her relatives, especially actual or potential offspring to whom disease may be transmitted. Some genetic diseases are different in women than in men. In others, the only difference is in transmission; the offspring of an affected woman being at different risk than those of an affected man. In still others, notably the sex-linked disorders, both the disease and transmission pattern are different in men and women.

EXPRESSION OF GENETIC DISEASES IN WOMEN

Gender differences in disease phenotype are either sex-linked, the underlying gene(s) being located on a sex chromosome, or sex-limited autosomal disorders, such as male-pattern baldness. In theory, sex-linked disorders could result from alterations of either the X or the Y chromosome. However, the Y chromosome is not only small but also has a low density of genes (1). Its known contribution to human neurogenetic disorders appears to be limited to a behavioral and mildly dysmorphic phenotype, the XYY syndrome (2). In practice, virtually all sex-linked disorders are encoded by genes on the X chromosome.

Sex-Linked Disorders

Recognized X-linked disorders are slightly more frequent than would be predicted by the ratio of one X chromosome to 22 autosomes. As of this writing, of the 14,561 entries in the catalog of human genes and genetic disorders, Online Mendelian Inheritance in Man (OMIM), 810 (5.56% of the total) are in the X chromosome catalog (1). Indeed, 101 of the 1,348 phenotype descriptions in OMIM are in the X chromosome catalog, representing 7.49% of the total number of all phenotypic descriptions in the entire catalog. This is a higher percentage than would be expected from the relative size of the X chromosome, the 151,567,156 base pairs (bp) of which represent only 4.67% of the 3,242,415,757 bp that constitute the haploid human genome. Indeed, Ensembl, a joint project between the European Bioinformatics Institute and the Sanger Institute, currently predicts the existence of 24,847 human genes, of which 869 (only 3.49%) are on the X chromosome (3). Thus, there are roughly twice as many known human X-linked traits as would be predicted by the proportion of human genes that is currently estimated to be located on this chromosome. This disproportion is largely technical and historical. For almost a century it has been known that X-linked inheritance can be recognized by the simple inspection of a pedigree, whereas a specific autosomal assignment requires linkage analysis (4,5). Early studies of X-linked genes were also facilitated by such useful generalizations as Ohno's law: If a gene were on the X chromosome in one species, it would be X-linked in others (6).

X-linked disorders might be expected to be more common in women, who have two X chromosomes and are thus twice as likely to carry an X-linked mutation, than in men, who have only one. The opposite is true, however. Most X-linked disorders are seen more often in men than in women. This apparent paradox is resolved by consideration of the protection afforded by having two allelic copies of each gene, only one of which is likely to be mutant. In classic mendelian theory, an individual with one copy of a recessive mutation appears normal because of compensation from the wild-type allele on the other chromosome. Classic theory also has it that an individual with one copy of a dominant mutation is affected as severely as is an individual with both copies mutant. That is to say, a dominant always completely trumps a recessive. Contrary to classical theory, no completely recessive or completely dominant alleles exist: Having a normal allele always ameliorates the effect of a mutant allele, albeit often very modestly. If phenotypes are examined with sufficient precision, all mutations are thus semidominant. The only known human exception is that of Huntington disease, possibly the only human disorder dominant in Mendel's sense of the word; that is, the phenotype of the homozygote is indistinguishable from that of the heterozygote for the mutant allele (7). This having been said, recessive and dominant remain very useful simplifications for physicians. In clinical practice, the term *recessive* refers to a clinical phenotype overtly detectable only when both alleles are mutant; the term *dominant* refers to phenotypes detectable when only one allele is mutant.

Furthermore, although Mendel recognized dominant and recessive phenotypes, X-linked inheritance was not recognized until half a century later, by Thomas Hunt Morgan (5). Later, Mary Lyon discovered that women are mosaics: In some cells, the paternal X chromosome is active; in others, the maternal (8). This pattern of inactivation of one of the X chromosomes—named *lyonization* in her honor—is established approximately 5 to 6 days after fertilization, when each somatic cell randomly inactivates either the maternal or paternal X chromosome, a pattern that is stably transmitted by each somatic cell to its daughters and their progeny (8). Although each cell expresses only one X chromosome or the other, compensation is frequently possible. Most recessive mutations encode soluble enzymes, normally synthesized in sufficient excess to compensate for haploinsufficiency—that

is, deficiency of that half of gene product that should have been contributed by the mutant allele. In certain metabolic pathways, such compensation can only occur within the same cell in which a block has occurred. In other diseases, a cell that has lyonized (stably inactivated) an X chromosome with a normal gene can be rescued by other cells that have lyonized the X with the mutant gene—so-called metabolic cooperation (9). In certain disorders, there is selective pressure against those cells that have lyonized the normal allele: As the heterozygote ages, abnormal cells drop out of the mosaic (10). The strength of this selective pressure can vary from tissue to tissue, sometimes influencing the course of the disease and sometimes restricting biopsy choices for diagnostic testing.

From these basic considerations we can derive clinically useful generalizations. The effects of X-linked mutations are milder in women than in men, often negligible. Furthermore, the degree of clinical and biochemical involvement in heterozygote women can vary in space and time, depending on the patch size of lyonized clones and the degree of selection against one of the lyonized populations. I will refrain from presenting a longer list of dry generalities at this juncture lest we unnecessarily try the patience of the reader. Instead, I will let other potentially useful generalizations emerge in the discussion of specific disorders.

Sex-Linked Disorders Seen (Almost) Exclusively in Females

Some X-linked disorders are seen only in female heterozygotes because they are lethal to hemizygous males in utero. Spontaneous abortions of affected male fetuses can occur early enough in pregnancy to be inapparent. A careful analysis of multiple families segregating such mutations discloses an excess of female births because of the failure of male conceptuses with the mutation to come to term. Given the small size of sibships in the industrialized world, such distorted birth ratios may not be apparent in an individual family. Such disorders are referred to as X-linked dominant or semidominant, male-lethal.

In many of these disorders, affected females show severe involvement of the nervous system with mental retardation—a useful starting point for the construction of a differential diagnosis, but a virtually worthless tool for its advancement. Specific clinical diagnosis is permitted by characteristic systemic findings. A striking example is provided by what had been called *incontinentia pigmenti type II*, considered by an increasing number of investigators the classic and only authentic form of incontentia pigmenti, not deserving the suffix "II" (11). This disorder results from mutations of the gene on Xp28 (12) encoding NEMO (13), a factor essential for the activation of the transcription factor, NF-kappa-B. Complete absence of this critical factor in affected males leads to death in utero, presumably because all their cells are vulnerable to pro-apoptotic signals. In half of the cells of a heterozygous female, however, intact NEMO is expressed from the normal X chromosome, permitting her survival. Shortly after birth, heterozygous females develop erythema, vesicles, and pustules that become verrucous and hypertrophic. In adolescence, these skin lesions become atrophic, hypopigmented linear streaks. They disappear by the age of 20 years, presumably because of selection against cells expressing the mutant NEMO allele and survival of only those cells expressing the normal, wild-type allele (14). Alopecia, retinal vascular changes with cicatrization, peg-shaped teeth, unilateral breast aplasia, and dystrophic nails have also been observed accompanying the mental retardation, spastic tetraparesis, and microcephaly. There are varying degrees of involvement, even within the same pedigree, where all affected individuals must have the same allele, presumably because of variations in the pattern of lyonization. The vast majority of cases are in females, although incontinentia pigmenti type II was once observed in an XX male (15) and was once transmitted to paternal half sisters by an asymptomatic father, presumably a gonadal mosaic (16).

Other syndromes of pigmentary cutaneous abnormalities and mental retardation can cause diagnostic confusion. Chief among these are a sporadic *Xp11-autosomal translocation disorder*, incorrectly named incontinentia pigmenti type I (17), and *hypomelanosis of Ito*, a syndrome associated with chromosomal mosaicism, in which the hypopigmented skin lesions (best seen under a Wood lamp) do not undergo a prodromal phase (18).

With rare exceptions, *oral-facial-digital dysplasia (OFD) type I* (19) has only been observed in females. In this disorder, malformation of the brain results in a static encephalopathy with mental retardation, a nonspecific neurologic finding. This results from a variety of mutations in the previously uncharacterized chromosome X open reading frame 5 (*CXORF5*) (20), thereby establishing the important role of this presumed microtubular regulator in human development (21). Diagnosis is made by recognition of characteristic facial and hand anomalies. There are abnormal oral frenulae, with clefting of the jaw and tongue in the area of lateral incisors and canines, as well as irregular, asymmetric clefts of the palate. Hand abnormalities include syndactyly (incompletely separated fingers), clinodactyly (curved fingers), brachydactyly (short fingers), and occasional postaxial polydactyly (extra fingers on the ulnar side). Radiographs of hands and feet show irregular mineralization, distinguishing this disorder from *OFD II* (22), a disorder that is also associated with heart defects. Later in life, some individuals develop polycystic kidneys and renal failure (23), an important consideration in the management of these patients and a possible source of diagnostic confusion with classic autosomal dominant *polycystic kidney—*

berry aneurysm disease, resulting from mutation in either the membrane-bound polycystin I (24) or polycystin 2, with which it heterodimerizes (25) to form an active signalling complex.

With rare exceptions, the CHILD syndrome (congenital hemidysplasia with ichthyosiform erythroderma and limb defects) is seen only in females (26). This is one of a growing list of developmental defects associated with mutations affecting cholesterol synthesis, resulting from mutations in the NSDHL gene at Xq28 (27). The hallmark of this X-linked disorder is an ichthyotic erythroderma with ipsilateral malformations, particularly absence or dysplasia of a limb (28). The hemidysplasia can affect not only the limbs but also parts of the central nervous system (CNS)—brain stem, cerebellum, and spinal cord, with unilateral absence of the trigeminal, facial, auditory, glossopharyngeal, and vagus nerves (29). As indicated by its name, a hallmark of CHILD syndrome is its extreme lateralization.However, it may exceptionally result in almost symmetric skin lesions (27). In one reported case, there was also a myelomeningocele (30).

Another developmental disorder of cholesterol metabolism is associated with a deficiency of 3-beta-hydroxysteroid-delta(8), delta(7)-isomerase (31), the *X-linked dominant chondrodysplasia punctata 2* (Conradi-Hunermann-Happle syndrome; CDPX2). CDPX2 accounts for about one-quarter of the cases of this group of skeletal dysplasias associated with linear or whorled pigmentary skin lesions. It is the only form that is X-linked dominant, lethal in utero to males (32), with only affected females surviving to manifest the syndrome. Unlike the CHILD syndrome, CDPX2 typically shows mild to moderate assymmetry, but occasionally may be extremely lateralized. Another striking feature of CDPX2 is anticipation, perhaps resulting from skewed gene methylation rather than the more widely recognized mechanism of triplet repeat expansion (33). Linear skin defects are also seen in *microphthalmia with linear skin defects (MIDAS syndrome: microphthalmia, facial dermal hypoplasia, sclerocornea)*, a male-lethal disorder associated with the absence of the Xp22 band, in which is encoded mitochondrial holocytochrome c synthase (34). In addition to the linear skin defects and microphthalmia with sclerocornea, agenesis of the corpus callosum occurs. An exceptional case was reported in two phenotypically male twins with an XX karyotype. The male phenotype was conferred by the abnormal presence of the Sry gene, the result of a subtle XY translocation (35).

The best known X-linked male-lethal disorder associated with agenesis of the corpus callosum is *Aicardi syndrome* (36), for which lacunar choreoretinopathy and infantile spasms complete the diagnostic triad. Evidence for X-linked inheritance comes from family studies that show a high spontaneous abortion rate in mothers of affected girls, as well as a skewed ratio of unaffected male to female siblings (37). Presumably, affected females result from the new onset of an X-linked dominant mutation that is lethal to male fetuses. After presentation with infantile spasms, affected females continue with lifelong mental subnormality and an epilepsy that is quite difficult to control. The characteristic anatomic findings are agenesis (72%) or hypoplasia (28%) of the corpus callosum (37) and chorioretinal lacunae in a highly specific pattern. Costovertebral defects such as hemivertebrae, scoliosis, and malformed or absent ribs are also common. The degree of psychomotor retardation is variable, apparently reflecting the pattern of lyonization (38), further evidence for X-linked dominant inheritance. In addition to brain heterotopias, there have been several reports of Aicardi syndrome in association with benign or malignant tumors of the CNS or periphery—choroid plexus papilloma and gastric polyps (39) and scalp lipomas as well as malignant cavernous hemangioma of the leg with angiosarcomatous metastases (40).

Unlike the previously described X-linked male-lethal disorders, in which characteristic systemic features permit clinical diagnosis, abnormalities in periventricular heterotopia are confined to the nervous system (41). Multiple uncalcified nodules appear on the lateral ventricular walls, sometimes causing diagnostic confusion with tuberous sclerosis, which differs from this disorder by the presence of depigmented ash-leaf spots, periungual fibromas, and mental retardation. Some females with characteristic MRI scans are asymptomatic, whereas others have seizures, sometimes severe (42).

Several other disorders of girls appear in which X-linked male-lethal inheritance had long been suggested but in which proof of such a mechanism proved elusive. The best known of these disorders is the *Rett syndrome*, a distinctive progressive encephalopathy characterized by autism, loss of purposeful hand movements, and an acquired microcephaly (43). Characteristically, these girls show normal development until 7 to 18 months of age, an essential criterion for clinical diagnosis (44). Deceleration of linear growth is the first sign of a 1.5-year period of illness, during which time the affected girl develops microcephaly, severe dementia, truncal ataxia, and peculiar wringing hand movements. After this period of decline, the course stabilizes, resulting in a profound but subsequently nonprogressive encephalopathy. Other features include seizures, spastic paraparesis, and vasomotor abnormalities of the lower limbs. By analogy to the Aicardi syndrome, it had been proposed that most girls with Rett syndrome harbor new mutations of an unspecified gene on the X-chromosome that is lethal to males (43). A few instances of affected sisters in which inheritance from a germinally mosaic mother could be posited (43), and reports exist of two patients with a balanced translocation involving the X chromosome (45,46). Other

pedigree and studies of lyonization, however, had argued against a simple X-linked hypothesis (47).

The X-linked model was finally confirmed by demonstrating pathogenic mutations in the gene in Xp28 encoding methyl-CpG-binding protein-2, a regulator of chromatin structure. Mutations in the same gene have been found responsible for about half the cases of the preserved speech variant (PSV) of Rett syndrome (48,49). Further evidence for the importance of the MECP2 gene is provided by independent reports of severe neurodevelopmental defects, including a case of otherwise typical Rett syndrome in boys with normal karyotypes and somatic mosaicism for MECP2 (50,51).

Sex-linked male-lethal inheritance has been proposed for the *Wildervanck cervicooculoacoustic syndrome*, the juxtaposition of congenital perceptive deafness with bony abnormalities of the inner ear, the Klippel-Feil anomaly, and Duane abducens palsy with retractor bulbi (52). Abducens palsy appears to be the most variable part of this syndrome, but Klippel-Feil cervical vertebral anomalies are more common. Indeed, such vertebral anomalies occur in 1% of deaf women. Similar inheritance has been proposed for the less common *CODAS syndrome* (cerebral, ocular, dental, auricular, and skeletal anomalies), thus far reported in only two unrelated females (53), a segregation pattern for which autosomal inheritance is equally plausible. Further, but as yet inconclusive, evidence against X-linked inheritance, is provided by reports of typically affected males (54). A slowly progressive *limb-girdle form of muscular dystrophy* limited to females has been reported in several families (55). The observed pattern of inheritance is compatible with either X-linked male-lethal or a sex-limited autosomal dominant trait.

Sex-Linked Disorders with Milder Manifestations in Females

Most sex-linked disorders are present in men, with only minor if any manifestations in females. In certain circumstances, however, the clinical phenotype in women can be significant, sometimes differing from the classic phenotype in males and thus causing diagnostic confusion.

Duchenne Muscular Dystrophy: The Best Studied Example

The most common X-linked single gene disorder in humans is Duchenne muscular dystrophy (DMD). Boys affected with DMD develop gait difficulty and calf hypertrophy as toddlers, need wheelchairs by the end of the first decade of life, and succumb by the end of the second decade. In the allelic disorder, Becker muscular dystrophy (BMD), onset and progression of symptoms is significantly delayed, and affected individuals survive into middle age. The gene encoding dystrophin—mutant in Duchenne and in Becker muscular dystrophy—enjoys pride of place as the first gene discovered by the now commonplace process of positional cloning, then called reverse genetics (56). For these two reasons, the expression of this gene in female heterozygotes has been studied more carefully than has that of any other. Lessons learned from DMD and BMD illuminate our understanding of less well characterized X-linked diseases and are considered in some depth.

Duchenne muscular dystrophy affects 1 in 3,300 live-born males, most of whom neither have had, nor will have, another case in their families (57). Because affected males virtually never survive into reproductive years, the half-life of a given DMD mutation is only one generation. The disorder remains common in all populations despite this strong selection pressure only because of the high rate of new mutations. DMD and BMD carrier females are more common than are affected heterozygote males, but most have no detectable muscle weakness. Thus, for women, the most common clinical problem posed by DMD or its milder allelic variant, BMD, is the birth of an affected son. If the son represents a new mutation, the risk to future pregnancies is negligible. If, however, the woman is an unaffected carrier, half of her sons will be affected by this devastating disorder. Determining carrier status is therefore a matter of considerable importance.

Approximately 70% of female heterozygotes for DMD have an elevated level of creatine kinase in the serum. The creatine kinase levels tend to be higher in younger carriers and to decrease with age (58). Efforts to improve the accuracy of carrier prediction have been only partially successful. The most convenient of these methods is DNA analysis, which demonstrates a detectable deletion or insertion in the dystrophin gene in 90% of affected males (59). Once detected in an affected hemizygous male, the deletion or insertion can be searched for in female relatives, albeit often with considerable technical difficulty because of the normal allele present on the other X chromosome.

An alternative method, staining for dystrophin protein with antibodies in muscle biopsies of many heterozygote females, has demonstrated dystrophin-negative myofiber segments (60). The majority of myofibers in heterozygotes, however, have no detectable deficiency of dystrophin. Each myofiber is a multinucleated syncytium derived from the fusion of hundreds of mononuclear myoblasts, some of which have lyonized the paternal X chromosome, others the maternal. In the majority of myofiber segments, dystrophin produced by normal nuclei is sufficient to compensate for segments served by mutant nuclei. Indeed, a mosaic of dystrophin-negative myofibers has only been detected in those obligate carriers who have an elevation of serum creatine kinase. Thus, staining of muscle sections is no more sensitive than mea-

surement of creatine kinase in the serum. Improvement in the accuracy of carrier detection is only afforded by the clonal analysis of myoblasts cultured from biopsied muscle from putative carriers (61). Although highly accurate, this tissue culture procedure is very expensive.

In a small proportion of women, DMD not only poses a concern for their offspring, but also affects their own health. Approximately 2.5% of DMD heterozygotes have symptoms, usually a limb-girdle weakness of later onset, sometimes asymmetric and usually much milder than that of affected boys (62). Although the proportion of manifesting heterozygotes is low, the frequency of DMD mutations in most populations is much higher than that of autosomal recessive limb-girdle dystrophies. Thus, a girl with a limb-girdle dystrophy is as likely to have DMD as an autosomal recessive sarcoglycanopathy. In a large survey of myopathic women with negative family history, elevated levels of serum creatine kinase, and myopathic muscle biopsy, 10% were found to have a dystrophinopathy (63).

Although most manifesting carriers have a mild limb-girdle phenotype, a small proportion have a severe progressive classic DMD phenotype. In all severely affected females, there has been a radical departure from the expected 50–50 pattern of lyonization. Typical DMD has been described in a phenotypic female with Turner syndrome, thus an XO hemizygote (64), and in approximately a dozen women with X-autosomal translocations. These translocations inactivated the dystrophin gene in the Xp21 band of one of the X chromomes, but also stuck on a piece of autosome that effectively required that the derivative chromosome be expressed in order for the cell to survive. Only the cells that lyonized the normal X chromosome survived in the mosaic. Thus, the only X chromosome active in these girls was the one that had disrupted the dystrophin gene. Such translocation females were instrumental in the search for the dystrophin gene (65) because the translocation points proved easy targets for molecular biologists.

More commonly, women with a typical severe DMD phenotype are one of a pair of discordant monozygotic twins. All monozygotic female twins heterozygous for a DMD mutation are discordant—one twin severely affected, the other one completely well. In all reported cases, the manifesting twin has disproportionately lyonized the normal X chromosome. The normal twin has had skewed X-inactivation in the opposite direction (66) or a normal pattern of inactivation (67). These findings suggest that twinning takes place after lyonization, with a small proportion of the inner cell mass breaking off and then catching up with the normal twin, albeit with a skew resulting from small initial sampling (68). Another pattern of skewed X-inactivation appears to result not from twinning, but from an as yet obscure mechanistic interaction between paternal inheritance and the development of new dystrophin mutations (69).

Another manifestation of DMD in females is cardiomyopathy. Unlike the multinucleated myofibers of skeletal muscle, cardiac myocytes are mononuclear; a cardiac monocyte expressing mutant dystrophin from its active X chromosome receives no protection from neighbors that have lyonized in the opposite direction. From 6.6% to 16.4% of DMD carrier females have electrocardiographic abnormalities. A smaller proportion have frank cardiomyopathy in the presence or absence of limb weakness (70). Similarly, certain mutations affecting the amino terminal end of the dystrophin molecule result in X-linked dilated cardiomyopathy—congestive heart failure in teenaged males and older women (71).

Other X-Linked Myopathies

Similar patterns have been seen in other X-linked myopathies not related to the dystrophin gene. Men affected with *Dreifuss-Emery muscular dystrophy* develop a characteristic syndrome of delayed weakness with early contractures of the elbows, Achilles tendons, and posterior cervical muscles (72). Additionally, the men have pectus excavatum and a cardiomyopathy beginning with atrioventricular block. In contrast, the only manifestation in females is cardiac disease with atrial arrhythmia, which is sometimes lethal (73). Cardiac involvement had been thought to result from selective localization of emerin, the protein primarily affected in this disorder, in the intercalated discs of cardiomyocytes. Subsequent studies with better antibodies, however, demonstrated emerin only in the nuclear member of cardiomyocytes (74).

A similar mechanism probably underlies selective cardiac involvement in female carriers of yet another X-linked disorder, the exceedingly rare syndrome of *scapuloperoneal muscular dystrophy, mental retardation, and lethal cardiomyopathy* reported by Bergia. Affected boys begin mental deterioration at the age of 5 years, followed by humeroperoneal muscular dystrophy and lethal hypertrophic cardiomyopathy when they are teenagers. In contrast, the female carriers have a cardiomyopathy without skeletal muscle involvement (75).

Another type of difference between multinucleated skeletal myotubes and mononucleated cells is suggested by the X-linked deficiency of *phosphoglycerate kinase* (PGK1). Affected men have recurrent myoglobinuria brought on by exercise-induced rhabdomyolysis, as well as mental retardation, epilepsy, and hemolysis (76). In contrast, reported women show only hemolytic anemia (77). Alternatively, these differences may be attributed to unique properties of individual PGK mutants. No reports appear of clinical abnormalities in females heterozygous for mutations of the *alpha subunit of phosphorylase kinase*, responsible for a rare X-linked muscle glycogenesis in hemizygous males (78).

A different pattern of mildly affected females is seen in other X-linked muscle diseases. *Myotubular* or *centronuclear myopathy* exists in several different forms: a very well documented X-linked recessive neonatal form that is lethal in infancy, a less well documented mild autosomal dominant form, and an autosomal recessive form of intermediate severity that begins in late infancy or early childhood (79). Males affected with the X-linked type [now known to result from a mutation affecting a putative tyrosine phosphatase, myotubularin (80)] are born as floppy infants with polyhydramnios, external ophthalmoplegia, weakness of facial and cervical muscles, and respiratory insufficiency leading to death in infancy. The clinical presentation is similar to that of neonatal myotonic dystrophy. Unlike mothers with the autosomal dominant myotonic dystrophy, however, mothers of male infants with X-linked myotubular myopathy do not show facial weakness, cataracts, or myotonia, although they may show mild abnormalities on muscle biopsy (81). An interesting possible exception to the general rule of non-manifesting carriers was related by Torres, who reported a mixed brain stem, peripheral nerve, and myopathic disorder in a mother of boys with neonatal lethal centronuclear myopathy (82).

In other X-linked myopathies, the only manifestation in female heterozygotes is minimal nonspecific changes on muscle biopsy. Asymptomatic female carriers of *fingerprint myopathy* have such changes rather than the characteristic fingerprint bodies found in the periphery of the sarcoplasm in hemizygote boys (83).

X-Linked Peripheral Neuropathies

Several forms of X-linked neuropathy exist, distinguishable by clinical features, map position, or both. Several of these X-linked forms have been referred to as Charcot-Marie-Tooth disease. Thus, just like myotubular myopathy, spastic paraplegia, and retinitis pigmentosa, Charcot-Marie-Tooth disease(s) can be either autosomal or X-linked. In *X-linked dominant Charcot-Marie-Tooth disease* (CMTX1), women are affected less severely than are men. Careful inspection of pedigrees demonstrates that this is a true sex-linked disorder rather than a sex-limited expression of an autosomal dominant Charcot-Marie-Tooth disease. Affected men transmit the disorder to all of their daughters but to none of their sons. Affected mothers transmit to half of their sons and to half of their daughters, a classic pattern of X-linked transmission. This map location has been confirmed and refined to Xq13 by linkage studies using DNA markers. This is primarily an axonal degeneration with secondary changes in peripheral myelin, with some affected males showing deafness. Affected women show mild clinical signs, including decreased nerve conduction velocities but no functional disability (84). In an exceptional family segregating a mutation in the same locus as CMTX1, episodes of transient paraparesis, monoparesis, tetraparesis, dysarthria, aphasia, and cranial nerve palsies occured associated with reversible white matter lesions on MRI (85). In addition to this disorder, which is now demonstrated to be caused by mutations affecting connexin-32 (86), there is also linkage evidence for two separate loci—CMTX2 at Xp22.2 and CMTX3 at Xp26—encoding X-linked recessive forms of Charcot-Marie-Tooth disease, so called because heterozygous women usually do not show signs of the disease (87).

Unfortunately, Charcot-Marie-Tooth disease has also been applied to several other more complex neurologic diseases with severe involvement in men and mild involvement in women. In the *Cowchock variant* of Charcot-Marie-Tooth (CMT2D), male infants are severely weak and most are either deaf or mentally retarded. Obligate heterozygote females are asymptomatic, although some show minor inconsistent alterations in hearing, on sensory nerve conduction studies, and on electromyography (88). Earlier speculations to the contrary, linkage studies clearly demonstrate that the so-called Cowchock variant is not an allelic variant of CMTX1 (89) because it maps to Xq24-q26. In another so-called X-linked recessive CMT variant, a Schwann-cell form of *sensorimotor neuropathy associated with aplasia cutis congenita* of the scalp, with underlying bony defects of the calvarium in affected males, but only minor distal wasting and denervation in asymptomatic female heterozygotes (90). In the *Rosenberg-Chutorian syndrome*, affected males have a sensorimotor neuropathy reminiscent of Charcot-Marie-Tooth disease as well as sensorineural deafness and optic atrophy (91). In contrast, heterozygous women show only slowly progressive hearing loss (92).

A small-fiber neuropathy quite distinct from Charcot-Marie-Tooth disease is a cardinal manifestation of *Fabry disease*, an X-linked multisystem disorder resulting from a deficiency of ceramide trihexosidase (also known as alpha-galactosidase) and the resultant vascular deposition of lipid (93). In addition to a painful small-fiber neuropathy with autonomic involvement and abdominal crises, the full syndrome includes a characteristic whorl-like corneal dystrophy, as well as infarctions in the retina and in the kidney. Whereas renal failure had previously led to death by the third decade, longer survival resulting from renal transplantation has permitted survival to a later stage manifesting multiple large- and small-vessel infarctions of the CNS. Affected males are easily recognized by a purpuric skin rash for which the disorder was given its other name, angiokeratoma diffusa. Corneal dystrophy is of similar severity in heterozygotes as in hemizygous males (94), but affected women almost never have the characteristic skin rash. Without the rash, the diagnosis is frequently overlooked. Although women tend to survive longer than do affected men, clinical involvement can be very severe, including debilitating autonomic neuropathy (95), renal failure, cardiomyopathy (96), and involvement of the CNS (97). A study of 60 obligate carrier females demonstrated painful neuropathy in 70% and other serious systemic manifestations in 30%, including renal failure and stroke (98).

In other X-linked disorders, peripheral neuropathy or sensory ganglionopathy may be the only manifestation in female heterozygotes of a more complex multisystem disorder in males. In the *myopia-ophthalmoplegia syndrome*, some carrier women have only areflexia, but not the ophthalmoplegia, pupillary abnormalities, chorioretinal degeneration, and cardiac and spinal malformations that are seen in affected male relatives (99).

X-Linked Motor Neuron Disorders

The first motor neuron disease in which the underlying biochemical defect was discovered genetically is X-linked *Kennedy spinobulbar atrophy*, which is caused by expansions of triplet repeats at one end of the gene encoding the androgen receptor (100). This was also the first demonstration of expansions of triplet repeats as a pathogenic mechanism, now demonstrated in half a dozen other human disorders, all of which affect the nervous system. Mutations at the other end of the androgen receptor cause the distinct syndrome of testicular feminization—normal female secondary sexual characteristics in XY males, who are infertile but have no motor neuron disease. Men with Kennedy syndrome develop gynecomastia in their teens and are usually impotent, but sometimes are fertile (101). Atrophy and fasciculations of the bulbar muscles begin anywhere from the twenties to forties. We have seen one phenotypic XY woman with testicular feminization and a bulbar spinal muscular atrophy. There is an increased frequency of the Kennedy triplet repeat expansion in women with polycystic ovary syndrome as well as preferential expression of the expanded triplet repeat, compared with that seen in the general population (102). [However, there has been no report of clinical or subclinical neurologic involvement in true female carriers in this disorder or in the other X-linked motor neuron disease, *lethal infantile sex-linked spinal muscular atrophy* (SMAX2) (103).]

Motor neuron disease may underly some forms of *distal infantile arthrogryposis*, of which there may be as many as three distinct X-linked types (104). In one such family, the disease was transmitted to severely affected male infants by female carriers, who themselves had milder manifestations such as minimal muscle weakness, kyphosis, contractures, and clubfoot (105).

X-Linked Spastic Parapareses

As in the case of Charcot-Marie-Tooth disease, myotubular myopathy, and retinitis pigmentosa, hereditary spastic paraparesis can segregate as either an autosomal dominant, autosomal recessive, or X-linked trait. Three well-characterized X-linked spastic parapareses exist, all of which can have significant clinical impact on heterozygous women. *Adrenoleukodystrophy* (ALD) and the milder *adrenomyeloneuropathy* (AMN) are alternate manifestations of mutations affecting a recently discovered peroxisomal transport protein encoded by a gene near the distal tip of the long arm of the X chromosome. The differences between ALD and AMN—one a leukodystrophy of childhood, the other a neuronopathy of adults—are not manifestations of different alleles at the same locus (106), but of an epistatic interaction from an as yet unidentified autosomal modifier gene. In the presence of one form of this putative modifier, affected boys develop rapidly progressive ALD, which is lethal in mid-childhood, beginning with markedly inflammatory demyelination, typically beginning in the occipital corona radiata and advancing frontally. In the absence of this modifier, a more slowly progressive AMN develops in late adolescence and progresses over a decade. Both disorders can coexist in the same pedigree, indicating that the same allele at Xp28 can give rise to either syndrome (106). In hemizygous males, adrenal insufficiency can occur as part of either syndrome, or as an isolated Addisonism. Approximately 15% of female heterozygotes develop a moderately severe spastic paraparesis (107), sometimes in association with a peripheral neuropathy (108) and sphincter disturbance (109). As is the case in all X-linked disorders, heterozygote females are mosaics of cells that have lyonized either the normal or mutant gene. Uniquely among X-linked disorders, there is a selective advantage for cells expressing the mutant ALD allele, resulting in their gradual outnumbering of their normal fellows in the mosaic as she grows older. Unlike affected men, heterozygous women are unlikely to have severe adrenocortical insufficiency, but they may be presdisposed to hypoaldosteronism when taking non-steroidal anti-inflammatory drugs (110).

Certain mutations affecting proteolipid protein give rise to a classic *Pelizaeus-Merzbacher* phenotype with a leukodystrophy limited to the CNS, resulting in oculomotor apraxia, spastic ataxia, and parkinsonian features that can present as early as 8 days of life and progress so slowly as to permit survival into middle age (111). Other mutations of the same X-linked gene give rise to a classic *spastic paraparesis* (X-linked, type 2, SPPX2) without involvement of eye movements. Some of these segregate as strict recessives; others are expressed frequently in females (112).

Similarly, three disparate syndromes, *MASA* (mental retardation, aphasia, shuffling gait, adducted thumbs), *X-linked aqueductal stenosis* with hydrocephalus, and an *X-linked spastic paraplegia*, can result from different mutations in L1CAM gene, which encodes a neural cell adhesion molecule (113). The clinical phenotype in heterozygous females from one such MASA family ranged from adducted thumbs, learning abnormalities, or mild mental retardation, to hydrocephalus that was lethal shortly after birth (114).

In addition to these three well-characterized X-linked spastic parapareses, there have been isolated reports of possible others. Mild spastic paraparesis was the only sign in a girl whose brothers also had Kallman syndrome—hypogonadotrophic hypogonadism and arrhinencephaly (115). The relevance of this isolated report is not clear, however. In autosomal Kallman syndrome, associated with mutations in KAL1 of a secreted protease inhibitor with repeats (116–117), no spastic paraparesis occurs, but both transmitting females and fully affected male heterozygotes have partial or complete anosmia. In a study of X-linked Kallman syndrome that was confirmed by a demonstration of mutations in anosmin, a regulator of migration of GnRH neurons and olfactory nerves to the hypothalamus, there was no discernible phenotype in female obligate carriers (118).

X-Linked Ataxias and Movement Disorders

Gene mutations do not always observe the tidy anatomic categories favored by neurologists. Nowhere is this muddle more evident than in those neurodegenerative disorders in which pyramidal, extrapyramidal, and cerebellar signs coexist, often with spectacularly different degrees of relative severity, even within members of the same sibship. For example, a rare X-linked neurodegenerative disorder described by Malamud and Cohen begins with cerebellar ataxia and is later characterized by extrapyramidal signs (119). Both clincial and anatomic involvement of the cerebellum and basal ganglia are evident in a recently reported X-linked disorder with iron deposition in the basal ganglia and neuroaxonal dystrophy similar to *Hallervorden-Spatz-Pettigrew syndrome* (120). Hemizygous boys show a Dandy-Walker malformation of the cerebellum as well as choreoathetosis, severe mental retardation with seizures, and marked hypotonia that evolves into spasticity. Although autopsy studies in a female carrier have shown iron deposition and neuroaxonal dystrophy, the clinical manifestations were limited to a presenile dementia in one woman and mild intellectual impairment in others.

Pelizaeus-Merzbacher disease, which was discussed in the previous section in relationship to mutations of the proteolipid protein gene and a form of X-linked spastic paraparesis, would actually fit as nicely into this section as the previous one. Although Pelizaeus-Merzbacher disease is much more commonly observed in boys, an otherwise typical case occurred in a girl with no obvious chromosomal abnormality (121).

Similarly, *Menkes kinky-hair disease* typically spares girls but affects hemizygous boys, with severe cerebellar and cerebral degeneration beginning in the first months of life, with concomitant growth failure, and death by the second year (122). The disease is named because of the characteristic fragile, microscopically twisted and fractured hair shafts of variable diameter—pili torti—present in all affected boys and in 43% of carrier women (123), usually the only clinical indicator of heterozygosity. A few women, however, have had typical neurologic involvement. Among these are girls with a balanced translocation X-autosomal translocation through Xp13 (124–126), the site of the gene encoding the alpha polypeptide of an adenosine triphosphate–dependent copper transporter, mutant in this disorder. Otherwise typical Menkes progressive encephalopathy was described in three additional girls, one a Turner mosaic and the others without demonstrable chromosomal alterations (127). Mild manifestations of the *cutis laxa/occipital horn syndrome*, recently shown to be allelic to Menkes (128), are frequently seen in female relatives (129) of males affected with mild mental retardation, hyperelasticity of the skin, and characterisitic bony projections of the occipital bone pointing caudally from the foramen magnum.

Two X-linked neurodegenerative disorders are associated with hyperuricemia: *Lesch-Nyhan syndrome*, a movement and behavioral disorder resulting from inactivation of hypoxanthine-guanine phosphoribosyl transferase (HGPRT), and a less well known ataxia syndrome due to superactivity of *phosphoribosylpyrophosphate synthetase-I* (PRPS). Some mutations of either enzyme produce only gout and uric acid kidney stones, whereas others produce a characteristic neurologic syndrome as well. The well-known *Lesch-Nyhan syndrome*—choreoathetosis, self-mutilation, mental retardation, and spasticity—has been reported virtually exclusively in males (130). Clinically unaffected heterozygous girls can be shown to have two populations of red blood cells—one defective in HGPRT, the other normal—but similar tests of adult heterozygote women demonstrate only one population, with normal HGPRT activity, indicating positive selection for those red blood cell precursors that had lyonized the mutant X chromosome (9,131). The one exceptional case of a girl with a typical Lesch-Nyhan syndrome had a deletion of the entire HGPRT gene on the maternally derived X chromosome and selective lyonization of normal paternal X chromosome (132).

In contrast, full or partial clinically evident involvement of women is more frequent in families segregating an abnormality of PRPS. In addition to hyperuricemia, affected boys in some sibships develop sensorineural high-tone deafness, ataxia, peripheral neuropathy with axonal and demyelinating features, as well as renal failure (independent of hyperuricemia), sometimes leading to death in early childhood (133). In some families, there are distinctive facial features—hypertelorism (widely spaced eyes) with a prominent forehead, beaked nose, and broad mouth (134). In some family members, there is only early-onset gout, whereas others develop the full syndrome. Curiously, heterozygous females are on average no less severely affected than are hemizygous males (135).

The extent of clinical involvement of female heterozygotes differs in a variety of less well characterized X-linked cerebellar ataxias. Cerebellar atrophy and self-limited episodes of ataxia were observed in mothers of boys with the *ataxia-deafness syndrome*: infantile hypotonia, developmental delay, esotropia, optic atrophy, and ataxia progressing to death in childhood (136). In contrast, clinical manifestations in women heterozygous for *Arts fatal X-linked ataxia and deafness* appear to be limited to mild hearing impairment in adulthood (137). Even less involvement of women is seen in the more commonly observed *X-linked cerebellar ataxia*, for which the only reported manifesting female was an XO Turner hemizygote (138).

It is distinctly unusual for women to be affected by X-linked extrapyramidal disorders. The rare exceptions include cytogenetically normal, presumably heterozygote females as well as two women with balanced X-autosomal translocations (139), variably affected with the *Goeminne TKCR syndrome*—torticollis, keloids, cryptorchidism, and renal dysplasia (140). No affected carriers have been reported in the *deafness-dystonia syndrome*, a progressive dystonia of boys with dysarthria and hyperactivity that leads to severe disability and death in the teenage years (141). Only one woman has been affected with *X-linked torsion-dystonia 3* (142), in which parkinsonian features are an early feature of a syndrome that begins in the thirties, often with spasmodic eye blinking, and evolves into generalized dystonia within seven years. Two women were mildly affected in a family segregating the X-linked *Waisman early-onset parkinsonism with mental retardation*, a syndrome that includes persistent frontal release signs as a large neurocranium with frontal bossing and, in some individuals, strabismus or seizures (143). Variable expression was seen in some female relatives of men affected with congenital hemiparesis and athetosis of the paretic upper extremity—hereditary hemihypotrophy, hemiparesis, and hemiathetosis. It is not clear from the single published pedigree if this is an X-linked trait or a sex-modified expression of an autosomal trait, as suggested by the authors (144).

X-Linked Metabolic Encephalopathies

As a general rule, metabolic disorders segregate as recessive genetic traits, whether the gene encoding the relevant enzyme lies on an autosome or on the X chromosome. The reason for this pattern lies in the large margin of error built into most metabolic pathways. The flux of metabolites permitted by the half-normal amount encoded by the unaffected allele on the other chromosome is usually sufficient for homeostasis. The exceptions to this remarkably durable clinical rule of thumb are few: (i) mutations of key regulatory enzymes and/or of enzymes normally working near their maximum velocity; and (ii) allosteric mutations affecting components of multisubunit enzyme assemblies, in which a few mutant protein chains can allosterically poison a disproportionate number of normal subunits.

In addition to the two relentlessly progressive disorders of uric acid metabolism described in the previous section, there are two major X-linked enzymopathies with profound, but often intermittent, metabolic consequences in women—*pyruvate dehydrogenase* (PDH) deficiency, the most common form of primary lactic acidosis in either sex, and *ornithine transcarbamylase* (OTC) *deficiency*, the most commonly occurring disorder of the urea cycle.

PDH is a massive multimer, visible on electron micrographs as a particle about the size of a ribosome, containing multiple copies of three subunits, one of which, the E1-alpha subunit, is encoded on the X chromosome. The majority of cases of PDH deficiency result from mutations of this X-linked subunit (145). This enzyme is the gatekeeper for partially metabolized products of the cytoplasmic Embden-Meyerhoff pathway seeking entry into mitochondria for completion of metabolism through the Krebs tricarboxylic acid cycle and subsequently the electron transport chain. In the brain, PDH typically is operating at approximately 75% capacity, leaving little margin for error for such a key metabolic step. Phenotypes resulting from mutation of the E1-alpha subunit range from lactic acidosis that is lethal in infancy, to a Leigh's polioencephalopathy in toddlers, to intermittent ataxia in adults, depending on the nature of the mutation and the sex of the patient. Curiously, even though PDH deficiency has been reported approximately as often in boys as in girls, almost all reported girls have had deletions or insertions, whereas most of the presumably milder missense mutations were reported in males. It seems likely that females with mild missense mutations tend to be overlooked, whereas boys with more severe deletion or insertion mutations die in utero (146). Unlike many metabolic disorders, PDH deficiency can be associated with malformations of the brain, ranging from cortical heterotopias and partial agenesis of the posterior corpus callosum to an olivopontocerebellar atrophy (147).

Although ornithine transcarbamylase (OTC) is not present in the brain (it functions mostly in the liver to convert waste nitrogen exported from the brain and elsewhere into excretable urea), the clinical phenotype associated with its deficiency is a profound encephalopathy (148). The disease is usually recognized by neonatologists in hemizygous males, who typically present in the first days of life with an alkalotic hyperammonemia, which, if left undiagnosed and untreated, leads to coma with massive brain swelling and death over a period of days

(149). Many heterozygous girls are unaffected. Others develop a lifelong habit of avoiding meat and other protein-rich foods. Some heterozygotes decompensate at times of fasting, viral infections, or other catabolic stresses into intermittent episodes of personality change and ataxia that can evolve over hours into stupor or even death from increased intracranial pressure. Initial episodes of hyperammonemic coma can occur quite late in life, as postpartum coma (150) and after initiation of valproic acid therapy (151). More commonly, metabolic decompensation in heterozygote females is self-limited. There appears, however, to be a strong correlation between long-term decrease in intellectual performance in heterozygotes and the number of such spells of metabolic decompensation that were left undiagnosed and untreated (152). In a given sibship, the phenotype of affected males can be so much more severe than that of affected sisters that neither parents nor physicians appreciate that they are suffering from the same disorder. The availability of effective dietary and pharmacologic treatment for this disorder makes failure of diagnosis particularly tragic (153,154), especially given a heterozygote frequency of 1:25,000 that makes it at least as common as Guillain-Barré syndrome. Metabolic competence of female OTC heterozygotes can be assessed noninvasively, without recourse to a liver biopsy (155).

In other X-linked enzymopathies, female involvement has only been observed in exceptional circumstances. *Hunter syndrome (MPS II)*, the only X-linked mucopolysaccharidosis, is a dwarfing dysostosis with atlantoaxial instability and hydrocephalus, coarse facies, intimal cardiac defects, and deafness in hemizygous boys. The full syndrome has been observed in a girl who was one of a pair of discordant identical twins (156) [strongly reminiscent of the assymetric lyonization seen in DMD female twins, as discussed above (68)] and also in a girl with a deletion of band Xq25, resulting in consistent lyonization of that chromosome, with active expression only from the other X chromosome, inherited from her mother, a biochemically proven heterozygote for iduronate 2-sulfatase (157).

X-Linked Nonprogressive Encephalopathies

A large number of disorders present with nonprogressive mental retardation, either with or without obvious structural malformations of the nervous system. More males are mentally retarded than are females (158). Although this disproportion may result in part from sex-limited or sex-modified expression of well-established autosomal traits, it seems likely that much of it results from mutations of an as yet unspecified number of genes located on the X chromosome, which give rise to phenotypes that segregate for the most part as recessives, with no detectable abnormality in women. However, in a few of these disorders, phenotypic expression occurs in females, usually quite minor compared with that of hemizygous males.

X-linked mental retardation can conveniently be divided into two general classes: (i) syndromic mental retardation, in which associated clinical or anatomic features permit a specific diagnosis; and (ii) nonspecific mental retardation syndromes, in which mental retardation segregates through a pedigree in a sex-linked pattern, but with no clinical features other than genetic linkage relationships to permit distinguishing one from another. There are currently 105 such mental retardation syndromes, which likely will collapse to 10 to 12 loci encoding multiple allelic syndromes after all the relevant genes have been identified and used to classify reported kinships (159).

The most common of the X-linked mental retardation syndromes is the *Martin-Bell fragile X-A syndrome*, representing 560 cases in a survey of 682 cases of syndromic X-linked mental retardation made by Fryns (1). FRAX-A is a syndrome of mental retardation, mild facial dysmorphism, and testicular enlargement, associated with expansions of an extragenic triplet repeat that leads to fragility of the chromosome in folate-deficient tissue culture medium. This chromosomal fragility previously served as the basis of a diagnostic test before more convenient and reliable DNA-based tests became available. Unlike many of the other X-linked mental retardation syndromes, involvement of women is frequent and can be severe. A large majority of female heterozygotes have an IQ of less than 85 (160) and a clinically unexpected decrease in the size of the posterior cerebellar vermis (161). The severity of mental impairment correlates with the proportion of active fragile X chromosomes. Other features of the fragile X syndrome are seen less frequently in heterozygous women. Approximately 40% of affected adult women show other phenotypic characteristics, including the typical square-jawed face, irregular teeth, and ligamentous laxity in the fingers (160). Typical facial characteristics are more noticeable in women than in girls. Two additional fragile sites appear on the X chromosome (as well as dozens on autosomes), *FRAX-E* (162) and *FRAX-F*; the former has been implicated by some studies as another cause of X-linked mental retardation. Cryptic deletions at the FRAX-E site appear to be associated with *premature ovarian failure* (163).

The next most common form of syndromic X-linked mental retardation, albeit mild, is the dysmorphic *Aarskog-Scott faciogenital dysplasia syndrome*, representing 60 of 682 cases in Fryns's survey (1). This results from mutations of a Cdc42 guanine nucleotide exchange factor, possibly a regulator of the subcortical actin cytoskeleton and Golgi complex (164). Serious mental deficiency is unusual in this syndrome, but mild impairment of cognitive function is frequently seen in males. Identifying stigmata in affected boys are a peculiar "shawl scrotum," moderate short stature with brachydactyly, and a distinctive facial appearance consisting of ocular hypertelorism with slight upslanting "antimongoloid" palpebral fissures, anteverted nares, a broad upper lip, and a "peculiar curved linear dimple of the inferior lower lip" (165). Typically, this dimple is one of the facial stigmata seen along with other facial and hand abnormalities as the sole manifestation in females. The full syndrome, however, was reported in a woman with an X-autosome translocation and consistent inactivation of the normal X (166). A significant cause of preventable neurologic deficit in this syndrome is atlantoaxial instability resulting from an abnormal dens and unusual laxity of the cruciate ligament.

The next most frequent syndromic X-linked mental retardation syndrome (representing 20 of Fryns's 682 cases) is the *Coffin-Lowry syndrome*, the distinguishing features of which are tapering fingers and coarse facial features, with patulous lips, bulbous nose, prominent brow, and downslanting "mongoloid" palpebral fissures (166), resulting from mutation of the RSK2 kinase gene (167), a regulator of chromatin structure, as is the gene product underlying Rett syndrome (168). Some affected individuals develop a compressive myelopathy form of excessive calcification of the ligamentum flavum (169) as well as extensive diverticular disease from a visceral neuropathy (170). Unlike in the Aarskog-Scott males, mental deficiency in Coffin-Lowry males is usually severe, the IQ of affected hemizygote males being 43.2, and of heterozygous females, 65 (171). There have also been several reports of mildly affected females with a depressive mood disorder (172) as well as the distinctive hand, facial, and visceral manifestations.

Facies sufficiently similar to cause diagnostic confusion with the Coffin-Lowry syndrome are seen in the nondeletion type of alpha-thalassemia mental retardation syndrome (173), most conveniently diagnosed by demonstration of hemoglobin H inclusions on a blood smear of affected boys. Similar inclusions were seen in very rare erythrocytes of female carriers, who were otherwise unaffected except for some similarity of facial features. Although intellectual impairment of true genotypic females has not been described, one can easily be misled. Abnormalities of external genitalia commonly seen in this syndrome have led to female sex rearing of affected XY individuals (174).

A disorder of similar frequency to that of Coffin-Lowry syndrome, 18 of 682 syndromic mental X-linked retardation cases in Fryns's survey (1), was his own *Lujan-Fryns syndrome* of mental retardation, psychosis, marfanoid habitus, as well as a distinctive long, narrow face with a high-arched palate and small mandible. Only one manifesting carrier female has been described (175).

Several X-linked static encephalopathies without distinguishing systemic or dysmorphic features can be diagnosed because of characteristic neuroanatomic abnormalities, recognizable by scanning or at post mortem. There have been reports of families segregating an apparently X-linked migration disorder in which males are lissencephalic and women have band heterotopias (176)—failure of migration of neurons comprising layers 5 and 6, particularly in the frontal and parietal lobes—detectable by scanning (177). This has been called the *double cortex syndrome*. Most affected women are mentally retarded and all have epilepsy, some severely so.

Several other rarer syndromic X-linked mental retardation syndromes exist in which karyotypically normal female carriers have normal intelligence, but do show some of the associated noncerebral manifestations typical of affected males. These minor anomalies are usually trivial, of no clinical importance to the affected woman except, of course, as sentinel signs warning of carrier status for a disorder that will be devastating to half of her male offspring. With few exceptions, including a woman with a balanced X-autosome translocation (178), the only manifestation in female carriers of *Lowe oculocerebrorenal syndrome* are mild "snowflake" lenticular opacities, which are asymptomatic but provide a sensitive and specific method of carrier detection (179). Similarly, some female carriers of the gene for *syndromic X-linked mental retardation-type 4* with congenital contractures and low fingertip arches usually have only a fingerprint pattern of low digital arches (180); carriers of the *Fitzsimmons mental retardation-spastic paraplegia-palmoplantar hyperkeratosis syndrome* have only palmoplantar hyperkeratosis (181); female carriers of the *Christian mental retardation abducens palsy and skeletal dysplasia syndrome* may have fusion of cervical vertebrae and short middle phalanges (182); female relatives of boys with the *FG syndrome* of mental retardation, large head, and imperforate anus, have normal intelligence but can have lateral displacement of the inner canthi and anterior displacement of the anus (183); the only manifestation in a mother of a boy severely affected with *Lenz dysplasia* (microphthalmia, mental retardation, and skeletal anomalies), was a deformity of the fifth finger (184).

SEX-LIMITED DISEASES

A difference in disease expression in men and women does not imply that the disorder results from a mutation of a gene located on an X chromosome. A variety of anatomic, hormonal, and behavioral differences between the sexes can alter the expression of autosomally encoded and nongenetic disorders. Indeed, this is the subject matter of this entire book. In this section, I confine my comments to effects of pregnancy on common autosomal disorders affecting the nervous system.

Toxemia of Pregnancy

Among the most serious disorders encountered during pregnancy or shortly after delivery are pre-eclampsia, which is characterized by hypertension, edema, and proteinuria, and the more severe condition of eclampsia, in which there are superimposed neurologic symptoms of seizures and coma (see also Chapter 16). Studies of mother-daughter pairs have given evidence of a possible genetic susceptibility to this spectrum of disorders (185). Multiple studies have suggested that eclampsia occurs in women who are homozygous for a relatively common susceptibility gene(s) (186). At least one factor in such susceptibility appears to be a common variant in the gene encoding angiotensin (187).

Exacerbations of Preexisting Hereditary Disorders during Pregnancy

A question that frequently arises in the management of women with genetic disorders is whether pregnancy will further jeopardize the affected woman's health. In some disorders, this important question has been studied systematically; in others, answers to this important question are anecdotal. In *type IV Ehlers-Danlos syndrome*, the form associated with fragility of intracerebral and systemic blood vessels, there is a 25% mortality rate associated with each pregnancy. Death occurs from a variety of causes including rupture of the aorta, vena cava, uterus, or bowel (188). We have observed intracranial hemorrhage during pregnancy in women with *familial intracranial cavernous hemangiomas* (189). Others have observed development of large extracerebral cavernous malformations with subsequent high-output cardiac failure during pregnancy, followed by rapid resolution after delivery (190). Rupture of aortic aneurysms during pregnancy has been observed in the *Marfan syndrome* (191), with some survivors suffering infarction of the spinal cord. Epidural anesthesia, which is commonly used in delivery, poses a significant risk of persistent leakage of cerebrospinal fluid in marfanoid women, who have very thin, often ectatic dural sacs. Serious thrombotic disease in either the arterial or venous circulation, systemically or in the CNS, has been observed in patients with *antithrombin III deficiency* (192), and this problem is exacerbated by pregnancy.

A single case has been reported of intraspinal hemorrhage from a hemangioblastoma in a pregnant woman with *von Hippel Lindau* (VHL) syndrome (193). Another consideration in managing pregnancies in women with VHL is the presence of pheochromocytomas, which occur in 5.2% of all affected individuals (194). Pheochromocytomas occur in lower frequency in *von Recklinghausen neurofibromatosis* (NF I). These are but one of several factors contributing to a higher caesarean section rate (36%) in NF I than in the general population (9.1% to 23.5%). Other contributing factors include kyphoscoliosis, pelvic neurofibromata, and spinal cord neurofibromas. Eighty percent of women reported an increase in number or size of neurofibromata during pregnancy, with 33% noting a subsequent decrease in size after delivery (195). In contrast, a systematic study of *bilateral acoustic neurofibromatosis (NF II)* found no adverse effects on acoustic schwannomas or other tumors from either pregnancy or the use of contraceptives (196). There have been anecdotal reports of worsening during pregnancy with *Charcot-Marie-Tooth disease IB* (198) and in *familial brachial neuritis* (198).

Pregnancy can unmask metabolic deficiencies that are otherwise inapparent in female carriers of certain autosomal recessive enzymopathies. Infants homozygous for mutations of the alpha subunit of *trifunctional enzyme* (hydroxyacyl-CoA dehydrogenase/3-ketoacyl-CoA thiolase/Enoyl-CoA hydratase) succumb to a Reye-like metabolic encephalopathy, cardiomyopathy, and skeletal myopathy. Their heterozygous mothers are at risk for acute fatty liver of pregnancy (199,200). Acute fatty liver of pregnancy also has been associated with heterozygosity for the beta subunit of trifunctional enzyme, long chain 3-hydroxyacyl-CoA dehydrogenase (201). Similar mutations more commonly give rise to hyperemesis gravidarum or to the *HELLP syndrome*, consisting of hypertension or hemolysis, elevated liver enzymes, and low platelets (202). Pregnancy has been reported to induce photosensitivity, neurobehavioral manifestations, and jaundice in hereditary coproporphyria (203). Weakness of the intrinsic hand muscles recurred in the seventh month of pregnancy and resolved 6 months later in a woman affected with a newly described autosomal dominant neuronopathy associated with cataracts and skeletal abnormalities (204).

TRANSMISSION OF GENETIC DISEASES BY WOMEN

Chromosomal Abnormalities

In the general population, the major concern about the maternal transmission of neurogenetic disease comes from chromosomal abnormalities—additional or missing copies of an entire chromosome (aneuploidy). Anywhere from 15% to 50% of all pregnancies are lost in the first 12 weeks, approximately half of them from chromosomal abnormalities. Only a few aneuploidies permit survival of the fetus until birth: (i) aneuploidies of sex chromosomes, including approximately 1% of Turner cases (presumed mosaics); (ii) partial autosomal trisomies or monosomies, in which only a part of an autosome is duplicated or missing; and (iii) complete trisomy of the smaller autosomes, with 21 causing Down syndrome, 18 causing Edward syndrome, and 13 causing Patau syndrome (2). All such autosomal aneuploidies cause profound neurologic deficits, intrauterine growth retardation, characteristic patterns of dysmorphism, and malformation. Complete aneuploidies result from nondisjunction, or errors of chromosome segregation during meiosis, particularly in the first meiotic division. A dramatic increase in the rate of nondisjunction corresponds with advanced maternal age, with a sharp increase at age 35 years.

X-Linked Inheritance

Sexual differences in disease transmission arise by any of several mechanisms, not all of which are genetic. X-linked inheritance has been extensively considered earlier in this chapter. To recapitulate, men transmit their single X chromosome to their daughters, and their single Y chromosome to their sons. Male-to-male transmission of a disorder rules out X-linked inheritance. Mothers transmit either their maternal or paternal X chromosome at random to either their daughters or their sons.

Mitochondrial Inheritance

Mothers exclusively provide mitochondrial DNA to offspring of either sex. Not all mitochondrial DNA disorders are maternally transmitted, however (205). The pattern of transmission relates in part to the severity of the mitochondrial mutation. Point mutations of protein-coding genes that minimally disrupt enzymatic activity underlie all known forms of *Leber's optic atrophy* (206). Such mutations typically are present in homoplasmic (i.e., identical mitochondrial DNA in every cell) form in affected individuals and are transmitted by affected mothers to all their children of either sex, all of whom develop peripapillary telangiectasias of the retina. For reasons that are not yet understood, however, homoplasmic men are seven times as likely to develop optic atrophy as are women. A hypothesized X-linked modifier gene has recently been disproved (207). Point mutations of intermediate severity, such as those disrupting tRNA genes in *MELAS* (208) or *MERRF* (209) syndromes, or the ATPase subunit 6 gene in one form of *Leigh's disease* (210) are only tolerated in heteroplasmic form, with survival only permitted by the compensatory presence of at least some normal mitochondrial DNA in each cell. Therefore, mosaic women transmit these mutations to their children in different proportions, with resultant differences in phenotypic severity. The deletion mutations of mitochondrial DNA, responsible for the *Kearns-Sayre syndrome* and the closely related *chronic progressive external ophthalmoplegia* (211), are the most severe. They, too, are present in heteroplasmic form, but with rare exceptions appear as de novo mutations in affected individuals and are not transmitted from mother to child. Although a specific mitochondrial DNA deletion mutation has never been transmitted from generation to generation, a tendency to generate new mitochondrial DNA deletions segregates as an autosomal dominant trait, the *multiple mitochondrial DNA deletion syndrome* (212), the result of mutation of an as yet unidentified nuclear-encoded protein that in some way disrupts mitochondrial DNA. Being autosomal dominant, this disorder can be transmitted by either an affected father or mother.

Genomic Imprinting

Other sexual differences in disease transmission result from genomic imprinting—the epigenetic inactivation of certain autosomal regions in a pattern that differs between spermatogenesis and oogenesis. As a result of such imprinting, certain autosomal regions inherited from the mother are not equivalent to those inherited from the father. Although well-established in animals, the evidence for imprinting in humans is still indirect, coming mostly from the observations of two neurogenetic syndromes that result from similar mutations in 15q11-13 (213).

The *Prader-Willi syndrome* of moderate mental retardation, hypotonia, and failure to grow in infancy, followed by hypothalamic hyperphagia and obesity, results either from deletions of 15q11-13 of the paternally derived chromosome or from isodisomy for maternal chromosome 15. Another more profound and easily distinguishable neurologic syndrome of profound mental retardation and cerebellar ataxia, the *Angelman syndrome*, can also result from isodisomy 15 or deletions of 15q11-13. Angelman syndrome cases, however, have paternal isodisomy or deletion of maternal 15q11-13, the reverse of the Prader-Willi syndrome.

Expansion of Triplet Repeats

An increasing number of neurogenetic disorders result from the instability of those stretches of DNA that contain multiple copies of the same trinucleotide, which are referred to as triplet repeats. A certain amount of repetition is tolerable, but beyond a certain length, deleterious effects occur. The triplet repeats underlying FRAX-A and myotonic dystrophy lie in noncoding regions and appear to exert their effects by altering the transcription of the neighboring gene(s). In contrast, the triplet repeats in the olivopontocerebellar atrophies and Huntington disease are intragenic and encode polyglutamine tracts that directly disrupt the function of the protein into which they are inserted. In both cases, the greater the length of the triplet repeat, the more deleterious its effect. The number of trinucleotides in a repeat tends to increase each time the DNA is replicated, particularly during the formation of gametes. This causes "anticipation"—greater severity and earlier onset of disease in subsequent generations. For reasons not yet understood, the tendency of such triplet repeats to increase in length can be different in oogenesis than during spermatogenesis. This inequality explains why the severe childhood-onset *Westphal variant of Huntington disease* only occurs when the mutation is inherited from the father (214). In contrast, the *severe infantile form of myotonic dystrophy* only occurs when the transmitting parent is the mother, but for a different reason. Sperm are sensitive to the genes affected in myotonic dystrophy, with a resultant censoring of extreme expansions of paternal mutations; sperm with large expansions in this region do not keep up with their fellows that have a smaller repeat length. By default, extreme expansions of the myotonic dystrophy type are only observed when the original mutation is transmitted by the mother (215).

Neural Tube Defects (NTDs)

Both genetic and nongenetic factors contribute to the formation of *spina bifida*, which ranks with chromosomal abnormalities as a major cause of neurologic malformations detectable before birth. The major identified nongenetic factor is maternal deficiency in folic acid at the time of conception. All women of childbearing age at risk for pregnancy are advised to take dietary supplements. The U.S. Department of Agriculture is undertaking a program of folate supplementation of common foodstuffs to ensure that women are not deficient in folate at the time of unplanned conception. Risk from both dietary and genetic factors can be calculated from the experience in previous pregnancies. In the absence of previously affected siblings, the risk of anencephaly and spina bifida is 0.3% to 0.87% (216,217); with one affected sibling, the risk is from 4.4% to 5.2%; with two affected siblings, the risk increases to 10%; and with three, to 25% (218).

Nongenetic Transmission

The transmission of neurologic or psychiatric disorders from one generation to another is not always mediated by DNA. A well-studied example of nongenetic maternal transmission of neurologic disease is *phenylketonuria* (PKU). Irrespective of their own genotype, children whose mothers were not in good metabolic control during their pregnancies have a much higher frequency of hypoplasia of the corpus callosum, microcephaly, intrauterine growth retardation, and congenital heart disease than do those whose mothers were in good control (219). Indeed, all children born to PKU mothers, well-controlled or not, suffer some degree of hyperactivity and other behavioral disorders (220). Metabolic abnormalities in mothers affected with other genetic enzymopathies are anecdotally reported to be harmful to genetically normal fetuses. For example, maternal hypoglycemia in a woman affected with *von Gierke glycogen storage disease* was suggested to be responsible for unexpected fetal death at 33 weeks' gestation (221).

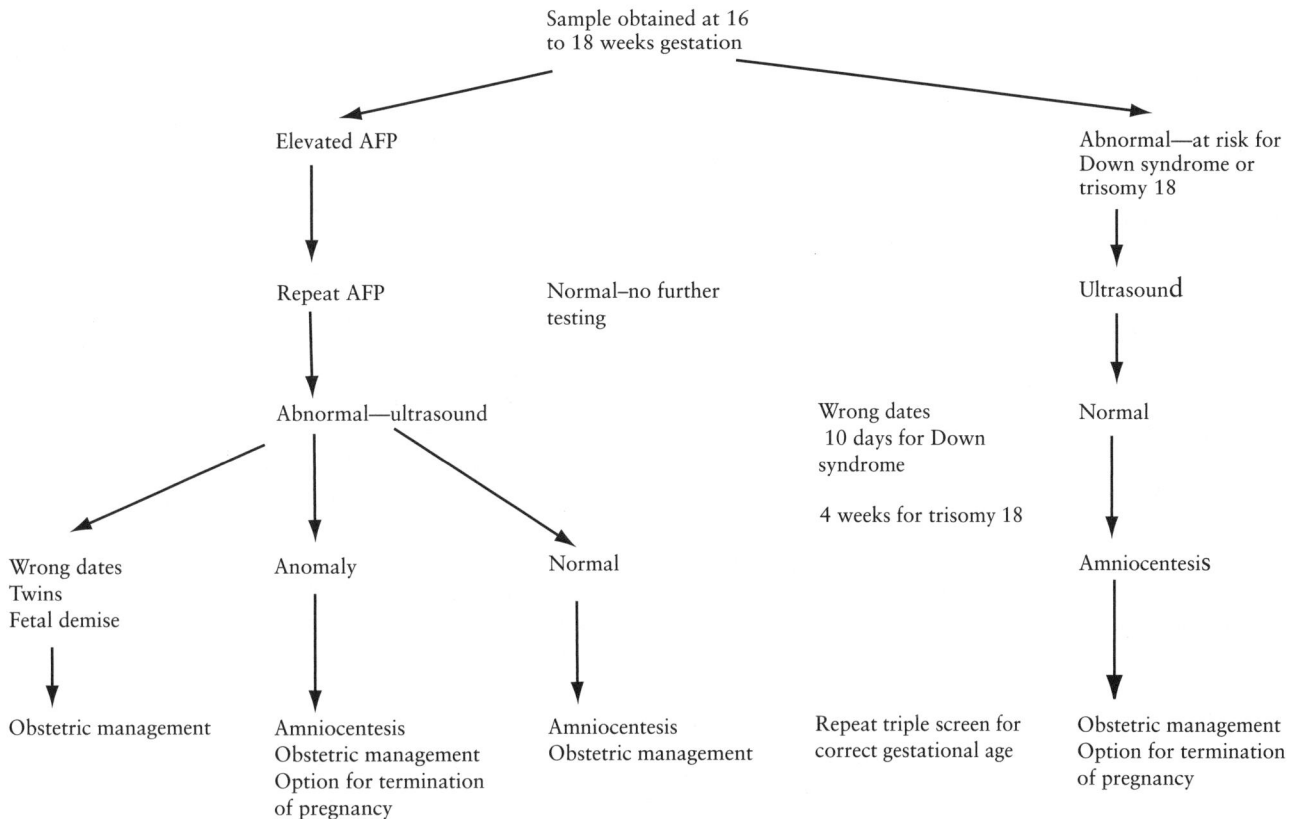

FIGURE 7.1

Triple screen procedure.

In addition to mitochondrial DNA and small metabolites, mothers exclusively provide the developing fetus with other important nongenetic, cytoplasmic factors, such as drugs, immunoglobulins, and transmissible pathogens, among them *toxoplasmosis*, *cytomegalovirus*, and the *AIDS retrovirus*. Furthermore, in most societies, there are significant differences in postnatal interaction with offspring, many of which have substantial influence on the transmission or expression of disease. These myriad, potentially sex-specific influences range from breast milk and subsequent choice of diet to language, other learned behaviors, and socioeconomic status.

Genetic Counseling

Screening for NTDs and chromosomal abnormalities has become standard obstetric care. Special testing is advised in cases of advanced maternal age and in women who had previously given birth to children with aneuploidy or NTDs. In many states, all pregnant women undergo "triple screening," which consists of testing of a venous blood specimen for alpha-fetoprotein, estriol, and human chorionic gonadotropin, at 16 to 18 weeks' gestational age. Abnormalities in this initial screening lead to rec-

ommendations for repeat testing, sonography, or amniocentesis, according to a protocol such as the one depicted in Figure 7.1. Such protocols have been devised to offer a meaningful balance of risk, cost, and provision of meaningful information from which the mother can make an informed decision about continuation of the pregnancy.

Other neurogenetic disorders can be of concern either because of a positive family history or if parents come from ethnic backgrounds in which heterozygosity for certain recessive disorders is frequent. In the latter category is Tay-Sachs disease, for which approximately 1 of 30 Ashkenazim and a similar number of French-Canadians are heterozygotes (1). Testing for heterozygosity by biochemical testing has been widely sought by prospective spouses to inform their choice of marriage partner and other reproductive options.

A positive family history for other neurogenetic disorders can lead to special counseling and testing that would not otherwise be part of routine obstetric care. Central to such endeavors is the accurate diagnosis of affected family members. Although some of these disorders can be detected biochemically or by determination of DNA markers (Table 7.1 and 7.2), for the majority the diagnosis must be made clinically. Indeed, given the

TABLE 7.1

X-Linked Neurogenetic Disorders Seen (Almost) Exclusively in Females

Definite
- Aicardi syndrome
- CHILD syndrome (congenital hemidysplasia, ichthyosiform erythroderma, and limb defects)
- Chondrodysplasia punctata, X-linked dominant form
- Incontinentia pigmenti, type II
- Microphthalmia with linear skin defects
- Periventricular heterotopias
- Rett syndrome

Probable
- Wildervanck syndrome (deafness, Klippel-Feil anomaly, and Duane syndrome)

Possible
- CODAS syndrome (cerebral, ocular, dental, auricular, skeletal)
- Hemizygous lethal muscular dystrophy

current high costs of biochemical and DNA tests, "shotgun" laboratory testing for neurogenetic disorders is not a viable option; an informed clinician must choose what tests are appropriate in a given circumstance. Once the diagnosis of the affected relative(s) is secure, the genetic counselor uses this information along with a knowledge of the pattern of inheritance to calculate the risk to the fetus. In many circumstances, the risk may be sufficient to advise special diagnostic testing by amniocentesis or chorionic villus sampling.

The list of disorders for which such testing is available is growing monthly (1). Some of these tests are available commercially, others only through special arrangement with research laboratories. Other changes in this rapidly evolving technology may soon include sampling of rare fetal cells in the maternal circulation, avoiding some of the cost and the 1 in 300 complication rate associated with amniocentesis. However the technology changes, certain things will remain constant. As in all branches of medicine, the obligation of the physician is to inform, not to coerce. The recognition of risk for a neu-

TABLE 7.2

X-Linked Neurogenetic Disorders Seen in Males and Females

MUSCLE DISORDERS

DISORDER	OMIM	LOCUS	GENE PRODUCT
Duchenne/Becker muscular dystrophy	310200	Xp21.1	Dystrophin
Emery-Dreifuss tardive dystrophy with contractures	310300	Xq28	Emerine, serine-rich vesicular transport protein
Scapuloperoneal muscular dystrophy, mental retardation, and lethal cardiomyopathy	309660	X	
Myotubular myopathy	310400	Xq28	MTM1 myotubularin, putative tyrosine phosphatase
Fingerprint myopathy	305550	X	
Phosphoglycerate kinase deficiency	311800	311800	PGK-I

PERIPHERAL NEUROPATHIES

DISORDER	OMIM	LOCUS	GENE PRODUCT
Charcot-Marie-Tooth, X-linked dominant (CMTX1)	302800	XP11.3	Connexin 32, gap junction protein
Charcot-Marie-Tooth, X-linked recessive (CMTX2)	302801	Xp22.2	
Charcot-Marie-Tooth, X-linked recessive (CMTX3)	302802	Xp26	
Charcot-Marie-Tooth, 2D (Cowchock variant with deafness and mental retardation)	310490	Xq24-q26. 1	
Charcot-Marie-Tooth, with deafness and optic atrophy (Rosenberg-Chutorian disease)	311070	X	
Charcot-Marie-Tooth, with aplasia cutis congenita	302803	X	
Fabry disease (angiokeratoma diffusa)	301500	Xq22	Alpha galactosidase

(continued)

TABLE 7.2

X-Linked Neurogenetic Disorders Seen in Males and Females (Continued)

DISORDER	OMIM	LOCUS	GENE PRODUCT
External ophthalmoplegia and myopia in women	311000	X	

ANTERIOR HORN CELL DISORDERS

DISORDER	OMIM	LOCUS	GENE PRODUCT
Spinal muscular atrophy, X-linked	301830	Xp11.3-q11.2	
Lethal infantile (distal arthrogryposis multiplex congenita)		X	

SPASTIC PARAPARESES

DISORDER	OMIM	LOCUS	GENE PRODUCT
Adrenomyeloneuropathy	300100	Xq28	Peroxisomal ATP-binding transport protein
MASA syndrome	303350	Xq28	L-CAM cell adhesion molecule
Spastic paraplegia 2	312920	Xq22	Proteolipid protein
Spastic paraplegia/Kallman syndrome	308750	X ?	

PROGRESSIVE ATAXIAS

DISORDER	OMIM	LOCUS	GENE PRODUCT
Menkes kinky-hair disease	309400	Xq13.2-q13.3	Cu(2+)-transporting ATPase, alpha polypeptide
Pelizaeus-Merzbacher	312080	Xq28	Proteolipid protein
PRPS deficiency	311850	Xq22-q24	Phosphoribosyl pyrophosphate synthetase
X-linked cerebellar ataxia (X-linked OPCA included)	302500	X	
X-linked ataxia-deafness syndrome	301790	X	
Arts fatal X-linked ataxia syndrome	301835	X	

MOVEMENT DISORDERS

DISORDER	OMIM	LOCUS	GENE PRODUCT
Lesch-Nyhan syndrome	308000	X	Hypoxanthine-guanine phosphoribosyl-transferase
Torsion-dystonia 3 with parkinsonism, Filipino type	314250	Xq12-q13.1	
Waisman early-onset parkinsonism and mental retardation	311510	Xq28	
Pettigrew MRXSS syndrome: basal ganglia disease, Dandy-Walker malformation with mental retardation and seizures	304340	Xq25-q27	
HHHH syndrome (hereditary hemihypotrophy hemiparesis hemiathetosis)	306960	X?	
Goeminne TKCR syndrome (torticollis, keloids, cryptorchidism, renal dysplasia)	314300	Xq28	

(continued)

TABLE 7.2

X-Linked Neurogenetic Disorders Seen in Males and Females (Continued)

METABOLIC ENCEPHALOPATHIES

DISORDER	OMIM	LOCUS	GENE PRODUCT
Lesch-Nyhan syndrome	308000	X	Hypoxanthine-guanine phosphoribosyl-transferase
PRPS deficiency	311850	Xq22-q24	Phosphoribosyl pyrophosphate synthetase
Pyruvate dehydrogenase deficiency	312170	Xp22.2-p22.1	Pyruvate dehydrogenase subunit
Ornithine transcarbamylase deficiency	311250	Xp21.1	Ornithine/transcarbamylase
Hunter syndrome	309900	X	Iduronate 2-sulfatase

NONPROGRESSIVE ENCEPHALOPATHIES

DISORDER	OMIM	LOCUS	GENE PRODUCT
Fragile X-A mental retardation and macroorchidism (Martin-Bell syndrome)	309550	Xq27.3	FMR-1 ribosome RNA binding associated protein
Fragile X-E mental retardation	309548	Xq28	Transcript with expanded triplet repeat
Miles-Carpenter X-linked MR (syndromic 4), with congenital contractures and low fingertip arches	309605	Xq13-q22	

NONPROGRESSIVE ENCEPHALOPATHIES

DISORDER	OMIM	LOCUS	GENE PRODUCT
X-linked MR (syndromic 5), with Dandy-Walker malformation, basal ganglia disease, and seizures	304340	Xq25-q27	
Occipital horn/cutis laxa syndrome	304150	Xq12-q13	Copper transporting ATPase
Aarskog-Scott faciogenital dysplasia syndrome	305400	Xp11.21	FGDl putative signal transduction protein with RAS-like RHO/RAC guanine nucleotide exchange factors
Coffin-Lowry syndrome	303600	Xp22.2-22.1	RSK 2 gene
Alpha-thalassemia/ MR; ATR-X syndrome: MR with characteristic face, genital anomalies, and alpha-halassemia	301040	Xq13.1-q21.1	Helicase 2
Lujan-Fryns MR with marfanoid habitus	309520	X	
Fitzsimmons MR with spastic paraplegia and palmoplantar hyperkeratosis	309560		
Lowe oculocerebrorenal syndrome	309000	X26.1	
Christian syndrome (MR, skeletal dysplasia and abducens palsy)	309620	Xq28	
FG syndrome (MR, macrocephaly, imperforate anus, partial agenesis of corpus callosum)	305450	X	
Lenz dysplasia (MR, microphthalmia, and associated anomalies)	309800	X	
MASA syndrome (MR, clasped thumbs)	303350	Xq28	L1 cell adhesion molecule LCAM [308840]
X-linked MR-skeletal dysplasia	309620	Xq28	

rogenetic disorder in her offspring requires that the woman be informed. What is done with that information is her choice.

Acknowledgments

I thank Mrs. Cathleen Escallon for information about triple screening, and Dr. Steven Hawes for bioinformatic information.

References

1. Online Mendelian Inheritance in Man OMIM (TM). Center for Medical Genetics, Johns Hopkins University (Baltimore, MD) and National Center for Biotechnology Information, National Library of Medicine (Bethesda, MD), 1996. World Wide Web URL: http://www3.ncbi.nlm.nih.gov/omim/.
2. Smith DW. *Recognizable patterns of human malformation.* Philadelphia, Pa: WB Saunders, 1981.
3. Ensembl Human release 11.31.1, http://www.ensembl.org/Homo_sapiens/mapview?chr=X and http://www.ensembl.org/Homo_sapiens/stats/, March 31, 2003.
4. Murphy EA, Chase GA. *Principles of genetic counselling.* Chicago, Il: Yearbook Medical Publishers, 1975.
5. Morgan TH. Sex limited inheritance in Drosophila. *Science* 1920;32:120–122.
6. Ohno S. *Sex-chromosomes and sex-linked genes.* Berlin: Springer, 1967.
7. Myers RH, Leavitt J, Farrer LA, et al. Homozygote for Huntington disease. *Am J Hum Genet* 1989;45:615–618.
8. Lyon MF. X-chromosome inactivation and developmental patterns in mammals. *Biol Rev* 1972;47:1–35.
9. Migeon BR. Selection and cell communication as determinants of female phenotype. In: Subtelny S, Sussex IM, (eds.) *The clonal basis of development.* New York, NY: Academic Press, 1978:205–218.
10 Prachal JT, Carroll AJ, Prachal JF, et al. Wiskott-Aldrich syndrome: cellular impairments and their implication for carrier detection. *Blood* 1980;56:1048–1054.
11. Happle, R. Incontinentia pigmenti versus hypomelanosis of Ito: the whys and wherefores of a confusing issue. (Letter) *Am J Med Genet* 1998;79:64–65.
12. Smahi A, Hyden-Granskog C, Peterlin B, et al. The gene for the familial form of incontinentia pigmenti (Ip2) maps to the distal part of Xp28. *Hum Mol Genet* 1994;3:273–278.
13. The International Incontinentia Pigmenti Consortium. Genomic rearrangement in NEMO impairs NF-kappa-B activation and is a cause of incontinentia pigmenti. *Nature* 2000;405:466–472.
14. Parrish JE, Scheuerle AE, Lewis RA, et al. Selection against mutant alleles in blood leukocytes is a consistent feature in incontinentia pigmenti type 2. *Hum Molec Genet* 1996;5:1777–1783.
15. Garcia-Dorado J, de Unamuno P, Fernandez-Lopez E, et al. Incontinentia pigmenti: XX male with a family history. *Clin Genet* 1990;38:128–138.
16 Kirchman TTT, Levy ML, Lewis RA, Kanzler MH, Nelson DL, Scheuerle AE. Gonadal mosaicism for incontinentia pigmenti in a healthy male. *J Med Genet* 1995;32:887–890.
17. Hodgson SV, Neville B, Jones RWA, et al. Two cases of X/autosome translocation in females with incontinentia pigmenti. *Hum Genet* 1985;71:231–234.
18. Happle R. Tentative assignment of hypomelanosis of Ito to 9q33-qter. *Hum Genet* 1987;75:98–99.
19. Gorlin RJ, Psaume J. Orodigitofacial dysostosis—a new syndrome. *J Pediat* 1962;61:520–530.
20. Selicorni A, Gammaro L, Scolari F, et al. Identification of the gene for oral-facial-digital type I syndrome. *Am J Hum Genet* 2001;68:569–576.
21. Emes RD, Ponting CP. A new sequence motif linking lissencephaly, Treacher Collins and oral-facial-digital type 1 syndromes, microtubule dynamics and cell migration. *Hum Molec Genet* 2001;10:2813–2820.
22. Anneren G, Arvidson B, Gustavson KH, et al. Oro-facio-digital syndromes I and II: radiological methods for diagnosis and the clinical variations. *Clin Genet* 1984;26:178–186.
23. Salinas CF, Pai GS, Vera CL, et al. Variability of expression of the orofaciodigital syndrome type I in black females: six cases. *Am J Med Genet* 1991;38:574–582.
24. Gillespie GA J, Somlo S, Germino GG, et al. CpG island in the region of an autosomal dominant polycystic kidney disease locus defines the 5-prime end of a gene encoding a putative proton channel. *Proc Natl Acad Sci* 1991;88:4289–4293.
25. Bhunia AK, Piontek K, Boletta A, et al. PKD1 induces p21-waf1 and regulation of the cell cycle via direct activation of the JAK-STAT signaling pathway in a process requiring PKD2. *Cell* 2002;109:157–168.
26. Wettke-Schafer R, Kantner G. X-linked dominant inherited diseases with lethality in hemizygous males. *Hum Genet* 1983;64:1–23.
27. Konig A, Happle R, Bornholdt D, et al. Mutations in the NSDHL gene, encoding a 3-beta-hydroxysteroid dehydrogenase, cause CHILD syndrome. *Am J Med Gene* 2000;90:339–346.
28. Happle R, Koch H, Lenz W. The CHILD syndrome: congenital hemidysplasia with ichthyosiform erythroderma and limb defects. *Eur J Pediat* 1980;134:27–33.
29. Tang TT, McCreadie SR. Congenital hemidysplasia with ichthyosis. *Birth Defects Orig Art Ser* 1974;10:257–261.
30. Hebert AA, Esterly NB, Holbrook KA, et al. The CHILD syndrome: histologic and ultrastructural studies. *Arch Derm* 1987;123:503–509.
31. Kelley RI, Wilcox, WG, Smith M, et al. Abnormal sterol metabolism in patients with Conradi-Hunermann-Happle syndrome and sporadic lethal chondrodysplasia punctata. *Am J Med Genet* 1999;83:213–219.
32. Manzke H, Christophers E, Weidemann HR. Dominant sex-linked inherited chondrodysplasia punctata: a distinct type of chondrodysplasia punctata. *Clin Genet* 1980;17:97–107.
33. Mabuchi A, Kura H, Yokoyama Y, et al. Skewed X-chromosome inactivation causes intra-familial phenotypic variation of an EBP mutation in a family with X-linked dominant chondrodysplasia punctata. *Hum Genet* 2003;112:78–83.
34. Schaefer L, Ballabio A, Zoghbi HY. Cloning and characterization of a putative human holocytochrome c-type synthetase gene (HCCS) isolated from the critical region for microphthalmia with linear skin defects (MLS). *Genomics* 1996;34:166–172.
35. Anguiano A, Yang X, Felix JK, et al. Twin brothers with MIDAS syndrome and XX karyotype. *Am J Med Genet* 2003;119A:47–49.
36. Aicardi J, Chevrie JJ, Rousselie F. Le syndrome des spasmes en flexion, agénésie calleuse, anomalies chorio-rétiniennes. *Arch Franc Pediat* 1969;26:1103–1120.

37. Donnenfeld AE, Packer RJ, Zackai EH, et al. Clinical, cytogenetic, and pedigree findings in 18 cases of Aicardi syndrome. *Am J Med Genet* 1989;32:461–467.

38. Neidich JA, Nussbaum RL, Packer RJ, et al. Heterogeneity of clinical severity and molecular lesions in Aicardi syndrome. *J Pediat* 1990;116:911–917.

39. Trifiletti RR, Incorpora G, Polizzi A, et al. Aicardi syndrome with multiple tumors: a case report with literature review. *Brain Dev* 1995;17:283–285.

40. Tsao CY, Sommer A, Hamoudi AB. Aicardi syndrome, metastatic angiosarcoma of the leg, and scalp lipoma. *Am J Med Genet* 1993;45:594–596.

41. Kamuro K, Tenokuchi Y. Familial periventricular nodular heterotopia. *Brain Dev* 1993;15:237–241.

42. Eksioglu YZ, Scheffer IE, Cardenas P, et al. Periventricular heterotopia: an X-linked dominant epilepsy locus causing aberrant cerebral cortical development. *Neuron* 1996;16:77–87.

43. Hagberg B, Aicardi J, Dias K, et al. A progressive syndrome of autism, dementia, ataxia, and loss of purposeful hand use in girls: Rett's syndrome: Report of 35 cases. *Ann Neurol* 1983;14:471–479.

44. Hagberg BA, Skjeldal OH. Rett variants: a suggested model for inclusion criteria. *Pediat Neurol* 1994;11:5–11.

45. Zoghbi HY, Ledbetter DH, Schultz R, et al. A de novo X;3 translocation in Rett syndrome. *Am J Med Genet* 1990;35:148–151.

46. Journel H, Melki J, Turleau C, et al. Rett phenotype with X/autosome translocation: possible mapping to the short arm of chromosome X. *Am J Med Genet* 1990;35:142–147.

47. Migeon BR, Dunn MA, Thomas G. Studies of X inactivation and isodisomy in twins provide further evidence that the X chromosome is not involved in Rett syndrome. *Am J Hum Genet* 1995;56:647–653.

48. De Bona C, Zappella M, Hayek G, et al. Preserved speech variant is allelic of classic Rett syndrome. *Europ J Hum Genet* 2000;8:325–330.

49. Zappella M, Meloni I, Longo I, et al. Preserved speech variants of the Rett syndrome: molecular and clinical analysis. *Am J Med Genet* 2001;104:14–22.

50. Clayton-Smith J, Watson P, Ramsden S, et al. Somatic mutation in MECP2 as a non-fatal neurodevelopmental disorder in males. *Lancet* 2000;356:830–832.

51. Topcu M, Akyerli C, Sayi A, et al. Somatic mosaicism for a MECP2 mutation associated with classic Rett syndrome in a boy. *Europ J Hum Genet* 2002;10:77–81.

52. Wildervanck LS. The cervico-oculo-acusticus syndrome. In: Vinken PJ, Bruyn GW, Myranthopoulos NC, (eds.) *Handbook of clinical neurology*. Amsterdam: North Holland, 1978;123–130.

53. Cabral de Almeida JC, Vargas FR, Barbosa-Neto JG, et al. CODAS syndrome: a new distinct MCA/MR syndrome with radiological changes of spondyloepiphyseal dysplasia: Another case report. *Am J Med Genet* 1995;55:19–20.

54. Innes AM, Chudley AE, Reed MH, et al. Third case of cerebral, ocular, dental, auricular, skeletal anomalies (CODAS) syndrome, further delineating a new malformation syndrome: first report of an affected male and review of literature. *Am J Med Genet* 2001;102:44–47.

55. Henson TE, Muller J, DeMyer WE. Hereditary myopathy limited to females. *Arch Neurol* 1967;17:238–247.

56. Monaco AP, Neve RL, Colletti-Feener C, et al. Isolation of candidate cDNAs for portions of the Duchenne muscular dystrophy gene. *Nature* 1986;323:646–650.

57. Edwards JH. The population genetics of Duchenne: natural and artifical selection in Duchenne muscular dystrophy. *J Med Genet* 1986;23:521–530.

58. Moser H, Vogt J. Follow-up study of serum creatine-kinase in carriers of Duchenne muscular dystrophy. *Lancet* 1974;ii:291–292.

59. Beggs AH, Koenig M, Boyce FM, et al. Detection of 98 percent of DMD/BMD gene deletions by polymerase chain reaction. *Hum Genet* 1990;86:45–48.

60. Minetti C, Chang HW, Medori R, et al. Dystrophin deficiency in young girls with sporadic myopathy and normal karyotype. *Neurology* 1991;41:1288–1292.

61. Hurko O, McKee L, Zuurveld J, et al. Comparison of Duchenne and normal myoblasts from a heterozygote. *Neurology* 1987;37:675–681.

62. Norman A, Harper P. A survey of manifesting carriers of Duchenne and Becker muscular dystrophy in Wales. *Clin Genet* 1989;36:31–37.

63. Hoffman EP, Arahata K, Minetti C, et al. Dystrophinopathy in isolated cases of myopathy in females. *Neurology* 1992;42:967–975.

64. Chelly J, Marlhens F, Le Marec B, et al. De novo DNA microdeletion in a girl with Turner syndrome and Duchenne muscular dystrophy. *Hum Genet* 1986;74:193–196.

65. Lindenbaum RH, Clarke G, Patel C, Moncrieff M, Hughes JT. Muscular dystrophy in an X;1 translocation female suggests that Duchenne locus is on X chromosome short arm. *J Med Genet* 1979;16:389–392.

66. Richards CS, Watkins SC, Hoffman EP, et al. Skewed X inactivation in a female MZ twin results in Duchenne muscular dystrophy. *Am J Hum Genet* 1990;46:672–681.

67. Lupski JR, Garcia CA, Zoghbi HY, et al. Discordance of muscular dystrophy in monozygotic female twins: evidence supporting asymmetric splitting of the inner cell mass in a manifesting carrier of Duchenne dystrophy. *Am J Med Genet* 1991;40:354–364.

68. Nance WE. Do twin lyons have larger spots? (Editorial). *Am J Hum Genet* 1990;46:646–648.

69. Pegoraro E, Schimke RN, Arahata K, et al. Detection of new paternal dystrophin gene mutations in isolated cases of dystrophinopathy in females. *Am J Hum Genet* 1994;54:989–1003.

70. Mirabella M, Servidei S, Manfredi G. Cardiomyopathy may be the only clinical manifestation in female carriers of Duchenne muscular dystrophy. *Neurology* 1993;43:2342–2345.

71. Towbin JA, Hejtmancik JF, Brink P, et al. X-linked dilated cardiomyopathy: molecular genetic evidence of linkage to the Duchenne muscular dystrophy (dystrophin) gene at the Xp21 locus. *Circulation* 1993;87:1854–1865.

72. Emery AEH. X-linked muscular dystrophy with early contractures and cardiomyopathy (Emery-Dreifuss type). *Clin Genet* 1987;32:360–367.

73. Dickey RP, Ziter FA, Smith RA. Emery-Dreifuss muscular dystrophy. *J Pediat* 1984;104:555–559.

74. Manilal S, Sewry CA, Pereboev A, et al. Distribution of emerin and lamins in the heart and implications for Emery-Dreifuss muscular dystrophy. *Hum Molec Genet* 1999;8:353–359.

75. Bergia B, Sybers HD, Butler IJ. Familial lethal cardiomyopathy with mental retardation and scapuloperoneal muscular dystrophy. *J Neurol Neurosurg Psychiatry* 1986;49:1423–1426.

76. Sugie H, Sugie Y, Tsurui S, Ito M. Phosphoglycerate kinase deficiency. *Neurology* 1994;44:1364–1365.

77. Kraus AP, Langston MF Jr, Lynch BL. Red cell phosphoglycerate kinase deficiency: a new cause of non-spherocytic hemolytic anemia. *Biochem Biophys Res Commun* 1968;30:173–177.

78. Clemens PR, Yamamoto M, Engel EG. Adult phosphorylase b kinase deficiency. *Ann Neurol* 1990;28:529–538.

79. Wallgren-Pettersson, C, Clarke, A, Samson, F. The myotubular myopathies: differential diagnosis of the X-linked recessive, autosomal dominant, and autosomal recessive forms and present state of DNA studies. *J Med Genet* 1995;32:673–679.

80. Taylor GS, Maehama T, Dixon JE. Myotubularin, a protein tyrosine phosphatase mutated in myotubular myopathy, dephosphorylates the lipid second messenger, phosphatidylinositol 3-phosphate. *Proc Natl Acad Sci* 2000;97:8910–8915.

81. Van Wijngaarden GK, Fleury P, Bethlem J, et al. Familial 'myotubular' myopathy. *Neurology* 1969;19:901–908.

82. Torres CF, Griggs RC, Goetz JP. Severe neonatal centronuclear myopathy with autosomal dominant inheritance. *Arch Neurol* 1985;42:1011–1014.

83. Fardeau M, Tome FMS, Derambure S. Familial fingerprint body myopathy. *Arch Neurol* 1976;33:724–725.

84. Fryns JP, Van den Berghe H. Sex-linked recessive inheritance in Charcot-Marie-Tooth disease with partial manifestation in female carriers. *Hum Genet* 1980;55:413–415.

85. Hanemann CO, Bergmann C, Senderek J, et al. Transient, recurrent, white matter lesions in X-linked Charcot-Marie-Tooth disease with novel connexin 32 mutation. *Arch Neurol* 2003;60:605–609.

86. Bergoffen J, Scherer SS, Wang S, et al. Connexin mutations in X-linked Charcot-Marie-Tooth disease. *Science* 1993;262:2039–2042.

87. Ionasescu VV, Trofatter J, Haines JL, et al. X-linked recessive Charcot-Marie-Tooth neuropathy: clinical and genetic study. *Muscle Nerve* 1992;15:368–373.

88. Cowchock FS, Duckett SW, Streletz LJ, et al. X-linked motor-sensory neuropathy type-II with deafness and mental retardation: a new disorder. *Am J Med Genet* 1985;20:307–315.

89. Priest JM, Fischbeck KH, Nouri N, et al. A locus for axonal motor-sensory neuropathy with deafness and mental retardation maps to Xq24-q26. *Genomics* 1995;29:409–412.

90. Castle D, Isaacs H, Ramsay M, et al. Hereditary motor and sensory neuropathy type I associated with aplasia cutis congenita: possible X-linked inheritance. *Clin Genet* 1992;41:108–110.

91. Rosenberg RN, Chutorian A. Familial opticoacoustic nerve degeneration and polyneuropathy. *Neurology* 1967;17:827–832.

92. Pauli RM. Sensorineural deafness and peripheral neuropathy. *Clin Genet* 1984;26:383–384.

93. Hasholt L, Sorensen SA, Wandall A, et al. A Fabry's disease heterozygote with a new mutation: Biochemical, ultrastructural, and clinical investigations. *J Med Genet* 1990;27:303–306.

94. Franceschetti AT, Philippart M, Franceschetti A. A study of Fabry's disease. I. Clinical examination of a family with cornea verticillata. *Dermatologica* 1969;138:209–221.

95. Mutoh T, Senda Y, Sugimura K, et al. Severe orthostatic hypotension in a female carrier of Fabry's disease. *Arch Neurol* 1988;45:468–472.

96. Broadbent JC, Edwards WD, Gordon H, et al. Fabry cardiomyopathy in the female confirmed by endomyocardial biopsy. *Mayo Clin Proc* 1981;56:623–628.

97. Bird TD, Lagunoff D. Neurological manifestations of Fabry disease in female carriers. *Ann Neurol* 1978;4:537–540.

98. MacDermot KD, Holmes A, Miners AH. Anderson-Fabry disease: clinical manifestations and impact of disease in a cohort of 60 obligate carrier females. (Letter) *J Med Genet* 2001;38:769-807.

99. Ortiz de Zarate JC. Recessive sex-linked inheritance of congenital external ophthalmoplegia and myopia coincident with other dysplasia. *Br J Ophthal* 1966;50:606–607.

100. La Spada AR, Wilson EM, Lubahn DB, et al. Androgen receptor mutations in X-linked spinal and bulbar muscular atrophy. *Nature* 1991;352:77–79.

101. Guidetti D, Motti L, Marcello N, et al. Kennedy disease in an Italian kindred. *Eur Neurol* 25:188–196.

102. Hickey T, Chandy A, Norman RJ. The androgen receptor CAG repeat polymorphism and X chromosome inactivation in Australian Caucasian women with infertility related to polycystic ovary syndrome. *J Cli Endocr Metab* 2002;87:161–165.

103. Baumbach L, Best B, Edwards J. X-linked lethal infantile spinal muscular atrophy: From clinical description to molecular mapping. *Am J Hum Genet* 1994;55:(suppl):A211.

104. Hall JG, Reed SD, Scott CI, et al. Three distinct types of X-linked arthrogryposis seen in six families. *Clin Genet* 1982;21:81–97.

105. Hennekam RCM, Barth PG, Van Lookeren Campagne W, et al. A family with severe X-linked arthrogryposis. *Eur J Pediat* 1991;150:656–660.

106. Davis LE, Snyder RD, Orth DN, et al. Adrenoleukodystrophy and adrenomyeloneuropathy associated with partial adrenal insufficiency in three generations of a kindred. *Am J Med* 1979;66:342–347.

107. Moser HW, Moser AB, Naidu S, et al. Clinical aspects of adrenoleukodystrophy and adrenomyeloneuropathy. *Dev Neurosci* 1991;13:254–261.

108. Holmberg BH, Hagg E, Hagenfeldt L. Adreno-myeloneuropathy—report on a family. *J Intern Med* 1991;230:535–538.

109. O'Neill BP, Moser HW, Marmion LC, et al. Adrenoleukodystrophy: elevated C26 fatty acid in cultured skin fibroblasts and correlation with disease expression in three generations of a kindred. *Neurology* 1982;32:540–542.

110. El-Deiry SS, Naidu S, Blevins LS, et al. Assessment of adrenal function in women heterozygous for adrenoleukodystrophy. *J Clin Endocr Metab* 1997;82:856–860.

111. Tyler HR. Pelizaeus-Merzbacher disease: a clinical study. *Arch Neurol Psychiatry* 1958;80:162–169.

112. Hodes ME, Pratt VM, Dlouhy SR. Genetics of Pelizaeus-Merzbacher disease. *Dev Neurosci* 1993;15:383–394.

113. Jouet M, Rosenthal A, Armstrong G, et al. X-linked spastic paraplegia (SPG1), MASA syndrome and X-linked hydrocephalus result from mutations in the L1 gene. *Nature Genet* 1994;7:402–407.

114. Kaepernick L, Legius E, Higgins J, et al. Clinical aspects of the MASA syndrome in a large family, including expressing females. *Clin Genet* 1994;45:181–185.

115. Tuck RR, O'Neill BP, Gharib H, et al. Familial spastic paraplegia with Kallmann's syndrome. *J Neurol Neurosurg Psychiatry* 1983;46:671–674.

116. Parenti G, Rizzolo MG, Ghezzi M, et al. Variable penetrance of hypogonadism in a sibship with Kallmann syndrome due to a deletion of the KAL gene. *Am J Med Genet* 1995;57:476–478.

117. Rugarli EI, Ghezzi C, Valsecchi V, et al. The Kallmann syndrome gene product expressed in COS cells is cleaved on the cell surface to yield a diffusible component. *Hum Molec Genet* 1996;5:1109–1115.

118. Oliveira LMB, Seminara SB, Beranova M, et al. The importance of autosomal genes in Kallmann syndrome: genotype-phenotype correlations and neuroendocrine characteristics. *J Clin Endocr Metab* 2001;86:1 532–1538.

119. Malamud N, Cohen P. Unusual form of cerebellar ataxia with sex-linked inheritance. *Neurology* 1958;8: 261–266.

120. Pettigrew AL, Jackson LG, Ledbetter DH, et al. New X-linked mental retardation disorder with Dandy-Walker malformation, basal ganglia disease, and seizures. *Am J Med Genet* 1991;38:200–207.

121. Hodes ME, DeMyer WE, Pratt VM, et al. Girl with signs of Pelizaeus-Merzbacher disease heterozygous for a mutation in exon 2 of the proteolipid protein gene. *Am J Med Genet* 1995;55:397–401.

122. Menkes JH, Alter M, Steigleder GK, et al. A sex-linked recessive disorder with retardation of growth, peculiar hair and focal cerebral and cerebellar degeneration. *Pediatrics* 1962;29:764–779.

123. Moore CM, Howell RR. Ectodermal manifestations in Menkes disease. *Clin Genet* 1985;28:532–540.

124. Kapur S, Higgins JV, Delp K, et al. Menkes syndrome in a girl with X-autosome translocation. *Am J Med Genet* 1987;26:503–510.

125. Sugio Y, Sugio Y, Kuwano A, et al. Translocation t(X;21)(q13.3;p11.1) in a girl with Menkes disease. *Am J Med Genet* 1998;79:191–194.

126. Abusaad I, Mohammed SN, Ogilvie CM et al. Clinical expression of Menkes disease in a girl with X;13 translocation. *Am J Med Genet* 1999;87:354–359.

127. Gerdes AM, Tonnesen T, Horn N, et al. Clinical expression of Menkes syndrome in females. *Clin Genet* 1990;3 8:452–459.

128. Das S, Levinson B, Vulpe C, et al. Similar splicing mutations of the Menkes/mottled copper-transporting ATPase gene in occipital horn syndrome and the blotchy mouse. *Am J Hum Genet* 1995;56:570–576.

129 Herman TE, McAlister WH, Boniface A, et al. Occipital horn syndrome: additional radiographic findings in two new cases. *Pediat Radiol* 1992;22:363–365.

130. Lesch M, Nyhan WL. A familial disorder of uric acid metabolism and central nervous system function. *Am J Med* 1964;36:561–570.

131. Migeon BR, Der Kaloustian VM, Nyhan HK et al. X-linked hypoxanthine-guanine phosphoribosyl transferase deficiency: heterozygote has two clonal populations. *Science* 1968;160:425–427.

132. Ogasawara N, Stout JT, Goto H, et al. Molecular analysis of a female Lesch-Nyhan patient. *J Clin Invest* 1989;84:1024–1027.

133. Simmonds HA, Webster DR, Wilson J, et al. An X-linked syndrome characterised by hyperuricaemia, deafness, and neurodevelopmental abnormalities. *Lancet* 1982; II:68–70.

134. Christen H-J, Hanefeld F, Duley JA, et al. Distinct neurological syndrome in two brothers with hyperuricaemia. *Lancet* 1992;340:1167–1168.

135. Rosenberg AL, Bergstrom L, Troost BL, et al. Hyperuricemia and neurological deficits: a family study. *N Engl J Med* 1970;282:992–997.

136. Schmidley JW, Levinsohn MW, Manetto CV, et al. Infantile X-linked ataxia and deafness: a new clinicopathologic entity. *Neurology* 1987;37:1344–1349.

137. Arts WFM, Loonen MCB, Sengers RCA, et al. X-linked ataxia, weakness, deafness, and loss of vision in early childhood with a fatal course. *Ann Neurol* 1993;33: 535–539.

138. Shokeir MHK. X-linked cerebellar ataxia. *Clin Genet* 1970;1:225–231.

139. Zuffardi O, Fraccaro M. Gene mapping and serendipity: the locus for torticollis, keloids, cryptorchidism and renal dysplasia (31430, McKusick) is at Xq28, distal to the G6PD locus. *Hum Genet* 1982;62:280–281.

140. Goeminne L. A new probably X-linked inherited syndrome: congenital torticollis, multiple keloids, cryptorchidism and renal dysplasia. *Acta Genet Med Gemellol* 1968;17:439–467.

141. Scribanu N, Kennedy C. Familial syndrome with dystonia, neural deafness, and possible intellectual impairment: clinical course and pathological findings. *Adv Neurol* 1976;14:235–243.

142. Kupke KG, Lee LV, Muller U, et al. Assignment of the X-linked torsion dystonia gene to Xq21 by linkage analysis. *Neurology* 1990;40:1438–1442.

143. Laxova R, Brown ES, Hogan K, et al. An X-linked recessive basal ganglia disorder with mental retardation. *Am J Med Genet* 1985;21:681–689.

144. Haar F, Dyken P. Hereditary nonprogressive athetotic hemiplegia: a new syndrome. *Neurology* 1977;27: 849–854.

145. Lissens W, De Meirleir L, Seneca S, et al. Mutations in the X-linked pyruvate dehydrogenase (E1) alpha subunit gene (PDHA1) in patients with a pyruvate dehydrogenase complex deficiency. *Hum Mutat* 2000;15:209–219.

146. Matthews PM, Brown RM, Otero LJ, et al. Pyruvate dehydrogenase deficiency: clinical presentation and molecular genetic characterization of five new patients. *Brain* 1994;117:435–443.

147. Shevell MI, Matthews PM, Scriver CR, et al. Cerebral dysgenesis and lactic acidemia: an MRI/MRS phenotype associated with pyruvate dehydrogenase deficiency. *Pediat Neurol* 1994;11:224–229.

148. Hopkins IJ, Connelly JF, Dawson AG, et al. Hyperammonaemia due to ornithine transcarbamylase deficiency. *Arch Dis Child* 1969;44:143–148.

149. Campbell AGM, Rosenberg LE, Snodgrass PJ, et al. Ornithine transcarbamylase deficiency: a cause of lethal neonatal hyperammonemia in males. *N Engl J Med* 1973;288:1–6.

150. Arn PH, Hauser ER, Thomas GH, et al. Hyperammonemia in women with a mutation at the ornithine carbamoyltransferase locus: a cause of postpartum coma. *N Engl J Med* 1990;322:1652–1655.

151. Honeycutt D, Callahan K, Rutledge L, et al. Heterozygote ornithine transcarbamylase deficiency presenting as symptomatic hyperammonemia during initiation of valproate therapy. *Neurology* 1992;42:666–668.

152. Batshaw ML, Roan Y, Jung AL, et al. Cerebral dysfunction in asymptomatic carriers of ornithine transcarbamylase deficiency. *N Engl J Med* 1980;302:482–485.

153. Maestri NE, Brusilow SW, Clissold DB, et al. Long-term treatment of girls with ornithine transcarbamylase deficiency. *N Engl J Med* 1996;335:855–859.

154. Maestri NE, Hauser ER, Bartholomew D, et al. Prospective treatment of urea cycle disorders. *J Pediat* 1991;119:923–928.

155. Yudkoff M, Daikhin Y, Nissim I, et al. In vivo nitrogen metabolism in ornithine transcarbamylase deficiency. *J Clin Invest* 1996;98:2167-2173.

156. Winchester B, Young E, Geddes S, et al. Female twin with Hunter disease due to nonrandom inactivation of the X chromosome: a consequence of twinning. *Am J Med Genet* 1992;44:834–838.

157. Broadhead DM, Kirk JM, Burt AJ, et al. Full expression of Hunter's disease in a female with an X chromosome deletion leading to non-random inactivation. *Clin Genet* 1986;30:392–398.

158. Priest JH, Thuline HC, Laveck GD, et al. An approach to genetic factors in mental retardation. Studies of families containing at least two siblings admitted to a state institution for the retarded. *Am J Mental Deficiency* 1961;66:42–50.

159. Lubs HA, Chiurazzi P, Arena JF, et al. XLMR genes—Update 1996. *Am J Hum Genet* 1996;64:147–157.

160. Loesch DZ, Hay DA. Clinical features and reproductive patterns in fragile X female heterozygotes. *J Med Genet* 1988;25:407–414.

161. Reiss AL, Aylward E, Freund LS, et al. Neuroanatomy of fragile X syndrome: the posterior fossa. *Ann Neurol* 1991;29:26–32.

162. Mulley JC, Yu S, Loesch DZ, et al. FRAXE and mental retardation. *J Med Genet* 1995;32:162–169.

163. Murray A, Webb J, Dennis N, et al. Microdeletions in FMR2 may be a significant cause of premature ovarian failure. *J Med Genet* 1999;36:767–770.

164. Estrada, L, Caron E, Gorski JL. Fgd1, the Cdc42 guanine nucleotide exchange factor responsible for faciogenital dysplasia, is localized to the subcortical actin cytoskeleton and Golgi membrane. *Hum Molec Genet* 2001;10:485–495.

165. Scott CI Jr. Unusual facies, joint hypermobility, genital anomaly and short stature: a new dysmorphic syndrome. *Birth Defects Orig Art Ser* 1971;VII(6):240–246.

166. Coffin GS, Siris E, Wegienka LC. Mental retardation with osteocartilaginous anomalies. *Am J Dis Child* 1966; 112:205–213.

167. Trivier E, De Cesare, D, Jacquot S, et al. Mutations in the kinase Rsk-2 associated with Coffin-Lowry syndrome. *Nature* 1996;384:567–557.

168. Hendrich B, Bickmore W. Human diseases with underlying defects in chromatin structure and modification. *Hum Molec Genet* 2001;10:2233–2242.

169. Miyazaki K, Yamanaka T, Ishida Y, et al. Calcified ligamenta flava in a patient with Coffin-Lowry syndrome: biochemical analysis of glycosaminoglycans. *Jpn J Hum Genet* 1990;35:215–221.

170. Machin GA, Walther GL, Fraser VM, et al. Autopsy findings in two adult siblings with Coffin-Lowry syndrome. *Am J Med Genet* 1987;(suppl 3):303–309.

171. Simensen R J, Abidi F, Collins JS, et al. Cognitive function in Coffin-Lowry syndrome. *Clin Genet* 2002;61: 299–304.

172. Sivagamasundari U, Fernando H, Jardine P, et al. The association between Coffin-Lowry syndrome and psychosis: a family study. *J Intellect Disabil Res* 1994;38: 469–473.

173. Weatherall DJ, Higgs DR, Bunch C, et al. Hemoglobin H disease and mental retardation: a new syndrome or a remarkable coincidence? *N Engl J Med* 1981;305:607–612.

174. McPherson EW, Clemens MM, Gibbons RJ, et al. X-linked alpha-thalassemia/mental retardation (ATR-X) syndrome: a new kindred with severe genital anomalies and mild hematologic expression. *Am J Med Genet* 1995;55:302–306.

175. Gurrieri F, Neri G. A girl with the Lujan-Fryns syndrome. *Am J Med Genet* 1991;38:290–291.

176. Reznik M, Alberca-Serrano R. Forme familiale d'hypertélorisme avec lissencephalie se presentant cliniquement sous forme d'une arrieration mentale avec epilepsie et paraplegie spasmodique. *J Neurol Sci* 1964;1:40–58.

177. Barkovich A, Jackson D, Boyer R. Band heterotopias: a newly recognized neuronal migration anomaly. *Radiology* 1989;171:455–458.

178. Hodgson SV, Heckmatt JZ, Hughes, et al. A balanced de novo X/autosome translocation in a girl with manifestations of Lowe syndrome. *Am J Med Genet* 1986;23:837–847.

179. Gardner RJM, Brown N. Lowe's syndrome: identification of carriers by lens examination. *J Med Genet* 1976;13:449–464.

180. Miles JH, Carpenter NJ. Unique X-linked mental retardation syndrome with fingertip arches and contractures linked to Xq21.31. *Am J Med Genet* 1991;38:215–223.

181. Fitzsimmons JS, Fitzsimmons EM, McLachlan JI, et al. Four brothers with mental retardation, spastic paraplegia and palmoplantar hyperkeratosis: a new syndrome? *Clin Genet* 1983;23:329–335.

182. Christian JC, DeMyer WE, Franken EA, et al. X-linked skeletal dysplasia with mental retardation. *Clin Genet* 1972;11:128–136.

183. Keller MA, Jones KL, Nyhan WL, et al. A new syndrome of mental deficiency with craniofacial, limb, and anal abnormalities. *J Pediat* 1976;88:589–591.

184. Dinno ND, Lawwill T, Leggett AE, et al. Bilateral microcornea, coloboma, short stature and other skeletal anomalies—a new hereditary syndrome. *Birth Defects Orig Art Ser* 1976;XII(6):109–114.

185. Humphries JO. Occurrence of hypertensive toxemia of pregnancy in mother-daughter pairs. *Bull Johns Hopkins Hosp* 1960;107:271–277.

186. Hayward C, Livingstone J, Holloway S, et al. An exclusion map for preeclampsia: assuming autosomal recessive inheritance. *Am J Hum Genet* 1991;50:749–757.

187. Ward K, Hata A, Jeunemaitre X, et al. A molecular variant of angiotensinogen associated with preeclampsia. *Nature Genet* 1993;4:59–61.

188. Rudd NL, Nimrod C, Holbrook KA, et al. Pregnancy complications in type IV Ehlers-Danlos syndrome. *Lancet* 1983;1:50–53.

189. Polymeropoulos MH, Hurko O, Hsu F, et al. Linkage of the locus for cerebral cavernous hemangiomas to human chromosome 7q in four families of Mexican American descent. *Neurology* 1997;48:752–757.

190. Norwood OT, Everett, MA. Cardiac failure due to endocrine dependent hemangiomas. *Arch Derm* 89: 759–760.

191. Massumi RA, Lowe EW, Misanik LF, et al. Multiple aortic aneurysms (thoracic and abdominal) in twins with Marfan's syndrome: fatal rupture during pregnancy. *J Thorac Cardiovasc Surg* 1967;53:223–230.

192. Johnson EJ, Prentice CRM, Parapia LA. Premature arterial disease associated with familial antithrombin III deficiency. *Thromb Haemost* 1990;63:13–15.

193. Ogasawara KK, Ogasawara EM, Hirata G. Pregnancy complicated by von Hippel-Lindau disease. *Obstet Gynecol* 1995;85:829–832.

194. Harries RW. A rational approach to radiological screening in von Hippel-Lindau disease. *J Med Screen* 1994;1: 88–95.

195. Dugoff L, Sujansky E. Neurofibroamatosis type 1 and pregnancy. *Am J Med Genet* 1996;66:7–10.

196. Evans DGR, Huson SM, Donnai D, et al. A clinical study of type 2 neurofibromatosis. *Quart J Med* 1992;84: 603–618.

197. Pollock M, Nukuda H, Kritchevsky M. Exacerbation of Charcot-Marie-Tooth disease in pregnancy. *Neurology* 1982;32:1311–1314.

198. Thomas PK, Ormerod IEC. Hereditary neuralgic amyotrophy associated with a relapsing multifocal sensory neuropathy. *J Neurol Neurosurg Psychiatry* 1993;56: 107–109.

199. Sims HF, Brackett JC, Powell CK, et al. The molecular basis of pediatric long chain 3-hydroxyacyl-CoA dehydrogenase deficiency associated with maternal acute fatty liver of pregnancy. *Proc Nat Acad Sci* 1995;92: 841–845.

200. Isaacs JD, Sims HF, Powell CK, et al. Maternal acute fatty liver of pregnancy associated with fetal trifunctional protein deficiency: molecular characterization of a novel maternal mutant allele. *Pediat Res* 1996;40:393–398.

201. Wilcken B, Leung K-C, Hammond J, et al. Pregnancy and fetal long-chain 3 hydroxyacyl coenzyme A dehydrogenase deficienncy. *Lancet* 1993;341:407–408.

202. Treem WR, Rinaldo P, Hale DE, et al. Acute fatty liver of pregnancy and long-chain hydroxyacyl-coenzyme A dehydrogenase deficiency. *Hepatology* 1994;19:339–345.

203. Hunter JAA, Khan, SA, Hope E, et al. Hereditary coproporphyria. Photosensitivity, jaundice and neuropsychiatric manifestations associated with pregnancy. *Brit J Derm* 1971;84:301–310.

204. Slavotinek AM, Pike M, Mills K, Hurst JA. Cataracts, motor system disorder, short stature, learning difficulties, and skeletal abnormalities: a new syndrome? *Am J Med Genet* 1996;62:42–47.

205. Wallace DC. Maternal genes: mitochondrial inheritance. In: McKusick VA, Roderick, TH, Mori J, Paul NW, (eds.) *Medical and experimental mammalian genetics: a perspective.* New York, NY: Alan R. Liss, 1988;137–190.

206. Singh G, Lott MT, Wallace DC. A mitochondrial DNA mutation as a cause of Leber's hereditary optic neuropathy. *N Engl J Med* 1989;320:1300–1305.

207. Chalmers RM, Davis MB, Sweeney MG, Wood NW, Harding AE. Evidence against an X-linked visual loss susceptibility locus in Leber hereditary optic neuropathy. *Am J Hum Genet* 1996;59:103–108.

208. Goto Y, Nonaka I, Horai S. A mutation in the tRNA(Leu[UUR]) gene associated with the MELAS subgroup of mitochondrial encephalo–myopathies. *Nature* 1990;348:651–653.

209. Wallace DC, Zheng XX, Lott MT, et al. Familial mitochondrial encephalomyopathy (MERRF): a genetic, pathophysiological and biochemical characterization of a mitochondrial DNA disease. *Cell* 1988;55:601–610.

210. Tatuch Y, Christodoulou J, Feigenbaum A, et al. Heteroplasmic mtDNA mutation (T-to-G) at 8993 can cause Leigh disease when the percentage of abnormal mtDNA is high. *Am J Hum Genet* 1991;50:852–858.

211. Holt IJ, Harding AE, Morgan-Hughes JA. Deletions of muscle mitochondrial DNA in patients wtih mitochondrial myopathies. *Nature* 1988;331:717–719.

212. Zeviani M, Servidei S, Gellera C, et al. An autosomal dominant disorder with mutiple deletions of mitochondrial DNA starting at the D-loop region. *Nature* 1989;339:309–311.

213. Magenis RE, Toth-Fejel S, Allen LJ, et al. Comparison of the 15q deletions in Prader-Willi and Angelman syndromes: specific regions, extent of deletions, parental origin, and clinical consequences. *Am J Med Genet* 1990; 35:333–349.

214. Huntington's Disease Collaborative Research Group. A novel gene containing a trinucleotide repeat that is expanded and unstable on Huntington's disease chromosomes. *Cell* 1993;72:971–983.

215. Harley HG, Brook JD, Rundle SA, et al. Expansion of an unstable DNA region and phenotypic variation in myotonic dystrophy. *Nature* 1992;355:545–546.

216. Carter O, Evans K. Spina bifida and anencephalus in Greater London. *J Med Genet* 1993;5:81–106.

217. Elwood JH, Nevin NC. Factors associated with anencephalus and spina bifida in Belfast. *Brit J Prev Soc Med* 1973;27:73–80.

218. Nevin NC, Johnson WP. Risk of recurrence after two children with central nervous system malformations in an area of high incidence. *J Med Genet* 1980;17(2):87–92.

219. Rouse B, Azen C, Koch R, et al. Maternal phenylketonuria collaborative study (MPKUCS) offspring: facial anomalies, malformations, and early neurological sequelae. *Am J Med Genet* 1997;69:89–95.

220 Levy HL, Lobbregt D, Barnes PD, et al. Maternal phenylketonuria: magnetic resonance imaging of the brain in offspring. *J Pediat* 1996;128:770–775.

221. Ryan IP, Havel RJ, Laros RK Jr. Three consecutive pregnancies in a patient with glycogen storage disease type IA (von Gierke's disease). *Am J Obstet Gynec* 1994;170: 1687–1691.

8 Women, Law, and Neurologic Disease

H. Richard Beresford

Certain laws have special relevance for women regardless of whether neurologic disorders are at issue. Some examples are laws that affect reproductive choice, the care of infants and children, and gender discrimination. For women with neurologic disease, generally applicable laws concerning autonomy, liberty, competency, and the limits of governmental power may come into play as well. No attempt is made here to survey the gamut of legal issues that might arise with respect to women and neurologic disorders. For example, I do not discuss certain matters of potential interest, such as social legislation that enables women to secure disability benefits for neurologic impairment or liability laws that permit women to recover damages for neurologic harms from nonphysicians (e.g., breast implant manufacturers, negligent automobile drivers). Instead, the focus of this chapter is on aspects of law that raise particularly compelling issues for women who have neurologic disorders or who are concerned with preventing or treating such disorders in their offspring.

In this context, the chapter addresses selected issues that relate to informed consent, coercive approaches to preventing fetal harm, and difficult treatment choices that have major neurologic overtones.

INFORMED CONSENT TO MEDICAL TREATMENT

The informed consent doctrine holds that competent individuals are entitled to make a voluntary choice about medical treatment after an adequate disclosure of its nature, risks, benefits, and reasonable alternatives. The doctrine developed through judge-made law in the tradition of the "common law." In recent years, however, several state legislatures have enacted statutes to codify the doctrine more explicitly. For example, New York's informed consent law allows an action against physicians for failure to obtain informed consent to nonemergency treatment or invasive diagnostic testing. It defines lack of informed consent as the "failure...to disclose...such alternatives...and the reasonably foreseeable risks and benefits involved as a reasonable medical practitioner under similar circumstances would have disclosed, in a manner permitting the patient to make a knowledgeable evaluation (1)." Georgia's medical disclosure law requires that a patient undergoing surgery or other invasive procedures be informed of the diagnosis requiring intervention, the nature of the procedure involved, and "the material risks generally recognized and accepted by reasonably prudent physicians ... which, if disclosed to a reasonably prudent person in the patient's position, could reasonably be expected to cause such prudent person to decline" the intervention (2).

Although the informed consent doctrine seems clear enough, there are nuances that sometimes complicate its application. For example, what constitutes decisional competency? Is it merely the ability to register assent after disclosure is made? Or must there be some indication that a person comprehends the disclosure and can weigh its content? Similar issues may surround the extent to which consent is voluntary. Is a consent provided while a person is in pain or under time pressure truly voluntary? Or does an intense desire for relief of symptoms prevent weighing of information about major risks of treatment? Moreover, an ostensibly comprehensive disclosure of risks and benefits might simply overwhelm the understanding of some individuals, rendering the adequacy of the disclosure highly suspect. Finally, in assessing the adequacy of a disclosure, is the test whether it satisfies the information needs of a particular individual, no matter how idiosyncratic, or whether it meets a more "objective" standard?

None of these concerns about application of the informed consent doctrine are particularly gender-sensitive on their face. Still it may be important to allow for the possibility that some male physicians—even today— might consciously or unconsciously derogate the capacity of their female patients to engage in dialogues about treatment. Such physicians may approach consent in a paternalistic or hierarchical fashion, thereby raising questions about the adequacy of disclosure or the voluntariness of consent.

It may also be that women who are acculturated to deferring to men in making important decisions may either waive their right to be informed or simply agree to accept whatever treatment is recommended. Considerations of gender politics aside, two state high court decisions serve to illustrate important elements of the law of informed consent. The first concerns what constitutes a relevant disclosure about the teratogenic risk of antiepileptic drugs to a woman with epilepsy. The second case, although it has no neurologic dimensions, is an apt example of current judicial thinking about the content of an adequate disclosure of risks and benefits of treatment.

1. The duty to make a relevant disclosure. In Harbeson v Parke-Davis Inc. (3), the supreme court of the state of Washington decided that the parents of two children with "fetal hydantoin syndrome" and the children themselves were entitled to recover damages because their physicians failed to adequately disclose the risks of that entity. The mother, Mrs. Harbeson, had developed epilepsy in 1970 while she was pregnant with her first child, Michael. Dilantin was prescribed for her, and Michael was born free of any defects. In 1972 and 1973,

she told three different physicians at an Army hospital that she was considering having more children but was concerned about the risks to her fetus if she took Dilantin during pregnancy. Each physician noted the potential risks of hirsutism and cleft palate, but none specifically mentioned the fetal hydantoin syndrome. She elected to continue Dilantin during subsequent pregnancies with daughters Elizabeth and Christine. Both were ultimately diagnosed as having fetal hydantoin syndrome, manifested as growth and developmental retardation, hypoplastic digits, and craniofacial dysmorphism.

The parents then sued the U.S. government in federal court, citing the alleged misconduct of the Army physicians. They also named the manufacturer of Dilantin as a defendant. As to the physicians, the central allegation was that they were careless in determining the fetal risks of Dilantin. The asserted harmful consequences were the neurologic and other impairments of the two daughters and infringement of the right of the parents to make an informed choice about childbearing. As remedies for the alleged wrongs, the parents sought damages for themselves for the "wrongful birth" of Elizabeth and Christine and for the children for their "wrongful life."

After hearing testimony from the parents' medical experts to the effect that the fetal hydantoin syndrome is a known risk of taking Dilantin during pregnancy, the federal court concluded that the physicians were negligent in not disclosing this risk to the parents. The court then asked the Washington supreme court to rule on whether state law permitted the type of damages the parents were seeking for themselves and for their affected children. The court thereupon concluded that the parents were entitled to "wrongful birth" damages. It underscored the failure of the Army physicians to adequately inform themselves of the risks of Dilantin and the adverse impact of this failure on the parents' reproductive choice. The court saw this as a breach of duty to potential parents who were relying on the physicians for assistance in making a decision about future childbearing.

In calculating damages, the court ruled that the parents should recover medical and special educational expenses to the extent that they exceeded what the parents would have spent had Elizabeth and Christine been normal children. The court also decided that the parents should recover damages for their own pain and suffering. With respect to the children's wrongful life claims, the court limited recovery to the costs of treatment and training beyond those required for normal children after they reach adulthood. It viewed an award of damages to the children for pain and suffering as incalculable because it would necessarily entail a comparison between the quality of impaired life and no life at all.

The *Harbeson* decision offers several insights with respect to the doctrine of informed consent. Perhaps the most important insight derives from the court's determination that the physicians carelessly infringed on the fundamental liberty of the parents to make informed choice about reproduction. Were it not for *Roe v Wade* (4) and its progeny, the Washington court might have viewed the parents' claim as less compelling. But because reproductive choice now has constitutional stature, conduct that impairs its exercise has potent overtones. The Harbeson case is not an abortion rights case, of course. At issue was a parental decision whether to have more children, not whether to terminate a pregnancy. However, the state court recognized implications of *Roe v Wade* for evaluating conduct that influences the "difficult moral choice" to avoid the birth of a defective child. The court's reasoning parallels that of courts in other states, which have permitted wrongful birth actions for negligent failure to diagnose or predict disorders amenable to prenatal diagnosis, such as chromosomal trisomies, neural tube defects, and Tay-Sachs disease (5).

Because such claims raise the divisive issue of abortion, some legislatures have limited or flatly banned claims for wrongful birth or wrongful life. For example, a Minnesota statute bars claims based on an allegation that but for a wrongful act or omission, a defective child would have been aborted (6). In *Hickman v Group Health Plan* (7), the Minnesota supreme court upheld the constitutionality of this law as applied to a suit by parents of a child with Down syndrome. The parents had alleged that the physician-defendants negligently failed to perform amniocentesis despite the mother's advanced age. They also asserted that if 21-trisomy had been confirmed by amniocentesis, the mother would have terminated the pregnancy. The court concluded that the statute did not directly burden her constitutional right to seek an abortion; in the court's view, the statute only limited the grounds on which a civil claim for damages could be asserted.

The *Harbeson* case also highlights what constitutes an appropriate standard of care for pregnant women. Both federal and state courts faulted the physicians for not informing themselves more completely about the potential teratogenicity of Dilantin. Merely communicating what they did know was held insufficient. In the opinion of the court, they should have reviewed the relevant literature or consulted more knowledgeable colleagues. On the issue of the causal relationship between the physician's nonfeasance and the parental choice to proceed with pregnancy, the court apparently credited the parents' assertion that they would have deferred future childbearing if adequate disclosure had been made. However, other parents have opted to proceed with pregnancy after being advised of the potential teratogenicity of antiepileptic drugs. Thus, one can question whether the court's seemingly easy reliance on what the parents said they would have done is an objective reading of the situation. On the other hand, parents may differ in risk-aver-

siveness, and courts may take this into account when weighing assertions made with the benefit of hindsight. Also, the *Harbeson* court might have believed that reasonable parents would have deferred further childbearing if confronted with the small risk of fetal hydantoin syndrome in their offspring.

As to the proper measure of damages in a case of this nature, the *Harbeson* court decided to compensate the parents for the incremental economic costs of caring for their affected children and for their own pain and suffering. The children were also granted the projected incremental costs of their care as adults, but were denied recovery for their own pain and suffering. The court conceded they had been harmed to the extent of being born with a condition that necessitated special care and that the law ordinarily allows damages for pain and suffering that attends physical harms. But it could not reduce the pain and suffering to monetary terms because it believed that this would require a comparison between impaired life and the void of nonexistence.

Other courts faced with calculating damages in cases similar to *Harbeson* have taken different tacks (5). One is to award damages only to parents and only for their pain and suffering. The rationale here is that the essential harm is the infringement of parental liberty, a moral harm rather than an economic one. Children are not compensated because the calculation of damages for being born in a defective state is too speculative or reflects a socially intolerable notion that life with disability is less worthy than "normal" life. A contrasting approach recognizes the imponderables of calculating noneconomic damages and limits damages to parental economic costs attributable to the impairments. Courts that permit children to recover damages on their own account for wrongful life generally follow *Harbeson* in limiting the recovery to economic damages. These contrasting judicial approaches to calculating damages highlight an ongoing controversy over whether awards of damages for wrongful birth or wrongful life should be compensatory only or if they should serve a deterrent function as well.

2. The content of disclosure. In Arato v Avedon (8), the California supreme court addressed the issue of how detailed a disclosure must be to satisfy the requirements of the informed consent doctrine. There was little controversy over whether the physician-defendants had attempted a broad and well-grounded disclosure. The dispute centered on the alleged inadequacy of the defendants' failure to take into account a patient's particular needs for information. The patient was a 42-year-old electrical contractor who had pancreatic cancer. After the diagnosis was established, the patient was referred by his surgeon to an oncologist (later defendant). The oncologist asked the patient if he wished to be "told the truth" about his condition. He indicated that he did and was offered the option of a three-drug chemotherapy regimen plus irradiation. He was told that most patients with pancreatic cancer die of the disease, that the risk of recurrence after treatment was "serious" or "great," that the efficacy of the proposed regimen was unproved, that the treatment would be difficult and painful, and that there was the option to forgo further therapy. Following this disclosure, the patient opted for treatment. He was not told of statistical data indicating that he had no greater than a 5 to 10% chance of a 5-year survival, but neither he nor his wife ever requested such specific information before treatment or during its course.

For several months, he was free of disease, but the tumor recurred and he died approximately one year after the diagnosis of pancreatic cancer. His wife and two children then brought suit against the surgeon and the oncologist. Their claim was that the physicians' prognosis and the prospects of benefit from the proposed treatment were incomplete, most significantly in their failure to provide statistical probabilities concerning outcome. They argued further that the allegedly incomplete disclosure created a false hope in the patient and led him to neglect the ordering of important financial affairs, which resulted in failure of his contracting business and substantial and avoidable real estate and tax losses after his death. In their defense, the physicians contended that their disclosure was appropriate, that a direct and specific disclosure of the high mortality rate of his condition would be countertherapeutic, and that the patient and his wife had overlooked many opportunities to ask more pointed questions about his prognosis.

After the evidence in the case was presented to the jury, the trial judge instructed the jury that:

- The duty of a physician is "to disclose…all material information to enable the patient to make an informed decision…."
- "Material information" is that which "the physician knows or should know would be regarded as significant by a reasonable person in the patient's position…."
- A physician "has no duty of disclosure beyond that required of physicians of good standing in the same or similar locality when he or she relied upon facts which would demonstrate to a reasonable person that the disclosure would seriously upset the patient that the patient would not have been able to rationally weigh the risks of refusing to undergo the recommended treatment."
- A physician is subject to liability "if a reasonably prudent person in the patient's position would not have consented to the treatment if he or she had been adequately informed of the likelihood of his premature death."

After deliberating, the jury concluded that none of the physicians was negligent and that they disclosed "all relevant information which would have enabled him to make an informed decision regarding the proposed treatment…." Claimants then appealed, and an intermediate appeals court reversed the trial court decision and ordered a new trial. Defendants then appealed to the California supreme court, which reversed the appellate court and reinstated the judgment of the trial court in favor of the physicians.

In reaching its decision that the jury had been properly instructed and had reached an appropriate verdict, the California high court observed as follows:

> …The contexts and clinical settings in which physician and patient interact and exchange information material to therapeutic decisions are so multifarious, the informational needs and degree of dependency of individual patients so various, and the professional relationship itself is such an intimate and irreducibly judgment-laden one, that we believe it is unwise to require "as a matter of law" that a particular species of information be disclosed….
>
> This sensitivity to context seems all the more appropriate in the case of life expectancy projections for cancer patients based on statistical samples…. In declining to endorse the mandatory disclosure of life-expectancy probabilities, we do not mean to signal a retreat from the patient-based standard of disclosure explicitly adopted in *Cobbs v Grant* (502 P 2d 1 [CA Sup Ct 1973]). We reaffirm the view taken in *Cobbs* that, because the "weighing of these risks (i.e., those inherent in a proposed procedure) against the individual subjective fears and hopes of the patient is not an expert skill," the test "for determining whether a potential peril must be divulged is its materiality to the patient's decision." In reaffirming the appropriateness of that standard, we can conceive of no trier of fact more suitable than lay jurors to pronounce judgment on those uniquely human and necessarily situational ingredients that contribute to a specific doctor-patient exchange of information relevant to treatment decisions; certainly this is not territory in which appellate courts can usefully issue "bright line" guides….

Here the evidence was more than sufficient to support the jury's finding that defendants had reasonably disclosed to Mr. Arato information material to his decision whether to undergo the proposed chemotherapy/irradiation treatment.

This important decision underscores the unique and fact-sensitive nature of informed consent dialogues between the patient and physician. It also displays the explicit reluctance of a court at the forefront of informed consent doctrine to micromanage how much disclosure is necessary to meet the test of materiality, at least where, as in the *Arato* case, an obviously substantial disclosure had been made. The particular disclosure surely must have conveyed the severity of Mr. Arato's plight.

Strictly speaking, the *Arato* decision is legally binding only in California. But it offers guidance to other courts faced with assertions that particular disclosures were legally flawed because they failed to address singular subjective concerns of patients. Thus, it encourages courts to allow jurors to sort out the question of whether patients' concerns are reasonable enough to require physicians to disclose more than they ordinarily do and argues against courts trying to formulate blanket rules about the specifics of disclosure. Although this approach may discomfit those who firmly believe that patients are often seriously underinformed about their therapeutic options, Arato hardly stands for the proposition that physicians can ignore concerns that are likely to concern the average patient.

What does this mean for women with neurologic disease? The most immediate conclusion is that physicians are legally obligated to disclose to their female patients who have neurologic disorders facts that the patients as women consider "material" or important to their decisions about treatment. Thus, women with epilepsy are lawfully entitled to an accurate account of the fetal risks of antiepileptic drugs; women with multiple sclerosis are entitled to learn about the effects of pregnancy on their disease or the effects of therapy on their fertility; women with cerebrovascular disease are entitled to hear about risks and benefits of estrogens; and women at risk for bearing neurologically impaired children are entitled to a full explanation of these risks. Another dimension of Arato, however, is its recognition that not everything a patient regards as material will satisfy an objective standard of materiality. For example, because a postmenopausal woman is quietly concerned that she might develop Alzheimer's disease, it does not necessarily follow that her physician has a legal obligation to inform her about preliminary studies suggesting that estrogen may delay onset of the disease in persons at risk.

COERCING WOMEN TO PREVENT FETAL HARM

Public concerns about the adverse effects of maternal substance abuse or HIV infection on offspring have fueled coercive legal strategies. These include expanded criminal prosecution, civil detention, and mandatory testing and treatment. Opponents of such measures often contend that a medical model that emphasizes counseling and treatment will ultimately yield better fetal protection. But there is an undeniable popular and political fascination with the notion that some difficult social problems can be solved by applying the blunt instrument of law. Although most neurologists probably take a detached view of the ongoing debate about the utility of maternal coercion to prevent fetal harm, those who treat infants and children who have been harmed by maternal substance abuse or maternally transmitted HIV disease are likely to be more engaged. In addition, policymakers may occasionally call on neurologists for advice or consultation about the neurologic harms attending maternal substance abuse or HIV infection. In this context, the following discussion addresses some of the legal and policy issues that arise out of the use of coercive legal measures against women in order to protect the health of their offspring.

Contrasting Paradigms

How one views the relationship between a woman and her fetus may influence the choice between coercive and therapeutic strategies. One paradigm is to envision mother and fetus as separate persons, one a potential wrongdoer and the other an innocent victim. In this construct, the mother becomes a target of social control, and physicians are cast as protectors of the fetus, even if this means violating maternal confidentiality or personal preferences. A second paradigm envisions mother and fetus as a single entity, too closely joined to generate a conflict between maternal and fetal interests. In this formulation, a physician's role is to assure that mother and child together receive optimal treatment. Social control considerations are not of paramount concern. Because the first paradigm evokes the more troubling legal issues, it is the focus of attention in the following discussion.

Coercive Strategies

Various legal strategies have been applied or proposed to implement social control of maternal behavior. These include criminal prosecution for conduct that endangers children, civil detention, removal of custody, mandatory testing for substance abuse or infection, and enforced treatment.

Criminal Prosecution

In a much publicized case, Pamela Stewart was charged with felony child abuse for violating a California statute that criminalized the willful failure to provide medical care to a minor child (9). The essence of the charge was that Ms. Stewart used amphetamines during her pregnancy, despite her physician's counsel that she abstain. Her newborn son had evidence of brain injury at birth and died at two months of age. The prosecutor contended that her fetus was legally equivalent to a minor child and that her drug abuse during pregnancy amounted to a willful failure to provide necessary care to such child. The court dismissed the charge, finding no evidence of a legislative intention to extend child abuse laws to cover conduct that endangers a fetus.

Although the prosecution failed in the Stewart case, it harmonizes with an effort in other states to enact laws to establish a separate crime of "fetal abuse" that could be invoked to punish women who engaged in conduct during pregnancy that they knew could endanger their unborn child (10).

Another strategy directed at women who abuse drugs is to invoke existing narcotics laws and charge pregnant women with the crime of unlawful delivery of controlled substances. The rationale is that maternal drug use equates to transplacental "delivery" of the unlawful agent to the person of the fetus and is therefore prosecutable in the same manner as other person-to-person transfers. Most prosecutions to date have targeted women using crack-cocaine. In a much-publicized Florida case, a conviction was obtained applying the foregoing rationale, but the verdict was reversed on appeal (11). Appellate courts have generally taken the position that antidrug laws, like other criminal laws, should be strictly construed and have not found evidence of express legislative intent to criminalize transplacental "delivery" of unlawful drugs (12).

Civil Detention

Civil commitment laws generally permit involuntary detention of mentally ill persons who are dangerous to self or others, and some laws permit confinement of such persons on a showing that they require treatment in order to prevent serious deterioration of their condition. If maternal drug use is viewed as a form of mental illness, these laws could conceivably be used to keep women drug-free during the term of pregnancy. There are formidable obstacles to such an approach, however. Substance abuse is not ordinarily considered the sort of mental illness that justifies involuntary confinement; if it were, the current orgy of prison-building would be outstripped by construction of new mental hospitals. Moreover, even if substance abuse is a qualifying mental illness, existing constitutional doctrine requires that detained persons be offered meaningful treatment as a condition of continuing confinement (13). Unless a confined substance abuser actually receives treatment other than being removed from access to drugs, she could plausibly assert that her confinement is unconstitutional.

Removal of Custody

Some child abuse and neglect laws may empower public officials to take custody of newborns away from their mothers on proof that the mothers exposed the babies to unlawful drugs during pregnancy (10). Some form of judicial hearing is ordinarily necessary to accomplish such a drastic step. In the hearing, the issue may arise as to whether maternal drug abuse in itself justifies removal of custody. A court that is strongly motivated by a desire to punish the mother as a drug user or to send a deterrent signal to other pregnant women may not carefully address the question of whether the mother is fit to care for her child. But if a court's focus is on the more traditional test of whether removal of custody is in the best interests of the child, it may consider a variety of factors other than the mother's drug use during pregnancy. Courts may also be tempted to draw medically unsupportable distinctions between use of lawful drugs, such as alcohol, and unlawful drugs, such as crack-cocaine. In the matter of fetal or infant health, an alcohol-abusing mother may be just as dangerous as a crack-using mother. Yet some courts may be inclined to remove custody more quickly from the crack-using mother than from the alcoholic mother because the former is violating narcotics laws whereas the latter is abusing a "lawful" drug.

Commentary on Coercive Strategies

Addressing maternal substance abuse in a coercive fashion raises contentious constitutional and public policy issues.

Constitutional Considerations

The constitutional questions center on achieving a balance between the rights of individuals and the power of the state to protect vulnerable persons. *Roe v Wade* and subsequent Supreme Court decisions have affirmed the liberty of women to make reproductive choices while recognizing that the state has an interest in protecting the fetuses. The balance remains an uneasy one. But it is clear that the state has a constitutionally legitimate interest in the outcome of pregnancy, which it can express through appropriate legislation. Laws that are rational in the sense of articulating a goal of fetal protection and providing the least restrictive effective means of achieving that goal can satisfy constitutional norms, provided they do not place an "undue burden" on the mother's exercise of her constitutional rights (14). Certainly there is no constitutionally protected liberty to abuse drugs during pregnancy. And the right to unconstrained abortion in early pregnancy does not logically include freedom to willfully or recklessly endanger one's fetus. Thus, it would seem that a carefully drafted law that aims to deter or constrain pregnant women who recklessly endanger their fetuses could survive constitutional challenge.

Public Policy Considerations

Whether such a law is wise social policy is another question. Any harm to a fetus from maternal misconduct may have already occurred by the time legal coercion is considered or applied. An obvious exception is the situation of the HIV-infected mother who, if appropriately treated, will be much less likely to transmit infection to her baby during pregnancy or delivery if antiretroviral therapy is initiated during pregnancy (15). This exception aside, the major social utility of a coercive law could be its signal to women that certain behaviors during pregnancy may trigger unpleasant personal consequences. A potential drawback of such a law is that it could actually deter some pregnant women from seeking prenatal care or undergoing testing that could lead to beneficial treatment.

Another social policy dimension of coercive laws is the potential for conscripting physicians as agents of social control. For example, if child abuse laws are extended to cover fetal abuse, physicians could incur a statutory duty to report instances of maternal drug usage or HIV-infection to public enforcement agencies. And if narcotics laws are amended to allow prosecution for transplacental delivery of unlawful drugs, physicians may incur a duty to report this "crime" when they undertake the care of pregnant drug users. Even if draconian new laws are not actually enacted, public clamor for them might persuade some physicians that they have an ethical duty to report some women to public officials. The "*Tarasoff* doctrine" may protect some physicians who violate confidentiality of their patients in order to protect endangered fetuses or children (16). But not all violations of confidentiality are necessarily justifiable enough to ensure immunity from suits by aggrieved patients. Federal narcotics laws and some state HIV confidentiality laws, for example, broadly and stringently prohibit nonconsensual disclosures of information by physicians.

DIFFICULT CHOICES: NEUROLOGIC IMPLICATIONS

In the context of this chapter, women may face two types of decisions in which neurologic disorders are pivotal factors. One concerns the right of a woman to make personal treatment decisions that put her offspring at risk for neurologic disease or harm. The other concerns withholding or withdrawing life-sustaining treatment from a neurologically impaired neonate or child. The first sort of decision may or may not have neurologic connotations and will be considered, but briefly. But it raises issues that may become more compelling as techniques for prenatal diagnosis of genetic disease become more reliable and available.

Choices that Risk Fetal Harm

A pair of recent state appellate court decisions indicate that a woman can lawfully decline invasive treatments, even if the consequence of the refusal is death or severe neurologic harm to her unborn child.

In one case, an Illinois court considered whether a pregnant woman could be compelled to undergo cae-sarean section in order to protect her fetus from hypoxic brain injury or death (17). Both her attending physician and a consulting university-based obstetrician concluded that the 35-week fetus was receiving insufficient oxygen because of a placental defect and recommended immediate caesarean section. Citing strong religious beliefs, the woman declined this option, a decision in which her husband concurred. At the request of the physicians, the state attorney's office asked a juvenile court to appoint the state as custodian of the fetus so that it could authorize a caesarean section. The court rejected the request, concluding that the fetus was not a "minor" person within the meaning of the statute authorizing appointment of custodians and that there was no precedent for ordering such an intrusive procedure over the objection of a competent woman. A state appellate court upheld this decision, emphasizing that the constitutionally protected right to refuse invasive treatment is retained throughout pregnancy and that a "woman is under no duty to guarantee the mental and physical health of her child at birth, and thus cannot be compelled to do or not do anything merely for the benefit of her unborn child."

The *Baby Boy Doe* decision is consistent with an earlier decision of the District of Columbia Court of Appeals that involved an attempt to force a dying woman to undergo a caesarean section in order to give her fetus a chance of survival (18). The woman had advanced cancer and declined surgery if it would hasten her own death. The court underscored that the mother's competent decision is the crucial determinant and that it would be legally inappropriate to balance the interests of the fetus against the interests of the mother. Although a New Jersey court has held that a pregnant Jehovah's Witness can be forced to have a blood transfusion in order to protect her unborn child (19), this is a minority view. Moreover, as stressed by the court in *Baby Boy Doe* (17), the intrusiveness of surgery is much greater than that of blood transfusion.

The thrust of these cases is that a competent pregnant woman can lawfully decline invasive treatments designed to protect her fetus from neurologic or other harms. This is true whether the reason for declining treatment is her own neurologic affliction, her fear of invasive treatment, or her personal religious beliefs. By the same token, a competent woman can also lawfully consent to an invasive, medically appropriate treatment designed to benefit her fetus, even if the treatment puts her at grave personal risk. In short, from the perspective of law, she can be as altruistic as she wishes to be with respect to invasive treatments so long as she is deemed competent. Obviously, debates can arise about whether a particular treatment is sufficiently invasive to afford a pregnant woman an absolute right of refusal. An example is antiretroviral therapy with protease inhibitors. The complexity of the treatment regimens and the range and severity of side effects are such that one could plausibly argue that the therapy is *invasive*, even if no cutting or other mechanical intrusions are involved.

Withholding or Withdrawing Neonatal Life Support

Parents and physicians can become enmeshed in difficult decisions about how much care to offer neonates with severe neurologic impairment. Although many seem to believe that these decisions are so intimate and personal that outsiders should play little or no role, legal developments in recent years contemplate a measure of social control in this area. The reasons are complex, including a pervasive belief that all life is sacred, no matter how impaired or unpromising, and coupled with a concern among some members of the public that parents and physicians may conspire to deny life to some impaired infants to spare parents the emotional and financial burdens of caring for gravely disabled children. In any case, proponents of greater social control have sought to expand the reach of antidiscrimination and child protection laws as a way of constraining such actions, whereas supporters of a stronger role for physicians in decision-making have argued that there should be no legal obligation to provide care that is medically futile.

Handicap-Based Discrimination

An informative example of an attempt to use antidiscrimination law to impede a parental choice is the federal court case of *United States v University Hospital* (20). The technical legal issue in the case was whether section 504 of the federal Rehabilitation Act of 1973, a precursor of the Americans with Disabilities Act, authorized the Department of Health and Human Services (DHHS) to obtain the hospital records of a neurologically impaired neonate known as Baby Jane Doe. At birth she had meningomyelocele, microcephaly, hydrocephalus, paraplegia, and impaired bowel and bladder functions. Her physicians informed her parents of therapeutic options, including operative repair of the meningomyelocele and a shunting procedure. They also disclosed that the infant was at high risk for mental retardation if she survived. After discussions with other physicians, religious counselors, and a social worker, the parents opted for conservative measures that included continuing nutrition, antibiotics, and local care of the exposed dural sac.

Litigation arose when a right-to-life advocate filed suit in a New York state court seeking appointment of a guardian for the baby and an order directing the hospital to have corrective surgery performed. After a hearing, the court decided that surgery was indicated and ordered the hospital to have it done. An intermediate state appeals court reversed this decision, concluding that the parental decision was informed, reasonable, and supported by "responsible medical authority." New York's highest court upheld this decision, but based on a different rationale. It concluded that the plaintiff in the case had no legal standing to bring the suit and that it was an abuse of discretion for the lower court to name him as guardian or to order specific medical treatment.

As the litigation was proceeding in the state court system, an anonymous person complained to DHHS that Baby Jane Doe was being discriminated against on the basis of handicap, an alleged violation of the Rehabilitation Act. The DHHSs thereupon asked the hospital to produce the infant's medical records so that it could determine whether she was in fact a victim of handicap-based discrimination. The hospital refused this request, asserting parental refusal to consent to release of the records and its own reservations about the lawful authority of DHHS to make the request. The DHHS then asked a federal district court to compel the hospital to produce the records. The district court rejected the request. It concluded that access to the records was barred by a New York law protecting confidentiality of medical records and that the federal statute did not apply to the hospital merely because it received payments from federal health benefit programs (i.e., Medicare, Medicaid).

The DHHS appealed this ruling to a federal circuit court, contending that the parents' choice of conservative treatment was based solely on the handicap of microcephaly—and the implicit prospect of mental retardation. To support its contention, DHHS asserted that the medically appropriate treatment for an infant without microcephaly would have been surgery and that the only reason surgery was withheld was because of her likely mental retardation.

After an extensive review of the complex legislative history of the federal law and relevant judicial precedents, the appeals court ruled in favor of the hospital. It concluded that Congress had not contemplated that the federal law would be applied to treatment decisions concerning impaired neonates. Moreover, it found no support in prior case law for the government's argument. The court noted that the hospital had been "even-handed" in treating the infant and remained willing to offer surgery if the parents requested it. The court further observed that requiring the hospital to provide surgery or to override the preferences of the parents "would pose a particularly onerous affirmative action burden."

This decision, and the later Supreme Court decision in *Bowen v American Hospital Association* (21), which invalidated DHHS regulations designed to force hospitals to report instances of nontreatment of impaired newborns to federal officials, effectively put an end to attempts to use federal antidiscrimination law to intrude on parental decisions about the care of impaired neonates.

Child Abuse

After the judicial rebuffs described, supporters of governmental oversight of the treatment of impaired neonates sought help from Congress. Its response was an amendment to the federal child abuse law (22) that is designed to encourage states to use their child protection agencies to regulate care of impaired neonates. The basic structure of the federal law is to condition grants to states for child protection services upon the states' agreement to apply federally prescribed standards to detect and prevent child abuse.

As amended, section 5102 of the federal law defines child abuse to include the withholding of "medically indicated treatment...for life-threatening conditions." The term *medically indicated treatment* is defined as treatment that is "likely to be effective in ameliorating or correcting all such conditions." Except for "appropriate nutrition, hydration or medication," the statute does not require treatment for infants who are "chronically ill and irreversibly comatose," for infants in whom treatment would "merely prolong dying," would be ineffective in ameliorating or correcting the life-threatening conditions, would "otherwise be futile in terms of survival," or would be "virtually futile" in the sense of being "inhumane."

The amendment hardly qualifies as a model of coherent legislation, but it serves to put state child protection agencies on notice that they must do at least two things if they want federal monies for their programs. First, they should implement measures to prevent parents and physicians from agreeing to withhold "appropriate" nutrition, hydration, and medication from impaired neonates. Second, they should try to limit the range of conditions for which withholding life-sustaining treatment might be considered to only those neonates who have extraordinarily severe impairments. The problems of interpretation with respect to the amendment are too numerous to detail, but pernicious effects are easy to envision. For example, the law could deter parents and physicians from making medically and ethically justifiable decisions concerning infants who do not fit neatly into the categories set forth in the statute. Moreover, the opaqueness of the law could either lead caregivers to throw up their hands and conclude that all impaired neonates must receive maximal care or could render it useless as an enforcement tool. At this juncture, however, it is extremely difficult to draw conclusions as to whether the law has, in and of itself, actually caused caregivers to make different decisions than they would have otherwise made concerning the care of infants with severe neurologic impairment.

Futility

The amendment to the child abuse law contemplates clinical circumstances in which treatment may be "futile" or "virtually futile" in the sense of being "inhumane." What Congress had in mind in using these terms is unclear. There is, of course, a rich debate about the definition of futility as it applies to medical treatment. However, no attempt is made here to revisit this debate other than to note that futility is an elusive concept. For some, treatment that prolongs nonsentient life is futile, whereas for others protecting human existence, no matter how compromised, is anything but futile. But however the word futility is defined, physicians obviously have an important role in giving it content because they are best situated to diagnose morbid conditions and to make predictions about their outcome. Still, a medical judgment that treatment is futile is not necessarily dispositive in a legal forum. An example is a recent federal appeals court ruling concerning the level of care owed an anencephalic child.

At issue in *Matter of Baby K* (23) was whether hospital-based physicians were required to provide care that they regarded as futile. The mother of an anencephalic infant wanted the physicians to use a mechanical ventilator when and if it was necessary to keep the baby alive.

This led the physicians to seek a ruling from a federal district court in Virginia that would shield them from liability if they opted not to use a ventilator if the child presented in respiratory distress. Invoking the federal emergency treatment law (24), the district court denied the request. Its ruling was affirmed by a federal court of appeals, and the Supreme Court declined further review.

The appellate court reasoned that the plain language of the federal statute required physicians to respond to an "emergency medical condition," such as life-threatening respiratory distress, by providing treatment that would "stabilize" that condition by preventing "material deterioration." In the court's eye, respiratory distress in an anencephalic child is an "emergency medical condition" and requires that physicians provide treatment to alleviate that condition, including a mechanical ventilator. The court rejected the physicians' assertion that they were not lawfully bound to use a ventilator because it was not a standard treatment in anencephaly. The court also determined that the federal law pre-empted a Virginia law that would excuse physicians from an obligation to prescribe care that they determine is "medically or ethically inappropriate." A dissenting judge faulted the majority for failing to recognize that the relevant medical condition here was anencephaly, not respiratory distress, and that the standard medical treatment for anencephaly does not encompass use of a ventilator.

Baby K obviously does not stand for the proposition that physicians must always provide care that neurologically impaired patients, or their parents or other lawful proxies, ask for, no matter how useless the treatment may seem. What it does seem to say is that if a treatment is capable of staving off an immediate threat to life in the context of emergency care, physicians cannot entirely rely on their own determination that the treatment is ultimately futile in the neurologic sense as a lawful justification for withholding treatment. In other words, certain therapeutic decisions call for physicians to take into account the values of patients or their lawful proxies, as well as the requirements of particular laws. Most physicians probably behave this way anyhow. *Baby K* merely stands as a reminder that this is a dimension of their professional role today.

References

1. NY Public Health Code Section 2805(d)(1) (1986).
2. GA Code Annotated Section 31-9-6.1(a) (1990).
3. *Harbeson v Parke-Davis Inc*, 656 P 2d 483 (WA Sup Ct 1983).
4. *Roe v Wade*, 410 US 113 (Sup Ct 1973).
5. Furrow BR. Impaired children and tort remedies: The emergence of a consensus. *Law, Medicine & Health Care* 1983;11:148–154.
6. MN Stat 145.424 (1987 Supp).
7. *Hickman v Group Health Plan*, 396 NW 2d 10 (MN Sup Ct 1986).
8. *Arato v Avedon*, 858 P 2d 598 (CA Sup Ct en banc 1993).
9. *People v Stewart*, Mun Ct San Diego Cty CA, #M508197 (1987).
10. Note: maternal rights and fetal wrongs: The case against the criminalization of "fetal abuse." *Harvard Law Rev* 1988;101:994–1012.
11. *Johnson v State*, 602 So 2d 1288 (FL Sup Ct 1992).
12. Phillips M. Umbilical cords: The new drug connection. *Buffalo Law Rev* 1992;40:525–566.
13. *O'Connor v Donaldson*, 422 US 563 (Sup Ct 1975).
14. *Planned Parenthood v Casey*, 505 US 833 (Sup Ct 1992).
15. Connor EM, et al. Reduction of maternal-infant transmission of human immunodeficiency virus type I with zidovudine treatment. *N Engl J Med* 1994;331:1173–1180.
16. Stone A. The Tarasoff decisions: Suing psychotherapists to safeguard society. *Harvard Law Rev* 1976;90:358–385.
17. *In re Baby Boy Doe*, 632 NE 2d 326 (IL App 1994), cert den 114 S Ct 1198 (1994).
18. *In re AC*, 573 A 2d 1235 (DC App 1990).
19. *Raleigh-Fitkin Hospital v Anderson*, 201 A 2d 537 (NJ Sup Ct 1964), cert den 84 S Ct 1894 (1964).
20. *United States v University Hospital*, 729 F 2d 144 (2d Cir 1984).
21. *Bowen v American Hospital Association*, 476 US 610 (Sup Ct 1986).
22. Child Abuse Prevention and Treatment Act, 42 US Code Annotated Section 5102 (West 1984).
23. *Matter of Baby K*, 116 F 3d 590 (4th Cir 1994).
24. Emergency Medical Treatment and Active Labor Act, 42 US Code Annotated Section 1395dd (West 1993).

II

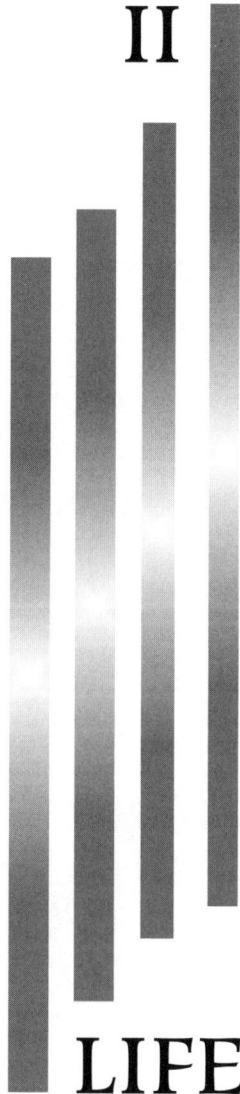

LIFE STAGES AND NEUROLOGIC DISEASE EXPRESSION IN WOMEN

9 Neurologic Disease in Girls

S. Lane Rutledge

Neurologic disease in children differs significantly from neurologic disease in adults. Disease may be specific for a developmental period (Rett syndrome, absence epilepsy, autism) or actually affect physical development of the nervous system (neuronal migration disorders, pyruvate dehydrogenase deficiency). For some disease entities, only children are affected, because life span is shortened. For others, life expectancy is normal, and disease may be diagnosed in childhood and continue into adulthood (Tourette syndrome, ornithine transcarbamylase deficiency). Children may experience the same disease as adults but with differing symptomatology (migraine). It is important to recognize the specific disease entities seen in childhood to provide appropriate genetic and prognostic counseling.

Some pediatric neurologic diseases are seen only in girls, others are more common or differentially expressed in girls. Those seen primarily in girls are usually X-linked or related to menses. Differential expression may be seen throughout childhood or exacerbated by puberty (migraine) and are related to gender but do not necessarily directly involve the X chromosome. In some, the disease is so differentially expressed that ascertainment by classical clinical criteria may not recognize disease in girls (Tourette syndrome presenting as obsessive compulsive disorder). These differences are important with regard to diagnosis, treatment, and prognosis.

(For a discussion of individual diseases and genetic counseling issues, see the chapters addressing these topics.)

X-LINKED DISEASE

The distinction between recessive and dominant inheritance in X-linked diseases is not as clear as for autosomal disease. The diseases discussed (Table 9.1) will be classified as dominant or recessive based on prevailing literature. Many X-linked diseases exist, but only those with significant neurologic manifestations are discussed here.

X-linked dominant diseases are seen only in girls, or primarily in girls, with the very rare case in males due to Klinefelter syndrome (XXY male), half chromatid mutation, or post-zygotic mutation (1–3). Otherwise, these diseases have apparent lethality in males. Thomas (4) postulates that higher numbers of affected females are also due to higher mutations rates in males, who only pass their X chromosome to their daughters (4); this has been reported in incontinentia pigmenti, Pelizaeus-Merzbacher syndrome, and Rett syndrome (5–8). The X chromosome location is known for some X-linked diseases, but only theorized for others. Although clinical disease is not limited to children, most present in childhood. Ascertainment of cases may continue into adulthood.

Recessive X-linked disorders are heritable diseases with differing risks of clinical expression between males

TABLE 9.1
X-linked Neurologic Disease in Girls

X-LINKED NEUROLOGIC DISEASE IN GIRLS	SYSTEMIC MANIFESTATIONS	NEUROLOGIC MANIFESTATIONS	GENETIC LOCATION/MECHANISM
Aicardi syndrome	Ocular, bone, orofacial	Seizures, malformations, agenesis of corpus callosum	Xp22
Goltz syndrome	Skin, bone, ocular, orofacial	Mental retardation, microcephaly	Xp22
MIDAS syndrome	Skin, ocular, bone	Malformations, mental retardation, seizures	Xp22
Rett syndrome	Cardiac, growth	Developmental arrest, hand stereotypies, microcephaly, breathing irregularities	MECP2
Bilateral periventricular nodular heterotopias	None	Neuronal migration abnormalities, seizures	Filamin 1
X-linked lissencephaly/ subcortical band heterotopia	None	Neuronal migration abnormalities, seizures, mental retardation	Double cortin
Incontinentia pigmenti	Skin, teeth, ocular	Seizures, mental retardation, microcephaly	NEMO gene
Oral-facial-digital syndrome	Bone, orofacial	Mental retardation, malformations	Xp22.2-22.3
Fragile X	Orofacial, skin, ocular	Mental retardation, seizures	Trinucleotide repeat FMR1
Charcot-Marie-Tooth	None	Peripheral neuropathy	Connexin 32 protein
Duchenne muscular dystrophy	Cardiac	Myopathy	Dystrophin
Pelizeus merzbacher	None	Leukodystrophy	Proteolipid protein
Adrenoleukodystrophy	Adrenal (rare)	Spinal cord	Xq28 ABCD1
Fabry disease	Cardiac, renal, skin	Painful crises	Xq22 α-galactosidase A
Pyruvate Dehydrogenase deficiency	Lactic acidosis	Malformations, episodic ataxia, progressive cortical involvement	Xq22
Ornithine transcarbamylase deficiency	Hyperammonemia	Psychiatric, mental retardation, coma	Xp

and females. The mutant genes are located on the X chromosome, and transmission from male to male does not occur. Females are heterozygous for the mutant allele. Females with Turner syndrome (45X), or females with X-autosome translocations who possess an abnormal allele on the X chromosome, can also demonstrate the typically male-only spectrum of disease (9,10).

Although a single female with Duchenne muscular dystrophy due to uniparental disomy has been reported (11), the presence of symptoms of X-linked disease in heterozygous 46XX females is largely dependent on X inactivation patterns. Early in the gestation of female fetuses, one X chromosome in each somatic cell is randomly inactivated—the process of *lyonization* (12). As a consequence of this phenomenon, all subsequent daughter cells retain the same inactivated X chromosome. Theoretically, in each tissue, approximately half of cells express the X chromosome derived from the father and half express the X chromosome derived from the mother. If a female bears a mutant allele on one X chromosome, half of the cells in each tissue transcribe only the diseased gene. X chromosome inactivation is not always random, however. In fact, examination of the fibroblasts and leukocytes of normal females demonstrates significantly skewed X inactivation in 20% (13–15). In addition, X inactivation ratios may vary among tissues in the same individual (16). Therefore, depending upon the X inactivation ratio in a vulnerable tissue, a female heterozygous for an X-linked recessive disorder may be asymptomatic, asymptomatic but with biochemical abnormalities, mildly symptomatic, or severely symptomatic.

The causes of apparent nonrandom X inactivation are poorly understood but include stochastic effects and selective advantages of mutant or wild type cells; in some cases, skewed X inactivation may be familial (17). The X inactivation center is located in band Xq13 (18). Alterations in this region could explain the occurrence of multiple symptomatic heterozygous females in families affected with Duchenne muscular dystrophy (19) and Fabry disease (20).

Nonrandom X inactivation nearly always occurs in the presence of a structurally abnormal X chromosome (14). In the presence of an unbalanced X:autosome translocation, the translocated X is preferentially inactivated (21). If a mutant allele is present on the remaining X chromosome, the carrier state is unmasked and the female exhibits the full syndrome. Conversely, in the event of a balanced X:autosome translocation, selective inactivation of the normal X chromosome and preservation of the two translocated pieces occurs (21). If the breakpoint disturbs a disease-causing gene, the female may express the full syndrome. The location of X chromosome breakpoints in females with Duchenne dystrophy and X:autosome translocations led to the discovery of the gene position at Xp21 (22). Similar occurrences aided the discovery of the genes for Menkes disease (23), Hunter syndrome (24), and Lowe oculocerebrorenal syndrome (25).

In several of the X-linked recessive disorders, a significant number of karyotypically normal females partially or completely express the disorder. These conditions are adrenoleukodystrophy (ALD), Fabry disease, ornithine transcarbamylase (OTC) deficiency, pyruvate dehydrogenase (PDH) E1α subunit deficiency, fragile X mental retardation, and the X-linked form of Charcot-Marie-Tooth disease. In the majority of such cases, skewed X chromosome inactivation most likely underlies disease expression in females. In the case of PDH E1α subunit deficiency Fabry disease, and OTC deficiency, the mutant allele, rather than behaving in a typically X-linked recessive manner, may in fact possess incomplete dominance (14).

Mechanisms other than skewed X inactivation may also play a role in the phenotypic variability in X-linked disease. Infrequent manifestations among girls heterozygous for mutations of the hypoxanthine phosphoribosyl transferase (hprt) allele, the Lesch-Nyhan gene, may be a result of in vivo selection against hprt-deficient cells. This phenomenon has been observed in lymphocytes and red blood cells (26,27). In Duchenne muscular dystrophy, dystrophin-negative cells that die may be replaced by dystrophin-positive cells, thus producing fewer symptoms with age.

A second phenomenon observed in Lesch Nyhan disease has been termed "metabolic cooperation." When fibroblasts lacking an active normal hprt allele come in close contact with hprt-expressing fibroblasts, the mutated fibroblasts are able to behave in a metabolically normal fashion (28). Apparently, a substance can be transmitted between cells that repairs the metabolic derangement. Females, because they exhibit a mosaic of hprt-positive and negative cells could, through metabolic cooperation among cells, lessen the effect of the heterozygous state.

X-LINKED DOMINANT DISEASE

Aicardi Syndrome

Aicardi first described the syndrome that now bears his name (29). Clinical diagnosis is based on a triad of features: agenesis of the corpus callosum, chorioretinal abnormalities, and infantile spasms. The mean onset of seizures is less than 3 months of age. Over two-thirds of affected females present with infantile spasms and hypsarrhythmia-like pattern on EEG; almost all develop spasms and hypsarrhythmia-like pattern (30,31). The diagnosis of Aicardi syndrome is usually made when the child presents with infantile spasms and should be suspected in any girl with infantile spasms. Seizures are often difficult to control, using an average of four antiepileptic drugs per patient (30).

The corpus callosum is completely or partially absent (Figure 9.1). Other brain malformations include neuronal migration defects, choroid plexus papillomas and cysts, and Dandy-Walker malformations (30,32,33). Ocular fundus abnormalities are classically described as punched out chorioretinal lacunae, but also include colobomas and microphthalmia. Other clinical manifestations are seen in most patients and include costovertebral malformations (hemivertebra, scoliosis, absent ribs; Figures 9.2A and 9.2B) and cleft lip and palate. Development is adversely affected to a pronounced degree, and most patients never reach a developmental level of greater than 12 months, although some patients develop speech and ambulation (30,32). Life expectancy is limited; only 40% survive to age 15 years (32).

The severity of the disease prohibits reproduction, thus all new cases are sporadic. At least four patients with a partial Aicardi phenotype and an X/3 translocation with a breakpoint at Xp22 have been described, but no mutations or deletions have yet been reported (30,33,34).

Goltz syndrome, or *focal dermal hypoplasia* (35), includes atrophy and linear pigmentation of the skin, fat herniation through dermal defects, striated bones, multiple papillomas, digital and oral anomalies, and mental retardation. *Microphthalmia with linear skin defects (MLS syndrome)* also known as *MIDAS syndrome* (microphthalmia, dermal aplasia, and sclerocornea) includes linear skin defects and ocular abnormalities. Features of Goltz, Aicardi, and MLS syndromes have been described in females with deletions of Xp22.3 (34,36,37). This may be due to a contiguous gene syndrome or a sin-

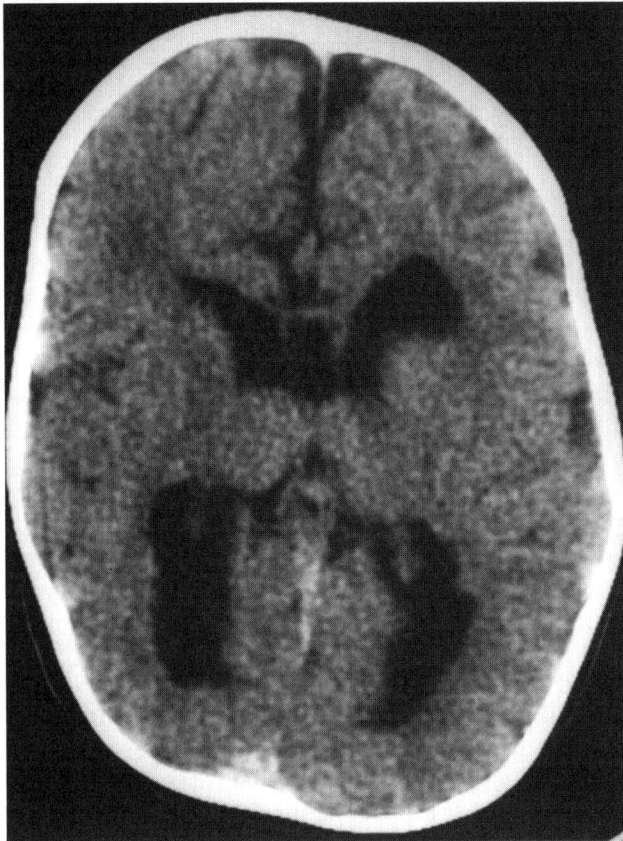

FIGURE 9.1

CT scan in a young girl with Aicardi syndrome demonstrates abnormal separation of the anterior horns of the lateral ventricles and superior displacement of the third ventricle, consistent with agenesis of the corpus callosum.

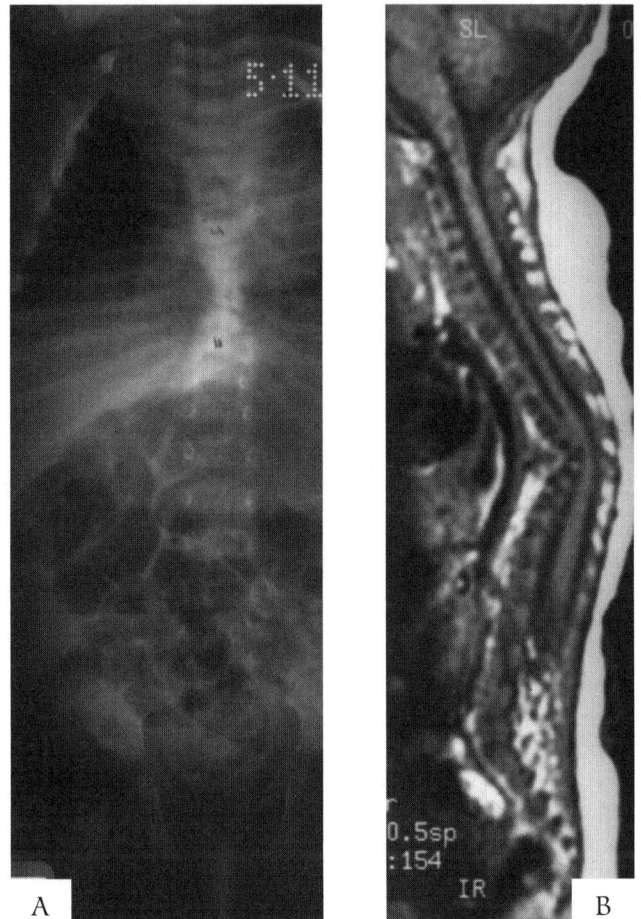

FIGURE 9.2

(A) Sharp kyphosis in Aicardi syndrome due to vertebral body anomalies. (B) Significant decrease in diameter of spinal cord due to the kyphosis seen in (A).

gle gene disorder with differential expression based on different patterns of X chromosome inactivation (36–38). The overlap of these syndromes may explain some atypical cases of Aicardi syndrome.

Rett Syndrome

Rett syndrome is a neurodevelopmental disorder described initially almost exclusively in girls. It was first recognized independently by Rett (39) and Hagberg (40) in the early 1960s. Rett syndrome is characterized by an arrest in motor, mental, and behavioral development in early childhood, deceleration in the rate of head and somatic growth, hand stereotypies, and gait apraxia without features of a progressive neurodegenerative process. The syndrome is seen in all ethnic groups, with a prevalence of 1:12,500 to 1:20,000, a rate exceeding that for phenylketonuria in females. Rett syndrome is due to mutations in the methyl CpG binding protein 2 gene (MECP2). This gene encodes a protein that affects the transcription of other genes (41).

In classic Rett syndrome, following normal pre- and perinatal periods, early development appears normal through the first 6 to 18 months, even though some deviations may be suspected (42). Deceleration in the rate of head growth, however, is already evident by 3 months of age. Then, language and fine motor development regress and typical hand stereotypies (hand-wringing, hand-washing, hand-knitting) appear. Subsequently, cognitive and behavioral function plateau or actually improve somewhat during later childhood and adolescence. Motor function tends to decline slowly, the majority remaining ambulatory into adulthood. Precise data on longevity are not available; however, survival beyond 30 years appears likely.

Associated features include breathing irregularities (hyperventilation, breath-holding, air swallowing) during wakefulness, bruxism (teeth grinding), scoliosis, seizures and cold, dystrophic, cyanotic feet. Scoliosis may progress and require surgical correction. Seizures may be difficult to differentiate from some of the unusual behaviors described above and may require video monitoring. EEG shows typical but nondiagnostic features of background slowing, little or no waking dominant rhythm, multifocal spike and slow spike and wave activity, and loss of normal sleep patterns.

Brain imaging (CT/MRI) reveals only mild to moderate atrophy. Neuropathologic studies show no evidence of progressive neurodegeneration but rather suggest an arrest in early development with smaller, more densely packed neurons and primitive dendritic arborizations with a sharp reduction in pigmented neurons in the substantia nigra.

Now that the genotype is known, the phenotype is expanding. Mutations in MECP2 are known to cause atypical Rett syndrome with preserved language in girls, Rett-like syndrome in boys, and X-linked mental retardation in boys (6,43). A poor genotype-phenotype correlation exists, probably due to X inactivation patterns. Random inactivation is typical in Rett syndrome, and nonrandom X inactivation is usually beneficial, producing milder or asymptomatic disease (44). Interestingly, in only one-quarter of familial cases has a mutation in MECP2 been found; there may be another genetic locus for the syndrome (43–45).

Treatment is symptomatic, and emphasis should be directed toward physical, communicative, and occupational therapies to optimize function and minimize physical disabilities (46).

Neuronal Migration Disorders

The normal six-layered cerebral cortex is formed by neurons that migrate from subependymal regions to their appropriate cortical locations. This migration is a very precise process in which immature neurons migrate along glial cell processes, with deeper cortical layers formed first and superficial neurons in layer 2 migrating last (47). The genetic basis of this process is not fully elucidated but at least two X-linked disorders of neuronal migration are known and others are suspected (48).

Bilateral periventricular nodular heterotopia is a neuronal migration disorder caused by mutations in filamin 1 (FLN1), an actin binding protein (49,50). It is expressed in females and has prenatal or perinatal lethality in males. MRI reveals bilateral continuous bands or discontinuous nodules of heterotopias with typical characteristics of gray matter (Figure 9.3; 49,51,52). Microscopically, these are composed of differentiated well-innervated neurons that appear normal except for being abnormally oriented (multiple directions) (49). The genetic defect appears to be highly penetrant, and the heterotopias are present as early as 6 months of age and are stable with time. Affected females are neurologically intact except for seizures, which only occur in some, but

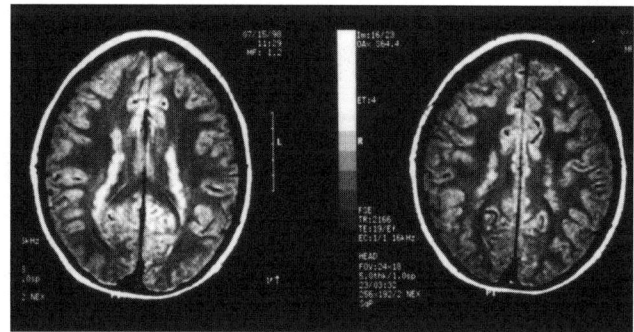

FIGURE 9.3

MRI imaging of a 15-year-old girl with normal intelligence, seizures, and bilateral periventricular nodular heterotopia.

not all, females with the heterotopias. Epilepsy, when present, may be of multiple seizure types, and EEG findings are nonspecific. Literature reviews of older, isolated cases of periventricular heterotopias reveal a female preponderance (52).

A second syndrome, *X-linked lissencephaly/subcortical band heterotopia* or the *double cortex syndrome*, was first described by Barkovich (53) and Marchal (54). MRI reveals an extensive band of subcortical gray matter separated from the overlying cortex by a band of white matter, most obvious in frontocentroparietal regions (55). Neuropathology shows preservation of cortical layers 1 to 4 but layers 5 and 6 are poorly differentiated and merge with white matter U fibers (54,55). All patients have seizures, ranging in severity from infantile spasms and Lennox-Gastaut to partial seizures. Most are mentally retarded, although the severity varies and some are functional in society (55,56). Affected daughters of affected mothers also have double cortex, but affected sons have lissencephaly with more devastating neurologic consequences (48). The gene responsible for this syndrome is double cortin (DCX) (57,58). DCX functions as a microtubule-associated protein, and normal microtubular function is crucial to neuronal migration (59). Women with two populations of X chromosomes have normal and abnormal neuronal migration, so two bands of cortex; males with only one X chromosome only have abnormally migrated cells, lissencephaly (59).

Three families with *aplasia of the cerebellar vermis* with a female:male ratio of 6:1 have been described (60). Affected women had ataxia, dysmetria, and nystagmus, and males were more severely affected.

Incontinentia Pigmenti

Incontinentia pigmenti is a disorder of the ectoderm involving skin, teeth, eyes, and the central nervous system (CNS). It shows X-linked dominant inheritance, usually with male lethality, but affected males have survived with subsequent father to daughter transmission possible (61,62). Familial incontinentia pigmenti is due to mutations in the NEMO gene (nuclear factor κB essential modulator) at Xq28 (8). This gene produces a transcription factor that regulates multiple genes in immune, inflammatory, and apoptotic pathways (8,7). Seventy to eighty percent of patients have an identical large genomic deletion (7,8). Milder mutations occur and may produce surviving males (63). There has been considerable debate over a second nonfamilial incontinentia pigmenti site at Xp11. Sybert (64) and Berlin (65) suggest that these patients do not satisfy the criteria for incontinentia pigmenti. Extremely skewed X chromosome inactivation is common and crucial to disease expression, as cells with the abnormal X activated are replaced by cells with the normal X activated (66,65)

Intrafamilial variability is the rule. Typical skin lesions progress through stages, with initial blistering (blisters, pustules, and erythema) presenting in a typically linear distribution (up to 4 months of age), followed by verrucous and hyperkeratotic lesions (up to 6 months of age) (Figure 9.4). These early lesions occur primarily on the extremities and are found at birth in 40% of patients; they occur in almost 95% of cases (67). In an individual patient, not all stages may occur, or some may occur simultaneously. Later, affected women develop truncal hyperpigmentation often following Blaschko's lines (developmental skin pattern due to proliferation of two different clonal cell lines during early embryogenesis) (up to 20 years of age), and pale hairless patches of skin (adulthood). Dental anomalies occur in 65%, and features include delayed eruption and dental malformations. Conical and pegged teeth are the most common findings (67). Ocular manifestations (retinal vascular abnormalities with secondary retinal detachment) may be absent or severe enough to cause visual loss (68). Neurologic involvement includes seizures, mental retardation, and microcephaly. CNS involvement in the neonatal period is a poor prognostic sign (69). CNS imaging in seven patients with incontinentia pigmenti revealed abnormalities consistent with small vessel occlusion in five patients with concordance of imaging and clinical involvement (70). A few patients with periventricular white matter abnormalities have been reported (Figure 9.5; 71,72).

Oral-Facial-Digital Syndrome I

OFD syndrome type I is another probable X-linked dominant disease with male lethality. Marked clinical variability occurs in heterozygous females (1). Extraneural manifestations include skull malformations (basilar kyphosis with steep anterior fossa and downsloping posterior fossa), digital anomalies (polydactyly, brachydactyly, and syndactyly), oro-facial involvement (lobu-

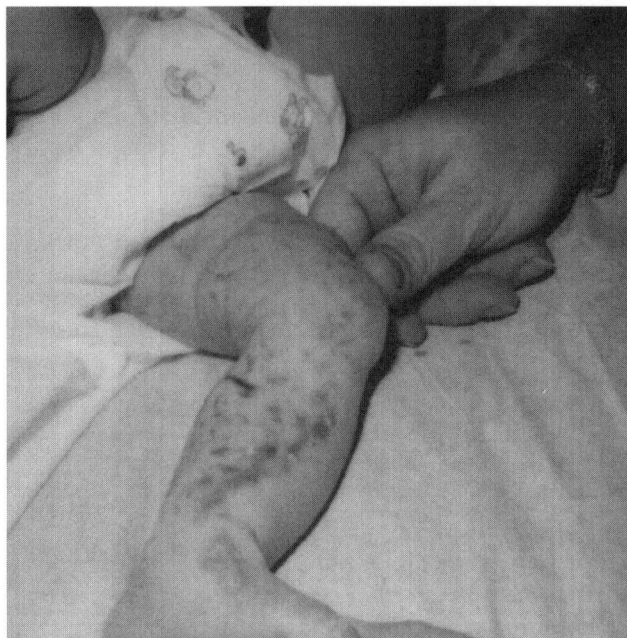

FIGURE 9.4

Three-month-old female with lesions of incontinentia pigmenti.

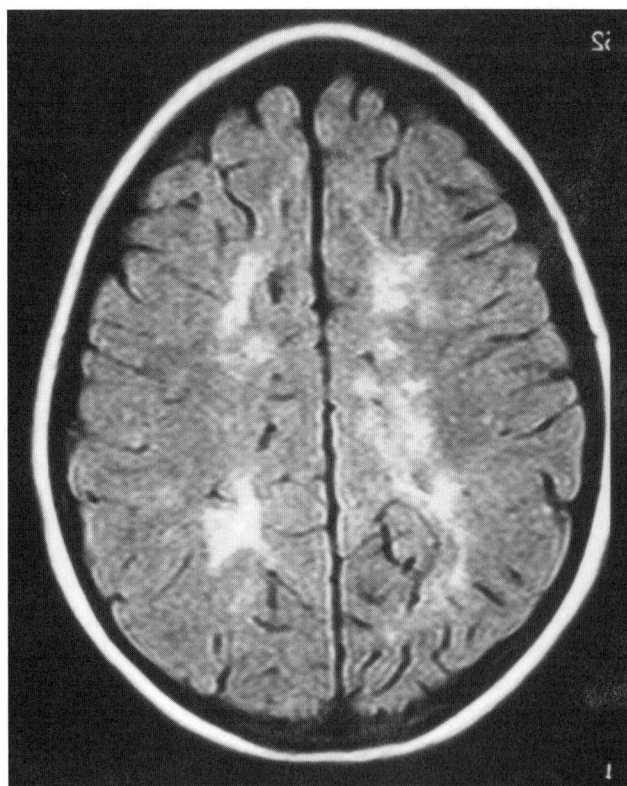

FIGURE 9.5

Axian T1-fast spin echo MRI demonstrates periventricular white matter abnormalities in a 6-year-old with incontinentia pigmenti.

lated tongue, dental malformations, cleft palate, hypertrophic frenula), and polycystic kidneys (73,74). Mental retardation occurs in 30 to 50% of heterozygous females. Speech delay due to the marked oral pathology in this disorder should not be misinterpreted as mental retardation. The incidence is approximated to be at least 1% of cleft palate cases (73).

CNS malformations may be severe and include agenesis of the corpus callosum, abnormal gyri (polymicrogyria), ependymal-lined cysts, and widespread heterotopias that involve the cortex, brainstem, and spinal cord (75,76). As many as one-third of affected girls may die in the first year of life (74). The gene responsible for OFD1 maps to Xp22.2-p22.3 (77) and mutations have been found (78), but gene function remains unknown.

Mental Retardation

It has been known for over a century that mental retardation is more common in males (79). One etiology is *Fragile X syndrome* but there are many other forms of X-linked mental retardation. This diagnosis is usually based on inheritance patterns, and the genetic loci for many are unknown (79). Skewed X-inactivation is common in X-linked mental retardation carriers (80). Many affected pedigrees are small but in some larger ones, affected females are found (79,81).

Fragile X Syndrome

Fragile X syndrome is the most common form of inherited mental retardation (82). In the hemizygous male, the phenotype is characterized by early delays in motor and speech development followed by hyperactivity, autistic or aggressive behavior, varying degrees of mental retardation in childhood, and macroorchidism in puberty. Characteristic dysmorphic features, which may be inapparent prior to adolescence, consist of a long face with prominent forehead and jaw and large ears. Additional variable features include strabismus, hyperextensible joints, mitral valve prolapse, and smooth skin (83).

The fragile X syndrome is most appropriately classified as an X-linked dominant condition with reduced penetrance in females. The gene, FMR1, carries a CGG trinucleotide. Among normal individuals, the number of CGG copies is less than 52. Individuals harboring the meiotically unstable premutation exhibit between 52 and slightly greater than 200 copies (84). Individuals with the full mutation of greater than 200 CGG copies will, under culture conditions depriving the cells of pyrimidine nucleotide precursors, demonstrate a fragile site (FRAXA) of some but not all of their metaphase X chromosomes (85). The FMR-1 gene protein product is an RNA binding protein that is absent or severely reduced in symptomatic males (86). The CGG repeat is located in the 5'

untranslated region, but apparently the expanded repeat sequence leads to abnormal methylation of another untranslated region upstream which, in turn, inhibits transcription of the gene (87).

Males and females who possess the intermediate length premutation are often phenotypically normal. Subtle expression of the fragile X phenotype may occur in such individuals, however, with a significant lowering of intellectual scores in males and females and minor facial dysmorphism in some males (88). Twenty-one percent of female permutation carriers will have premature ovarian failure (89). All hemizygous males with the larger full mutation express some fragile X characteristics and the threshold for full expression of the phenotype appears to be slightly greater than 200 copies. Additionally, both the premutation and full mutation are mitotically unstable, possibly leading to mosaicism of the number of repeats between and among tissues (84). The risk of complete phenotype expression increases in subsequent generations, a phenomenon termed *genetic anticipation*, and depends upon the sex of the parent from whom the defect is inherited. Although the intermediate length premutation is stable during spermatogenesis, it is markedly unstable during oogenesis, producing symptomatic sons and daughters of an asymptomatic carrier female (90).

Symptomatology among heterozygous females bearing the full mutation is variable (91–93). In heterozygous females, the repeat length, if within the full mutation range, does not correlate with the degree of mental impairment (93,94). Rather, X chromosome inactivation ratios favoring the normal FMR1 allele have been detected in higher functioning females bearing the full mutation (91). The neuropsychologic profiles of young girls with the full mutation show that as many as 85% demonstrate mild intellectual impairment and 50% are mentally retarded. These girls may demonstrate avoidant, autistic, and hyperactive behaviors, and mood disorders (95–97). Specific deficits may be apparent in math achievement; longitudinal studies are underway to determine neuropsychologic profiles (97). Females may also exhibit a subtle facial dysmorphism similar to that observed in affected males (90).

Charcot-Marie-Tooth Disease

A second disorder inherited in a semidominant fashion is the X-linked form of Charcot-Marie-Tooth (CMTX) disease. Abnormalities of the connexin 32 protein, a gap junction protein involved in the intercellular transfer of ions and small molecules, have been established in CMTX families (98). In hemizygous males, the disorder manifests during childhood or adolescence as a severe, diffuse demyelinating neuropathy with resultant distal weakness, atrophy and sensory loss, pes cavus, and areflexia (99). Heterozygous females often have milder clinical features with later onset, less severe slowing of nerve conduction velocity, and slower progression than their affected male relatives. However, 15% of females will present before 10 years of age (100). In some families, heterozygous females may be asymptomatic (101). The presence of symptoms in females depends on unfavorable X inactivation ratios but also on specific mutations (100). Families bearing frame shift mutations causing a complete lack of the connexin 32 protein may demonstrate a more severe phenotype among both hemizygous males and heterozygous females (101). A female with onset of symptoms at 1 year of age is probably the result of the specific mutation she carries (100).

Other Possible X-Linked Dominant Conditions

CHILD syndrome consists of unilateral ichthyosiform erythroderma with ipsilateral limb malformations. This syndrome may include unilateral hypoplasia of cranial nerves, brain stem, and cerebellum (1). A single family has been described in which affected females have a slowly progressive spastic paraparesis, IgG2 deficiency, and reduced night vision, while males died in infancy of severe hypotonia (102). *Cervico-oculo-acusticus syndrome (Wildervanck syndrome)* includes congenital sensorineural deafness, Klippel-Feil anomaly (cervical vertebrae fusion and short neck), and Duane syndrome (abducens nerve paralysis), dysmorphic features, and mental retardation (1). Affected females outnumber males by a ratio of 10:1.

X-LINKED RECESSIVE DISEASE

Muscular Dystrophy

Duchenne muscular dystrophy is an X-linked recessive muscular dystrophy caused by mutations within the dystrophin gene that lead to an absence of dystrophin at the sarcolemma membrane (103). The absence of dystrophin causes muscle fiber degeneration and loss. Hemizygous males present with progressive skeletal muscle weakness with calf hypertrophy. Creatine phosphokinase (CPK) levels are markedly elevated. Mental retardation and cardiomyopathy occur in many. Although persistent elevations of CPK are present in approximately 70% of carrier females (104), only 10 to 15% exhibit clinically evident weakness (104). Common complaints in symptomatic carrier females are cramping and enlargement of the calves and mild to moderate proximal muscle weakness that may mimic limb-girdle muscular dystrophy (104,105). In a study of muscle biopsies in females (106), 4% of isolated cases of neuromuscular disease in females (limb-girdle dystrophy, myopathy) had dystrophinopathies and another 4% were symptomatic carri-

ers of Duchenne muscular dystrophy, having a positive family history. Abnormalities in dystrophin are a not uncommon cause of neuromuscular disease in females. With advancing age, symptomatic carrier females may experience an improvement of muscle symptoms and normalization of CPK (107). This is produced by constant selective pressure for dystrophin-negative myofibers to become increasingly dystrophin-positive through the diffusion of dystrophin to affected areas. Also, the regeneration of necrotic dystrophin-negative areas by dystrophin-expressing satellite cells will increase the number of dystrophin-positive cells (108). Girls with moderate weakness, however, may experience progression as the rate of fiber necrosis exceeds the rate of fiber regeneration (104,108). Dilated cardiomyopathy has also been reported in females (109,110). With advancing age, its incidence and severity increase. The compensatory replacement of dystrophin-negative cells by dystrophin-positive cells seen in skeletal muscle does not occur in cardiac muscle (111). In almost all symptomatic carrier females, skewed X inactivation underlies the presence and severity of symptoms (108,112). A single female with Duchenne muscular dystrophy and uniparental disomy of the X chromosome (two copies of one of the parental chromosomes) with a deletion in the dystrophin gene has been described (11), and some girls are symptomatic due to X-autosome translocations.

A second X-linked disorder of muscle, *Emery-Dreifuss syndrome*, is characterized in the hemizygous male by a clinical triad of early contractures, scapulo-humeroperoneal distribution of weakness, and cardiac conduction defects that may precipitate sudden death (113). Among heterozygous females, significant and persistent elevations of CPK do not occur (114), but cardiac conduction abnormalities may appear during adulthood (113,115).

Leukodystrophies

Two X-linked forms of leukodystrophy are recognized, *Pelizaeus-Merzbacher* and *X-linked adrenoleukodystrophy*. The Pelizaeus-Merzbacher disease phenotype in males ranges from onset in infancy or early childhood of eye movement abnormalities, profound hypotonia, and choreoathetosis followed by spasticity and early death, to later onset with more static CNS disease to spastic parapareis (5). Imaging in the early onset forms show a profound lack of myelin. This X-linked recessive leukodystrophy results from abnormalities of proteolipid protein (PLP), a major constituent of myelin. Mutations in the PLP gene include duplications in 60 to 70%, null or point mutations in 10 to 20%, and no mutation found in 10 to 20%. The gene is dosage sensitive, and Pelizaeus-Merzbacher is one of few diseases produced by increase in gene function (116).

Symptomatic females are reported, some with detectable mutations and some without (117–119). Symptoms range from an infantile-onset of encephalopathy with nystagmus and decreased central myelin to spastic paraparesis to adult-onset leukodystrophies (120). In general, female carriers of duplications and other mutations that produce a severe phenotype in males are asymptomatic, whereas female carriers of milder mutations are more often symptomatic. X-inactivation may play a role, but more important, in severe mutations, the affected population of oligodendrocytes may die, leaving only the normal population of cells, while in milder mutations, the cells survive and produce abnormal myelin and symptoms (120). Two exceptions to this have been reported by Inoue (120): two girls with duplications presented with CNS dysmyelinating disorder with marked improvement with time. He postulated that skewed inactivation of the X chromosome was responsible for symptoms, but affected oligodendrocytes failed to differentiate and were gradually replaced by cells with the normal X activation, and symptoms gradually improved. If most symptomatic girls do not have a duplication, then testing by fluorescent in-situ hybridization (FISH) to detect the duplication will not detect most affected females.

X-linked adrenoleukodystrophy (ALD) is a heterogeneous disorder producing five distinct phenotypes in the hemizygous male: rapidly progressive childhood form; adolescent and adult cerebral forms; adrenomyeloneuropathy (AMN), primarily a spinal cord disease; and isolated adrenal insufficiency (121). The variability of phenotype among family members presumably carrying the same mutation is most likely explained by the presence of modifying autosomal genes (122). A striking elevation of saturated very long chain fatty acids in tissues and body fluids is present in all affected and presymptomatic males (121). Concentrations of very long chain fatty acids are increased in the plasma of 88% of obligate female heterozygotes. Sensitivity improves to 94% when levels in skin fibroblasts are also assayed (121).

AMN is the most common phenotype observed in adult heterozygous females (121). Its presence has not been recorded in childhood. It is characterized by an insidious onset of weakness, spasticity, and vibration loss affecting the lower extremities (123). Although 15 to 20% of heterozygous females eventually develop overt signs and symptoms of AMN, as many as 60% will demonstrate abnormalities on neurologic examination (121). Rarely, heterozygous females may experience progressive cerebral symptoms, and occasionally these symptoms occur in childhood and adolescence. Three adolescent females with seizures, encephalopathic symptoms, and adrenal dysfunction have been reported (124). Adrenal dysfunction is very rare in adult heterozygotes. Childhood onset of the cerebral phenotype has been

reported in a female with monosomy of Xq27-terminus (125). All affected females have elevated blood levels of very long chain fatty acids. The presence of neurologic symptoms in heterozygous females is probably due to skewed X inactivation (126).

Ornithine Transcarbamylase Deficiency

Ornithine transcarbamylase (OTC) deficiency is an X-linked disorder of urea synthesis that classically presents as hyperammonemia in hemizygous newborn males, with lethargy progressing to coma and, without treatment, death at 1 to 5 days of life.

Approximately 20% of female heterozygotes will be symptomatic during their lifetime (127). Females can present at any age; a few cases of typical neonatal onset disease in females have been described (128). More commonly, symptomatic female heterozygotes present with later onset disease. Patients may have a lifelong history of protein avoidance and poor growth. There may have been no or many episodes of altered mental status, and early symptoms may be mistaken for behavioral or psychiatric disturbances. During hyperammonemic episodes, hyperactivity and behavioral changes precede ataxia and vomiting, which are followed by lethargy and coma. Among heterozygous females, diagnosis is often delayed, and a significant number die or are left with serious neurologic sequelae (127). Hyperammonemic episodes in heterozygous females may be precipitated by infection, high protein intake, valproate therapy, and the puerperium (127,129,130). Because of the risk of serious symptoms among carrier females, a detailed search of affected family members is required if a case of OTC deficiency is identified. Effective dietary and medical treatment is available. Symptomatic females have undergone curative liver transplantation (131). The presence of symptoms in such a large proportion of female carriers may be due to skewed X inactivation in the liver, as was recently demonstrated in OTC-deficient mice (132).

Mutations in the gene coding for OTC have been found in approximately 75% of patients with confirmed enzymatic deficiency; most are private mutations (133). Symptomatic females have mutations seen in neonatal onset males, mutations that severely affect gene function (134). Allopurinol loading and the measurement of urinary orotate has been used in the past to diagnose carriers, but may not be sensitive or specific (135). Measurement of 15N labeled urea to glutamine ratio may be a more sensitive and specific test of carrier status (136).

Pyruvate Dehydrogenase Deficiency

Pyruvate dehydrogenase is a multienzyme complex that catalyzes the conversion of pyruvate to acetyl CoA. PDH is the rate limiting step connecting glycolysis with the tri-

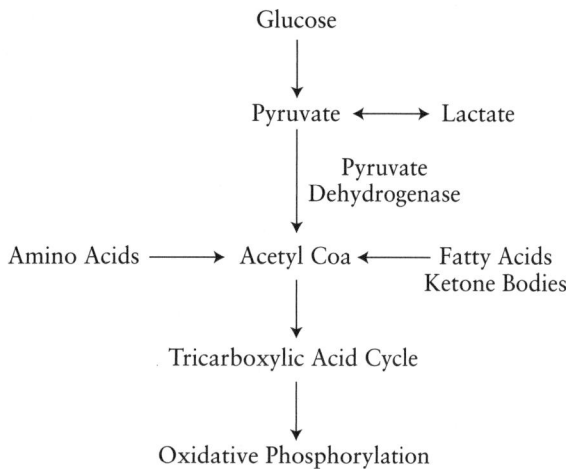

Glucose

$\downarrow$

Pyruvate $\longleftrightarrow$ Lactate

Pyruvate
Dehydrogenase

Amino Acids $\longrightarrow$ Acetyl Coa $\longleftarrow$ Fatty Acids
                                                Ketone Bodies

$\downarrow$

Tricarboxylic Acid Cycle

$\downarrow$

Oxidative Phosphorylation

FIGURE 9.6

Glucose metabolism.

carboxylic acid cycle (TCA) and oxidative phosphorylation (Figure 9.6). A deficiency of PDH is the most common cause of congenital lactic acidosis. With deficiency of PDH, cells have decreased ATP production and accumulate pyruvate (and, therefore lactate, since the two are in equilibrium). If severe deficiency is present, cell death may ensue. Clinical symptoms relate to a cell's dependence on glycolysis as an energy source and a tissue's energy demands. The brain is completely dependent on glycolysis for its high energy needs. Enzyme function is nearly maximal normally (137). Thus, the CNS is the primary structure affected in PDH deficiency. Both structural malformations and destructive cystic lesions are found, probably reflecting the timing of the insult. Regions affected are those with the highest levels of PDH (138,139).

The three components of the multienzyme complex are pyruvate decarboxylase (E1, EC1.2.4.1), dihydrolipoyl transacetylase (E2, EC2.3.1.12), and dihydrolipoyl dehydrogenase (E3, EC 1.8.14). The E1 enzyme is a heterotetramer of two α and two β subunits. Most cases of PDH deficiency are due to E1α subunit deficiency and are sporadic (139). The E1-α subunit has been localized to Xq22. Patterns of disease expression make it difficult to classify as simple X-linked recessive or X-linked dominant. Although X-linked, an equal incidence of disease occurs in males and females (140,141). This equal ratio is the result of several factors: prenatal lethality in some affected males, skewed X inactivation, and a very low threshold of enzyme deficiency required to produce CNS disease in heterozygous females (142).

Enzyme activity is measured in cells (fibroblasts) other than the affected tissue (brain). X-inactivation in the cells in which PDH is measured may not correlate with X-inactivation in the affected tissue; measured enzyme activity in the fibroblasts of affected women may

not correlate with, or even be diagnostic of, PDH deficiency in the CNS (139).

The phenotype of PDH deficiency in females is extremely variable, ranging from fatal neonatal lactic acidosis to progressive neurologic disease with CNS malformations, to carbohydrate-induced mild lactic acidosis and episodic ataxia (138,140). Affected girls may present with infantile spasms, but this is rarely seen in affected males (143). In females, a broad spectrum of disease is probably produced by variations in residual enzyme activities and X-inactivation patterns. The role that X-inactivation plays in PDH deficiency is further evidenced by the phenotypic variation in women with identical mutations (144). Three females with the same point mutation (R302C) had phenotypes ranging from mild mental retardation and seizures to severe systemic acidosis and death by age 5 months. Two of these females were mother and child but the mother was only able to be diagnosed by mutational analysis after the diagnosis was made in her child. In the mother's fibroblasts (the tissue tested for enzyme activity), over 90% of cells expressed the normal X chromosome, and enzyme analysis was normal. Diagnosis in a female suspected of PDH deficiency may require mutational screening, determination of X-inactivation patterns by analysis of methylation patterns, or monoclonal antibody staining for mosaicism in fibroblasts (13,145–147).

Disease should be suspected in females with systemic or central lactic acidosis and characteristic CNS involvement. Typical clinical neurologic involvement may present as profound neonatal hypotonia, infantile spasms and other seizure types, a neurodegenerative course, or episodic ataxia. Structural involvement includes destructive lesions and malformations. Malformations include agenesis of the corpus callosum, abnormal inferior olives and medullary pyramids, and ectopic gray matter (138,140,144,148). Cerebral atrophy and cystic lesions in cortex, basal ganglia, brain stem, and cerebellum are evidence of cell death and tissue loss. Features of *Leigh syndrome* may be seen on imaging (Figure 9.7). Milder cases in females may be missed if the course or lesions are not typical. Treatment is a high-fat, low-carbohydrate (ketogenic) diet. Rare cases respond to thiamine (140).

Fabry Disease

Fabry disease, resulting from a deficiency of the lysosomal enzyme α-galactosidase A (149), typically manifests in the young male hemizygote as painful crises involving the palms and soles. The presence of characteristic skin lesions (telangiectases of the back, buttocks, umbilicus, and scrotum) often leads to the correct diagnosis in adolescence. With advancing age, cardiac (cardiomyopathy), cerebral (stroke), and renal vascular abnormalities appear (150).

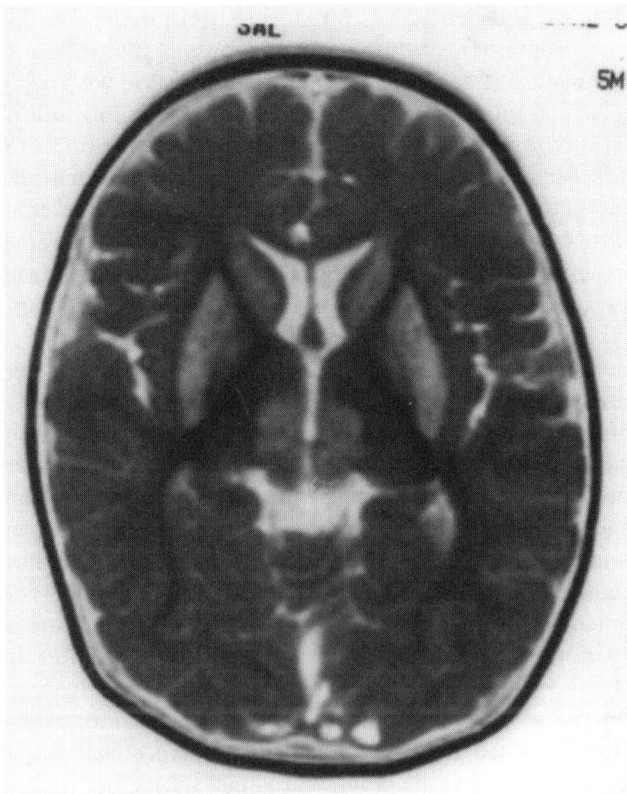

FIGURE 9.7

Axial T2-weighted MRI demonstrates typical features of Leigh syndrome with abnormal high signal in basal ganglia and brainstem representing primary areas affected by the disease.

In the past, Fabry disease was considered X-linked recessive, but reports documenting symptoms in carrier females are common, and the deficiency may function more as a dominant trait (151). All symptoms seen in males may also occur in carrier females, although at a later age (151,152). In females, the mean age of onset of neuropathic pain is 9.3 years, and renal failure has been reported in patients as young as 19 years old (151).

Other X-Linked Recessive Diseases

Several neurodegenerative disorders of infancy and early childhood are transmitted in an X-linked recessive manner. *Menkes disease* is an X-linked recessive disorder of copper transport marked by intractable seizures, progressive neurodegeneration, and an unusual malformation of hair termed *pili torti* (153). Among female heterozygotes, low copper and ceruloplasmin levels are not present, although patchy areas of poorly pigmented skin and pili torti (kinky hair) have been reported (154,155). Rarely, severe symptoms have appeared in girls with a normal karyotype (156). A defect of X-linked creatine transporter has been recently described (157). Affected males have mental retardation, severe language deficits, and hypotonia. Some female carriers have been reported to have low IQ and learning disabilities, and magnetic resonance spectroscopy has demonstrated low creatine levels throughout the brain in a young infant carrier female (158). Neurologic symptoms have only rarely been documented among females heterozygous for *myotubular myopathy* (159), *Hunter syndrome* (160,161), and *Lesch-Nyhan disease* (162,163). Again, extremes of lyonization, Turner syndrome, and X chromosome translocations appear to be responsible.

DISEASE DIFFERENTIALLY EXPRESSED IN GIRLS

A number of common pediatric neurologic diseases are differentially expressed in males and females. This differential expression may simply be an increased incidence of the disease in girls (absence seizures, lupus) (Table 9.2), but often involves clinical symptomatology (Tourette syndrome) and disease severity (autism). The basis of the differential expression may be hormonal and exacerbated by puberty (migraine, menstrual-related disorders) or due to a varying threshold for disease presentation (autism) or unknown (multiple sclerosis). The practitioner should be aware of these differences because they may play an important role not only in treatment and prognosis, but also in their own perception of the patient and her disease.

Tourette Syndrome

Tourette syndrome remains a fascinating disease both phenotypically and genotypically. Phenotypically, it is a disease with varied expression ranging from classic Tourette syndrome (onset less than 18 years of age, motor and vocal tics present for more than 1 year), to chronic tic disorder (usually a single type of tic, motor or vocal), to obsessive compulsive disorder (170–172). The male-to-female ratio in children is 3:1 to 4:1 when only classic Tourette syndrome is considered (172,173). In family studies, however,

TABLE 9.2 *Neurologic Diseases More Commonly Seen in Girls*
Absence epilepsy (164)
Myasthenia gravis (165)
Sydenham chorea (166)
Occult spinal dysraphism (167)
Systemic lupus erythematosus (168)
Dopa-responsive dystonia (169)
Dermatomyosistitis (168)

if all three components of the phenotype (Tourette syndrome, chronic tic disorder, obsessive compulsive disorder) are included, this ratio drops to 1.6:1. Female relatives of Tourette syndrome probands are more likely to have obsessive compulsive disorder without tics and male relatives to have a tic disorder (170,172). Gender influence on disease expression is seen structurally in magnetic resonance imaging studies of patients with Tourette syndrome; changes seen in the corpus callosum and basal ganglia of boys are not seen in girls (174,175). Assuming autosomal dominant transmission (as yet unproven), penetrance of the gene is lower for females for all three expressions of the disease, and gender plays a role in the type of disease expressed (172,176).

More is at play here than just gender-based expression, however. In classic Tourette syndrome, males and females have a similar mean age at onset of tics with similar severity, but females have a later age at diagnosis by 7 to 9 years (171,173). A comparison of ratios between childhood and adulthood found an almost even ratio in adults with Tourette syndrome. Santangelo (171) postulates that gender-based behavioral and socialization differences and physician awareness of increased incidence in boys may play a role in later age at diagnosis in females. In most studies, proband ascertainment is through the diagnosis of Tourette syndrome and, if the disease has a significant gender-based expression, with females presenting with non-Tourette syndrome symptoms, then clearly there is ascertainment bias (170).

When the disease expression is Tourette syndrome, some gender differences in symptoms occur. Females are more likely to have sensory tics, to have onset with complex tics (reproducible set of tics) or compulsive tics, and to experience uninhibited anger and aggression (rage) during the course of the disease (but males are more likely to present with rage) (171). Copralalia may be more common in females (39% vs. 28%) (173). In general, however, disease experience is similar for males and females with Tourette syndrome.

Headache

Headaches are common in children, with 35 to 40% of 5- to 7-year-olds and 68% of 14-year-olds reporting some type of headache (177,178). The prevalence of headache in the pediatric population increases with age. The two most frequent headache diagnoses in children and adolescents are migraine and tension-type headaches and, with increasing age, both are more frequent in girls (178–182).

Any discussion of migraine in children must be prefaced by some comments about definition. The International Headache Society criteria were not developed for children and are not always appropriate for use in children. Most pediatric practitioners have modified the criteria for children, sometimes formally (183).

Migraine without aura (common migraine) is more frequent and has a later onset than migraine with aura (classical migraine) in all children. The onset for both is later in girls, with a peak for classical migraine of 12 to 13 years in girls and 4 to 7 years in boys, and for common migraine, 13 to 17 years in girls and 8 to 12 years in boys (180,183). Many epidemiologic studies of migraine in children have been performed (184), but stratification by age and migraine type vary considerably. In prepubertal children, migraine is probably more frequent in males, but the trend is reversed in pubertal and postpubertal children and adolescents (178–181,183). Although some authors (181,185) report no gender difference in common migraine incidence, these studies are not stratified by age or do not include patients older than 14 years of age. When age stratification is incorporated, the incidence of common migraine increases throughout adolescence in females but remains relatively steady in males, producing a male-to-female ratio of 1:2 by age 15 years. Classical migraine is more frequent in adolescent females, a reversal of early childhood findings (180,181,183). Basilar artery migraine (migraine with symptoms referable to the posterior circulation) is much more common in girls, and most have onset by 5 to 6 years of age (186,187). Attacks sometimes begin in infancy but can only be diagnosed in retrospect. Other types of headache seen more frequently in girls include cyclic migraine, chronic paroxysmal hemicrania, and hemicrania continua (188). Children with recurrent abdominal pain are more likely to have headache, significantly so in girls (189).

Pediatric female migraneurs have a higher relapse rate of migraine in adulthood (182). Females are more likely to have aggravation of the headache by physical activity and are less likely to vomit with headache (181). They are more likely to report stress as a precipitant (190) and to have panic attacks (191). They are more likely to miss school, and to miss more days, than males, and somewhat more likely to report severe headache, longer duration of headache, and a higher frequency of headache than males (192). In our experience, status migrainosis is more common in adolescent females than in any other pediatric population. There are little data regarding treatment outcome and gender in pediatric migraine, but Linder (193) reported a 91% response rate of boys to subcutaneous sumitriptan but only a 68% response in girls. There are increasing data regarding the interaction of hormone levels, the menstrual cycle, and headache in females, with possible implications for treatment, but these data do not extend to pediatric females. The increased incidence of migraine in pubertal and postpubertal female children would seem to argue for a hormonal role in pediatric migraine as well, once again with implications for treatment.

Chronic daily headache and chronic daily headache with migraine may be slightly increased in female adolescents (193,194). Females with chronic daily headache have fewer coping skills, more parental negative responses to headache, and fewer solicitous parental responses (194). See also Chapter 14.

Multiple Sclerosis

Multiple sclerosis (MS) is usually considered an adult onset disease but 0.2 to 6.0% of cases have childhood onset, with 20% of those presenting at less than 10 years of age (195,196). The female preponderance seen in adult cases is even more pronounced in childhood-onset cases, with a female-to-male ratio of 3:1 to 5:1 (195,197). Peak age of onset (11 to 14 years) is similar for males and females. Childhood onset cases in general are likely to present with purely sensory symptoms, to recover completely from the initial episode, and to have a remitting or relapsing-remitting course and slower progression of disease (195,196,198). Cerebrospinal fluid (CSF) findings are similar to those of the adult population.

The risk of developing MS after a bout of optic neuritis is higher in adult women than men (74% vs. 34%) (199), but gender does not seem to affect the risk of developing MS after optic neuritis in childhood (200). See also Chapter 18.

Autism

Autism is a syndrome that is usually diagnosed by age 3 years because of characteristic abnormalities in language and social development. Affected children have a marked impairment in social behaviors (eye contact, peer relationships, spontaneous interactions) and ability to interact socially. There is severe impairment in language abilities (delayed language development, little spontaneous language, and abnormal use of language) and repetitive stereotyped behaviors (self-stimulatory behaviors, rituals and compulsions). Known etiologies account for 10 to 30% of cases and include chromosomal defects (particularly Fragile X), metabolic disturbances, tuberous sclerosis, structural brain malformations, and Rett syndrome (201,202). Males and females have a fairly equal chance (56% vs. 65%) of having an identifiable organic condition (202). Males are affected with autism three to four times more frequently than females, but females are more severely affected. In classic autism, affected females have a significantly lower mean IQ than males (42 vs. 57), with few females having an IQ greater than 50 (203). In children with IQs greater than 70 and pervasive developmental disorder (PDD), females are more common (204). Affected females have more impaired receptive and expressive language skills, poorer social development, and fewer self-help skills (203). When studies control for IQ, other authors report few gender differences (204). Girls are more likely to have seizures (201,205).

Tsai and Beisler (203) hypothesize a genetic load model. A higher threshold for disease in females requires a higher genetic load to cause autism in females, thus producing more severe disease. Other hypotheses include more genetic variation in males for autistic characteristics, and constitutional gender differences that make females less vulnerable to language loss, but also less able to compensate for language loss (206).

Periodic Hypersomnia

Three forms of sleep disorder are associated with menses: premenstrual insomnia, menstruation-linked hypersomnia, and insomnia associated with menopause (207). Menstruation-linked hypersomnia has sometimes been called a female Kleine-Levin syndrome (periodic hypersomnia in teenage boys) (208,209). Onset is within 2 to 3 years of the onset of menses. The hypersomniac episodes may begin a few days before menses and last up to 7 days. Episodes begin with personality change; affected girls become hostile and withdrawn. During the episode, they are pale and do not get up to eat or drink but only to void. No consistent neurotransmitter or hormonal abnormalities have been described, but with suppression of ovulation, the hypersomniac episodes resolve. Of 94 women presenting to a sleep clinic for excessive daytime sleepiness, two had menstruation-linked hypersomnia (210).

Catamenial Seizures

The onset of seizures with menarche or the exacerbation of seizures with menses does occur, but the etiology and incidence remain obscure. Many seizure types may exacerbate with puberty in males and females, but females who are later determined to have catamenial epilepsy often present at menarche. A review by Newmark and Penry (211) finds no predominant seizure type and inconsistent hormonal data, although seizures may respond to hormonal therapy. See also Chapter 15.

TREATMENT ASPECTS OF NEUROLOGIC DISEASE IN GIRLS

Most treatments in pediatric neurologic disease are not affected by gender. When hormonal status affects disease (catamenial seizures, migraines), however, then specific hormonal therapy (estrogen and progesterone) may play a role. Treatment in postpubertal girls must always take potential pregnancies into account. The side effects of drugs that may be common in both males and females, may be more cosmetically apparent and bothersome for females (hirsutism in phenytoin therapy).

The most common association of gender with treatment is that of valproate and polycystic ovary syndrome

(212). Valproate may increase the risk of not just poly-cystic ovaries but polycystic ovary syndrome, which includes hyperandrogenism, hirsutism, obesity, and poly-cystic ovaries, although there is controversy about actual increased risk (213).

PSYCHOSOCIAL ASPECTS OF NEUROLOGIC DISEASE IN GIRLS

Many studies of psychosocial illness in children with chronic disease have been performed, but little data are given on the effects of gender. Isolated examples of gen-der differences can be found; for example, parental response to females with chronic daily headache are more negative than toward boys (194). An excellent review of much of this data by Pless and Nolan (214) reports that girls are less likely than boys to have emotional malad-justment with chronic disease. In general, children with chronic disorders have a twofold increased risk for an emotional handicap (214). This risk is increased if the CNS is involved in the chronic disorder (215). The risk may be further increased by medications used to treat the underlying disorder, because these medications may actu-ally worsen cognitive or behavioral functions. Diagnoses in these children include depression, anxiety disorders, and conduct and behavior disorders.

If the disease affects appearance, there may be sig-nificantly abnormal self-esteem. The occurrence of seizures, tics, compulsions, or other disease manifestations in school or in the presence of other children often leads to ridicule. Many children are in an inappropriate class-room setting where they are consistently the poorest stu-dents. A positive correlation exists between headache and school absence (216), and children with more school absences have poorer psychologic adjustment (215).

Children often fear visits to their physician. There is anxiety about tests such as imaging studies or blood draw-ing. There may be fears not verbalized by the patient; thoughts that they are dying or have a brain tumor. Edu-cation of parents and children is crucial to addressing these fears. Children should be reassured when appropriate.

Adolescence and puberty may be a particularly dif-ficult time. At this time when most adolescents are strug-gling to become more independent, those with chronic disease must incorporate the fact of their disease in this struggle. Parents are fearful of too much independence for the child because they fear a negative impact on the child's condition. The patient may also be afraid of increasing independence and its effects on their condition. The iso-lation experienced by many adolescents may be com-pounded by a chronic disease. Patients should be allowed as much freedom as is reasonable with regard to the ill-ness. The patient should be included in the decision mak-ing process.

Of course, several of the diseases discussed in this chapter affect mental functioning so severely that emo-tional adjustment to the disease is usually not an issue for the child. These are the children whose families are most affected by the severity of the child's impairment and the intensive care these children require. There may appear to be intense, sometimes pathologic, focus on the affected child, sometimes at the expense of parental rela-tionships or parent–nonaffected sibling relationships. This may stem from parental guilt over the disease, espe-cially in genetic disease. These issues should be addressed by the practitioner early and often, and recommendation for more counseling may be needed.

Physicians are often less aware of psychosocial issues. In visits with patients, only 25% of parental expec-tations of psychosocial issues were addressed by the physician (217).

References

1. Wettke-Schafer R, Kantner G. X-linked dominant inher-ited diseases with lethality in hemizygous males. *Hum Genet* 1983;64:1–23.
2. Happle R, Effendy I, Megahed M, Orlow SJ, Kuster W. CHILD syndrome in a boy. *Am J Med Genet* 1996;62: 192–194.
3. Lenz W. Half chromatid mutations may explain incon-tinentia pigmenti in males. *Am J Hum Genet* 1975;27: 690–691.
4. Thomas GH. High male:female ratio of germ-line muta-tions: an alternative explanation for postulated gesta-tional lethality in males in X-linked dominant disorders. *Am J Hum Genet* 1996;58:1364–1368.
5. Inoue K, Osaka H, Imaizumi K, et al. Proteolipid pro-tein gene duplications causing Pelizaeus-Merzbacher dis-ease: molecular mechanism and phenotypic manifesta-tions. *Ann Neurol* 1999;45:624–632.
6. Percy AK, Dragich J, Schanen C. Rett Syndrome: Clini-cal-Molecular Correlates. In: Fisch G, (ed.) *Genetics and neurobehavioral disorders*. Totowa, NJ: Humana Press, 2003.
7. Aradhya S, Woffendin H, Jakins T, et al. A recurrent deletion in the ubiquitously expressed NEMO (IKK-gamma) gene accounts for the vast majority of inconti-nentia pigmenti mutations. *Hum Mol Genet* 2001;10: 2171–2179.
8. Smahi A, Courtois G, Vabres P, et al. Genomic rearrange-ment in NEMO impairs NF-kB activation and is a cause of incontinentia pigmenti. *Nature* 2000;45:466–472.
9. Turner. A syndrome of infantilism, congenital webbed neck, and cubitus valgus. *Endocrinology* 1938;23: 566.
10. Ferrier P, Bamatter F, Klein D. Muscular dystrophy (Duchenne) in a girl with Turner's syndrome. *J Med Genet* 1965;2:38–46.
11. Quan F, Janas J, Toth-Fejel S, Johnson DB, Wolford JK, Popovich BW. Uniparental disomy of the entire X chro-mosome in a female with Duchenne muscular dystrophy. *Am J Hum Genet* 1997;60:160–165.
12. Lyon MF. X-chromosome inactivation and develop-mental patterns in mammals. *Biol Rev Camb Philos Soc* 1972;47:1–35.

13. Brown R M, Brown GK. X chromosome inactivation and the diagnosis of X linked disease in females. *J Med Genet* 1993;30:177–184.

14. Willard H. The sex chromosomes and X chromosome inactivation. In: Beaudet A, (eds.) 7th ed. *The metabolic and molecular bases of inherited disease*. New York, NY: McGraw-Hill, 1995.

15. Gale RE, Wheadon H, Linch DC. X-chromosome inactivation patterns using HPRT and PGK polymorphisms in haematologically normal and post-chemotherapy females. *Br J Haematol* 1991;79:193–197.

16. Brown RM, Fraser NJ, Brown GK. Differential methylation of the hypervariable locus DXS255 on active and inactive X chromosomes correlates with the expression of a human X-linked gene. *Genomics* 1990;7:215–221.

17. Van den Veyver IB. Skewed X inactivation in X-linked disorders. *Semin Reprod Med* 2001;19:183–191.

18. Brown CJ, Lafreniere RG, Powers VE, et al. Localization of the X inactivation centre on the human X chromosome in Xq13. *Nature* 1991;349:82–84.

19. Kaladhar Reddy B, Anandavalli TE, Reddi OS. X-linked Duchenne muscular dystrophy in an unusual family with manifesting carriers. *Hum Genet* 1984;67:460–462.

20. Ropers HH, Wienker TF, Grimm T, Schroetter K, Bender K. Evidence for preferential X-chromosome inactivation in a family with Fabry disease. *Am J Hum Genet* 1977;29:361–370.

21. Mattei MG, Mattei JF, Ayme S, Giraud F. X-autosome translocations: cytogenetic characteristics and their consequences. *Hum Genet* 1982;61:295–309.

22. Boyd Y, Buckle VJ. Cytogenetic heterogeneity of translocations associated with Duchenne muscular dystrophy. *Clin Genet* 1986;29:108–115.

23. Verga V, Hall BK, Wang SR, Johnson S, Higgins JV, Glover TW. Localization of the translocation breakpoint in a female with Menkes syndrome to Xq13.2-q13.3 proximal to PGK-1. *Am J Hum Genet* 1991;48:1133–1138.

24. Roberts SH, Upadhyaya M, Sarfarazi M, Harper PS. Further evidence localising the gene for Hunter's syndrome to the distal region of the X chromosome long arm. *J Med Genet* 1989;26:309–313.

25. Mueller OT, Hartsfield JK Jr, Gallardo LA, et al. Lowe oculocerebrorenal syndrome in a female with a balanced X;20 translocation: mapping of the X chromosome breakpoint. *Am J Hum Genet* 1991;49:804–810.

26. Dancis J, Berman PH, Jansen V, Balis ME. Absence of mosaicism in the lymphocyte in X-linked congenital hyperuricosuria. *Life Sci* 1968;7:587–591.

27. McDonald JA, Kelley WN. Lesch-Nyhan syndrome: absence of the mutant enzyme in erythrocytes of a heterozygote for both normal and mutant hypoxanthineguanine phosphoribosyl transferase. *Biochem Genet* 1972;6:21–26.

28. Cox RP, Krauss MR, Balis ME, Dancis J. Evidence for transfer of enzyme product as the basis of metabolic cooperation between tissue culture fibroblasts of Lesch-Nyhan disease and normal cells. *Proc Natl Acad Sci USA* 1970;67:1573–1579.

29. Aicardi J, Lefebvre J, Lerique-Koechlin A. A new syndrome: spasms in flexion, callosal agenesis, ocular abnormalities. *Electroencephalograph Clin Neuophysiol* 1965;19:609–610.

30. Donnenfeld AE, Packer RJ, Zackai EH, et al. Clinical, cytogenetic, and pedigree findings in 18 cases of Aicardi syndrome. *Am J Med Genet* 1989;32:461–467.

31. Ohtsuka Y, Oka E, Terasaki T, Ohtahara S. Aicardi syndrome: a longitudinal clinical and electroencephalographic study. *Epilepsia* 1993;34:627–634.

32. Menezes AV, MacGregor DL, Buncic JR. Aicardi syndrome: natural history and possible predictors of severity. *Pediatr Neurol* 1994;11:313–318.

33. Nielsen KB, Anvret M, Flodmark O, Furuskog P, Bohman-Valis K. Aicardi syndrome: early neuroradiological manifestations and results of DNA studies in one patient. *Am J Med Genet* 1991;38:65–68.

34. Ropers HH, Zuffardi O, Bianchi E, Tiepolo L. Agenesis of corpus callosum, ocular, and skeletal anomalies (X-linked dominant Aicardi's syndrome) in a girl with balanced X/3 translocation. *Hum Genet* 1982;61:364–368.

35. Goltz RW. Focal dermal hypoplasia syndrome. An update. *Arch Dermatol* 1992;128:1108–1111.

36. Naritomi K, Izumikawa Y, Nagataki S, et al. Combined Goltz and Aicardi syndromes in a terminal Xp deletion: are they a contiguous gene syndrome? *Am J Med Genet* 1992;43:839–843.

37. Lindsay EA, Grillo A, Ferrero GB, et al. Microphthalmia with linear skin defects (MLS) syndrome: clinical, cytogenetic, and molecular characterization. *Am J Med Genet* 1994;49:229–234.

38. Wapenaar MC, Bassi MT, Schaefer L, et al. The genes for X-linked ocular albinism (OA1) and microphthalmia with linear skin defects (MLS): cloning and characterization of the critical regions. *Hum Mol Genet* 1993;2:947–952.

39. Rett A. A cerebral atrophic syndrome in hyperammonemia (German). *Monatsschrift fur Kinderheikunde* 1966;116: 310–311.

40. Hagberg B, Aicardi J, Dias K, Ramos O. A progressive syndrome of autism, dementia, ataxia, and loss of purposeful hand use in girls: Rett's syndrome: report of 35 cases. *Ann Neurol* 1983;14:471–479.

41. Amir RE, Van den Veyver IB, Wan M, Tran CQ, Francke U, Zoghbi HY. Rett syndrome is caused by mutations in X-linked MECP2, encoding methyl-CpG-binding protein 2. *Nat Genet* 1999;23:185–188.

42. Hagberg B. Clinical peculiarities, diagnostic approach, and possible cause. *Pediatr Neurol* 1989;5:75–83.

43. Hoffbuhr KC, Moses LM, Jerdonek MA, Naidu S, Hoffman EP. Associations between MeCP2 mutations, X-chromosome inactivation, and phenotype. *Ment Retard Dev Disabil Res Rev* 2002;8:99–105.

44. Hammer S, Dorrani N, Dragich J, Kudo S, Schanen,C. The phenotypic consequences of MECP2 mutations extend beyond Rett syndrome. *Ment Retard Dev Disabil Res Rev* 2002;8:94–98.

45. Dure IV, LS, Percy AK. The Rett syndrome: An overview. In: *Disorders of Movement in Psychiatry and Neurology*, Joseph AB, Young RR (eds.) 2nd ed. Blackwell Scientific Publiscation, Cambridge, 1999, 613–622.

46. Percy AK. Rett syndrome: current status and new vistas. *Neurol Clin N Am* 2002;20:1125–1141.

47. Sarnat H. Neuroembryology. In: Berg B, (ed.) Principles of child neurology. New York, NY: McGraw-Hill, 1996.

48. Dobyns WB, Truwit CL. Lissencephaly and other malformations of cortical development: 1995 update. *Neuropediatrics* 1995;26:132–147.

49. Eksioglu YZ, Scheffer IE, Cardenas P, et al. Periventricular heterotopia: an X-linked dominant epilepsy locus causing aberrant cerebral cortical development. *Neuron* 1996;16:77–87.

50. Fox JW, Lamperti Ed, Eksioglu YZ, et al. Mutations in filamin 1 prevent migration of cerebral cortical neurons in human periventricular heterotopia. *Neuron* 1999;21: 1315–1325.

51. Kamuro K, Tenokuchi Y. Familial periventricular nodular heterotopia. *Brain Dev* 1993;15:237–241.

52. Huttenlocher PR, Taravath S, Mojtahedi S. Periventricular heterotopia and epilepsy. *Neurology* 1994;44: 51–55.

53. Barkovich AJ, Jackson DE Jr, Boyer S. Band heterotopias: a newly recognized neuronal migration anomaly. *Radiology* 1989;171:455–458.

54. Marchal G, Andermann F, Tampieri D, et al. Generalized cortical dysplasia manifested by diffusely thick cerebral cortex. *Arch Neurol* 1989;46:430–434.

55. Palmini A, Andermann F, Aicardi J, et al. Diffuse cortical dysplasia, or the 'double cortex' syndrome: the clinical and epileptic spectrum in 10 patients. *Neurology* 1991;41:1656–1662.

56. Pinard JM, Motte J, Chiron C, Brian R, Andermann E, Dulac O. Subcortical laminar heterotopia and lissencephaly in two families: a single X linked dominant gene. *J Neurol Neurosurg Psychiatry* 1994;57:914–920.

57. Gleeson JG, Allen KM, Fox JW, et al. Doublecortin, a brain-specific gene mutated in human X-linked lissencephaly and double cortex syndrome, encodes a putative signaling protein. *Cell* 1998;92:63–72.

58. Des Portes V, Pinard JM, Smadja D, et al. Dominant X linked subcortical laminar heterotopia and lissencephaly syndrome (XSCLH/LIS): evidence for the occurrence of mutation in males and mapping of a potential locus in Xq22. *J Med Genet* 1997;34:177–183.

59. Leventer RJ, Mills PL, Dobyns WB. X-linked malformations of cortical development. *Am J Med Genet* 2000;97:213–220.

60. Fenichel GM, Phillips JA. Familial aplasia of the cerebellar vermis. Possible X-linked dominant inheritance. *Arch Neurol* 1989;46:582–583.

61. Emery MM, Siegfried EC, Stone MS, Stone EM, Patil SR. Incontinentia pigmenti: transmission from father to daughter. *J Am Acad Dermatol* 1993;29:368–372.

62. Kirchman TT, Levy ML, Lewis RA, Kanzler MH,Nelson DL, Scheuerle AE. Gonadal mosaicism for incontinentia pigmenti in a healthy male. *J Med Genet* 1995;32: 887–890.

63. Mansour S, Woffendin H, Mitton S, Jeffery I, Jakins T, Kenwrick S, Murday VA. Incontinentia pigmenti in a surviving male is accompanied by hypohidrotic ectodermal dysplasia and recurrent infection. *Am J Med Genet* 2001;99:172–177.

64. Sybert VP. Incontinentia pigmenti nomenclature. *Am J Hum Genet* 1994;55:209–211.

65. Berlin AL Paller AS Chan LS. Incontinentia pigmenti: a review and update on the molecular basis of pathophysiology. *J Am Acad Dermatol* 2002;47:169–187; quiz 188–190.

66. Wieacker P, Zimmer J, Ropers HH. X inactivation patterns in two syndromes with probable X-linked dominant, male lethal inheritance. *Clin Genet* 1985;28: 238–242.

67. Gorski JL, Burright EN. The molecular genetics of incontinentia pigmenti. *Semin Dermatol* 1993;12:255–265.

68. Goldberg MF. The blinding mechanisms of incontinentia pigmenti. *Ophthalmic Genet* 1994;15:69–76.

69. Landy SJ, Donnai D. Incontinentia pigmenti (Bloch-Sulzberger syndrome). *J Med Genet* 1993;30:53–59.

70. Lee AG, Goldberg MF, Gillard JH, Barker PB, Bryan RN. Intracranial assessment of incontinentia pigmenti using magnetic resonance imaging, angiography, and spectroscopic imaging. *Arch Pediatr Adolesc Med* 1995;149: 573–580.

71. Mangano S, Barbagallo A. Incontinentia pigmenti: clinical and neuroradiologic features. *Brain Dev* 1993;15: 362–366.

72. Aydingoz U, Midia M. Central nervous system involvement in incontinentia pigmenti: cranial MRI of two siblings. *Neuroradiology* 1998;40:364–366.

73. Gorlin R, Psaume J. Orodigitofacial dysostosis - a new syndrome. *J Pediatr* 1962;61:520–530.

74. Connacher AA, Forsyth CC, Stewart WK. Orofaciodigital syndrome type I associated with polycystic kidneys and agenesis of the corpus callosum. *J Med Genet* 1987; 24:116–118.

75. Wood BP, Young LW, Townes PL. Cerebral abnormalities in the oral-facial-digital syndrome. *Pediatr Radiol* 1975;3:130–136.

76. Towfighi J, Berlin CM Jr, Ladda RL, Frauenhoffer EE, Lehman RA. Neuropathology of oral-facial-digital syndromes. *Arch Pathol Lab Med* 1985;109:642–646.

77. Feather SA, Woolf AS, Donnai D, Malcolm S, Winter RM. The oral-facial-digital syndrome type 1 (OFD1), a cause of polycystic kidney disease and associated malformations, maps to Xp22.2-Xp22.3. *Hum Mol Genet* 1997;6:1163–1167.

78. Ferrante MI, Giorgio G, Feather SA, et al. Identification of the gene for oral-facial-digital type I syndrome. *Am J Hum Genet* 2001;68:569–576.

79. Tariverdian G, Vogel F. Some problems in the genetics of X-linked mental retardation. *Cytogenet Cell Genet* 2000;91:278–284.

80. Plenge RM, Stevenson RA, Lubs HA, Schwartz CE, Willard HF. Skewed X-chromosome inactivation is a common feature of X-linked mental retardation disorders. *Am J Hum Genet* 2002;71:168–173.

81. Christianson AL, Stevenson RE, van der Meyden CH, et al. X linked severe mental retardation, craniofacial dysmorphology, epilepsy, ophthalmoplegia, and cerebellar atrophy in a large South African kindred is localised to Xq24-q27. *J Med Genet* 1999;36:759–766.

82. Webb TP, Bundey SE, Thake AI, Todd J. Population incidence and segregation ratios in the Martin-Bell syndrome. *Am J Med Genet* 1986;23:573–580.

83. Tarleton JC, Saul RA. Molecular genetic advances in fragile X syndrome. *J Pediatr* 1993;122:169–185.

84. Fu YH, Kuhl DP, Pizzuti A, et al. Variation of the CGG repeat at the fragile X site results in genetic instability: resolution of the Sherman paradox. *Cell* 1991;67: 1047–1058.

85. Sutherland GR. Fragile sites on human chromosomes: demonstration of their dependence on the type of tissue culture medium. *Science* 1977;197:265–266.

86. Siomi H, Siomi MC, Nussbaum RL, Dreyfuss G. The protein product of the fragile X gene, FMR1, has characteristics of an RNA-binding protein. *Cell* 1993;74:291–298.

87. Oberle I, Rousseau F, Heitz D, et al. Instability of a 550-base pair DNA segment and abnormal methylation in fragile X syndrome. *Science* 1991;252:1097–1102.

88. Loesch DZ, Hay DA, Mulley J. Transmitting males and carrier females in fragile X—revisited. *Am J Med Genet* 1994;51:392–399.

89. Sherman SL. Premature ovarian failure in the fragile X syndrome. *Am J Med Genet* 2000;97:189–194.

90. Laxova R. Fragile X syndrome. *Adv Pediatr* 1994;41: 305–342.

91. de Vries BB, Wiegers AM, Smits AP, et al. Mental status of females with an FMR1 gene full mutation. *Am J Hum Genet* 1996;58:1025–1032.

92. Rousseau F, Heitz D, Tarleton J, et al. A multicenter study on genotype-phenotype correlations in the fragile X syndrome, using direct diagnosis with probe StB12.3: the first 2,253 cases. *Am J Hum Genet* 1994;55:225–237.

93. Taylor AK, Safanda JF, Fall MZ, et al. Molecular predictors of cognitive involvement in female carriers of fragile X syndrome. *JAMA* 1994;271:507–514.

94. Reiss AL, Freund LS, Baumgardner TL, Abrams MT, Denckla MB. Contribution of the FMR1 gene mutation to human intellectual dysfunction. *Nat Genet* 1995;11: 331–334.

95. Thompson NM, Gulley ML, Rogeness GA, et al. Neurobehavioral characteristics of CGG amplification status in fragile X females. *Am J Med Genet* 1994;54: 378–383.

96. Freun LS, Reiss AL, Abrams MT. Psychiatric disorders associated with fragile X in the young female. *Pediatrics* 1993;91:321–329.

97. Keysor CS, Mazzocco MM. A developmental approach to understanding Fragile X syndrome in females. *Microsc Res Tech* 2002;57:179–186.

98. Bergoffen J, Scherer SS, Wang S, et al. Connexin mutations in X-linked Charcot-Marie-Tooth disease. *Science* 1993;262:2039–2042.

99. Fairweather N, Bell C, Cochrane S, et al. Mutations in the connexin 32 gene in X-linked dominant Charcot-Marie-Tooth disease (CMTX1). *Hum Mol Genet* 1994; 3:29–34.

100. Dubourg O, Tardieu S, Birouk N, et al. Clinical, electrophysiological and molecular genetic characteristics of 93 patients with X-linked Charcot-Marie-Tooth disease. *Brain* 2001;124:1958–1967.

101. Ionasescu V, Searby C, Ionasescu R, Meschino W. New point mutations and deletions of the connexin 32 gene in X-linked Charcot-Marie-Tooth neuropathy. *Neuromuscul Disord* 1995;5:297–299.

102. Woods G, Black G, Norbury G. Male neonatal death and progressive weakness and immune deficiency in females: an unknown X linked condition. *J Med Genet* 1995;32:191–196.

103. Hoffman EP, Brown RH Jr, Kunkel LM. Dystrophin: the protein product of the Duchenne muscular dystrophy locus. *Cell* 1987;51:919–928.

104. Moser H, Vogt J. Follow-up study of serum creatine-kinase in carriers of Duchenne muscular dystrophy. *Lancet* 1974;2:661–662.

105. Minetti C, Chang HW, Medori R, et al. Dystrophin deficiency in young girls with sporadic myopathy and normal karyotype. *Neurology* 1991;41:1288–1292.

106. Hoffman EP, Arahata K, Minetti C, Bonilla E, Rowland LP. Dystrophinopathy in isolated cases of myopathy in females. *Neurology* 1992;42:967–975.

107. Moser H, Emery AE. The manifesting carrier in Duchenne muscular dystrophy. *Clin Genet* 1974;5:271–284.

108. Pegoraro E, Schimke RN, Garcia C, et al. Genetic and biochemical normalization in female carriers of Duchenne muscular dystrophy: evidence for failure of dystrophin production in dystrophin-competent myonuclei. *Neurology* 1995;45:677–690.

109. Kinoshita H, Goto Y, Ishikawa M, et al. A carrier of Duchenne muscular dystrophy with dilated cardiomyopathy but no skeletal muscle symptom. *Brain Dev* 1995;17:202–205.

110. Politano L, Nigro V, Nigro G, et al. Development of cardiomyopathy in female carriers of Duchenne and Becker muscular dystrophies. *JAMA* 1996;275:1335–1338.

111. Kamakura K. Cardiac involvement of female carrier of Duchenne muscular dystrophy. *Intern Med* 2000;39:2–3.

112. Azofeifa J, Voit T, Hubner C, Cremer M. X-chromosome methylation in manifesting and healthy carriers of dystrophinopathies: concordance of activation ratios among first degree female relatives and skewed inactivation as cause of the affected phenotypes. *Hum Genet* 1995;96: 167–176.

113. Emery AE. Emery-Dreifuss syndrome. *J Med Genet* 1989;26:637–641.

114. Bialer MG, Bruns DE, Kelly TE. Muscle enzymes and isoenzymes in Emery-Dreifuss muscular dystrophy. *Clin Chem* 1990;36:427–430.

115. Dickey RP, Ziter FA, Smith RA. Emery-Dreifuss muscular dystrophy. *J Pediatr* 1984;104:555–559.

116. Woodward K, Malcolm S. CNS myelination and PLP gene dosage. *Pharmacogenomics* 2001;2:263–272.

117. Hodes ME, DeMyer WE, Pratt VM, Edwards MK, Dlouhy SR. Girl with signs of Pelizaeus-Merzbacher disease heterozygous for a mutation in exon 2 of the proteolipid protein gene. *Am J Med Genet* 1995;55: 397–401.

118. Raskind WH, Williams CA, Hudson LD, Bird TD. Complete deletion of the proteolipid protein gene (PLP) in a family with X-linked Pelizaeus-Merzbacher disease. *Am J Hum Genet* 1991;49:1355–1360.

119. Ziereisen F, Dan B, Christiaens F, Deltenre P, Boutemy R, Christophe C. Connatal Pelizaeus-Merzbacher disease in two girls. *Pediatr Radiol* 2000;30:435–438.

120. Inoue K, Tanaka H, Scaglia F, Araki A, Shaffer LG, Lupski JR. Compensating for central nervous system dysmyelination: females with a proteolipid protein gene duplication and sustained clinical improvement. *Ann Neurol* 2001;50:747–754.

121. Moser H. X-Linked adrenoleukodystrophy. In: Beaudet A, Scriver C, Sly W, Valle D, (eds.) *The metabolic and molecular bases of inherited disease*. New York, NY: McGraw Hill, 1995.

122. Moser HW, Moser AB, Smith KD, et al. Adrenoleukodystrophy: phenotypic variability and implications for therapy. *J Inherit Metab Dis* 1992;15:645–664.

123. Schaumburg HH, Powers JM, Raine CS, et al. Adrenomyeloneuropathy: a probable variant of adrenoleukodystrophy. II. General pathologic, neuropathologic, and biochemical aspects. *Neurology* 1977;271114–1119.

124. Heffungs W, Hameister H, Ropers HH. Addison disease and cerebral sclerosis in an apparently heterozygous girl: evidence for inactivation of the adrenoleukodystrophy locus. *Clin Genet* 1980;18:184–188.

125. Hershkovitz E, Narkis G, Shorer Z, et al. Cerebral X-linked adrenoleukodystrophy in a girl with Xq27-Ter deletion. *Ann Neurol* 2002;52:234–237.

126. Naidu S, Washington C, Thirumalai S. X-chromosome inactivation in symptomatic heterozygotes in x-linked adrenoleukodystrophy. *Ann Neurol* 1997;42:498.

127. Batshaw ML, Msall M, Beaudet AL, Trojak J. Risk of serious illness in heterozygotes for ornithine transcarbamylase deficiency. *J Pediatr* 1986;108:236–241.

128. Girgis N, McGravey V, Shah BL, Herrin J, Shih VE. Lethal ornithine transcarbamylase deficiency in a female neonate. *J Inherit Metab Dis* 1987;10:274–275.

129. Arn PH, Hauser ER, Thomas GH, Herman G, Hess D, Brusilow SW. Hyperammonemia in women with a mutation at the ornithine carbamoyltransferase locus. A cause of postpartum coma. *N Engl J Med* 1990;322:1652–1655.

130. Honeycutt D, Callahan K, Rutledge L, Evans B. Heterozygote ornithine transcarbamylase deficiency presenting as symptomatic hyperammonemia during initiation of valproate therapy. *Neurology* 1992;42:666–668.

131. Hasegawa T, Tzakis AG, Todo S, Reyes J, Nour B, Finegold DN, Starzl TE. Orthotopic liver transplantation for ornithine transcarbamylase deficiency with hyperammonemic encephalopathy. *J Pediatr Surg* 1995; 30:863–865.

132. Mrozek JD, Holzknecht RA, Butkowski RJ, Mauer SM, Tuchman M. X-chromosome inactivation in the liver of female heterozygous OTC-deficient sparse-furash mice. *Biochem Med Metab Biol Jun* 1991;45:333–343.

133. Tuchman M, Morizono H, Rajagopal BS, Plante RJ, Allewell NM. The biochemical and molecular spectrum of ornithine transcarbamylase deficiency. *J Inherit Metab Dis* 1998;2(suppl 1):40–58.

134. Tuchman M, McCullough BA, Yudkoff M. The molecular basis of ornithine transcarbamylase deficiency. *Eur J Pediatr* 2000;159:(suppl 3)S196–198.

135. Bonham JR, Guthrie P, Downing M, et al. The allopurinol load test lacks specificity for primary urea cycle defects but may indicate unrecognized mitochondrial disease. *J Inherit Metab Dis* 1999;22:174–184.

136. Scaglia F, Zheng Q, O'Brien WE, et al. An integrated approach to the diagnosis and prospective management of partial ornithine transcarbamylase deficiency. *Pediatrics* 2002;109:150–152.

137. Brown RM, Dahl HH, Brown GK. X-chromosome localization of the functional gene for the E1 alpha subunit of the human pyruvate dehydrogenase complex. *Genomics* 1989;4:174–181.

138. Robinson BH, MacMillan H, Petrova-Benedict R, Sherwood WG. Variable clinical presentation in patients with defective E1 component of pyruvate dehydrogenase complex. *J Pediatr* 1987;111:525–533.

139. Dahl HH. Pyruvate dehydrogenase E1 alpha deficiency: males and females differ yet again. *Am J Hum Genet* 1995;56:553–557.

140. Brown GK, Otero LJ, LeGris M, Brown RM. Pyruvate dehydrogenase deficiency. *J Med Genet* 1994;31:875–879.

141. Matthews PM, Brown RM, Otero LJ, et al. Pyruvate dehydrogenase deficiency. Clinical presentation and molecular genetic characterization of five new patients. *Brain* 1994;117(Pt3):435–443.

142. Robinson B. Lactic Acidosis. In: Beaudet A, Scriver C, Sly W, Valle D, (eds.) *The metabolic and molecular bases of inherited disease.* New York, NY: McGraw-Hill, 1995.

143. Naito E, Ito M, Yokota I, Saijo T, Ogawa Y, Shinahara K, Kuroda Y. Gender-specific occurrence of West syndrome in patients with pyruvate dehydrogenase complex deficiency. *Neuropediatrics* 2001;32:295–298.

144. Dahl HH, Hansen LL, Brown RM, Danks DM,Rogers JG, Brown GK. X-linked pyruvate dehydrogenase E1 alpha subunit deficiency in heterozygous females: variable manifestation of the same mutation. *J Inherit Metab Dis* 1992;15:835–847.

145. Lib MY, Brown RM, Brown GK, Marusich MF, Capaldi RA. Detection of pyruvate dehydrogenase E1 alpha-subunit deficiencies in females by immunohistochemical demonstration of mosaicism in cultured fibroblasts. *J Histochem Cytochem* 2002;50:877–884.

146. Lissens W, DeMeirleir L, Seneca S, et al. Mutation analysis of the pyruvate dehydrogenase E1 alpha gene in eight patients with a pyruvate dehydrogenase complex deficiency. *Hum Mutat* 1996;7:46–51.

147. Matsuda J, Ito M, Naito E, Yokota I, Kuroda Y. DNA diagnosis of pyruvate dehydrogenase deficiency in female patients with congenital lactic acidaemia. *J Inherit Metab Dis* 1995;18:534–546.

148. Michotte A, DeMeirleir L, Lissens W, et al. Neuropathological findings of a patient with pyruvate dehydrogenase E1 alpha deficiency presenting as a cerebral lactic acidosis. *Acta Neuropathol* (Berl) 1993;85:674–678.

149. Kint JA. Fabry's disease: alpha-galactosidase deficiency. *Science* 1970;167:1268–1269.

150. Desnick R, Ioannov Y, Eng C. a-Galactosidase A deficiency: Fabry disease. In: Beaudet A, Scriver CR, Sly WS, Valle D, (eds.) *The metabolic and molecular bases of inherited disease.* New York, NY: McGraw-Hill, 1996.

151. Whybra C, Kampmann C, Willers I, et al. Anderson-Fabry disease: clinical manifestations of disease in female heterozygotes. *J Inherit Metab Dis* 2001;24:715–724.

152. Kampmann C, Baehner F, Whybra C, et al. Cardiac manifestations of Anderson-Fabry disease in heterozygous females. *J Am Coll Cardiol* 2002;40:1668–1674.

153. Vulpe C, Levinson B,Whitney S, Packman S, Gitschier J. Isolation of a candidate gene for Menkes disease and evidence that it encodes a copper-transporting ATPase. *Nat Genet* 1993;3:7–13.

154. Volpintesta EJ. Menkes kinky hair syndrome in a black infant. *Am J Dis Child* 1974;128:244–246.

155. Moore CM, Howell RR. Ectodermal manifestations in Menkes disease. *Clin Genet* 1985;28:532–540.

156. Gerdes AM, Tonnesen T, Horn N, et al. Clinical expression of Menkes syndrome in females. *Clin Genet* 1990; 38:452–459.

157. Salomons GS, van Dooren SJ, Verhoeven NM, et al. X-linked creatine-transporter gene (SLC6A8) defect: a new creatine-deficiency syndrome. *Am J Hum Genet* 2001; 68:1497–1500.

158. Cecil KM, DeGrauw TJ, Salomons GS, Jakobs C, Egelhoff JC, Clark JF. Magnetic resonance spectroscopy in a 9-day-old heterozygous female child with creatine transporter deficiency. *J Comput Assist Tomogr* 2003; 27:44–47.

159. Dahl N, Hu LJ, Chery M, et al. Myotubular myopathy in a girl with a deletion at Xq27-q28 and unbalanced X inactivation assigns the MTM1 gene to a 600-kb region. *Am J Hum Genet* 1995;56:1108–1115.

160. Winchester B, Young E, Geddes S, et al. Female twin with Hunter disease due to nonrandom inactivation of the X-chromosome: a consequence of twinning. *Am J Med Genet* 1992;44:834–838.

161. Clarke JT, Greer WL, Strasberg PM, Pearce RD, Skomorowski MA, Ray PN. Hunter disease (mucopolysaccharidosis type II) associated with unbalanced inactivation of the X chromosomes in a karyotypically normal girl. *Am J Hum Genet* 1991;49:289–297.

162. Ogasawara N, Stout JT, Goto H, Sonta S, Matsumoto A, Caskey CT. Molecular analysis of a female Lesch-Nyhan patient. *J Clin Invest* 1989;84:1024–1027.

163. Aral B, de Saint Basile G, Al-Garawi S, Kamoun P, Ceballos-Picot I. Novel nonsense mutation in the hypoxanthine guanine phosphoribosyltransferase gene and nonrandom X-inactivation causing Lesch-Nyhan syndrome in a female patient. *Hum Mutat* 1996;7:52–58.

164. Loiseau P. Childhood absence epilepsy. In: Bureau M, Roger J, Dravet C, Dreifuss F, Perret A, Wolf P, (eds.) *Epileptic syndromes in infancy and childhood and adolescence*, 2nd ed. London: John Libbey & Company, 1992.

165. Penn A. Neuromuscular junction. In: Rowland L, (ed.) *Merritt's textbook of neurology*, 8th ed. Philadelphia, Pa: Lea & Febiger, 1989.

166. Carter S. Movement disorders. In *Merritt's Textbook of Neurology*, Rowland L (ed.): Philadelphia, PA: Lea & Febiger, 1989.

167. Carter CO, Evans KA, Till K. Spinal dysraphism: genetic relation to neural tube malformations. *J Med Genet* 1976;13:343–350.

168. Behrman R, Kliegman R, Nelson W, Vaughan V. Nelson T*extbook of Pediatrics*. Philadelphia, Pa: W.B. Saunders, 1992.

169. Tuite P and Lang A. Syndromes of disordered posture and movement. In: Berg B, (ed.) *Principles of child neurology*, 1st ed. New York, NY: McGraw-Hill, 1996.

170. Pauls DL, Raymond CL, Stevenson JM, Leckman JF. A family study of Gilles de la Tourette syndrome. *Am J Hum Genet* 1991;48:154–163.

171. Santangelo SL, Pauls DL, Goldstein JM, Faraone SV, Tsuang MT, Leckman JF. Tourette's syndrome: what are the influences of gender and comorbid obsessive-compulsive disorder? *J Am Acad Child Adolesc Psychiatry* 1994;33:795–804.

172. Pauls DL, Leckman JF. The inheritance of Gilles de la Tourette's syndrome and associated behaviors. Evidence for autosomal dominant transmission. *N Engl J Med* 1986;315:993–997.

173. Comings DE, Comings BG. Tourette syndrome: clinical and psychological aspects of 250 cases. *Am J Hum Genet* 1985;37:435–450.

174. Zimmerman AM, Abrams MT, Giuliano JD, Denckla MB, Singer HS. Subcortical volumes in girls with tourette syndrome: support for a gender effect. *Neurology* 2000;54:2224–2229.

175. Mostofsky SH, Wendlandt J, Cutting L, Denckla MB, Singer HS. Corpus callosum measurements in girls with Tourette syndrome. *Neurology* 1999;53:1345–1347.

176. Pauls DL, Pakstis AJ, Kurlan R, et al. Segregation and linkage analyses of Tourette's syndrome and related disorders. *J Am Acad Child Adolesc Psychiatry* 1990;29:195–203.

177. Scheller JM. The history, epidemiology, and classification of headaches in childhood. *Semin Pediatr Neurol* 1995;2:102–108.

178. Sillanpaa M, Piekkala P. Prevalence of migraine and other headaches in early puberty. *Scand J Prim Health Care* 1984;2:27–32.

179. Pascual J, Berciano J. Clinical experience with headaches in preadolescent children. *Headache* 1995;35:551–553.

180. Stewart WF, Linet MS, Celentano DD, Van Natta M, Ziegler D. Age- and sex-specific incidence rates of migraine with and without visual aura. *Am J Epidemiol* 1991;134:1111–1120.

181. Wober-Bingol C, Wober C, Karwautz A, et al. Diagnosis of headache in childhood and adolescence: a study in 437 patients. *Cephalalgia* 1995;15:13–21; discussion 14.

182. Bille B. Migraine in childhood and its prognosis. *Cephalalgia* 1981;1:71–75.

183. Mortimer MJ, Kay J, Jaron A. Epidemiology of headache and childhood migraine in an urban general practice using Ad Hoc, Vahlquist and IHS criteria. *Dev Med Child Neurol* 1992;34:1095–1101.

184. Stewart WF, Shechter A, Lipton RB. Migraine heterogeneity. Disability, pain intensity, and attack frequency and duration. *Neurology* 1994;44:S24–39.

185. Raieli V, Raimondo D, Cammalleri R, Camarda R. Migraine headaches in adolescents: a student population-based study in Monreale. *Cephalalgia* 1995;15:5–12; discussion 14.

186. Golden GS, French JH. Basilar artery migraine in young children. *Pediatrics* 1975;56:722–726.

187. Bickerstaff E. Basilar artery migraine. *Lancet* 1961:15–17.

188. Rothner AD. Miscellaneous headache syndromes in children and adolescents. *Semin Pediatr Neurol* 1995;2:159–164.

189. Mortimer MJ, Kay J, Jaron A. Clinical epidemiology of childhood abdominal migraine in an urban general practice. *Dev Med Child Neurol* 1993;35:243–248.

190. Gladstein J, Holden EW, Peralta L, Raven M. Diagnoses and symptom patterns in children presenting to a pediatric headache clinic. *Headache* 1993;33:497–500.

191. Stewart W, Breslau N, Keck PE, Jr. Comorbidity of migraine and panic disorder. *Neurology* 1994;44:S23–27.

192. Stewart WF, Shechter A, Rasmussen BK. Migraine prevalence. A review of population-based studies. *Neurology* 1994;44:S17–23.

193. Linder SL. Subcutaneous sumatriptan in the clinical setting: the first 50 consecutive patients with acute migraine in a pediatric neurology office practice. *Headache* 1996;36:419–422.

194. Holden EW, Gladstein J, Trulsen M, Wall B. Chronic daily headache in children and adolescents. *Headache* 1994;34:508–514.

195. Duquette P, Murray TJ, Pleines J, et al. Multiple sclerosis in childhood: clinical profile in 125 patients. *J Pediatr* 1987;111:359–363.

196. Boiko A, Vorobeychik G, Paty D, Devonshire V, Sadovnick D. Early onset multiple sclerosis: a longitudinal study. *Neurology* 2002;59:1006–1010.

197. Millner MM, Ebner F, Justich E, Urban C. Multiple sclerosis in childhood: contribution of serial MRI to earlier diagnosis. *Dev Med Child Neurol* 1990;32:769–777.

198. Izquierdo G, Lyon-Caen O, Marteau R, et al. Early onset multiple sclerosis. Clinical study of 12 pathologically proven cases. *Acta Neurol Scand* 1986;73:493–497.

199. Rizzo JF 3rd, Lessell S. Risk of developing multiple sclerosis after uncomplicated optic neuritis: a long-term prospective study. *Neurology* 1988;38:185–190.

200. Lucchinetti CF, Kiers L, O'Duffy A, et al. Risk factors for developing multiple sclerosis after childhood optic neuritis. *Neurology* 1997;49:1413–1418.

201. Elia M, Musumeci SA, Ferri R, Bergonzi P. Clinical and neurophysiological aspects of epilepsy in subjects with autism and mental retardation. *Am J Ment Retard* 1995;100:6–16.

202. Mason-Brothers A, Ritvo ER, Pingree C, et al. The UCLA-University of Utah epidemiologic survey of autism: prenatal, perinatal, and postnatal factors. *Pediatrics* 1990;86:514–519.

203. Tsai LY, Beisler JM. The development of sex differences in infantile autism. *Br J Psychiatry* 1983;142:373–378.

204. Volkmar FR, Szatmari P, Sparrow SS. Sex differences in pervasive developmental disorders. *J Autism Dev Disord* 1993;23:579–591.

205. Volkmar FR, Nelson DS. Seizure disorders in autism. *J Am Acad Child Adolesc Psychiatry* 1990;29:127–129.

206. Wing L. Sex ratios in early childhood autism and related conditions. *Psychiatry Res* 1981;5:129–137.

207. DCS Committee. *The International Classification of Sleep Disorders*. Lawrence, Kansas: Allen Press, 1990.

208. Billiard M, Guilleminault C, Dement WC. A menstruation-linked periodic hypersomnia. Kleine-Levin syndrome or new clinical entity? *Neurology* 1975;25:436–443.

209. Sachs C, Persson HE, Hagenfeldt K. Menstruation-related periodic hypersomnia: a case study with successful treatment. *Neurology* 1982;32:1376–1379.

210. Guilleminault C, Dement WC. 235 cases of excessive daytime sleepiness. Diagnosis and tentative classification. *J Neurol Sci* 1977;31:13–27.

211. Newmark ME, Penry JK. Catamenial epilepsy: a review. *Epilepsia* 1980;21:281–300.

212. Vainionpaa L. Valproate-induced hyperandrogenism during pubertal maturation in girls with epilepsy. *Ann Neurol* 1999;45:444–450.

213. Genton P. Controversies in Epilepsy: 1 of 3 articles on the association between valproate and polycystic ovary syndrome. *Epilepsia* 2001;42:295–304.

214. Pless IB, Nolan T. Revision, replication and neglect—research on maladjustment in chronic illness. *J Child Psychol Psychiatry* 1991;32:347–365.

215. Midence K. The effects of chronic illness on children and their families: an overview. *Genet Soc Gen Psychol Monogr* 1994;120:311–326.

216. Carlsson J, Larsson B, Mark A. Psychosocial functioning in schoolchildren with recurrent headaches. *Headache* 1996;36:77–82.

217. Lau RR, Williams HS, Williams LC, Ware JE Jr, Brook RH. Psychosocial problems in chronically ill children: physician concern, parent satisfaction, and the validity of medical records. *J Community Health* 1982;7:250–261.

10 Menstruation and Pregnancy: Interactions with Neurologic Disease

James O. Donaldson

Pregnancy may affect the course and complicate the management of pre-existing neurologic disorders. Additionally, some conditions are uniquely or particularly apt to occur during the pregnancy and the puerperium. Although muscle cramps, nocturnal acroparesthesiae, back pain, and restless legs are common nuisances that are familiar to obstetricians, the presentation of a serious problem engenders anxiety because any one physician's personal experience is limited. Expect more hubbub when parents or in-laws arrive on the scene, ready to take charge of things for their grown child and probably demanding a second opinion before hearing your advice.

This chapter provides an overview of the physiologic changes that accompany menstruation and pregnancy, as illustrated by their effects on neurologic diseases.

ESTROGEN EFFECTS ON PHYSIOLOGY AND METABOLISM

Estrogen is produced by two mechanisms. In nonpregnant ovulatory women, estradiol is synthesized by ovarian thecal cells, and estrone is produced from the extraglandular conversion of androstenedione, mainly by fat cells. In ovulatory women, this extraglandular mechanism provides a relatively constant estrogen level to which is added ovarian estradiol, which fluctuates during the menstrual cycle. For prepubertal children and post-menopausal women, it is the main source of estrogens. Because the percent of androstenedione converted to estrone is a function of body weight and the surface area of adipocytes, this author has suggested that the extraglandular production of estrogen is involved with the pseudotumor cerebri syndrome of obese young women and perhaps the growth of meningiomas in overweight women (1).

There is a marked increase in estrogen production during pregnancy. During a full-term pregnancy, a gravid woman produces more estrogen than a ovulatory woman would in more than 100 years! After the first few weeks of pregnancy, the placenta becomes another source of extraglandular estrogen. As pregnancy progresses, maternal steroids and dihydroisoandrostene from developing fetal adrenal glands are converted to estriol, and to lesser amounts of estradiol and estrone. The fetal adrenal gland is a "steroid factory," estimated to produce several times more steroids than the adrenal glands of a nonstressed, resting adult. Women carrying an anencephalic fetus, which typically does not develop a fetal zone in its adrenal glands, have one-tenth the expected estrogen excretion during pregnancy (2).

Increased estrogen levels during pregnancy have protean effects in addition to breast development and myometrial hyperplasia, which may directly or indirectly affect neurologic conditions.

Effects on Seizures and Epilepsy

High estrogen concentrations lower the seizure threshold. Conversely, high progesterone levels lessen the propensity to convulse. The ratio of estrogen and progesterone levels is important, as has been determined in women with catamenial epilepsy who convulse around the time of menstruation (3). During pregnancy, both estrogen and progesterone increase and may partially cancel the epilepsy-threshold modifying effects of each other (4). Nevertheless, there are some women with true gestational epilepsy who convulse only while pregnant, presumably due to the effect of estrogen on the seizure threshold.

In addition to whatever effect hormones may have, the effect of pregnancy on the course of epilepsy is determined by altered metabolism of antiepileptic drug metabolism, compliance, and sleep deprivation, among other factors. A pattern of catamenial exacerbation of epilepsy with more seizures does not predict the effect of pregnancy on epilepsy.

Effects on Tumors

Catamenial sciatica is recurrent sciatic pain and later weakness that typically begins a few days before menstruation, when estrogen levels are at their highest during an ovulatory cycle (5). The cause is an ectopic endometrioma implanted in the sciatic nerve. Estrogen replacement after oophorectomy worsens this neuropathy.

Stimulation of estrogen and progesterone receptors on brain tumors—meningiomas, neurofibromas, and to a lesser extent gliomas—may accelerate tumor growth, which may regress post partum, at least temporarily (6). Rarely, symptoms of meningiomas recur days before menstruation, corresponding to the highest levels of estrogen during the ovulatory cycle (7).

Stimulation of prolactin secretion during pregnancy increases the volume of the pituitary gland by 50 percent (8). Pituitary adenomas have produced visual field deficits during successive pregnancies, with regression of symptoms between pregnancies (9).

Effects on Movement Disorders

Understanding the effect of estrogens on the basal ganglia is in its infancy. Catamenial exacerbations of action myoclonus have been reported, but the responsible mechanism is unclear (10). Chorea gravidarum, chorea associated with oral contraceptives, and some experimental data suggest that estrogen enhances dopamine activity (11). The incidence of the chorea induced by oral contraceptives has declined as the estrogen content of the pill has decreased.

Effects on Blood Vessels

Increased estrogen levels dilate vascular shunts, which is visibly apparent as palmar erythema and spider nevi that fade within days after delivery (12). A similar effect presumably affects cerebral and spinal cord arteriovenous malformations. Neurosurgeons prefer to operate on benign tumors several weeks after delivery to minimize blood loss and provide a clearer operative field.

Effect on Headache

It should be noted that catamenial classic migraine is associated with perimenstrual estrogen withdrawal. The majority of classic migraineurs are protected during pregnancy.

CARDIOVASCULAR EFFECTS

There appears to be an effect of pregnancy on the media of arterial walls, which becomes clinically significant for women who have vascular Ehlers-Danlos syndrome (type IV) and a predisposition to develop aneurysms. It may also predispose some women to develop dissecting aneurysms of the extracranial arteries after violent neck movements that occur during the throes of childbirth. The incidence of aneurysms at all sites—cerebral, aortic, splenic, and renal—increases with the duration of pregnancy.

As pregnancy proceeds, cardiac output increases approximately 50 percent. This may cause decompensation in patients who have pre-existing vascular disease and increase the risk of emboli. The click-murmur of mitral valve prolapse typically becomes inaudible, thus eliminating a clue for the neurologist who is looking for a cause of an episode of cerebral ischemia. Another cause of emboli may be peripartum cardiomyopathy.

Pregnant women are at risk for air embolism, which is often fatal. Air has access to the uterine veins during complicated vaginal deliveries and caesarean sections. Forceful insufflation of the vagina as a sexual activity is not safe during pregnancy (13). Similarly, air trapped within a patulent vagina when the patient lies down after postpartum knee-chest exercises may be squeezed, as if by a bellows, into the uterus and the uterine veins (14).

The pelvic bed of veins is a source of pulmonary emboli and paradoxical cerebral emboli, especially after caesarean section. Straining during labor increases right atrial pressure and may open a usually physiologically closed, yet anatomically patent foramen ovale. This may be a factor in the higher than expected incidence of carotid artery occlusions in the first week postpartum.

MECHANICAL FACTORS

Even in healthy women, the simple bulk of an enlarging uterus can change posture, alter gait, and cause back pain. These problems are magnified for women who have multiple sclerosis and other diseases that cause weakness and difficulty walking. Additionally, management of a neurogenic bladder becomes ever more difficult and the risk of infection increases.

In the second half of pregnancy, the enlarging uterus elevates the diaphragm and changes chest configuration. Functionally, it decreases functional residual capacity, the volume in the lungs at their resting position (15). However, because the diaphragm and chest wall continue to work, vital capacity is unchanged. Thus, pregnancy does not alter guidelines based on vital capacity for intubating patients with myasthenic crisis and Guillain-Barré syndrome.

Meralgia paresthetica is a condition associated with enlarging abdominal girth, which presumably traps the lateral femoral cutaneous nerve at the lateral inguinal ligament. This nuisance typically remits within a few months of childbirth.

Intrapelvic nerves may be entrapped during labor by the descending fetal head. Sorting out the pathogenesis of these neuropathies was a hot topic in the late nineteenth century. Around 1900, 3.2% of deliveries in three large series of consecutive births were complicated by femoral neuropathy, and undoubtedly more had a postpartum footdrop (16). More accurate estimation of the size of both the fetal head and the pelvic outlet, coupled with the frequency of delivery by caesarean section, has markedly reduced the incidence of these neuropathies.

METABOLIC CHANGES

Pregnancy often alters drug compliance, absorption, protein binding, distribution, metabolism, and excretion. Additionally, fetal metabolism must be considered. Generally, drugs that cross the blood-brain barrier can be expected to cross the placenta. However, binding and metabolism of drugs by the fetus and neonate may be different. For instance, diazepam and its active N-dimethyl derivative accumulate in the fetus. Thus, infants whose mothers took 10 mg to 15 mg diazepam daily for one to three weeks before delivery still had a significant plasma level 10 days after birth (17).

One example of the clinical importance of biochemistry is maternal carbon monoxide poisoning. Carbon monoxide intoxication may affect the fetus more than the mother because fetal hemoglobin, which has a greater affinity for oxygen than does adult hemoglobin, also has a greater affinity for carbon monoxide (18).

Another rarer example is the lipid storage myopathy carnitine deficiency, which may deteriorate during and after pregnancy (19). Even in normal women, plasma carnitine levels decrease during pregnancy to levels approximating the levels seen in patients who have inborn carnitine deficiency (20).

IMMUNOLOGY

In humans, the fetus and neonate are passively immunized by maternal immunoglobulin G (IgG) that has crossed the placenta (21). Larger globulins and immune complexes do not cross the placenta. The fetus and newborn baby can produce macroglobulin but do not make IgG antibodies. Unlike primates, rodents transfer maternal antibodies postnatally via milk.

In 1960 John Simpson advanced his notion that myasthenic weakness was due to an antibody to a "receptor substance" blocked neuromuscular transmission by acetylcholine in large part because infants of some women with myasthenia gravis developed transient neonatal myasthenia gravis (22). Transplacental antibodies also proved to be responsible for neonatal Graves disease and neonatal immunogenic thrombocytopenic purpura (ITP). Conversely, it should be noted that Guillain-Barré syndrome does not affect the fetus and neonate.

Pregnancy often is associated with a remission in autoimmune diseases during pregnancy, often with a subsequent exacerbation. Evidence for immunosuppression during pregnancy includes susceptibility to infections and prolongation of graft rejection. The list of possible factors is long and includes pregnancy-associated immunoregulatory proteins, including alpha-fetoprotein (21).

For all the information this book contains, there is much more to learn. Careers will be spent exploring the effect of estrogen on the nervous system and the immunobiology of pregnancy. Physicians and scientists in many fields focus on the unsolved mystery of eclampsia, which still causes at least 50,000 maternal deaths per year around the world.

References

1. Donaldson JO. The endocrinology of pseudotumor cerebri. *Neurol Clin* 1986; 4:919–927.
2. Frandsen VA, Stakemann G. The site of production of oestrogenic hormones in human pregnancy: Hormone excretion in pregnancy with anencephalic foetus. *Acta Endocrinol* 1961; 38:383–391.
3. Backstrom T. Epileptic seizures in women related to plasma estrogen and progesterone during the menstrual cycle. *Acta Neurol Scand* 1976; 54:321–347.
4. Holmes GL, Donaldson JO. Effect of sexual hormones on the electroencephalogram and seizures. *J Clin Neurophysiol* 1987; 4:1–22.
5. Torkelson SJ, Lee RA, Hildahl DB. Endometriosis of the sciatic nerve: A report of two cases and a review of the literature. *Obstet Gynecol* 1988; 71:473–477.

6. Markwalder TM, Zava DT, Goldhirsch A, et al. Estrogen and progesterone receptors in meningiomas in relation to clinical and pathologic features. *Surg Neurol* 1983;20:42–47.

7. Bickerstaff ER, Small JM, Guest IA. The relapsing course of certain meningiomas in relation to pregnancy and menstruation. *J Neurol Neurosurg Psychiatry* 1958; 21:89–91.

8. Elster AD, Sanders TG, Vines FS, Chen MY. Size and shape of the pituitary gland during pregnancy and post partum: Measurement with MR imaging. *Radiology* 1991;181:531–535.

9. Enoksson P, Lundberg N, Sjöstedt S, et al. Influence of pregnancy on visual fields in suprasellar tumours. *Acta Psychiat Neurol Scand* 1961;36:524–538.

10. Goetting MG. Catamenial exacerbation of action myoclonus. *J Neurol Neurosurg Psychiatry* 1985;40: 1304–1305.

11. Nausieda PA, Koller WC, Weiner WJ, Klawans HL. Chorea induced by oral contraceptives. *Neurology* 1979; 29:1605–1609.

12. Bean WB, Cogswell R, Dexter M, et al. Vascular changes in the skin in pregnancy: Vascular spiders and palmar erythema. *Surg Obstet Gynecol* 1949;88:739–752.

13. Bray P, Myers RAM, Cowley RA. Orogenital sex as a cause of nonfatal air embolism in pregnancy. *Obstet Gynecol* 1983;61:653–657.

14. Redfield RL, Bodine HR. Air embolism following knee-chest position. *JAMA* 1939;113:671–673.

15. Prowse CM, Gaensler EA. Respiratory and acid-base changes during pregnancy. *Anesthesiology* 1965;26: 381–392.

16. Donaldson JO, Wirz D, Mashman J. Bilateral postpartum femoral neuropathy. *Connecticut Med* 1985;49: 496–498.

17. Kanto J, Erkkola R, Sellman R. Perinatal metabolism of diazepam. *Br Med J* 1974;1:641–642.

18. Koren G, Sharav T, Pastuszak A, et al. A multicenter, prospective study of fetal outcome following accidental carbon monoxide poisoning in pregnancy. *Reprod Toxicol* 1991;5:397–403.

19. Angelini C, Govoni E, Bragaglia MM, Vergani L. Carnitine deficiency: Acute postpartum crisis. *Ann Neurol* 1978;4:558–561.

20. Marzo A, Cardace G, Corbelletta C, et al. Plasma concentration, urinary excretion and renal clearance of L-carnitine during pregnancy: A reversible secondary L-carnitine deficiency. *Gynecol Endocrinol* 1994; 8:115–120.

21. Hunt JS. Immunobiology of pregnancy. *Curr Opin Immunol* 1992; 4,591–596.

22. Simpson JA. Myasthenia gravis: A new hypothesis. *Scott Med J* 1960; 5:419–436.

11 Obstetric Issues in Women with Neurologic Diseases

Errol R. Norwitz, MD, PhD and John T. Repke, MD

Neurologic diseases occur during pregnancy as they do in the non-pregnant state. During pregnancy, the investigation and management of neurologic conditions may be complicated by concern for the safety of the fetus. This chapter is designed as a clinical reference for the practicing neurologist. It is written from the point of view of the obstetrician, and focuses primarily on issues pertinent to pregnancy, delivery, the puerperium, and breast-feeding in patients with specific neurologic ailments. Some topics are not included, or are dealt with only briefly, because details of individual neurologic diseases are discussed in detail elsewhere in this book. The chapter concludes with discussions of neurologic emergencies during pregnancy and other situations specific to obstetric practice, such as drugs and breast-feeding, genetic counseling, and antenatal diagnosis for inherited neurologic diseases.

OBSTETRIC MANAGEMENT OF SELECTED NEUROLOGIC DISORDERS

Seizure Disorders and Epilepsy

Seizure disorders are the most frequent major neurologic complication encountered during pregnancy, affecting 0.3 to 0.6% of all pregnancies (1–4). The incidence of obstetric complications is increased in women with idiopathic seizure disorders, including hyperemesis gravidarum (1.6-fold), preterm delivery (3-fold), pregnancy-induced hypertension or preeclampsia (1.7-fold), cesarean delivery, placental abruption (2- to 3-fold), and perinatal mortality (1–7). However, the majority of pregnant women with seizure disorders will have an uneventful pregnancy and good outcome (8).

Ideally, patients with seizure disorders should be seen before conception. The withdrawal of medication altogether should be considered in patients who have been seizure-free for 2 years or more, although 25 to 40% of such women will have a recurrence of their seizures during pregnancy (9,10). In patients on anticonvulsant therapy, folic acid supplementation (4 mg daily) should be administered for at least 3 months before conception and continued throughout the first trimester of pregnancy to prevent folic acid deficiency-induced malformations, most notably neural tube defects (NTDs) (discussed subsequently) (3,8,11). Genetic counseling should be offered if both parents have an unexplained seizure disorder, or if the disease is inherited (3,8,12).

Generalized seizures in pregnancy may cause significant maternal hypoxemia, with resultant fetal injury and even spontaneous abortion (12). If a woman is prone to convulsions off medication, treatment during pregnancy

TABLE 11.1

Recommended Therapy for Acute Seizures in Pregnancy

DRUG	LOADING DOSE	MAINTENANCE DOSE	THERAPEUTIC LEVEL
Magnesium sulfate#	4–6 g IV over 10–20 minutes	2–3 g/h IV infusion	4–8 mEq/L*
	10 g IM (given as 5 g IM into each buttock)	5 g IM every 4 hours alternating buttocks	As above
Phenytoin	15–20 mg/kg IV at a rate of ≤50 mg/min (usually 1–1.5 g IV over 1 hour)	Depending on serum level (usually 250–500 mg every 10–12 hours IV or PO)	10–20 µg/mL
Diazepam	—	10 mg/h IV infusion	—

\# Only indicated in the setting of preeclampsia/eclampsia.
* Not tested prospectively.

is mandated. The aim of therapy during pregnancy should be to control convulsions with a single agent, using the lowest possible dose (3,8,12–15). It is recommended that drug levels be followed periodically in pregnant patients, although this has yet to be shown to be useful in the absence of symptoms of toxicity or seizure activity. Given the risk of structural anomalies, prenatal diagnosis should include genetic counseling, maternal serum alpha-fetoprotein (AFP), and multiple serum marker screening for aneuploidy at 15 to 20 weeks' gestation (discussed subsequently), and possible amniocentesis if such results are equivocal. Additionally, a careful sonographic structural survey of the fetus is recommended at approximately 18 to 22 weeks. Traditional teaching has suggested that women with unexplained seizure disorders are more likely to deliver a fetus with a congenital structural abnormality, even if they did not take anticonvulsant drugs during the pregnancy. Several recent reports, however, have failed to demonstrate any such association (13–15).

Labor and delivery are usually uneventful. Anticonvulsant medication may need to be given intravenously instead of orally if labor is prolonged. If a seizure does occur, it may be necessary to give a second agent, such as phenytoin (Table 11.1). Benzodiazepines should be used with caution because they have been associated with maternal apnea as well as early neonatal depression. The possibility of an eclamptic seizure should always be considered.

All the commonly used anticonvulsant drugs cross into breast milk. The ratio of transmission varies with the drug used (2% for valproic acid; 30 to 45% for phenytoin, phenobarbital, and carbamazepine; 90% for ethosuximide). The use of such medications, however, is not a contraindication to breast-feeding unless the infant develops signs of toxicity (3,13,14,16). Certain drugs (phenobarbital, benzodiazepines, primidone) are more likely to sedate the infant. See Chapter 15 for more information on epilepsy in women.

Cerebrovascular Disease

Stroke

Stroke is responsible for approximately 5 to 10% of all pregnancy-related maternal deaths in the United States each year (17,18). The overall incidence of cerebrovascular accident is approximately 1 in 6,000 pregnancies (19–21). It is not yet clear whether the risk of stroke is increased during pregnancy; however, the risk of both cerebral infarction and intracerebral hemorrhage does appear to be increased during the puerperium (relative risk 8.7 and 28.3, respectively) (19,22,23). The reported mortality rate of pregnancy-related stroke varies between 5 and 20%. Of those women who survive, 50% are left with substantial neurologic sequelae (19,23).

Hemorrhagic stroke, which complicates 1 in 10,000 to 1 in 45,000 pregnancies, has a poorer prognosis as compared with other categories of stroke, because these strokes tend to be intraparenchymal and more extensive (19,21,24,25). In general, such patients tend to be older with underlying chronic hypertension. Cocaine use has also been associated with hemorrhagic stroke. Cerebral lesions, such as arterial aneurysms and arteriovenous malformations (AVMs), predispose to hemorrhagic stroke. In both obstetric and nonobstetric populations, aneurysms (which rupture most commonly into the subarachnoid space and present as a sudden severe headache) have a threefold increased incidence of bleeding as compared with AVMs (which usually leak into the parenchyma) (26). The literature suggests that the overall incidence of bleeding complications in such patients does not increase during pregnancy (27,28). Without surgical repair, approximately 3.5% of AVMs will bleed during pregnancy, as compared with 5 to 7% over a 12-month period in the nonpregnant population (29). Bleeding complications appear to be more common in the latter half of pregnancy, with approximately 80% of such events occurring after 20 weeks' gestation (22,26). The most concerning observation, however, and the reason why most authors recommend surgical clipping and/or resection of cerebral vascular lesions prior to conception, is that a bleed during pregnancy carries a far more guarded prognosis than if the patient were not pregnant, with the mortality rate increasing from 10% (29) to approximately 28 to 35% (26). In patients who do have a bleed during pregnancy, some evidence suggests that early surgery for cerebral aneurysm may be associated with a decreased maternal and fetal mortality. Aggressive evaluation, including cerebral angiography, is therefore appropriate. The benefit of early surgery for bleeding AVMs, on the other hand, is less clear. At the time of surgery, care should be taken to avoid hypotension, which could result in fetal compromise and ultimately fetal death; hypothermia is relatively well tolerated by the fetus. Alternatives to operative treatment (including embolization) should be explored.

No contraindication exists to vaginal delivery in patients who have had their aneurysm or AVM surgically corrected. In patients with unrepaired cerebral vascular lesions, however, especially those who have survived a previous intracerebral hemorrhage, the recommendations regarding route of delivery remain uncertain (30–33). In a retrospective review of 142 patients with previously symptomatic cerebral aneurysms, Hunt and associates (32) showed no benefit to cesarean over vaginal delivery. Most clinicians agree however, that cesarean delivery prior to labor is probably prudent in women who have already had a bleed in the third trimester (33). If a vaginal delivery is to be attempted, early epidural for optimal pain control and an assisted second-stage delivery have been advocated to minimize Valsalva pressures and dangerous elevations in intracranial pressure, but no clinical data support this approach. See Chapter 17 for more information on stroke in women.

Hypertensive Encephalopathy

Hypertensive encephalopathy is a subacute neurologic syndrome that occurs in patients with sustained elevated systemic blood pressure (usually diastolic blood pressure ≥150 mm Hg) over a period of a few days (34). It is characterized by rapidly progressive signs and symptoms including headache, seizures, visual disturbances, altered mental status, and/or focal neurologic signs. Other evidence of end-organ damage may be evident, such as myocardial ischemia, renal failure, or pulmonary edema. Preeclampsia is a common cause of hypertensive encephalopathy and may manifest with a diastolic blood pressure as low as 100 mm Hg (35). Regardless of the cause, the clinical course seems to be the same. Prognosis is excellent if the hypertension is treated early and effectively, but may be fatal if unrecognized or if treatment is delayed.

Whether the cerebral manifestations of this disorder result from vasospasm or from forced vasodilatation of the cerebral vasculature is as yet unclear (36–38). The brain is normally protected from extremes of pressure by an autoregulatory mechanism that ensures constant perfusion over a wide range of systemic pressures. In response to systemic hypertension, for example, cerebral arterioles normally constrict to maintain adequate perfusion. Hypertensive encephalopathy represents a breakdown in this autoregulatory mechanism in the setting of severe hypertension. The end result is the focal overdistention of cerebral arterioles with disruption of the blood–brain barrier and leakage of fluid and proteins into the surrounding tissues (36,38). Infarcts and significant hemorrhage are rarely seen. The posterior cerebral circulation is more susceptible to such vasogenic edema, hence the predilection for visual symptoms. These pathologic findings appear to result from an acute process, known collectively as *reversible posterior leukoencephalopathy syndrome* (39). Some investigators have suggested that the pathologic basis for hypertensive encephalopathy in the setting of preeclampsia is not due to a disruption in vascular autoregulation, but to barotrauma and vessel injury caused by an increase in cerebral perfusion pressure (40).

The immediate goal of therapy is to reduce the mean arterial pressure (MAP) gradually over the first hour by no more than 20 to 25% or to a diastolic blood pressure of 100 mm Hg, whichever value is higher. Rapid reduction in MAP of 50% or more within the first hour may precipitate cerebral ischemia or infarction and may decrease placental perfusion, resulting in fetal compromise. Sodium nitroprusside (0.5 to 1.0 μg/kg/ min IV infusion) is considered the drug of choice for the treatment of hypertensive encephalopathy in the nonobstetric population. Animal studies, however, have suggested that this drug may selectively decrease placental perfusion (41), so it is reserved as a second-line agent. During pregnancy, hydralazine (5-10 mg IV bolus every 15 to 20 min) is our drug of choice to control blood pressure. Acceptable alternatives include labetalol (20 to 80 mg IV bolus every 5 to 10 minutes up to 300 mg, or 0.5 to 2 mg/min IV infusion); diazoxide (50 to 100 mg IV bolus every 5 to 10 min up to 600 mg, or 10 to 30 mg/min IV infusion); nicardipine (5 mg/h IV infusion increased by 1 to 2 mg/h every 15 minutes to a maximum of 15 mg/h); and oral nifedipine (10 to 20 mg PO repeated at intervals of 5 to 15 minutes). Central-acting agents such as α-methyldopa and clonidine have the effect of depressing the central nervous system, which may confuse the clinical picture; these should therefore be avoided in this setting. Beta-adrenergic antagonists (which reduces uteroplacental blood flow) and trimethaphan (which is associated with meconium ileus) are not recommended in pregnancy. Fluid restriction and diuretic therapy also should be avoided, since many of these patients are intravascularly depleted (see also Chapter 16).

Paraplegia

Approximately 11,000 new spinal cord injuries are reported in the United States per year. The majority of these are traumatic in origin. Approximately 15 to 30% of such injuries occur in women of reproductive age. Fertility is usually unaffected. Anemia (63%), urinary tract infections (UTI) (80%), and pressure sores (26%) may complicate antepartum obstetric management (42,43). Suppressive antibiotic therapy should be considered in patients with recurrent UTIs and/or in patients who self-catheterize. Baseline pulmonary and renal function studies should be carried out, if appropriate. Routine supportive care, including the prevention of decubitus ulcers and contractures, should not be neglected during pregnancy. On occasion, patients with high thoracic or cervical lesions may require ventilatory support during the latter part of pregnancy and labor.

Regarding intrapartum care, the majority of women can deliver vaginally. Cesarean delivery should be reserved for routine obstetric indications. Women with cord transections above the T10 segment will have painless labors, but they will also be unable to appreciate premature uterine contractions should they occur. The recommendation in such patients is therefore to perform weekly cervical exams after 28 weeks' gestation to exclude premature labor (44). Direct abdominal palpation techniques by the patient and home uterine monitors have been used in this setting with some success.

Autonomic dysreflexia is a rare but potentially life-threatening complication of spinal cord injury. It is characterized by acute-onset throbbing headache, hypertension, reflex bradycardia, sweating, flushing, tingling, nasal congestion, and occasionally cardiac dysrhythmias and respiratory distress. Eighty-five percent of women with lesions at or above T5/6 segment (either complete or incomplete transections) are subject to autonomic dysreflexia syndrome (45). Autonomic dysreflexia results from a loss of hypothalamic control over sympathetic spinal reflexes through viable segments of cord below the level of transection and is most often triggered by an afferent stimulus (a full bladder, a bimanual examination, or a simple manipulation, such as changing the urinary catheter). Uterine contractions can also trigger such activity. The severity of this syndrome varies from symptomatic annoyance to hypertensive encephalopathy, stroke, intraventricular and retinal hemorrhage, and death. Uteroplacental vasoconstriction may result in fetal asphyxia. In patients with a history of such an event, continuous blood pressure monitoring via an arterial line is recommended during labor. Bladder and bowel overdistention should be avoided, and pelvic manipulations and examinations should be kept to a minimum and should be preceded by the application of topical anesthetic agents. In susceptible patients, the placement of an epidural catheter and the establishment of a T10 anesthesia level in an attempt to block afferent stimuli arising from the pelvic area should prevent autonomic dysreflexia. If autonomic dysreflexia does occur, delivery should be expedited and blood pressure must be brought under control with fast-acting agents (such as sodium nitroprusside or nitroglycerin). Emergent cesarean section is indicated if symptoms and/or blood pressure cannot be well controlled. All patients with spinal cord injuries require adequate anesthesia for cesarean delivery (46).

Backache

Backache is particularly common in pregnancy as a result of the increased postural and mechanical stress placed on the spine, coupled with hormonal factors that render the intervertebral discs more vulnerable to stress (47). Benign conditions should be distinguished from more sinister causes such as lumbosacral disc disease, bone disease, infections [spinal tuberculosis (Pott's disease), meningitis, herpes zoster], and tumors.

In a review of 347 consecutive cases of surgically proved lumbar disc herniations in women, in which 39% of the women experiencing symptoms either during or immediately after pregnancy, O'Connell (48) concluded that pregnancy predisposes to disc prolapse. Prolapse is usually lateral, involving spinal segments L4 to S1. Lesions above L4 should raise suspicion of an alternative cause. The symptoms and signs of lumber disc protrusion during pregnancy are similar to those in the nonpregnant patient (low back pain, paraspinous rigidity, and tenderness with or without lower extremity weakness and sensory deficit). Bed rest and simple analgesics for symptomatic relief are usually all that is required. Imaging studies and surgery can usually be deferred until after delivery. Bilateral signs of leg weakness, however, especially if associated with sphincter disturbance, may suggest significant central herniation that requires laminectomy and excision of the protruding disc.

Back pain developing in the puerperium may represent new-onset disc disease, temporary palsy due to compressive injury to the lumbosacral plexus during labor, or to a complication of regional anesthesia. Neurologic complications of epidural anesthesia (including epidural hematoma, epidural abscess, and "spinal nerve mass") are exceedingly rare (49–51). Epidural hematomas may be more common in patients on aspirin or with known bleeding disorders (50) and may preclude the use of regional anesthesia in such patients.

Myasthenia Gravis

Myasthenia gravis (see also Chapter 21) is a disease that is characterized by weakness and fatigability of the voluntary muscles (52). Smooth muscles, including the myometrium, are relatively unaffected. Myasthenia gravis is not associated with infertility (53). However, some studies have suggested an increased incidence of spontaneous abortion in these patients (54). The effect of pregnancy on myasthenia gravis is unpredictable, and the course of the disease in a prior pregnancy cannot be used to reliably predict the course in a current or future pregnancy. Overall, pregnancy does not appear to alter the course of the disease. Myasthenia gravis in and of itself is therefore not an indication for pregnancy termination. Indeed, the disease may exacerbate following therapeutic abortion (55). In general, one-third of patients experience definite remission during pregnancy, one-third show evidence of relapse and/or exacerbation, and one-third remain stable (56). Symptomatic relapse appears to be more likely during the puerperium and may be quite sudden and severe (57). No data suggest an increase in the incidence of either preterm delivery or pregnancy-induced hypertension in these patients (53,58).

The management of myasthenia gravis during pregnancy, including myasthenic crises, should be similar to that in the nonpregnant patient (59). Anticholinesterase medications (pyridostigmine, neostigmine) in a pregnant myasthenic patient are administered in doses identical to those given to the nonpregnant patient. Some authors have suggested that corticosteroids and azathioprine be reserved only for pregnant myasthenic patients unresponsive to anticholinesterase therapy (60). Plasmapheresis (61) and thymectomy (62) should be used only in emergency situations. The key to preventing symptomatic exacerbation during pregnancy is adequate rest, avoidance of stress, and aggressive early management of infection.

During labor, consideration should be given to substituting oral doses of anticholinesterase medication with an equivalent intravenous or intramuscular dose. Periodic clinical evaluation of the patient should be performed, looking for evidence of increasing muscle weakness or exhaustion. Myasthenic patients may have a shortened labor due to generalized muscle relaxation (63). A marked contrast may be evident between the strength of the uterine contractions and the generalized muscle weakness exhibited by the patient. Some authors have advocated the use of outlet forceps to shorten the second stage, thereby minimizing the muscle fatigue associated with expulsive efforts (64). Cesarean delivery should be performed only for standard obstetric indications. In the setting of preeclampsia/eclampsia, intrapartum magnesium sulfate therapy should be replaced by phenytoin, phenobarbital, or diazepam for seizure prophylaxis (59,65).

Because the autoantibodies in patients with myasthenia gravis are mostly IgG, they do cross the placenta and may affect the fetus. Neonatal myasthenia syndrome is a transient form of myasthenia gravis that occurs in approximately 12 to 15% of babies born to myasthenic mothers (66). Symptoms (including lethargy, poor suck, feeble cry, generalized muscle weakness, and difficulty swallowing and breathing) usually develop within the first 4 days of life in untreated patients, and up to 80% of cases will be evident within the first 24 hours (67). Term infants are generally delivered with normal Apgar scores. Maternal anticholinesterase medications cross the placenta and may protect the neonate for a few days, which results in delayed diagnosis. The duration and severity of the disease in the mother is not predictive of which fetuses will go on to develop neonatal myasthenia syndrome. Treatment of the neonate includes anticholinesterase medications and supportive care. This syndrome is self-limiting and completely subsides within 2 to 6 weeks. It should not be confused with congenital myasthenia gravis, in which a neonate born to normal parents develops the adult form of the disorder shortly after birth (68). In such cases, the condition is usually permanent.

Despite the presence of anticholinesterase medications and antiacetylcholine receptors in maternal milk, there is no evidence that breast-feeding adversely affects either mother or child.

Disorders of Muscle

Muscle cramping is a very common complaint during pregnancy. Support stockings and calcium supplementation may be useful. This is a benign condition, and reassurance may be all that is needed. The differential diagnosis of a more global muscle weakness includes metabolic myopathies and, rarely, degenerative disorders (motor neuron disease, spinal muscular atrophy). Primary disorders of muscle are rare. Some conditions are reviewed below.

Myotonic muscular dystrophy is a slowly progressive disease characterized by weakness of the facial, sternomastoid, and distal limb muscles. Transmission is autosomal dominant, and the disorder usually manifests in early adulthood. Pregnancy may accelerate the course of the disease, with rapidly worsening weakness and muscle stiffness (myotonia) usually in the latter half of pregnancy (69,70). The reason for this is unclear. Although fecundity is unaffected, pregnancies in women with myotonic dystrophy appear to be at increased risk of spontaneous abortion (69). Affected fetuses are unable to swallow effectively in utero (71), which results in a high incidence of polyhydramnios and preterm labor. Labor may be dysfunctional because of the inability of the uterus to contract normally (69,72) and because of weakness of the skeletal muscles and resultant poor voluntary expulsive effort in the second stage. Assisted vaginal delivery may be necessary. Retained placenta and postpartum hemorrhage are common complications and should be anticipated. Regional anesthesia is preferred, because some IV anesthetic agents (pentothal) are liable to further depress respiration, whereas others (depolarizing muscle relaxants) can cause myotonic spasm.

Just as in myotonic dystrophy, the symptoms of myotonia congenita may be aggravated by pregnancy, especially in the latter half of gestation. Symptoms may improve postpartum (70,73). The effect of pregnancy on the course of pre-existing polymyositis and dermatomyositis is not well described, but the data that do exist suggest that these conditions are rarely exacerbated by pregnancy. If an exacerbation does occur, it is more likely to develop in later pregnancy (74).

Wilson's Disease

An autosomal recessive disorder of copper metabolism, Wilson's disease is characterized by an accumulation of copper in the brain, liver, and other organs. In treated patients, pregnancy does not appear to be affected. Despite initial concerns over the teratogenic potential of penicillamine (75), this has not been borne out in subsequent clinical trials (76), and treatment may be continued throughout pregnancy. It may be prudent, however, to decrease the dose of penicillamine close to term (to 250 mg daily) to avoid potential interference with wound healing (76). Untreated patients have a high rate of spontaneous abortion.

Restless Leg Syndrome

Restless leg syndrome is the most common movement disorder in pregnancy. It usually occurs in the third trimester and has been reported in up to 11 to 12% of all pregnancies. This condition is characterized by an unpleasant "crawling" feeling in the legs (and occasionally in the arms) that occurs most often at night when the patient is relaxed, resulting in an irresistible urge to move about. Symptoms appear to settle down after delivery (77). The cause of this disorder is not known. Neurologic examination is almost always normal. Occasionally, correction of coexisting anemia or iron deficiency may cause the symptoms to abate. Treatment with carbidopa/levodopa, pergolide, or opiates (codeine, propoxyphene) may be useful if the symptoms are severe (77).

NEUROLOGIC EMERGENCIES DURING PREGNANCY

Status Epilepticus

Status epilepticus, defined as a series of repeated generalized convulsions with no intervening periods of consciousness, is a medical emergency for both mother and baby. It may occur during pregnancy without any preceding increase in seizure frequency (78) and is often pre-

cipitated by discontinuation of medication because of concern over the safety of the fetus. Teramo and Hiilesmaa (79) described 29 cases of pregnancy complicated by status epilepticus. The overall maternal mortality rate during or shortly after the event was 31% (9 of 29), and the fetal/infant mortality rate was 48% (14 of 29). Thus, the aggressive management of status epilepticus is mandated.

Intravenous diazepam (5 to 10 mg IV push repeated as required to a maximum of 50 mg) rapidly enters the central nervous system (CNS), where it can achieve anticonvulsant levels within 1 minute and will control seizures in more than 80% of patients within 5 minutes (80). Alternatively, lorazepam (2 to 3 mg IM or IV push repeated as required to a maximum of 4 mg) can be administered to good effect. Such medications have the potential to profoundly depress the fetus, however, and may cause maternal apnea (81). Intravenous phenytoin has a long duration of action (half-life approximately 24 hours) and has a low incidence of serious side effects. If seizures persist, the patient may require intubation and the administration of phenobarbital (20 mg per kg IV), pentobarbital, propofol, or other anesthetic agents.

The differential diagnosis of an acute seizure is detailed in Table 11.2. Eclamptic seizures are almost always brief and rarely last longer than 3 to 4 minutes. The administration of an agent to abort the seizure is seldom necessary. Magnesium sulfate (2 to 3 g IV push repeated every 20 minutes to a maximum of 6 g) is the drug of choice for eclamptic seizures, both for the treatment (82) and prevention of recurrent seizures (83). Magnesium appears to selectively increase cerebral blood flow and oxygen consumption in patients with preeclampsia/eclampsia (84), whereas this does not appear to be the case for phenytoin (85).

TABLE 11.2
Differential Diagnosis of an Acute Seizure during Pregnancy

- Eclampsia
- Cerebrovascular accident (e.g., intracerebral hemorrhage, cerebral venous thrombosis)
- Acute hypertension (e.g., malignant hypertension)
- Space-occupying lesions of the CNS (e.g., brain tumor, abscess)
- Metabolic disorders (e.g., hypoglycemia, uremia, inappropriate antidiuretic hormone secretion resulting in water intoxication)
- Infectious etiology (e.g., meningitis, encephalitis)
- Drug-related seizures (e.g., theophylline toxicity, alcohol and cocaine withdrawal)
- Epilepsy

Transient fetal bradycardia is a common finding after a seizure and does not necessitate immediate delivery. Every attempt should be made to stabilize the mother and resuscitate the fetus in utero before making a decision about delivery. In most cases, pregnancy can continue to term. Prolonged seizure activity (>5 minutes) has been associated with placental abruption (86). See also Chapter 15.

MISCELLANEOUS NEUROLOGIC CONDITIONS SPECIFIC TO PREGNANCY

Obstetric Nerve Injuries

A number of peripheral nerve or plexus injuries may develop during an obstetric surgical procedure or during labor due to compression or stretching of the nerve. Such injuries are more common in anesthetized patients.

The lithotomy position (derived from the Greek: *lithos*, meaning stone, and *otomy*, meaning to cut) evolved from the position that elderly men were placed in for surgical removal of obstructing bladder stones. This is not a natural position for childbirth. Flexion and abduction of the hip can result in compression of the femoral nerve (L2–L4) by Poupart's ligament or by the iliopsoas muscle (87), causing weakness and wasting of the quadriceps, depression of the knee jerk, and sensory impairment over the anteromedial aspect of the lower extremity. Similarly, the obturator nerve (L2–L4) may be stretched as it exits the obturator foramen in the pelvis (87), resulting in gait disturbance due to weakness of the adductor muscles of the leg as well as sensory impairment or pain over the medial part of the thigh. Obturator neuropathies may also result from pudendal regional anesthesia. Lumbosacral plexus palsy is due to compression of the roots of the sciatic nerve within the pelvis, either by the fetal head or by instrumentation (forceps). Involvement of the common peroneal fibers (derived from the posterior divisions of L4–S2) may result in leg weakness, paresthesias and numbness over the dorsum of the foot and lateral aspect of the leg, and even foot drop. The incorrect placement of a patient in obstetric stirrups may result in the compression of the saphenous branch of the femoral nerve (leading to numbness and paresthesias over the medial aspect of the leg below the knee) or of the common peroneal nerve in the region of the head of the fibula (causing weakness of dorsiflexion and eversion of the foot) (88). Traction injury to the sciatic nerve may also occur in this position, but a misplaced deep intramuscular injection should also be considered as a possible iatrogenic cause of sciatic neuropathy. (For other details regarding nerve injuries, see also Chapter 20).

The symptoms of such neuropathies are usually mild and unilateral, and complete recovery can be expected in the majority of cases. Physical therapy may be useful in the short-term. The careful positioning of the obstetric patient during labor or surgical procedures is important to prevent such injuries.

Neurologic Birth Injury

Neurologic birth injuries include intracranial hemorrhage, skull fracture, neck and spinal cord injuries, and facial nerve and brachial plexus injuries. A small number of these occur prior to labor and may be associated with underlying conditions such as maternal alloimmune thrombocytopenia or the intrauterine fetal demise of one twin. The majority occur intrapartum.

Intracranial Hemorrhage

Although bleeding into the fetal head can occur at several anatomic sites (subdural, subarachnoid, cerebral, periventricular), hemorrhage into the germinal matrix within the ventricles—so-called *intraventricular hemorrhage* (IVH)—occurs most frequently. The greatest risk factor for IVH is prematurity. Although the incidence of IVH is debated, Hayden and colleagues (89) reported that 4.6% (23 of 505) of otherwise healthy term infants have sonographic evidence of subepidymal germinal matrix hemorrhage unrelated to obstetric factors. Because of the mechanical forces on the fetus during labor, therapeutic anticoagulation of the mother at the time of delivery has been associated with severe hemorrhage in the fetus. For both maternal and fetal indications, anticoagulation should be discontinued prior to labor.

Birth trauma is an uncommon cause of intracranial hemorrhage. Tearing of the bridging veins from the cerebral cortex to the sagittal sinus or, even less commonly, rupture of the internal cerebral veins or vein of Galen where it joins the straight sinus may occur at the time of spontaneous vaginal delivery due to excessive molding of the parietal bones. It has been suggested that forceps delivery may exacerbate the molding and therefore predispose to intracranial hemorrhage, but this remains theoretical. Early retrospective studies suggesting an association between prophylactic low forceps delivery for small fetuses and IVH (90,91) have been countered by more recent reports showing no significant difference in outcome in neonates weighing 500 to 1,500 g delivered spontaneously or by outlet forceps (92,93). Indeed, the study by Shaver and associates (94) suggested a protective effect of low forceps delivery in neonates weighing ≤1,750 g.

Commonly, the clinical condition of an infant with IVH begins to deteriorate at around 12 hours of life, at which time the infant becomes drowsy, apathetic, fails to feed, develops a feeble cry, and may become cyanotic and dyspneic. Seizure activity may follow. With the advent of sonography and computed tomographic (CT) imaging, diagnosis has become relatively straightforward. Treatment is primarily supportive. Surgical intervention is rarely necessary. The prevention of peripartum intracranial hemorrhage depends on the elimination of difficult forceps deliveries, correct management of breech presentation in labor, and appropriate and timely cesarean delivery for cephalopelvic disproportion. All infants should receive vitamin K (1 mg IM) within 1 hour of birth to prevent hemorrhagic disease of the newborn.

Prognosis depends largely on gestational age at delivery, and the extent and anatomic location of the intracranial bleed (parenchymal and subdural hemorrhages are associated with a poor prognosis in up to 90% of cases, and IVH cases have a poor prognosis in 45% of infants). Other proposed prognostic factors include the etiology of the hemorrhage, the presence or absence of ventriculomegaly, and the degree of ventriculomegaly (>15 mm) suggests a poor outcome. Using these factors, a prognostic scoring system has been developed (95). Overall, intracranial hemorrhage is associated with poor outcome in approximately 68% of cases (95).

Shoulder Dystocia and Brachial Plexus Injury

Shoulder dystocia (defined as impaction of the anterior shoulder of the fetus behind the pubic symphysis following delivery of the head) is an obstetric emergency, occurring in 0.15 to 2.1% of all vaginal deliveries (96–99). It has been associated with neonatal birth trauma (including neurologic injuries and fractures of the humerus, skull, and/or clavicle) in up to 20% of cases (99). Its immediate identification at the time of delivery and prompt and appropriate intervention can prevent neonatal birth trauma in some cases. Can shoulder dystocia be predicted? A number of risk factors for shoulder dystocia have been identified. These include fetal macrosomia (estimated fetal weight ≥4,500 g) (100–104), a history of a previous shoulder dystocia (103–106), diabetes mellitus (including gestational diabetes) (103,104,106,107), midcavity operative vaginal delivery (101,106,108,109), and an abnormal labor pattern (prolonged second stage) (103,106,107). The majority of shoulder dystocias, however, occur in nondiabetic women with fetuses weighing less than 4,000 g (103,104).

First described by Smellie in 1764 (110), brachial plexus paralysis is the second most common neurologic birth injury (after facial nerve palsy), occurring in 0.5 to 2.6 per 1,000 live births (101,103). It is due to "excessive" lateral traction on the head and neck at the time of delivery, with resultant damage to the brachial plexus, usually to cervical nerve roots C5 and C6 (Erb-Duchenne's palsy) (111,112). The end result is paralysis of the ipsilateral deltoid and infraspinatus muscles and the flexor muscles of the forearm. The arm therefore falls limply at the side of the body with the forearm extended and internally rotated, the classic "waiter's tip" deformity.

The function of the fingers is usually retained. The lower brachial plexus (nerve roots C8 and T1) may also be involved, resulting in paralysis of the hand. Isolated lower plexus injuries (Klumpke's palsy) (113) are rare, however, comprising only 2 to 3% of all brachial plexus palsies. Bilateral brachial plexus injuries have been reported, as well as associated unilateral paralysis of the diaphragm and Horner's syndrome (due to injury to the sympathetic fibers of nerve roots C8–T1). The vast majority of traction injuries to the brachial plexus (93 to 95%) resolve completely within 2 years with the help of physical therapy (103,105). Prognosis is especially good if recovery has started within 3 months (114). Overall, only approximately 1 to 5% of brachial plexus palsies result in long-term neurologic compromise (105,115).

Recommendations regarding the route of delivery for women with risk factors for shoulder dystocia remain controversial. Cesarean delivery, especially elective cesarean delivery, is believed to protect the fetus from birth injury. However, there have been reports of neurologic injuries following elective cesarean delivery (103) as well as spontaneous vaginal deliveries in the absence of dystocia (116,117). It has been postulated that in some cases, brachial plexus injury may occur early in the delivery, with stretching and tearing of the nerve roots as the head descends into the pelvis. Brachial plexus injury should therefore not be taken as prima facie evidence of birth process injury. Given the difficulty in predicting and preventing shoulder dystocia, the inconsistent relationship between shoulder dystocia and neurologic injuries, and the rarity of long-term neonatal morbidity, along with the fact that cesarean delivery may not completely prevent such injuries, elective cesarean delivery cannot be recommended for all women with risk factors for shoulder dystocia (103,104).

Fetal Acidosis and Cerebral Palsy

Despite advances in perinatal medicine, the overall prevalence of cerebral palsy remains unchanged at 1.5 to 2.5 per 1,000 live births. Only approximately 10% of children born at term who subsequently go on to develop cerebral palsy had an identified intrapartum hypoxic ischemic event. It seems clear that severe hypoxic ischemic injury to the fetus, such as that seen after a large placental abruption or uterine rupture, may lead to fetal demise or long-term neurologic handicap, including cerebral palsy. Whether milder forms of fetal acidosis or hypoxemia can cause cerebral palsy, however, is a question of considerable debate. Using rhesus monkeys, Myers and associates (118) demonstrated that partial asphyxia may eventually lead to long-term cerebral lesions that resemble, but are not identical to, the lesions of cerebral palsy seen in the human infant. In a retrospective, case-control study, Richmond and colleagues (119) found that abnormal fetal heart rate recordings were identified more frequently in children with subsequent cerebral palsy. The authors concluded, however, that "optimal management of fetal distress" would be expected to decrease the prevalence of cerebral palsy by "only 16%." Other investigators have been unable to demonstrate any association between fetal heart rate patterns and subsequent neurologic development (120). Before intrapartum hypoxic acidemia can be considered as the cause of neurologic injury, a set of specific criteria, defined by both the American College of Obstetricians & Gynecologists (121) and the American Academy of Pediatrics (122), must be met. These include (i) profound metabolic or mixed acidemia (pH <7.00) in an umbilical cord arterial blood sample, if obtained; (ii) persistent Apgar score of 0 to 3 for longer than 5 minutes; (iii) evidence of neonatal neurologic sequelae (seizures, coma, or hypotonia); and (iv) neonatal multiorgan system dysfunction. The bulk of evidence indicates that intrapartum hypoxic ischemic encephalopathy is an infrequent cause of cerebral palsy.

Although the pathophysiologic mechanisms that underlie most of the cerebral palsy syndromes remain poorly understood, recent data suggest that antepartum magnesium sulfate administration may be associated with a decreased incidence of cerebral palsy (123–127). This association was initially noted by Kuban and co-workers (123) in very low birth weight infants born to women who were given magnesium for seizure prophylaxis in the setting of preeclampsia/eclampsia. This finding has more recently been confirmed in a number of other retrospective analyses (124–126), with a reported crude odds ratio of 0.11 (95% CI: 0.02–0.81) (126). This effect appears to be independent of steroid therapy (126,127). Moreover, the effect is also observed in infants born of pregnancies not complicated by preeclampsia (124). The latter finding is important because preeclampsia itself, for reasons that are not well understood, is protective against the development of cerebral palsy (128). The proposed mechanism of action is speculative, but magnesium may act to increase the threshold and decrease the excitability in membranes of neurons and muscle cells. Some investigators have suggested that magnesium may reduce the prevalence of cerebral palsy simply by increasing the death rate among susceptible fetuses and infants. Indeed, during the Magnesium and Neurologic Endpoints Trial (MagNET), a large randomized clinical trial designed to test the neuroprotective effect of magnesium sulfate in the setting of preterm labor (not preeclampsia), the occurrence of excess total pediatric mortality in the children exposed to magnesium (10 of 75 fetuses randomized to magnesium or saline control versus 1 of 75 infants randomized to "other" tocolytics or saline control; P=0.02) led to the early termination of the trial (127,129). The authors concluded that, despite the alarming findings in MagNET, it is conceivable that exposures to doses of

magnesium sulfate less than those used for aggressive tocolysis may be neuroprotective without being lethal (129). This conclusion may be supported by the recently published Magpie Trial (130), a clinical study of 10,141 women with preeclampsia randomized in 33 countries to receive either magnesium sulfate or placebo for seizure prophylaxis. This study showed no substantive short-term harmful effects of magnesium sulfate on the fetus.

The risk factors for newborn encephalopathy are summarized in Table 11.3 (131–133). Intrauterine infection (chorioamnionitis) (134) and maternal fever in labor (131,133) have been strongly associated with the subsequent development of cerebral palsy. It is possible that the association with newborn encephalopathy may be mediated directly by fetal infection or indirectly through inflammatory cytokines (134–136). Evidence also suggests that perinatal brain injury following an intrapartum hypoxic ischemic event may evolve, at least in part, over a period of hours or days, thereby providing a possible window of opportunity for early intervention. Indeed, preliminary studies on the use of neonatal hypothermia treatment suggest that such an approach may provide some neuroprotective effect (137,138). Until further studies are available, such treatment should be regarded as investigational.

Other Congenital Neurologic Injuries

Facial nerve paralysis resulting from pressure to the facial nerve as it exits the stylomastoid foramen is the most common neurologic birth injury. The reported incidence varies from 0.07 to 7.5 per 1,000 live births (97,105,115). These injuries have been associated with operative vaginal (forceps) delivery, although up to a third of cases follow spontaneous vaginal delivery. Facial paralysis may be immediately apparent or may develop within hours of birth. Resolution is usually complete within a few days.

Injuries to the neck and spine are rare and usually result from excessive traction on the spinal cord at the time of vaginal delivery, such as during a difficult breech extraction or operative vaginal delivery. Actual fracture or dislocation of the vertebrae may occur, and such injuries may prove fatal (139). The true incidence of spinal injuries is not known.

Multicystic encephalomalacia is a pathologic condition most commonly seen in multiple gestations, in which cerebral damage develops in the surviving fetus (or fetuses) following an intrauterine demise in the second half of pregnancy. It may result in mental retardation and/or cerebral palsy in the surviving infant. The mechanism of cerebral injury is not clear. Embolization of tissue thromboplastin through placental anastomoses to the surviving twin has been suggested as a possible explanation. This is supported by findings that encephalomalacia is more common in monochorionic as compared with

TABLE 11.3
*Risk Factors for Newborn Encephalopathy**

PRECONCEPTIONAL FACTORS	ANTEPARTUM FACTORS	INTRAPARTUM FACTORS
• Increased maternal age • Primiparity • Unemployed, unskilled laborer, or housewife • No private health insurance • Infertility treatment • Family history of seizures • Family history of neurologic disorders	• Male fetus • Maternal thyroid disease • Severe preeclampsia/eclampsia • Bleeding in pregnancy • Viral illness during pregnancy • Prematurity • Postterm pregnancy • Placental abnormalities • Intrauterine growth restriction in the fetus • Structural anomalies in the fetus	• Intrapartum fever • Prolonged rupture of membranes • Thick meconium • Malpresentation and malposition • Intrapartum hypoxia • Acute intrapartum events (including cord prolapse, abruptio placentae, uterine rupture, maternal seizures) • Forceps delivery • Emergency cesarean delivery

* Data from Badawi et al. *Br Med J* 1998;317:1554 (131); Ellis et al. *Br Med J* 2000;320:1229 (132); and Adamson et al. *Br Med J* 1995;311:598 (133).

dichorionic twin gestations (4 to 5% versus 20%, respectively) (140,141). In dichorionic twin pregnancies, the surviving twin may be protected from injury by the rarity of placental vascular communications. Other possible mechanisms of neurologic injury include fetal hypotension, with hypoxemia resulting in ischemic injury and/or fetal exsanguination. Unfortunately, immediate delivery does not appear to prevent encephalomalacia in the surviving twin (142). Clinical management should be dictated by the gestational age, chorionicity of the conception, fetal lung maturity, and the presence or absence of maternal disseminated intravascular coagulopathy [which occurs in up to 25% of cases of singleton intrauterine fetal demise within 3 to 5 weeks (143), but is rarely seen in the presence of a surviving fetus].

Neurologic Disorders in the Fetus

Many factors may put a fetus at increased risk of having a genetic disorder or neurologic birth defect. A comprehensive questionnaire (inquiring about heritable diseases, birth defects in the family, underlying medical conditions, medications, maternal age, consanguinity, racial and ethnic background, and potential teratogen exposure) should be given to all women at their first prenatal visit to detect pregnancies at risk. Genetic counseling by trained professionals should be offered to all women deemed to be at increased risk for fetal anomaly.

Preconceptional Genetic Counseling

Ideally, genetic counseling for couples at high risk of a congenital anomaly should take place prior to conception. The incidence of congenital abnormalities in the general population is on the order of 2 to 3% (144). Over

and above this background risk, each pregnancy brings with it additional risks specific to that couple. Depending on the problem, a number of preventative measures may ameliorate this risk if they are taken before pregnancy. For example, meticulous glucose control in insulin-dependent diabetic patients prior to conception can significantly decrease the risk of structural anomalies in the fetus [which include anencephaly or neural tube defect (NTD), caudal regression, and spinal anomalies] (145). Similarly, couples who have had a previous fetus affected by NTD are at increased risk of having a fetus with an NTD in a subsequent pregnancy (0.3 to 1% compared with the general population risk of 0.1 to 0.2%). In such couples, periconceptional folic acid supplementation (4 mg daily) has been shown to decrease the NTD recurrence risk by approximately 71% (146). Evidence also suggests that lower doses of supplemental folic acid (0.4 to 0.8 mg daily, similar to that in prenatal vitamins) may decrease the incidence of a first occurrence of NTD (147). Additionally, the genetic screening of potential parents before conception may detect couples at risk for having a fetus with one of the more common autosomal recessive disorders, such as Tay-Sachs disease, cystic fibrosis, sickle cell disease, and the thallasemias.

Postconceptional Genetic Counseling

A number of antenatal screening tests are currently available to modify a patient's a priori age-related risk of having a pregnancy complicated by fetal aneuploidy. Detection of AFP in maternal serum (a fetal glycoprotein produced early in gestation by the yolk sac and later by the fetal gastrointestinal tract and liver), forms the basis of AFP screening for both open NTD (elevated levels) and trisomy 21 [Down syndrome (low levels)]. A positive screening test at 15 to 20 weeks' gestation should be followed by more definitive testing. Amniotic fluid AFP and acetylcholinesterase activity should be measured in women with elevated maternal serum AFP (148), and a targeted sonographic examination looking for a spinal defect should be performed. Low maternal serum AFP can be used in conjunction with maternal age to predict risk for Down syndrome. Fetal karyotyping by amniocentesis or chorionic villus sampling is generally recommended when the risk of aneuploidy approaches that of a 35-year-old woman (i.e., 1 in 270) (149). Using this approach to screen a population of over 77,000 pregnant women under 35 years of age, the New England Regional Genetics Prenatal Collaborative Group could only detect 25% of infants with Down syndrome (150). To increase the sensitivity of this test, two further maternal serum markers have been included, unconjugated estriol (low levels) and β-human chorionic gonadotropin (elevated levels) (151). Up to 60% of Down syndrome can be detected using this so-called maternal serum "triple screen" at 15 to 20 weeks of gestation (151–154). Other maternal serum markers have been evaluated in conjunction with the triple screen in an attempt to improve the detection of fetal aneuploidy. The most promising new second-trimester analyte is dimeric inhibin A (155), which is already being used by some commercial laboratories. The addition of inhibin A to the standard "triple screen" increases the detection rate of Down sydnrome from 50 to 60% to over 80% with a halving of the false-positive rate (from 14 to 7%) (156,157). Maternal serum marker screening can also be used to screen for trisomy 13 and 18, but the sensitivity of such testing has yet to be clearly delineated (150,154,158). A level II sonographic examination may be able to increase the overall sensitivity of antenatal screening for Down syndrome. A normal fetal anatomic survey will decrease a woman's age-related risk of having a fetus with Down syndrome by approximately 50%.

Recent attention has focused on first-trimester screening for fetal aneuploidy, including maternal serum analytes [primarily free β-human chorionic gonadotropin and pregnancy-associated plasma protein A (PAPP-A)] and fetal nuchal lucency measurements (154,159). An increased nuchal translucency measurement in the first trimester, in combination with maternal age, has been reported to identify 27 to 89% of Down syndrome pregnancies, with a screen-positive rate of 2.8 to 9.3% (154,160,161). Several large clinical trials are currently in progress to assess the utility of first-trimester screening for fetal aneuploidy. Until these data are available, such screening should not be regarded as the standard of care (154).

In couples with a previous chromosomally abnormal infant, an abnormal fetus on sonographic examination, or in whom one or both of the partners have a known chromosomal abnormality, a more focused evaluation is indicated. The genetic testing of the parents may be useful in couples with a previously affected infant, looking for a balanced translocation. Careful imaging of the fetus using x-ray, ultrasound, or magnetic resonance imaging (MRI) may be indicated. However, definitive genetic testing for this pregnancy requires harvesting either placental cells (by chorionic villus sampling) or fetal cells (by amniocentesis, percutaneous umbilical blood sampling, or, rarely, fetal skin or liver biopsy). The details and complications of such procedures have been reviewed in detail elsewhere (153,154). The identification of specific genetic abnormalities is now available for a number of inherited neurologic disorders (Table 11.4) (see also Chapter 7).

All states have laws governing newborn screening for conditions that can be effectively treated or even prevented by early intervention. These include conditions such as phenylketonuria, congenital hypothyroidism, sickle cell disease, galactosemia, and homocysteinuria.

Radiologic Imaging during Pregnancy

The diagnosis of CNS lesions has been revolutionized by advances in imaging technology. In general, the use of diagnostic techniques should not be restricted because the patient is pregnant. The effect of ionizing radiation on the fetus depends on both the dose of radiation that reaches the fetus and the gestational age at the time of exposure. Shielding of the pregnant abdomen is recommended, if possible, especially during fluoroscopy. Although most of the fetal exposure during radiologic procedures results from the scatter of ionizing radiation off the maternal axial skeleton, every attempt should be made to reduce potential exposure. Such efforts are usually greatly appreciated by the parents. The potential injury to the fetus from ionizing radiation is threefold: (i) an increased risk of spontaneous abortion, especially if exposure occurs during the preimplantation stage (162); (ii) an increased risk of congenital anomalies, specifically microcephaly and/or mental retardation after exposure to >5–10 rads (163,164); and (iii) an increased risk of subsequent childhood leukemia (relative risk 1.5–2.0 after exposure to ≥1–2 rads) (163,164). It is generally accepted that exposure of the fetus to less than 5 rads is incapable of producing any detectable teratogenic effect. Exposure of the fetus to x-radiation from routine diagnostic tests is low [from a maternal chest x-ray ± 0.02–0.07 mrad; from a skull x-ray <0.05 mrad; from a head or chest CT (10 slices × 10 mm thickness) ± 0.05–0.1 rad; from an abdominal CT (10 slices × 10 mm) ± 1.7–2.6 rad; from a lumbar spine CT (5 slices × 10 mm) ± 2.3–3.5 rad]. The potential for germ cell mutations and genetic disorders in subsequent generations remains a theoretical concern; however, in animal models, acute exposure to at

TABLE 11.4

Prenatal Diagnosis of Common Inherited Neurologic Disorders

NEUROLOGIC DISORDER	INHERITANCE PATTERN	PRENATAL DIAGNOSIS
Chromosomal Abnormalities		
• Down syndrome (trisomy 21)	C (mosaicism, non-disjunction)	Screen using maternal age and serum screening Karyotyping of fetal cells; FISH; ultrasound may be useful
• Other autosomal trisomies		
– Edward's syndrome (trisomy 18)	C	As above
– Patau's syndrome (trisomy 13)	C	As above
• Unbalanced translocations	C	As above
• Cri-du-chat syndrome	C (deletion)	Karyotyping (deletion of 5p)
• Prader-Willi syndrome	C (deletion, UPD)	Microdeletion of 15q11-15q13 (60–70%), deletion is paternal in origin
• Angelman's syndrome	C (deletion, UPD)	Deletion of 15q11, associated with loss of maternal genes (UPD)
• Fragile X syndrome	XR	Identification of triplet repeats on chromosome X by DNA analysis
Inborn Errors of Metabolism		
• Aminoacidurias		
– Phenylketonuria	AR	DNA analysis; ↓ phenylalanine hydroxylase activity in fetal cells#
– Maple syrup urine disease	AR	↑↑Amino acid levels
– Homocystinuria	AR	↑ Serum methionine; ↑ cystathionine-β-synthase activity in fetal cells
– Hartnup's disease	AR	None
• Mucopolysaccharidoses		
– Hunter's syndrome	XR	↓ Iduronate sulfatase activity in fetal cells
– Hurler's syndrome	AR	↓ α-iduronidase enzyme activity in fetal cells
• Lipidoses		
– Tay-Sachs disease	AR	↓ Hexosaminidase A activity (useful for detecting carrier status); DNA analysis
– Niemann-Pick disease	AR	↓ Spingomyelinase enzyme activity in fetal cells
• Carbohydrate metabolism		
– Galactosemia	AR	↓ Galactose-1-phosphate uridyl transferase activity in fetal cells
• Purine metabolism		
– Lesch-Nyhan syndrome	XR	↓ Guanine phosphoribosyltransferase activity in fetal cells
Hereditary Degenerative Disorders		
• Myotonic dystrophy	AD	DNA analysis identifying amplified trinuleotide repeats in a protein kinase gene on chromosome 19q
• Muscular dystrophy	XR, ?AD, ?AR	Linkage analysis and fetal DNA analysis; detection of dystrophin in fetal muscle biopsy can identify carrier status for Duchenne's, but is rarely used

(continued)

TABLE 11.4
Prenatal Diagnosis of Common Inherited Neurologic Disorders (Continued)

NEUROLOGIC DISORDER	INHERITANCE PATTERN	PRENATAL DIAGNOSIS
Primary CNS Defects		
• Primary microcephaly	Variable, ?AR	Ultrasound
• Congenital hydrocephalus		
– Stenosis of Aqueduct of Sylvius	XR, variable	Ultrasound; DNA analysis
– Dandy-Walker syndrome	Variable	Ultrasound
• Anencephaly/NTD	MF, variable	Screen using MS-AFP ($\uparrow$); amnio for AF-AFP and presence of acetylcholinesterase activity ($\uparrow$); ultrasound
• Ataxia telangectasia	AR	DNA analysis (often 14/14 or 7/14 translocations)
• Color blindness	XR	None
• Ocular albanism	XR	None
• Huntington's chorea	AD	Analysis of DNA triplet repeats
• Frederich's ataxia	AR	DNA analysis in selected families (genetic defect in region 9q)
• Familial epilepsy	AD, ?AR	None
Neuroectodermatosis		
• Tuberous sclerosis	AD	DNA analysis in selected families if genetic defect is known; ultrasound or MRI may help in selected cases
• Neurofibromatosis	AD (type I)	DNA linkage analysis in selected families (only for type I)
Neuromuscular Disorders		
• Myasthenia gravis	MF	None
• Charcot-Marie-Tooth disease	AD (type I)	Linkage analysis in selected families (genetic defects localized mainly to 1q, 17p, Xq); gene analysis in informative families
• Werdnig-Hoffman disease	AR	DNA analysis available in selected families (genetic defect in region 5q)
Miscellaneous		
• Autism	Unknown	None
• Sickle cell disease	AR	Hemoglobin electrophoresis (useful to identify carrier status in parents); gene mutation analysis of fetal cells
• Wilson's disease	AR	DNA linkage analysis in selected families (genetic defect localized to region 13q14)
• Alzheimer's disease	Variable, AD	None

= Fetal cells can be trophectoderm cells from CVS, amniocytes from amniocentesis, fetal blood from PUBS, or endothelial cells from fetal skin biopsy.

C = chromosomal; AR = autosomal recessive; AD = autosomal dominant; XR = X-linked recessive; XD = X-linked dominant; MF = multifactorial; UPD = uniparental disomy; CVS = chorionic villus sampling; amnio = amniocentesis; FISH = fluorescent in-situ hybridization; PCR = polymerase chain reaction; AFP = α-fetoprotein; MRI = magnetic resonance imaging least 140 rads is necessary to produce any measurable increase in cellular mutation rate.

MRI does not employ radiation and is thought to be devoid of fetal risks (167,168). If available, it is the preferred technique for CNS imaging during pregnancy. Contraindications to the use of MRI include the presence of mechanically, electrically, or magnetically activated implants or devices, but these are rarely encountered in reproductive-age women. MRI is especially useful for diagnosing demyelinating diseases, posterior fossa and spinal cord lesions, and screening for AVMs. It is also the imaging technique of choice to evaluate lesions in the abdomen and retroperitoneum, such as adrenal tumors, some gastrointestinal lesions, and intra-abdominal malignancies. Other applications of MRI in pregnancy include MR pelvimetry for planned breech deliveries (168) and MRI of the fetus to further define fetal anatomy when a structural anomaly is suspected and sonographic evaluation is suboptimal. The limited space available within the MR scanner has to some degree restricted its use, because it is often difficult to continuously monitor critically ill patients during the procedure and because some pregnant women are unable to tolerate the claustrophobic conditions. Furthermore, movement of the fetus in utero during scanning may create images that are blurred and difficult to interpret. For this reason, some authors have advocated sedating the fetus prior to pelvis MRI, but this is not routinely done.

In certain clinical situations (such as an acute hemorrhagic injury), cranial CT may be superior to MR both in terms of greater accessibility and improved resolution. Cerebral angiography with contrast injection may be invaluable in this setting. Iodinated contrast agents are physiologically inert and pose little risk to the fetus. Maternal hydration should be maintained during the administration of iodinated contrast to avoid the possibility of fetal dehydration.

Positron emission tomography (PET) is a relatively new technique that uses positron-emitting radioisotopes to evaluate cerebral blood flow and glucose metabolism. The need for radioisotope administration, however, severely limits its use during pregnancy.

Drugs and Breastfeeding

The benefits of breast-feeding are well established. With few exceptions—the most important of which are chronic hepatitis B or C, cytomegalovirus, and human immunodeficiency virus (HIV) infection—breast-feeding should be encouraged. Diuretics, bromocriptine, and combined oral contraceptives (but not the progestin-only pill) may suppress lactation and decrease the volume of milk production. Such agents are not absolutely contraindicated in lactating women, but patients should be made aware of this potential complication. Smoking has also been shown to adversely affect lactation. It is interesting that combined oral contraceptives do not appear to affect milk production if they are started after lactation is established.

Most drugs given to the mother are excreted to some extent into breast milk. The concentration is usually no higher than that in maternal serum, however. The result is that the amount of drug ingested by the infant is typically small, and this is rarely a contraindication to breastfeeding. However, breast-feeding is contraindicated with some drugs. These include drugs of abuse [cocaine, heroin, phencyclidine (PCP)], cytotoxic drugs that are known to be immunosuppressive even in low concentrations (cyclophosphamide, doxorubicin, methotrexate), and drugs that are biologically active in the infant at much lower serum levels than in the adult (such as lithium and possibly ergotamine) (16). Breast-feeding should probably be suspended for 24 to 48 hours if the mother receives radioisotopes such as ^{67}gallium, ^{111}indium, ^{125}iodine, ^{131}iodine, or ^{99}technetium. A number of drugs exist (e.g., antidepressants, anxiolytic drugs, antipsychotics, metoclopramide, metronidazole) whose effect on the nursing infants is unknown, but may be of concern. The recommendation of the Committee on Drugs of the American Academy of Pediatrics (16) in this setting is to monitor the nursing infants carefully and, if the clinical situation dictates, measure blood levels of the drug in both mother and infant before making a decision.

SUMMARY

The successful management of pregnancy in women with neurologic disorders requires a team approach, incorporating recommendations from specialists in both neurology and maternal–fetal medicine/perinatology. In general, most chronic neurologic disorders are compatible with normal pregnancy outcome and should be managed as if the patient were not pregnant. Diagnostic investigations (including imaging studies) should be undertaken if indicated. Our primary responsibility as physicians is to "do no harm." With few exceptions, the potential to "do harm" to both mother and fetus by failing to detect or adequately manage a neurologic condition during pregnancy far outweighs the potential risk to the pregnancy.

References

1. Bjerkedal T, Bahna SL. The occurrence and outcome of pregnancy in women with epilepsy. *Acta Obstet Gynecol Scand* 1973;52:245.
2. Nelson KB, Ellenberg JH. Maternal seizure disorder, outcome of pregnancy, and neurologic abnormalities in the children. *Neurology* 1982;32:1247.
3. Nulman I, Laslo D, Koren G. Treatment of epilepsy in pregnancy. *Drugs* 1999;57:535.

4. Pschirrer ER, Monga M. Seizure disorders in pregnancy. *Obstet Gynecol Clin North Am* 2001;28:601.

5. Yerby M, Koepsell T, Daling J. Pregnancy complications and outcomes in a cohort of women with epilepsy. *Epilepsia* 1985;26:631.

6. Wilhelm J, Morris D, Hotham N. Epilepsy and pregnancy—a review of 98 pregnancies. *Aust N Z J Obstet Gynaecol* 1990;4:290.

7. Hiilesmaa VK, Bardy A, Teramo K. Obstetric outcome in women with epilepsy. *Am J Obstet Gynecol* 1985;152:499–504.

8. Delgado-Escueta AV, Janz D. Consensus guidelines: preconception counseling, management, and care of the pregnant woman with epilepsy. *Neurology* 1992;42:149.

9. Pedley TA. Discontinuing antiepileptic drugs. *N Engl J Med* 1988;318:982.

10. Browne TR, Holmes GL. Epilepsy. *N Engl J Med* 2001;344:1145.

11. Bruno MK, Harden CL. Epilepsy in pregnant women. *Curr Treat Options Neurol* 2002;4:31.

12. Schupf N, Ottman R. Risk of epilepsy in offspring of affected women: association with maternal spontaneous abortion. *Neurology* 2001;57:1642.

13. Yerby MS. The use of anticonvulsants during pregnancy. *Semin Perinatol* 2001;25:153.

14. Holmes LB, Harvey EA, Coull BA, et al. The teratogenicity of anticonvulsant drugs. *N Engl J Med* 2001;344:1132.

15. Matalon S, Schechtman S, Goldzweig G, Ornoy A. The teratogenic effect of carbamazepine: a meta-analysis of 125 exposures. *Reprod Toxicol* 2002;16:9.

16. American Academy of Pediatrics. Committee on Drugs. Transfer of drugs and other chemicals into human milk. *Pediatrics* 1989;84:924.

17. Kaunitz AM, Hughes JM, Grimes DA, Smith JC, Rochat RW, Kafrissen ME. Causes of maternal mortality in the United States. *Obstet Gynecol* 1985;65:605.

18. Rochat RW, Koonin LM, Atrash HK, Jewett JJ, and the Maternal Mortality Collaborative. Maternal mortality in the United States: report from the Maternal Mortality Collaborative. *Obstet Gynecol* 1988;72:91.

19. Simolke GA, Cox SM, Cunningham FG. Cerebrovascular accidents complicating pregnancy and the puerperium. *Obstet Gynecol* 1991;78:37.

20. Lanska DJ, Kryscio RJ. Stroke and intracranial venous thrombosis during pregnancy and puerperium. *Neurology* 1998;51:1622.

21. Jaigobin C, Silver FL. Stroke and pregnancy. *Stroke* 2000;31:2948.

22. Kittner SJ, Stern BJ, Feeser BR, et al. Pregnancy and the risk of stroke. *N Engl J Med* 1996;335:768.

23. Lamy C, Hamon JB, Coste J, Mas JL. Ischemic stroke in young women: risk of recurrence during subsequent pregnancies. French Study Group on Stroke in Pregnancy. *Neurology* 2000;55:269.

24. Noronha A. Neurologic disorders during pregnancy and the puerperium. *Clin Perinatol* 1985;12:695.

25. Minielly R, Yuzpe AA, Drake CG. Subarachnoid hemorrhage secondary to ruptured cerebral aneurysm in pregnancy. *Obstet Gynecol* 1979;53:64.

26. Dias MS, Sekhar LN. Intracranial hemorrhage from aneurysms and arteriovenous malformations during pregnancy and the puerperium. *Neurosurgery* 1990;27:855.

27. Horton JC, Chambers WA, Lyons SL, Adams RD, Kjellberg RN. Pregnancy and the risk of hemorrhage from cerebral arteriovenous malformations. *Neurosurgery* 1990;27:867.

28. Parkinson D, Bachers G. Arteriovenous malformations: summary of 100 consecutive supratentorial cases. *J Neurosurg* 1980;53:285.

29. Itoyama Y, Uemura S, Ushio Y, Carazzi J, Nonaka N. Natural course of unoperated intracranial arteriovenous malformation: study of 50 cases. *J Neurosurg* 1989;71:805.

30. Witlin AG, Mattar F, Sibai BM. Postpartum stroke: a twenty-year experience. *Am J Obstet Gynecol* 2000;183:83.

31. Lanska DJ, Kryscio RJ. Risk factors for peripartum and postpartum stroke and intracranial venous thrombosis. *Stroke* 2000;31:1274.

32. Hunt HB, Schrifin BS, Suzuki K. Ruptured berry aneurysms and pregnancy. *Obstet Gynecol* 1974;43:827.

33. Wiebers DO. Subarachnoid hemorrhage in pregnancy. *Semin Neurol* 1988;8:226.

34. Gifford RW Jr, Westbrook E. Hypertensive encephalopathy: mechanism, clinical features, and treatment. *Prog Cardiovasc Dis* 1974;17:115.

35. Finnerty FA Jr. Hypertensive encephalopathy. *Am J Med* 1972;52:672.

36. Schwartz RB, Jones KM, Kalina P, et al. Hypertensive encephalopathy: findings on CT, MR imaging, and SPECT imaging in 14 cases. *Am J Radiol* 1992;159:379.

37. Apollon KM, Robinson JN, Schwartz RB, Norwitz ER. Cortical blindness and severe preeclampsia: computed tomography, magnetic resonance imaging, and single-photon-emission computed tomography findings. *Obstet Gynecol* 2000;95:1017.

38. Schwartz RB, Feske SK, Polak JF, et al. Preeclampsia-eclampsia: clinical and neuroradiographic correlates and insights into the pathogenesis of hypertensive encephalopathy. *Radiology* 2000;217:371.

39. Mabie WC. Management of acute severe hypertension and encephalopathy. *Clin Obstet Gynecol* 1999;42:519.

40. Belfort AM, Varner MW, Dizon-Townson DS, Grunewald C, Nisell H. Cerebral perfusion pressure, and not cerebral blood flow, may be the critical determinant of intracranial injury in preeclampsia: a new hypothesis. *Am J Obstet Gynecol* 2002;187:626.

41. Naulty J, Cefalo RC, Lewis PE. Fetal toxicity of nitroprusside in the pregnant ewe. *Am J Obstet Gynecol* 1981;139:708.

42. Verduyn WH. Spinal cord injured women, pregnancy and delivery. *Paraplegia* 1986;24:231.

43. Mitish VA, Svetukhin AM, Glyantsev SP. Pressure sores in pregnancy. *Br J Plast Surg* 1998;51:573.

44. Robertson DNS. Pregnancy and labour in the paraplegic. *Paraplegia* 1972;10:209.

45. Wanner MB, Rageth CJ, Zach GA. Pregnancy and autonomic hyperreflexia in patients with spinal cord lesions. *Paraplegia* 1987;25:482.

46. Agostoni M, Giorgi E, Beccaria P, Zangrillo A, Valentini G. Combined spinal-epidural anaesthesia for caesarean section in a paraplegic woman: difficulty in obtaining the expected level of block. *Eur J Anaesthesiol* 2000;17:329.

47. O'Connell JEA. Maternal obstetrical paralysis. *Surg Gynecol Obstet* 1944;79:374.

48. O'Connell JEA. Lumbar disc protrusions in pregnancy. *J Neurol Neurosurg Psychiatry* 1960;23:138.

49. Crawford JS. Maternal complications of epidural analgesia. *Anaesthesia* 1985;40:1219.

50. Sage DJ. Epidurals, spinals and bleeding disorders in pregnancy: a review. *Anaesth Intensive Care* 1990;18: 319.

51. Mack PF, Gurvitch DL, Gadalla F. Transient paraplegia after epidural anesthesia in a parturient. *Anesth Analg* 2000;90:114.

52. Willis T. *De anima brutorum*. Oxford, England: Theatro Sheldoniano, 1672;404–406.

53. Duff GB. Preeclampsia and the patient with myasthenia gravis. *Obstet Gynecol* 1979;54:355.

54. Foldes FF, McWall PG. Myasthenia gravis: a guide for anesthesiologists. *Anesthesiology* 1967;23:837.

55. Perry CP, Hilliard GD, Gilstrap LC, Harris RE. Myasthenia gravis in pregnancy. *Ala J Med Sci* 1975;12:219.

56. Osserman KE. Pregnancy in myasthenia gravis and neonatal myasthenia gravis. *Am J Med* 1955;19:718.

57. Fraser D, Turner JWA. Myasthenia gravis and pregnancy. *Proc Royal Soc Med* 1963;56:379.

58. Cohen BA, London RS, Goldstein PJ. Myasthenia gravis and preeclampsia. *Obstet Gynecol* 1976;48:355.

59. Repke JT. Myasthenia gravis in pregnancy. In: Goldstein PJ, Stern BJ, (eds.) *Neurological Disorders of Pregnancy*. 2nd ed. Mount Kisco, NY: Futura Publishing Co., 1992;269–291.

60. Plauche WC. Myasthenia gravis in pregnancy: an update. *Am J Obstet Gynecol* 1979;135:691.

61. Fennell DF, Ringel SP. Myasthenia gravis and pregnancy. *Obstet Gynecol Surv* 1987;41:414.

62. Ip MSM, So SY, Lam WK, Tang LCH, Mok CK. Thymectomy in myesthenia gravis during pregnancy. *Postgrad Med J* 1986;62:473.

63. Chambers DC, Hall JE, Boyce J. Myasthenia gravis and pregnancy. *Obstet Gynecol* 1967;29:597.

64. McNall PG, Jafarnier MR. Management of myasthenia gravis in the obstetrical patient. *Am J Obstet Gynecol* 1965;92:518.

65. Repke JT. Clinical dialogue: treating preeclampsia with phenytoin. *Contemp Obstet Gynecol* 1989;34:57.

66. Namba T, Brown SB, Grob D. Neonatal myasthenia gravis: report of 7 cases and review of the literature. *Pediatrics* 1970;45:488.

67. Fenichel GM. Clinical syndromes of myasthenics in infancy and childhood. *Arch Neurol* 1978;35:97.

68. Namba T. Familial myasthenia gravis. *Arch Neurol* 1971;25:49.

69. Shore RN, MacLachlan TB. Pregnancy with myotonic dystrophy: course, complications and management. *Obstet Gynecol* 1971;38:448.

70. Rudnick-Schôneborn S, Glauner B, Rôhrig D, Zerres K. Obstetric aspects in women with facioscapulohumeral muscular dystrophy, limb-girdle muscular dystrophy, and congenital myopathies. *Arch Neurol* 1997;54:888.

71. Dunn LJ, Dierker LJ. Recurrent hydramnios in association with myotonia dystrophica. *Obstet Gynecol* 1973; 42:104.

72. Sciarra JJ, Steer CM. Uterine contractions during labor in myotonic muscular dystrophy. *Am J Obstet Gynecol* 1961;82:612.

73. Hakim CA, Thomlinson J. Myotonis congenita in pregnancy. *J Obstet Gynaecol Br Commonw* 1969;76:561.

74. Rozenweig BA, Rotmensch S, Binnette SP, Phillippe M. Primary idiopathic polymyositis and dermatomyositis complicating pregnancy: diagnosis and management. *Obstet Gynecol Surv* 1989;44:162.

75. Marsh L, Fraser FC. Chelating agents and teratogenesis. *Lancet* 1973;2:846.

76. Scheinberg IH, Sternlieb I. Pregnancy in penicillamine-treated patients with Wilson's disease. *N Engl J Med* 1975;293:1300.

77. Earley CJ. Sleep disorders. In: Johnson RT, Griffen JW, (eds.) *Current therapy in neurologic disease* (4th ed.) St. Louis, Mo: Mosby, 1993.

78. Knight AH, Rhind EG. Epilepsy and pregnancy: a study of 153 pregnancies in 59 patients. *Epilepsia* 1975;16:99.

79. Teramo K, Hiilesmaa VK. Pregnancy and fetal complications in epileptic pregnancies: review of the literature. In: Janz D, Dam M, Richens A, Bossi L, Helge H, Schmidt D, (eds.) *Epilepsy, pregnancy, and the child*. New York, NY: Raven Press; 1982:53-59.

80. Delgado-Escueta AV, Wasterlain C, Treiman DM, Porter RS. Current concepts in neurology: Management of status epilepticus. *N Engl J Med* 1982;306:1337.

81. Yerby MS. Problems and management of the pregnant woman with epilepsy. *Epilepsia* 1987;28:29.

82. The Eclampsia Trial Collaborative Group. Which anticonvulsant for women with eclampsia? Evidence from the Collaborative Eclampsia Trial. *Lancet* 1995;345: 1455.

83. Lucas MJ, Leveno KJ, Cunningham FG. A comparison of magnesium sulphate with phenytoin for the prevention of eclampsia. *N Engl J Med* 1995;333:201.

84. Belfort MA, Moise KJ Jr. Effect of magnesium sulfate on maternal brain blood flow in preeclampsia: a randomized, placebo-controlled study. *Am J Obstet Gynecol* 1992;167:661.

85. Gerthoffer WT, Shafer PG, Taylor S. Selectivity of phenytoin and dihydropyridine calcium channel blockers for relaxation of the basilar artery. *J Cardiovasc Pharmacol* 1987;10:9.

86. American College of Obstetricians and Gynecologists. *Seizure disorders in pregnancy*. ACOG Educational Bulletin No. 231. Washington, DC: ACOG, 1996.

87. Sunderland S. *Nerves and nerve injuries*. Edinburgh: Churchill Livingstone, 1968.

88. Slocum HC, O'Neal KC, Allen CR. Neurovascular complications of malposition on the operating table. *Surg Gynecol Obstet* 1948;86:729.

89. Hayden CK Jr, Shattuck KE, Richardson CJ, Ahrendt DK, House R, Swischuk LE. Subependymal germinal matrix hemorrhage in full-term neonates. *Pediatrics* 1985;75:714.

90. Richardson DA, Evans MI, Cibils LP. Midforceps delivery: a critical review. *Am J Obstet Gynecol* 1983;145: 621.

91. O'Driscoll K, Meagher D, MacDonald D, Geoghegan F. Traumatic intracranial hemorrhage in first born infants and delivery with obstetric forceps. *Br J Obstet Gynecol* 1981;88:577.

92. Tejani N, Verma U, Hameed C, Chayen B. Method and route of delivery in the low birth weight vertex presentation correlated with early periventricular/intraventricular hemorrhage. *Obstet Gynecol* 1987;69:1.

93. Schwartz DB, Miodovnik M, Lavin JP Jr. Neonatal outcome among low birth weight infants delivered spontaneously or by low forceps. *Obstet Gynecol* 1983;62:283.

94. Shaver DC, Bada HS, Korones SB, Anderson GD, Wong SP, Arheart KL. Early and late intraventricular hemorrhage: the role of obstetric factors. *Obstet Gynecol* 1992;80:831.

95. Vergani P, Strobelt N, Locatelli A, et al. Clinical significance of fetal intracranial hemorrhage. *Am J Obstet Gynecol* 1996;175:536.

96. Benedetti TJ, Gabbe SG. Shoulder dystocia: a complication of fetal macrosomia and prolonged second stage of labor with midpelvic delivery. *Obstet Gynecol* 1978; 52:526.

97. Levine MG, Holroyde J, Woods JR, Siddiqi TA, Scott M, Miodovnik M. Birth trauma: incidence and predisposing factors. *Obstet Gynecol* 1984;63:792.

98. Jackson ST, Hoffer MM, Parrish N. Brachial-plexus palsy in the newborn. *J Bone Joint Surg* 1988;70:1217.

99. McCall JO. Shoulder dystocia: a study after effects. *Am J Obstet Gynecol* 1962;83:1486.

100. Spellacy WN, Miller S, Winegar A, Peterson PQ. Macrosomia, maternal characteristics and infant complications. *Obstet Gynecol* 1985;66:158.

101. McFarland LV, Raskin M, Daling JR, Benedetti TJ. Erb/Duchenne's palsy: a consequence of fetal macrosomia and method of delivery. *Obstet Gynecol* 1986; 68:784.

102. Modanlou HD, Dorchester WL, Thorosian A, Freeman RK. Macrosomia: maternal, fetal and neonatal implications. *Obstet Gynecol* 1980;55:420.

103. American College of Obstetricians and Gynecologists. *Fetal macrosomia*. ACOG Practice Bulletin No. 22. Washington, DC: ACOG, 2000.

104. Ecker JL, Greenberg JA, Norwitz ER, Nadel AS, Repke JT. Birth weight as a predictor of brachial plexus injury. *Obstet Gynecol* 1997;89:643.

105. Gordon M, Rich H, Deutschberger J, Green M. The immediate and long-term outcome of obstetric birth trauma. I: Brachial plexus paralysis. *Am J Obstet Gynecol* 1985;68:784.

106. Acker DB, Sachs BP, Friedman EA. Risk factors for shoulder dystocia. *Obstet Gynecol* 1985;66:762.

107. Boyd ME, Usher RH, McLean FH. Fetal macrosomia: prediction, risks and proposed management. *Obstet Gynecol* 1983;61:715.

108. Gabbe SG, Niebyl JR, Simpson JL. *Obstetrics: Normal and problem pregnancies*. New York, NY: Churchill Livingstone, 1986;477.

109. Hernandez C, Wendel GD. Shoulder dystocia. *Clin Obstet Gynecol* 1990;33:526.

110. Smellie W. *A collection of cases and observations in midwifery*, 4th ed. Vol. 2. London, 1768.

111. Erb W. Ueber eine eigenthümliche localisation von Lähmengen im plexus brachialis. Heidelberg: *Verhandl der Naturhist-Med*, 1874;2:130.

112. Duchenne GBA. *De l'eléctrisation localiseé at de son application à la pathologie at à la therapeutique*, 3rd ed. Paris: JB Ballière, 1872.

113. Klumpke A. Contribution á l'etude des paralysies radiculaires du plexus brachial. *Rev Med* (Paris) 1885;5:591.

114. Boome RS, Kaye JC. Obstetric traction injuries of the brachial plexus. *J Bone Joint Surg* 1988;70:571.

115. Curran JS. Birth-associated injury. *Clin Perinatol* 1981;8:111.

116. Jennett RJ, Tarby TJ, Kreinick CJ. Brachial plexus injury: an old problem revisited. *Am J Obstet Gynecol* 1992; 166:1673.

117. Rubin A. Birth injuries and incidence, mechanism and end results. *Obstet Gynecol* 1964;23:218.

118. Myers RE, Beard R, Adamsons K. Brain swelling in the newborn rhesus monkey following prolonged partial asphyxia. *Neurology* 1969;19:1012.

119. Richmond S, Niswander K, Snodgrass CA, Waystaff I. The obstetric management of fetal distress and its association with cerebral palsy. *Obstet Gynecol* 1994;83:643.

120. Thacker SB, Stroup DF, Peterson HB. Efficacy and safety of intrapartum electronic fetal monitoring: an update. *Obstet Gynecol* 1995;86:613.

121. American College of Obstetricians & Gynecologists. *Fetal distress and birth asphyxia*. ACOG Committee Opinion No. 137. Washington, DC: ACOG, 1994.

122. American Academy of Pediatrics. Use and abuse of the Apgar score. *Pediatrics* 1986;7:1148.

123. Kuban KCK, Leviton A, Pagano M, et al. Maternal toxemia is associated with reduced incidence of germinal matrix hemorrhage in premature babies. *J Clin Neurol* 1992;7:70.

124. Nelson KB, Grether JK. Can magnesium sulphate reduce the risk of cerebral palsy in very low birthweight infants? *Pediatrics* 1995;95:263.

125. Hauth JC, Goldenberg RL, Nelson KG, DuBard MB, Peralta MA, Gaudier FL. Reduction of cerebral palsy with maternal MgSO4 treatment in newborns weighing 500-1000 g. *Am J Obstet Gynecol* 1995;172:419.

126. Schendel DE, Berg CJ, Yeargin-Allsopp M, Boyle CA, Decoufle P. Prenatal magnesium sulphate exposure and the risk of cerebral palsy or mental retardation among very low-birth-weight children aged 3 to 5 years. *JAMA* 1996;276:1805.

127. Pryde PG, Besinger RE, Gianopoulos JG, Mittendorf R. Adverse and beneficial effects of tocolytic therapy. In: D'Alton ME, Gross I, Robinson JN, Norwitz ER, (eds.) *Seminars in perinatology: current concepts in the management of preterm labor* (part 2). Philadelphia, Pa: WB Saunders, 2001;25(5):316–340.

128. Spinillo A, Capuzzo E, Cavallini A, et al. Preeclampsia, preterm delivery and infant cerebral palsy. *Eur J Obstet Gynaecol Reprod Biol* 1998;77:151.

129. Mittendorf R, Pryde PG. An overview of the possible relationship between antenatal pharmacologic magnesium and cerebral palsy. *J Perinat Med* 2000;28:286.

130. The Magpie Trial Collaborative Group. Do women with pre-eclampsia, and their babies, benefit from magnesium sulphate? The Magpie Trial: a randomised placebo-controlled trial. *Lancet* 2002;359:1877.

131. Badawi N, Kurinczuk JJ, Keogh JM, et al. Intrapartum risk factors for newborn encephalopathy: the Western Australian case-control study. *Br Med J* 1998;317:1554.

132. Ellis M, Manandhar N, Manandhar DS, et al. Risk factors for newborn encephalopathy in Kathmandu, Nepal, a developing country: unmatched case-control study. *Br Med J* 2000;320:1229.

133. Adamson SJ, Alessandri LM, Badawi N, et al. Predictors of newborn encephalopathy in full-term infants. *Br Med J* 1995;311:598.

134. Dammann O, Leviton A. Maternal intrauterine infection, cytokines, and brain damage in the preterm infant. *Pediatr Res* 1997;42:1.

135. Yoon BH, Romero R, Park JS, et al. Fetal exposure to an intra-amniotic inflammation and the development of cerebral palsy at the age of three years. *Am J Obstet Gynecol* 2000;182:675.

136. Berger R, Garnier Y, Jensen A. Perinatal brain damage: underlying mechanisms and neuroprotective strategies. *J Soc Gynecol Invest* 2002;9:319.

137. Battin MR, Dezoete JA, Gunn TR, Gluckman PD, Gunn AJ. Neurodevelopmental outcome of infants treated with head cooling and mild hypothermia after perinatal asphyxia. *Pediatrics* 2001;107:480.

138. Whitelaw A, Thoresen M. Clinical trials of treatments after perinatal asphyxia. *Curr Opin Pediatr* 2002;14:664.

139. Menticoglou SM, Perlman M, Manning FA. High cervical spinal cord injury in neonates delivered with forceps: report of 15 cases. *Obstet Gynecol* 1995;86:589.

140. Fusi L, Gordon H. Twin pregnancy complicated by single intrauterine death: problems and outcome with conservative management. *Br J Obstet Gynecol* 1990;97:511.

141. Burke MS. Single fetal demise in twin gestation. *Clin Obstet Gynecol* 1990;33:69.

142. D'Alton ME, Newton ER, Cetrulo CL. Intrauterine fetal demise in multiple gestation. *Acta Gen Med Gemell* 1984;33:43.

143. Landy HJ, Weingold AB. Management of a multiple gestation complicated by an antepartum fetal demise. *Obstet Gynecol Surv* 1989;44:171.

144. American College of Obstetricians and Gynecologists. Teratology. ACOG Educational Bulletin No. 233. Washington, DC: ACOG, 1997.

145. Reece EA, Hobbins JC. Diabetic embryopathy: pathogenesis, prenatal diagnosis and prevention. *Obstet Gynecol Surv* 1986;41:325.

146. MRC Vitamin Study Research Group. Prevention of neural tube defects: results of the Medical Research Council Vitamin Study. *Lancet* 1991;338:131.

147. Czeizel AE, Dudás I. Prevention of the first occurrence of neural tube defects by periconceptional vitamin supplementation. *N Engl J Med* 1992;327:1832.

148. American College of Obstetricians and Gynecologists. *Prenatal detection of neural tube defects.* ACOG Technical Bulletin No. 99. Washington, DC: ACOG, 1986.

149. American College of Obstetricians and Gynecologists. *Alpha-fetoprotein.* ACOG Technical Bulletin No. 154. Washington, DC: ACOG, 1991.

150. New England Regional Genetics Group Prenatal Collaborative Study of Down Syndrome Screening. Combined maternal serum AFP and age to screen in pregnant women under age 35. *Am J Obstet Gynecol* 1989;160:575.

151. Wald NJ, Cuckle HS, Densem JW, et al. Maternal serum unconjugated oesteriol as an antenatal screening test for Down syndrome. *Br J Obstet Gynaecol* 1988;95:334.

152. MacDonald ML, Wagner RM, Slotnick RN. Sensitivity and specificity of screening for Down syndrome with alphafetoprotein, HCG, unconjugated estriol, and maternal age. *Obstet Gynecol* 1991;77:63.

153. Prenatal diagnosis and invasive techniques to monitor the fetus. In: Cunningham FG, MacDonald PC, Leveno KJ, Gant NF, Gilstrap LC III, (eds.) *Williams obstetrics.* 19th ed. Stamford, Ct: Appleton & Lange, 1993; 939–957.

154. American College of Obstetricians and Gynecologists. *Prenatal diagnosis of fetal chromosomal abnormalities.* ACOG Practice Bulletin No. 27. Washington, DC: ACOG, 2001.

155. Aitken DA, Wallace EM, Crossley JA, et al. Dimeric inhibin A as a marker for Down syndrome in early pregnancy. *N Engl J Med* 1996;334:1231.

156. Wald NJ, Huttly WJ, Hackshaw AK. Antenatal screening for Down's syndrome with the quadruple test. *Lancet* 2003;361:835-836.

157. Benn PA, Fang M, Egan JF, et al. Incorporation of inhibin-A in second-trimester screening for Down syndrome. *Obstet Gynecol* 2003;101:451-454

158. American College of Obstetricians and Gynecologists. *Maternal serum screening.* ACOG Educational Bulletin No. 228. Washington, DC: ACOG, 1996.

159. Haddow JE, Palomaki GE, Knight GJ, Williams J, Miller WA, Johnson A. Screening of maternal serum for fetal Down syndrome in the first trimester. *N Engl J Med* 1998;338:955.

160. Wald NJ, Kennard A, Hackshaw A, McGuire A. Antenatal screening for Down syndrome. *Health Technol Assess* 1998;2:1.

161. Hafner E, Schuchter K, Leibhart E, Philipp K. Results of routine fetal nuchal translucency measurement at weeks 10–13 in 4233 unselected pregnant women. *Prenat Diagn* 1998;18:29.

162. Russell WL. Effect of the interval between irradiation and conception on mutation frequency in female mice. *Proc Natl Acad Sci USA* 1965;54:1552.

163. Brent RL. Clinicial teratology counseling and consultation case report: exposure to diagnostic radiation early in pregnancy. *Teratology* 1992;46:31.

164. Dekaban AS. Abnormalities in children exposed to x-radiation during various stages of gestation: tentative timetable of radiation injury to the human fetus. *J Nucl Med* 1968;9:471.

165. MacMahon X. Prenatal x-ray exposure and childhood cancer. *J Natl Cancer Inst* 1962;28:1173.

166. Bithell J, Stewart A. Prenatal irradiation and childhood malignancy: a review of British data from Oxford survey. *Br J Cancer* 1975;31:271.

167. Schwartz JL, Crooks LE. NMR imaging produces no observable mutations or cytotoxicity in mammalian cells. *Am J Radiol* 1982;139:5.

168. Stark DD, McCarthy SM, Filly RA, Parer JT, Hricak H, Callen PW. Pelvimetry by magnetic resonance imaging. *Am J Radiol* 1985;144:947.

12 The Menopausal Transition: Changing Physiology, Symptoms, and Hormone Therapy

Nancy Fugate Woods, PhD, RN

As the Baby Boomer cohort of women began experiencing the transition to menopause,they demanded increasing attention to menopause, itself, and to the health consequences associated with menopause. Although the science of menopause lags far behind women's and clinicians' need for accurate information, recently published studies begin to fill the void in our knowledge about this important portion of the lifespan. This chapter considers:

- The menopausal transition and related endocrine changes
- Changing physiology following menopause
- Implications of the menopausal transition for symptoms and diseases of advanced age
- Therapies for symptom management and prevention of diseases of advanced age

MENOPAUSAL TRANSITION: A MULTISTAGE PROCESS

Serious attention of researchers to understanding the transition to menopause as part of women's developmental trajectory is relatively recent. In 1991, the National Institute on Aging convened a workshop of clinicians and researchers to develop a system for staging reproductive aging, analogous to that for staging puberty, that could be incorporated into clinical research as well as practice. The purposes of the staging system are to standardize research and practice with respect to the nomenclature used to describe the menopausal transition; allow researchers and clinicians to compare results across studies; and help clinicians and women themselves assess their progression through the transition to menopause (1).

As seen in Figure 12.1, menopause is defined as the cessation of menses and is marked by a woman's last menstrual period, which anchors the stages. Looking back in time from the final menstrual period, the menopausal transition occurs prior to the menopause and includes two stages, early and late transition. The early menopausal transition stage (−2) is characterized by increased variability in menstrual cycle length that exceeds a difference of 7 days from cycle to cycle. The late stage of the menopausal transition (−1) is characterized by skipping of menses, in which the typical menstrual cycle length is doubled or longer. Prior to the menopausal transition, the late reproductive stage (−3) is characterized by rising FSH levels and shortening of menstrual cycle length. Moving forward in time from the final menstrual period, early postmenopause (+1) encompasses the first 5 years after the final menstrual period, and the late postmenopause (+2) extends throughout the remainder of the lifespan. The perimenopause encompasses the early and late menopausal transition and 1 year postmenopause.

					Final Menstrual Period (FMP)		
Stages	–5	–4	–3	–2	–1	0 ▼	+1	+2
Terminology	Reproductive			Menopausal Transition			Postmenopause	
	Early	Peak	Late	Early	Late*		Early*	Late
				Perimenopause				
Duration of Stage	Variable			Variable		1 Year	4 Years	Until demise
Menstrual Cycles	Variable to Regular	Regular — Length Decreases ~2 Days		Variable Cycle Length (>7 Days Different from Normal)	Intervals of Amenorrhea (>4 Days)		None	
Endocrine	Normal FSH		↑FSH	↑FSH			↑FSH	

FIGURE 12.1

Proposed staging system and revised nomenclature.

During the menopausal transition, women also frequently report spotting (bloody discharge that does not require use of a napkin or tampon) before, after, and between episodes of menstrual bleeding, and longer and heavier episodes of bleeding (menorrhagia or flooding) that may cause them to seek health care (2).

The transition to menopause, as estimated from U.S. women's menstrual bleeding patterns recorded daily on menstrual calendars, has been timed to occur during the mid-forties, at a median age of 45.5 years for a population of Midwestern white women (3) and 47.5 years as reported in telephone interviews by participants in the Massachusetts Women's Health Study (MWHS) (4). The duration of the menopausal transition averages 4 years, but varies widely, with a range of 2 to 7 years and a median of 4.5 years in the Minnesota (3) and 3.5 years in the MWHS samples (4).

The Study of Women across the Nation (SWAN) is a multisite longitudinal study of a multiethnic population of U.S. women as they make the transition to menopause. SWAN is designed to characterize the physical and psychosocial changes that occur around the time of the menopausal transition and to observe their effects on later risk factors for age-related diseases and health (5). Over 16,000 women between the ages of 40 and 55 years were screened from 1995–1997, and subsequently 3,302 women 42 to 52 years of age were enrolled in a longitudinal cohort studied through annual visits and other data collection efforts for 6 years of follow-up. Of these, 900 women are participating in a daily hormone study. The data being collected in SWAN include ovarian markers, lifestyle and behavior indicators, and markers of cardiovascular and bone health. SWAN, as well as other longitudinal studies such as the Seattle Midlife Women's Health Study and the Melbourne Women's Health Project (6,7) will elucidate features of the menopausal transition stages (5).

Altered Hypothalamic-Pituitary-Ovarian Function during the Menopausal Transition

Changing cycle regularity patterns are indicators of menopausal transition; these changes result from a logarithmic decrease in the number of ovarian follicles as women age. Comparing women aged 45 to 55 years who were menstruating regularly with women having irregular cycles and postmenopausal women, Richardson found that follicle counts decreased dramatically among the groups, and were nearly absent in the postmenopausal group (8).

In addition to changes in bleeding patterns and cycle regularity, elevated gonadotropins are commonly used indicators of changing ovarian function associated with the transition to menopause. Sustained increases of follicle stimulating hormone (FSH) occur on average 5 to 6 years and luteinizing hormone (LH) 3 to 4 years before the last period (9,10). Elevated gonadotropins have been attributed to both ovarian aging (loss of follicles and therefore reduced estrogen and the reduction in inhibin levels that provide negative feedback to FSH) and central regulation aging (decrease in sensitivity to feedback at the hypothalamus and/or pituitary). Klein and colleagues (11) found that accelerated follicular development was asso-

TABLE 12.1

Ranges of Hormonal Values from Daily First Voided Urine Samples: Comparison of Younger Menstruating, Perimenopausal, and Postmenopausal Women*

ENDOCRINE LEVELS	YOUNGER MENSTRUATING WOMEN 19–38 YEARS OLD (N=11)	PERIMENOPAUSAL WOMEN, CYCLING, 47 YEARS AND OLD (N=11)	POSTMENOPAUSAL WOMEN 50 YEARS AND OLDER (N=5)
Estrone – mean ng/mgCr	23–60	13–135	3–6
Estrone – peak ng/mgCr	58–237	47–278	—
Pregnanediol µg/mgCr	1.6–12.7	1.0–8.4	—
FSH – mean mIU/mgCr	3–7	4–32	24–85
LH – mean mIU/mgCr	1.1–4.2	1.4–6.8	4.3–14.8

*From Santoro et al, 1996 (13).

ciated with a monotropic rise in FSH in women between 40 and 45 years who were still cycling. As women near the end of regular ovulation, their estradiol levels obtained during the early follicular phases are higher and their estradiol levels rise earlier in the follicular phase than those measured among younger women. As reproductive age advances, progesterone levels diminish.

Inhibin B levels, but not inhibin A, fall in perimenopausal women as FSH levels rise (12). The dramatic increases in FSH may be responsible for elevated levels of estrogens during the later phase of the menopausal transition, producing periods of hyperestrogenism (13).

In a longitudinal study of endocrine changes during the perimenopause, Rannevik and associates (14) measured FSH, LH, estrogens, progesterone, testosterone, and androstenedione every 6 months, over a 12-year period from premenopause to postmenopause, in 152 women. Their findings yielded estimates based on variable numbers of observations (24 to 152) and indicated that the ratio between estrone and estradiol increased, reflecting the declining follicular steroidogenesis. A marked decrease in estrogen (particularly estradiol) and progesterone levels occurred during the 6-month period around the menopause. Both estrone and estradiol levels decreased slowly following menopause. Also testosterone and androstenedione levels decreased around the menopause.

Women produce androgens in the ovary and adrenal cortex. Using radio-labeled steroids, Longcope and Johnston (15) measured metabolic clearance rates, the interconversions of androgens to estrogens, and the peripheral aromatization of androgens. When measured twice at 2-year intervals in the same midlife women (n=54), no differences were found in metabolic clearance for testosterone, androstenedione, estrone, and estradiol for women regardless of their menopausal status. The conversion of estrone to estradiol decreased in women who continued to menstruate over the 2-year period (n=15). The peripheral aromatization of androstenedione to estrone increased in all women regardless of their menopausal status (menstruating to menopausal, and menopausal at both occasions). These findings suggest that metabolic changes occur prior to menopause, resulting in a lower production of estradiol with increasing production of estrone.

The adrenal gland secretes a number of androgen precursors, such as dehydroepiandrosterone sulfate (DHEAS) and dehydroepiandrosterone (DHEA), androstenedione, and testosterone (16).

Data from the Melbourne Women's Health Project, a longitudinal study of an Australian cohort of women followed across the menopausal transition, revealed no significant changes in total testosterone in relation to changes in menopausal status (17). The free androgen index [testosterone: sex hormone binding globulin ratio (SHBG) ratio] increased by 80% from measures 4 years prior to menopause to 2 years after menopause due to a decrease in SHBG levels across the period. DHEAS levels declined gradually with age, but did not change in relation to the final menstrual period in this cohort. However, DHEAS levels rose transiently in the late perimenopause in the SWAN cohort (18).

Because of the marked fluctuations in endocrine levels during the menopausal transition, single measurements of FSH or estradiol are not likely to be useful as indicators of the menopausal transition. To date, menstrual calendar data remain the most accurate basis for staging the menopause transition.

THE MENOPAUSE TRANSITION AS A TIME OF REREGULATION

Although some authors have emphasized the disregulation of the hypothalamic-pituitary-ovarian (HPO) axis functions occurring with the menopausal transition, it is useful to consider this period as a time of reregulation of endocrine function. With the cessation of ovulation, the ovary produces lower levels of estradiol as the ovarian follicles are diminished, but this is punctuated by higher levels of estradiol in response to increasing levels of FSH. There is disagreement in the literature about the ovarian production of testosterone and androstenedione during the transition to menopause. A compensatory increase in the peripheral aromatization of the androgens androstenedione to estrone and testosterone to estradiol may occur during the perimenopausal period, thus supporting reregulation of the HPO axis to a new pattern not dependent on the ovarian production of higher levels of estrogen.

Physiologic Consequences of Menopause

Given the widespread physiologic effects of estrogens, progesterone, and androgens, compensatory changes in their production necessitate reregulation of the HPO axis and produce changes in physiologic functioning. In their extreme form, some of these changes may be associated with pathology. The physiologic effects of estrogen and progesterone seen in menstruating women change over the course of the menopausal transition as estradiol production diminishes, progesterone production linked to ovulation ceases, testosterone and androstenedione levels fluctuate, and the proportion of estrone to estradiol increases.

Estrogens and progesterone each have physiologic effects on an array of functions, including those of the uterus, fallopian tubes, vagina, and breast tissue. In addition, gonadal steroids influence bone, lipid, carbohydrate, and protein metabolism. Both alpha and beta receptors for estrogen and progesterone mediate hormonal effects. The cell types in which each type of receptor is functional have not been clearly demonstrated (19). Some estrogenic effects are mediated by effects on hepatic protein secretion. In addition, estrogen and progesterone have widespread effects on bone, adipose tissue, and muscle; on blood clotting, blood pressure, electrolytes, and respiration; and on nervous system and immune system functions, as outlined in Table 12.2.

Contemporary concerns related to the diminished levels of estrogen following menopause focus on changing physiology that may be linked to pathology in some women. To date, extensive research has been conducted on the effects of hormone therapy on bone, body composition, cardiovascular system, lipid metabolism, hemostasis, blood pressure, central and autonomic nervous system activity, and uterine and breast tissue.

Concern about osteoporosis has prompted some to link the decreased production of estrogen after menopause to changes in bone density. Evidence suggests that women with higher estrone and estradiol levels have greater bone density. Moreover, women who have a higher body mass index (BMI) have greater bone mass density (BMD). They may also produce higher postmenopausal levels of estrone and estradiol through aromatization (22). Studies of the SWAN cohort revealed that bone density varies across ethnic groups of women, with highest BMD levels among African American women and lowest in Caucasians (23). Serum FSH, but not serum estradiol, testosterone, or SHBG were significantly associated with BMD in this population (24).

The *metabolic syndrome* (also known as *insulin resistance syndrome* or *syndrome X*) is a clustering of metabolic abnormalities consisting of glucose intolerance, high blood pressure, high triglyceride levels, high LDL levels, hyperuricemia, adiposity, and insulin resistance. Many aspects of this syndrome are being studied as they appear or intensify with the transition to menopause.

Weight gain is a concern to most U.S. women, and during the menopausal transition, women in the Healthy Women Study experienced an average weight gain of 5 pounds. Nearly 20% gained 10 or more pounds (25). Women in the SWAN cohort reported similar weight gains, adjusted for height regardless of whether they had experienced natural menopause or were premenopausal. Those who had a hysterectomy were heavier, and those using hormone therapy were lighter than their counterparts. Physical activity and ethnicity had greater effects on weight than menopausal status or hormone use (26). Whether weight gain is due to changing ovarian function, aging, lifestyle factors, or to a combination of these has yet to be determined. Whether there is a change in body fat distribution (e.g., an increase in intra-abdominal fat) is known (27). Postmenopausal women with higher BMI produce higher levels of estrone and estradiol (28). Therefore, understanding the metabolic changes during the natural menopausal transition may provide an important key to disease prevention efforts.

Rising blood insulin levels during the transition to menopause appear to be related to weight gain and to changes in the distribution of body fat. An increase in waist circumference and upper body fat occurs during the transition (25,27). Levels of blood insulin are highest in women with both a higher BMI and increased upper body fat (27).

Substantial increases in LDL-C levels occur among women from the pre- to postmenopausal period, but no effects are apparent on estrogen or testosterone levels and HDL-C either early or late in the menopausal transition (29). In studies of women making the transition to postmenopause, only women with dramatic changes in estradiol levels also had changes in LDL and HDL-C (22). Although the dietary intake of fats and genotype influence risk of heart disease, data about changes in these factors over the menopausal transition are incomplete. The Healthy Women Study results indicated that lipoprotein

TABLE 12.2
*Comparison of Physiologic Effects of Estrogen and Progesterone**

PHYSIOLOGIC EFFECTS	ESTROGEN	PROGESTERONE
Effects on Sexual Organs		
Uterus	• Proliferation of endometrium	• Stimulates development of secretory endometrium
	• Contractile activities of myometrium	• Maintains placental implantation
	• Upregulates uterine progesterone receptor	• Relaxes smooth muscle
	• Enhances vascularity of cervix	• Downregulates progesterone receptor
	• Secretion of cervical mucus, clear, thin, spinbarkheit	
Fallopian tubes	• Promotes normal contractile activities	• Relaxes smooth muscle
Vagina	• Proliferation of epithelium with glycogen deposition in superficial cells	
Breast	• Promotes breast development and maintenance, especially ductal system	• Stimulates lobulo-alveolar growth along with estrogen
	• Increases breast mass	
Effects on Metabolism		
Liver function	• Increased hepatic protein secretion (including lipoproteins, clotting factors, renin substrate, and binding proteins)	
	• Increased binding proteins, including: sex hormone binding globulin, corticosteroid binding globulin, thyroxin-binding globulin, growth hormone binding proteins, and ceruloplasmin	
	• Excretory capacity for BSP, bilirubin, bile salts	
	• Changes in serum transaminase, alkaline phosphatase	
Lipids	• Increases secretion of lipoproteins, VLDL, LDL, and HDL	• Diminishes secretion of certain hepatic proteins, VLDL, HDL
	• Decreases serum cholesterol	
	• Increases phospholipids	
Carbohydrates	• Increased insulin secretion	• Diminishes insulin action, produces insulin resistance
	• Decreases blood sugar	
	• Decreases glucose tolerance	
Proteins	• Increases hepatic protein secretion:	• Enhances nitrogen wasting
	• Lipoproteins, VLDL, LDL, HDL	
	• Increases thyroxin and cortisol binding globulin	
	• Increases copper and iron binding plasma proteins	
	• Changes tryptophan metabolism	
Bone	• Inhibition of bone resorption	
General Physiologic Effects		
Respiration	• Decreases metabolic rate	• Enhances hypothalamic respiratory center, stimulates respiration
Blood clotting	• Increases clotting factors, I, II, VI, VII, VIII, IX, X	
	• Accelerates platelet aggregation	

(continued)

TABLE 12.2

Comparison of Physiologic Effects of Estrogen and Progesterone* (Continued)

PHYSIOLOGIC EFFECTS	ESTROGEN	PROGESTERONE
Blood pressure and electrolytes	• Increases renin substrate (angiotensinogen) and renin activity • Increases aldosterone, sodium retention • Elevates blood pressure	• Increases sodium excretion by kidney, decreases proximal tubular absorption • Lowers blood pressure by relaxing arterioles
Adipose tissue	• Increases adipose tissue mass	• Enhances fat breakdown
Muscle		• Relaxes smooth muscle of the gut and arterioles
Endocrines	• Stimulates pituitary secretion of prolactin • Increases serum growth hormone	
Nervous system	• Excites neurons	• Sedates neurons
Immune system	• Modulates immune response • Estrogen receptors on T-lymphocytes, inhibits cell-mediated immunity in some T lymphocytes, e.g., low E_2 stimulates, CD8+ suppressor, hi E_2 inhibits CD4+ helper cells • Cytokines and growth factors: low E_2 stimulates interleukin-1 (along with low P4) E_2 inhibits interleukin-1 production and TNFα	

• Data are from Dyrenfurth (20) and Patton et al. (21).
• E_2 = Estradiol
• P4 = Progesterone
• TNFα = Tumor Necrosis Factor
• HDL = High-Density Lipoprotein
• LDL = Low-Density Lipoprotein
• VLDL = Very Low-Density Lipoprotein
• BSP = Bromsulphalein

(a) levels [LP(a)] increase after menopause (30). Relatively little change in HDL-C levels occurs during the transition to menopause (31). Obesity and fat distribution, physical activity, cigarette smoking, and alcohol intake influenced HDL-C and its changes during the menopausal transition (32). Changes in hemostatic factors are of concern due to their relationship to heart disease. Among participants in the Healthy Women Study, factor VIIc and fibrinogen levels increased across the menopausal transition (33). The ongoing SWAN study will provide data on the cardiovascular changes (lipids, blood pressure, insulin resistance, clotting changes) occurring as women experience early and late stages of the menopausal transition and reach postmenopause.

Changes in blood pressure are of concern due to their relationship to stroke. Little evidence supports an effect of menopause on blood pressure. Attention to the specific effects of estrogen on the arterial wall (e.g., stiffness), is one focus of the ongoing SWAN study.

The effects of menopause on cognitive function are of interest owing to concern about dementia in aged

women, particularly dementia of the Alzheimer's type. (Please also see Chapter 30.) To date, no longitudinal studies have tracked changes in cognition across the menopause transition. One component of the ongoing SWAN study will focus on cognitive changes across the transition to menopause using measures of verbal memory, working memory, and cognitive processing speed.

Evidence suggests that estrogen has excitatory effects on the brain and progesterone has the opposite effect, diminishing human cortical excitability (33,34). Little is known about the effects of testosterone on neuronal excitability in women. Animal studies demonstrate changes in synaptic and dendritic plasticity, with development of, and loss of, apical dendritic spine density in the CAI hypocampal area and ventrimedial hypothalamus over the course of the estrus cycle (also see Chapter 6. These changes are mediated by estrogen in the presence of progesterone (34). Sherwin (35) cites evidence that estrogen can affect mood by means of: i) reducing monoamine oxidase (MAO) levels, which leads to increased serotonin (5HT) levels, ii) displacing tryptophan, a precursor of 5HT, from binding sites to plasma albumin, iii) increasing levels of choline acetyl transferase and reducing choline acetyl transferase associated with impaired memory in rats, and iv) enhancing central norepenephrine availability, sensitizing dopamine receptors, and reducing alpha-adrenergic receptors in rat cortex. Whether the natural menopausal transition produces clinically significant changes in cognitive function in humans remains to be determined.

Changes in autonomic nervous system function across the menopausal transition have begun to be investigated. To date, investigators have demonstrated differences in stress response when comparing premenopausal and postmenopausal women. Postmenopausal women exhibited greater increases in heart rate during all laboratory stressors when compared to premenopausal women, with a pronounced increase during a speech task stressor deemed to be socially relevant to middle-aged women. Postmenopausal women exhibited greater increases in systolic blood pressure and epinephrine during the speech task, but not in response to other stressors (36). Subsequent experiments confirmed this effect and demonstrated that women receiving estrogen therapy had an attenuated stress response (37).

Concerns about changes in the immune response are of interest owing to the greater prevalence of autoimmune diseases among women compared with men. Among these are thyroid disease, lupus erythematosus, scleroderma, and rheumatoid arthritis. The role of estrogen changes in menopause and immune response is not yet clear. Evidence suggests that estradiol can modulate immune response via estrogen receptors on T lymphocytes and by modulating cytokines and growth factors (38–40). To date, no studies document the effects of menopausal transition on immune function.

Breast cancer increases in prevalence as women age. Postmenopausal obesity is associated with breast cancer, and obesity is associated with higher blood estrogen levels (41). Understanding how changes in body weight, dietary intake, and estrogen levels are related to breast cancer incidence is needed. Following menopause, breast tissue becomes less dense.

Symptoms during the Menopausal Transition

The most prevalent symptoms during the menopausal transition are vasomotor symptoms (hot flashes and sweats). Between 23 and 38% of U.S. and Canadian women experience hot flashes and sweats during the transition to menopause (2,4). In addition, midlife women experience depressed moods, somatic, neuromuscular, and insomnia symptoms that are not exclusive to menopausal transition (42–44). Dysphoric mood and neuromuscular and insomnia symptoms were stable over 3 years in a predominantly premenopausal sample,

whereas vasomotor and somatic symptoms varied across time (43). Vaginal dryness occurs in some women following menopause and is related to thinning of the estrogen-dependent vaginal tissue. Some women may experience post-coital spotting or painful intercourse, which can be prevented with a water-soluble lubricant.

Some evidence suggests that menopausal symptoms are a culture-bound phenomenon, with women from cultures not influenced by Western medicine reporting few symptoms or different symptoms (44). For example, Lock's work (45) with Japanese women revealed that their most frequently reported symptom was shoulder pain, not hot flashes. Moreover, the infrequent reporting of hot flashes by Japanese women may be attributable to the high phytoestrogen content of their diets.

Findings from the SWAN study revealed no universal menopause syndrome consisting of a variety of vasomotor and psychologic symptoms. Instead, perimenopausal women, hormone users, and women who had surgical menopause reported more vasomotor symptoms but no more psychologic symptoms than their counterparts. Caucasian women reported more psychomatic symptoms than other ethnic groups, and African-American women reported more vasomotor symptoms than other ethnic groups of women. These findings suggest that observations of a "menopausal syndrome" of vasomotor and psychologic symptoms are largely confined to women seeking care in menopause clinics or consulting health care providers for distressing symptoms (46). Nonetheless, for some women, the menopausal transition may precipitate severe distress. Studies of women attending menopause clinics reveal a high frequency of symptom-related visits. In a California study, 79% of visits by perimenopausal women were for physical symptoms such as vasomotor symptoms and 63% were for depression (47).

Longitudinal studies of symptoms and their endocrine correlates have been published recently. Matthews and associates (48) found that women who developed hot flashes had lower estradiol levels than those without hot flashes, but Rannevik and associates (14) found no correlation between estradiol and vasomotor symptoms or psychic symptoms. These inconsistent findings may be attributable to reliance on single measures of endocrine levels (estrogen) in cross-sectional studies or measures repeated at infrequent intervals in longitudinal studies that fail to capture a changing trajectory and thus produce unreliable estimates. The results of longitudinal studies of menopause suggest that the rate of change in ovarian hormone levels may be an important factor in symptom distress. Women in the Massachusetts Women's Health Study who had a shorter menopausal transition (transition from premenopause to postmenopause occurred over fewer months) were more likely to experience hot flashes than those with a longer menopausal transition (4), but women who had a longer menopausal transition and who had more severe vasomotor symptoms were more likely to experience depressed mood during the transition and after menopause (44). Rannevik and associates (14) did find that women who experienced a greater drop in estradiol around the time of menopause were more likely to have more vasomotor symptoms, but the symptom measures in this study were measured once in an initial interview during 1977–1978 and not assessed regularly throughout the study. Thus, the temporal link between hormone levels and symptoms during the menopausal transition is difficult to interpret. Data from the Massachusetts Women's Health Study indicate that both lower estrone and estradiol levels were correlated with women's experiences of hot flashes (15).

Studies of psychologic symptoms during the transition to menopause indicate a possible transient increase in symptoms, but the endocrine effects on mood are less clear. Early findings from the Massachusetts Women's Health Study suggested that if menopause were related to depression, the period of vulnerability would occur during the transition to menopause, especially when it was prolonged. Women experiencing long transitions to menopause (greater than 27 months) were at greater risk of depression than those having short transitions, and the relationship seemed to be explained by increased menstrual symptoms. In subsequent analyses, the prevalence of depressed mood (CES-D scores higher than 16) was slightly greater in the phase during which women were skipping periods than in the premenopause or postmenopause (49). Data from the Melbourne Women's Health Study (50) demonstrated no relationship between menopausal status and negative affect when stress, health status, premenstrual syndrome (PMS) history, marital, and lifestyle variables were controlled. They did find a slightly higher negative affect in the early and late transition (perimenopause in their terminology) and 1 to 2 years postmenopause when compared with premenopause. For women who were 2 or more years postmenopausal, the negative affect scores were not significantly different from the women in premenopause. These analyses suggest that if there is a change in the prevalence of dysphoric mood across the transition, it is likely to be transient. The Southeast England Study also revealed a higher incidence of depressed mood in a group of women who had changed to perimenopause or postmenopause from an earlier stage. In addition, vasomotor symptoms were related to the higher depression scores (51). Analyses of CES-D data from the Manitoba Women's Health Study did not support an increased prevalence of depressed mood during this phase of the transition to menopause (52). Likewise, the Seattle Midlife Women's Health Study data did not reflect a menopause-related change in patterns of depressed mood over a period as long as 10 years in some women (53).

In several studies of depressed or dysphoric mood, minimal evidence associated endocrine changes or endocrine levels with depressed mood. Rannevik and associates (14) found no correlation between estradiol and psychic symptoms. The results of longitudinal studies of menopause suggest that the rate of change in ovarian hormone levels, not merely the level, may be an important factor in symptom distress. Rannevik and associates (14) did find that women who experienced a greater drop in estradiol around the time of menopause were not more likely to have dysphoric mood or depression.

Participants (n=309) in the Massachusetts Women's Health Study who provided data about depressed mood, estradiol levels, and other factors over three occasions 9 months apart did not provide evidence of an association between depressed mood and menopause transition stage or with the annual change in estradiol levels. Although the unadjusted association between estradiol levels and CES-D scores was negative and statistically significant, when the adjustment was made for symptoms, the association was not statistically significant. Instead, hot flushes, night sweats, and trouble sleeping were each positively associated with the CES-D scores. The results of this study provided strong support for the domino hypothesis, which posits that depressed mood is caused by vasomotor symptoms and sleep problems associated with changing estrogen levels. This study adds to the body of literature suggesting that any association found between menopause and depression is most likely to be explained by other factors, such as vasomotor symptoms and sleep problems. Findings also highlight the importance of studying the complex relationship between hormone levels, sleep problems, and vasomotor symptoms during the menopausal transition (49).

In the recently reported SWAN cohort data, a higher rate of psychologic distress was reported (feeling tense, depressed, and irritable in the previous 2 weeks) among women in the early transition stage when compared with women who were premenopausal or postmenopausal (54). Whether this pattern persists as more women make the transition to the late menopause transition stage and postmenopause remains to be seen.

Little information exists about the relationship between symptoms and endogenous androgen (ovarian and adrenal) levels during the menopausal transition. There are current studies of androgen therapy for low sexual desire (55).

Studies of women with PMS link androgens (testosterone and DHA) to irritability and other dysphoric mood symptoms (56), and postmenopausal women treated with more androgenic progestins [as part of hormone replacement therapy (HRT)] experience more dysphoric mood symptoms (57). Androgen is currently prescribed for women with low sexual desire, but data are limited about its clinical effectiveness and long-term risks.

Given the association of stress with symptoms, a reasonable explanation for symptoms, particularly dysphoric mood symptoms, could be found in the stressful nature of some women's lives. Longitudinal studies revealed that women exposed to more stressful events in their lives were those most likely to experience subsequent dysphoric mood and vasomotor symptoms (45,51,52,58,59). Women with the most negative attitudes toward menopause and aging reported the most perceived stress and most severe vasomotor and dysphoric mood symptoms during subsequent years of follow-up (58–60). What remains to be determined is whether perceived stress is related to symptoms through the physiologic mechanisms of stress arousal and/or through altered ovarian function during the menopausal transition.

The relationship of physiologic stress arousal to symptoms during the menopausal transition has been rarely addressed in the literature. Ballinger (61) found that chronically stressed women seeking health care had lower estradiol and cortisol levels than less stressed women. She attributed the lower cortisol levels to the fact that women had sought health care for their problems and were coping with them. Alternatively, women who were highly stressed could have reached the phase of exhaustion in which cortisol levels actually declined. Also, measures may have been obtained at different times of day, thus introducing the effects of diurnal variation. Although exposure to stressors that provoke high levels of stress hormones like cortisol (including starvation, novel environments, and intense physical activity) can induce or interfere with ovulation (62–64), we do not know the consequences of physiologic stress arousal on ovarian function and symptoms among women during the menopausal transition.

Longitudinal studies of midlife women demonstrated that those with diagnosed chronic illnesses were at increased risk of depression (4,52). Midlife women with chronic conditions who rate their health as fair or poor have more perceived stress and dysphoric mood (59).

Symptoms not related to the menopausal transition, but relevant to women with neurologic problems include headache, seizures, cognition, and autoimmune changes affecting the nervous system. For particular changes in the clinical expression of these entities, please refer to the relevant chapters.

HORMONE THERAPY FOR SYMPTOM MANAGEMENT

Symptom management refers to women's attempts to relieve symptoms by initiating self-care and practicing health-related behaviors as well as by using health services and prescriptives from health professionals. Few investigators have collected data about women's attempts at self-treatment. A recent national survey sponsored by the North American Menopause Society revealed that women tried exercise, nutritional modification, vitamin supplementation, relaxation, and alteration of mental attitude to manage their symptoms (64). Despite women's apparent reluctance to use HRT for long periods, no data indicate the strategies women use for varying types of symptoms.

Health behaviors also affect HPO axis-hormones and may accelerate the rate of change in ovarian hormones over the menopausal transition and, in turn, increase symptom distress. Smoking has been associated with earlier menopause and thus lower estrogen levels (4). Single measures of endogenous hormones in serum and the dietary intake of alcohol, fats, fiber, and caffeine among 325 healthy Massachusetts women aged 50 to 60 who had menstruated within the past 12 months revealed that caffeine was inversely related to estradiol and positively correlated with SHBG (65). In experimental studies manipulating dietary intake in premenopausal women, alcohol consumption was associated with increased total estrogen levels (66), and dietary fiber and fat had individual and joint effects on estrogen concentrations. When diet was changed to low fat (20–25% of calories as fat) and high fiber (40 g/day) significant decreases occurred in serum concentrations of estrone, estrone sulfate, testosterone, androstenedione, and SHBG, with a trend toward significant decreases in estradiol. High fiber alone produced a drop in estradiol and SHBG, whereas fat and fiber together caused a decrease in estrone sulfate. Dietary fat independently influenced androstenedione levels. Increased fiber caused a lengthening of the menstrual cycle by nearly 1 day and a lengthening of the follicular phase (67). Exercise has been shown to be associated with lower hot flash frequency (68) and to have a positive effect on mood in some studies (69).

Overall fat accumulation increases with age and with menopause for women (25). Because adipose tissue can aromatize steroids for the synthesis of estrogen, fat accumulation may reduce symptoms in women for whom ovarian estradiol production is declining but also may increase endometrial hyperplasia and associated bleeding. Dual-energy, x-ray absorptiometry revealed that postmenopausal women have greater total fat mass, trunk mass, and proportion of android fat than premenopausal women (70). Increased waist:hip ratio, a more specific indicator of android fat deposition than BMI, has been associated with increased androgenic hormone profiles (71) and with elevated cortisol (72) in postmenopausal women.

Prospective studies show that midlife women use health services for multiple purposes, often combining visits for prevention and screening with symptom management (73). In addition, midlife women are likely to seek health care for bleeding problems associated with the perimenopause (2). The use of hormone therapy for menopausal symptoms and prevention is of increasing interest to health professionals and policy-makers as the proportion of the population in middle-age increases, reflecting the large number of baby-boomers.

Prevention of Diseases of Advanced Age

Estrogen (E) was first approved for use by post-menopausal women during the 1940s, but the prevalence of estrogen use did not increase substantially until the 1960s, when clinicians prescribed it for relief of menopausal hot flashes and urogenital symptoms. During the early 1970s, evidence of an increased incidence of endometrial cancer associated with estrogen therapy and worries about possible associations with increased risk of vascular disease (as had occurred with the use of oral contraceptives) led to a decrease in prescription of estrogen therapy (74). In the 1980s, clinicians added a progestin (P) to prescriptions of estrogen therapy to reduce the risk of endometrial cancer (75). In 1986, the Food and Drug Association (FDA) approved the use of postmenopausal estrogen for the prevention and management of osteoporosis based on evidence supporting the effectiveness of estrogen in reducing hip and vertebral fractures (76). Evidence linking the use of estrogen therapy to a reduction in the incidence of heart disease has introduced yet another indication for hormone therapy: the prevention of heart disease by use of estrogen or estrogen/progestin (E + P) therapy (77).

Despite the promise of new evidence for the protective effects of estrogen and combined hormone therapy, caution pervaded the discussion of recommendations for its use. In 1992, the American College of Physicians (ACP) advocated careful and separate consideration of the benefits of the short-term use of hormone therapy for managing menopausal symptoms and disease prevention in their "Guidelines for Counseling Postmenopausal Women about Preventive Hormone Therapy" (78). The ACP advised a limited course of therapy (1 to 5 years) for women seeking relief from symptoms such as hot flashes associated with menopause and recommended that women of all races should consider carefully using preventive hormone therapy. At that time, they advised that those women who had had a hysterectomy would be likely to benefit from estrogen therapy and have no need for combined hormone therapy (estrogen and a progestin). Based on retrospective studies of coronary heart disease, the ACP recommended that women who had coronary heart disease or who were at increased risk of coronary heart disease would be likely to benefit from hormone therapy and should receive combined therapy if they had a uterus, unless careful endometrial monitoring was performed (e.g., endometrial biopsies, aspirations). Women without a uterus could be treated with estrogen

only. The ACP cautioned that risks of hormone therapy may outweigh benefits for women at increased risk of breast cancer. Similar counsel has been offered by the U.S. Preventive Services Task Force (79), which concluded that there was insufficient evidence to recommend for or against hormone therapies for all women.

Over the past decade, three large NIH-sponsored clinical trials, the Postmenopausal Estrogen and Progestin Intervention (PEPI) study, the Heart and Estrogen/Progestin Replacement Study (HERS), and the Women's Health Initiative (WHI) Trial, have altered dramatically the information about the relative benefits and risks of hormone therapy for preventing diseases of advanced age. The PEPI trial examined the effects of estrogen and progestin on LDL and HDL cholesterol levels and other risk factors. The trial included 875 healthy postmenopausal women aged 45 to 64 years who had no known contraindication to hormone therapy. Those women were randomized to placebo, conjugated equine estrogen (CEE), 0.625 mg, CEE 0.625 mg plus cyclic medroxyprogesterone acetate (MPA) 10 mg/day for 12 days per month; CEE 0.625 mg plus consecutive MPA 2.5 mg per day; or CEE 0.625 mg plus cyclic micronized progesterone (MP) 200 mg/day for 12 days per month. Results indicated that estrogen alone or in combination with a progestin improved lipoproteins and lowered fibrinogen levels without adverse effects on postchallenge insulin or blood pressure. Unopposed estrogen was the optimal regimen for elevating HDL-C. A high rate of endometrial hyperplasia occurred in the groups that used unopposed estrogen, thus restricting recommendations for its use to women without a uterus (80). Women with a uterus who took unopposed estrogen developed simple/cystic (27.7%), complex/adenomatous (22.7%), and atypical hyperplasia (11.8%) more frequently than those in the placebo group. Ninety-four percent of the women with hyperplasia reverted to a normal endometrial biopsy after progestin therapy (81). Women treated with estrogens or estrogen and progestin gained bone mass at the hip and spine (from 3.5–5%) over a 3-year period (81). In women who had a uterus, CEE with cyclic micronized progesterone had the most favorable effect on HDL-C and with no excess increased risk of endometrial hyperplasia. MPA had no detrimental effects on lipids compared with the risk for those not taking hormones (80). These findings, suggesting the beneficial effects of hormone therapy for cardiovascular risk factors, would contrast sharply with the effects of hormone therapy in two later clinical trials focusing on disease outcomes.

The HERS study was a randomized, blinded, placebo-controlled trial of E + P therapy in postmenopausal women with documented heart disease (n=2,763). Women ranged from 55 to 79 years of age, with a mean of 67 years. After 4 years of follow-up, researchers noted a higher risk of coronary events during the first year, with unclear benefit after years 3 to 5. The study was extended in an open-label design (HERS II) by asking the participants to stay on their study medications (E + P or placebo) after consulting with their health care providers. A total of 93% of the original HERS participants continued treatment for an additional 2.7 years, for a mean total of 6.8 years of study (83).

The WHI began in 1993, and includes a set of three interrelated clinical trials and an observational study in an apparently healthy postmenopausal sample. At entry to the study, 7.7% of women had prior cardiovascular disease. The randomized, blinded, controlled hormone therapy study included two arms, one using estrogen alone for women without a uterus (n=10,739) and one using combined conjugated estrogen and progesterone therapy (n=16,608). Postmenopausal women between 50 and 79 years old were enrolled (mean age 63.2). The combined conjugated estrogen and progesterone therapy arm was terminated in July 2002, after an average of 5 years of follow-up because the overall risks exceeded benefits (83). The estrogen only arm, the dietary modification arm, and the calcium and vitamin D arms of the clinical trials was terminated in 2004.

To date several findings from the HERS and WHI studies have modified the thinking about the risks versus benefits of hormone therapy (conjugated estrogens with a progestin). The WHI revealed a significant increase in the risk of coronary heart disease, whereas the HERS study showed a nonsignificant decreased risk with the increased risk apparent only in year 1 of the study. The WHI demonstrated a significant increased risk of stroke with use of E + P, but the HERS study showed a nonsignificant increased risk. Both the HERS and the WHI study revealed a significant increased risk of venous thromboembolism and both showed a nonsignificant increase in the risk of breast cancer. HERS showed a significant increased risk of gallbladder disease. WHI demonstrated a significant decreased risk of colon cancer and HERS a nonsignificant decreased risk. WHI results indicated a significantly decreased risk of hip, vertebral, and total osteoporotic fractures, whereas HERS showed a nonsignificant increased risk of hip fracture and a nonsignificant decreased risk of vertebral fracture, but a nonsignificant increased risk of total fractures. The increased risks and benefits of E + P therapy persisted throughout the duration of the WHI and HERS trials. Breast cancer risk was related to the duration of therapy. Risk for coronary heart disease and venous thromboembolism was observed during the first year of therapy (82–85). The estrogen therapy arm of the trial was terminated based on no observed preventive effect on heart disease in 2004. There were significant increases in the risk of stroke and significant benefits in osteoporotic fractures. There was no significant difference in other disease outcomes (86). The WHI ancillary studies, the WHI

Memory Study (WHIMS), and the WHI Study of Cognitive Aging (WHISCA) have indicated that there is no significant benefit of estrogen and progestin or estrogen alone on either dementia or mild cognitive impairment. Indeed, there was a significant increase in the incidence of dementia among women using E + P and a nonsignificant increase among women using E along (87–89).

Based on data from the WHI trial, the HERS studies, and other clinical trials, the North American Menopause Society Advisory Panel on Postmenopausal Hormone Therapy (90–92) recommended that:

- Treatment of menopause-related symptoms (vasomotor symptoms, urogenital symptoms such as vaginal dryness) remains the primary indication for estrogen therapy.
- The only menopause-related indication for progestin treatment appears to be protecting women from endometrial hyperplasia induced by estrogen therapy (women without a uterus who use estrogen do not need to use a progestogen).
- No estrogen or estrogen-plus-progestin therapy regimen should be used for primary or secondary prevention of heart disease; instead, proven heart disease prevention regimens should be considered.
- Although estrogen and estrogen-plus-progestin are FDA approved for the prevention of postmenopausal osteoporosis, other alternatives should be considered.
- The use of estrogen or estrogen and progesterone should be considered only for the shortest possible duration consistent with the treatment goals, risks, and benefits of individual women.
- Lower than standard doses should be considered; the Women's Health Osteoporosis Progestin Estrogen (HOPE) trial demonstrated that symptom relief and preservation of bone density without increased endometrial hyperplasia could be achieved with lower estrogen-plus-progestin doses (93–95).
- For women who have severe symptoms, such as hot flashes, or are nonresponsive to alternative treatments, estrogen or estrogen-plus-progestin can be considered carefully.
- Alternate routes for the administration of estrogen and progestin carry unknown risks.
- Individual risk profiles for each woman contemplating estrogen or estrogen-plus-progestin should be considered, and women should be informed about unknown risks.

In January 2003, the FDA recommended that a warning be included on all products containing estrogen advising that extended use could lead to increased risk of heart attacks, stroke, breast cancer, and life-threatening blood clots with either estrogen alone or estrogen plus progesterone. This warning stresses the importance of the individual decisions made by women and their health care providers, and may assist them in weighing the risks and benefits of such therapy.

Many questions remain to be answered. Among these are the definition of short- vs. long-term treatment, the length of treatment for symptom management for vasomotor symptoms, justification for any long-term use of estrogen or estrogen and a progestin, use of hormones for women with premature menopause, methods for weaning women from hormone therapy, and which agents other than those tested in the recently reported large clinical trials are likely to have the same outcomes.

The WHI will continue to assess the long-term consequences of estrogen therapy (E and E + P) in postmenopausal women for heart disease, osteoporosis, and breast cancer. (In addition, the use of a low-fat diet and calcium and vitamin D supplementation will be compared with the effects of hormone therapy on several disease endpoints.) Women will be followed for a 10-year period to assess the effects of hormone therapy along with or in conjunction with dietary modification and use of calcium and vitamin D supplementation on a host of disease endpoints, including heart disease, cancer, and osteoporotic fractures. Ancillary studies will assess the effects of hormone therapy on cognitive function and Alzheimer's disease. The science in this field is changing rapidly and bears close monitoring.

SUMMARY

Menopause is the cessation of menstruation, one component of the perimenopausal period, which encompasses the years of the menopausal transition and the 5 years following menopause. This transition in women's menstrual cycles is a marker for physiologic reregulation. Some of the changes associated with menopause include symptoms such as hot flashes and night sweats. A subset of women may experience more extreme health problems, such as depression. To date, researchers have focused on the use of hormone therapies (estrogen and progestin) for symptom management and more recent work has focused on the use of hormones to prevent the diseases of advanced age. Information is incomplete about the long-term risks and benefits and alternative symptom management approaches and preventive interventions.

References

1. Soules M, Sherman S, Parrott E, et al. Stages of Reproductive Aging Workshop (STRAW). *Menopause* 2001; 8:402–407.
2. Kaufert PA. Menstruation and menstrual change: women in midlife. *Health Care for Women International* 1986; 7(1-2):63–76.
3. Treloar AE. Menstrual cyclicity and the pre-menopause. *Maturitas* 1981;3(3-4):249–264.
4. Mc Kinlay S, Brambilla D, Posner J. The normal menopause transition. *Maturitas* 1992;14:103–115.
5. Sowers M, Crawford S, Sternfeld B, et al. SWAN: A multicenter, multiethnic community-based cohort study of women and the menopausal transition. In: Lobo R, Kelsey J, Marcus R. *Menopause: biology and pathobiology*. San Diego, Calif: Academic Press, 2000;175–188.
6. Woods NF, Mitchell ES. Anticipating menopause: observations from the Seattle Midlife Women's Health Study. *Menopause* 1999;6:167–163.
7. Dennerstein L, Dudley E, Burger H. Well-being and the menopausal transition. *J Psychosom Obstet Gynecol* 1997;18(2):95–101.
8. Richardson SJ. The biological basis of the menopause. *Balliere's Clinical Endocrinol Metabol* 1993;7:1–16.
9. Lenton EA, Sexton L, Lee S, Cooke ID. Progressive changes in LH and FSH and LH: FSH ratio in women throughout reproductive life. *Maturitas* 1988;10:35–43.
10. Metcalf MG. The approach of menopause: a New Zealand study. *New Zealand Medical Journal* 1988; 101(841):103–106.
11. Klein N, Battaglia D, Fujimoto V, Davis G, Bremner W, Soules M. Reproductive aging: accelerated follicular development associated with a monotropic follicle simulating hormone rise in normal older women. *J Clin Endocrinol Metabol* 1996;81:1038–1045.
12. Burger H, Dudley E, Hopper J, et al. Prospectively measured levels of serum FSH, estradiol and the dimeric inhibins during the menopausal transition in a population-based cohort of women. *J Clin Endocrin Metabol* 1999;84:11:4025–4030.
13. Santoro N, Rosenberg Brown J, Adel T, Skurnick JH. Characterization of reproductive hormonal dynamics in the perimenopause. *J Clin Endocrinol Metabol* 1996;81: 1495–1501.
14. Rannevik G, Jeppsson S, Johnell O, Bjerre Y, Laurell-Borulf B, Svanberg L. A longitudinal study of the perimenopausal transition: altered profiles of steroid and pituitary hormones, SHBG and bone mineral density. *Maturitas* 1995;21:103–113.
15. Longcope C, Johnston CCJ. Androgen and estrogen dynamics: stability over a two-year interval in perimenopausal women. *J Steroid Biochem* 1990;35:91–95.
16. Longcope C. Hormone dynamics at the menopause. In: Flint M, Kronenberg F, Utian W, eds. *Multidisciplinary perspectives on menopause*. New York, NY: New York Academy of Sciences; 1990.
17. Burger H, Dudley E, Cui J, Dennerstein L. Hopper J. A prospective longitudinal study of serum testosterone dehydroepiandrosterone sulphate and sex hormone binding globulin levels through the menopause transition. *J Clin Endocrinol Metabol* 2000;85:2832–2938.
18. Lasley B, Santoro N, Gold E, et al. The relationship of circulating dehydroepiandrosterone, testosterone, and estradiol to stages of the menopausal transition and ethnicity. *J Clin Endocrinol Metabol*. (In press.)
19. Mc Donnell D. Molecular pharmacology of Estrogen and Progesterone Receptors. In: Lobo R, Kelse J, Marcus R, eds. *Menopause biology and pathobiology*. New York, NY: Academic Press; 2000.
20. Dyrenfurth I, Endocrine Function in the Women's Second Half of Life. In: Voda A, Dennerstein M, O'Donnell S, eds. *Changing perspective on menopause*. Austin, Tx: University of Texas Press; 1982;307–334.

21. Patton H, Fuchs A, Hille B, Scher A, Steiner R. *Textbook of Physiology*, Vol. 2. Philadelphia, Pa: WB Saunders; 1989.

22. Kuller LH, Meilahn EN, Cauley JA, Gutai JP, Matthews KA. Epidemiologic studies of menopause changes in risk factors and disease. *Exper Gerontol* 1994;29:495–509.

23. Finkelstein J, Lee M, Sowers M, et al. Ethnic variation in bone density in premenopausal and early perimenopausal women: effects of anthropometric and lifestyle factors. *J Clin Endocrinol Metabol* 2002;87(7):3057–3067.

24. Sowers M, Finkelstein J, Geendale G, et al. Study of women's health across the nation. The association of endogenous hormone concentrations in bone mineral density (BMD) and bone mineral apparent density (BMAD) in pre- and perimenopausal women. *Osteoporosis Internat* 2003;14(1):44–52.

25. Wing RR, Matthews KA, Kuller LH, Meilahn EN, Plantinga PL. Weight gain at the time of menopause. *Arch Intern Med* 1991;151(1):97–102.

26. Matthews K, Abrams B, Crawford S, et al. Body mass index in midlife women: relative influence of menopause, hormone use, and ethnicity. *Internat J Obesity Related Metabolic Dis* 2001;25:863–873.

27. Wing RR, Jeffery RW, Burton LR, Thorson,C, Kuller LH, Folsom AR. Change in waist-hip ratio with weight loss and its association with change in cardiovascular risk factors. *Amer J Clin Nutrition* 1992;55:1086–1092.

28. Cauley JA, Gutai JP, Kuller LH, Powell JG. The relation of endogenous sex steroid hormone concentrations to serum lipid and lipoprotein levels in postmenopausal women. *Am J Epidemiol* 1990;132:884–894.

29. Meilahn EN, Kuller LH, Matthews KA, Stein EA. La (a) concentrations among pre- and postmenopausal women over time: The Healthy Women Study (abstract No. 2170). *Circulation* 1991;84:II-546.

30. Matthews KA, Meilahn EN, Kuller LH, Kelsey SF, Caggiula AW, Wing RR. Menopause and risk factors for coronary heart disease. *N Engl J Med* 1989;321:641–646.

31. Meilahn EN, Kuller LH, Matthews KA, Wing RR, Caggiula AW, Stein EA. Potential for increasing high-density lipoprotein cholesterol, subfraction HDL2-C and HDL3-C, and apoprotein A1 among middle-age women. *Prevent Med* 1991;20:462–473.

32. Meilahn EN, Kuller LH, Matthews KA, Kiss JE. Hemostatic factors according to menopausal status and use of hormone replacements therapy. *Ann Epidemiol* 1992;2:445–455.

33. Backstrom T, Sanders D, Leask R, Davidson D, Warner P, Bancroft J. Mood, sexuality, hormones and the menstrual cycle: hormone levels and their relationship to the premenstrual syndrome. *Psychosomatic Med* 1983;43:503–507.

34. McEwen BS, Woolley CS. Estradiol and progesterone regulate neuronal structure and synaptic connectivity in adult as well as developing brain. *Experim Gerontol* 1994;29:431–436.

35. Sherwin BB. Sex hormones and psychological functioning in postmenopausal women. *Experim Gerontol* 1994;29(3/4):423–430.

36. Saab PG, Matthews KA, Stoney CM, McDonald RH. Premenopausal and postmenopausal women differ in their cardiovascular and neuroendocrine responses to behavioral stressors. *Psychophysiology* 1989;26:270–280.

37. Lindheim SR, Legro RS, Bernstein L, et al. Behavioral stress responses in premenopausal and postmenopausal women and the effects of estrogen. *Am J Obstet Gynecol* 1992;167:1831–1836.

38. Polan ML, Daniele A, Kuo A. Gonadal steroids modulate human monocyte interleukin-1 (IL-1) activity. *Fertility Sterility* 1988;49:964–968.

39. McKane WR, Khosla S, Peterson JM, et al. Circulating levels of cytokines that modulate bone resorption: effects of age and menopause in women. *J Bone Min Res* 1994;9:1313–1318.

40. Stimson WH. Estrogen and human T lymphocytes: presence of specific receptors in T-suppressor/cytotoxic subset. *Scand J Immunol* 1988;28:345–350.

41. Cauley JA, Lucas FL, Kuller LH, Vogt MT, Browner WS, Cummings SR. Bone mineral density and risk of breast cancer in older women: the study of osteoporotic fractures. *JAMA* 1996;276:1404–1408.

42. Mitchell ES, Woods NF. Symptom experiences of midlife women: observations from the Seattle Midlife Women's Health Study. *Maturitas* 1996;25:1–10.

43. Shaver J, Giblin E, Lentz M, Lee K. Sleep patterns and sleep stability in perimenopausal women. *Sleep* 1988;11(6):556–561.

44. Avis NE, Kaufert PA, Lock M, McKinlay S, Vass K. The evolution of menopausal symptoms. In: Burger H, (ed.) *Ballière's Clinical Endocrinology and Metabolism*, Vol. 7. London: Harcourt Brace Jovanovich Publishers; 1993.

45. Lock M, Kaufert P, Gilbert P. Cultural construction of the menopausal syndrome: the Japanese's case. *Maturitas* 1988;10:317–322.

46. Avis N, Stellato R, Crawford S, et al. Is there a menopause syndrome? Menopause status and symptoms across ethnic groups. *Soc Sci Med* 2001;52:345–356.

47. Anderson E, Hamburger S, Lin JH, Rebar RW. Characteristics of menopausal women seeking assistance. *Am J Obstet Gynecol* 1987;156:428–433.

48. Matthews KA, Wing RR, Kuller LH, Meilahn EN. Plantinga P. Influence of the perimenopause on cardiovascular risk factors and symptoms of middle-aged healthy women. *Arch Intern Med* 1994;154:2349–2355.

49. Avis N, Crawford S, Stellato R, Longcope C. Longitudinal study of hormone levels and depression among women transitioning through menopause. *Climacteric* 2001;4:243–249.

50. Dennerstein L, Dudley E, Hopper J, Guthrie J, Burger H. A prospective population-based study of menopausal symptoms. *Obstet Gynecol* 2000;96:351–358.

51. Hunter M. The Southeast England Longitudinal Study of the climacteric and postmenopause. *Maturitas* 1992;14:117–126.

52. Kaufert PA, Gilbert P, Tate R. The Manitoba Project: a re-examination of the link between menopause and depression. *Maturitas* 1992;14:143–155.

53. Woods N, Mariella A, Mitchell E. Patterns of depressed mood across the menopausal transition: approaches to studying patterns in longitudinal data. *Acta Obstetrica Gynecol Scandnavica* 2002;81:623–632.

54. Bromberger J, Meyer P, Kravitz H, et al. Psychological Distress and Natural Menopause: A Multi-ethnic Community Study. *Am J Pub Health* 2001;91:1435–1442.

55. Shifren J, Braunstein G, Simon J, et al. Transdermal testosterone treatment in women with impaired sexual function after oophorectomy. *N Engl J Med* 2000;343(10):682–688.

56. Eriksson E, Sundblad C, Lisjo P, Modigh K, Andersch B. Serum levels of androgens are higher in women with pre-

menstrual irritability and dysphoria than in controls. *Psychoneuroendocrinology* 1992;17(2/3):195–204.

57. Smith RNJ, Holland EFN, Studd JWW. The symptomatology of progestogen intolerance. *Maturitas* 1994;18:87–91.

58. Woods NF, Mitchell ES. Patterns of depressed mood in midlife women: observations from the Seattle Midlife Women's Health Study. *Res Nursing Health* 1996;19:111–123.

59. Woods NF, Mitchell ES. Pathways to depressed mood for midlife women: observations from the Seattle Midlife Women's Health Study. *Res Nursing Health* 1997;20:119–129.

60. Matthews KA, Wing RR, Kuller LH, et al. Influences of natural menopause on psychological characteristics and symptoms of middle-aged healthy women. *J Consult Clin Psychol* 1990;58:345–351.

61. Ballinger S. Stress as a factor in lowered estrogen levels in the early postmenopause. *Ann NY Acad Sci.* 1990;592:95–113.

62. Rabin DS, Johnson EO, Brandon DD, Liapi C, Chrousos GP. Glucocorticoids inhibit estradiol-mediated uterine growth: possible role of the uterine estradiol receptor. *Biol Reprod* 1990;42(1):74–80.

63. Shively CA, Knox SS, Sherwin BB, Walsh BW, Wilson PW. Sex steroids, psychosocial factors, and lipid metabolism. *Metabol Clin Experiment* 1993;42:16–24.

64. Utian WH, Schiff I. NAMS-Gallup survey on women's knowledge, information sources, and attitudes to menopause and hormone replacement therapy. *Menopause* 1994;1:39–48.

65. London S, Willett W, Longcope C, Mc Kinlay S. Alcohol and other dietary factors in relation to serum hormone concentrations in women at climacteric. *Am J Clin Nutrit* 1991;53:166–171.

66. Reichman M, Judd J, Longcope C, et al. Effects of alcohol consumption on plasma and urinary hormone concentrations in premenopausal women. *J Nation Cancer Instit* 1993;85:722–727.

67. Goldin BR, Woods MN, Spiegelman DL, et al. The effect of dietary fat and fiber on serum estrogen concentrations in premenopausal women under controlled dietary conditions. *Cancer* 1994;74(suppl 3):1125–1131.

68. Hammar M, Berg G, Lindgren R. Does physical exercise influence the frequency of post-menopausal hot flashes? *Acta Obstetrica Gynecol Scandnavica* 1990;69:409–412.

69. Owens JF, Matthews KA, Wing RR, Kuller LH. Can physical activity mitigate the effects of aging in middle-aged women? *Circulation* 1992;85:1265–1270.

70. Ley CJ, Lees B, Stevenson JC. Sex-and menopause-associated changes in body-fat distribution. *Am J Clin Nutrit* 1992;55:950–954.

71. Kaye SA, Folsom AR. Is serum cortisol associated with body fat distribution in postmenopausal women? *Internat J Obesity* 1991;15:437–439.

72. Marin P, Darin N, Amemiya T, Andersson B, Jern S, Bjorntorp P. Cortisol secretion in relation to body fat distribution in obese premenopausal women. *Metabol Clin Experim* 1992;41(8):882–886.

73. Morse CA, Smith A, Dennerstein L, Green A, Hopper J, Burger H. The treatment-seeking woman at menopause. *Maturitas* 1994;18:161–173.

74. Bush T. Feminine forever revisited: menopausal hormone therapy in the 1990s. *J Women's Health* 1991;1:1–4.

75. Hemminki E, Kennedy D, Baum C, McKinlay M. Prescribing of noncontraceptive estrogens and progestins in the United States, 1974–1986. *Am J Public Health* 1988;78:1479–1481.

76. Weiss N, Ure C, Ballard J, Williams A, Daling J. Decreased risk of fractures of the hip and lower forearm with postmenopausal use of estrogen. *N Engl J Med* 1980;303:1195–1198.

77. Bush T, Barrett-Connor E, Cowan L, et al. Cardiovascular mortality and noncontraceptive use of estrogen in women: results from the Lipid Research Clinics Program Follow-up Study. *Circulation* 1987;75:1102–1109.

78. American College of Physicians. Guidelines for counseling postmenopausal women about preventive hormone therapy. *Ann Intern Med* 1992;117:1038–1041.

79. U.S. Preventive Services Task Force. Postmenopausal hormone prophylaxis. In: *Guide to clinical preventive services*, 2nd ed. Baltimore, Md: Williams & Wilkins; 1996.

80. The Writing Group for the PEPI Trial. Effects of estrogen or estrogen/progestin regimens on heart disease risk factors in postmenopausal women. The postmenopausal estrogen/progestin interventions (PEPI) trial. *JAMA* 1995;273(3):199–208.

81. The Writing Group for the PEPI Trial. Effects of hormone therapy on bone mineral density: results from the postmenopausal estrogen/progestin interventions (PEPI) trial. *JAMA* 1996;276:1389–1396.

82. Hulley S, Grady D, Bush T, et al. for the Heart and Estrogen/progestin Replacement Study (HERS) Research Group. Randomized trial of estrogen plus progestin for secondary prevention of coronary heart disease in postmenopausal women. *JAMA* 1998;280:605–613.

83. Writing Group for the Women's Health Initiative Investigators. Risks and benefits of estrogen plus progestin in healthy postmenopausal women: principal results from the Women's Health Initiative randomized controlled trial. *JAMA* 2002;288:321–333.

84. Grady D, Herington D, Bittner V, et al, for the HERS Research Group. Cardiovascular disease outcomes during 6.8 years of hormone therapy: Heart and Estrogen/Progestin Replacement Study follow-up (HERS II). *JAMA* 2002;288:49–57.

85. Hulley S, Furberg C, Barrett-Connor E, et al, for the HERS Research Group. Noncardiovascular disease outcomes during 6.8 years of hormone therapy: Heart and Estrogen/Progestin Replacement Study follow-up (HERS II). *JAMA* 2002;288:58–66.

86. Anderson GL, Limacher M, Assaf AR, et al., for the Somen's Health Initiative Steering Committee. Effects of conjugated equine estrogen in postmenopausal women with hysterectomy: the Women's Health Initiative randomized controlled trial. *JAMA* 2004;291:1701–1712.

87. Shumaker SA, Legault C, Thal L, et al, for the WHIMS Investigators. Estrogen plus progestin and the incidence of dementia and mild cognitive impairment in postmenopausal women: the Women's Health Initiative Memory Study: a randomized controlled study. *JAMA* 2003;289:2651–2662.

88. Rapp SR, Espeland MA, Shumaker SA, et al, for the WHIMS Investigators. Effect of estrogen plus progestin on global congitive function in postmenopausal women: the Women's Health Initiative Memory Study: a randomized controlled trial. *JAMA* 20-03;289:2663–2672.

89. Espeland MA, Rapp SR, Shumaker SA, et al., for the Women's Health Initiative Memory Study Investigators. Conjugated equine estrogens and global cogtnitive function in postmenopausal women: the Women's Health Initiative Memory Study. JAMA 2004;291:2959–2968.

90. The North American Menopause Society. Amended report from the NAMS Advisory Panel on Postmenopausal Hormone Therapy. *Menopause* 2003;10:6–12.

91. The North American Menopause Society. Estroen and progestogen use in peri- and postmenopausal somen: September 2003 position statement of The North American Menopause Society. *Menopause* 2003, 10:497–506.

92. North American Menopause Society. Recommendations for estrogen and progestogen use in peri- and postmenopausal women: October 2004 position statement of The North American Menopause Society. *Menopause* 2004:11:589–600.

93. Utian W, Shoupe D, Bachmann G, Pinkerton J, Pickar J. Relief of vasomotor symptoms and vaginal atrophy with lower doses of conjugated equine estrogens and medroxyprogesterone acetate. *Fertility Sterility* 2001;75:1065–1079.

94. Archer D, Dorin M, Lewis V, Schneider D, Pickar J. Effects of lower doses of conjugated equine estrogens and medroxyprogesterone acetate on endometrial bleeding. *Fertil Steril* 2001;75:1080–1087.

95. Lindsay R, Gallagher J, Kleerekoper M, Pickar J. Effect of lower doses of conjugated equine estrogens with and without medroxyprogesterone acetate on bone in early postmenopausal women. *JAMA* 2002;287:2668–2676.

13 Frailty in Elderly Women

E. Jeffrey Metter

Aging and diseases of the nervous system are among the most important contributors to physical disability and nursing home admissions in elderly women. At age 65, the average woman can expect to live another 19.2 years, whereas at age 85, the expectation is 6.7 years. In fact, the fastest growing age group in the United States is that of individuals over 85 years of age, with approximately 70% being women. In the 2000 census, 48% of the 35 million elderly individuals were more than 75 years of age (1). This age group has the highest rates of disability and requirements for assistance [Figure 13.1, data from (2)], and the rates are higher in women than in men. According to the 2000 census, however, a decline occurred in individuals 65 and older who were living in nursing homes from 5.1% in 1990 to 4.5% in 2000. The greatest decline occurred in those over 85 years, where 18% were living in nursing homes in 2000, as compared with 24.5% in 1990 (1).

Aging is associated with greater susceptibility to physical disability and frailty. Frailty has been defined as those losses of strength, mobility, balance, and endurance that lead to decreased ability for self-care in the elderly (3). Frailty is an expansion of the concept of disability as applied to the elderly. Disability refers to losses in functional performance that result from diseases and alteration in health. It includes the lack of ability to perform activities in a normal manner, and is concerned with abilities that are generally accepted as essential components of everyday life—personal care, activities of daily living (ADLs; dressing, washing, eating, toileting, bathing), and locomotor activities (4).

The disability model is important to the concept of frailty, because it is based on an orderly development of the physical problem. Disability develops over time, starting from risk factors that lead to pathology or impairment, causing functional limitations and disability that result in handicap within society. Frailty adds the additional element of age. Increasing age leads to a decreasing capacity for the adaptation to and compensation for existing problems. As an example, an older woman who fractures a hip may not be able to use crutches and may have trouble using a manual wheelchair to get around, which would not be the case for a younger individual. Age-associated changes including less strength, slower reactions, and poorer posture, among others, adversely affect the process of recovery. Young individuals have enormous functional capacities and reserves for their activities. Illness or disability can usually be overcome by using part or all of that reserve. In the elderly, the reserve is diminished, thus permitting a narrower range of adaptation to illness, injury, changing health, or environmental factors. Aging of the nervous system makes a substantial contribution to the loss of functional reserves and declining adaptability. Greater focus on these declines can minimize the long-term consequences of aging and potentially prevent or treat the development of frailty.

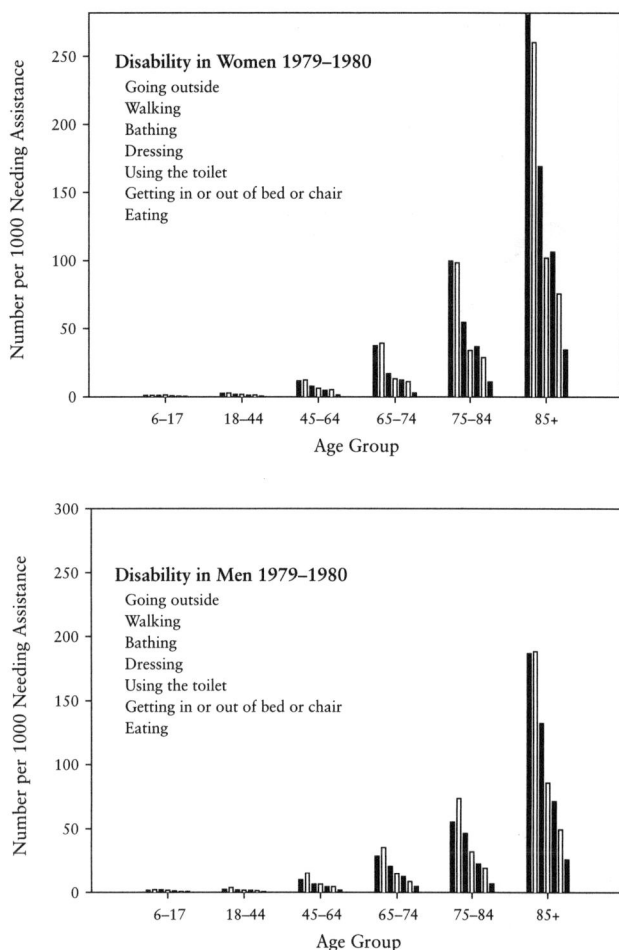

FIGURE 13.1

Disability rates in women and men from 1979–1980 (from reference 2) for a variety of activities including going outside, walking, bathing, dressing, using the toilet, getting in and out of bed or chair, and eating. The rate of disability rises rapidly after age 75, to where over 25% of women over the age of 85 have difficulties going outside.

A clear concept of disability is required to understand the neurology of frailty. Neurologists typically consider disease processes by systems: pyramidal, extrapyramidal, cerebellar. For frailty, it is necessary to examine broader functional concepts that reflect how the elderly perform, e.g., gait, ADLs, falls, and incontinence. This functional orientation is important because disability is seldom a result of a single problem, but reflects multifactorial dysfunction from multiple medical and neurological abnormalities that may or may not be related to disease. Age is an added consideration because it leads to declining function in essentially all body organs, including the nervous system. In some situations, the distinction between disease and aging can be difficult to determine. For this reason, gerontologists often will distinguish between primary and secondary aging, in which the latter considers the impact of disease on the aging process (5).

Women have a greater rate of frailty with increasing age than men. In part, this can be attributed to the longer life expectancy of women, particularly in the presence of chronic diseases including neurologic disorders. Verbrugge (6) has noted that women tend to have more chronic diseases, whereas men succumb to acute disease. The distinction implies that whereas women are more robust, men who survive tend to be somewhat healthier.

A number of factors contributes to functional disability and the development of frailty, as shown in Table 13.1. The table is not complete, nor is it meant to be. I have divided contributing factors based on how they impact on functional capability. The nervous system has important impacts at each of the levels described. The divisions are somewhat arbitrary, but are an attempt at an orderly sequence of factors that contribute to frailty. Environmental and social factors have an enormous impact on functioning in elderly women. During a long life, friends and family die or move away, so that an older woman may live by herself with little public contact. At the same time, she will develop chronic diseases that will further limit her ability to interact with others and her environment. Similarly, aging is associated with gradual declines in homeostatic mechanisms that maintain most body systems and directly affect functional capability. An example of a homeostatic mechanism is the role of the autonomic and cardiovascular systems for the maintenance of blood pressure in the upright position, a necessary position for mobility. In addition, the mechanisms are directly dependent on the pressor and depressor actions of the ventral lateral medulla, which are dependent on the maintenance of peripheral nervous system afferent nerve fibers, more rostral nuclei, and cortical functions (95). In general, the nervous system is directly involved with aging in most homeostatic systems. Body systems involved directly with movement change with age, with loss of muscle mass, declining nervous system ability to sense the environment, alteration in postural balance and stability, and changes in bone structure with greater risks of fracture. Together, these systems allow the body to develop strength, coordination, endurance, and movement. Each patient must be understood in regard to the factors that led to her disability. In some women, the treatment of disease is what is needed. In others, social, environmental, or the address of aging changes will be more important. This chapter reviews aspects of neurologic changes with age, particularly those neurologic diseases that contribute to increased risk for frailty.

AGING IN WOMEN

With increasing age, most neurologic systems show changes in both women and men. Data from the National

TABLE 13.1
Factors and Diseases Associated with Frailty

Environment
 Lighting
 Noise
 Driving
 Ground composition
 Temperature
 Trauma
Social
 Isolation
 Depression
 Economics
Disease
 Arthritis
 Heart disease
 Stroke
 Alzheimer's disease
 Parkinson's disease
 Peripheral neuropathy
 Pulmonary disease
Homeostatic Mechanisms
 Cardiovascular
 Pulmonary
 Autonomic
 Endocrine
 Nutrition/metabolic
 Inflammatory
Body Systems Involved with Movement
 Muscle
 Nervous system
  Central nervous system
  Peripheral nervous system
 Bone/cartilage
 Joint
 Sensation
  Vision
  Hearing
  Proprioception
  Vestibular
Physical Abilities
 Strength
 Coordination
 Movement speed
 Endurance
Consequences
 Frailty
 Falls
 ADL
 IADL

Physiological Changes with Age in Women—
Baltimore Longitudinal Study of Aging

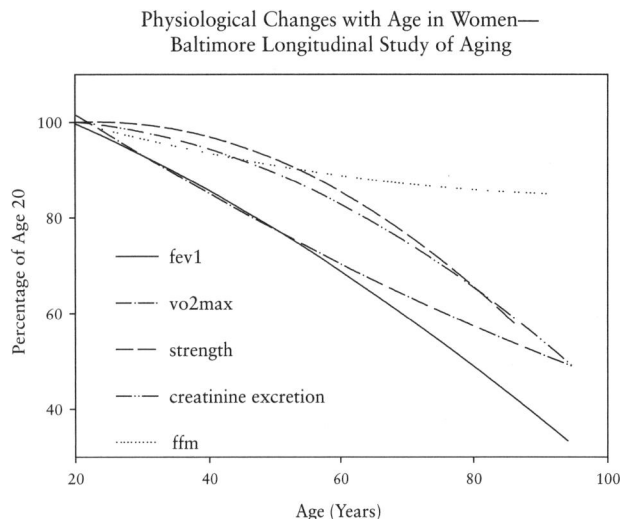

FIGURE 13.2

Physiologic changes with age in women from the Baltimore Longitudinal Study of Aging referenced to levels observed in 20- to 30-year-old women.

pendence (Figure 13.2). The age changes occur at varying rates and are not necessarily linear. Thus, different body systems age at different rates, and different parts of the nervous system age differently. Even within the auditory system, the physiologic consequences of aging are different in different parts of the organ of Corti (7), and are different according to gender (8). This can be seen by differences in the rate of hearing loss for different frequencies. The hearing of high frequency tones begins to decline in the thirties, with only small changes in the speech frequencies. The speech frequencies become involved in the fifties and sixties. Women lose their hearing at a somewhat later age than men, but the time course of change is similar. A great deal of variability occurs in the rate and extent of presbycusis. In fact, as individuals age, these variations become increasingly diverse. This is true for hearing and other physiologic, psychologic, and biochemical functions. The age changes shown in Figure 13.2 affect each woman at a different rate and to a different extent, and do not uniformly affect all systems to the same extent. For most measures, the best performing elderly woman cannot achieve the maximal levels of young adults. In most, there is an associated alteration in motor performance and in the ability to perceive the environment.

Age Changes in Muscle Strength

Women tend to be 30 to 40% weaker than men at all ages. Age-associated losses of strength are not confined to the elderly but may begin at relatively young ages

Institute on Aging's Baltimore Longitudinal Study of Aging (BLSA), a 45-year longitudinal study of men and women across the adult life span, shows that increasing age is associated with physiologic and biochemical changes in the many systems critical for functional inde-

(9–17). The rate of decline increases with age, particularly after 50 years. In six studies that measure either concentric strength (strength generated during muscle shortening) or isometric strength (strength generated without muscle shortening) (Figure 13.3), there is a trend towards strength declines by the mid forties. By this age, 10% of the muscle strength observed in 20-year-olds was already lost. Up to 60% or more of strength was lost by age 80 to 90 years.

The effects of such losses are greater in women, since women start at a lower strength level. The relationship between muscle strength and function in healthy individuals shows a linear relationship up to a certain strength level and then plateaus. Kwon et al. (96) found that women occupy the linear part of this relationship, so that their functional capability is directly dependent on their mus-

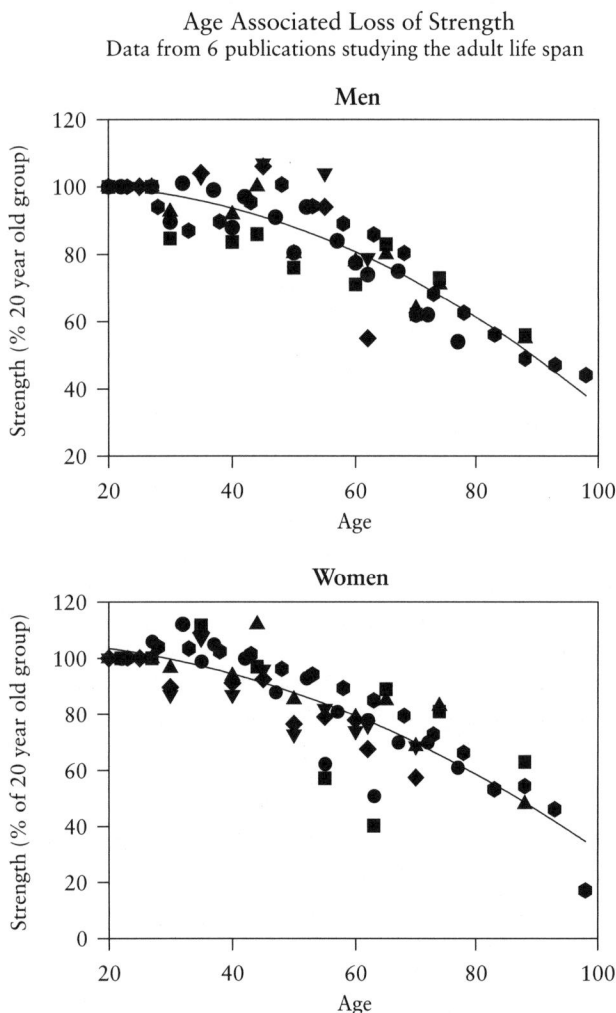

Phases of Changing Muscle Strength in Adult Women

FIGURE 13.4

Phases of changing muscle strength in adult women. Cross-sectional arm and leg strength measurements from women who participate in the BLSA are plotted by age. We observe four phases of changes in muscle strength during the adult lifespan. Phase 1 is characterized by reaching maximal strength and performance. During Phase 2, subtle declines in strength begin to appear and may differ by muscle groups and extremities. Phase 3 shows clear declines, but the rate of loss may be slower than in Phase 4, where the rates of decline accelerate.

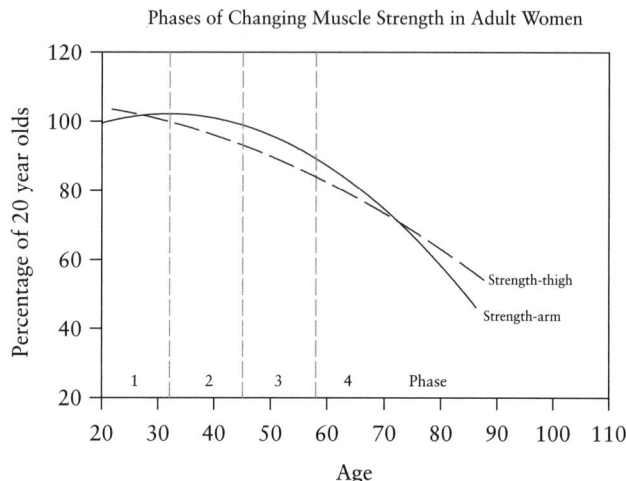

Age Associated Loss of Strength
Data from 6 publications studying the adult life span

FIGURE 13.3

Age-associated loss of strength (from references 10,13–17), where strength was expressed as the percentage of what was observed in 20-year-olds in each study.

cle strength. The plateauing of performance in relationship to strength or fitness has been called *functional reserve*, which is defined as a level of physical fitness (frequently considered in relation to muscle strength) beyond which further increases in fitness do not lead to further improvements in physical function (97). Since muscle mass and strength decline by as much as 50 to 60% with increasing age, functional reserve should decline, thus contributing to increased frailty. The 60% loss may put many women at a level where functional disability occurs as a function of strength (18), leaving little reserve when other processes, such as illness, intervene.

The strength loss results from muscle mass loss, which has been called *sarcopenia*. Sarcopenia emphasizes changes in the elderly (19) and ignores changes that may occur across the adult lifespan. Baumgartner et al. (98) define sarcopenia as having muscle mass greater than two standard deviations below the average mass for young adults; they found that approximately one-third of women 70 to 80 years of age, and 45% of women greater than 80 years of age were sarcopenic. In addition to muscle mass, muscle composition changes with age, with a decline in the number of muscle fibers. Associated with this are losses of type 2 muscle fibers in some studies (20–22) but not in others (23,24). These type 2 fibers are the fast twitch fibers required for explosive power (as illustrated by their higher percentage in sprinters and power lifters) (25,26). They are larger than type 1 fibers and generate relatively more force per fiber. Type 2 fibers tend to be recruited late in the development of strength, when maximal levels of force generation are required.

The alteration in muscle structure and neural innervation (see next section) lead to changes in muscle quality, which is characterized as the force generated per unit of muscle mass. Age changes in fiber type composition can result in differences in strength per unit of muscle and could potentially explain some aspects of decreasing muscle responsiveness, strength, and power, and changing movement control with age. The changes can result in a loss of fine movement control, gait and posture instability, and alterations in other physical functions.

In our work from the BLSA (27), age-associated loss of strength in women seems to be directly tied to the level of muscle mass, whereas in men, other age factors are also important. Recently, the role of estrogen on maintaining strength has been raised. Phillips et al. (28) found that postmenopausal women on hormonal replacement were stronger and showed less change in strength than untreated postmenopausal women, but the direct effect of menopause on strength is unclear. Two points against the hypothesis are that the time course of change is similar in both genders and begins before the menopause, and most studies do not find a specific acceleration in strength in women at or immediately after the menopause. Our studies of concentric isokinetic strength in the BLSA women, found declines beginning in the twenties and thirties in concentric strength in elbow flexors and extensors and knee flexor and extensors. The rate of change with age was similar in both genders through middle and old age.

Based on an examination of the time course of strength loss, muscle mass, peripheral nerve function, and changes in reaction and movement times, the adult life span can be divided into at least four phases (Figure 13.4).

- *Phase 1: Early Adulthood: Attaining maximal physical potential.* This phase is reached between 20 and 35 years of age, when maximal strength and performance is achieved. Routine daily activities are easily done and with no limitations.
- *Phase 2: Late Early Adulthood: The beginning of change.* This phase occurs between 30 and 45 years of age. Subtle changes begin in functional capability, with slight losses in muscle strength and slowing of reaction and movement times. The changes are most apparent in maximal performance. High levels of performance can often be maintained by compensating through altered mechanics of performance. Causes of the declines are not clear and are related primarily with aging. Diseases are not important factors during this phase.
- *Phase 3: Middle Age: Slow declines.* This phase occurs between 40 and 65 years of age. Declines are

clearly apparent in the maximal functional performance, even in the fittest individuals and even with the greatest degree of compensation by using alternative strategies to maximize capabilities. Some individuals begin to experience functional difficulties with daily routines. During this phase, woman go through menopause. Diseases become apparent, contributing to functional incapacity.

- *Phase 4: Older age: Dramatic and large losses of muscle strength, which may reach significant levels.* This phase begins between 60 and 70 years of age. Muscle strength losses are more rapid. In women, the extent of strength loss may be enough to lead to functional disability. The changes in this phase are related to sarcopenia and intercurrent disease. Disease becomes increasingly important as functional capability and compensation become limited.

The time course of change suggests that different factors are at play during the different phases of a woman's life. Furthermore, the expectations for performance are different. In young healthy women, there are few issues regarding ADLs and instrumental IADLs. By middle age, performance is not as good, and work-related injuries can have a major impact on continued occupation. In old age, the focus becomes ADLs and IADLs. In general, there is little concern about high-level performance in the elderly. Such differences in performance and expectation lead to differing focuses by physicians on what type and level of interventions are valuable.

Nerve Function

With age, a decrease in the number and size of the motor neurons, along with a slowing of nerve conduction velocity occurs (99). Nerve conduction velocity declines by about 10% from the twenties through the eighties (29,30). The age changes in nerve conduction velocity are directly related to muscle strength, which in part is independent of muscle mass and age (105). Since the measured velocity is determined by the largest alpha motor neurons that innervate muscle, the decline implies losses of, or changes in the largest neurons.

More recent techniques allow for the direct examination of the motor unit. Campbell, McComas, and Petito (31) reported that after age 60 years, a marked decline occurred in the number of motor units. In the biceps brachii, Brown, Strong, and Snow (32) estimated that individuals less than 60 years of age had an average of 911 motor units, whereas in older subjects, the average was 479 (a 47% decline). Doherty and Brown (33) found a 52% decline in thenar units over the adult life span. Doherty, Vandervoort, and Brown (34) summarized the changes in motor units with age and found declines of 50 to 80% in thenar muscles, 50% in hypothenar muscles, and declines in extensor digitorum brevis of more than 40% over the adult life span (although most of the studies do not include subjects over 80 years of age).

The effect of the loss of motor units on the central nervous system (CNS), and vice versa, is not understood, nor are the effects on functional performance. It is clear that the number of functional motor units will change after primary damage to the CNS, as may be seen with the loss of functional motor units in hemiplegic patients after stroke. The importance of the CNS on the nerve–muscle interactions is also reflected in developmental biology, where the isolation of the motor units from spinal influences alters the development of slow but not fast muscle fibers (35).

Taken together, the evidence suggests an important role for a changing nerve–muscle relationship in the development of sarcopenia. Reorganization of the motor units results in fewer but larger motor units, and may cause the shift in the proportion from fast to slow muscle fibers. Together, the nerve reorganization is likely a contributing factor to the loss of muscle mass and changes in fine motor coordination.

Age Changes in Movement

Slowing of reaction and movement times occurs throughout the adult life span. Women have longer reaction times than men throughout their adult life for both simple (tap a button when you hear a sound) and complex responses (tap the button when you hear a lower pitched sound) (36). One possible explanation is the appearance of parkinsonian features in elderly subjects with the appearance of decreasing spontaneous movement, a forward bend in the posture with kyphosis, a decreasing arm swing, and gait irregularities. No consistent pattern is observed. In general, these changes are not felt to be Parkinson's disease because the clear clinical features of the disease are not consistently present. Increasing age is associated with losses in the nigrostriatal dopamine system (101). These changes begin in young adulthood and linearly decline with age. The parkinsonian-like features are likely to represent manifestation of the lifelong change in the basal ganglia.

An alternate explanation is that changes occur as a result of a changing cortical control of movement. Older subjects, and particularly women, are more concerned with the accuracy of their movements. In a simple tapping task, where subjects were required to go back and forth between two circles, Brogmus (37) found that women tend to have slower and more accurate movements trying to touch the center of each circle to minimize errors, whereas men are willing to sacrifice accuracy to gain time by touching just inside the circumference. The planning strategies in this test were clearly different based on gender. In a somewhat different task, however, Morgan et al. (38) found that the accuracy of movement was the same in the elderly whether movements were slow or fast, and that movements were associated with a jerkiness not present in younger subjects. Thus, changes in movement accuracy in part are task dependent and in part are associated with age-associated changes that slow and reduce the accuracy of the movements. These findings suggest differential gender- and age-determined strategies for patterned or predetermined movements. From a practical level, the changes in movement speed and accuracy further restrict the ability of elderly women to adjust in the presence of chronic health problems. Health problems that would be minor for younger women can lead to major functional incapacity in older women.

Gait and Postural Stability

In aggregate, the previous discussion suggests that older women are weak, have slowed reaction to environmental factors, and slow deliberate movements. Together, such changes may impair gait and balance. Both activities are complex motor control processes that utilize several neurologic systems, so that multiple factors can contribute to age-associated changes. Gait disturbances are common in the elderly: one-quarter of a 79-year-old cohort in Göteborg, Sweden required mechanical aids in walking (39), and 40 to 50% of nursing home residents had gait difficulties (40). Changes in gait are easily demonstrated using a *timed gait*—the time required to walk a given distance. In our experience, changes begin in the early fifties in healthy women and men (Figure 13.5). Guralnik et al. (41) have shown that a timed 8-foot walk is a strong predictor of functional disability in elderly subjects. Imms and Edholm (42) found that the slowing of gait is related to a variety of diseases to a greater degree than advancing age, but the changes also occur in healthy elderly women (43). These studies focused on the elderly and do not explain the changes in gait speed occurring in middle age. The diminution in speed was associated with a shorter stride, broader base of support, more time spent with both feet on the floor, and less time in a one-footed stance, although Rubino (44) noted that *senile gait* in women is characterized by a narrow gait with increased side-to-side movement. Wolfson et al. (45) have reported that gait differences in stride length and walking speed differed between those nursing home residents who do or do not fall. Most gait disorders in the elderly are attributed to neurologic or orthopedic disorders (46,47) but these problems cannot explain the decrease in speed seen during middle age.

The changes in gait can be explained in part by loss of muscle strength (48), but other factors are also contributing. The basal ganglia may play a central role. Studies of the basal ganglia suggest that loss of dopaminergic neurons in the substantia nigra begins early in adult life

Normal Gait Speed over 50 Feet

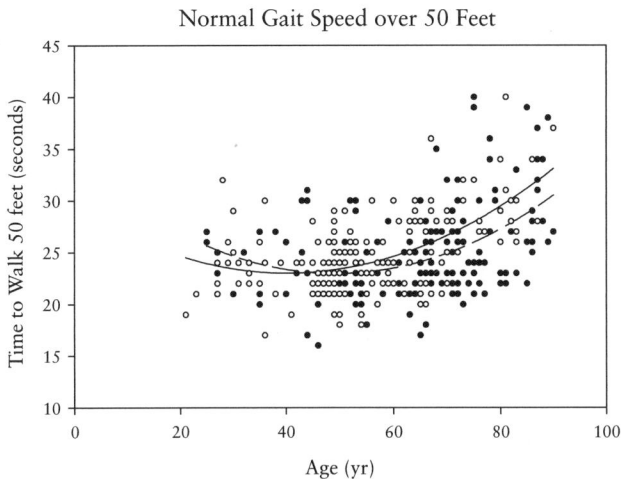

FIGURE 13.5

Time to walk 50 feet at a normal gait speed from participants in the BLSA. Subjects were asked to walk 25 feet in a hospital corridor, turn around, and walk back. The dashed line and solid circles are data from women and the solid line and open circles are data from men.

and continues through adulthood (49,50). This may explain many of the behavioral changes in motor performance that begin in the twenties and thirties. The dopaminergic model of motoric aging has been advanced by Joseph et al. (51), based on animal models. Such changes may result in senile gait that has been described in the elderly. This pattern of movement is characterized by its parkinsonian quality with a stooped posture, elevation of arms, and short steps. The gait pattern usually appears in the sixties and seventies, but is not universal. It is distinguished from Parkinson's disease by the absence of rigidity, prominent bradykinesia, and tremor. The time course for the development of senile gait has not been studied. Using a simple timed gait, the decreases beginning in the speed of movement starting in the fifties for both women and men are associated with a decrease in stride length. Neurologic disorders that can lead to gait disorders include bilateral frontal lobe disease with apraxia of gait, pyramidal disorders with spasticity, extrapyramidal disorders with Parkinson's disease, cerebellar disorders with gait ataxia, myopathy, neuropathy, and hysteria (44).

Balance is the ability to maintain an upright posture. It is essential for standing, sitting, turning, reaching, walking, and running. Balance is multifaceted and includes maintenance of posture and control of the center of gravity (52). The orderly process of maintaining balance requires at least the following: detecting body sway, determining appropriate corrective movements, and actively bringing the body back to a stable position (53). These steps require the integration of vestibular, visual, proprioceptive, tactile afferent systems, spinal and supraspinal integration of the incoming information, and appropriate activation of motor responses to meet these demands. Most of these actions are time-dependent, yet each of the sensory systems becomes less sensitive with age, and the motor systems are slower to respond (54). Taken together, elderly individuals, both women and men, show increasing body sway, a less secure base of support, and greater dependence on sensory cues from vision (55), vestibular, and somatosensory systems. Simoneau et al. (56) showed the importance of visual cues on postural steadiness in 55 to 70-year-old women. Some gender differences have only been observed in older subjects. For example, Wolfson et al. (57) found that older women performed poorly on the initial dynamic posturography trial, with inaccurate visual and somatosensory inputs, but by the third trial, they performed similarly to men. In addition to changing motor control, loss or alteration of multiple sensory inputs are an important contributor to the changes in balance that occur with increasing age (58).

Age Changes in Sensory Perception

Age changes in sensory perception occur along with those seen in the peripheral motor nerve. All senses may be affected, but the extent of deficit or rate of deterioration differs among sensory modalities. Gender differences have been found in the rate of loss of hearing. Increasing age is associated with a gradual sensorineural impairment in hearing that starts with the higher frequencies and involves the speech frequencies in older ages. Women tend to retain their hearing better with age than men, but by age 80, almost half of women have mild to moderate hearing losses. The cause of presbycusis (sensorineural hearing loss that occurs with age, independent of disease) is not entirely understood. Most interest has focused on the organ of Corti, where changes occur in the structure and function of the hair cells. Changes also occur in the efferent pathways, as reflected by changes in acoustic reflex. The acoustic reflex threshold measures the relative changes in middle ear compliance by reflexive contraction of the stapedius muscle to an auditory stimulus (59). At present, most of the deterioration is believed to be peripheral rather than central in origin. Four types of presbycusis have been described:

- *Sensory loss* begins in middle age and shows slow progression with a high-tone deficit. The primary pathology is atrophy of the organ of Corti.
- *Neural loss* occurs at any age and is characterized by poor speech discrimination compared to pure tone thresholds.
- *Vascular loss* occurs between the third and sixth decade and is progressive, resulting in a flat audio-

gram and preserved speech discrimination. The stria vascularis shows partial or diffuse atrophy.

- *Mechanical loss* is caused by loss of elasticity in the basilar membrane (60).

Vision appears to be more stable in the absence of pathology (cataracts, retinal degeneration), but changes in vision typically begin in the forties with the need for reading glasses, greater luminence and declines in contrast sensitivity. Analysis from the Longitudinal Study of Aging found that visual impairment in the elderly (average age 75 years) was associated with a 1.37 times probability of increasing disability in ADLs over a 4-year period, compared with subjects without visual impairment. In the same study, hearing impairment was associated with increased disability in ADLs (RR=1.34), but not after adjusting for chronic health conditions (e.g., hypertension, vascular disease, arthritis) and demographic variables (61). The causes of senile changes in vision are primarily related to the eye and include change in color of the cornea, cataracts, glaucoma, and retinal degeneration, diabetic retinopathy, and age-related declines in the pupil diameter. Neurologic disorders also include ischemic and compressive injuries to the optic and oculomotor nerves.

Changes in vision and hearing adversely affect physical and emotional stability in elderly women to a greater extent than men. Since women tend to outlive their spouses, they often live alone and become socially isolated. Hearing and visual losses compound the problem by restricting the elderly individual's ability to adapt to her environment, particularly when it changes. In some instances, increasing social interactions can have a positive effect on functional ability.

Age Changes in Cognition and Memory

Cognitive declines are frequent with aging, although some cognitive processes improve with healthy aging. For example, vocabulary scores on the Wechsler Adult Intelligence Scale continue to increase as individuals become 70 or even 80 years of age. Most cognitive processes show some decline. In particular, verbal and spatial memory functions tend to decline. In addition, there is a slowing in the time it takes for older subjects to search and retrieve memories, which is often referred to as bradyphrenia. Such slowing can adversely affect functional independence in IADLs and mobility and may limit driving ability.

The time course of cognitive performance has been found to differ between healthy subjects, and those who will subsequently develop Alzheimer's disease. In one study, Zonderman et al. (62) found that BLSA subjects who subsequently developed Alzheimer's disease began to show early measurable cognitive changes 10 to 20 years prior to the diagnosis. This suggests that transitions from normal to pathologic cognitive performance have a long and slow process.

Evidence from observational studies suggested that estrogen replacement therapy in postmenopausal women can be associated with improvements in memory, reaction time, attention, and a reduced risk for the development of Alzheimer's disease in postmenopausal women (63–67). However, results from the recent randomized trial, Women's Health Initiative Memory Study (WHIMS) did not find estrogen to be protective against cognitive changes or dementia (68–70). However, Henderson et al. (71) have found that early use of estrogen following menopause may be advantageous, a question not addressed in the WHIMS.

Hormones and Other Circulating Factors

Circulatory mediators act on muscle to maintain and modulate homeostasis. These include hormones, growth factors, inflammatory factors, and protein synthesis activators that function separately but not necessarily independently from the neuromuscular system. Hormones important to this process include growth hormone (72), corticosteroids (73), and androgenic steroids (74,75). These factors are important for the maintenance as well as hypertrophy and hyperplasia of the muscle, whereas the neuromuscular system is responsible for the movement. Phillips and colleagues (28) have recently noted that, as women go through menopause, the use of hormone replacement helps to maintain muscle strength. Currently, there is interest in the potential use of growth hormone to increase muscle strength in the elderly (76). Blackman et al. (102), in a randomized trial, found that, in women, growth hormone or growth hormone plus estrogen replacement increased lean body mass and decreased body fat, but did not affect strength or endurance. As more information becomes available, hormonal replacement strategies may prove useful in modulating functional loss in the elderly.

The interest in the role of inflammatory and blood clotting factors in the development of frailty has increased in recent years. A direct relationship has been observed between the level of serum inflammatory and clotting markers (e.g., C-reactive protein, factor VIII) and frailty status in the elderly (103). At what point in the process of frailty and sarcopenia that inflammation becomes important and is, at present, not known. The inflammatory process is likely to represent a set of common end pathways that are activated by a variety of disease processes. With advancing age, a decline in the body's capability to manage any deleterious effects from these pathways is likely impaired.

DISEASES

Many neurologic disorders can contribute to the development of frailty. The most common are stroke, dementia, and Parkinson's disease (77). Frailty can occur with any one of these processes, but as a general rule, these diseases represent only one part of a complex of health-related problems that lead to disability. The complexity can be seen in the factors that contribute to falls (78,79). Myers et al. (78), in a comprehensive review, list nine categories associated with falls, including general physical functioning; gait, balance, and physical performance; musculoskeletal and neuromuscular measures; demographic factors; sensory impairments; medical conditions; indicators of general health; medication; and psychologic, behavioral, social, and environmental factors. Although diseases, including stroke, dementia, and Parkinson's disease, are important to the occurrence of falls, the physician cannot restrict her investigations to just the medical issues to maximize the plan to prevent future falls. Similar issues occur for many of the frailty-related medical conditions that occur in elderly women.

Stroke

Stroke is a leading cause of disability in elderly women. The incidence and prevalence of stroke increase with age in both women and men. It is the third leading cause of death in people over age 65, and the second leading cause over 85 years of age. Throughout much of the twentieth century, the incidence and death rates have been on the decline, and the decline has been greatest in women (80). Increasing age is associated with a greater likelihood to develop a severe disability (81), and older individuals are at a higher risk to develop dementia than are stroke-free individuals of the same age (82). See also Chapter 17.

Depression

Depression is frequently seen in the elderly and has been reported in 12 to 15% of community-dwelling women and a higher percentage of nursing home patients (83). The dysphoric mood characteristic of depression is often not recognized or reported by elderly patients and can be characterized by subtle changes that are easily missed on examination. Part of the difficulty in its recognition is that depression in the aged is associated with increasing health, cognitive, and functional problems (84) that frequently mask the underlying dysphoric mood. The presence of depression can have a major contribution to frailty by impairing mobility, functional independence, and cognitive performance (85). The concurrence of depression and cognitive dysfunction can lead to a diagnosis of dementia, but with treatment, the cognitive dysfunction may reverse and produce a positive influence on functional disability. See also Chapter 31.

Dementia

Dementia is the most common cause of nursing home admission in elderly women. Associated with the cogni-

tive problems, functional disabilities become manifest in ADLs, IADLs, and mobility. Changes in mobility typically occur late, so that during early and moderate stages, the woman must be watched because of poor judgments in their actions, which can result in injuries to themselves and others. Such problems require close supervision from caregivers and eventually lead to nursing home placement. See also Chapter 30.

Parkinson's Disease

Parkinson's disease is another common neurologic condition that adversely affects functional independence in elderly women. The prevalence rate is about 2% of the elderly population, and 2.4% of women who have shown moderate or greater impairment in the Women's Health and Aging Study, and 7% for those women receiving help with ADLs (86). The diagnosis can be particularly difficult in elderly women who may have extrapyramidal features related to aging and is complicated by other health problems. Furthermore, the physical examination may underestimate or overestimate the functional capabilities of the Parkinson's disease patient. See also Chapter 23.

PREVENTION

The prevention of frailty in any woman requires addressing one or more factors that can contribute to the development of disability. Table 13.1 contains a partial list of these factors. Current directions in frailty prevention have focused on habits, diet, bone maintenance, fall prevention, and physical activity, but a number of other factors are equally important, including prevention and control of acute and chronic diseases.

Diet recommendations have focused primarily on cardiovascular risk through low fat diets, weight control, and dietary calcium. A low fat, calorically controlled, low salt diet can decrease heart disease, hypertension, and possibly stroke. The same diet can also reduce the risk for some cancers. Dietary calcium is important for bone maintenance and may decrease hip fracture risk. The current recommendation for dietary calcium for women has been increased to 1,500 mg. In elderly women, an added problem can be loss of appetite and malnutrition. The malnutrition can result from social problems including depression, isolation, and poverty. However, loss of the hunger drive and early satiety limit caloric intake, resulting in loss of body weight, protein, and lean body mass, and increasing frailty.

The role of hormonal replacement therapy (HRT) in postmenopausal women (see Chapter 12) has taken a dramatic change over the last several years. HRT was thought to be effective in decreasing the risk for cardiovascular diseases, improving the lipid profile, maintaining bone density with decreased risk of hip fracture, and decreasing the risk of Alzheimer's disease. Recent reports have found that estrogen with progesterone increases the risk for breast cancer, is associated with an increased risk of thrombosis, and does not protect against coronary artery disease. It has been shown to decrease the risk of hip fractures, although other treatments appear to be safer (104).

A growing body of literature shows the value of exercise and increased physical activity for the prevention of disability and frailty. Fiatarrone et al. (87,88) have demonstrated that exercise in 90-year-old nursing home residents can lead to significant improvements in mobility and self-care. Exercise programs using both aerobic and resistive (weight lifting) methods have been shown to have in community-dwelling elderly women and men (89–91) a positive impact on quality of life and improvement in cardiovascular fitness (92). Furthermore, exercise leads to an overall increase in quality of life and well-being. Neither improvement in strength nor cardiovascular fitness are required for an exercise program to improve quality of life, as has been seen with the use of tai chi (93) and yoga (92). None of these approaches leads to overly trained elderly, but rather they help to maintain a woman at minimal to moderate strength levels while promoting independence. The key is to encourage physical activity at all ages. Increasing physical activity leads to improved mobility, independence, and quality of life. Prolonged bed rest without physical therapy adversely affects muscle strength and tone, particularly in the elderly. Early rehabilitation should be considered by the neurologist and other health providers in planning care for the wide range of neurologic problems that beset the elderly.

Smoking, alcohol, and drug abuse can have a negative health impact that increases the susceptibility to disease, decreases recovery, and increases disability and frailty. Smoking has declined in the United States over the past 30 years, but many individuals continue with this habit. Likewise, alcohol abuse leads to increased rates of liver disease and to traumatic injuries across the age span. Strategies exist for overcoming each problem, but these programs are only partially successful.

Injury is a major contributor to disability and frailty. The elderly have a high incidence of falling, particularly on uneven surfaces and in decreasing light. Stairways and high shag rugs can be a particular problem. Stopping driving leads to a marked dependence on others in our mobile society, and disproportionately occurs in women. Six conditions lead to about half of the decisions to stop driving: macular degeneration, retinal hemorrhage, ADL deficits, Parkinson's disease, stroke, and syncope (94). Driving injuries, although not necessarily more frequent in the elderly, can have devastating effects. The elderly often have limitations because of slower reaction times and poorer vision and hearing, and thus drive at slower speeds and in a more cautious manner. This can be dangerous when they are unable to keep up with the flow of traffic. The elderly often have trouble driving at night and particularly at dusk, when glare becomes a major problem—automobiles and roads are not designed with the elderly in mind.

SUMMARY

Frailty is a common problem that adversely affects elderly women. Age is a particularly important contributor that lowers the reserve capacity of most body systems and decreases a woman's ability to overcome the disability caused by chronic diseases (18). Many disease processes contribute to the development of frailty, but management also must consider psychologic, social, and environmental factors that can adversely affect functional capability. Changes in neurologic function are frequent and important contributors to the development of frailty in elderly women. Some neurologic changes are directly related to aging and (at least at present) cannot be prevented. The adverse effects of neurologic aging can be modified through a healthy lifestyle including exercise, diet, weight control, and environmental adaptations. The prevention and management of neurologic diseases can limit functional disability and the necessity of nursing home placement.

References

1. Hetzel L, Smith A. The 65 years and over population: 2000. *U.S. Census Bureau Brief C2KBR/01-10*, 2001.
2. LaPlante MP. Disability in basic life activities across the life span. *National Institute on Disability and Rehabilitation Research. Disability Statistics Report* 1, 1991.
3. Hadley EC, Ory MG, Suzman R, Weindruch R. Foreward. *J Gerontol* 1993;48(special issue):vii-viii.
4. World Health Organization. *International classification of impairments, disabilities, and handicaps.* Geneva: World Health Organization, 1980.
5. Fozard JL, Metter EJ, Brant LJ. Next steps in describing aging and disease in longitudinal studies. *J Gerontol Med Sci* 1990;45:P116–127.
6. Verbrugge LM. The twain meet: empirical explanations of sex differences in health and mortality. *J Health Soc Behav* 1989;30:282–304.
7. Brant LJ, Fozard JL. Age change in pure-tone hearing thresholds in a longitudinal study of normal human aging. *J Acoust Soc Am* 1990;88:813–820.
8. Pearson JD, Morrell CH, Gordon-Salant S, et al. Gender differences in a longitudinal study of age-associated hearing loss. *J Acoust Soc Am* 1995;97:1196–1205.
9. Larsson L, Grimby G, Karlsson J. Muscle strength and speed of movement in relation to age and muscle morphology. *J Appl Physiol* 1979;46:451–456.
10. Mathiowetz V, Kashman N, Volland G, Weber K, Dowe M, Rogers S. Grip and pinch strength: normative data for adults. *Arch Phys Med Rehabil* 1985;66:69–74.

11. Kallman EA, Plato CC, Tobin JD. The role of muscle loss in the age-related decline of grip strength: cross-sectional and longitudinal perspectives. *J Gerontol Med Sci* 1990; 45:M82–88.

12. Christ CB, Boileau RA, Slaughter MH, Stillman RJ, Cameron JA, Massey BH. Maximal voluntary isometric force production characteristics of six muscle groups in women aged 25 to 74 years. *Am J Human Biol* 1992; 4:537–545.

13. Vandervoort AA, McComas AJ. Contractile changes in opposing muscles of the human ankle joint with age. *J Appl Physiol* 1986;61:361–367.

14. Fugl-Meyer AR, Gustafsson L, Burstedt Y. Isokinetic and static plantar flexion characteristics. *Eur J Appl Physiol* 1980;45:221–234.

15. Clement FJ. Longitudinal and cross-sectional assessments of age changes in physical strength as related to sex, social class, and mental ability. *J Gerontol* 1974; 29:423–429.

16. Stanley SN, Taylor NAS. Isokinematic muscle mechanics in four groups of women of increasing age. *Eur J Appl Physiol* 1993;66:178–184.

17. Borges O. Isometric and isokinetic knee extension and flexion torque in men and women aged 20-70. *Scand J Rehab Med* 1989;21:45–53.

18. Pendergast DR, Fisher NM, Calkins E. Cardiovascular, neuromuscular, and metabolic alterations with age leading to frailty. *J Gerontol* 1993;48(special issue):61–67.

19. Dutta C, Hadley EC. The significance of sarcopenia in old age. *J Gerontol Series A* 50(special issue):1995;1–5.

20. Larsson L, Sjodin B, Karlsson J. Histochemical and biochemical changes in human skeletal muscle with age in sedentary males, age 22-65 years. *Acta Physiol Scand* 1978;103:31–39.

21. Larsson L, Edstrom L. Effects of age on enzyme-histochemcial fibre spectra and contractile porperties of fast- and slow-twitch skeletal muscles in the rat. *J Neurol Sci* 1986;76:69–89.

22. Lexell J, Henriksson-Larsen K, Winblad B, Sjostorom M. Distribution of different fiber types in human skeletal muscles: effects of aging studied in whole muscle cross sections. *Muscle Nerve* 1983;95:142–154.

23. Essen-Gustavsson B, Borges O. Histochemical and metabolic characteristics of human skeletal muscle in relation to age. *Acta Physiol Scand* 1986;126:107–114.

24. Lexell J, Taylor CC, Sjostrom M. What is the cause of the ageing atrophy? Total number, size and proportion of different fibre types studied in whole vastus lateralis muscle from 15-83-years-old men. *J Neurol Sci* 1988;84: 275–294.

25. Gollnick PD, Armstrong RB, Saubert IV CW, Piehl K, Saltin B. Enzyme activity and fiber composition in skeletal muscle of untrained and trained men. *J Appl Physiol* 1972;33:312–319.

26. Staron RS, Hikidi RS, Hagerman FC, Dudley GA, Murray TF. Human skeletal muscle fiber type adaptability to various workloads. *J Histochem Cytochem* 1984;32: 146–152.

27. Shock NW, Gruelich RC, Andres RA, et al. *Normal human aging. The Baltimore Longitudinal Study of Aging.* Washington, DC: U.S. Government Printing Office, 1984.

28. Phillips SK, Rook KM, Siddle NC, Bruce SA, Woledge RC. Muscle weakness in women occurs at an earlier age than in men, but strength is preserved by hormone replacement therapy. *Clin Sci* 1993;84:95–98.

29. Wagman IH, Lesse H. Maximum conduction velocities of motor fibers of ulnar nerve in human subjects of various ages and size. *J Neurophysiol* 1952;15: 235–242.

30. Norris AH, Shock NW, Wagman IH. Age changes in the maximum conduction velocity of motor fibers of human ulnar nerves. *J Appl Physiol* 1953;5:589–593.

31. Campbell MJ, McComas AJ, Petito F. Physiological changes in aging muscles. *J Neurol Neurosurg Psychiat* 1972;35:845–852.

32. Brown WF, Strong MJ, Snow R. Methods for estimating numbers of motor units in biceps-brachialis muscles and losses of motor units with aging. *Muscle Nerve* 1988;11:423–432.

33. Doherty TJ, Brown WF. The estimated numbers and relative sizes of thenar motor units as selected by multiple point stimulation in young and older adults. *Muscle Nerve* 1993;16:355–366.

34. Doherty TJ, Vandervoort AA, Brown WF. Effects of aging on the motor unit: a brief review. *Can J Appl Physiol* 1993;18:331–358.

35. Buller AJ, Eccles JC, Eccles RM. Interaction between motoneurones and muscles in respect of the characteristic speeds of their responses. *J Physiol* 1960;150:417–439.

36. Fozard JL, Vercruyssen M, Reynolds SL, Hancock PA, Quilter RE. Age differences and changes in reaction time: The Baltimore Longitudinal Study of Aging. *J Gerontol Psychol Sci* 1994;49:179–189.

37. Brogmus GE. Effects of age and gender on speed and accuracy of hand movements and the refinements they suggest for Fitt's Law. Unpublished Masters' thesis, University of California, 1991.

38. Morgan M, Phillips JG, Bradshaw JL, Mattingley JB, Iansek R, Bradshaw JA. Age-related motor slowness: simple strategic? *J Gerontol Med Sci* 1994;49:M133–139.

39. Lundgren-Lindquist B, Aniansson A, Rundgren Å. Functional studies in 79-year-olds. III. Walking performance and climbing capacity. *Scand J Rehabil Med* 1983;15: 125–131.

40. Tinetti ME, Speechley M. Prevention of falls among the elderly. *N Engl J Med* 1989;320:1055–1059.

41. Guralnik JM, Ferrucci L, Simonsick EM, Salive ME, Wallace RB. Lower-extremity function in persons over the age of 70 years as a predictor of subsequent disability. *N Engl J Med* 1995;332:556–561.

42. Imms FJ, Edholm OG. Studies of gait and mobility in the elderly. *Age Aging* 1981;10:147–156.

43. Hageman PA, Blanke DJ. Comparison of gait of young women and elderly women. *Physical Therapy* 1986;66: 1382–1387.

44. Rubino FA. Gait disorders in the elderly: distinguishing between normal and dysfunctional gait. *Postgraduate Med* 1993;93:185–190.

45. Wolfson L, Whipple R, Amerman P, Tobin JN. Gait assessment in the elderly: a gait abnormality rating scale and its relation to falls. *J Gerontol Med Sci* 1990;45: M12–M19.

46. Sudarsky L, Ronthal M. Gait disorders among elderly patients. *Arch Neurol* 1983;40:740–743.

47. Alexander NB. Gait disorders in older adults. *J Am Geriatr Soc* 1996;44:434–451.

48. Bassey EJ, Bendall MJ, Pearson M. Muscle strength in the triceps surae and objectively measured customary walking activity in men and women over 65 years of age. *Clin Sci* 1988;74:85–89.

49. Wong DF, Wagner H, Dannals R, et al. Effects of age on dopamine and serotonin receptors measured by positron

tomography in the living human brain. *Science* 1984; 226:1391–1395.

50. Antonini A, Leenders KL, Reist H, Thomann R, Beer HF, Locher J. Effect of age on D2 dopamine receptors in normal human brain measured by positron emission tomography and 11C-raclopride. *Arch Neurol* 1993;50:474–480.

51. Joseph JA, Roth GS. Hormonal regulation of motor behavior in senescence. *J Gerontol* 1993;48 (Spec No):51–55.

52. King MB, Judge JO, Wolfson L. Functional base of support decreases with age. *J Gerontol: Med Sci* 1994;49: M258–M263.

53. Quoniam C, Hay L, Roll JP, Harlay F. Age effects on reflex and postural responses to propriomuscular inputs generated by tendon vibration. *J Gerontol Biol Sci* 1995; 50A:B155–B165.

54. Era P, Schroll M, Ytting H, Gause-Nilsson I, Heikkinen E, Steen B. Postural balance and its sensory-motor correlates in 75-year-old men and women: A cross-national comparative study. *J Gerontol Med Sci* 1996;51A:M53–M63.

55. Sundermier L, Woollacott MH, Jensen JL, Moore S. Postural sensitivity to visual flow in aging adults with and without balance problems. *J Gerontol Med Sci* 1996; 51A:M45–M52.

56. Simoneau GG, Leibowitz HW, Ulbrecht JS, Tyrrell RA, Cavanagh PR. The effects of visual factors and head orientation on postural steadiness in women 55 to 70 years of age. *J Gerontol Med Sci* 1992;47:M151–M158.

57. Wolfson L, Whipple R, Derby CA, Amerman P, Nashner L. Gender differences in the balance of healthy elderly as demonstrated by dynamic posturography. *J Gerontol Med Sci* 1994;49:M160–M167.

58. Teasdale N, Stelmach GE, Breunig A. Postural sway characteristics of the elderly under normal and altered visual and support surface conditions. *J Gerontol Biol Sci* 1991;B238–B244.

59. Moller MB. Audiological evaluation. *J Clin Neurophysiol* 1994;11:309–318.

60. Fisch L, Brooks DN. Disorders of hearing. In: Brocklehurst JC, Tallis RC, Fillit HM, (eds.) *Textbook of geriatric medicine and gerontology*, 4th ed. Edinburgh: Churchill Livingstone, 1992;480–493.

61. Rudberg MA, Furner SE, Dunn JE, Cassel CK. The relationship of visual and hearing impairments to disability: an analysis using the Longitudinal Study of Aging. *J Gerontol Med Sci* 1993;48:M261–M265.

62. Zonderman AB, Giambra LM, Arenberg D, Resnick S, Costa PT Jr, Kawas CH. Changes in immediate visual memory predict cognitive impairment. *Arch Clin Neuropsychol* 1995;10:111–123.

63. Paganini-Hill A, Henderson VW. Estrogen deficiency and risk of Alzheimer's disease in women. *Amer J Epidemiol* 1994;140:256–261.

64. Henderson VW, Paganini-Hill A, Emanuel CK, Dunn ME, Buckwalter JG. Estrogen replacement therapy in older women: comparison between Alzheimer's disease cases and nondemented control subjects. *Arch Neurol* 1994;51:896–900.

65. Tang MX, Jacobs D, Stern Y, et al. Effect of oestrogen during menopause on risk and age at onset of Alzheimer's disease. *Lancet* 1996;17;348:429–432.

66. Kawas C, Resnick S, Morrison A, et al. A prospective study of estrogen replacement therapy and the risk of developing Alzheimer's disease: The Baltimore Longitudinal Study of Aging. *Neurology* 1997;48:1517–1521.

67. Resnick SM, Metter EJ, Zonderman AB. Estrogen replacement therapy and longitudinal decline in visual memory: A possible protective effect? *Neurology* 1997;49:1491–1497.

68. Rapp SR, Espeland MA, Shumaker SA, et al.; WHIMS Investigators. Effect of estrogen plus progestin on global cognitive function in postmenopausal women: the Women's Health Initiative Memory Study: a randomized controlled trial. *JAMA* 2003;289(20):2663–2672.

69. Shumaker SA, Legault C, Keller L, et al.; Women's Health Initiative Memory Study. Conjugated equine estrogens and incidence of probable dementia and mild cognitive impairment in postmenopausal women: Women's Health Initiative Memmory Study. *JAMA* 2004;291)24):2947–2958.

70. Espeland MA, Rapp SR, Shumaker SA. Conjugated equine estrogens and global congnitive function in postmenopausal women: Women's Health Initiative Memory Study. JAMA 2004;291:2859–2968.

71. Henderson VW, Benke KS, Green RC, Cupples LA, Farrer LA for the MIRAGE Study Group. Postmenopausal hormone therapy and Alzheimer's disease risk: interaction with age. *J Neurol Neurosurg Psychiatry* 2005;76:103–1154.

72. Corpas E, Harman SM, Blackman MR. Human growth hormone and human aging. *Endo Rev* 1993;14:20–39.

73. Rebuffe-Scrive M, Krotkiewski M, Elfverson J, Bjorntopr P. Muscle and adipose tissue morphology and metabolism in Cushing's syndrome. *J Clin Endocrinol Metab* 1988;67:1122–1128.

74. Gutmann E, Hanzlikova V. Effect of androgens on histochemical fibretype. Differentiation in temporal muscle of the guinea pig. *Histochem* 1970;24:287–291.

75. Krotkiewski M, Kral JG, Karlsson J. Effects of castration and testosterone substitution on body composition and muscle metabolism in rats. *Acta Physiol Scand* 1980; 109:233–237.

76. Rudman D, Feller AG, Nagraj HS, et al. Effects of human growth hormone in men over 60 years old. *N Engl J Med* 1990;323:1–6.

77. Rockwood K, Stolee P, McDowell I. Factors associated with institutionalization of older people in Canada: testing a multifactorial definition of frailty. *J Am Geriatr Soc* 1996;44:578–582.

78. Myers AH, Young Y, Langlois JA. Prevention of falls in the elderly. *Bone* 1996;18(suppl):87S–101S.

79. Tinetti M, Speechley M, Ginter SF. Risk factors for falls among elderly persons living in the community. *N Engl J Med* 1988;319:1701–1707.

80. Garraway WM, Whisnant JP, Furlan AJ, et al. The declining incidence of stroke. *N Engl J Med* 1979;300: 449–452.

81. Pohjasvaara T, Erkinjuntti T, Vataja R, Kaste M. Comparison of stroke features and disability in daily life in patiens with ischemic stroke aged 55 to 70 and 71 to 85 years. *Stroke* 1997;28:729–735.

82. Prencipe M, Ferretti C, Casini AR, Santini M, Giubilei F, Culasso F. Stroke, disability, and dementia: results of a population survey. *Stroke* 1997;28:531–536.

83. Bond J. Psychiatric illness in later life. A study of prevalence in a Scottish population. *Int J Geriatr Psychiatry* 1987;2:39–57.

84. Blazer D, Burchett B, Service C, George LK. The association of age and depression among the elderly: an epidemiologic exploration. *J Gerontol Med Sci* 1991;46: M210–M215.

85. Wells KB, Stewart A, Hays RD, et al. The functioning and well-being of depressed patients: results from the Medical Outcomes Study. *JAMA* 1989;261:914–919.

86. Ferrucci L, Kittner S, Corti MC, Guralnik JM. Neurologic conditions. The women's health and aging study. National Institutes of Health, *NIH Publication* 95-4009, 1995;140–145.

87. Fiatarone MH, Mark SEC, Ryan ND, Meredith CN, Lipsitz LA, Evans WJ. High intensity strength training in nonagenarians. *JAMA* 1990;263:3029–3034.

88. Fiatarone MA, O'Neill EF, Ryan ND, et al. Exercise training and nutritional supplementation for physical frailty in very elderly people. *N Engl J Med* 1994;330: 1769–1775.

89. Svanborg A. A medical-social intervention in a 70-year-old Swedish population: is it possible to postpone functional decline in aging? *J Gerontol* 1993;48(special issue):84–88.

90. Morey MC, Cowper PA, Feussener JR, DiPasquale RC, Crowley GM, Sullivan RJ Jr. Two-year trends in physical performance following supervised exercise among community-dwelling older veterans. *J Am Geriatr Soc* 1991;39:549–554.

91. McCartney N, Hicks AL, Martin J, Webber CE. Long-term resistance training in the elderly: effects on dynamic strength, exercise capacity, muscle, and bone. *J Gerontol Biol Sci* 1995;50A:B97–B104.

92. Blumenthal JA, Emery CF, Madden DJ, et al. Cardiovascular and behavioral effects of aerobic exercise training in healthy older men and women. *J Gerontol Med Sci* 1989;44:M147–M157.

93. Wolf SL, Barnhart HX, Kutner NF, McNeely E, Coogler C, Xu T, and the Atlanta FICSIT Group. Reducing frailty and fals in older persons: an investigation of Tai Chi and computerized balance training. *J Am Geriatr Soc* 1996; 44:489–497.

94. Campbell MK, Bush TL, Hale WE. Medical conditions associated with driving cessation in community-dwelling ambulatory elders. *J Gerontol Soc Sci* 1993;48:S230–S234.

95. Ally A. Ventrolateral medullary control of cardiovascular activity during muscle contraction. *Neurosci Biobehav Rev* 1998;23:65–86.

96. Kwon IS, Oldaker S, Schrager M, Talbot LA, Fozard JL, Metter EJ. The relationship between muscle strength and the time taken to complete a standardized walk-turn-walk test. *J Gerontol Biol Sci* 2001;56A:B398–B404.

97. Buchner DM, deLateur BJ. The importance of skeletal muscle strength to physical function in older adults. *Ann Behav Med* 1991;13:91–98.

98. Baumgartner RN, Koehler KM, Gallagher D, et al. Epidemiology of sarcopenia among the elderly in New Mexico. *Am J Epid* 1998;147:755–763.

99. Conwit RA, Metter EJ. Age related changes in peripheral and central conduction. In: Brown WF, Bolton CF, Aminoff MJ, (eds.) *Neuromuscular function and disease, basic, clinical and electrodiagnostic aspects*. New York, NY: Saunders, 2002;602–617.

100. Metter EJ, Conwit R, Metter B, Pacheco T, Tobin J. The relationship of peripheral motor nerve conduction velocity to age-associated loss of grip strength. *Aging Clin Exp Res* 1998;10:471–478.

101. van Dyck CH, Seibyl JP, Malison RT, et al. Age-related decline in dopamine transporters, analysis of striatal subregions, nonlinear effects, and hemispheric asymmetries. *Am J Geriatr Psychiatry* 2002;10:36–43.

102. Blackman MR, Sorkin JD, Munzer T, et al. Growth hormone and sex steroid administration in healthy aged women and men, a randomized controlled trial. *JAMA* 2002;288:2282–2292.

103. Walston J, McBurnie MA, Newman A, et al. Frailty and activation of the inflammation and coagulation systems with and without clinical comorbidities: results form the Cardiovascular Health Study. *Arch Intern Med* 2002; 162:2333–2341.

104. Nelson HD, Humphrey LL, Nygren P, Teutsch SM, Allan JD. Postmenopausal hormone replacement therapy: scientific review. *JAMA* 2002;288:872–881.

105. Metter EJ, Conwit R, Metter B, Pacheco T, Tobin J. The relationship of peripheral motor nerve conduction velocity to age-associated loss of grip strength. *Aging Clin Exp Res* 1998;10:471–478.

III

NEUROLOGIC DISORDERS
IN WOMEN

14 Migraine

Ramesh K. Khurana, MD, FAAN, FAHS

Simply put, migraine is an episodic headache with or without aura. In women, it is often associated with menstruation, frequently remits during pregnancy, and sometimes decreases following menopause. In reality, however, there is nothing simple about this disorder, and a precise definition is somewhat elusive. Clinically, it is not a biphasic neural and/or vascular disorder, but a multiphasic disorder with cerebral and systemic components. Pathophysiologically, genetics and plasma serotonin may differ between migraine with and without aura, raising doubts about whether these are two true subtypes of the same entity. The number and location of the migraine generators and modulators in the central nervous system (CNS) are subject to debate. The influence of female sex hormones on migraine is undisputed, but how female hormones influence migraine is incompletely understood.

DEFINITION

Moritz H. Romberg (1853) described hemicrania or "la migrène," including premonitory symptoms, headache characteristics, aggravating and relieving factors, associated autonomic and somatic features, and postictal state (1). In 1988, Gowers defined migraine as "an affliction characterized by paroxysmal nervous disturbance, of which headache is the most constant element. The pain is seldom absent...commonly accompanied by nausea and vomiting; and it is often preceded by some disorder of the sense of sight. The symptoms are frequently one-sided" (2).

A standard definition was necessary. Based partly on symptomatology and partly on assumed pain mechanisms, the Ad Hoc Committee on Classification of Headaches (1962) included migraine (classic, common, hemiplegic, ophthalmoplegic, and lower-half headache), along with cluster, toxic-vascular, and hypertensive headaches under the rubric of vascular headache. Migraine was therefore too loosely defined as "recurrent attacks of headache, widely varied in intensity, frequency, and duration, commonly unilateral in onset, usually associated with anorexia, sometimes with nausea and vomiting; and some are preceded by, or associated with, conspicuous sensory, motor, and mood disturbances; and are often familial." The terms *classic* and *common* were subsequently confused with the terms *typical* and *most prevalent* respectively (3).

The International Headache Society classification system for headache, developed in 1988 and revised in 2004, proposed a hierarchically constructed classification (Table 14.1). Cluster headache was designated as a separate major category, whereas *common migraine* was replaced by "migraine without aura," and *classic migraine*, by "migraine with aura" (4). Migraine was classified into six subtypes:

TABLE 14.1
International Classification of Migraine

1.1 Migraine without aura
1.2 Migraine with aura
    1.2.1 Typical aura with migraine headache
    1.2.2 Typical aura with non-migraine headache
    1.2.3 Typical aura without headache
    1.2.4 Familial hemiplegic migraine (FHM)
    1.2.5 Sporadic hemiplegic migraine
    1.2.6 Basilar-type migraine
1.3 Childhood periodic syndromes that are commonly precursors of migraine
    1.3.1 Cyclical vomiting
    1.3.2 Abdominal migraine
    1.3.3 Benign paroxysmal vertigo of childhood
1.4 Retinal migraine
1.5 Complications of migraine
    1.5.1 Chronic migraine
    1.5.2 Status migrainosus
    1.5.3 Persistent aura without infarction
    1.5.4 Migrainous infarction
    1.5.5 Migraine-triggered seizure
1.6 Probable migraine
    1.6.1 Probable migraine without aura
    1.6.2 Probable migraine with aura
    1.6.3 Probable chronic migraine

Migraine without aura, per International Headache Society (IHS) classification, is defined as five or more headache attacks of 4 to 72 hours in duration. The headache has at least two of the following four characteristics: unilateral location, pulsating quality, moderate or severe intensity, and aggravation by physical activity. The headache is associated with one or more of the following: nausea, vomiting, photophobia, and phonophobia. Under IHS classification, migraine with aura should have at least two attacks with fully reversible aura symptoms of focal cerebral and/or brainstem dysfunction. Aura symptoms should develop gradually over more than 4 minutes and last no more than 60 minutes, and headache should follow, with a free interval of less than 60 minutes. In both types of migraines, structural disease should be excluded clinically or by neuroimaging studies.

These operational diagnostic criteria improved the reliability of migraine diagnosis for research purposes but were believed to be too complex and too restrictive to be used by primary care physicians (5,6). Furthermore, the IHS definitions of migraine imply that it is only a uniphasic or biphasic disorder with gastrointestinal symptoms.

CLINICAL FEATURES

For more than a century, clinical investigators have observed that migraine involves a widespread dysfunction of the central and autonomic nervous systems and other systems as well (1,2). Among the clinical features of migraine, Kinnier Wilson included anxiety, a "twilight state," incoherence, anger and violence, behavior change from reserve to loquacity, vasovagal fits, pseudoangina, and palpitations (7). Wolff noted that headache is but part of a widespread disturbance that includes abdominal distension, cold cyanosed extremities, vertigo, tremors, pallor, dryness of the mouth, excessive sweating, and "chilliness" (8). Selby suggested that migraine has three phases: aura or prodromal phase, headache, and post-headache phase (9). Blau recognized five phases of migraine: premonitory symptoms, aura, headache and associated symptoms, sleep resolution, and recovery phase (10). Recently, Barbiroli, Montagna, and colleagues have demonstrated abnormal muscle mitochondrial function in patients with migraine, suggesting a systemic component (11,12).

Premonitory symptoms may occur in migraine with or without aura and may precede the headache attack by several hours or days. The incidence of these symptoms varies from 12 to 88% in different studies (13). The symptoms are usually brought out by careful questioning. The range of premonitory symptoms is large, but a particular set of symptoms may be characteristic for the individual patient. These symptoms include psychic disturbances, gastrointestinal manifestations, and changes in fluid balance. The patient usually experiences a sullen mood and depression, but elation and associated hyperactivity may occur. Other psychic disturbances include irritability, impaired concentration, poor judgment, impulsivity, and altered behavior. Physical and emotional fatigue are common. Gastrointestinal symptoms include loss of appetite, increased appetite with a craving for sweet foods, and altered bowel frequency. Patients may feel inappropriately cold, yawn excessively, and feel drowsy. An increase in weight, occasionally up to 17 pounds, with or without signs of generalized edema, and altered urinary frequency have been noted. Wolff's attempts at precipitating migraine by inducing weight gain and preventing migraine by reducing weight were without success (8–10,13–15).

The various aura symptoms may occur in isolation, in succession, or in various combinations. Visual symptoms are more frequent (99%), followed by sensory (31%), aphasic (18%), and motor (6%) symptoms (16). Visual symptoms may occur alone or with other aura symptoms. The aura symptoms commonly display the following characteristics: positive symptoms followed by negative symptoms, gradual onset, gradual spread, persistence for a duration, and reversibility. Visual symptoms start at or near the center of fixation as flickering zig-zag lines (positive symptom); march toward the periphery of one hemifield, increasing in size and shape; and leave behind a scotoma (negative symptom) (16). Lashley mapped the progress of his own scotomas as they drifted toward the periphery of the visual field at a rate of 3 mm/min (17). Visual symptoms are usually homonymous and symmetric in both eyes. Focal paraesthesias and numbness usually develop in the fingers and ascend over minutes to the hands and forearm before involving the circumoral region, including both sides of the tongue (Cheiro-oral syndrome of Bruyn). The upper arm, shoulder, side of the nose, and face are usually spared. Examination when symptoms are present demonstrates the impairment of touch and pain whereas proprioception, discriminative sensation, and stereognosis are rarely involved, suggesting the thalamus as a possible site of origin. Speech disturbances may occur as the spreading paraesthesias reach the face or the tongue. The typical motor aura affects the hand and arm. Other aura manifestations include neglect, alexia, acalculia, anxiety, depersonalization, automatic behavior, and gustatory hallucinations (9,17).

When aura symptoms appear to be of brainstem or bilateral occipital lobe origin, the term *basilar migraine* is used. This entity, originally described by Bickerstaff (18,19), includes two or more of the following aura symptoms: bilateral visual symptoms affecting temporal and nasal fields, dysarthria, vertigo, tinnitus, decreased hearing, diplopia, ataxia, bilateral paraesthesias, bilateral paresis, and a decreased level of consciousness (19).

The visual, sensory, or aphasic auras usually last less than 60 minutes, whereas the motor aura has a mean duration of 13 ± 18 hours. When the aura symptoms last from 1 hour to 1 week and neuroimaging is normal, the term prolonged aura migraine is applied. Familial hemiplegic migraine is a variety of *prolonged aura migraine* in which some degree of hemiparesis may be prolonged and at least one first-degree relative has identical attacks (18).

The next phase of migraine begins with headache after several hours of premonitory symptoms or after an aura. Pain, hemicranial or holocranial, increases slowly in intensity, reaches a peak, lasts for several hours, and then recedes slowly. Nausea and photophobia are the most frequently associated symptoms (13). Graham has aptly described this phase of migraine: "its talismans are the iceberg and emesis basin; its habitat, the silent, darkened room with the shades down; its victim, the pallid, sweating, prostrate, pain-wracked sufferer" (20). Various neurologic symptoms associated with this phase include photophobia, sonophobia, generalized irritability, hypersensitivity to smell, yawning, temperature lability, diarrhea, slowed pulse rate, polyuria, blurred vision, and sluggish thought processes (9,10,20). Violent pains in the limbs are not rare; these pains may be ipsilateral to headache or alternating sides (7,21).

A disturbance of alertness during the headache phase extends into the sleep resolution phase, and sleep helps resolve the attack (10). Gowers observed that the termination of headache paroxysm is attended not only by vomiting but also by copious diuresis or perspiration (2). The recovery phase may be characterized by anorexia, tiredness, yawning, mood changes, diuresis, prostration, and malaise (9,10).

PATHOPHYSIOLOGY

Migraine is a multiphasic, "episodic," and self-limited neurophysiologic disorder. No current hypothesis of its pathophysiology explains all migrainous phenomena. Progress in the last decade suggests that it may be a combination of genetic susceptibility with a superimposed influence of internal and external factors.

What constitutes genetic susceptibility is not clear; altered cortical function, impaired hypothalamic function, pain dysmodulation, abnormal vascular reactivity, neuro-vegetative dysfunction, or a combination of these or other factors have been suggested. A tendency to develop migraine shows familial aggregation, as pointed out by Liveing as early as 1873 (22). This observation has been supported by the most recent genetic research. Twin studies show a higher concordance for migraine in monozygotic twins than in dizygotic twins (23). Familial studies reveal that the first-degree family members of probands of migraine with aura show nearly four times the risk of migraine with aura, and first-degree family members of probands with migraine without aura show an increased risk of both migraine without aura (1.9 quotient) and migraine with aura (1.4 quotient) (24,25). The discovery of a genetic locus for certain patients with familial hemiplegic migraine on chromosome 19p13 has rekindled interest in the genetics of migraine. (23) Other susceptibility loci for familial hemiplegic migraine have been identified on chromosomes 1q21–q23 and 1q31. The loci for migraine with and without aura have been mapped to 19p13, x q24–28, 4q24, 6 p12.2–p21.1, and 14q 21.2–14q 22.3. (26–28). Unfortunately, the confounding variables of a wide range of age of onset, chance occurrence due to a high incidence in the general population, and the lack of a biological marker have affected the studies.

The migrainous brain has been extensively studied between attacks. Changes in electrophysiology, metabolism, and blood flow in the cerebral cortex; neurophysiologic changes in the brainstem; and overexcitation in the trigeminal pathways have been noted and are summarized in this paragraph. A higher amplitude and prolonged latency of visual evoked potentials and an increased amplitude of the contingent negative variation, which fails to habituate, have been interpreted as evidence for the increased excitability of the occipital cortex (29–32). Magnetoencephalographic studies have shown the presence of large-amplitude wave forms over the temporal-parietal-occipital region (33). Magnetic resonance spectroscopy has disclosed low magnesium and a low phosphocreatine content, accompanied by high adenosine diphosphate concentration (34,35). In 1996, Facco and colleagues demonstrated abnormal regional cerebral blood flow in patients with migraine (36). Brainstem auditory evoked responses displayed a significant increase of side differences of all peak latencies except IV and V in migraine patients compared with controls, suggesting impairment of brainstem functions (27). Drummond and Lance observed frequent occurrence of ice-pick pains in migraine patients coincident with the site of the customary headache, indicating excessive activation of trigeminal pathways (38).

Two theories of migraine pathophysiology, vascular and neurogenic, were proposed more than a century ago. Vascular distension as the primary cause of headache was described by Willis (39). The vascular theory considers vasomotor disturbance as a primary event, with early symptoms being due to arterial spasm, and headache then being due to the subsequent dilatation and inflammation of cephalic vessels. This theory gained prominence by the 1930s, when Wolff and associates reported the amelioration of the aura with inhalation of carbon dioxide or amyl nitrite, suggesting the role of intracranial vasoconstriction in the production of aura. Furthermore, ergotamine terminated the migraine headache by vasoconstricting the dilated extracranial vessels. They postulated vascular dilatation in the branches of the external carotid artery, including the middle meningeal artery, increased capillary hydrostatic pressure, and the release of pain threshold-lowering substances such as bradykinin and prostaglandins into perivascular tissues. Although observations by Wolff added weight to the vascular hypothesis, he did not conceive migraine as a dichotomy, but saw the headache as a late phenomenon in a cascade of neurologic and biochemical events (8). Heyck suggested that during the headache phase, blood was shunted away from the cutaneous capillaries directly into veins by deeply situated arterial-venous anastomosis. In support of this idea, he demonstrated high levels of oxygen saturation in jugular venous blood during attacks (40). Goadsby and colleagues demonstrated the simultaneous occurrence of constriction in the cerebral vessels and dilatation in the extracranial vessels secondary to the stimulation of the ipsilateral locus coeruleus (41). Vascular involvement in migraine headaches is still implicated in the painful phase of migraine, but it is now considered a secondary event to the neuronal process. Moskowitz has suggested that the antidromic release of substance P

and other neuropeptides from trigeminal nerve terminals may cause pain and vasodilatation in the head (42).

Liveing proposed the neurogenic hypothesis, which states that "nerve-storm" is a primary event and that vasomotor disturbance is of secondary origin (22). Gowers supported this view because of the localized involvement of the same region of the brain each time and because of the simultaneous occurrence of symptoms attributable to excitation and inhibition (2). Recent studies of aura, trigeminal-vascular mechanisms, and serotonin agonists have revived the neurogenic hypothesis.

Three years after Lashley plotted the progression of his own visual auras, Leao described cortical spreading depression (CSD) in rodents (43). He observed a brief wave of hyperexcitation followed by a short-term depression after local cortical injury. Cortical spreading depression reflects a transient breakdown of brain-ion homeostasis with transient depolarization and subsequent changes in microcirculation that last for hours. In rats, CSD induces contralateral sensory neglect and motor impairment of the forepaw that lasts for 15 to 30 minutes. However, this phenomenon has never been proven in humans, and no known pain is associated with CSD (34). Milner proposed that CSD might underlie the migraine aura (44).

The episodic nature and short duration of the migraine aura have precluded organized clinical studies in humans. Indirect evidence has been gathered from cerebral blood flow and magnetoencephalographic studies. In the 1980s, Xenon blood flow studies during attacks of angiography-provoked migraine revealed oligemia beginning in the occipital region and propagating anteriorly at the rate of 2 to 3 mm per min, independent of arterial territories (45). A loss of CO_2 reactivity and reduced cortical blood flow during functional activation, with preservation of autoregulation, characteristic of CSD, were demonstrated. Subsequently, similar findings were observed during spontaneous attacks of migraine with aura (46,47). Focal hypoperfusion is the most consistent finding, but the band of hyperperfusion that should precede oligemia has not been identified, presumably due to the narrow width of the band and to the limitations of current imaging techniques (48). The most convincing demonstration of hypoperfusion was recorded in a patient with migraine and atypical visual disturbance (difficulty focusing vision) who, by chance, experienced an attack while lying in the positron emission tomographic (PET) scanner. The attack was accompanied by bilateral hypoperfusion on the order of 40% and a slow anterior spread (49).

Berkley and colleagues performed magnetoencephalographic studies in migraine patients and observed a long duration decrement in spontaneous electrical activity, similar to that seen in rabbits with CSD (33). These findings have been recorded in a few patients and do not occur universally. Thus, symptomatic patients without disturbance in cerebral blood flow have been observed (50). It is postulated that migraine with aura differs from migraine without aura only in that, with aura, all layers of the cortex are involved and reduction in blood flow is more severe (34). It is unclear how aura is linked to head pain, but it is speculated that dural ischemia or direct stimulation of the c-nociceptive fibers by CSD initiates the head pain (51,52). Moskowitz and associates have shown that CSD promotes the expression of C-fos, a biological marker for cellular memory, within laminae I and II of the ipsilateral trigeminal nucleus caudalis in rats (52). This indicates that a process originating in the cortex can activate brain stem neurons involved in the transmission of head pain.

Experimental and clinical studies have implicated the brain stem in the pathophysiology of migraine. Electrical stimulation of the locus ceruleus in monkeys at frequencies of 1 to 10 Hz reduced blood flow in the ipsilateral internal carotid artery by 20%, whereas an increase in stimulation frequency beyond 10 Hz resulted in progressive ipsilateral dilatation of the extracranial vessels (41). The localization of binding sites for dihydroergotamine in the cat brainstem provides additional evidence (53). Raskin and colleagues reported the development of migraine-like headaches in a series of nonmigraineurs who had undergone surgical stimulatory intervention of ventral lateral periaqueductal gray area for the relief of chronic pain syndrome. These headaches even responded to specific serotonergic agonists (54). Afridi and colleagues used PET in 24 patients with migraine with and without aura to examine changes in brain blood flow during migraine attack induced by glyceryl trinitrate infusion. The patients were divided into three groups according to the location of their headache: right, left, or bilateral. During attacks, increased blood flow was found in the rostral medulla, the dorsal pons, bilateral cerebellar hemispheres, the putamen, the insula, the anterior cingulate, and the prefrontal cortex. The dorsolateral pontine activation was ipsilateral in the right-sided and left-sided groups and bilateral in the bilateral headache group with a left-sided preponderance. This activation persisted after the successful termination of migraine with sumatriptan injection. These studies suggest that the brain stem is the generator and/or modulator of migraine and its unilaterality.

There is agreement that trigeminovascular system participates in the generation of migraine, but the source of headache pain has not been conclusively determined. Graham and Wolff observed a decrease in the amplitude of pulsation of the superficial temporal artery concurrently with a decrease in the intensity of headache following the injection of ergotamine (56). This suggested a major contribution of extracranial circulation to the pain of migraine. A referral of pain to the trigeminal nerve

distribution during intracranial-endovascular procedures and relief of the pain in only approximately one-third of the patients with compression of extracranial circulation suggests that the pain may be of intracranial vascular origin in one-third of the patients. The remaining one-third of patients presumably have pain of nonvascular origin (57–59). Regional cerebral blood flow studies have shown that the headache may begin during the oligaemic phase, the blood flow changes may be bilateral, and the headache may disappear before the onset of hyperperfusion, suggesting that it is unlikely that the pain arises from a primary vascular abnormality (48,49). A sterile inflammation of the extracranial vessels, as an important source of pain, has attracted attention since Chapman and co-workers found a bradykinin-like substance in the periarterial fluid (60). A recent observation that electrical stimulation of the trigeminal ganglion in animals can induce plasma extravasation supports this view (61). An increase in calcitonin-gene-related peptide (CGRP) in the external jugular vein blood of migraine patients also indicates the activation of trigeminovascular system (62).

The side of headache usually corresponds to the side of CSD, suggesting that the same process triggers the blood flow changes and stimulates perivascular nociceptors directly or through the release of neuropeptides (34). Pain is transmitted via trigeminal afferents to the trigeminal nucleus caudalis, quintothalamic tract, ventrobasal complex of the thalamus, and cerebral cortex (63). Pain perception is controlled by interneurons that modulate synaptic transmission from trigeminal afferents. These interneurons are regulated, in turn, by monoaminergic pathways descending from the brainstem, a serotonergic pathway from the periaqueductal gray matter of the midbrain, and a noradrenergic pathway from the locus ceruleus (64).

The involvement of serotonin in migraine was suggested more than 30 years ago. Methysergide, a serotonin antagonist, prevented migraine. Intramuscular reserpine, which releases serotonin, induced a typical headache in migraineurs (65,66), and prior methysergide administration prevented these headaches (67). Moreover, increased urinary 5-hydroxyindole acetic acid, a metabolite of serotonin, was found during migraine attacks (68). Based on these observations, serotonin was administered to the patients. This relieved migraine but caused multiple side effects, including flushing, faintness, and parasthesias (69). It is thought that serotonin is released from platelets at the onset of an attack, with an associated increase in free plasma serotonin, and the later stages of attack are characterized by low levels of serotonin. In 1989, Ferrari and associates demonstrated that platelet serotonin content fell only in patients who had migraine without aura, thus adding to the speculation that migraine with aura is a different condition (70). The role of serotonin has been further augmented by the recent introduction of serotonin agonists in the treatment of acute migraine attacks (71). Recently, the gene for hemiplegic migraine on chromosome 19p13 has been found to be close to the gene for hereditary paroxysmal cerebellar ataxia, an acetazolamide-responsive channelopathy. It is postulated that P/Q calcium channels in the brain, which govern serotonin release, may be affected (72).

A unifying model of migraine pathophysiology hypothesizes a genetic predisposition with neuronal hyperexcitability. Factors such as menstruation or excessive afferent stimulation lower the threshold so that triggers precipitate migraine by activating brainstem nuclei, especially the locus ceruleus, via a hypothalamic connection. This initiates cortical neuronal depolarization, followed by "spreading depression." This may activate the trigemino-vascular system and lead to a stimulation of perivascular nociceptors, pain transmission via trigeminal afferents, and headache. Central dysnociception of the endogenous pain pathways further contributes to the pain (73–75). Furthermore, the central neurons become sensitized as a migraine attack progresses, thus leading to the intensification of head pain and an increased sensitivity to convergent sensory stimuli from extracranial tissues such as scalp and periorbital skin (76,77).

SEX HORMONES AND MIGRAINE

Epidemiologic data highlight a link between migraine and sex hormones. Bille observed that in children between 7 and 9 years, the frequency of migraine sufferers was 2.5%, similar for girls and boys; but between 10 to 12 years of age, the boys' percentage was 3.9%, whereas girls scored 5.4% (78). Stewart and associates used data from a nationwide sample of more than 20,000 respondents between 12 and 80 years of age and found a migraine prevalence of 17.6% in females and 5.7% in males. At age 12 years, the female–male ratio was below 2.0, increasing sharply in the second decade and peaking at 3.3 between 40 and 45 years. Even after the age of menopause, the sex ratio continued to be elevated above 2.0 (79). As is evident from these figures, migraine disproportionately affects women, and the changing hormonal environment plays a significant role in gender difference. The normal female life cycle includes at least three hormonal milestones: menarche, pregnancy, and menopause. Additionally, exogenous hormones are often prescribed for contraceptive use during the reproductive years and for hormone replacement during menopause. These physiologic events or therapeutic interventions may affect migraine.

The specific mechanisms underlying the influence of hormonal changes remain uncertain. Estrogen is believed to influence the susceptibility to migraine as well as the perception and processing of pain. By the combined methods of autoradiography and flouorescence biochemistry, Heritage and associates observed catecholamine neurons with concentrations of [3H] estradiol in the regions of nucleus tractus solitarii and the nucleus locus ceruleus (80). These nuclei participate in the pathogenesis of migraine. In adult ovariectomized rats, pregnancy and the use of contraceptive pills increase the plasma CGRP concentration, a neuropeptide regulating the vascular tone (81). The data suggest that ovarian hormones alter the size of the receptive fields of trigeminal mechonoreceptors (82). Additionally, majority of enkephalin-producing neurons in the spinal cord, trigeminal ganglia, and dorsal horn of female rats have intracellular estradiol receptors. When these neurons are supplemented with estradiol, enkephalin levels increase (83). Moreover, ovariectomized female rats are far less likely to develop tactile allodynia following partial sciatic nerve ligation than the ovary-intact animals (84). These studies suggest an important role of estradiol as a pain modulator.

Menarche

Limited information exists on the impact of menarche on migraine. The incidence of migraine rises at the onset of menarche. In a survey of 131 female migraineurs, Epstein and associates found that the highest concentration of onset of migraine coincided with the onset of menarche (24 of 131). However, in 18 patients, it began before the menarche, and in 67 patients, it occurred 5 or more years after menarche. The patients with migraine onset at menarche were more likely to have menstrual migraine (85).

Menstruation

A complex sequence of interactions between the hypothalamus, pituitary gland, ovary, and endometrium occurs during the menstrual cycle. A neuronal oscillator or "clock" located in the arcuate nucleus of the hypothalamus fires at regular intervals, resulting in the periodic release of gonadotropin-releasing hormone, which causes the release of luteinizing hormone (LH) and follicle-stimulating hormone (FSH) from the anterior pituitary. LH and FSH are responsible for the growth and maturation of the graafian follicle in the ovary and for the production of estrogen and progesterone.

The estrogen and progesterone produced by the ovary exert feedback on the pituitary and hypothalamus. Women menstruate regularly at approximately 28-day intervals and ovulate on the 14th day of the cycle (86).

Ovulatory migraine, with migraine attacks occurring only during ovulation, is rare, whereas an association between menstruation and migraine is common. Nattero observed a chronologic connection with menstruation in 55% of patients (87,98).

A standard definition is lacking for menstruation-associated or *catamenial migraine*. The prevalence of this entity, therefore, varies depending on the defined criteria. The Ad Hoc Committee suggested in its comments about "common migraine" that this type of headache may show exacerbation in relation to the menstrual cycle (3). The IHS criteria do not characterize it as a separate entity but include it within code 1.1, migraine without aura. The feature required for the definition is that 90% of migraine attacks occur on or between days –2 to +3 in at least two-thirds of cycles (4). It is suggested that an increase in migraine activity several days before or during menstruation should be called "menstrually related migraine," whereas occurrence of migraine just before or at the time of menstruation (88) should be called "menstrual migraine." MacGregor proposes that the term menstrual migraine should be restricted to attacks exclusively starting between days 1 and 2 of the menstrual cycle, because this period coincides with low estrogen and high prostaglandin levels (89). The incidence of "menstrually related migraine" varies from 52 to 70%, whereas the incidence of strictly defined "menstrual migraine" varies from 8% to 25% (88). In a study of 232 menstruating patients comparing the relationship between menstruation and migraine, the menstrual migraine (from 2 days before to 3 days after menstruation) was significantly more common in migraine without aura than in migraine with aura (90).

The precipitating factors implicated in the pathogenesis of menstrual migraine include the sudden release of 5-hydroxytryptamine from the platelets or its serotonergic neurons, the rise of plasma catecholamines, the opioid dysregulation, and abnormalities of prolactin release (91). The two mechanisms most compatible with MacGregor's proposed definition are estrogen withdrawal and the release of prostaglandins.

The estrogen withdrawal is by far the most accepted hypothesis. Somerville studied hormone levels and administered estrogen or progesterone to women with menstrual migraine. He demonstrated that progesterone administration delayed menstruation without affecting the timing of the migraine attack. In contrast, estrogen given premenstrually delayed the onset of migraine but not menstruation. He suggested that estrogen primes cranial vessels before withdrawal induces headache. He administered long-acting estradiol valerate to four women and short-acting estradiol benzoate to two women. Estrogen-withdrawal migraine occurred in three of the four women treated with the long-acting preparation but in neither of the two women treated with the short-acting preparation. He proposed that a prolonged exposure, followed by a reduction of the circulating estradiol, was required to cause migraine (92–94). A role for progesterone, however, has not been entirely excluded (95).

Prostaglandin E1, infused into healthy nonmigrainous humans, can produce migraine-type headache (96). The plasma concentrations of PGF2 and PGE2 are significantly higher during the attack of menstrual migraine (91,97). The maximum entry of prostaglandin and its metabolites into the systemic circulation occurs during the first 48 hours of menstruation. Prostaglandins inhibit adrenergic transmission, sensitize nociceptors, promote the development of neurogenic inflammation, and modulate the descending noradrenergic pain control system (42,98,99). Thus, prostaglandin excess may contribute to menstrual migraine. See also Chapter 12.

Treatment

A careful history will bring forth a frequent association between menstruation and migraine. A prospective diary kept by the patient for 3 months is essential (i) to differentiate between menstrually related migraine and menstrual migraine; (ii) to observe cycle regularity; (iii) to define the perimenstrual time window; and (iv) to note the predictability of headache with each cycle.

There is no single, universally effective treatment for menstrual migraine. Studies reporting on the various pharmacologic treatments do not adhere to the same definition of menstrual migraine, so figures are not strictly comparable. Furthermore, placebo-controlled studies are lacking. Despite these limitations, nonpharmacologic as well as pharmacologic treatments have been used to provide relief to these patients. The most significant nonpharmacologic treatment is to identify triggers and avoid them at key times in the cycle. Reassurance and sleep hygiene are helpful. Solbach and colleagues studied the usefulness of no treatment, autogenic phrases, electromyographic feedback, and thermal feedback in 136 subjects with menstrual migraine (3 days before menstruation, during the time of flow, or 3 days after). There was a tendency for all groups to improve but overall usefulness was limited (100).

Table 14.2 provides an algorithm for the management of menstrual migraines (101). For the menstrually related aggravation of migraine, acute and prophylactic treatments are the same as those used for other migraineurs (102–104). In my experience, some of these patients show improvement in their regular migraine headache, but perimenstrual and menstrual components persist and may even be refractory to treatment. In these patients, raising the dose of prophylactic drugs or adding acute attack therapy in the perimenstrual period can be beneficial (97).

Patients who suffer only from menstrual migraine benefit from cyclical prophylaxis, which involves the perimenstrual administration of drugs from 2 days before the expected onset until 1 to 5 days after the headache relief (Table 14.3). Nonsteroidal anti-inflammatory drugs

TABLE 14.2
Management of Menstrual Migraine

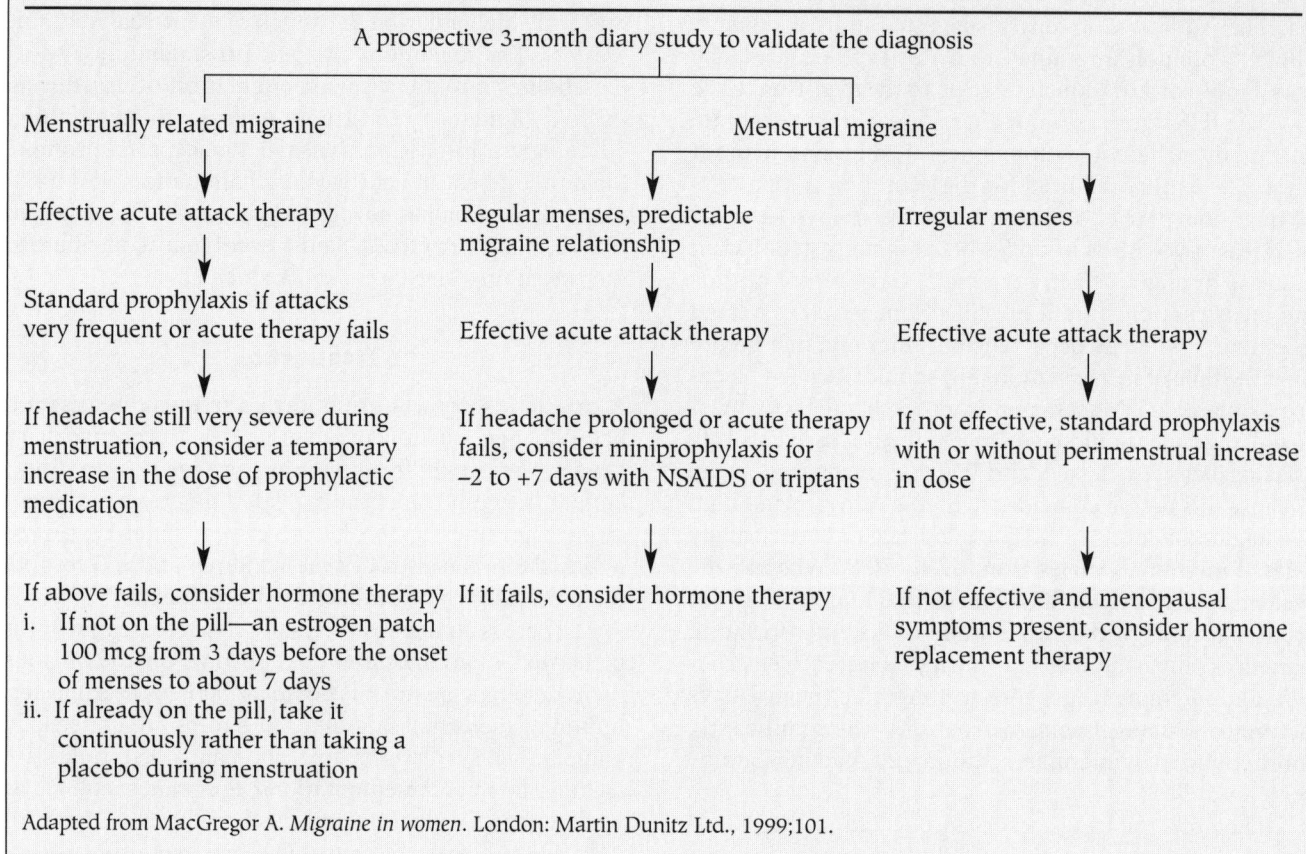

A prospective 3-month diary study to validate the diagnosis

Menstrually related migraine	Menstrual migraine	
↓		
Effective acute attack therapy	Regular menses, predictable migraine relationship	Irregular menses
↓	↓	↓
Standard prophylaxis if attacks very frequent or acute therapy fails	Effective acute attack therapy	Effective acute attack therapy
↓	↓	↓
If headache still very severe during menstruation, consider a temporary increase in the dose of prophylactic medication	If headache prolonged or acute therapy fails, consider miniprophylaxis for −2 to +7 days with NSAIDS or triptans	If not effective, standard prophylaxis with or without perimenstrual increase in dose
↓	↓	↓
If above fails, consider hormone therapy i. If not on the pill—an estrogen patch 100 mcg from 3 days before the onset of menses to about 7 days ii. If already on the pill, take it continuously rather than taking a placebo during menstruation	If it fails, consider hormone therapy	If not effective and menopausal symptoms present, consider hormone replacement therapy

Adapted from MacGregor A. *Migraine in women*. London: Martin Dunitz Ltd., 1999;101.

(NSAIDs) have been recommended to inhibit the prostaglandin production that may be enhanced in menstrual migraine. Sances and colleagues found naproxen sodium to be an effective prophylactic medication (105). Mathew compared ergotamine alone, beta-blocker nadolol alone, naproxen alone, nadolol and ergotamine, and naproxen and ergotamine. He found the combination of naproxen and ergotamine to be most effective (106). Gallagher administered ergonovine maleate, which acts on alpha-adrenergic and dopaminergic receptors, in 40 patients with menstrual migraine. He observed that 65% of the patients reported improvement over 3 months and 50% over 6 months (107). Silberstein found DHE-45 to be an effective therapy (108). Facchinetti and co-workers performed a double-blind, placebo-controlled study of the effect of sumatriptan in menstrual migraine. Headache relief was reported in 73% of patients compared with 31% of placebo-controlled subjects (109). Other triptans have also demonstrated good efficacy (110–113).

For refractory cases that cannot be controlled with abortive treatment, cyclical prophylaxis or regular prophylaxis, hormone therapy, or bromocriptine treatment may be beneficial. The aim of hormone therapy is to stabilize estrogen levels during the late luteal phase of the menstrual cycle. This can be achieved by maintaining plasma estrogen levels at a high or low range. Estrogen replacement with percutaneous estradiol gel or estradiol implant may elevate estrogen levels and provide a mild to moderate improvement. Magos and associates suppressed ovarian activity using a subcutaneous estradiol implant in 24 patients with menstrual migraine for a mean duration of 2.5 years; 83% became headache-free. Regular monthly periods were induced with cyclical oral progestogens (114). Diminished estrogen activity can be achieved by the use of tamoxifen, an antiestrogen, or by the administration of danazol, an androgen derivative. Tamoxifen, 10 to 20 mg per day, given to eight women in an open trial, produced improvement in seven cases (115). Danazol acts by suppressing the pituitary-ovarian axis. The administration of 200 to 600 mg per day, given in the perimenstrual time window, can improve menstrual migraine (97,116). Continuous bromocriptine therapy with 2.5 mg three times a day, in a prospective but open trial, was shown to reduce headache in 62.5% of 24 women (117).

TABLE 14.3
Acute Attack Therapy of Menstrual Migraine

MEDICATION / DOSE	MODE OF ACTION
1. Nonsteroidal anti-inflammatory drugs	
• Naproxen sodium 550 mg twice a day	Inhibition of prostaglandin synthesis by reversible binding to cyclooxygenase
2. Triptans—once or twice a day	5-HT 1B/1D agonist at the peripheral and central sites
• Sumatriptan 6 mg subcutaneous injection or 100 mg oral	
• Rizatriptan 5 or 10 mg oral	Rizatriptan and zolmitriptan display faster onset of action
• Zolmitriptan 2.5 or 5 mg oral	
• Naratriptan 1 mg oral	
• Eletriptan 40 mg oral	
• Frovatriptan 2.5 mg oral	
• Almotriptan 12.5 mg oral	
3. Ergotamine suppository 2 mg, half a suppository once or twice a day or Dihydroergotamine mesylate nasal spray, one metered dose in each nostril every 8 hours	Binds to 5-HT 1D λ and 5-HT 1Dβ, noradrenaline and dopamine receptors
4. Transdermal estradiol 100 mcg patch for 7 days beginning with day −3. Change patch depending on the prescribed product	Delays headache onset by providing a sustained low level of estrogen
Initiate treatment at day −3 or −2 and continue up to 7 days.	
Once medication is effective, adjust the dosing schedule to the lowest dose, the fewest days, and reduced frequency.	
Supplement with nondrug therapy and avoid triggers.	

Hysterectomy as a treatment for hormonally influenced migraine is a relic of the past (118).

PREGNANCY

A high proportion of women become free of migraine attacks during pregnancy. The improvement in headache begins gradually in the third or fourth month of pregnancy and is not related to social or emotional status (20). The patients with menstrually related migraine are more likely to have relief of their migraine during pregnancy (85,119). Lance and Anthony studied 120 migrainous women who had a total of 252 pregnancies and reported relief of migraine in 57.5% of pregnancies (120). Somerville reported improvement in 24 of 31 women migraineurs during pregnancy (121). Ratinahirana and associates, in a prospective study of 703 women, reported improvement in 69.4% (119). In a retrospective study of 1,300 migraineurs, Granella reported complete remission in 17.4% and significant improvement in 49.2% (122). In a study of 428 women, Maggioni and co-workers noted at least a 50% decrease in headache frequency in 80% of the pregnant migraineurs (123). These observations received experimental evidence support from Hardebo and Edvinnson, who demonstrated a reduced sensitivity of intracranial and extracranial vessels to adrenergic stimulation during late pregnancy in cats and rabbits (124). Critchley and associates found high levels of serum β-endorphin-like immunoreactivity and held it responsible for hyponociception in pregnant women (125).

Often overlooked, however, are the cases that do not improve during pregnancy. Graham observed an aggravation of migraine with aura (20). Somerville found that 23% of his case series either failed to improve or worsened (121). Granella observed worsening in 3.5% of 1,300 migraineurs (122). Although uncommon, migraine may develop for the first time during pregnancy, usually in the first trimester (121,126). Other authors have described the occurrence of migraine with focal symptoms during pregnancy (127–130). These cases are difficult to explain if one believes that sustained high estrogen levels in pregnancy are responsible for an improvement in migraine.

Migraineurs have no increased risk of complications during pregnancy, and their children have no increased incidence of birth defects. In a retrospective study of 777 women migraineurs, Wainscott found that the incidence of miscarriage, toxemia, congenital malformations, and stillbirths was similar in the migraineurs compared with the 182 nonmigrainous controls (131).

Headaches may return in the first postpartum week or on return of menstruation. In a study by Stein, 15 of 40 women on a postnatal ward had headaches in the first postpartum week, particularly between days 3 and 6. It was ascribed to the withdrawal of estrogen and progesterone (132). Lactation, which entails both vascular and neurohumoral alterations, also influences migraine. Dooling and Sweeney reported a 25-year-old woman with occurrence of familial hemiplegic migraine in relation to breast-feeding and use of a breast pump, and postulated a complex effect of oxytocin on cerebral vessels (133). Askmark and Lundberg reported a case of a woman experiencing brief but intense headaches with breast-feeding. She received no relief from propranolol but became symptom-free after weaning her baby (134).

DIAGNOSIS

Headache may be a disabling symptom of a primary condition such as migraine or a reflection of an underlying neurologic disorder. An accurate diagnosis is a prerequisite to appropriate management.

The single most important diagnostic step in the evaluation of a headache is obtaining an accurate history. Age at the time of onset, frequency, periodicity, and progression of headache indicate the temporal relationship and assist in the differential diagnosis. A set of standard questions is used to elicit a profile of an individual attack, including onset, premonitory symptoms, prodrome, location of pain, character and duration of pain, associated symptoms, precipitating and aggravating factors, and relieving factors (135). An acute, severe, new-onset headache with neurologic deficit would include in the differential diagnosis intracranial hemorrhage, temporal arteritis, internal carotid artery dissection, cerebral venous thrombosis, and pituitary apoplexy, whereas a subacute onset would encompass a wider diagnostic spectrum (136).

A thorough general and neurologic examination not only is reassuring to patients with migraine, but also may suggest appropriate tests. Examination is usually normal in patients with migraine but one should be wary of the "migraine mimics." New-onset migraine with aura can be caused by an underlying disorder, such as vasculitis, brain tumor, or occipital arteriovenous malformation. Neurologic abnormalities may be present in patients with traction and inflammatory headaches. Exhaustive tests are usually unnecessary in patients with chronic, constant, and nonprogressive headache. Laboratory and radiologic tests are usually indicated if the headaches are of recent onset, if there has been a recent change in a previously stable headache pattern, or if neurologic examination is abnormal (136).

Radiologic investigations on pregnant patients should be performed only when absolutely necessary, and if possible, they should be delayed until the third trimester or postpartum. Magnetic resonance imaging (MRI) is a useful test, especially for posterior fossa examination. The potential risk of MRI in pregnancy remains controversial. Gadolinium should be avoided because it crosses the placental barrier. Cranial computed tomographic (CAT) scan, used especially for the diagnosis of intracranial hemorrhage, provides significant information with the least risk. Total radiation exposure to the uterus is less than 1 mrad. Electroencephalography without the administration of drugs is a harmless procedure of low diagnostic yield that may demonstrate abnormalities in patients with suspected focal lesions. Lumbar puncture is necessary in patients with severe rapid-onset headache, progressive headache, and chronic intractable headache. It is without major complications in patients who do not have raised intracranial pressure from focal lesions. Lumbar puncture is definitely indicated in patients with suspected meningitis or encephalitis. Cerebral angiography is useful in the evaluation of aneurysm or arteriovenous malformation. When medically necessary, radiologic studies should be performed with the abdomen appropriately shielded and field size as limited as possible (136,137).

DIFFERENTIAL DIAGNOSIS

Traction and inflammatory headaches enter the differential diagnosis in patients who develop headache for the first time during pregnancy. Because migraine headache often improves after the first trimester of pregnancy, severe headache persisting into the third trimester may be a warning sign of an underlying structural disease. A 10-year study of maternal mortality during pregnancy and up to 6 months postpartum disclosed that 23% of all maternal deaths were due to CNS complications. Of these, the majority were caused by intracranial tumors, subarachnoid hemorrhage, intracranial hemorrhage, and arterial and venous occlusions. Brain tumors, especially meningiomas, choriocarcinoma, and pituitary tumors may grow rapidly in pregnancy, probably due to hormonal stimulation or fluid retention. Intracranial hemorrhage from arteriovenous malformation and subarachnoid hemorrhage demands definitive treatment. A retrospective study of 146 patients found the incidence of arteriovenous malformations to be four times greater in association with pregnancy. These tended to bleed during the middle and end of pregnancy. Aneurysms were more likely to bleed between weeks 30 and 40 of pregnancy.

Strokes from major arterial occlusions are more common than venous occlusions and carry a higher mortality. Most of them occur during the puerperium (136,137). Cerebral venous thrombosis may present with migraine-like visual disturbance and progressive headache. Although it can occur in the first and second trimesters, it usually occurs around labor, possibly due to a hypercoagulable state.

PHARMACOTHERAPY

Pharmacotherapy, which has otherwise been the mainstay of migraine treatment, is limited in the pregnant patient because of its potential effects on the fetus. Nonpharmacologic treatments constitute an extremely useful alternative to drug therapy. The nonpharmacologic approach includes:

- Reassurance after a detailed and sympathetic evaluation with an explanation of the mechanisms of migraine.
- Identification and removal of trigger factors to diminish susceptibility. These trigger factors may include emotional stress, bright sunlight, fatigue, poor sleep hygiene, and fasting for more than 5 hours during the day or 13 hours overnight (138). The patient should avoid alcohol and vasoactive foods such as cured meats, aged cheese, monosodium glutamate, and chocolate.
- Physical measures such as local use of ice packs for at least 12 minutes (139) and rest in dark and quiet surroundings. Physiotherapy to cervical muscles, use of a cervical collar, trigger point injections, dental treatment for uneven bite, and correction of refractory error may be useful.
- Psychophysiologic methods, including biofeedback and relaxation therapy (140). Schraft and colleagues demonstrated the beneficial effects of physical therapy, relaxation training, and biofeedback in 80% of 30 pregnant women for up to 1 year following delivery (141).

Pharmacotherapy (Table 14.4) in a pregnant patient should be used only when absolutely necessary and with full understanding of the risks and benefits, especially during the most teratogenic period of 6 weeks, lasting from approximately 4 weeks through 10 weeks from the last menstrual period. The patient should be made aware of the incidence of major and minor malformations in the general population, which may be as high as 7 to 10%. The side effects of various medications to the patient and the fetus should be explained, and advice should be duly documented in the progress notes. The prescription of medications should preferably be limited to FDA risk categories A (no risk) and B (no evidence of risk to humans

---

TABLE 14.4
Pharmacologic Treatment of Pregnant Women with Migraine Guidelines

- Avoid drugs during the first trimester
- Use drugs only when absolutely necessary
- Make patient aware of the side effects to her and the fetus
- Use drugs in minimal but effective doses
- Avoid the use of multiple drugs
- Recommend management as "high-risk pregnancy"
- Discontinue drugs 2 weeks before delivery

Acute Attack
- Acetaminophen
- Meperidine
- Codeine
- Prochlorperazine
- Prednisone

Prophylaxis
- Propranolol
- Verapamil?
- Fluoxetine?

---

but no control studies available). Drugs in category C (risk to humans not ruled out) should be used with some trepidation. Drugs in category D (positive evidence of risk) and category X (contraindicated) should not be prescribed. The treatment of migraine in a pregnant patient is directed toward control of an acute attack and prophylaxis for recurrent attacks (136,137).

For acute episodes, ergotamine, an effective medication, is contraindicated during pregnancy because of its oxytocic potential (142). Sumatriptan (category C) has been reported to cause embryo lethality in rabbits, at three times human plasma concentration (137). Meperidine and acetaminophen, which both belong to FDA risk category B, can be used to treat acute attacks (143). Codeine and butalbital, category C drugs, and a component of many pain pills, should be used with caution. For severe acute attacks, intravenous hydration, intravenous rectal administration of prochlorperazine (category C), and prednisone (category B) may be effectively employed (137). For prophylaxis, use drugs in minimal but effective doses and avoid the use of multiple drugs. These patients should be managed as high-risk pregnancies, and longitudinally followed with ultrasonography of the fetus; prophylactic drugs should be discontinued 2 weeks before delivery. The beta adrenergic blocking agent propranolol (category C), the calcium channel blocker verapamil (category C), and serotonin uptake inhibitor fluoxetine (category B) may be used in severe and refractory cases. Fluoxetine and verapamil, although safer, have not been extensively used in the treatment of migraine headache. The ter-

TABLE 14.5
Teratogenicity of Antimigraine Drugs

Drugs	Risk categories		Lactation	Remarks
Acute Attack	FDA	TERIS		
Acetaminophen	B	N	Compatible	Best choice
Meperidine	B	N-min	Compatible	Sporadic use
Codeine	C	N-min	Compatible	Sporadic use
Caffeine	B	N-min	Compatible	<300 mg/day
Prochlorperazine	C	N	Compatible	
Prednisone	B	N-min	Compatible	Occasional use
Prophylaxis				
Propranolol	C	U	Compatible	In severe cases
<160 mg/day				
Verapamil	C	U	Compatible	
Fluoxetine	B	N	Caution	

TERIS = Teratogenic risk based on consensus of expert opinion and literature evidence.
N: None; N-min: none to minimal; min: minimal; H: high; U: undetermined.

atogenic potential and relative safety of these drugs have been substantiated in various studies (Table 14.5) (144–150).

Breast-feeding has regained popularity in the United States. A mother suffering from severe migraine may not comply with the recommendation that she should either not nurse her baby or not take medication. Several antimigraine drugs are excreted into breast milk. During lactation, acetaminophen, caffeine, narcotics, and prochlorperazine can be used for the treatment of acute attacks (Table 14.5). Beta-blockers and verapamil may be relatively safe choices for prophylaxis (151,152).

MENOPAUSE

"Hemicrania generally diminishes in advanced age, or entirely ceases; in females it often terminates at the period of decrepitude," said Romberg in 1853 (1). In contrast to this traditional view, migraine may regress, worsen, or show no change with menopause. In some women, migraine may become a problem only after menopause. The type of menopause seems to be important. The women with surgical menopause following bilateral oophorectomy are more likely to get worse (153–155). Lichten and colleagues gave 5 mg depoestradiol injection to 16 postmenopausal women with previous history of menstrual migraine and 12 postmenstrual women without any history of headache. Control subjects reported no migraine during the month. All 16 women with a history of migraine developed severe migraines 18.5 ± 2.8 days after the injection. Thus, in postmenopausal patients, estrogen withdrawal precipitated migraine (156).

ORAL CONTRACEPTIVES

Oral contraceptives (OCs) produce a state of pharmacologic anovulation by interfering with the midcycle gonadotropin surge at both the hypothalamic and pituitary levels. OCs are used by women at the prime of their reproductive life, coincident with the peak prevalance of migraine. Therefore, the twin issues of the effect of OCs on the migraine headache and the stroke risk imposed by OCs on female migraineurs are important (157).

Headache is a common side effect of oral contraceptive use. In a study of 1,800 women using three different low-dose OC preparations, Ramos and associates noted that headache was a predominant reason for termination of treatment. The incidence of headache varied between 8.3 and 11.5% (158). There are conflicting data regarding the relationship of OC use to the occurrence of migraine. The studies are not comparable because of the variable dosages of synthetic estrogens, small sample size, and the selection bias. Furthermore, evidence concerning risk or benefit is based primarily on observational epidemiologic studies.

It has been generally accepted that migraine worsens when the patient uses OCs. The first such report was probably made by Mears and Grant in 1962 (159). Kudrow studied 239 women, of whom 60 used OCs, 87 used replacement or supplemental estrogen, and 92 used no hormone. Of the 60 OC users, 42% had migraine headache before starting the OC. Fifty-eight percent of the women, however, developed migraine only after starting the OC. The withdrawal of OCs resulted in a marked improvement in 70% of the women (160). Dalton observed that of the women with menstrual migraine, 81% reported an increase in migraine while on the OCs, as opposed to 57% of women with sporadic migraine (150). In a retrospective study of 1,676 women from Uppsala, taking combined, sequential, or low-dose gestagen OCs, 10.3% of women without a prior history of headache developed headache. However, of 362 women with pretreatment migraine, 87 experienced a reduction of their symptoms, 42 had no headaches, and 66 had more headaches (162). At present, the various effects of OCs on female migraineurs include (163,164):

- No change in migraine pattern in the majority of women
- Worsening of migraine in terms of frequency and severity, and reversal following discontinuation
- Onset of migraine for the first time within days or weeks of starting the OCs, usually in the early cycles of usage but occasionally after prolonged use
- Change of migraine without aura into migraine with aura
- Distinct improvement in some patients

Strong evidence suggests that migraine itself increases the risk of ischemic stroke (163). Tzourio and associates investigated this relationship by studying 72 women under 45 years of age with ischemic stroke and 173 randomly selected controls. Ischemic stroke was associated with history of migraine without aura (odds ratio 3:0) as well as with migraine with aura (odds ratio 6:2) (165). A significantly increased risk of ischemic stroke in women migraineurs was also observed by Lidegaard, who reported an odds ratio for stroke at 2.9 in users of combined OCs containing 50 μg synthetic estrogen, 1.8 in OCs containing 30–40 μg of estrogen, but no excess risk for progestogen-only OCs (166). This has been attributed to vasoconstriction, dehydration, and platelet activation during migraine attack (163).

OCs increase the risk of stroke in young women. A 1973 collaborative study revealed a ninefold increase of stroke risk among OC users (167). Stroke risk from migraine and OCs may be additive. Tzourio and colleagues observed a fourfold increased risk of ischemic stroke in female migraineurs who used OCs (165).

The use of OC in migraine patients is controversial, but recommendations outlined by Becker should be helpful (163).

General Recommendations

- Individualize the risk–benefit ratio for each patient. Weigh the risk of stroke against medical, psychological, social, and economic benefits to the patient.
- When patients with migraine are prescribed OCs, monitor them carefully for an increase in migraine headache and the development of focal symptoms.

- Prescribe OCs that contain low-dose estrogens and progestins in women with migraine without aura.

Specific Recommendations

- Avoid OCs if the patient is older than 34 years or has additional risk factors, such as smoking and hypertension.
- Discontinue OCs if headache attacks become severe in frequency or severity or if they change into migraine with aura.
- In women with migraine with aura, avoid OCs except in younger women with short-lasting visual aura and discontinue OCs if aura is prolonged.
- Avoid OCs in patients who have prolonged aura, multiple aura symptoms, recurrent aura symptoms, complicated migraine, and transient ischemic attacks.

HORMONE REPLACEMENT THERAPY

Vasomotor symptoms or osteoporosis prophylaxis may necessitate hormone replacement therapy (HRT). In a study of 112 women receiving HRT, 50 women reported improvement, 52 believed their migraine worsened, and 10 noted no change (168). HRT may result in a new onset "migraine" in approximately 3% of patients (169–171). The association between HRT and stroke risk remains controversial. The Framingham study found an increased risk of stroke in postmenopausal women who used estrogens (relative risk = 2.3). Recent studies show either no effect or an adverse effect on stroke risk (172,173). In patients with migraine exacerbation, Silberstein suggests reducing estrogen dose, changing estrogen type (from conjugate estrogen to pure estradiol, to synthetic ethinyl estradiol, or to pure estrase), and converting from interrupted to continuous dosing or from oral to parental dosing. Rarely, androgen addition may be beneficial (97,174).

References

1. Romberg MH. *A Manual of the nervous disease of man*, vol. 1. Translated and edited by EM Sieverking. Printed for the Syndenham Society, London 1853;176–191.
2. Gowers WR. *A manual of disease of the nervous system.* Philadelphia, Pa: P. Blakistan Son, 1888;1171–1189.
3. Ad Hoc Committee on Classification of Headache. Classification of headache. *JAMA* 1962;179:717–718.
4. Headache Classification Subcommittee of the International Headache Society. The Interanational Classification of Headache Disorders, 2nd ed. *Cephalalgia* 2004;24 (suppl 1):1–160.
5. Solomon S, Lipton RB. Criteria for the diagnosis of migraine in clinical practice. *Headache* 1991;31:384–387.
6. Solomon S. Diagnosis of primary headache disorders. *Neurol Clin* 1997;15:15–26.

7. Kinnier Wilson SA. *Neurology*. (2nd ed.), vol. 3. Baltimore, Md: Williams & Wilkins, 1955;1704–1725.
8. Dalessio DJ, ed. *Wolff's headache and other head pain*. New York, NY: Oxford University Press, 1972;225–347.
9. Selby G. Migraine and its variants. Sydney: Adis Health Science Press, 1983.
10. Blau JN. Migraine pathogenesis: the neural hypothesis reexamined. *J Neurol Neurosurg Psychiatry* 1984;47:437–442.
11. Barbiroli B, Montagna P, Cortelli P, et al. Abnormal brain and muscle energy metabolism shown by 31-P magnetic resonance spectroscopy in patients affected by migraine with aura. *Neurology* 1992;42:1209–1214.
12. Montagna P, Cortelli P, Monari L, et al. 31-P magnetic resonance spectrocopy in migraine without aura. *Neurology* 1994;44:666–669.
13. Olesen J, Tfelt-Hansen P, Welch KMW, (eds.) *The headache*. New York, NY: Raven Press, 1993;225–262.
14. Bing R, Haymaker W. *Textbook of nervous diseases*. St. Louis, Mo: Mosby, 1939;722–737.
15. Critchley M, Friedman KP, Gorini S, Sicuteri F, (eds.) *Headache: physiopathological and clinical concepts*. New York, NY: Raven Press, 1982;21–26.
16. Russell MB, Olesen J. A nosographic analysis of the migraine aura in a general population. *Brain* 1996;119:355–361.
17. Lashley KS. Patterns of cerebral intergration indicated by the scotomas of migraine. *Arch Neurol Psychiat* 1941;46:331–339.
18. Olesen J, Tfelt-Hansen P, Welch KMW, (eds.) The headache. New York, NY: Raven Press, 1993;263–275.
19. Bickerstaff ER. Basilar artery migraine. *Lancet* 1961;1:15–17.
20. Vinken PJ, Bruyn GW, (eds.) *Handbook of clinical neurology, vol.5. Headache and cranial neuralgias*. Amsterdam: North-Holland Publishing, 1968;45–48.
21. Guiloff RJ, Fruns M. Limb pain in migraine and cluster headache. *J Neurol Neurosurg Psychiat* 1988;51:1022–1031.
22. Liveing E. On Megrim. *Sick-headache and some allied disorders: a contribution to the pathology of nerve storms*. London: J & A Churchill, 1873.
23. Haan J, Gisela M, Ferrari MD. Genetics of migraine. *Neurol Clin* 1997;15:43–60.
24. Russell MB, Olesen J. Increased familial risk and evidence of genetic factor in migraine. *Br Med J* 1995;311:541–544.
25. Stewart WF, Staffa J, Lipton RB, Ottman R. Familial risk of migraine: a population-based study. *Ann Neurol* 1997;41:166–172.
26. Sàndor PS, Ambrosim A, Agosti RM, et al. Genetics of migraine: possible links to neurophysiological abnormalities. *Headache* 2002;42:365–377.
27. Carlsson A, Foregren L, Nylander PO, et al. Identification of a susceptibility locus for migraine with and without aura on 6p12.2–21.1. *Neurology* 2002;59:1804–1807.
28. Soragna D, Vettori A, Carravo G, et al. A locus for migraine without aura maps on chromosome 14 q 21.2–q 22.3. *Am J Human Genet* 2003;72:161–167.
29. Diener H-C, Scholz E, Dichgans J, et al. Central effects of drugs used in migraine prophylaxis evaluated by visual evoked potentials. *Ann Neurol* 1989;25:125–130.
30. Gawel M, Connolly JF, Rose FC. Migraine patients exhibit abnormalities in the visual evoked potentials. *Headache* 1983;23:49–52.
31. Van Dijk JF, Dorresteign M, Haan J, et al. Visual evoked potentials and background EEG activity in migraine. *Headache* 1991;31:392–395.
32. Kropp P, Gerber WD. Is increased amplitude of contingent negative variations in migraine due to cortical hyperactivity or to reduced habituation? *Cephalalgia* 1993;13:37–41.
33. Barkley GL, Tepley N, Nagel-Leiby S, et al. Magnetoencephalographic studies of migraine. *Headache* 1990;30:428–434.
34. Lauritzen M. Pathophysiology of the migraine aura. *Sci Med* July-August 1996;32–41.
35. Welch KMW, Barkley GL, Tepley N, et al. Central neurogenic mechanisms of migraine. *Neurology* 1993;43(suppl 3):521–525.
36. Facco E, Munari M, Behr AV, et al. Regional cerebral blood flow (rCBF) in migraine during the interictal period: different rCBF patterns in patients with and without aura. *Cephalalgia* 1996;16:161–168.
37. Schlake HP, Grotemeyer KH, Hoffer Berth B, et al. Brainstem auditory evoked potentials in migraine—evidence of increased side differences during the pain-free interval. *Headache* 1990;30:129–132.
38. Drummond PD, Lance JW. Neurovascular disturbance in headache patients. *Clin Exp Neurol* 1984;20:93–99.
39. Lance JW. *Mechanisms and management of headache*. London: Butterworth Scientific, 1982.
40. Heyck H. Vascular shunt mechanisms and migraine pathogenesis. *Neurology* 1981;31:1203–1203.
41. Goadsby PJ, Lambert GA, Lance JW. Differential effects on the internal and external carotid circulation of the monkey evoked by locu coeruleus stimulation. *Brain Res* 1982;249:247–254.
42. Moskowitz MA. The neurobiology of vascular head pain. *Ann Neurol* 1984;16:157–168.
43. Leao AA. Spreading depression of activity in cerebral cortex. *J Neurophysiol* 1944;7:359–390.
44. Milner PM. Note on possible correspondence between the scotomas of migraine and spreading depression of Leao. *EEG Clin Neurophysiol* 1958;10:705.
45. Lauritzen M, Skyhoj Olsen T, Lassen NA, et al. Changes of regional cerebral blood flow during the course of classical migraine attacks. *Ann Neurol* 1983;13:633–641.
46. Olesen J, Friberg L, Olsen TS, et al. Timing and tomography of cerebral blood flow, aura and headache during migraine attacks. *Ann Neurol* 1990;28:791–798.
47. Lauritzen M, Losen J. Regional cerebral blood flow during migraine attacks by xenon-133 inhalation and emission tomography. *Brain* 1984;107:447–461.
48. Olesen J. Understanding the biologic basis of migraine. *N Engl J Med* 1994;331:1713–1714.
49. Woods RP, Iacoboni M, Maziotta JC. Bilateral spreading cerebral hypoperfusion during spontaneous migraine headache. *N Engl J Med* 1994;331:1689–1692.
50. Andersen AR, Friberg L, Olsen TS, et al. SPECT demonstration of delayed hypraemia following hypoperfusion in classic migraine. *Arch Neurol* 1988;45:154–159.
51. Lambert GA, Michalicek J. Cortical spreading depression reduced dural blood flow—a possible mechanism for migraine pain? *Cephalalgia* 1994;14:430–436.
52. Moskowitz MA, Nozaki K, Kraig RP. Neocortical spreading depression provokes the expression of C-fos protein-like immunoreactivitiy within trigeminal nucleus caudalis via trigeminovascular mechanisms. *J Neurosci* 1993;13(3):1167–1177.

53. Goadsby PJ, Gundlach AL. Localization of 3H-dihy-droergotamine binding sites in the cat CNS: relevance to migraine. *Ann Neurol* 1991;29:91–94.

54. Raskin NH, Hosobuchi Y, Lamb S. Headache may arise from perturbation of brain. *Headache* 1987;27:416–420.

55. Afridi SK, Matharu MS, Lee L, et al. A PET Study exploring the laterality of brainstem activation in migraine using glyceryl trinitrate. *Brain* 2005;128:932–939.

56. Graham JR, Wolff HG. Mechanism of migraine headache and action of ergotamine tartarate. *Arch Neurol Psychiat* 1938;39:737–763.

57. Blau JN, Dexter SL. The site of pain origin during migraine attacks. *Cephalalgia* 1981;1:143–147.

58. Martins IP, Baeta E, Paiva T, et al. Headaches during intracranial endovascular procedures: a possible model of vascular headache. *Headache* 1993;33:227–233.

59. Drummond PD, Lance JW. Extracranial vascular changes and the source of pain in migraine headache. *Ann Neurol* 1983;13:32–37.

60. Chapman LF, Ramos AO, Goodell H, Silverman G, Wolff HG. A humoral agent implicated in vascular headache of the migrainous type. *Arch Neurol* 1960;3:223–229.

61. Markowitz S, Saito K, Moskowitz MA. Neurogenically mediated leakage of plasma proteins occurs from blood vessels in dura mater but not brain. *J Neurosci* 1987;7:4129–4136.

62. Goadsby PJ, Edvinsson L, Ekman R. Vasoactive peptide release in the extracerebral circulation of humans during migraine headache. *Ann Neurol* 1990;28:183–187.

63. Zagami AS, Lambert GA. Stimulation of cranial vessels excites nociceptive neurons in several thalamic nuclei of the cat. *Exp Brain Res* 1990;81:552–566.

64. Goadsby PJ. Current concepts of the pathophysiology of migraines. *Neurol Clin* 1997;15:27–42.

65. Sicuteri F. Prophylactic and therapeutic properties of UML-491 in migraine. *Int Arch Allergy* 1959;15:300–307.

66. Curzon G, Barrie M, Wilkinson MIP. Relationship between headache and amino acid changes after administration of reserpine to migrainous patients. *J Neurol Neurosurg Psychiat* 1969;32:555–561.

67. Caroll JD, Hilton BP. The effects of reserpine injection on methysergide treated control and migrainous subjects. *Headache* 1974;14:149–156.

68. Sicuteri F, Testi A, Anselmi B. Biochemical investigations in headache: increase in the hydroxyindoleacetic acid excretion during migraine attacks. *Int Arch Allergy* 1961;15:55–58.

69. Kimball RW, Friedman AP, Vallejo E. Effect of serotonin in migraine patients. *Neurol* (Minneap) 1960;10:107–111.

70. Ferrari MD, Odink J, Tapparelli C, et al. Serotonin metabolism in migraine. *Neurol* 1989;39:1239–1242.

71. Moskowitz MA, Cutrer FM. Sumatriptan: a receptor-targeted treatment of migraine. *Ann Rev Med* 1993;44:145–154.

72. Ophoff RA, Terwindt GM, Vergouwe MN. Familial hemiplegic migraine and episodic ataxia type-2 are caused by mutations in Ca2+ channel gene CACNLA4. *Cell Tissue Res* 1996;87:543–552.

73. Lance JW. A concept of migraine and the search for the ideal headache drug. *Headache* 1990;30(suppl 1):17–23.

74. Welch KMW. Migraine: a biobehavioral disorder. *Arch Neurol* 1987;44:323–327.

75. Oleson J, Tfelt-Hanson P, Welch KMW, (eds.) *The headache*. New York, NY: Raven Press, 1993;247–253.

76. Burstein R. Yarnitsky D, Goor-Aryeh I, et al. An association between migraine and cutaneous allodynia. *Ann Neurol* 2000;47:614–624.

77. Burstein R, Yamamura H, Malick A, et al. Chemical stimulation of the intracranial dura induces enhanced responses to facial stimulation in brainstem trigeminal neurons. *J Neurophysiol* 1998;79:964–982.

78. Bille B. Migraine in school children. *Acta Paediat Scand* 1962;51(suppl 136):1–151.

79. Stewart WF, Lipton RB, Celentano DD, et al. Prevalence of migraine headache in the United States. Relation to age, income, race, and other sociodemographic factors. *JAMA* 1992;267:64–69.

80. Heritage AS, Stumpf WE, Sar M, et al. Brainstem catecholamine neurons as target sites for sex steroid hormones. *Science* 1980;207:1377–1379.

81. Gangula PRR, Wimalalawansa SJ, Yallampalli C. Pregnancy and sex steroid hormones enhance circulating calcitonin gene-related peptide concentrations in rats. *Human Reproduction* 2000;15:949–953.

82. Brieter DA, Stanfor LA, Barker DJ. Hormone-induced enlargement of receptive fields in trigeminal mechanoreceptive neurons. II possible mechanisms. *Brain Res* 1980;184:411–423.

83. Amandusson A, Hallbeck M, Hallbeck A-L, et al. Estrogen-induced alterations of spinal cord enkephalin gene expression. *Pain* 1999;83:243–248.

84. Coyle DE, Selhorst CS, Behbehani MM. Intact female rats are more susceptible to the development of tactile allodynia than ovariectomized female rats following partial sciatic nerve ligation (PSNL). *Neuroscience Letters* 1996;203:37–40.

85. Epstein MT, Hockaday JM, Hockaday TDR. Migraine and reproductive hormones throughout the menstrual cycle. *Lancet* 1975;1:543–547.

86. Hardman JG, Limbird LE, Molinoff PB, Ruddon RW, (eds.) *Goodman and Gilman's the pharmacological basis of therapeutics*, 9th ed. New York, NY: McGraw-Hill, 1996;1411–1440.

87. Critchley M, Friedman AP, Gorini S, Sicuteri F, (eds.) *Headache—physiopathological and clinical concepts*. New York, NY: Raven Press, 1982;215–226.

88. Lokken C, Holm JE, Myers TC. The menstrual cycle and migraine: a time-series analyses of 20 women migraineurs. *Headache* 1997;37:235–239.

89. MacGregor EA. Menstrual migraine: towards a definition. *Cephalalgia* 1996;16:11–21.

90. Cupini LM, Matteis M, Troisi E, et al. Sex-hormone-related events in migrainous females. A clinical comparative study between migraine with aura and migraine without aura. *Cephalalgia* 1995;15:140–144.

91. Benedetto C. Eicosanoids in primary dysmenorrhea, endometriosis, and menstrual migraine. *Gynecol Endocrinol* 1989;3:71–94.

92. Somerville BW. The role of progesterone in menstrual migraine. *Neurology* (Minneap) 1971;21:853–859.

93. Somerville BW. The role of estradiol withdrawal in the aetiology of menstrual migraine. *Neurology* (Minneap) 1972;22:355–365.

94. Somerville BW. Estrogen-withdrawal migraine. *Neurology* (Minneap) 1975;25:239–244.

95. Beckham JC, Krug LM, Penzien DB, et al. The relationship of ovarian steroids, headache activity and menstrual distress: a pilot study with female migraineurs. *Headache* 1992;32:292–297.

96. Carlson LA, Ekelund L, Oro L. Clinical and metabolic effects of different doses of prostaglandin E1 in man. *Acta Med Scand* 1968;183:423–430.

97. Silberstein SD, Merriam GR. Estrogens, progestins, and headache. *Neurology* 1991;41:786–793.

98. Nattero G, Alais G, DeLorenzo C, et al. Relevance of prostaglandins in true menstrual migraine. *Headache* 1989;29:232–238.

99. Taiwo Yo, Levine JD. Prostaglandins inhibit endogenous pain control mechanisms by blocking transmission at spinal noradrenergic synapses. *J Neurosci* 1988;8:1346–1349.

100. Solbach P, Sargent J, Coyne L. Menstrual migraine headache: results of a controlled, experimental, outcome study of non-drug treatments. *Headache* 1984;24:75–78.

101. MacGregor A, (ed.) *Migraine in women.* London: Martin Dunitz; 1999;33–46.

102. Wilkinson M. Treatment of acute migraine: The British experience. *Headache* 1990;30(suppl 2):545–549.

103. Welch KMA. Drug therapy of migraine. *N Engl J Med* 1993;329:1476–1483.

104. Tfelt-Hansen P. Prophylactic pharmacotherapy of migraine. *Neurol Clin* 1997;15:153–165.

105. Sances G, Martignoni E, Fiorini L, et al. Naproxen sodium in menstrual migraine prophylaxis: a double-blind placebo controlled study. *Headache* 1990;11:705–709.

106. Mathew NT. Cyclical prophylactic treatment of menstrual migraine using naproxen and ergotamine. *Headache* 1986;26:314.

107. Gallagher RM. Menstrual migraine and intermittent ergonovine therapy. *Headache* 1989;29:366–367.

108. Silberstein SD. DHE-45 in the prophylaxis of menstrually related migraine. *Cephalalgia* 1996;16:371.

109. Facchinetti F, Bonellie G, Kangasniemi P, et al. The efficacy and safety of subcutaneous sumatriptan in the acute treatment of menstrual migraine. *Obstet Gynecol* 1995;86:911–916.

110. Loder E. Prophylaxis of menstrual migraine with triptans: problems and possibilities. *Neurology* 2002;59:1677–1681.

111. Gross M, Barrie M, Bates D, et al. The efficacy of sumatriptan in menstrual migraine—a prospective study. *Cephalalgia* 1995;15(suppl14):227.

112. Solbach MP, Waymer RS. Treatment of menstruation-associated migraine headache with subcutaneous sumatriptan. *Obstet Gynaecol* 1993;82:769–772.

113. Silberstein SD, Massiou H, MacCarroll KA, Lines CR. Further evaluation of rizatriptan in menstrual migraine: retrospective analysis of long-term data. *Headache* 2002;42(9):917–923.

114. Magos AL, Zilkha KJ, Studd JWW. Treament of menstrual migraine by oestradiol implants. *J Neurol Neurosurg Psychiatr* 1983;46:1044–1046.

115. O'Dea JPK. Tamoxifen in the treatment of menstrual migraine. *Neurology* 1990;40:1470–1471.

116. Carlton GJ, Burnett JW. Danazol and migraine. *N Engl J Med* 1984;310:721–722.

117. Herzog AG. Continuous bromocriptine therapy in menstrual migraine. *Neurology* 1997;48:101–102.

118. Alvarez WC. Can one cure migraine in women by inducing menopause? Report on forty-two cases. *Mayo Clin Proc* 1940;15:380–382.

119. Ratinahirana H, Darbois Y, Bousser MG. Migraine and pregnancy: a prospective study in 703 women after delivery. *Neurology* 1990;40(suppl 1):437.

120. Lance JW, Anthony M. Some clinical aspects of migraine. *Arch Neurol* 1966;15:356–361.

121. Somerville BW. A study of migraine in pregnancy. *Neurology* 1972;22:824–828.

122. Granella F, Sances G, Zanferrari C, et al. Migraine without aura and reproductive life events: a clinical epidemiologic study in 1,300 women. *Headache* 1993;33:385.

123. Maggioni F, Alessi G, Maggino T, et al. Primary headaches and pregnancy (abstract). *Cephalalgia* 1995; 15:54.

124. Hardebo JE, Edvinsson L. Reduced sensitivity to alpha and beta-adrenergic receptor agonists of intra and extracranial vessels during pregnancy: relevance to migraine. *Acta Neurol Scand* 1977;56(suppl):204–205.

125. Critchley M, Friedman AP, Gorini S, Sicuteri F, (eds.) *Headache—Physiopathological and clinical aspects.* New York, NY: Raven Press, 1982;65–74.

126. Chancellor AM, Wroe SJ, Cull RE. Migraine occurring for the first time in pregnancy. *Headache* 1990;30:224–227.

127. Bending JJ. Recurrent bilateral reversible migrainous hemiparesis during pregnancy. *Can Med Assoc J* 1982; 127(6):508–509.

128. Wright GDS, Patel MK. Focal migraine and pregnancy. *Br Med J* 1986;293:1557–1558.

129. Mandel S. Hemoplegic migraine in pregnancy. *Headache* 1988;28:414–416.

130. Jacobson SL, Redman CWG. Basilar migraine with loss of consciousness in pregnancy. Case report. *Br J Obstet Gynaecol* 1989;96:494–495.

131. Wainscott G, Sullivan FM, Volans GN, et al. The outcome of pregnancy in women suffering from migraine. *Postgrad Med J* 1978;54:98–102.

132. Stein GS. Headaches in the first post partum week and their relationship to migraine. *Headache* 1981;21:201–205.

133. Dooling EC, Sweeney VP. Migrainous hemiplegia during breast-feeding. *Am J Obstet Gyneacol* 1974;118:568–570.

134. Askmark H, Lundberg PO. Lactation headache—a new form of headache? *Cephalalgia* 1989;9:119–122.

135. Diamond S. A headache history. The key to diagnosis. *Postgrad Med* 1974;56:69–73.

136. Goldstein PJ, Stern BJ, (eds.) *Neurological disorders of pregnancy,* 2nd ed. New York, NY: Futura Publishing, 1982:107–124.

137. Silberstein SD. Migraine and pregnancy. *Neurol Clin* 1997;15:209–231.

138. Rose FC, (ed.) *Progress in migraine research 2.* London: Pittman Press, 1984;18–29.

139. Robbins LD. Cryotherapy for headache. *Headache* 1989;29:598–600.

140. Diamond S. Biofeedback and headache. *Neurol Clin* 1983;1:479–488.

141. Schraft L, Marcus DA, Turk DC. Maintenance of effects in the nonmedical treatment of headaches during pregnancy. *Headache* 1996;36:285–290.

142. Davis ME, Adair FL, Rogers G, et al. A new active principle in ergot and its effect on uterine motility. *Am J Obstet Gynecol* 1935;29:155–167.

143. Rudolph AM. Effects of aspirin and acetaminophen on pregnancy and in the newborn. *Arch Intern Med* 1981; 141:358–363.

144. Pruyn SC, Phelan JP, Buchanan GC. Long-term propranolol therapy in pregnancy: maternal and fetal outcome. *Am J Obstet Gynecol* 1979;135:485–489.

145. Kaplan PW, (ed.) *Neurologic diseases in women.* New York, NY: Demos, 1998;25–44.

146. Hughes HE, Goldstein DA. Birth defects following maternal exposure to ergotamine, beta blockers and caffeine. *J Med Genet* 1988;25:396–399.

147. Redmond GP. Propranolol and fetal growth retardation. *Semin Perinatol* 1982;6:142–147.

148. Altschuler LL, Cohen L, Szuba MP, et al. Pharmacologic management of psychiatric illness during pregnancy: dilemmas and guidelines. *Am J Psychiat* 1996;153: 592–606.

149. Chambers CD, Johnson KA, Dick LM, et al. Birth outcomes in pregnant women taking fluoxetine. *N Engl J Med* 1996;335:1010–1015.

150. Nulman I, Rovet J, Stewart DE, et al. Neurodevelopment of children exposed in utero to antidepressant drugs. *N Engl J Med* 1997;336:258–262.

151. Wisner KL, Perel JM, Findling RL. Antidepressant treatment during breast-feeding. *Am J Psychiat* 1996;153: 1132–1137.

152. Miles CB. Treatment of migraine during pregnancy and lactation. *South Dakota J Med* 1995;48:373–377.

153. Whitty CWM, Hockaday JM. Migraine: a follow-up study of 92 patients. *Br Med J* 1968;1:735–736.

154. Critchley M, Friedman AP, Gorini S. Sicuteri E, eds. *Headache—physiopathological and clinical concepts.* New York, NY: Raven Press, 1982;377–390.

155. Neri I, Granella F, Nappi R, et al. Characteristics of headache at menopause. *Maturitas* 1993;17:31–37.

156. Lichten EM, Lichten JB, Whitty A, et al. The confirmation of a biochemical marker for women's hormonal migraine: the depo-estradiol challenge test. *Headache* 1996;36:367–371.

157. Silberstein SD, Merriam GR. Sex hormones and headache. *J Pain and Symptom Management* 1993;8: 98–114.

158. Ramos R, Apelo R, Osteria T, Vilar E. A comparative analysis of three different dose combinations of oral contraceptives. *Contraception* 1989;39:165–177.

159. Mears E, Grant ECS. Anovlar as a contraceptive. *Br Med J* 1962;2:75–79.

160. Kudrow L. The relationship of headache frequency to hormonal use on migraine. *Headache* 1975;15:36–49.

161. Dalton K. Migraine and oral contraceptives. *Headache* 1975;15:247–251.

162. Larsson-Cohn V, Lundberg PO. Headache and treatment with oral contraceptives. *Acta Neurol Scand* 1970; 46:267–278.

163. Becker WJ. Migraine and oral contraceptives. *Can J Neurol Sci* 1997;24:16–21.

164. Massiou H, MacGregor EA. Evolution and treatment of migraine with oral contraceptives. *Cephalalgia* 2000;20:170–174.

165. Tzourio C, Tehindrazanarivelo A, Iglesias S, et al. Case-control study of migraine and risk of ischaemic stroke in young women. *Br Med J* 1995;310:830–833.

166. Lidegaard O. Oral contraceptives, pregnancy and the risk of cerebral thromboembolism: the influence of diabetes hypertension, migraine and previous thrombolic disease. *Br J Obstet Gynecol* 1995;102:153–159.

167. Collaborative group for the study of stroke in young women. Oral contraception and increased risk of cerebral ischaemia or thrombosis. *N Engl J Med* 1973; 288:871–877.

168. MacGregor EA. Menstruation, sex hormones, and migraine. *Neurol Clin* 1997;15:125–141.

169. Martin PL, Burnier AM, Segre EJ, et al. Graded sequential therapy in the menopause: a double-blind study. *Am J Obstet Gynecol* 1971;111:178–186.

170. Greenblatt RB, Bruneteau DW. Menopausal headache—psychogenic or metabolic? *J Am Geriatr Soc* 1974;283: 186–190.

171. Kaiser HJ, Meienberg O. Deterioration or onset of migraine under oestrogen replacement therapy in the menopause. *J Neurol* 1993;240:195–197.

172. Wilson PWF, Garrison RJ, Castelli WP. Postmenopausal estrogen use, cigarette smoking, and cardiovascular morbidity in women over 50. The Framingham Study. *N Engl J Med* 1985;313:1038–1045.

173. Viscoli CM, Brass LM, Kernan WN, et al. A clinical trial of estrogen-replacement therapy after ischaemic stroke. *N Engl J Med* 2001;345:1243–1249.

174. Silberstein SD, de Lignires D. Migraine, menopause and hormone replacement therapy. *Cephalalgia* 2000;20: 214–221.

15 Seizures and Epilepsy in Women

Martha J. Morrell, MD

Epilepsy is a common neurologic disorder that affects 1 in every 100 individuals, both children and adults. With the exception of epilepsy related to head trauma, the incidence is equal for men and women. All persons with epilepsy live with the concern that a seizure could occur at any time, must take medications every day for years or even a lifetime, and endure the social and economic hardships that accompany this misunderstood condition (1,2).

Women with epilepsy face additional challenges. Neuroactive ovarian steroid hormones alter the clinical expression of seizures and of epilepsy syndromes over a woman's reproductive life. Some antiepileptic drugs (AEDs) reduce the levels of physiologic ovarian sex steroid hormones and may reduce the efficacy of contraceptive steroids. Women with epilepsy have a greater risk for syndromes associated with infertility, such as hypothalamic-pituitary axis disruption, polycystic ovary–like syndrome, and anovulatory cycles. Bone loss related to AEDs is more likely to lead to pathologic fracture in women. In addition, women with epilepsy taking AEDs are at higher risk for pregnancy complications related to seizures, morphologic abnormalities in offspring, and, perhaps, neurodevelopmental compromise. Unfortunately, most physicians are not knowledgeable about these health risks (3).

Women receiving AEDs for conditions other than epilepsy face challenges similar to women with epilepsy.

AEDs are used widely in the treatment of affective disorders such as bipolar disorder, migraine, and pain. AED effects on the metabolism of carbohydrates, hormones, and bone place these women at equal risk concerning long-term health consequences. Therefore, this topic is addressed in two chapters—one discussing issues that relate more specifically to women with epilepsy (to women receiving AEDs for other indications; see also Chapter 5).

EPIDEMIOLOGY OF SEIZURES AND EPILEPSY IN WOMEN

Seizures are transient alterations in neurologic function that arise because of excessive and/or hypersynchronous abnormal electrical discharges in neurons of the cerebral cortex. Approximately 10% of the population will experience a seizure in their lifetime. Epilepsy is defined as a chronic neurologic condition characterized by recurrent unprovoked epileptic seizures.

The incidence of epilepsy and of all unprovoked seizures in Rochester, Minnesota, from 1935 through 1984 was 44 per 100,000 person-years (4), and the incidence and prevalence rates for epilepsy are higher in men than in women (see Table 15.1).

The cumulative incidence of all epilepsy is also significantly higher in men than women. The cumulative

TABLE 15.1
*Incidence and Prevalence Rates
for Epilepsy by Gender*

	Male	Female
Incidence per 100,000 person-years[1]	49	41
Prevalence per 1,000 persons[2]	6	5.6

[1]Hauser et al., 1993.
[2]Hauser and Kurland, 1975.

TABLE 15.3
*Age-adjusted Incidence of Seizures
per 100,000 Person-Years by Gender[1]*

	Male	Female
Partial seizures	28	24
Generalized tonic-clonic	20	15
Absence	2	3

[1]Hauser et al., 1993.

incidence for men is 3.4% through age 74 years, compared with 2.8% in women through 74 years (4). After a single seizure, the risk of recurrence (second seizure) is no different for men and women (5,6) and the probability of remission in men and women with epilepsy is also not different (7). The higher prevalence and incidence rates for epilepsy in men is attributable to the greater frequency of neurologic disorders such as cerebral palsy (8), head trauma, cerebrovascular disease, and alcohol-related epilepsy in men (9).

Epileptic Seizures

Table 15.2 lists the classification of epileptic seizures, as established by the International League against Epilepsy (10).

Using the Rochester, Minnesota database, the age-adjusted incidence per 100,000 person-years for partial seizures is 25 years and for generalized seizures is 17 years. As shown in Table 15.3, the age-adjusted incidence for simple partial, complex partial, and generalized tonic-clonic seizures is higher in men than in women (4). Only absence seizures (petit mal) show a predilection for females.

Epilepsy Syndromes

An international classification for the epilepsies defines syndromes by seizure type and etiology and is provided in Table 15.4 (11).

Syndromic classification predicts the response to treatment and prognosis and is therefore a useful clinical

TABLE 15.2
International Classification of Epileptic Seizures[1]

Partial (focal, local) Seizures
    Simple partial seizures (consciousness not impaired)
        Motor signs
        Somatosensory or special sensory symptoms
        Autonomic symptoms or signs
        Psychic symptoms
    Complex partial seizures (consciousness impaired)
        Simple partial onset followed by impaired consciousness
        Consciousness impaired at onset
    Partial seizures evolving to generalized seizures (tonic, clonic, or tonic-clonic)
        Simple partial seizures evolving to generalized seizures
        Complex partial seizures evolving to generalized seizures
        Simple partial seizures evolving to complex partial seizures evolving to generalized seizures

Generalized Seizures (convulsive or nonconvulsive)
    Absence seizures
        Typical (brief stare, eye flickering, no motion)
        Atypical (associated with movement)

    Myoclonic seizures
        Clonic seizures
        Tonic seizures
        Tonic-clonic seizures
        Atonic seizures

Unclassified Epileptic Seizures

[1]From the Commission on Classification and Terminology of the International League Against Epilepsy, 1981.

TABLE 15.4

International Classification of Epilepsies, Epilepsy Syndromes, and Related Seizure Disorders[1]

(Syndrome defined by seizure type and other clinical features, including anatomic localization and etiology)

Localization-Related (focal, local, partial) Epilepsies:
Idiopathic
Benign childhood epilepsy with centrotemporal spikes
Childhood epilepsy with occipital paroxysms
Primary reading epilepsy
Symptomatic
Temporal lobe epilepsy
Frontal lobe epilepsy
Parietal lobe epilepsy
Occipital lobe epilepsy
Chronic progressive epilepsia partialis continua
Cryptogenic (presumed to be symptomatic but cause is unknown)
Temporal lobe epilepsy
Frontal lobe epilepsy
Parietal lobe epilepsy
Occipital lobe epilepsy
Chronic progressive epilepsia partialis continua
Generalized Epilepsies
Idiopathic
Benign neonatal convulsions (familial and nonfamilial)
Benign myoclonic epilepsy in infancy
Childhood absence epilepsy
Juvenile myoclonic epilepsy
Epilepsy with generalized tonic-clonic seizures on awakening

Cryptogenic
West's syndrome (infantile spasms)
Lennox-Gastaut syndrome
Epilepsy with myoclonic-astatic seizures
Epilepsy with myoclonic absences
Symptomatic
Nonspecific etiology
Early myoclonic encephalopathy
Early infantile epileptic encephalopathy with suppression burst
Other symptomatic generalized epilepsies
Undetermined Epilepsies
Generalized and focal features
Neonatal seizures
Severe myoclonic epilepsy of childhood
Epilepsy with continuous spike waves during slow-wave sleep
Acquired epileptic aphasia (Landau-Kleffner syndrome)
Other undetermined epilepsies
Without unequivocal generalized or focal features
Special Syndromes
Situation-related seizures
Febrile convulsions
Isolated seizures or status epilepticus
Seizures caused by an acute or toxic event, such as alcohol or drug overdose, eclampsia, or hyperglycemia

---

[1]From the Commission on Classification and Terminology of the International League Against Epilepsy, 1989.

TABLE 15.5

Epileptic Syndromes and Gender[1]

Syndromes Equally Common in Men and Women
Benign familial neonatal convulsions
Benign epilepsy with occipital paroxysms
Epilepsy with continuous spike and wave during slow sleep (ESES)
Juvenile myoclonic epilepsy
Syndromes More Common in men
Febrile seizures
Ohtahara syndrome
West syndrome (infantile spasms)
Benign and severe myoclonic epilepsy in infants
Lennox-Gastaut syndrome
Benign partial epilepsy with centrotemporal spikes (Rolandic epilepsy)
Juvenile absence epilepsy

Epilepsy with generalized tonic-clonic seizures upon awakening
Localization related epilepsy of frontal or temporal origin
Landau-Kleffner syndrome
Epilepsies associated with X-linked disorders:
Fragile-X
Menke's disease
Syndromes More Common in Women
Childhood absence epilepsy
Photosensitive epilepsy
Syndromes Occurring Exclusively in Females
Associated with Epilepsy
Retts syndrome
Aicardi syndrome

---

[1]Adapted from Wallace, 1991.

construct. As illustrated in Table 15.5, most epilepsies preferentially affect men.

Several epilepsy syndromes, however, are more likely to affect women. Childhood absence epilepsy is a relatively common genetic epilepsy of childhood characterized by absence seizures and, rarely, by generalized tonic-clonic seizures as well. Age of onset is between 3 and 5 years and puberty (12), and 60% of affected individuals are female (13). This epilepsy is not associated with other neurologic dysfunction and carries a favorable prognosis for remission by puberty (14). Photosensitive epilepsy is a rare form of epilepsy characterized by generalized seizures provoked by flickering light. Seizures are typically generalized tonic-clonic, although absence and myoclonic seizures may occur as well (15). Developmental and neurologic exams are normal, but the EEG displays a photoconvulsive response with photic stimulation (16). The ratio of affected women to men is 1.5 to 1 (15). Juvenile myoclonic epilepsy (JME) is a genetically mediated epilepsy syndrome that arises around puberty (17). The hallmark is myoclonic seizures. Persons with JME typically have infrequent generalized tonic-clonic seizures and may have absence seizures as well. Women are more often affected than men. This epilepsy syndrome does not remit but usually responds quite well to AED therapy.

Seizures occur in some neurologic syndromes that affect only females. Rett syndrome (18) is a genetic disorder that is lethal in males and is characterized by developmental arrest and regression at age 6 months, mental retardation, loss of purposeful use of hands, and hyperventilation. Approximately 75% of girls with Rett syndrome develop epilepsy. Aicardi syndrome (19) affects females only and is characterized by severe mental retardation, infantile spasms, agenesis of the corpus callosum, hypotonia or spasticity, and typical lesions in the optic fundus (lacunae). Seizures in Aicardi syndrome begin early in life and are rarely controlled.

Nonepileptic Seizures

Seizures manifest as paroxysmal, transient alterations in neurologic function. A number of clinical entities can mimic epileptic seizures (20). A differential diagnosis for seizures is provided in Table 15.6.

Within this category of events mimicking seizures in adults, the most commonly encountered entities are cardiogenic or vasovagal syncope, migraines, anxiety disorders, and psychogenic seizures. Nonepileptic psychogenic seizures affect women more often than men. Nonepileptic psychogenic seizures are also called *pseudoseizures* and represent the most frequent seizure-like event presenting to epilepsy centers (21), arising in between 20 and 30% of patients referred to epilepsy centers.

Nonepileptic psychogenic seizures may resemble epileptic seizures but do not arise as a result of abnormal paroxysmal discharge of cerebral neurons. Most psychogenic seizures are precipitated by psychologic factors, which, in many cases, remain subconscious. Patients with these spells are often young and female (22,23) and may suffer from somatoform, panic, or dissociative disorders, from psychosis, and less commonly, malingering (22).

TABLE 15.6
Differential Diagnosis of Epileptic Seizures

Syncope of Cardiac Origin
Arrhythmias
    Supraventricular and ventricular
    Stokes Adams attacks
    Heart block/asystole
Congenital heart disease
Cardiomyopathy
Atrial myxoma

Syncope of Noncardiac Origin
Vasovagal
    Micturition, tussive, carotid sinus disturbance
Valsalva
Medication induced (related to drop in systemic vascular resistance)
    Tricyclic antidepressants, levodopa, antihypertensives, phenothiazines
Orthostatic
    Shy Drager syndrome, Parkinson's disease
    Autonomic neuropathies
Hypovolemia
Hyperventilation
Breath-holding

Benign Paroxysmal Vertigo
Migraine
Transient global amnesia
Cerebrovascular disease
Toxic/metabolic disturbance
    Alcohol, strychnine, carbon monoxide poisoning, cyanide
    Hypoglycemia
    Porphyria
    Renal/hepatic disease
    Pheochromocytoma
Psychiatric disease
    Anxiety/panic disorder, conversion disorder, intermittent explosive disorder (episodic dyscontrol)
Sleep disorders
    Narcolepsy, parasomnias, paroxysmal nocturnal choreoathetosis
Movement disorders
    Paroxysmal dyskinesias
Psychogenic seizures

¹Adapted from Morrell, 1993.

No behaviors absolutely differentiate nonepileptic from epileptic seizures (21–23,24). Psychogenic seizures present with a wide spectrum of behaviors from subtle alterations in sensation mimicking simple partial seizures to generalized motor events that resemble tonic-clonic convulsions. Dramatic motor events such as fluctuating, arrhythmic, "struggling" type movements, pelvic thrusting, trunk and extremity extension, alternating to-and-fro head movements, bizarre facial grimacing, body posturing, and opisthotonos are more characteristic of psychogenic seizures. Prolonged nonresponsiveness with motor arrest (more than 5 minutes) is a common presentation in psychogenic seizures, as is a motionless collapse. Retained consciousness, despite bilateral motor manifestations, has been described as typical for psychogenic spells. The length of the episode may help differentiate between epileptic and nonepileptic events. Although most tonic-clonic seizures are less than 60 seconds in duration, psychogenic convulsive seizures may be considerably longer. Urinary incontinence and injury have been described in as many as 20% of patients with pseudoseizures and therefore does not serve as a useful distinguishing criterion.

These behavioral distinctions serve as guidelines only. Each of these behaviors can also arise with epileptic seizures, particularly seizures originating in the frontal lobe (20). Frontal lobe seizures may be brief and bizarre, containing many behaviors previously thought to suggest psychogenic seizures, such as back arching, pelvic thrusting, asynchronous movements, retained consciousness despite bilateral movements, and a brief or nonexistent post-ictal phase.

Although behaviors may not be specific, nonepileptic events can be suspected when behaviors are unusual and not stereotyped, when the events do not respond to appropriate AEDs, and when the events have a constant precipitant related to psychosocial stresses. The psychogenic seizure may bring secondary benefits such as increased attention from significant individuals, relief from home and work responsibilities, and disability insurance or other financial benefits.

Psychogenic seizures may be more likely to affect women because sexual and physical abuse appear to be risk factors, and women are more likely than men to experience such abuse. In one study of women presenting to two urban emergency departments, one in four had a history of physical or nonphysical partner violence in the previous year (25). It is estimated that 5 to 10% of the female population has experienced severe, penetrative sexual abuse (26). Individuals experiencing such significant life traumas are more likely to have psychogenic seizures that arise as a consequence of conversion disorders or dissociative disorders similar to posttraumatic stress disorder or multiple personality disorder. Other psychologic and psychodynamic mechanisms leading to psychogenic seizures include misinterpretation of other somatic events such as anxiety episodes or panic attacks, or of paroxysmal behaviors such as movement disorders, explosive behaviors, and even daydreaming. Less commonly, the psychogenic seizure represents malingering.

WHY EPILEPSY IS DIFFERENT IN WOMEN THAN IN MEN

Phenotypic Expression of Epilepsy

Ovarian sex steroid hormones alter neuronal excitability and affect seizure frequency (27). Gonadal and adrenal steroid hormones have immediate, short-term effects on neuronal excitability, as well as long-acting, delayed genomic effects. Estrogen acts at the cell membrane to increase net excitation, whereas progesterone enhances net inhibition. In experimental models of generalized and focal epilepsies, estrogen exerts a seizure activating effect. In contrast, progesterone elevates the seizure threshold and acts as a CNS depressant. Dynamic changes occur in neuronal excitability and morphology over the menstrual cycle. The seizure threshold in animal models of epilepsy is altered over the estrous cycle. It is presumed that the same phenomenon occurs in humans and explains the phenomenon of catamenial seizures and changes in seizure expression at puberty and menopause.

Molecular Mechanism of Action of Ovarian Steroids

Estrogen has both genomic and membrane effects that increase excitation and reduce inhibition (28). Estrogen exerts immediate effects on membrane excitability at the A receptor for gamma aminobutyric acid (GABA-A). When estrogen occupies a recognition site on the GABA-A receptor, chloride conductance is altered so that GABA-mediated inhibition is less effective. Estrogen also acts as an agonist at the N-methyl-D-aspartate (NMDA) receptor to mediate excitation in the CA-1 region of the hippocampus. This serves to increase excitation in this region of the medial temporal lobe. The genomic effects of estrogen include alteration of the messenger RNA that encodes for GABA amino decarboxylase (GAD), an enzyme that regulates the synthetic rate for the neurochemical GABA. Estrogen also reduces the rate of synthesis of the GABA-A receptor subunits. The net effect of estrogen is a reduction in numbers of GABA-A receptor subunits, a reduction in GABA concentration, and subsequently, less inhibitory effect.

Progesterone has the opposite effect of estrogen (28). The occupation of the GABA-A receptor subunit by progesterone results in increased inhibitory effect and reduced glutamate-mediated excitatory effect in the temporal lobe. Genomically, progesterone enhances GABA synthesis and increases the total number of GABA-A receptor subunits.

In animal models, estrogen is proconvulsive and progesterone is anticonvulsive. Estrogen reduces the electroconvulsive shock threshold in animals, which is thought to be a model for human generalized tonic-clonic seizures. Estrogen induces, aggravates, or prolongs seizures in animal models of epilepsy. In some women with epilepsy, estrogen increases the frequency of EEG epileptiform activity. The reduced metabolites of progesterone increase the seizure threshold and suppress seizures in animal models. In some women with epilepsy, progesterone reduces EEG epileptiform discharges.

The proconvulsant effect of estrogen was demonstrated by studies conducted by Woolley et al. (29,30). These investigators compared the effect of exposure to physiologic concentrations of estrogen on CA-1 neurons taken from ovariectomized animals to the effects of a control an oil vehicle (30). Estrogen exposure profoundly altered neuronal morphology; numerous dendritic spines were formed, representing potential synaptic connections. These morphologic changes were evident within 12 to 24 hours of estrogen exposure. Conversely, when estrogen levels fell, these changes reversed within a similar period. Recently, Woolley et al. (29) demonstrated the significance of these findings. In CA-1 neurons from ovariectomized animals, glutamate treatment resulted in a significant increase in excitatory outputs [input/output (I/O) slope] in CA-1 neurons that were pretreated with estrogen, compared with control neurons pretreated with oil. The increased height of the input/output slope with estrogen exposure represents an increased likelihood of a synaptic event and neural firing after glutamate exposure.

Responsiveness to steroid hormones may be more pronounced in the postpubertal than in the prepubertal brain. Hormonal influences on epilepsy may also be different in the premenopausal versus the postmenopausal woman.

Effect of Puberty on Epilepsy

The reported effects of puberty on epilepsy are contradictory. Niijima and Wallace (31) reported a transient worsening of localization-related epilepsy syndromes that they attributed to a reduction in AED plasma concentrations rather than a hormonally driven effect. Rosciszewska (32) found that generalized tonic-clonic and complex partial seizures were likely to worsen at puberty. In contrast, Diamantopoulos and Crumrine (33) reported a reduction in the frequency of complex partial seizures at puberty.

Catamenial seizures

The ovulatory phase of the human menstrual cycle is characterized by an estrogen peak, the perimenstrual or menstrual phase by progesterone withdrawal (decline), and menses by an increase in the estrogen to progesterone ratio. Catamenial seizures are influenced by these cyclical hormonal changes and occur in one-third to one-half of women with epilepsy (34). Seizures are more frequent perimenstrually and sometimes also at ovulation.

Indeed, research on seizure patterns finds a strong relationship between the stage of the menstrual cycle and seizures, with the majority of seizures occurring during the perimenstrual period (about 3 days before the onset of menstrual flow) and at ovulation (34). This seizure pattern is not seen in anovulatory cycles when the ovulatory estrogen surge and luteal progesterone peak do not occur. Rather, during an anovulatory cycle, the estrogen-to-progesterone ratio remains elevated and relatively constant. Not surprisingly, seizure distribution is more randomly distributed, and seizure frequency is greater, compared with ovulatory cycles (34).

Catamenial seizures may occur as a result of the reduced plasma concentration of AEDs. Current opinion, however, is that catamenial seizures arise because of cycle-related changes in neuroactive steroids. Elevated estrogen at ovulation, progesterone withdrawal at menses, and an elevated estrogen:progesterone ratio (anovulatory cycles) are the major proposed hormonal mechanisms (34).

Epilepsy at Menopause

Little is known about the effects of menopause on epilepsy. During the perimenopausal period, significant fluctuations in pituitary gonadotrophins and ovarian steroids may precede the menopausal ovarian failure by many years. In one retrospective descriptive study (32), seizures were likely to improve at menopause if seizure onset had been relatively later in life, there was a catamenial relationship, and seizures were already well controlled. Women with frequent partial or tonic-clonic seizures were likely to become worse. A recent survey in an epilepsy center in Maryland identified a small group of women in whom seizures appeared to arise in the menopausal period (35). Another retrospective study found that women often experienced a seizure exacerbation over the perimenopause (36).

Treatment of Hormonally Sensitive Seizures

No sufficient data exist to develop guidelines for the treatment of hormone-sensitive seizures. The results of small open trials (37) suggest that some women may benefit from sustained therapy with natural progesterone, but further research is needed to confirm this in clinical practice. Currently, these seizures are treated conventionally with AEDs and acetazolamide.

RESPONSE TO TREATMENT: AED EFFICACY AND TOLERABILITY BY GENDER

The treatment of epilepsy is directed towards suppression of seizures by AEDs. The most widely used drugs are phenobarbital, phenytoin, carbamazepine, and valproate—all released before 1978. These drugs have been evaluated for efficacy individually and in comparative trials (38,39) so that differential efficacy can be defined. The efficacy of the most commonly used AEDs by epilepsy syndrome and seizure type is listed in Table 15.7.

An analysis of efficacy by gender is mandated by the U.S. Food and Drug Administration (FDA) for each new pharmacologic product tested in the United States (40).

TABLE 15.7

Commonly Used Antiepileptic Drugs: Use by Seizure Type* and Pharmacokinetic Characteristics

Drug	Seizure types	Usual adult dose (mg/day)	Half-life (h)	Metabolism	Usual effective plasma concentration (μg/mL)	Effect on hepatic cytochrome P450 enzymes	Bound fraction (%)
Phenytoin (Dilantin)	Partial and GTC	300–400	22	>90% hepatic with induction	10–20	Induction	90–95
Carbamazepine (Tegretol, Carbatrol)	Partial and GTC	800–1600	8–22	>90% hepatic with induction	8–12	Induction	75
Phenobarbital	Partial and GTC	90–180	100	>90% hepatic with induction	15–40	Induction	45
Valproate (Depakote, Depakene)	Broad spectrum	1000–3000	15–20	>95% hepatic with inhibition	50–120	Inhibition	80–90
Ethosuximide (Zarontin)	Absence	750–1500	60	65% hepatic, no induction	40–100	No effect	<5
Felbamate (Felbatol)	Broad spectrum	2400–3600	14–23	60% hepatic	20–140[a]	No significant effect	25
Gabapentin (Neurontin)	Partial and GTC	1800–3600	5–7	>95% renal	4–16[a]	No effect	<5
Lamotrigine (Lamictal)	Broad spectrum	100–500	12–60[b]	>90% hepatic, no induction	2–16[a]	No effect	55
Topiramate (Topamax)	Broad spectrum	200–400	19–25	30% hepatic no induction	4–10	Induction at higher dosage	9–17
Tiagabine (Gabitril)	Partial	32–56	5–13	>90% hepatic, no induction	NE	No effect	95
Oxcarbazepine (Trileptal)	Partial and GTC	600–1800	8–10[c]	>90% hepatic, mild induction	10–35[c]	Induction at higher dosage	40[c]
Levetiracetam (Keppra)	Broad spectrum?	1000–3000	6–8	>65% renal excretion	5–45[a]	No effect	<10
Zonisamide (Zonegran)	Broad spectrum	100–400	63	70% hepatic no induction	10–40[a]	No effect	40

[a] Not established; represents usual concentration in patients receiving therapeutic dose.
[b] Varies with concomitant ASD (lower with enzyme inducers; higher with inhibitors).
[c] Of MHD, active metabolite.
GTC=generalized tonic–clonic; NE=not established.
*Use by seizure type represents expert opinion and practice and does not necessarily correspond to FDA approved indications.

In 1993, the FDA called for a careful characterization of drug effects by gender so that differences in efficacy and safety relative to physiological gender differences could be detected (41). "For Phase III trials… women and minorities and their subpopulations must be included such that valid analysis of differences in intervention effect can be accomplished. In order to detect efficacy and safety differences related to physiologic gender differences, such as the effects of hormones, substantial representation of both sexes is expected, as is analysis by gender of effectiveness, adverse-event rates and dose-response" (41).

The gender-specific analysis of AED efficacy and tolerability is indicated because the pharmacokinetic and pharmacodynamic effects of some drugs may be altered in women because of smaller body size, higher body fat, lower body water content, and a lesser muscle mass. Pharmacokinetic interactions with endogenous hormones and with therapeutic hormones—such as contraceptive sex steroid hormones and hormone replacement therapy (HRT), might also alter AED efficacy. The neuroactive steroids could also modulate the pharmacodynamic effects of the AEDs.

An analysis of efficacy by gender is available for the majority of the newly marketed and soon to be released AEDs, but has not been provided for the older AEDs. Gabapentin, felbamate, lamotrigine, tiagabine, and topiramate were as effective and well tolerated in women as in men during premarketing trials. Zonisamide was as efficacious in men as in women but was somewhat better tolerated by women (42). Further analysis of efficacy and tolerability over the menstrual cycle and with changes in reproductive status has not been provided.

Although federal guidelines encourage the inclusion of women of child-bearing potential in investigational drug trials, these same agencies assume that pregnant and lactating women will be excluded (43). DHHS regulation 46, Subpart B directs that pregnant women may not be research subjects except under two circumstances: either that the purpose of the activity is to meet the health needs of the mother, and the fetus will be placed at risk only to the minimum extent necessary to meet such needs, or the risk to the fetus is minimal. The consequence of this policy is that very little information is available regarding the safety of an AED in the pregnant and lactating woman, even though these drugs will be used by many women with epilepsy throughout gestation and while breastfeeding.

This policy has been re-examined recently by the National Institutes of Health (NIH) and FDA, which directed the Institute of Medicine (IOM) to examine policies regarding the inclusion of pregnant and lactating women in clinical trials. In 1994, The IOM committee on women in research made a controversial recommendation that pregnant and lactating women be considered eligible to be subjects in clinical research. The IOM report stated, "…the prevailing presumption regarding the par-

ticipation of pregnant women in clinical trials…(should) be shifted from one of exclusion to one of inclusion." The IOM felt that women who are, or may become pregnant during the course of a research study should be viewed as any other competent adult who is a potential research subject (44).

Health Concerns for Women with Epilepsy

Chronic illnesses often carry comorbidities. Health concerns for the woman with epilepsy who must receive AEDs include reproductive dysfunction, metabolism disturbances such as unfavorable lipid profiles, changes in carbohydrate metabolism, and bone disease. Metabolic disorders appear to be the consequence of AEDs, rather than epilepsy. This topic is discussed in Chapter 5. Only a brief summary regarding contraceptive choice and bone health is included here.

Family Planning

Contraceptive choice is limited for women who take an AED that induces the hepatic cytochrome P450 enzyme system. Because of AED induction, steroid hormone metabolism and binding are increased. The failure rate of hormonal contraception in women on cytochrome P450 enzyme–inducing AEDs may exceed 6% per year (45). A detailed discussion concerning the effect of AEDs on hormonally based contraception is included in Chapters 4 and 5.

Bone Health

Persons with epilepsy are at a greater risk for bone disease, which typically presents as pathologic fracture. Bone biochemical abnormalities described in people with epilepsy include hypocalcemia, hypophosphatemia, elevated serum alkaline phosphatase, elevated parathyroid hormone (PTH), and reduced levels of vitamin D and its active metabolites (46). The most severe bone and biochemical abnormalities are found in patients receiving AED polytherapy and in patients who have taken AEDs for a longer time. Further information regarding bone loss and diagnostic and treatment strategies is contained within Chapter 5.

Reproductive Health

Reproductive health may be compromised in women with epilepsy. Women with epilepsy are more likely to experience infertility, failure of hormonal contraception, and adverse pregnancy outcome. Anticipating these risks permits the clinician to provide treatment for the woman with epilepsy that is least likely to compromise reproductive health.

Women with epilepsy are at risk for reduced fertility and reproductive endocrine abnormalities (47,48). Women with epilepsy are only 37% as likely to have had a pregnancy as their nonepileptic sisters, independent of marital status (49–51). The cause of lower fertility rates is multifactorial. A study in Finland found that persons with epilepsy were less likely to marry and to have offspring (52). In part, this reflects a choice. Much of that choice comes from wrong information suggesting that women with epilepsy are not fit parents, the risk of transmission of epilepsy is very high, or the risk of birth defects in children born to mothers with epilepsy is higher than it really is. A recent survey of health care professionals likely to encounter women with epilepsy finds that there is a marked lack of knowledge regarding pregnancy and fetal risks associated with maternal epilepsy and that many physicians would not support the decision of a woman with epilepsy to become pregnant (3). In addition to psychosocial challenges to parenting, lower birth rates are a consequence of menstrual cycle abnormalities, anovulatory menstrual cycles, reproductive endocrine disorders, and sexual dysfunction.

Abnormalities in the basal concentrations of pituitary gonadotrophins and in ovarian steroids may be one mechanism for infertility in women with epilepsy. Hypogonadotrophic hypogonadism, hypergonadotrophic hypogonadism, and polycystic ovaries are described in women with partial and generalized seizures (53–56). Hypothalamic dysfunction is suggested by observations that the pituitary release of LH is altered spontaneously and in response to gonadotrophin-releasing hormone (56–58). These alterations in reproductive hormones are described in women both treated and not treated with AEDs.

Some AEDs, however, alter the risk for specific reproductive disturbances, in part by altering the concentration of sex steroid hormones. Hypothalamic-pituitary axis function is altered as a consequence of changes in sex steroid hormone feedback inhibition and excitation. Women receiving CYP450 enzyme–inducing AEDs have significant reductions in serum concentrations of estradiol, testosterone, and dihydroepiandrostenedione, as well as elevations in sex hormone binding globulin (SHBG) (5962). Women taking valproate (which does not induce liver cytochrome enzymes) have higher gonadal and adrenal androgen levels (53,59,63). Enhanced steroid metabolism and binding reduces the concentration of biologically active steroid. In contrast, adrenal and gonadal androgens are significantly elevated in women receiving the CYP450 enzyme inhibitor valproate. Women with epilepsy taking gabapentin or lamotrigine—two AEDs that do not alter CYP450 enzymes—have sex steroid hormone levels no different from those of nonepileptic controls not taking medications (59). See Table 15.8.

Infertility may also arise because of menstrual cycle irregularity, an inadequate luteal phase, and ovulatory

TABLE 15.8

Categorization of AEDs by Effects on CYP450 Liver Enzymes

Drugs that induce CYP450 enzymes	Drugs that inhibit or have no effect on CYP450 enzymes
Carbamazepine	Felbamate
Oxcarbazepine	Gabapentin
Phenobarbital	Lamotrigine
Phenytoin	Valproate
Topiramate	Vigabatrin

Drugs that induce this enzyme system can be anticipated to lower the concentration of biologically available hormone and therefore reduce efficacy of hormonally based contraception. Drugs that inhibit or have no effect on this enzyme system will not alter the efficacy of hormonal contraception.

failure (1). Women with epilepsy are more likely to experience menstrual cycles that are abnormally short (less than 23 days) or long (greater than 36 days). About one-third of menstrual cycles in women with epilepsy are anovulatory, compared with a rate of about 10% in women without epilepsy (1,64). Women with primary generalized epilepsy are more likely to have anovulatory cycles than women with localization-related epilepsy (1). The antiepileptic medication valproate, unlike carbamazepine, gabapentin, lamotrigine, phenobarbital, or phenytoin, was significantly associated with anovulatory cycles in two studies (1,64). Women with primary generalized epilepsy receiving valproate were at highest risk. In fact, 55% of menstrual cycles were anovulatory in this group of women with epilepsy (1). Ovulatory failure associated with epilepsy and some AEDs may be a result of endocrine and end organ disturbances. Hypothalamic-pituitary axis dysfunction is suggested by observations that pituitary release of lutenizing hormone (LH) in women with epilepsy is altered spontaneously and in response to gonadotrophin-releasing hormone (GnRH) (54,57,58).

Polycystic Ovary Syndrome

The polycystic ovary syndrome (PCOS) is a gynecologic disorder affecting approximately 7% of reproductive-age women. Polycystic appearing ovaries, while often present in women with this syndrome, are not required for diagnosis. In fact, asymptomatic polycystic ovaries may be relatively common in normal women of reproductive age, occurring in 21 to 23% of women (65–67).

The diagnostic requirements for PCOS are phenotypic or serologic evidence for hyperandrogenism and anovulatory cycles (68). Phenotypic signs of hyperandrogenism include hirsutism, truncal obesity, and acne. Hirsutism presents as increased facial and body hair, coarsening of pubic hair with extension down the inner thigh and male pattern scalp hair loss—temporal recession and thinning over the crown. Obesity is in an axial distribution. Acne tends to be cystic, involving the lower face and often the back. Women with this syndrome have frequent anovulatory cycles, may have elevated androgen levels, an abnormal ratio of pituitary LH to follicle-stimulating hormone (FSH), elevated cholesterol with abnormal lipid profiles, elevated fasting or postprandial insulin levels, and glucose intolerance. The health consequences of PCOS include infertility, accelerated atherosclerosis, diabetes, and endometrial carcinoma, thus underscoring the importance of detection and treatment.

Women with epilepsy appear to be at risk for developing features of this syndrome, although no study in a cohort of women with epilepsy is adequately designed to permit an accurate diagnosis of this syndrome. In a random sample of 20 women with epilepsy of temporal lobe origin, five had PCOS, characterized clinically by oligomenorrhea, hirsutism, and androgen and LH elevation, or by ovarian cysts visualized directly or by ultrasonography (69). Another evaluation of 50 women with partial seizures arising from the temporal lobe found that 28 had menstrual cycle disturbance and 19 had reproductive endocrine disorders and polycystic ovaries (56). Polycystic-appearing ovaries and hyperandrogenism are reported to arise in as many as 40% of women with epilepsy receiving valproate (1,53,64) and may be more likely to occur in women who first receive valproate at puberty (69) or before age 20 (53). Other studies have shown that valproate is more often associated with polycystic ovaries than are carbamazepine, phenytoin, gabapentin, and phenobarbital (1,53,70). However, one study found no difference in the frequency of polycystic appearing ovaries in 52 women taking valproate and 53 women taking carbamazepine for epilepsy (71).

In a prospective assessment of 94 reproductive-age women with epilepsy, polycystic ovaries were detected by transvaginal ultrasound in 26% of women with localization-related epilepsy, 41% of women with primary generalized epilepsy, and 16% of nonepileptic controls (1). Women receiving valproate within the preceding 3 years were more likely to have polycystic-appearing ovaries (38%) than women receiving other AEDs. Other investigators have similarly reported a higher frequency of anovulatory cycles and polycystic ovaries in women receiving valproate for epilepsy (64). This condition in women receiving valproate may be reversible when medication is changed to lamotrigine (70).

The relative effect of epilepsy versus AED therapy on reproductive physiology can be considered by evaluating reproductive health in persons receiving AEDs for conditions other than epilepsy. Two studies have assessed menstrual cycle regularity and ovarian morphology in women with bipolar disease (BPD). One study of women with bipolar disease treated with either valproate or lithium found no difference in the length of the menstrual cycle or appearance of polycystic ovaries, although both groups had a high prevalence of prolonged menstrual cycles (72). More than 40% had cycles longer that 35 days, suggesting that these cycles were anovulatory. However, another group of investigators evaluated the length of the menstrual cycle, ovarian morphology, and testosterone levels in women with bipolar disorder treated with valproate or other agents. Abnormally long menstrual cycles occurred in 47% of those receiving valproate, as compared with 13% of those not receiving valproate and none of the healthy controls. Polycystic ovaries and elevated androgens were found in 41% of women with BPD on valproate and in none of the other women with BPD or the controls (73).

Whether reproductive endocrine and reproductive cycle disturbances are primarily a consequence of the brain disorder or the AED has been addressed in a human study and a primate study. Menstrual cycle length, androgen status, and pituitary gonadotrophins were assessed in women with BPD receiving lithium or valproate, and in women with primary generalized epilepsy receiving valproate (74). Both groups of women receiving valproate had more frequent menstrual cycle abnormalities (20% of women with BPD and 47% of the women with epilepsy). Women treated with lithium or valproate for BPD, however, did not exhibit the phenotypic signs of hyperandrogenism such as hirsutism and truncal obesity, although serum androgens were elevated in this group. Pituitary hormone abnormalities, as represented by significantly lower FSH levels and an increased ratio of LH to FSH, were observed only in the women with epilepsy. The investigators conclude that the valproate-associated phenotype is influenced by the brain disorder.

Additional evidence that these reproductive health disturbances are a consequence of an underlying brain disorder comes from a study in female primates (75). Seven nonepileptic, regularly cycling healthy primates were treated with valproate over 1 year, achieving serum concentrations of valproate similar to those of adults with epilepsy. Over the prospective 1-year assessment, the primates did not develop abnormalities in menstrual cycle length, ovarian morphology, or response to GnRH stimulation.

These data suggest that epilepsy and some AEDs individually affect fertility and that these effects may be additive. This implies that the most sophisticated therapy for epilepsy will consider disease treatment effects on reproductive health.

Sexual Function

Many men and women with epilepsy have sexual dysfunction (76–78). Studies evaluating sexual attitude and behavior find an incidence of sexual dysfunction ranging from 30 to 66% of men with epilepsy and from 14 to 50% of women. The variability in these estimates reflects varying cultural norms for sexual behavior and differing methods for assessing sexual function.

Studies obtaining information by patient self-report have cataloged a variety of sexual complaints. Women with epilepsy are reported to experience a global hyposexuality (79). However, in one recent study of 116 women with epilepsy seen as outpatients in an epilepsy clinic (77) sexual desire and sexual experience were normal, but more than one-third experienced deficits in arousal such as dyspareunia, vaginismus, lack of lubrication, and arousal insufficiency—symptoms more often attributed to disorders of physiologic sexual arousal rather than a disorder of sexual desire. One quantitative study of sexual arousal in women with temporal lobe epilepsy found an impairment in the first phase of physiologic sexual arousal (increased genital blood flow) as measured by the relative increase in genital blood flow after presentation of erotic video stimuli (80). In this experimental model of sexual response, subjective sexual arousal was not diminished in the women with epilepsy. These results suggest an impairment in sexual arousal, with relative preservation of sexual desire.

Sexual behavior requires the normal and integrated function of the peripheral and central nervous system (CNS), peripheral vasculature, and hormones, as well as normal psychologic responsiveness. Areas of the CNS subserving sexual behavior in mammals include regions of the frontal lobe, hypothalamus, and limbic cortex. The hypothalamic-pituitary axis also mediates sexuality via the regulation of gonadotrophins, prolactin, and gonadal steroids. Extensive reciprocal connections between the amygdala and hypothalamus allow limbic structures to modulate the release of hypothalamic trophic factors. In addition, high-affinity uptake receptors for sex steroids in the amygdala provide a pathway by which hormones alter limbic function.

A number of mechanisms for sexual dysfunction are active in women with epilepsy (79). Social development and self-esteem may be impaired. Sexual feelings may elicit anxiety. Women with partial seizures were more likely to report anxiety associated with sexual activity (77). Although the basis for heightened sexual anxiety in this population is not known, sexual desire and arousal may be negatively reinforced when sexual activity precipitates seizures or when sexual sensations or behaviors become identified as part of the seizure or postictal period.

Epileptic discharges in limbic structures may also contribute to sexual dysfunction. Sexual dysfunction usually arises after the onset of seizures and may be most common in patients with partial, rather than generalized, seizures. Some patients treated for partial epilepsy with temporal lobectomy report postoperative improvement in sexual desire and arousal, with the greatest improvement seen in those patients achieving the best seizure control.

Sexuality in people with epilepsy may be adversely affected by abnormalities in the basal and pulsatile release of LH, elevations in prolactin, and alterations in gonadal and adrenal steroid hormones. AEDs may contribute to sexual dysfunction by direct cortical effects or secondarily through alterations in the hormones supporting sexual behavior. Treatment with enzyme-inducing AEDs reduces the biologically active fraction of gonadal and adrenal steroid hormone. These steroid alterations, as well as AED-induced changes in pituitary hormones could adversely impact sexual behavior. Elevated pituitary prolactin is recognized as a common cause of sexual dysfunction in nonepileptic men and women and is known to be elevated interictally in women and men receiving AEDs. Although the effect of individual AEDs on sexual function has not been evaluated, AED polytherapy appears to be more often associated with sexual dysfunction than is AED monotherapy (77).

A woman with epilepsy presenting with sexual dysfunction should be questioned about precipitating factors, such as acute or chronic life stresses, recent medications, illnesses, surgery, or symptoms of depression. A recommended evaluation strategy is provided in Table 15.9.

If no correctable organic cause of sexual dysfunction is identified, the patient can be referred for the most appropriate form of intervention, such as marriage therapy, primary psychiatric therapy, sex education, behavior

---

TABLE 15.9
Evaluation Strategy for Women with Epilepsy and Sexual Dysfunction

Past medical and psychiatric history
Detailed sexual and relationship history
Medication history
Physical, gynecologic, and neurologic examinations
Serum studies
   Complete blood count, liver function tests, and fasting glucose
   Thyroid function tests
   Pituitary hormones
      Luteinizing hormone and follicle stimulating hormone
      Prolactin
   Gonadal and adrenal steroids
      Estradiol, progesterone, testosterone, dihydroepiandrostenedione (DHEA)

therapy, or psychotherapy. A simple explanation that sexual dysfunction is an epiphenomenon of epilepsy may assuage guilt and relieve marital strain. Women with vaginismus and dyspareunia may benefit from relaxation techniques and graded dilation. Inadequate vaginal lubrication can be treated with products available for vaginal moisture replenishment and with lubricating agents.

PREGNANCY IN THE WOMAN WITH EPILEPSY

Pregnancy in the woman with epilepsy is most often uneventful. About 30% of women with epilepsy, however, will experience more frequent or more severe seizures during pregnancy, many will become noncompliant with AED treatment, others will experience changes in AED pharmacokinetics that lead to alterations in CNS concentrations of AEDs, and approximately 10% will experience a pregnancy complication. Of children born to epileptic mothers, 5 to 10% will have malformations, and 10 to 30% will have a congenital anomaly. Recent information regarding the mechanisms by which AEDs can act as teratogens encourages treatment strategies that will optimize pregnancy and fetal outcome.

Transmission of Epilepsy to Offspring

A family history of epilepsy places individuals at two to three times greater risk for developing epilepsy than individuals with no family history of epilepsy (81). In addition, a child born to a mother with epilepsy has twice the risk of developing epilepsy than does a child born to a father with epilepsy (82–84). These observations suggest that epilepsy "susceptibility" may be preferentially transmitted from the mother—perhaps by a mitochondrial gene or the imprinting of a nuclear gene (82).

If the mother's epilepsy syndrome can be classified, then the clinician can provide a better estimate of the risk of transmission. A symptomatic localization-related epilepsy with partial seizures is unlikely to be transmitted to the offspring, whereas idiopathic localization-related epilepsy, such as benign rolandic epilepsy with centrotemporal spikes, carries a higher likelihood of transmission. The primary generalized epilepsy syndromes, such as childhood absence and JME, are recognized to be genetically transmitted diseases and, as such, carry a higher likelihood of transmission (85).

Pregnancy Complications

Women with epilepsy taking AEDs are at greater risk for a pregnancy complicated by spontaneous abortion, miscarriage, and preterm delivery. In part, these adverse outcomes may be a consequence of maternal tonic-clonic seizures that are associated with fetal hypoxia and acidosis and may compromise placental perfusion (86,87). Abnormalities in the pulsatile release of LH in women with convulsive and nonconvulsive seizures may disrupt the formation of the uterine endometrium and compromise implantation.

Infants of mothers with epilepsy may be at risk for other adverse pregnancy outcomes, as well. Women with epilepsy are more likely to give birth to fetuses with low birth weight (88). Other literature suggests that the infants of epileptic mothers are more likely to have fetal head growth retardation, although this appears in part to be attributable to smaller parental head circumference (89).

AED Pharmacokinetics during Pregnancy

Seizure frequency may change during pregnancy. Approximately 35% of pregnant women with epilepsy experience an increase in seizure frequency, 55% have no change, and 10% have a decrease in seizure frequency (9,90). The factors that are believed to alter seizure frequency include changes in sex hormones, AED metabolism, sleep schedules, and medication compliance.

An increased volume of distribution and increased clearance reduces serum levels (91,92). A reduction in serum albumin and increased competition by sex steroid hormones for binding sites, however, leads to a relative increase in the free (non–protein bound) fraction of drug. For AEDs that are highly protein bound, such as valproate, a specific determination of the free level may be needed to accurately portray the CNS level. Another factor contributing to the decline in serum levels of AEDs is poor medication compliance, prompted by fears that medication will have adverse effects on the fetus. To optimize medical management during pregnancy, women must be counseled that uncontrolled seizures are deleterious to the fetus.

AED concentrations may change during pregnancy. Physiologic changes during pregnancy that can alter AED pharmacokinetics and total AED concentrations include decreased gastric tone and motility; nausea and vomiting, which arise in 40% of women during the first trimester; an increase in plasma volume of 40 to 50%; and an increase in renal clearance. The pharmacokinetics of some AEDs is more profoundly affected than others, probably because of the pregnancy-related differential effects on cytochrome P450 enzymes. Two cytochrome P450 enzymes, CYP2C9 and CYP2C19, are induced to a greater extent than is CYP3A4. This could account for the greater reduction in phenytoin compared to carbamazepine, which is principally metabolized by CYP3A4, and valproate, which is predominantly eliminated by glucuronidation and beta-oxidation (91,93). See also Chapters 4 and 5.

Although the total concentration falls for many AEDs, there tends to be an increase in the percentage of unbound or free drug because of a reduction in albumin and thus, in protein binding (92). Lamotrigine undergoes significant alterations in metabolism over the course of pregnancy. An increase in apparent clearance of more than 65% was observed between conception and the second and third trimesters and a decrease in apparent clearance occurred between the second and third trimesters, and postpartum (94). These data suggest that lamotrigine levels must be monitored throughout pregnancy, that dose increases to maintain steady serum levels can be anticipated, and that the dosage achieved over the pregnancy will need to be reduced after delivery.

Antiepileptic Drugs and Fetal Outcome

The AEDs are commonly divided into the "older drugs"—carbamazepine, phenobarbital, phenytoin, and valproate—and the "newer" drugs—gabapentin, levetiracetam, lamotrigine, tiagabine, topiramate, and zonisamide. Whereas the older AEDs are teratogenic in animal reproductive toxicology studies, the newer drugs are not. Nevertheless, the lack of direct human experience with many of the newer agents has made it difficult for clinicians to feel comfortable advocating their use during pregnancy. Also, it has not been clear how much the malformations and anomalies associated with gestational exposure to the older AEDs are due to medication exposure, and how much are due to the maternal trait of epilepsy and maternal seizures.

The children of women with epilepsy exposed in utero to AEDs have a risk of major malformations of 4 to 8%, in contrast to the rate in the general population of approximately 3%. Studies including women with epilepsy who have not taken AEDs during pregnancy indicate that these children do not have a higher risk for birth defects. Although it can be argued that untreated mothers with epilepsy probably do not have epilepsy as severe as mothers who have received AED treatment during pregnancy, these observations suggest that the elevated risk for birth defects in children of mothers with epilepsy is primarily a consequence of AED exposure. For that reason, a complete discussion of birth defects associated with individual AEDs, mechanisms for teratogenesis, and a review of data thus far available from prospective pregnancy registries for individual AEDs is included in Chapters 4 and 5. Nevertheless, it is important to mention strategies for managing pregnancy in the woman with epilepsy that may reduce the risk of adverse fetal outcome (95).

The management of epilepsy in reproductive-age women should focus on maintaining effective control of seizures while minimizing fetal AED exposure (96,97). This applies to dosage and to number of AEDs. Medication reduction or substitution should take place prior to conception. Altering medication during pregnancy increases the risk of breakthrough seizures and exposes the fetus to an additional AED. The recommended management during pregnancy is AED monotherapy at the lowest effective dose. The best drug to choose is the drug most likely to be effective and well tolerated for that woman's seizure type. At present, there is insufficient information to identify any particular AED as the drug of choice during pregnancy. In addition, if there is a family history of neural tube defects (NTDs), an agent other than carbamazepine or valproate might be considered. (See Table 15.10).

Guidelines for the medical management of the pregnant woman with epilepsy are:

- Reevaluate the need for AEDs.
- Choose the most effective drug for that woman's epilepsy and seizure type.
- Utilize AED monotherapy at the lowest effective dose.
- Provide periconceptional folate supplementation.
- Monitor the free (unbound) level of the AED.
- Provide prenatal diagnostic testing.
- Supplement vitamin K1 at 10 mg/day during the last month of pregnancy.

TABLE 15.10

U.S. Food and Drug Administration Pregnancy Risk Categories for Antiepileptic Drugs

Category C

Risk cannot be ruled out. Human studies are lacking, and animal studies show no evidence for fetal risk.

    Felbamate
    Gabapentin
    Lamotrigine
    Oxcarbazepine
    Tiagabine
    Topiramate
    Zonisamide

Category D

Positive evidence of risk in animals. Investigational or postmarketing data show risk to the fetus. Nevertheless, potential benefits may outweigh potential risk.

    Phenytoin
    Valproate
    Carbamazepine
    Phenobarbital

Not Categorized

    Ethosuximide
    Clonazepam
    Diazepam

Breast-feeding is, in general, encouraged for women with epilepsy taking AEDs. The benefits of breast-feeding are believed to outweigh the risks associated with further exposure of the neonate to AEDs (96,98). Exceptions to this recommendation are made when the infant appears lethargic or irritable, or if there is feeding difficulty or poor weight gain. Further discussion regarding the concentrations of individual AEDs in breast milk is provided in Chapter 5.

Concerns are mounting that exposure to AEDs in utero may confer long-lasting neurodevelopmental or neurocognitive deficits. Fetal head growth retardation and low intelligence (89,99) has been associated with the maternal use of AEDs. Although prospective trials are lacking, retrospective studies show that children exposed in utero to valproate in monotherapy or polytherapy are more likely to require special educational resources (100). Prospective studies are under way to better define the neurodevelopmental risks of AED exposure to the developing brain.

Recent efforts by the American Academy of Neurology (96) and the American College of Obstetric and Gynecologic Physicians (97) to highlight those issues relevant to the care of women with epilepsy will enhance clinician familiarity with these diverse health concerns. These professional efforts, as well as a large-scale professional and public initiative by the Epilepsy Foundation of America, provide the medical professional with information and educational resources to enhance the comprehensive care of women with epilepsy.

RESOURCES AVAILABLE FOR HEALTH CARE PROVIDERS AND WOMEN WITH EPILEPSY

Epilepsy Foundation of America
4351 Garden City Drive
Landover, MD 20785-2267
Telephone: 800-EFA-1000
Web site: www.efa.org

The Antiepileptic Drug Pregnancy Registry
Genetics and Teratology Unit
14CNY-MGH East
Room 5022A
Charlestown, MA 02129-2000
Telephone: 888-233-2334
Web site: neuro-www2.mgh.harvard.edu/aed/registry.nclk

The American Epilepsy Society
638 Prospect Avenue
Hartford, CT 06105-4240
Telephone: 860-586-7505
Web site: www.aesnet.com

References

1. Morrell MJ, Guidice L, Seale C, et al. Ovulatory dysfunction in women with epilepsy receiving antiepileptic drug monotherapy: an interaction of syndrome and treatment. Ann Neurol 2002;52(6):704–711.
2. Fisher RS, Vickrey BG, Gibson P, et al. The impact of epilepsy from the patient's perspective I. Descriptions and subjective perceptions. Epilepsy Res 2000;41:39–51.
3. Morrell MJ, Sarto GE, Osborne-Shafer P, Borda EA, Herzog A, Callanan M. Health issues for women with epilepsy: a descriptive survey to assess knowledge and awareness among healthcare providers. J Womens Health Gend Based Med 2000;9:959–965.
4. Hauser WA, Annegers JF, Kurland LT. Incidence of epilepsy and unprovoked seizures in Rochester, Minnesota: 1935–1984. Epilepsia 1993;34(3):453–468.
5. Hauser WA, Rich SS, Annegers JF, Anderson VE. Seizure recurrence after a first unprovoked seizure: an extended follow-up. Neurology 1990;40:1163–1170.
6. Hopkins A, Garman A, Clarke C. The first seizure in adult life: value of clinical features, electroencephalography, and computerized tomographic scanning in prediction of seizure recurrence. Lancet 1988;1:721–726.
7. Annegers JF, Hauser WA, Elveback LR. Remission of seizures and relapse in patients with epilepsy. Epilepsia 1979;20:729–737.
8. Nelson KB, Ellenberg JH. Epidemiology of cerebral palsy. Adv Neurology 1978;19:421–435.
9. Hauser WA, Hesdorffer DC. Risk factors. In: Hauser WA, Hesdorffer DC, (eds.) Epilepsy: frequency, causes and consequences. New York, NY: Demos, 1990; 53–100.
10. Commission on Classification and Terminology of the International League Against Epilepsy. Proposal for revised clinical and electroencephalographic classification of epileptic seizures. Epilepsia 1981:22:489–501.
11. Commission on Classification and Terminology of the International League Against Epilepsy. Proposal for revised classification of epilepsies and epileptic syndromes. Epilepsia 1989:30(4):389–399.
12. Pearl PL, Holmes GL. Absence seizures. In: Dodson WE, Pellock JM, (eds.) Pediatric epilepsy: diagnosis and therapy. New York: Demos, 1993;157–169.
13. Panayiotopoulos CP, Obeid T, Waheed G. Differentiation of typical absence seizures in epileptic syndromes: a video-EEG study of 224 seizures in 20 patients. Brain 1989;112:1039–1056.
14. Sato S, Dreifuss FE, Penry JK. Prognostic factors in absence seizures. Neurology 1976;26:788–796.
15. Harding GFA, Jeavons PM. Photosensitive epilepsy. London: MacKeith Press, 1994.
16. Zifkin BG, Andermann F. Epilepsy with reflex seizures. In: Wyllie E, (ed.) The treatment of epilepsy: principles and practice, 2nd ed. Baltimore, Md: Williams and Wilkins, 1996;573–583.
17. Janz and Christian, 1957.
18. Wallace H, Shorvon S, Tallis R. Age-specific incidence and prevalence rates of treated epilepsy in an unselected population of 2,052,922 and age-specific fertility rates of women with epilepsy. Lancet 1998;352:1970–1973.
19. Aicardi J, (ed.) Infantile spasms and related syndromes. In: Aicardi J. Epilepsy in children. New York, NY: Raven Press; 1986;17–38.
20. Morrell MJ. Differential diagnosis of seizures. Neurol Clin 1993;11(4):737–754.

21. Lesser RP. Psychogenic seizures. *Neurology* 1996;46: 1499–1507.

22. Gumnit RJ, Gates JR: Psychogenic seizures. *Epilepsia* 1986; 27(S2):S124–S129.

23. Gates JR, Ramani V, Whalen SM, Loewenson RB. Ictal characteristics of pseudoseizures. *Arch Neurol* 1985; 42:1183–1187.

24. Leis AA, Ross MA, Summers AK. Psychogenic seizures: ictal characteristics and diagnostic pitfalls. *Neurology* 1992;42:95–99.

25. Feldhaus KM, Koziol-McLain J, Amsbury HL, Norton IM, Lowenstein SR, Abbott JT. Accuracy of three brief screening questions for detecting partner violence in the emergency department. *JAMA* 1997;277:1357–1361.

26. Betts T, Boden S. Diagnosis, management and prognosis of a group of 128 patients with non-epileptic attack disorder. Part II. Previous childhood sexual abuse in the aetiology of these disorders. *Seizure* 1992;1(1):27–32.

27. Smith S, Woolley CS. Cellular and molecular effects of steroid hormones on CNS excitability. *Cleve Clinic J Med*, 2004;71(Suppl 2):S4–S10.

28. Woolley CS, Schwartzkroin PA. Hormonal effects on the brain. *Epilepsia* 1998;39(suppl 8):S2–S8.

29. Woolley et al. 1997.

30. Woolley et al. 1996.

31. Niijima and Wallace 1989.

32. Rosciszewska D. Epilepsy and menstruation. In: Hopkins A, (ed.) *Epilepsy.* London: Chapman and Hall, 1987;373–381.

33. Diamantopoulos N, Crumrine P. The effect of puberty on the course of epilepsy. *Arch Neurol* 1986;43(9): 873–876.

34. Herzog AG, Klein P. Three patterns of catamenial epilepsy. *Epilepsia* 1996;37:83.

35. Abbasi F, Krumholz A, Kittner SJ, Langenberg P. New onset epilepsy in older women is influenced by menopause. *Epilepsia* 1996;37(5):97.

36. Harden CL, Pulver MC, Ravdin L, Jacobs AR. The effect of menopause and perimenopause on the course of epilepsy. *Epilepsia* 1999;40(10):1402–1407.

37. Herzog AG. Progesterone therapy in women with epilepsy: a 3-year follow-up. *Neurology* 1999;52(9): 1917–1918.

38. Mattson RH, Cramer JA, Collins JF. A comparison of valproate with carbamazepine for the treatment of complex partial seizures and secondarily generalized tonic-clonic seizures in adults. The Department of Veterans Affairs Epilepsy Cooperative Study No. 264 Group. *N Engl J Med* 1992;10:327(11):765–771.

39. Mattson RH, Cramer JA, Collins JF, et al. Comparison of carbamazepine, phenobarbital, phenytoin and primidone in partial and secondarily generalized tonic clonic seizures. *N Engl J Med* 1985;313:145–151.

40. Merkatz RB, Temple R, Sobel S, Felden K, Working Group on Women in Clinical Trials. Women in clinical trials of new drugs: a change in Food and Drug Administration Policy. *N Engl J Med* 1993;329:292–296.

41. FDA/DHHS. Guidelines for the study of and evaluation of gender differences in the clinical evaluation of drugs. *Federal Register* 1993;58(139):39406–39416.

42. Morrell MJ. The new antiepileptic drugs and women: efficacy, reproductive health, pregnancy and fetal outcome. *Epilepsia* 1996;37(S6):S34–S44.

43. DHHS. Additional DHHS protections pertaining to research, developemnt and related activities involving fetuses, pregnant women and human in vitro fertiliza-tion. Title 45. Code of Federal Regulations. Part 46, Subpart B. March 15, 1994.

44. Institute of Medicine. Women and health research: ethical and legal issues of including women in clinical studies. Washington D.C.: National Academy Press; 1994; 1–25.

45. Mattson RH, Cramer JA, Darney PD, Naftolin F. Use of oral contraceptives by women with epilepsy. *JAMA* 1986;256:238–240.

46. Pack AM, Morrell MJ. Adverse effects of antiepileptic drugs on bone structure. Epidemiology, mechanisms and therapeutic implications. *CNS Drugs* 2001;15(8): 633–642.

47. Webber MP, Hauser WA, Ottman R, Annegers JF. Fertility in persons with epilepsy:1935–1974. *Epilepsia* 1986;27:746–752.

48. Morrell MJ. Stigma and epilepsy. *Epilepsy Behav* 2002;3(6):S21–S25.

49. Schupf N, Ottman R. Reproduction among individuals with idiopathic/cryptogenic epilepsy: risk factors for reduced fertility in marraige. *Epilepsia* 1996;37: 833–840.

50. Schupf N, Ottman R. Likelihood of pregnancy in individuals with idiopathic/cryptogenic epilepsy: social and biologic influence. *Epilepsia* 1994;35(4):750–756.

51. Dansky LV, Andermann E, Andermann F. Marriage and fertility in epileptic patients. *Epilepsia* 1980;21:261–271.

52. Jalava M, Sillanpaa M. Reproductive activity and offspring health of young adults with childhood-onset epilepsy: a controlled study. *Epilepsia* 1997;38(5): 532–540.

53. Isojarvi JIT, Laatikainen TJ, Pakarinen AJ, Juntunen KTS, Myllyla VV. Polycystic ovaries and hyperandrogenism in women taking valproate for epilepsy. *N Engl J Med* 1993;329:1383–1388.

54. Bilo L, Meo R, Valentino R, Buscaino GA, Straino S, Nappi C. Abnormal pattern of luteinizing hormone pulsatility in women with epilepsy. *Fertil Steril* 1991;55: 705–711.

55. Herzog AG, Seibel MM, Schomer DL, Vaitukaitis JL, Geschwind N. Reproductive endocrine disorders in men with partial seizures of temporal lobe origin. *Arch Neurol* 1986;43:347–350.

56. Herzog AG, Seibel MM, Schomer DL, Vaitukaitis JL, Geschwind N. Reproductive endocrine disorders in women with partial seizures of temporal lobe origin. *Arch Neurol* 1986;43:341–346.

57. Drislane FW, Coleman AE, Schomer DL, et al. Altered pulsatile secretion of luteinizing hormone in women with epilepsy. *Neurology* 1994;44:306–310.

58. Meo R, Bilo L, Nappi C, et al. Derangement of the hypothalamic GnRH pulse generator in women with epilepsy. *Seizure* 1993;2:241–252.

59. Morrell MJ, Flynn KL, Seale CG, et al. Reproductive dysfunction in women with epilepsy: antiepileptic drug effects on sex-steroid hormones. *CNS Spectrums* 2001;6:771–786.

60. Isojarvi JIT, Parakinen AJ, Rautio A, Pelkoren O, Myllyla VV. Serum sex hormone levels after replacing carbamazepine with oxcarbazepine. *Eur Clin Pharmacol* 1995;47:461–464.

61. Levesque LA, Herzog AG, Seibel MM. The effect of phenytoin and carbamazepine on serum dehydroepiandrosterone sulfate in men and women who have partial seizures with temporal lobe involvement. *J Clin Endocrinol Metab* 1986;63:243–245.

62. Stoffel-Wagner B, Bauer J, Flugel D, Brennemann W, Klingmuller D, Elger CE. Serum sex hormones are altered in patients with chronic temporal lobe epilepsy receiving anticonvulsant medication. *Epilepsia* 1998; 39:1164–1173.

63. Morrell MJ, Isojarvi J, Taylor A, et al. Higher androgens and weight gain with valproate compared with lamotrigine for epilepsy. *Epilepsy Res* 2003;54:189–199.

64. Murialdo G, Galimbertu CA, Magri F, et.al. Menstrual cycle and ovary alterations in women with epilepsy on antiepileptic therapy. *J Endocrinol Invest* 1997;20(9): 519–526.

65. Polson et al. 1988.

66. Farquhar et al. 1994.

67. Clayton et al. 1992.

68. American College of Obstetric and Gynecologic Physicians. Polycystic ovary syndrome. *Practice Bulletin #41.* 2002;100(6):1389–1402.

69. Vainionpaa LK, Rattya J, Knip M, et al. Valproate-induced hyperandrogenism during pubertal maturation in girls with epilepsy. *Ann Neurol* 1999;45(4):444–450.

70. Isojarvi JIT, Rattya J, Myllyla VV, et al. Valproate, lamotrigine, and insulin-mediated risks in women with epilepsy. *Ann Neurol* 1998;43:446–451.

71. Luef G, Abraham I, Haslinger M, et al. Polycystic ovaries, obesity and insulin resistance in women with epilepsy. A comparative study of carbamazepine and valproic acid in 105 women. *J Neurol* 2002;249(7): 835–841.

72. Rasgon NL, Altshuler LL, Gudeman D, et al. Medication status and PCO syndrome in women with bipolar disorder: a preliminary report *J Clin Psychiatry.* 2000;61(3):173–178.

73. O'Donovan C, Kusumakar V, Graves GR, Bird DC. Menstrual abnormalities and polycystic ovary syndrome in women taking valproate for bipolar mood disorder. *J Clin Psychiatry* 2002;63:322–330.

74. Akdeniz F, Taneli F, Noyan A, Yuncu Z, Vahip S. Valproate-associated reproductive and metabolic abnormalities: are epileptic women at greater risk than bipolar women? *Prog Neuropsychopharmacol Biol Psychiatry* 2003;27(1):115–121.

75. Ferin M, Morrell M, Xiao E, et al. Endocrine and metabolic responses to long-term monotherapy with the antiepileptic drug valproate in the normally cycling rhesus monkey. *J Clin Endocr Metab* 2003;88(6): 2908–2915.

76. Demerdash A, Shaalon M, Midori A, Kamel F, Bahri M. Sexual behavior of a sample of females with epilepsy. *Epilepsia* 1991;32:82–85.

77. Morrell MJ, Guldner GT. Self-reported sexual function and sexual arousability in women with epilepsy. *Epilepsia* 1996;37:1204–1210.

78. Guldner GT, Morrell MJ. Nocturnal penile tumescence and rigidity evaluation in men with epilepsy. *Epilepsia* 1996;37:1211–1214.

79. Morrell MJ. Sexuality in epilepsy. In: Engel J, Pedley TA, (eds.) *Epilepsy: a comprehensive textbook.* New York: Lippincott-Raven, 1997;2021–2026.

80. Morrell MJ, Sperling MR, Stecker M, Dichter MA. Sexual dysfunction in partial epilepsy: a deficit in physiological sexual arousal. *Neurology* 1994;44:243–247.

81. Annegers JF, Hauser WA, Anderson VE, Kurland LT. The risks of seizure disorders among relatives of patients with childhood onset epilepsy. *Neurology* 1982;32:174–179.

82. Ottman R, Annegers JF, Hauser WA, Kurland LT. Higher risk of seizures in offspring of mothers than of fathers with epilepsy. *Am J Hum Genet* 1988;43:257–264.

83. Ottman R, Hauser WA, Susser M. Genetic and maternal influences on susceptibility to seizures. An analytic review. *Am J Epidemiol* 1985;122:923–939.

84. Annegers JF, Hauser WA, Elveback LR, Anderson VE, Kurland LT. Congenital malformations and seizure disorders in the offspring of parents with epilepsy. *Int J Epidemiol* 1978;7:241–247.

85. Treiman LJ, Treiman DM. Genetic aspects of epilepsy. In: Wyllie E, (ed.) *The Treatment of epilepsy: principles and practice.* Baltimore, Md: Williams and Wilkins, 1997;151–164.

86. Swatjes JM, van Geijn HP, Meinardi H, Mantel R. Fetal heart rate patterns and chronic exposure to antiepileptic drugs. *Epilepsia* 1992;33(4):721–728.

87. Teramo K, Hiilesmaa V, Brady A, Saarikoski S. Fetal heart rate during a maternal grand mal epileptic seizure. *J Perinatal Med* 1979;7:3.

88. Battino D, Granata T, Binelli S, et al. Intrauterine growth in the offspring of epileptic mothers. *Acta Neurol Scand.* 1992;86:555–557.

89. Hiilesmaa VK, Teramo K, Granstrom ML, Bardy AH. Fetal head growth retardation associated with maternal antiepileptic drugs. *Lancet* 1981;2:165–167.

90. Schmidt D, Beck-Mannagetta G, Janz D, Koch S. The effect of pregnancy on the course of epilepsy: a prospective study. In: Janz D, Dam M, Richens A, (eds.) *Epilepsy, pregnancy and the child.* New York: Raven Press, 1982;39–49.

91. Tomson T, Lindbom U, Ekqvist B, Sundqvist A. Disposition of carbamazepine and phenytoin in pregnancy. *Epilepsia* 1994;35:131–135.

92. Yerby MS, Friel PN, McCormick K. Pharmacokinetics of anticonvulsants in pregnancy: alterations in plasma protein binding. *Epilepsy Res* 1990;5:223–228.

93. McAuley JW, Anderson GD. Treatment of epilepsy in women of reproductive age: pharmacokinetic considerations. *Clin Pharmacokinet.* 2002;41(8):559–579.

94. Tran TA, Leppik IE, Blesi K, Sathanandan ST, Remmel R. Lamotrigine clearance during pregnancy. *Neurology* 2002;59(2):251–255.

95. Zahn CA, Morrell MJ, Collins SD, Labiner DM, Yerby MS. Management issues for women with epilepsy: a review of the literature. American Academy of Neurology Practice Guidelines. *Neurology* 1998;51:949–956.

96. American Academy of Neurology. Quality Standards Subcommittee. Practice parameter: management issues for women with epilepsy (summary statement). *Neurology* 1998;51:944–948.

97. American College of Obstetric and Gynecologic Seizure disorders in pregnancy. *Physicians Educational Bulletin.* 1996;231:1–13.

98. American Academy of Pediatrics. The transfer of drugs and other chemicals into human milk. *Pediatrics* 1994;93:137–150.

99. Gaily E, Kantola-Sorsa E, Granstrom ML. Intelligence of children of epileptic mothers. *J Pediatr* 1988;113: 677–684

100. Adab N, Jacoby A, Smith D, Chadwick D. Additional educational needs in children born to mothers with epilepsy. *J Neurol Neurosurg Psychiatry* 2001;70:15–21.

16 Eclampsia

Peter W. Kaplan, MS, BS, FRCP

T oxemia of pregnancy (preeclampsia, or toxemia gravidarum) is a syndrome that is characterized by pregnancy-induced hypertension (PIH), proteinuria, and edema after week 20 of pregnancy. Although this complex disorder can involve a number of organ systems, its clinical presentation varies. Patients may present with multisystem failure that results in oliguria; disseminated intravascular coagulation (DIC); hemorrhages into the liver; Hemolysis, Elevated Liver enzymes and Low Platelets (HELLP) syndrome; pulmonary edema; and a number of neurologic problems. The neurologic presentation frequently includes confusion, headaches, visual hallucinations (from which the name eclampsia arises), and blindness. With the appearance of seizures or coma, the patient's condition is that of eclampsia. No constant relationship exists, however, between the various neurologic manifestations and the severity of preeclampsia. Seizures and ischemic events, for example, may appear with few heralding signs of preeclampsia (1).

Worldwide, preeclampsia and eclampsia are major causes of perinatal morbidity and death (2). In the United States, 6 to 8% of pregnancies have preeclamptic complications (3). This affects 5 to 10% of whites, 15 to 20% of black primigravidas, and up to 30% of twin pregnancies (4). The incidence of preeclampsia also has other demographic differences. It is most frequently seen in poorly nourished, nulliparous woman, multiparous women over the age of 35 with extrauterine pregnancies, and women with multiple pregnancies or hydatidiform mole. The American College of Obstetricians and Gynecologists proffers criteria for preeclampsia-eclampsia shown in Table 16.1 (5).

CLINICAL CHARACTERISTICS

Hypertension

Preeclampsia is characterized by hypertension. Although blood pressure values may vary, guidelines suggest a systolic pressure of 140 mm Hg or above; or 90 mm Hg or above, diastolic (5). A blood pressure above 160 to 180 mm Hg systolic, or 110 mm Hg diastolic during bed rest signals severe preeclampsia in the presence of proteinuria of (>5 g/24 h), or 3+ to 4+ by dipstick (5). The diagnosis is usually established by elevation in blood pressure on two occasions separated by 6 hours, but not infrequently, eclamptic seizures supervene over a shorter period and may occur in the absence of edema or proteinuria.

Edema

Normal pregnancy frequently results in edema of the legs. The edema of preeclampsia, however, is more marked in degree and affects not only the legs but also the hands and face.

TABLE 16.1

Clinical Manifestations of Severe Disease in Patients with Pregnancy-Induced Hypertension

Blood pressure >160–180 mm Hg systolic, >110 mm Hg diastolic
Proteinuria >5/g/24 h (normal <300 mg/24 h)
Elevated serum creatinine
Grand mal seizures (eclampsia)
Pulmonary edema
Oliguria <500 mL/24 h
Microangiopathic hemolysis
Thrombocytopenia
Hepatocellular dysfunction (elevated alanine aminotransferase, aspartase aminotransferase)
Intrauterine growth retardation or oligohydramnios
Symptoms suggesting significant end-organ involvement: headache, visual disturbances, or epigastric or right-upper quadrant pain

Adapted with permission from the Committee on Terminology of the American College of Obstetricians and Gynecologists, ACOG technical bulletin, #219, January 1996, p. 2.

TABLE 16.2

Causes of Seizures around Pregnancy

Epilepsy Toxins	Central stimulants (e.g., amphetamines cocaine); theophylline
Metabolic problems	Hyponatremia, hypocalcemia, hypoglycemia, hyperglycemia
Cerebrovascular problems	Cerebral infarction Cerebral edema Cerebral hemorrhage Cerebral venous sinus thrombosis Subarachnoid hemorrhage
Infections/infestations	Bacterial Viral Parasitic infestations HIV
Space-occupying lesions	Benign and malignant tumors Arterovenous vascular malformations Cerebral abscess

Proteinuria

Proteinuria in preeclampsia is defined as the accumulation of more than 300 mg of protein in a 24-hour urine collection, whereas severe preeclampsia induces >5 g/24h proteinuria (3+ to 4+ by dipstick).

Seizures

The exact nature of eclamptic seizures remains unclear, but increasing evidence suggests that focal neuronal excitability arises from cortical damage produced by a number of neuropathologic changes in preeclampsia and eclampsia. These include vasospasm with ischemia, hemorrhages of various sizes, and cerebral edema; these are discussed later. Epileptic seizures usually remit with delivery of the baby, treatment of the hypertension, or the use of magnesium sulfate. Focal seizures from a variety of etiologies may secondarily spread, resulting in a generalized tonic-clonic seizure. Because of the other neurologic abnormalities that may appear during pregnancy that may also result in seizures, consideration should be given to the differential diagnosis of peripartum seizures (Table 16.2).

Seizures in eclampsia may be focal or generalized tonic-clonic. Although they usually appear before childbirth, they frequently occur during or shortly after childbirth. In some patients, seizures occur more than a week postpartum, and there are case reports of seizures occurring up to 26 days postpartum (6,7). One series noted that 44% of eclampsia cases occurred postpartum; 12% within 48 hours, but 2% more than a week postpartum

(8). In another series, late postpartum seizures (those occurring >48 hours postpartum) accounted for up to 16% of cases of eclampsia (9) whereas others reported a 48% incidence for the same period (4). Late onset eclampsia may present without the heralding features of preeclampsia such as edema, proteinuria, or even hypertension (10,11). If untreated, approximately 10% of women with eclampsia have further seizures (12).

Visual Problems

Visual symptoms are common. They may involve different parts of the visual axis from the retina to the occipital cortex. There may be hypertension-induced retinal arteriolar dilatation, papilledema, occlusion of the central retinal artery, and vasospasm (13). Retinal edema, hemorrhages, and exudates (Figure 16.1) as well as retinal detachment can occur. Although some permanent visual changes may occur, most symptoms resolve with control of hypertension or in the postpartum period. In the posterior visual pathway, there may be microinfarctions, microhemorrhages, and edema of the visual cortex with cortical blindness (14) (Figure 16.2).

Other Clinical Features

Other problems with severe preeclampsia include a fall in urine output to below 400 mL/day; cyanosis or pulmonary edema and ARDS, upper abdominal quadrant pain, thrombocytopenia, or hemolysis (HELLP syndrome).

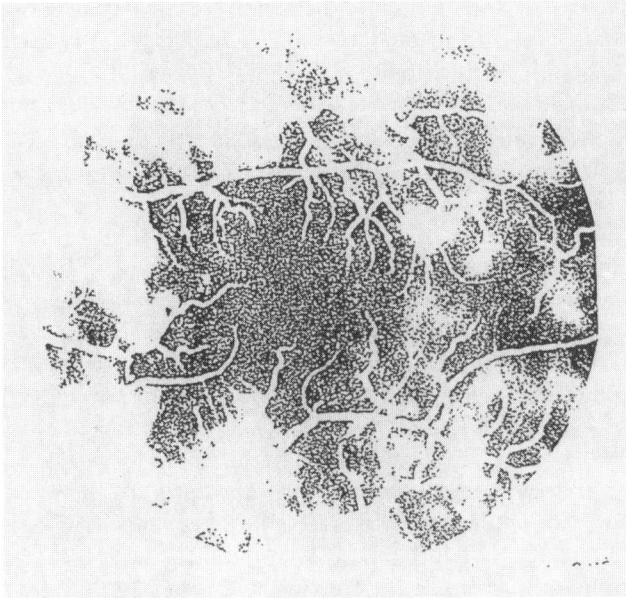

FIGURE 16.1

Fluorescein retinal angiography in eclampsia showing subretinal leakage. (Reproduced with permission from Oliver M, Uchenk D. Bilateral exudative retinal detachment in eclampsia without hypertensive retinopathy. *Am J Ophthalmol* 1980;90:794. Copyright by Ophthalmic Publishing Company.)

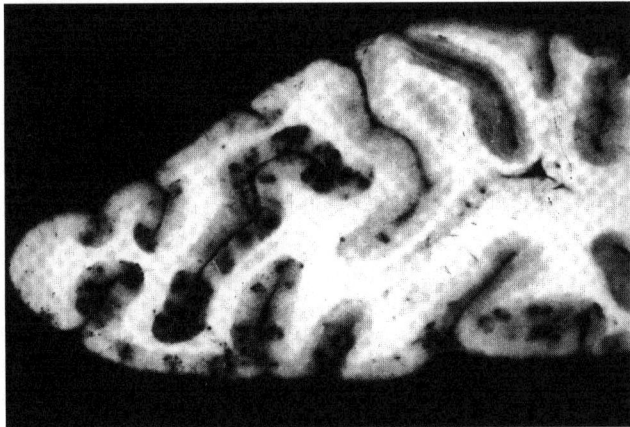

FIGURE 16.2

The occipital poles of a brain showing multiple cortical petechial hemorrhages that may cause cortical blindness. (Reproduced with permission from Sheehan HL, Lynch JB. *Pathology of toxaemia of pregnancy*. Edinburgh: Churchill Livingston, 1973.)

PATHOPHYSIOLOGY

Myriad pathophysiologic mechanisms have been invoked to explain the changes in preeclampsia-eclampsia, and it is probable that a number of these mechanisms contribute to the symptom complex (15–17) (Table 16.3). Some derive from the physiologic changes that occur during pregnancy,

with changes in immunologic tolerance between maternal tissues and paternal elements in the fetus, morphologic arterial changes in the uteroplacental bed, vasodilatation from prostaglandin secretion, and abnormalities of platelet aggregation. Particular fetal or uterine factors are not essential for the appearance of preeclampsia because it may occur following extrauterine or molar pregnancies. Data suggest that the vascular damage in the preeclamptic period arises from the interactions of neutrophils and activated macrophages, T-cell lymphocytes, and the interaction between complement, coagulation systems, and platelets. Endothelial dam-

---

TABLE 16.3
Mechanisms Suggested as Possible Etiologies for Preeclampsia

Abnormal Placentation
  Abnormal trophoblast invasion
  Increased trophoblast mass
  Abnormal uteroplacental location

Immunologic Dysfunction
  Primarily a disease of primigravida
  Immunologic complexes in placenta and various organs
  Immunologic complexes in maternal serum
  Multisystem involvement

Coagulation Abnormalities
  Abnormal prostaglandin metabolism
  Disseminated intravascular coagulopathy
  Platelet activation and consumption
  Low antithrombin III

Endothelial Damage
  Cytotoxic factors against endothelial cells
  Increased capillary permeability
  Damaged endothelium on electron microscopy
  Increased fibronectin levels

Dietary Factors
  Protein and caloric intake
  Magnesium, calcium, zinc deficiency
  Excessive sodium intake
  Essential fatty acids deficiency

Endocrine Abnormalities
  Activated renin-angiotensin-aldosterone system
  Abnormal catecholamines
  Abnormal progesterone metabolism

Genetic Predisposition
  Increased incidence in daughter and granddaughters
  Increased incidence in sisters
  Increased incidence in patients with previous disease

Vasospasm
  Sensitivity to vasoactive substances
  Reduced plasma volume in severe disease

Reproduced with permission from Sibai BM. Eclampsia. In: Goldstein PJ, Stern BJ, (eds.) *Neurological disorders of pregnancy*, 2nd ed. Mount Kisco, NY: Futura Publishing Co., Inc., 1992.

age may be produced by platelet consumption and increased platelet aggregation (18) and hypertension.

Pregnancy-induced hypertension appears to be a multifactorial process. No single mechanism can account completely for the rise in blood pressure; however, multi-organ vasospasm associated with endothelial dysfunction appears to be a significant contributor. Additionally, the increased vascular responsiveness to catecholamines and angiotensin adversely affect renal function, with consequent proteinuria, hypoalbuminemia, edema, and hypertension. A shrinking intravascular volume may result in decreased cardiac output and renal function, adversely affecting utero-placental profusion. Multi-organ, including central nervous system (CNS) morbidity, may arise from the HELLP syndrome, consisting of a number of clinical abnormalities, including hemolysis, elevated liver enzymes, and low platelets.

With the invasion of the muscular layer of the uterus by the endovascular trophoblast during the first trimester, deactivation of autonomic innervation of the spiral arteries occurs; these result in vascular changes in the inner third of the myometrium (19,20). The spiral arteries then transform into uteroplacental arteries, which release nitric oxide (NO) (21,22). Nitric oxide produces a low-pressure, low-resistance, uteroplacental circulation. In preeclampsia, however, an impaired transformation of the spiral arteries of the nonpregnant uterus to uteroplacental arteries occurs, only the decidual layers of the uteroplacental arteries are involved in the transformation, and fewer arteries are produced (23). There is failure of NO production, immunologic maladaptation of nondilating spiral arteries, increasing inactivation of NO, and further vasoconstriction from oxygen free radicals and lipid peroxides. The balance is shifted between the vasoconstrictor and platelet-aggregation promoting effects of platelet-derived thromboxane-A2 (TXA2) (24), and the vasodilator and platelet-aggregation inhibiting effects of prostacyclin (PGI2) elaborated in the maternal vascular walls. Decreases in PGI2 and NO decrease platelet activation and the production of circulating serotonin. Mild increases in serotonin in mild preeclampsia may restore vascular PGI2 and NO release, in turn improving uteroplacental perfusion by increasing perfusion pressure. Thus, an increase in maternal blood pressure satisfies the vascular needs of the fetus. Further increases in serotonin result in increased vasoconstriction and platelet aggregation, however, worsening the pathologic process. Other abnormalities include the renin-angiotensin-aldosterone system (25,26) and the prostacyclin-thromboxane-A2 systems (15).

Increasing evidence suggests a mitochronidal defect that impairs cytotrophoblastic differentiation and invasion (27). This involves the mitochondrial mutation of the nuclear or mitochondrial genomes, resulting in mutant mitochondria in the daughter cells. These impaired mitochondria in syncytial tissues are subject to high metabolic demands. The mitochondrial defects are thought to impair normal placentation in pregnancy. Higher incidences of the disease exist in immediate blood relatives, especially in a line from mother to daughter (28,29). Such lack of concordance could be explained by differing proportions of wild-type and mutant DNA segregating to twins or siblings, thus engendering different cytoplasmic phenotypes (30). These genetic differences are linked to changes in function and morphology, with loss of cristae in the mitochondria, indicating a systemic metabolic dysfunction associated with a decrease in cytochrome oxidase (31). The same chromosomal locus for pregnancy-induced hypertension is found for the mitochondrial production of endothelial NO synthetase (32).

More recent work by Redman and colleagues underscores the probable contribution of an intravascular inflammatory response to the preeclamptic process (33). Excessive inflammatory stimulation proportional to placental size (in keeping with the finding that preeclampsia is more frequently seen in multiple gestations and increasing placental size near term), is thought to activate leukocytes and stimulate proinflammatory cytokine production. In this fashion, the increasing placental size, with its concomitant proinflammatory role, generates signals that may stimulate a more generalized inflammatory response in the mother. This balance may decompensate possibly from excessive placental stimulus or excessive maternal response. As part of the normal pregnancy process, inflammatory response is shared in the states of normal pregnancy and preeclampsia, and the pathophysiologic processes are thought to reflect exaggerated responses in an otherwise normal pregnancy. The problem lies, therefore, not with pre-eclampsia per se, but the physiology of pregnancy itself. Intercurrent toxic, genetic, septic, or other factors may impair the normal downregulation of particular components of the immune activation system that normally keep the inflammatory reactions in check. This dynamic represents the normal maternal-fetal "genetic conflict" (34).

Hypertension, which accounts for many of the neurologic features seen with the resulting hypertensive encephalopathy and vasospasm, however, is not universally present in all patients with eclampsia. Hence, the reliance placed by a clinician on hypertension to make the diagnosis might result in a delay in management, even with patients manifesting other signs of preeclampsia, but without significant increase in blood pressure. HELLP syndrome, with its associated coagulopathy, may result in major neurologic sequelae and intracranial hemorrhage without hypertension (35) or indeed, proteinuria or edema.

Cerebral Pathology

A major contributing factor to the cerebral pathology in preeclampsia-eclampsia is cerebral edema supervening when the cerebral blood pressure exceeds the limits of cerebral autoregulation. Cerebral autoregulation is maintained by the modulation of cerebral arteriolar resistance in the face of the arterial pressure of the blood supply to the brain. This mechanism maintains the independence of cerebral perfusion pressure from the systemic arterial blood pressure. With the relative hypertension seen in preeclampsia, the autoregulation of the cerebral circulation is impaired, resulting at one extreme in hypertension and encephalopathy and at the other extreme in cerebral hypoperfusion (36,37). The ensuing damage to precapillaries and capillaries, disruption of the "tight junctions," and the extravasation of red cells and proteins in the perivascular spaces contribute to the blood–brain barrier disruption at particular areas of risk, which are the border zones between the larger cerebral arteries. There is local vulnerability to cortical petechiae, microinfarctions, and pericapillary brain hemorrhages. Some of these changes are due to the regional differences in the control of cerebral blood flow (38), with regions of alternating arteriolar dilatation and constriction resulting in capillary breakdown, extravasation of blood elements, increased platelet consumption, and the triggering of coagulation with fibrin deposition (39). When the protective precapillary arteriolar vasoconstriction fails, the increase in blood pressure exerts a direct effect on the capillary bed, resulting in hemorrhages.

The neurologic manifestations of preeclampsia-eclampsia, although sudden, may be transient. Progressively severe headache lasting days may occur with visual disturbances, hallucinations, or even the perception of "flashing lights" (from whence the name eclampsia is derived). Even the occipital blindness can be reversible. The pathologic processes may progress, presenting clinically with focal neurologic deficit, confusion, seizures, or even coma. The visual system may be affected by retinal arteriolar dilatation or spasm, retinal hemorrhages and exudates, or even retinal detachment. Papilledema may result from raised intracerebral pressure. The posterior cortical watershed zones, less protected by sympathetic vasoconstrictor tone, are particularly subject to microhemorrhages and infarctions, as well as to subcortical gray–white zone edema. Any part of the cerebral hemisphere can be involved, however, resulting, for example, in aphasia or pareses.

Eclampsia is a significant risk factor for stroke during pregnancy in the first 6 weeks postpartum (40) and accounts for about half of the case-related strokes (41).

PATHOLOGY

Pathologic changes affect various parts of the neuraxis (14). Aside from cerebral edema, hemorrhaging may occur in the subarachnoid, subcortical, and intraparenchymal areas. Small- to medium-sized infarctions can occur in the cerebral cortex, corona radiata, basal ganglia, and brainstem. Metabolic and hypertensive encephalopathy are also seen. Although damage predominantly affects the watershed zones in the parieto-occipital regions, vascular changes may also affect the parietal and frontal lobes. Many of these processes may be a source of seizures.

Subarachnoid hemorrhages may occur in circumscribed areas of cerebral cortex, whereas larger hemorrhages can be seen in the hemispheres, basal ganglia, and pons (14,42). Hemorrhages in the gray matter may then erupt into the ventricles or subarachnoid spaces (14). Smaller hemorrhagic areas, in the form of sulcal petechiae and microinfarctions appear in the precapillary and capillary areas as well as around arterioles (14,42–43). These result in splitting of the elastic fibers, necrosis of the arterial wall, and edema. Deep-seated hemorrhages in the corona radiata, basal ganglia, and brainstem may be seen along with larger cortical hemorrhages (14,43). A recent study of stroke in pregnancy, with eclampsia given as a leading cause, showed the incidence of intraparenchymal hemorrhages and ischemic strokes to be similar (hemorrhages usually account for approximately 15% of strokes), suggesting that pregnancy increases the risk of cerebral hemorrhage (44). Diffuse cerebral edema is associated with a rise in cerebrospinal fluid pressure and papilledema (45). On postmortem, there may be marked central or transverse herniation as well as gyral flattening (14,42).

A number of organ systems can be damaged because of the pathologic vascular changes that occur in preeclampsia and eclampsia. Platelet consumption and active coagulopathy may occur in various organs. There is an increasing literature of angiographic and transcranial Doppler studies attesting to the vasospastic component in cerebral pathology (46–48) (Figure 16.3).

DIAGNOSIS

Preeclampsia is characterized by variable weight gain, pregnancy-induced hypertension, and edema. An excessive weight gain is defined as more than 2 pounds per week. Pathologic edema is that which involves the hands and face. However, seizures may appear before the edema, weight gain, or proteinuria (10,11,49). Standard definitions of preeclampsia and hypertension are given in Table 16.1. The proteinuria may appear late in the course of preeclampsia. Neurologic features frequently include headache and photophobia, pain in the upper abdominal area, and brisk reflexes (Table 16.4).

LABORATORY STUDIES

Preeclampsia-eclampsia is a clinical diagnosis. Some accompanying laboratory abnormalities are the raised

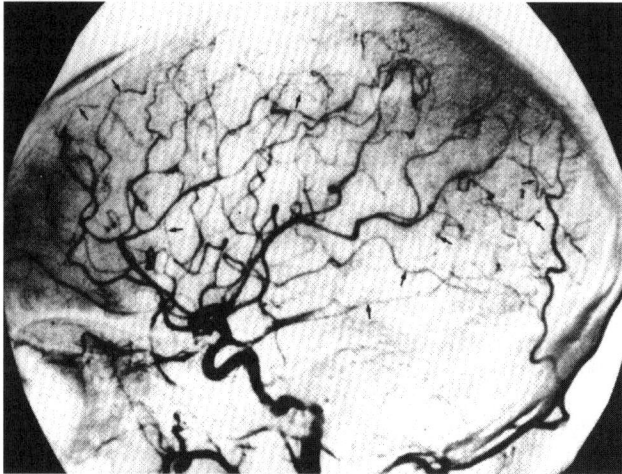

FIGURE 16.3

Left common carotid artery injection shows spasm of peripheral branches of left anterior and middle cerebral arteries. Arrows point to beaded appearance of these vessels. Paucity of peripheral branches is shown. (Reproduced with permission from Trommer BL, et al. Cerbral vasospasm and eclampsia. *Stroke* 1988;19:326–329.)

| TABLE 16.4 | |
Clinical Features Preceding Eclampsia	
Clinical Features	**Percent of Patients**
Headache	83
Hyperreflexia	80
Clonus	46
Visual signs	45
Epigastric pain	20

Adapted with permission from Sibai et al. *Obstet Gynecol* 1982; 57:199.

serum creatinine and uric acid that occur in approximately 60% of patients. In approximately one-third or fewer patients, a fall in platelets below 150,000 per mm^3 may occur; hemolysis from disseminated intravascular coagulation; and elevation of liver enzymes (HELLP syndrome), an entity that is associated with significant maternal morbidity (49,50).

IMAGING

In most cases of eclampsia, particularly those without focal neurologic findings, computed tomography (CT) head scans are usually normal, but magnetic resonance imaging (MRI) may still show T2-weighted abnormalities in watershed zones. Patients with focal neurologic findings and atypical cases warrant investigation to

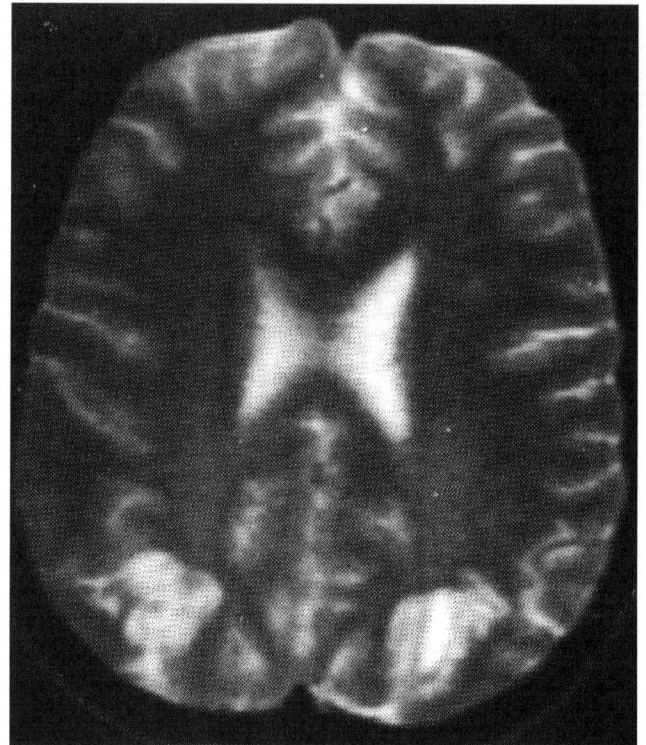

FIGURE 16.4

MRI scan. Hyperintense areas in the posterior parietal area on a higher section. (Reproduced with permission from Raroque HG, Orrison WW, Rosenberg GA. *Neurology* 1990;40:167–169.)

address neurologic complications. Various series of CT head scans have shown abnormalities in 29% to 75% of eclamptic patients (51). These changes include cerebral edema; hemorrhages in the brain stem, subependymal regions, subarachnoid spaces, and parenchymal areas; and infarction (52). Other large series have reported no abnormalities (12,53). MRI scans have documented hypodensities in the basal ganglia, border zone ischemia, and focal cerebral edema, which usually resolve on subsequent scanning (49, 54,55) (Figure 16.4). In eclampsia, there may be the characteristic multifocal curvilinear abnormalities at the gray–white junction of the posterior watershed zones. Such reversible angiopathy has been further documented using angiography (Figure 16.5), single photon emission computerized tomography (SPECT), and transcranial Doppler ultrasound (TCD) (46,48,54–57).

Most patients under obstetric care with eclampsia do not get head MRI or CT scans, and it is only after focal neurologic findings appear that a neurologic consult and imaging are requested. Women with focal neurologic findings warrant further investigation, but without it, clinical diagnosis usually leads to treatment with magnesium sulfate and expeditious delivery of the baby.

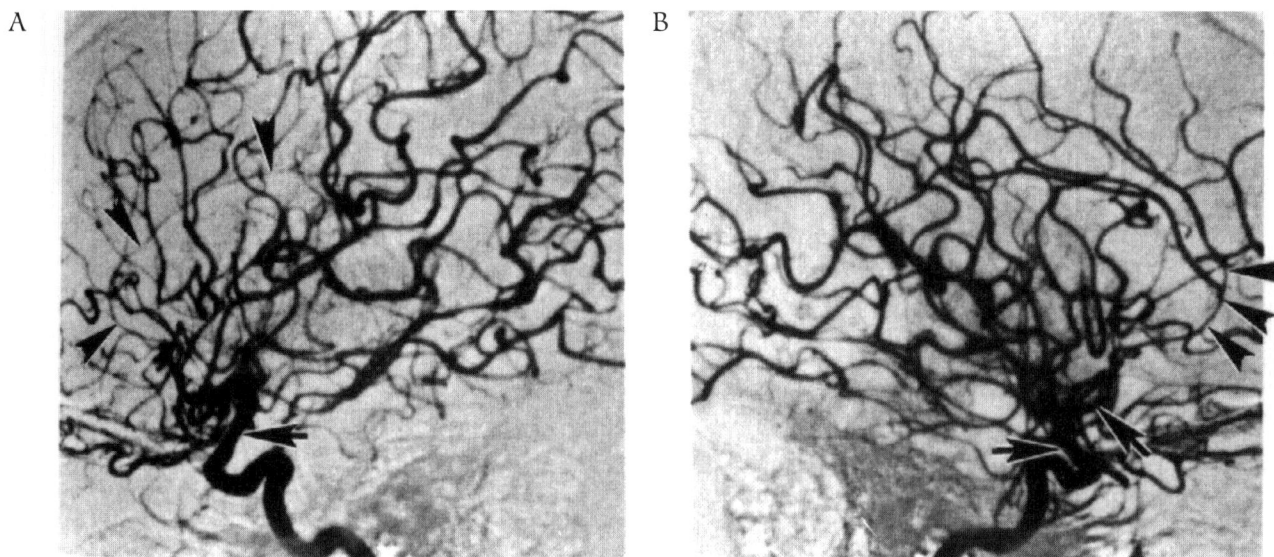

FIGURE 16.5

A cerebral angiogram with injection of contrast into the right (A) and left (B) internal carotid arteries. Diffuse narrowing of anterior cerebral arteries can be seen bilaterally (arrowheads). Focal areas of vasospasm are also seen (arrows). (Reproduced with permission from Geraghty JJ, et al. Fatal puerperal cerebral vasospasm and stroke in a young woman. *Neurology* 1991;41:1146–1147.)

ELECTROENCEPHALOGRAPHY

Electroencephalography is usually abnormal (49). There may be diffuse or focal slowing, and/or focal or generalized epileptiform activity (58,59).

THE MANAGEMENT OF ECLAMPSIA

The treatment of mild, moderate, or even severe eclampsia is usually handled by obstetricians, and only rarely are neurologists consulted for management. More frequently, neurologists are involved with the appearance of seizures, focal neurologic deficits, or coma. The treatment goal is the rapid delivery of a viable baby, with preservation of maternal health. Therapeutic strategies are directed at decreasing blood pressure to the autoregulatory range, preventing seizures or their recurrence, and preventing or minimizing cerebral edema. Preeclampsia and eclampsia represent a spectrum of neuropathologic change, and management should be directed at the process as a whole.

Treatment of Hypertension

Cerebral edema may rapidly resolve when hypertension is lowered to within the boundaries of cerebral perfusion autoregulation, usually a fall in 20 to 25% of the mean arterial pressure. Antihypertensive agents used have included diazoxide, sodium nitroprusside, nitroglycerin, and hydralazine (60–62). Nifedipine and labetalol are currently favored agents (61) (Table 16.5).

TABLE 16.5

Pharmacologic Management of Hypertensive Crisis Persistent Blood Pressure—160/110

Drug	Administration
Hydralazine	5 mg IV; repeat in 10 minutes; then 10 mg IV every 20 minutes until stable blood pressure (140–150/90–110 mm Hg) achieved
Labetalol	5–15 mg IV push; repeat every 10–20 minutes by doubling dose to a maximum of 300 mg total
Sodium nitroprusside[a,b] (best used for refractory hypertension)	Controlled infusion 0.5–3.0 mg/kg/min, not to exceed 800 mg/min
Nifedipine[b]	10 mg sublingual, repeat in 30 minutes; then 10–20 mg PO every 4–6 hours
Nitroglycerine	Should be used only by practitioners thoroughly familiar with its use in obstetrics

[a]Requires arterial line for continuous blood pressure monitoring.

[b]Avoid use in antepartum patients. Profound hypotension may result.

Reproduced with permission from Repke JT. A longitudinal approach. In: Moore TR, Reiter RC, Rebar RW, (eds.) *Gynecology and obstetrics. Hypertension and preeclampsia* 1993; 29:463–477.

With the appearance of intracranial hemorrhage, management should follow the guidelines for the monitoring and acute management of raised intracranial pressure. Intubation with hyperventilation, diuresis, and occasionally intracranial pressure monitoring in an intensive care setting may all be warranted.

Treatment of Seizures

The pathophysiologic changes underlying seizures and eclampsia remain unclear. Seizure activity arises from the abnormal excessive neuronal excitability and its subsequent spread, but the changes that precipitate neuronal excitability have been the subject of much discussion. In preventing epileptogenesis, management is directed both at treating the underlying cause of cerebral damage and at preventing the precipitation and spread of seizure activity. In the United States, the camps have been divided between the emphasis placed by obstetricians on magnesium sulfate as an "anticonvulsant," and the position taken by neurologists that the principal cause of epileptogenesis is the hypertensive encephalopathy and associated cerebrovascular abnormalities—with the seizures remaining a problem that is best treated by known anticonvulsants. Some evidence suggested that the aggressive treatment of hypertension diminished eclamptic seizures, but the controversy remained over how best to treat impending seizures and preeclampsia and prevent recurrence of seizures in eclampsia. The evolution of this controversy led to large multicentered trials that have answered the question of which treatment is best in preventing eclamptic seizures or their recurrence before the clear underpinnings or rationale for this treatment had been clearly established. In part motivated by the controversies regarding magnesium sulfate in eclampsia (63–65), a large multicenter trial in 1,680 women with eclampsia demonstrated that 4 g intravenous (IV) magnesium sulfate over 5 minutes, followed by 5 g intramuscular (IM) in each buttock and 5 g every 4 hours was superior to a loading dose of phenytoin 1 g or diazepam 10 mg IV over 2 minutes repeated if seizures recurred, followed by 40 mg in 50 mL of normal saline over 24 hours (66). Patients who received the magnesium sulfate treatment had a 67% lower risk of recurrent seizures than those who received phenytoin, and a 52% lower risk than those who were treated with diazepam (Figure 16.6). Some criticism could be leveled at this study for the absence of phenytoin levels and data showing only mean blood pressures in defining the diagnosis of eclampsia in both treatment arms. A subsequent multicenter trial that examined 2,138 patients with preeclampsia, however, clearly showed the superiority of magnesium sulfate at 10 g IM and 5 g every 4 hours to treatment with 1 g phenytoin (67). In this paper, none of the 1,049 patients who were given magnesium sulfate went on to have eclamp-

(i) Magnesium sulphate versus diazepam

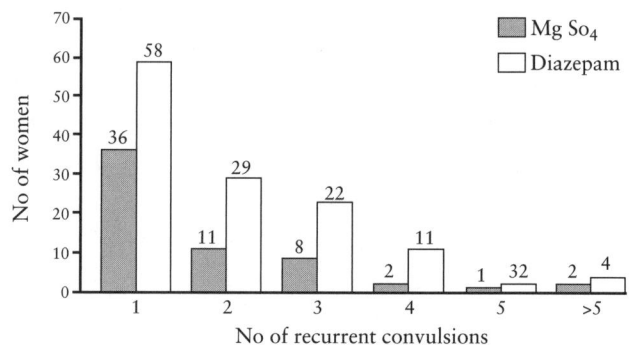

(ii) Magnesium sulphate versus phenytoin

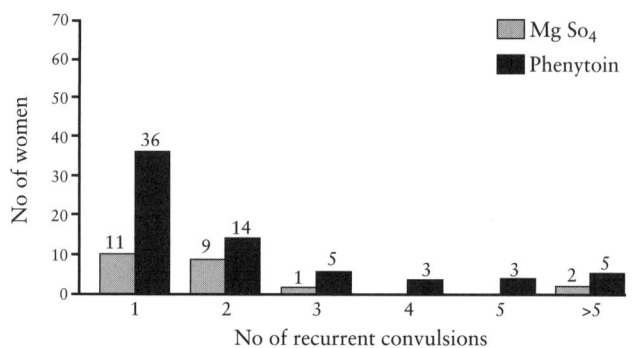

FIGURE 16.6

A study of 1,680 women with eclampsia showed a 52% lower risk of recurrent seizures with magnesium sulfate compared with diazepam, and a 67% lower risk compared with phenytoin. (Reproduced with permission from *Lancet* 1995;45:1455–1463.)

tic seizures, whereas 10 of the 1,089 patients treated with phenytoin had seizures. Phenytoin levels in nine of the ten women with seizures, however, were documented to be in the lower therapeutic range (<13.1 mg/mL). More recent data from the Magpie Trial, in over 10,000 pregnant women with hypertension, showed a decrease in maternal death (68). For a protocol for the administration of magnesium sulfate and advice on monitoring patients, see Tables 16.6 and 16.7.

The cellular and vascular mechanisms underlying eclamptic seizures are still unresolved, but some evidence suggests that the N-methyl D-asparate (NMDA) subtype of the glutamate receptor, which can be blocked by magnesium ions, is involved in neuronal firing thresholds (69,70). Magnesium blocks these receptors, thus preventing neuronal damage that would in turn lead to seizures. Animal models have shown that magnesium sulfate suppresses neuronal burst firing and interictal EEG spike generation (71), but other investigators using the same model failed to support these findings and revealed that the decrease in neuronal firing was a decay phe-

TABLE 16.6
Magnesium Sulfate Administration for Seizure Prophylaxis

Intramuscular
10 g (5 g deep IM in each buttock)
5 g deep IM every 4 hours alternating sides
Made up as 50% solution

Intravenous
6 g bolus over 15 minutes
1 to 3 g/h by continuous infusion pump
May be mixed in 100 mL of crystalloid; if given as intravenous push, make up as 20% solution; push at maximum rate of 1 g/min
40 g Mg SO$_4$ 7H$_2$O in 1000 mL Ringer's lactate; run at 25 to 75 mg/h (1 to 3 g/h)

Reproduced with permission from Repke JT. A longitudinal approach. In: Moore TR, Reiter RC, Rebar RW, et al., (eds.) *Gynecology and obstetrics. Hypertension and preeclampsia* 1993; 29:463–477.

TABLE 16.7
Monitoring the Patient Who Is Receiving Magnesium Sulfate

Assess patient vital signs, urine output, and reflexes every 2–4 hours
  Patellar reflexes >1+
  Respiratory rate >12 breaths per minute
  Monitor pulse for arrhythmia
  Watch for O$_2$ desaturation
  Watch for widening QRS or prolonged QT intervals on electrocardiogram
  If urine output <30 ml/h, check level, adjust infusion.
Laboratory
  Therapeutic levels accepted as 4–8 mEq/L
Toxicities
  Absence of deep tendon reflexes (>4–6 mEq/L)
  Somnolence (>8 mEq/L)
  Respiratory depression (>8 mEq/L)
Cardiotoxicity (>15 mEq/L)

Reproduced with permission from Repke JT. A longitudinal approach. In: Moore TR, Reiter RC, Rebar RW, et al., (eds.) *Gynecology and obstetrics. Hypertension and preeclampsia* 1993; 29:463–477.

nomenon (72). In vivo studies in animals and humans do not show evidence suggesting that magnesium sulfate infusion controls or prevents seizures. When given to rodents subjected to electroshock and pentylenetretazol, which are rodent models for epilepsy, magnesium sulfate had little effect in preventing seizures (73). Seizures outside the setting of eclampsia, in renal failure or porphyria, have occasionally been prevented by magnesium sulfate infusion, whereas in other situations it is either ineffective (74,75) or has not been tried. However, magnesium sulfate might act as a calcium antagonist, preventing cerebral vasoconstriction and the subsequent cortical injury that leads to seizures. Curiously, dietary supplementation with calcium decreases the incidence of preeclampsia in high-risk patients (76).

Magnesium sulfate is not without side effects. The higher serum levels of magnesium sulfate suppress patellar reflexes at 6 mEq/L, and at higher levels of 8 to 10 mEq/L it results in lethargy and respiratory depression, with cardiac arrest occurring at levels above 12 mEq/L. There are reports of women with eclampsia having seizures refractory to magnesium sulfate (12,60), and up to one-third of patients may have recurrent seizures (12,77). Phenytoin has been used with good effect (78–80) and may also control seizures that are resistant to magnesium sulfate (81).

Rapid Control of Seizures

Intravenous diazepam can rapidly control ongoing prolonged seizures, usually with minimal effect on the fetus. Diazepam may, however, result in neonatal hypothermia, lethargy, apnea, hypotonia, and poor sucking effort. Although phenobarbital is an effective antiepileptic drug, it is less often used because of its sedating effects.

PREVENTING ECLAMPSIA

Low-dose aspirin (60 to 100 mg) has been reported to decrease preeclampsia in women at risk but may not work in nulliparous women (82). Another study reported an increased risk of placental abruption (83). As mentioned previously, calcium supplements may also help forestall eclampsia (76).

SUMMARY

Neurologists can make an important contribution to the management of eclampsia. When consulted by their obstetric colleagues, they can provide input into the management of seizures and the intracerebral vascular events that occur with eclampsia and the peripartum period (Table 16.5). Much remains to be done in elucidating the pathophysiology of preeclampsia and eclampsia, particularly with regard to the vascular and antivasospastic effects of treatments such as magnesium sulfate on the cerebral circulation. The most recent studies have shown a benefit of magnesium sulfate over phenytoin in the prevention of seizures in preeclampsia and the prevention of recurrent seizures in eclampsia. A need exists for more basic and clinical research from both obstetric and neurologic perspectives in the optimal management of patients with eclampsia.

References

1. Porapakkam S. An epidemiologic study of eclampsia. *Obstet Gynecol* 1979;54:26–30.

2. MacGillivray I. *Preeclampsia: The hypertensive disease of pregnancy*. Philadelphia: WB Saunders, 1983:17.

3. Chesley LC. Hypertensive disorders in pregnancy. New York: Appleton-Century-Crofts, 1978:225.

4. Sibai BM. Preeclampsia-eclampsia In: Sciarra JJ, (ed.) *Gynecology and obstetrics*, vol. 2. Philadelphia: JB Lippincott, 1989;51:1–12.

5. American College of Obstetricians and Gynecologists. ACOG Technical Bulletin 216. Hypertension in pregnancy. Washington, D.C. 1996;1–8.

6. Brown CE, Cunningham FG, Pritchard JA. Convulsions in hypertensive, proteinuric primiparas more than 24 hours after delivery: eclampsia or some other cause? *J Reprod Med* 1987;32:499–503.

7. Sibai BM, Schneider JM, Morrison JC, et al. The late postpartum eclampsia controversy. *Obstet Gynecol* 1980;55:75–78.

8. Douglas K, Redman CW. Eclampsia in the United Kingdom. *Brit Med J* 1994;309:1395–1400.

9. Lubarsky SL, Barton JR, Friedman SA, et al. Late postpartum eclampsia revisited. *Obstet Gynecol* 1994;83:502–505.

10. Veltkamp, Kupsch A, Polasek J, Yousry TA, Pfister HW. Late onset postpartum eclampsia without pre-eclamptic prodromi: clinical and neuroradiological presentation in two patients. *J Neurol Neurosurg Psychiatry* 2000;69:824–827.

11. Dziewas R, Stögbauer, Freund M, Lüdemann, Imai T, Holzapfel C, Ringelstein EB. Late onset postpartum eclampsia: a rare and difficult diagnosis. *J Neurol* 2002;249:1287–1291.

12. Pritchard JA, Cunningham FG, Pritchard SA. The Parkland Hospital protocol for treatment of eclampsia: evaluation of 245 cases. *Am J Obstet Gynecol* 1984;148:951–963.

13. Hallum AV. Eye changes in hypertensive toxemia of pregnancy. *J Am Med Assoc* 1936;106:1649–1651.

14. Sheehan HL, Lynch JB. *Pathology of toxaemia of pregnancy*. Baltimore: Williams & Wilkins, 1973.

15. Friedman SA, Taylor RM, Roberts JM. Pathophysiology of preeclampsia. *Clin Perinatol* 1991;18:661.

16. Rappaport VJ, Hirata G, Kim Yap H, et al. Anti-vascular endothelial cell antibodies in severe preeclampsia. *Am J Obstet Gynecol* 1990;162:138.

17. Rodgers GM, Taylor RN, Roberts JM. Preeclampsia is associated with a serum factor cytotoxic to human endothelial cells. *Am J Obstet Gynecol* 1988;159:908.

18. Samuels B. Postpartum eclampsia. *Obstet and Gynecol* 1960;15:748–752.

19. Brosens J, Robertson WB, Dixon HG. The physiological response of the vessels of the placental bed to normal pregnancy. *J Pathol Bacteriol* 1967;93:569.

20. Pijnenborg R, Bland JM, Robertson WB, et al. Utero-placental arterial changes related to interstitial trophoblast migration in early human pregnancy. *Placenta* 1983;4:387.

21. Myatt L, Brewer A, Brockman DE. The action of nitric oxide in the perfused human fetal-placental circulation. *Am J Obstet Gynecol* 1991;164:687.

22. Furchgott RF. The discovery of endothelium-derived relaxing factor and its importance in the identification of nitric oxide. *JAMA* 1996;276:1186.

23. Khong TY, Dewolf F, Robertson WB, et al. Inadequate maternal vascular response to placentation in pregnancies complicated by preeclampsia and by small-for-gestational age infants. *Br J Obstet Gynaecol* 1986;93:1049.

24. Zeeman GG, Dekker GA. In: Brooks PG, Sibai BH, Pitkin RM, Scott JR (eds). Pathogenesis of preeclampsia: a hypothesis. *Clin Obstet Gynecol* 1992;35:317–337.

25. Gant NF, Daley GL, Chand S, et al. A study of angiotensin II pressor response throughout primigravid pregnancy. *J Clin Invest* 1973;52:2682.

26. Talledo OE, Chesley LC, Zuspan FP. Renin-angiotensin system in normal and toxemic pregnancies. III. Differential sensitivity to angiotensin II and norepinephrine in toxemia of pregnancy. *Am J Obstet Gynecol* 1968;100:218.

27. Widschwendter M, Schrocksnadel H, Mortl MG. Opinion: Pre-eclampsia: a disorder of placental mitochrondria? *Mol Med Today* 1998;4:286–291.

28. Cooper DW, Brennecke SP, Wilton AN. Genetics of preeclampsia. *Hypertens Pregn* 1993;12:1–23.

29. Cooper DW, Hill JA, Chesley LC, et al. Genetic control of susceptibility to eclampsia and miscarriage. *Br J Obstet Gynaecol* 1988;95:644–653.

30. Folgero T, Storbakk N, Torbergsen T, et al. Elimination of paternal mitochondrial DNA in intraspecific crosses during early mouse embryogenesis. *Proc Natl Acad Sci USA* 1995;92:4542–4546.

31. Furui T, Kurauchi O, Tanaka M, et al. Decrease in cytochrome c oxidase and cytochrome oxidase subunit 1 messenger RNA levels in preeclamptic pregnancies. *Obstet Gynecol* 1994;84:283–288.

32. Amgrimsson R, Hayward C, Nadaul S, et al. Evidence for a familial pregnancy-induced hypertension focus in the eNOS-gene region. *Am J Hum Genet* 1997;61:354–362.

33. Redman CWG, Sacks GP, Sargent IL. Preeclampsia: an excessive maternal inflammatory response to pregnancy. *Am J Obstet Gynecol* 1999;180:499–506.

34. Haig D. Genetic conflicts in human pregnancy. *Q Rev Biol* 1993;68:495–532.

35. Redman CWG, Roberts JM. Management of preeclampsia. *Lancet* 1993;341:1451–1454.

36. Auer L. The role of cerebral perfusion pressure as origin of brain edema in acute arterial hypertension. *Europ Neurol* 1978;15:153–156.

37. Strandgaard S. The lower and upper limit for autoregulation of cerebral blood flow. *Stroke* 1973; 4:323.

38. Baumbach GL, Heistad DD. Heterogeneity of brain blood flow and permeability during acute hypertension. *Am J Physiol* 1985;249:H629–H637.

39. Anderson G, Sibai B. Hypertension in pregnancy. In: Gabbe S, Niebyl J, Simpson J, (eds.) *Obstetrics: normal and problem pregnancies*. New York: Churchill Livingstone, 1986:819.

40. Lanska DJ, Kryscio RJ. Stroke and intracranial venous thrombosis during pregnancy and puerperium. *Neurology* 1998;51:1622–1628.

41. Sharshar T, Lamy C, Mas JL. Stroke in Pregnancy Study Group. Incidence and causes of strokes associated with pregnancy and puerperium. *Stroke* 1995;26:930–936.

42. Govan ADT. The pathogenesis of eclamptic lesions. *Pathologia et Microbiologia* 1961;24:561–575.

43. Parks J, Pearson JW. Cerebral complications occurring in the toxemias of pregnancy. *Am J Obstet Gynecol* 1943;45:774–785.

44. Lamy C, Sharshar T, Mas J-L. Pathologie vasculaire cérébrale au ours de la grossesse et du post-partum. *Rev Neurol* 1996;152:422–440.

45. Richards A, Graham D, Bullock R. Clinicopathological study of neurological complications due to hypertensive disorders of pregnancy. *J Neurol Neurosurg Psychiatry* 1988;51:416–421.

46. Call GK, Fleming MC, Sealfon S, et al. Reversible cerebral segmental vasoconstriction. *Stroke* 1988;19: 1159–1170.

47. Raps EC, Galetta SL, Broderick M, et al. Delayed peripartum vasculopathy: Cerebral eclampsia revisited. *Ann Neurol* 1993;33:222–225.

48. Qureshi AI, Frankel MR, Ottenlips JR, Stern BJ. Cerebral hemodynamics in preeclampsia. *Arch Neurol* 1996;53:1226–1231.

49. Sibai BM, McCubbin JH, Anderson GD, et al. Eclampsia I. Observation from 67 recent cases. *Obstet Gynecol* 1981;48:609.

50. Sibai BM, Ramadan MK, Chari RS, Friedman SA. Pregnancies complicated by HELLP syndrome (hemolysis, elevated liver enzymes, and low platelets): subsequent pregnancy outcome and long-term prognosis. *Am J Obstet Gynecol* 1995;172:125–129.

51. Brown CEL, Purdy P, Cunningham FG. Head computed tomographic scans in women with eclampsia. *Am J Obstet Gynecol* 1988;159:915.

52. Finelli PF. Postpartum eclampsia and subarachnoid hemorrhage. *J Stroke Cerebrovasc Dis* 1992;2:151–153.

53. Sibai BM, Spinnato JA, Watson DL, et al. Eclampsia IV. Neurological findings and future outcome. *Am J Obstet* 1985;152:184.

54. Raroque HG, Orrison WW, Rosenberg GA. Neurologic involvement in toxemia of pregnancy: reversible MRI lesions. *Neurology* 1990;40:167–169.

55. Schwartz RB, Jones KM, Kalina P, et al. Hypertensive encephalopathy: findings on CT, MR imaging, and SPECT imaging in 14 cases. *Am J Radiol* 1992;159: 379–383.

56. Crawford S, Varner MW, Digre KB, et al. Cranial magnetic resonance imaging in eclampsia. *Obstet Gynecol* 1985;70:474–477.

57. Trommer BL, Homer D, Mikhael MA. Cerebral vasospasm and eclampsia. *Stroke* 1988;19:326–329.

58. Kolstad P. The practical value of electro-encephalography in pre-eclampsia and eclampsia. *Acta Obstet Gynec Scand* 1961;40:127.

59. Sibai BM, Spinnato JA, Watson DL, et al. Effect of magnesium sulfate in electroencephalographic findings in preeclampsia-eclampsia. *Obstet Gynecol* 1984b;64: 261–266.

60. Editorial. Management of eclampsia. *Br Med J* 1976;2: 1485–1486.

61. Michael CA. Intravenous labetalol and intravenous diazoxide in severe hypertension complicating pregnancy. *Austral N Z J Obstet Gynaecol* 1986;26:26–29.

62. Morris JA, Arce JJ, Hamilton CJ, et al. The management of severe preeclampsia and eclampsia with intravenous diazoxide. *Obstet Gynecol* 1977;49:675–680.

63. Donaldson JO. The case against magnesium sulfate for eclamptic convulsions. *Intern J Obstet Anes* 1992;1: 159–166.

64. Kaplan PW, Lesser RP, Fisher RS, et al. No, magnesium sulfate should not be used in treating eclamptic seizures. *Arch Neurol* 1988;45:1361.

65. Donaldson JO. Does magnesium sulfate treat eclamptic convulsions? *Clin Neuropharmacol* 1986;9:37–45.

66. The Eclampsia Trial Collaborative Group. Which anticonvulsant for women with eclampsia? Evidence from the Collaborative Eclampsia Trial. *Lancet* 1995;45: 1455–1463.

67. Lucas M, Leveno K, Cunningham G. A comparison of magnesium sulfate with phenytoin for the prevention of eclampsia. *N Engl J Med* 1995;333:201–205.

68. The Magpie Trial Collaborative Group. Do women with pre-eclampsia, and their babies, benefit from magnesium sulphate? The Magpie Trial: a randomized placebo controlled trial. *Lancet* 2002;359:1877–1890.

69. Coan EJ, Collingridge GL. Magnesium ions block an N-methyl-D-aspartate receptor-mediated component of synaptic transmission in rat hippocampus. *Neurosci Lett* 1985;53:21–26.

70. Stasheff SF, Anderson WW, Clark S, et al. NMDA antagonists differentiate epileptogenesis from seizure expression in an in vitro model. *Science* 1985;245:648–651.

71. Borges LF, Gucer G. Effect of magnesium on epileptic foci. *Epilepsia* 1978;19:81.

72. Koontz WL, Reid KH. Effect of parenteral magnesium sulfate on penicillin-induced seizure foci in anesthetized cats. *Am J Obstet Gynecol* 1985;153:96.

73. Krauss GL, Kaplan P, Fisher RS. Parenteral magnesium sulfate fails to control electroshock and pentylenetetrazol seizures in mice. *Epilepsy Res* 1989;4:201–206.

74. Fisher RS, Kaplan PW, Krumholz A, et al. Failure of high-dose intravenous magnesium sulfate to control myoclonic status epilepticus. *Clin Neuropharmacol* 1988;11: 537–544.

75. Link MJ, Anderson RE, Meyer FB. Effects of magnesium sulfate on pentylenetetrazol-induced status epilepticus. *Epilepsia* 1991;32(4):543–549.

76. Bucher HC, Guyatt GH, Cook RJ, et al. Effect of calcium supplementation on pregnancy-induced hypertension and preeclampsia: a meta-analysis of randomized controlled trials. *JAMA* 1996;275:1113–1117.

77. Crowther C. Magnesium sulphate versus diazepam in the management of eclampsia: a randomized controlled trial. *Br J Obstet Gynaecol* 1990;97:110–117.

78. Dommisse J. Phenytoin sodium and magnesium sulphate in the management of eclampsia. *Br J Obstet Gynaecol* 1990;97:104–109.

79. Friedman SA, Lim KH, Baker CA, Repke JT. Phenytoin versus magnesium sulfate in preeclampsia: a pilot study. *Am J Perinat* 1983;10:233–238.

80. Ryan G, Lange IR, Naugler MA. Clinical experience with phenytoin prophylaxis in severe preeclampsia. *Am J Obstet Gynecol* 1989;161:1297–1304.

81. Combs CA, Walker C, Matlock BA. Transient diabetes insipidus in pregnancy complicated by hypertension and seizures. *Am J Perintol* 1990;7:287–289.

82. CLASP (Collaborative Low-Dose Aspirin Study in Pregnancy) Collaborative Group. CLASP: a randomized trial of low-dose aspirin for the prevention and treatment of pre-eclampsia among 9364 pregnant women. *Lancet* 1994;343:619–629.

83. Sibai BM, Caritis SN, Thom E, et al., and the National Institute of Child Health and Human Development Network of Materal-Fetal Medicine Units. Prevention of preeclampsia with low-dose aspirin in healthy, nulliparous pregnant women. *N Engl J Med* 1993;329: 1213–1218.

17 Cerebrovascular Disease in Women

Rafael H. Llinas, MD and Carla J. Weisman, MD

Stroke continues to be the third leading cause of death and the leading cause of disability in the United States. In women, stroke is the second leading cause of death, with 102,892 women dying of stroke in 2000, accounting for 61.4% of total stroke deaths (1). Interestingly, the overall rate of stroke among women is lower than that in men but women are more likely to die from stroke (1,2). Because women live longer and stroke rates increase with age, women have a higher incidence of stroke when over 85 years (2–4).

Furthermore, treatments geared toward the general population may not be applicable to women, because women may have different risk factors and may appear to respond differently to certain therapies. For women who are premenopausal, the stroke rate is low except when associated with hormonal contraception; smoking also clearly increases the stroke rate among women. Pregnancy does not increase stroke rates significantly until the last trimester, although pregnancy can complicate pre-existing cerebrovascular disease. Oral hormone replacement used by menopausal women may increase the stroke rate.

This chapter reviews the statistics, epidemiology, stroke presentation, and treatments directed to women. Issues related to stroke and pregnancy, oral contraception, and hormone replacement also are discussed.

STROKE PRESENTATION, TREATMENT DIFFERENCES IN WOMEN

Stroke is a word that refers to acute neurologic damage and dysfunction from vascular causes. Many types of strokes and etiologies exist. It is generally preferable to avoid acronyms like CVA (cerebral vascular accident). Strokes are not always cerebral, not necessarily primarily vascular, and they are never an accident.

Ischemic strokes are typically due to the thromboembolism of intra- or extracranial arteries. This is due to either local arterial disease with or without embolization, hypercoagulable states, or from aorto/cardiac embolization, which results in bland ischemia and cell death. Treating the cause of thromboembolism consequently reduces the risk of recurrent ischemic strokes. Such ischemic strokes are prevented by using antiplatelet agents or anticoagulation for emboli arising from medium and small vessels, carotid endarterectomy (CEA) for a carotid disease source, or anticoagulation for emboli of cardiac origin. The determination of etiology is important because it defines treatment. In general, those hypercoagulable states that mainly affect the venous system cause strokes by means of "paradoxical" emboli, which cross over from the right to the left side of the heart via anatomic deficits such as an atrial septal defect on a patent foramen ovale, often with an atrial septal aneurysm.

Hemorrhagic strokes can occur because of the hemorrhagic transformation of a previous bland ischemic infarct, and these have the same etiologies. Hemorrhagic strokes can occur due to cerebral venous thrombosis (CVT) or venous strokes. CVT causes strokes by slowing exiting blood flow and increasing intracerebral pressure. This results in bland and hemorrhagic infarcts in nonarterial vascular distributions. The classic triad of papilledema, seizures, and headache is a typical presentation. CVT is often caused by hypercoagulable states, similar to those that predispose to deep venous thrombosis, such as smoking and oral contraceptive use, or dehydration. Structural lesions such as meningiomas or congenital bony abnormalities can obstruct the venous outflow and predispose to venous thrombosis. Treatment often includes anticoagulation, despite the presence of hemorrhage.

Primary central nervous system (CNS) hemorrhages are often due to hypertension and can result in hemorrhages in the thalamus, basal ganglia, cerebellum, or pons. Treatment is mainly supportive and includes the reversal of bleeding disorders. Primary CNS hemorrhages can also occur due to trauma, blood dyscrasias, hypercoagulable states, and structural vascular lesions such as arteriovenous malformations, cavernous angiomata, or cerebral aneurysms. Structural vascular lesions are often best treated using surgical or interventional radiologic procedures.

Acute Stroke Presentation

It is unclear why women die more often from stroke than men do, while the stroke rate for men is higher (Figure 17.1). One study showed that women may experience a longer delay from arrival in emergency rooms to the time they are evaluated for stroke symptoms (5). This may be due to a possible sex difference in the reporting of acute stroke symptoms. One study looked at 1,189 admissions that ended with a validated stroke diagnosis in emergency rooms. The traditional stroke symptoms of postural imbalance (men 20% vs. women 15%) and hemiparesis (men 24% vs. women 19%) were more likely to be the presenting symptoms for men than for women. Women were more likely to present with symptoms that were somewhat atypical for stroke, including pain (men 8% vs. women 12%) and change in level of consciousness (men 12% vs. women 17%). Women reported nontraditional stroke symptoms 62% more often than men did (6). That this accounts for the gender difference in death from stroke seems unlikely. Although the use of intravenous for acute stroke is potentially life-saving and is highly time-dependent, a majority of active stroke centers probably treat only about 1.8% of stroke patients with this therapy (7).

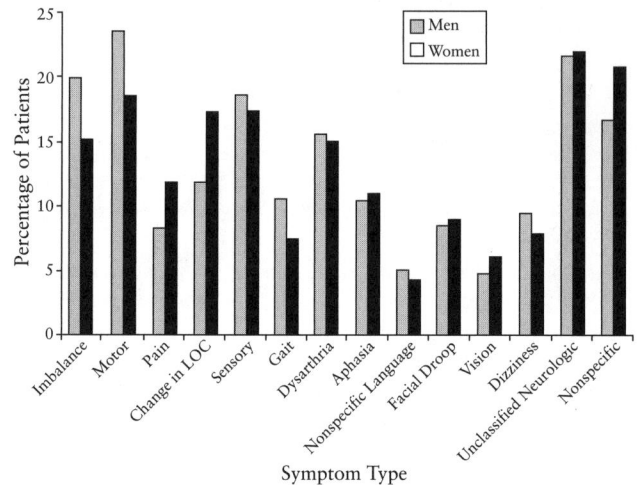

FIGURE 17.1

Women are more likely to present with nontraditional stroke symptoms. (Reproduced with permission from Labiche LA, Chan W, Saldin KR, Morgenstern LB. *Ann Emerg Med* 2002;40:453–460.)

Stroke Treatment in Women

Once the diagnosis of stroke in women has been made, how men and women are treated may be different (Table 17.1). Management of stroke may differ based on presumed differences in the efficacy of medications and procedures. In fact, this may be due to the comparatively greater age of women with stroke. Significant gender differences exist in the treatment of cardiac disease. Women are less likely to receive major diagnostic and therapeutic procedures for cardiac disease (8,9). Further, evidence suggests that men with stroke are more likely to have significant comorbidities, such as a higher rate of ischemic heart disease (men 18.1% vs. women 15.3%) and diabetes (men 20.1% vs. women 18.7%), but women have higher rates of hypertension (women 33.8% vs. men 30.0%) and higher rates of atrial fibrillation (women 12.9% vs. men 10.2%) (3). This study also showed that men 85 years and older were more likely to receive aspirin and ticlopidine for their strokes than did women aed 85 and older, although both groups received warfarin at the same rate; these problems of therapy were similar at younger ages. This may be because women with a lesser burden of cardiac disease or diabetes are less likely to have received preventive medications for these two disorders, and these medications may also protect against stroke.

Aspirin is an effective medication for stroke prevention in men and is most likely useful in stroke prevention in women. Some studies suggest little benefit, but may lack power to demonstrate efficacy, whereas others have shown benefit (3). Present recommendations are to use aspirin.

> **TABLE 17.1**
> *Workup/Treatment for Stroke by Etiology*
>
> **Evaluate Size and Location of Stroke**
> - CT or MRI of brain strokes may not appear for 6–24 hours unless diffusion MRI is done
> - Assess whether stroke is ischemic, hemorrhagic, or primary CNS hemorrhage
> - Assess whether stroke is in normal arterial vascular distribution
>
> **Evaluate Location of Arterial Occlusion**
> - Evaluation of intra- and extracranial vessels
> - MR angiography, CT angiography, transcranial Doppler of intracranial vessels
> - Warfarin may be required for high-grade symptomatic stenosis intracranially
> - Carotid imaging with duplex, CT angiography, MR angiography, or conventional angiography
> - Symptomatic carotid stenosis >70% should be treated surgically
>
> **Evaluate Possibility of Aortic or Cardiac Thrombus Embolization**
> - Transthoracic echocardiography—LVEF, valvular lesions, right to left shunts
> - Transesophageal echocardiography—aortic artherosclerosis, left atrial appendage clot
> - Warfarin often required for cardiac source emboli
>
> **Evaluate Risk Factors and Treat**
> - Antiplatelet agents for small- and medium-vessel disease
> - Warfarin for hypercoagulable states
> - Treat hypertension, diabetes, and hypercholesterolemia

A recent study showed that aspirin may be effective for primary prevention of stroke in women but not in men. The study suggests that while the data for aspirin use men has been poor for primary prevention of stroke aspirin tends to protect women from having their first stroke. Interestingly aspirin seems less effective at preventing myocardial infarction than in men. Presently women at risk for having their first stroke need to consider aspirin for prevention (3a).

Aspirin and dipyridamole in combination is a new treatment and is available in a combination pill. After the analysis of the European Stroke Prevention Study, it was found that women had lesser benefit from this combination therapy than men. Men had a risk reduction for stroke of 49% compared to 41% for women. Risk reduction for all vascular endpoints of the study showed a risk reduction for men of 39% compared to 30% for women. The combination medication is effective for both sexes, but seemingly less effective in women than in men (10).

Ticlopidine is an antiplatelet agent that is still in use, but has largely been supplanted by clopidogrel because of gastrointestinal and hematologic side effects. In the Canadian American Ticlopidine Study (CATS) trial, ticlopidine was found superior to aspirin 650 mg twice a day in both sexes, with a nonstatistically significant trend toward greater risk reduction in women for stroke or death (risk reduction of 27% for women; 19% for men over aspirin) (11). Other ticlopidine and clopidogrel trials have shown no difference between sexes. Both sexes had reductions in stroke and vascular death at similar rates (12).

Warfarin is probably as effective in women as in men. It is the treatment of choice for antiphospholipid antibody syndrome and stroke from cardiac source. Abnormalities of protein C, protein S, antithrombin III, and factor V Leiden are treated with warfarin if they are suspected to be the cause of stroke. In general, these factors lead to venous clots but may cause stroke when associated with right to left shunts, or a patent foramen ovale with an atrial septal aneurysm. A higher incidence of stroke occurs among women with coronary artery disease and atrial fibrillation (13), however, possibly giving women greater benefit from warfarin than men (3).

Carotid endarterectomy is an important treatment for the primary and secondary prevention of stroke in patients with significant carotid stenosis. Carotid disease is more common in men than women. A male to female prevalence ratio ranges from 3:2 to 8:1 (14). Studies lack congruence as to whether women have a higher postoperative stroke rate than men. Studies show a higher rate of postoperative complications in women: in one study, postoperative stroke was seen in women patients more often ($p=0.050$), the urgency of intervention ($p=0.026$), and carotid reoperation ($p=0.024$) (15,16). Other population studies have found no difference in morbidity and mortality (17,18). Cited causes for the higher complication rate in women have been old age of patient at presentation, presence of hypertension, and surgical issues regarding the smaller size of carotid arteries in women (14).

Stroke Risk Factors Specific to Women

Some specific differences have been found between men and women that may predispose them to stroke (Table 17.2). One study found that women with stroke had an elevated tissue plasminogen activator antigen, which was an independent risk factor for stroke in nondiabetic women aged 15 to 44 years old. It was suggested that impaired endogenous fibrinolysis might be a risk factor for stroke in women (19). This does not seem to be a modifiable risk factor.

Another study showed that a significant proportion of young women (13% of studied) have elevated total homocysteine serum levels, an independent risk factor for stroke and vascular disease. Increased serum homocys-

TABLE 17.2
Work-up for Uncommon Causes of Stroke in Selected Patients

Arterial Stroke
- MRI with MR angiogram evaluating Circle of Willis
- CT with either TCD, CT angiography, or conventional angiogram
- Carotid and transesophageal echocardiography
- Anti-thrombin III
- Antiphospholipid antibodies IgG/IgM
- Lupus anticoagulant
- Fasting homocysteine level
- Toxicology screen

Venous stroke
- MRI with MR venogram or CT with conventional angiography
- Protein C, Protein S
- Factor V Leiden, antithrombin III
- Phospholipid antibodies IgG/IgM
- Lupus anticoagulant
- Prothrombin gene mutation
- Can cause arterial stroke if right to left shunt present

Primary CNS hemorrhage
- MRI with contrast and MR venogram and arteriogram
- CT with contrast
- Conventional angiography

teine levels were correlated with increasing age, higher serum cholesterol levels, alcohol intake (more than 7 drinks a week), and cigarette smoking. Serum homocysteine levels were decreased in women who took daily multivitamins with vitamin B6, B12, and folate (20).

The drug phenylpropanolamine, commonly found in cough remedies and appetite suppressants, was associated with hemorrhagic strokes in women, but not in men. Most affected women were between the ages of 17 to 45 years. The FDA has also received reports of 22 cases of spontaneous intracranial hemorrhage in association with phenylpropanolamine. Most cases (16 patients) occurred when the drug was used as an appetite suppressant. In the study, no men had used phenypropanolamine as an appetite suppressant, and there was no association between men and cold remedy use of the drug and stroke. These women were also more likely to be African-American, to smoke, and to have recently used cocaine. Phenylpropanolamine appetite suppressants should thus be avoided in women (21).

For stroke and heart disease, the recognized risk factors of smoking, elevated cholesterol, a previous stroke, and large artery atherosclerotic disease hold true for both men and women. Workup for new strokes should be similar in both sexes and in the elderly. Hypertension and elevated cholesterol become more common in women as they age. Typically, cholesterol levels will increase after the age of 45, presumably due to the onset of menopause. Women should have routine checks of blood pressure and cholesterol after they become menopausal, even if previously normotensive with normal cholesterol levels (22). Strategies for lowering cholesterol with statin medications are similar for men and women.

AUTOIMMUNE AND COLLAGEN VASCULAR DISEASE

Autoimmune disorders and collagen vascular diseases are more common in women than in men; therefore, cerebrovascular diseases from these causes are also more common. The three major causes of stroke in women from collagen vascular diseases are from systemic lupus erythematosus (SLE), the antiphospholipid antibody (APLA) syndrome, and from large-, medium-, and small-vessel vasculitis.

Systemic Lupus Erythematosus

Systemic lupus erythematosus can cause neurologic disorders including psychosis, chorea, neuropathies, and stroke. SLE is found in a ratio of men to women of 1:7; it predisposes to stroke and therefore is a significant risk factor for stroke in women (23). Data regarding SLE and stroke are difficult to interpret because SLE is a systemic autoimmune disorder and may be associated with antiphospholipid antibodies, which cause a hypercoagulable state and lead to both venous and arterial disease. The presence of antiphospholipid antibodies with SLE is referred to as a secondary antiphospholipid antibody syndrome. In one study of patients with SLE, stroke occurred at an average age of 35 years, with the diagnosis of SLE being made on average 4.4 years previously; 86% of SLE patients had active SLE at the time of their stroke. Headache was common at onset (24). The presumed mechanisms of stroke were coagulopathy, cardiogenic embolism, large cerebral vessel vasculitis, occlusive vasculopathy, cervical arterial dissection, and premature atherosclerosis. On evaluation of the patients, findings included major intracranial or extracranial vessel occlusive processes from thrombus, dissection, fibromuscular dysplasia or vasculitis, and atherosclerosis (24). A vasculopathy is associated with SLE, but it is debatable whether an actual small- and medium-vessel vasculitis is associated with SLE, because autopsy studies have not found evidence of true vasculitis. Echocardiography studies show that a significant number of patients with SLE have Libman-Sacks endocarditis, which has the potential to generate emboli to the cerebral circulation and cause stroke (25,26). The treatment of stroke associated with SLE mirrors the treatment of SLE flares. Immunosupression is often required, and anticoagulation is recommended for occlusive events associated with antiphospholipid antibodies (as discussed in Chapter 22).

Antiphospholipid Antibody Syndrome

Antiphospholipid antibody represents a group of autoantibodies that present with thrombo-occlusions and include both anticardiolipin antibodies and the lupus anticoagulant. The syndrome of antiphospholipid antibody (APLA) syndrome occurs when the antibodies are found in the absence of SLE. Presence of these antibodies is an independent risk factor for stroke in young women (28) and is associated with early fetal loss. In one series of 93 patients with vascular occlusions and APLA syndrome, there occurred occlusions (59%), arterial occlusion (28%), and both arterial and venous occlusions (13%) (27). The Stroke Prevention in Women study is a population-based case-control study in which anticardiolipin antibody was found in 26.9% patients with stroke and in 18.2% of nonstroke controls. The lupus anticoagulant was found in 20.9% of stroke patients and in 12.8% of controls. The presence of either anticardiolipin antibody or lupus anticoagulant was found in 42% of patients with strokes and in only 27.9% of controls. Thus, the presence of either antibody leads to a relative odds ratio of stroke of 1.87 (1.25-2.83, p=0.0027) (28).

The APLA syndrome may present with strokes, death, cerebral vein thrombosis, or retinal occlusive syndromes. Diagnosis is made by finding elevations of activated partial thromboplastin time (aPTT). Confirmation can be made by finding prolongation of the dilute Russell viper venom time (dRVVT) (29). The presence of mildly elevated anticardiolipin antibodies, especially IgM, does not appear be associated with stroke, but elevations of IgG, especially in range above 40 GPL, is associated with stroke recurrence and death (30).

The treatment of APLA syndrome in patients with prior stroke involves long-term anticoagulation with an INR of 2.0 to 3.0. Low-dose aspirin is probably not helpful, and warfarin has been shown to be more effective than aspirin alone (29,30). Low molecular weight heparin or unfractionated subcutaneous heparin is used in pregnant women because warfarin is teratogenic (29,30).

Vasculitis

Takayasu's arteritis was originally described in young and middle-aged women. It is a large-vessel vasculitis affecting the aortic arch and the major branches. The majority of symptoms arise from the stenosis or occlusion of these great vessels. It causes stroke secondary to the malignant hypertension from arterial stenosis and stenosis of the major arterial blood supply to the brain. It presents with fever, malaise, anemia, and loss of peripheral pulses. Treatment includes immunosuppression and surgical and nonsurgical treatment of large artery stenosis (31).

Polyarteritis nodosa (PAN) is a medium- and small-vessel vasculitis that affects arteries. PAN patients presents with fever, malaise, and weight loss. The skin lesions may help to differentiate it from other vasculitides; lesions are erythematous, purpuric, and nodular (32). Renal involvement occurs in over 70% of patients. As with Takayasu's arteritis, the long-term morbidity is due to hypertension affecting the heart and cerebral vessels. Stroke usually occurs later in the course of disease. Frequent presentations of PAN include encephalopathy, multifocal strokes of the brain and spinal cord, and subarachnoid hemorrhage. It is treated by immunosupression with steroid and cyclophosphamide (Cytoxan®) (32–34).

Isolated angiitis of the CNS is a small-vessel vasculitis restricted to the brain, with few systemic symptoms or laboratory findings. It occurs in the fourth to sixth decades, more commonly in women. Strokes or subarachnoid hemorrhage are often the only symptom (32). Patricia Moore and colleagues set forth the following diagnostic criteria for the disorder: (i) patients must have clinical features consistent with recurrent, multifocal, or diffuse disease; (ii) a systemic inflammatory process or infection must be excluded; (iii) neuroradiographic studies, usually a cerebral angiogram, must indicate a vasculopathy; and (iv) brain biopsy is required to establish the presence of vascular inflammation and exclude infection, neoplasia, or alternate causes of vasculopathy (32,35). Mortality from angiitis of the CNS either may be due to strokes or hemorrhage over a short period of time, or occasionally the disorder can smolder for years. Therapy for isolated angiitis of the CNS is a combination of cyclophosphamide with a low dose of prednisone. Remission and cure have been reported (32).

Fibromuscular Dysplasia

Fibromuscular dysplasia (FMD) of the carotid or the intracranial arteries is a disorder of the arterial wall presenting with constricting bands of fibrous material alternating with smooth muscle (36); this results in alternating constriction and dilatation of the artery. A rare disorder, it is found in 0.6% of nonselective angiograms (37). It is most prevalent among middle-aged women. In one study where 70 patients were diagnosed with cerebrovascular FMD, 89% of the patients were women with a mean age of 64; 91% of these patients presented with transient ischemic attacks (TIAs), stroke, or pulsatile tinnitus (36). It is not thought to be an inflammatory disorder. Patients with FMD are at a higher rate of spontaneous carotid artery dissection. The etiology of the small strokes and TIAs is generally unknown.

Treatment of FMD depends on the symptoms. Asymptomatic FMD is often treated with aspirin only. Carotid endarterectomy alone does not effectively treat the disease, because the vascular disorder is not isolated to the extracranial carotid. Intra-arterial angioplasty and stenting have been performed successfully. The most important issue is that patients with intracranial FMD need screening for aneurysms that may bleed magnetic resonance angiography or computed tomography (CT) angiography for aneurysms that may bleed (36).

Moya-Moya

Moya-moya is Japanese for "puff of smoke." It is less of a disorder per se, than the normal response to large-vessel cerebral occlusions (Figure 17.2). The syndrome classically presents with unilateral or bilateral intracranial carotid stenosis or occlusions. Collateral vessels form to compensate for lost blood flow and form a myriad of small collateral vessels that are small and tangled in appearance and look like a "puff of smoke" on angiography (37).

Moya-moya is 50 times more likely to occur in women than men and is found more commonly in women who smoke and use oral contraceptives (38,39). It can present with headaches, seizures, and intracerebral hemorrhage as well as stroke. Angiography, which demonstrates the small perforating collaterals, is needed for diagnosis. The presumed etiology for the hemorrhage is the aneurysmal thinning of blood vessels and disease of the very small end vessels from atherosclerotic disease (37).

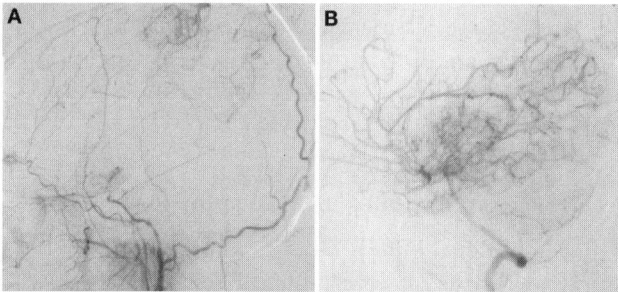

FIGURE 17.2

Cerebral angiograms. Lateral intracranial view of the left common carotid injection (A) shows occlusion of the distal intercranial carotid artery with a tuft of enlarged collaterals distal to the occulation. Lateral intercranial view after vertebral artery injection (B) shows extensive collateral vessels resembling 'puff of smoke' arising from the basilar artery and the posterior cerebral arteries. (Reproduced with permission from Wityk RJ, Hillis A, Beauchamp N, Barker PB, Rigamonti D. Perfusion-weighted magnetic resonance imaging in adult moya-moya syndrome: characteristic patterns and change after surgical intervention: case report. *Neurosurgery* 2002;51:1499–1506.)

Treatment is difficult because strokes are more common in children, but hemorrhage is more likely in adults. Aspirin or warfarin are thought to worsen the risk of hemorrhage. Abnormal cerebral blood perfusion has been demonstrated using SPECT or magnetic resonance imaging (MRI) perfusion and may account for the bland infarcts associated with the disease. Pial synangiosis or encephalomyosynangiosis surgery can be performed and has been shown to improve cerebral blood perfusion as measured by MRI (40) and may improve neurologic function in a very small number of patients (40). No improvement is gained in long-term morbidity or mortality.

CEREBRAL VASOSPASTIC DISORDERS

Migraine is a prevalent disorder affecting about 6% of men and 15 to 18% of women. It occurs most often between the ages of 25 and 55 years (41). Stroke is a known complication of migraine and has been shown to be an independent risk factor, especially in those less than 35 years of age. In one study, 160 patients were evaluated for migrainous strokes with other causes excluded. Migraine was found to be a significant risk factor for juvenile stroke, with an odds ratio for individuals under 35 of 3.26 and for women of 2.68 (42).

Not only are patients who have migraine at risk for stroke but also women of childbearing age who have migraine with aura are at greater risk. Another study followed 86 women with migrainous strokes and found that women were more likely to have strokes if they had migraine with aura instead of migraine without aura, and if they had 12 or more migraines with aura per year. No correlation was found among oral contraceptive use, migraine, and stroke (43).

Treatment for migrainous strokes has typically included prophylaxis, because the fewer migraines with aura, the lesser the chance of a stroke. Because of the vasospastic quality to the stroke etiology, a calcium channel blocker (verapamil) is used in combination with aspirin. Smoking should be discontinued. A careful workup for stroke etiology should always be done, including screening for antiphospholipid antibody; migrainous strokes are often thought of as a diagnosis of exclusion.

Reversible segmental vasoconstriction or Call's syndrome is a poorly understood disorder. It presents with headaches, seizures, lethargy, and strokes, typically in young women with a history of migraine. The stroke workup shows multifocal areas of vasodilation and vasoconstriction in multiple vascular territories in the Circle of Willis. Diffuse brain edema, hemorrhages, and death can also occur. Repeat angiography may show spontaneous resolution of vasoconstriction. It is treated using calcium blocking agents, corticosteroids, and increased intracranial pressure management; a functional outcome is variable (44,45).

Angiitis of pregnancy is a similar disorder that tends to present with hemorrhages and strokes in the postpartum period. It tends to present more often with hemorrhages. It occurs in the absence of typical clinical findings suggestive of eclampsia or preeclampsia. It also presents initially with diffuse and severe vasoconstriction on conventional angiography. How this disorder relates in etiology to reversible segmental vasoconstriction, migraine, and eclampsia or preeclampsia is not clear. Whether these are distinct vasospastic disorders or ends of the same spectrum is unclear. Angiitis of pregnancy is treated with corticosteroids, blood pressure control, and intensive care management; it generally has a good functional outcome (45,46).

CNS HEMORRHAGE

Cerebral Venous Thrombosis

Cerebral venous thrombosis (CVT) occurs more frequently in women than in men; pregnancy and oral contraceptive use are significant risk factors for the disease. CVT is often described as the deep venous thrombosis (DVT) of the brain. An occlusion of the cerebral veins causes a back-up of pressure and bland ischemic infarcts with hemorrhagic transformation. The infarcts from venous occlusions are often in nonclassic arterial vascular distributions and provide the clue to the diagnosis. It presents typically with a constellation of symptoms: headache, papilledema, seizures, and focal neurologic deficits. In the largest published series of 160 patients, headache occurred in 82%, papilledema occurred in 55.5%, focal deficits occurred in 42%, seizures occurred in 39%, and alteration of coma occurred in 30.5% (47). CVT can also present with isolated intracranial hypertension only. Pulsatile tinnitus and multiple cranial neuropathies have also been described.

CVT is caused by trauma, tumors compressing on the sagittal sinus, dehydration, and prothrombotic states. In general, those prothrombotic states that predispose to DVT can also predisposed to CVT and include sickle cell disease, factor V Leiden, prothrombin G20210A mutation, resistance to activated protein C, APLA syndrome, oral contraceptive use, and antithrombin III deficiency (47,48). These hypercoagulable factors predispose more to venous clots than arterial clots or stenosis. Hemorrhage in CVT may be cortically based and appear as a primary CNS hemorrhage; only with workup is a sagittal or cortical vein thrombosis noted. Workup includes brain imaging with CT and MRI. Finding of the "delta sign," in which a clot within the confluence of the sinuses is seen as a bright triangle, can be difficult to see on brain CT (Figure 17.3). New techniques of venograms using CT

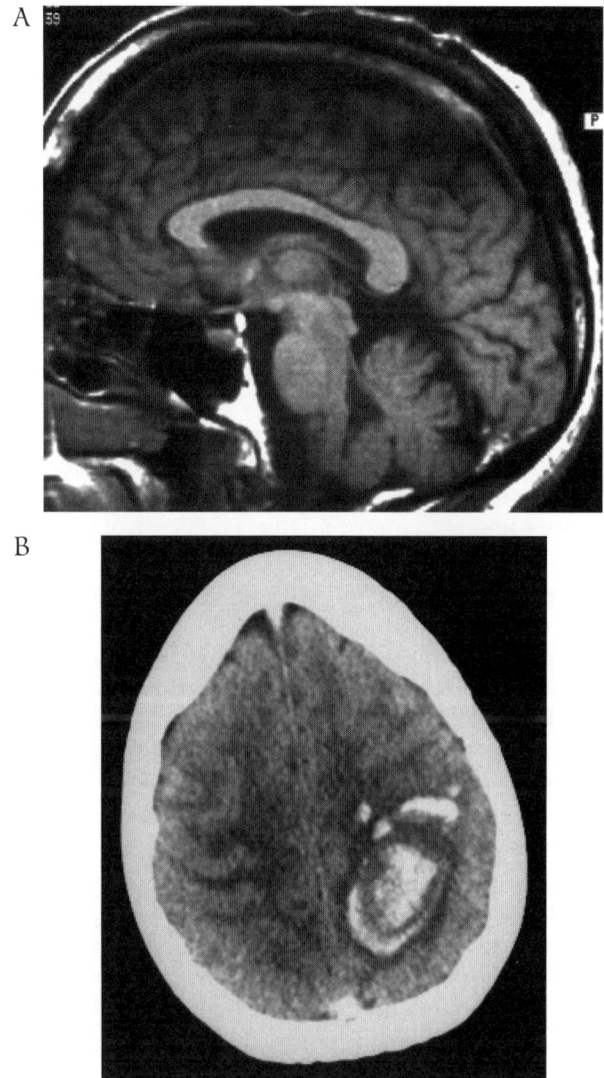

FIGURE 17.3

A. MRI with clot within the superior sagittal sinus see arrows. Blood will be bright in subaxute setting. B. CT scan with nonarterial distribution stroke. Arrow points to 'delta sign.' (Special thanks to Robert Wityk, Johns Hopkins Hospital, for providing these images.)

and MRI have made this easier to diagnose. The "gold standard" remains conventional angiography.

Treatment is with anticoagulation; therefore, diagnosis must be clear, because hemorrhage is often associated with the venous infarct. The studies showing benefit have few patients but the results are fairly robust. Heparin showed benefit in a randomized prospective trial in which 20 patients with CVT were studied. Eight patients in the heparin group recovered completely, whereas only one in the placebo group did; there were no deaths in the heparin group and three in the placebo group (49). Studies looking at low molecular weight heparin showed less robust findings. Heparin has been shown to provide an absolute risk reduction of 70% for mortality from CVT (50).

Newer techniques include rt-PA administered endovascularly and the use of vacuum catheters. Patients seem to suffer more often from new or progressive hemorrhages with endovascular thrombolytics but the occlusions resolve more quickly with endovascular techniques than with systemic anticoagulation. It is unclear at present whether patients do better with heparin alone or with endovascular treatment (47,51). Mortality is reduced with treatment, and 80% of patients were living independently after 3 years, although three out of four patients had residual symptoms including seizures, weakness, headaches, and visual field defects (52). Outcome is often poor without intervention.

Cerebral Aneurysms

Cerebral aneurysms are lesions consisting of weakening of the wall of a cerebral artery and thinning of the vessel wall. The aneurysm itself can compress local structures, but the most dangerous consequence is subarachnoid hemorrhage (SAH). The most common presentation is severe acute-onset headache, vomiting, focal neurologic findings, and meningeal signs. Cerebral aneurysms with subarachnoid hemorrhage are more common in women over 55 years of age than in age-matched men (53,54). Women are more likely to have multiple aneurysms, as shown in one study (281 women; 80 men). The proportion of patients with multiple aneurysms and subarachnoid hemorrhage was higher in women for all age categories (5.2%:15.2%). Women tended to have worse outcomes than men (54). There is no gender difference in outcome in SAH with a single aneurysm (55). Diagnosis is made based on head CT and lumbar puncture findings and confirmed with conventional angiography. Recently, MR angiography and CT angiography have become less invasive screening tests for both symptomatic and asymptomatic cerebral aneurysms. Treatment involves surgical clipping or endovascular coiling of the aneurysmal dilatation.

HORMONES AND STROKE

Oral Contraceptive Pills and Stroke

Oral contraceptive pills (OCPs) and hormonal contraception have been linked to an increased stroke risk in multiple studies (56–60). Much of this perceived increased stroke risk is based on early studies of higher dose preparations containing ≥50 mcg of estradiol (57,61,62). In normotensive, nonsmoking women, OCPs containing 35 mcg of estradiol or less do not increase the risk of stroke (63,66). The majority of studies of second- and third-generation OCPs containing these lower doses of estrogens did not find an increased risk of stroke (61,62,67–70). A pooled analysis of two large population case-control studies showed no increased risk of hemorrhagic or ischemic stroke in current users of OCPs containing less than 50 mcg of estradiol, compared with past users or "never-users" (71). One case-control study did report an increased risk of stroke using first-, second-, or third-generation OCPs, however, but the reasons for this discrepancy are unclear (72).

Among OCP users, cigarette smoking, hypertension, diabetes, migraine headache, and prior noncerebral thromboembolic events also increase the risk of stroke (64,65,67,71,73). Some data (71) suggest, however, that women with chronic hypertension can use combination OCPs containing 35 mcg of estradiol or less, provided that they are otherwise healthy nonsmokers under the age of 35, and that their blood pressure is well-controlled and monitored before beginning OCPs and for several months after starting use (74). The pooled analysis of two case-control studies found no elevation in stroke risk in OCP users who were over the age of 35, smokers, obese, or those with uncontrolled hypertension (71). The American College of Obstetricians and Gynecologists (ACOG) recommends that OCPs should be prescribed with caution, if ever, to women who are older than 35 and are smokers (74).

Migraine headaches are common in women of reproductive age. Some women with migraines experience an improvement in their headaches on OCPs but, in women on OCPs, most migraines occur during the hormone-free interval. A large case-control study found that women with a history of migraines and who were using OCPs did not have a significantly increased risk of ischemic stroke compared with women who were not using OCPs and were without migraines (75). Compared with women who did not smoke, did not use OCPs, and were without migraines, women who smoked, were using OCPs, and had a history of migraines had a 34-fold increased risk of stroke in this study. The pooled analysis of two large, U.S. population-based case-control studies also observed a statistically significant twofold increased risk of ischemic stroke among women on OCPs with migraine headaches (71). In a large Danish population-based case-control study, the risk of stroke was elevated approximately threefold among women with a history of migraines (73). Neither study categorized migraines by type, however. The additional risk of stroke attributable to OCPs for women with migraines has been estimated as 8 per 100,000 women at age 20 years, and 80 per 100,000 women at age 40 years (76). Because the absolute risk of a cerebrovascular event remains low among women of reproductive age, the use of OCPs may be considered for women with migraine headaches who do not have focal neurologic signs, do not smoke, are younger than age 35, and are otherwise healthy. OCPs should be discontinued in these women if the frequency or severity of headaches increases or focal neurologic signs or symptoms arise.

A strong association between CVT and use of oral contraceptives has been established in several case-control studies (77–79). Mutations in the prothrombin gene and the factor V Leiden gene are associated with CVT. The presence of both the prothrombin gene mutation and oral contraceptive use further increases the risk of CVT (77,78). Routine screening for the prothrombin gene mutation in young women is not currently recommended before prescribing them OCPs.

A recent meta-analysis concluded that the risk of ischemic stroke is increased in OCP users, but that the absolute increase in risk would be small due to the low stroke incidence in this young and healthy population (80). An individual's risk of stroke must be weighed against the benefits of effective contraception and the risks of unintended pregnancy. The impact of stroke in a woman of reproductive age is so devastating, though, that clinicians should consider alternative forms of contraception such as progestin-only (oral or injectable), barrier, or intrauterine contraceptives in the setting of the additional risk factors mentioned above (81). Stroke risk is not increased with the use of progestin-only OCPs or injectables, except among women with hypertension (82,83).

HORMONE REPLACEMENT THERAPY

Hormone replacement therapy (HRT) is commonly used for the treatment of vasomotor symptoms and urogenital atrophy, as well as for the prevention of osteoporosis and cardiovascular disease in women. Data on the association of postmenopausal HRT and stroke have been inconsistent. The impact of HRT on stroke risk is ill-defined due to a lack of well-designed, controlled studies; as a result, definitive conclusions cannot be reached. Since 1980, at least 18 studies have been published on this subject (84). The Framingham Heart Study found a 2.6-fold increase in the relative risk of atherothrombotic stroke among women receiving HRT versus nonusers (85). None of the other studies detected a large increase in stroke risk, and several reported a slight (but often insignificant) decrease in risk (86–92).

In the 20-year report from the Nurses' Health Study, the investigators noted for the first time an increased risk of stroke in women taking estrogen alone (35%) and in women taking combined therapy of estrogen and a progestin (93). However, the overall risk in current users for all HRT regimens was increased by only 13%. The risk of fatal stroke was decreased by 19% in women on estrogen alone, compared with an increase of 22% in those on combined HRT.

These findings conflict with those of previous observational reports. Neither estrogen alone nor combined therapy increased the risk of nonfatal stroke in a large Danish case-control study (94). In another prospective cohort, estrogen therapy was associated with a 46% overall reduction in stroke mortality, with a 79% reduction in current users (95). Finucane et al. showed a similar reduced risk for women who had used HRT compared with those who had never used HRT, with stroke incidence lower by 31% and stroke mortality by 63% (90). The Copenhagen City Heart Study, a case-control study of women aged 45 to 69 years in the United Kingdom, showed no effect of HRT on stroke incidence (86). The much-publicized Women's Health Initiative (WHI) trial revealed an excess of eight nonfatal strokes per 10,000 women per year in the combined therapy group, but, as in the Nurses' Health Study, the rate of fatal strokes was not increased (96). The limitations of this study include the older average age of enrolled patients, use of only one HRT regimen, and increased unblinding of the study patients on HRT.

The most compelling evidence for the benefit of HRT in stroke prevention are the data on mortality from stroke. As discussed above, the larger cohort studies that have assessed the impact of hormone use on stroke mortality have demonstrated a beneficial impact, with the exception of the Nurses' Health Study (89,90,95,97). These data are consistent with the possibility that hormone therapy decreases the severity of strokes and therefore the incidence of stroke-related mortality, if not stroke events. Hormone replacement therapy appears to influence stroke risk factors positively. The Copenhagen City Heart Study showed a reduced stroke risk for smokers taking HRT compared with smokers not taking HRT (86). The Lipid Research Clinics of North America revealed that HRT decreases cholesterol, decreases low-density lipoprotein, and raises high-density lipoprotein compared with women not receiving HRT after controlling for compounding risk factors (97). Therefore, HRT may be especially protective for women who smoke and/or have elevated cholesterol. Multiple case-control and cohort studies offer overwhelming evidence for at least a 40 to 50% reduction in the risk of primary coronary heart disease and myocardial infarction in estrogen users (98). The recently reported results of the randomized WHI trial would indicate the situation is otherwise, but this was not a primary prevention trial—the findings also may have been biased by the new and unreported statin and aspirin use in the placebo group after the trial started (96). The WHI data not withstanding, HRT may be particularly beneficial for reducing stroke risk in patients with preexisting occlusive vessel disease, even after adjusting for any "healthy-user" effect, although additional studies are necessary and ongoing.

For women who have already suffered a stroke, the Women's Estrogen for Stroke Trial (WEST) study was designed to evaluate estrogen and the secondary prevention of stroke. In this trial, no significant differences were found between treated and placebo groups in outcomes for fatal and nonfatal stroke, nonfatal myocardial infarctions, or coronary death (99). The risk was actually greater in the first year of estrogen exposure. The WEST group concluded that estrogen therapy was not effective for preventing a new or recurrent cerebrovascular event in stroke patients.

In 2003, the results of the Women's Health Initiative Study was published in *JAMA*. Specifically it looked at dementia and possible protective effects of estrogen plus progestin in postmenopausal women. A paper describing stroke risk in treatment and placebo groups was reviewed. The study found that of the there were significantly more strokes in the treatment group versus the placebo group. Looking at the article one finds that of 16,608 women there were 258 strokes of which almost 80% were ischemic strokes. There were 151 strokes in the treatment group and 107 strokes in the placebo group which constituted a hazard ratio for ischemic stroke (greater than 1 suggesting harm, less than one suggesting protection) of 1.44 (95% CI, 1.09–1.90) and for hemorrhagic stroke, 0.82 (95% CI, 0.43–1.56). This, despite similar background stroke risks in the women aged 50–79, there was greater risk of ischemic stroke. Admittedly the number needed to harm (the number of patients needed to put on therapy to cause one stroke) is approximately 226, still there is statistically significantly greater risk of stroke with HRT in this trial. care should be taken when HRT is considered as there is a small but significant risk of stroke (99a).

In summary, the risk of stroke associated with HRT appears low but requires further study. The existing data have methodologic limitations, including nonspecific endpoints, lack of control for prior HRT use or specific regimens, a lack of sufficient numbers of women from minority racial or ethnic groups, and possible confounding by a healthy-user effect. No healthy postmenopausal women should be denied the benefits of hormone therapy for fear of stroke alone; the other potential benefits, risks, and side effects of therapy must be considered and tailored to the individual patient.

Hormone Replacement Therapy and Subarachnoid Hemorrhage

The etiology of SAH is poorly understood. Because the incidence of SAH is highest in women after menopause (100), it has been hypothesized that estrogen might be protective for this condition (101,102). Unlike ischemic stroke, most of the epidemiologic data have shown that the risk of hemorrhagic stroke, including SAH, is not affected by either hormone replacement therapy or OCPs. A large population-based, case-control study of women with SAH showed significant independent associations between use of either HRT or OCPs and reduced risk of SAH (102). In this study, premenopausal women had a markedly reduced risk of SAH compared with postmenopausal women. The protective effect of HRT in postmenopausal women was highest in postmenopausal smokers receiving HRT compared with those not receiving HRT. The Nurses' Health Study (103) compared SAH risk in current versus former users of HRT; current users had a reduced risk compared with nonusers after adjusting for other variables. No protective effect was observed in women who had used HRT in the past.

The studies of HRT and risk of SAH have been difficult to interpret due to methodologic problems of small studies, incomplete data, differences in therapy, and potential confounding variables. A study of women in Sweden showed that SAH risk was reduced for users of combined estrogen and progestin therapy compared with those using estrogen alone (104). Additionally, there was no protective effect of former estrogen use, whereas former estrogen-progestin use may be beneficial. A recent prospective, multicenter, population-based, case-control study demonstrated that estrogen, either alone or in combination with a progestogen, reduces the risk of SAH (105). The inverse association was moderately strong for any use of HRT and risk of SAH, but only borderline when current or past use of HRT was considered separately. Data pertaining to the risk in relation to endogenous hormonal factors, such as menstrual patterns, are limited. One study (102) demonstrated that among premenopausal women with SAH, 74% were menstruating at the time of the event, suggesting that states of relative estrogen deficiency, such as menopause and the premenstrual period, may increase the risk of SAH in women.

HRT has been shown consistently to decrease the risk of fatal stroke (106,107). Stratification by fatal and nonfatal strokes may be important in clarifying the link between HRT and both ischemic and hemorrhagic stroke, because the majority of nonfatal strokes are ischemic, whereas approximately one- and two-thirds of fatal strokes are hemorrhagic, including SAH (108). The currently available data support a key role for hormonal therapy in the prevention of SAH among postmenopausal women.

STROKE AND PREGNANCY

Ischemic Stroke

Risk factors for stroke in pregnancy and the postpartum period (or puerperium) include all the established causes for any young nonpregnant stroke patient, such as vasculopathy, cardiogenic embolism, drug use, migraine, and hematologic disorders. Pregnancy and the puerperium (defined as up to 6 weeks postpartum) are states of hyper-coagulability (109) and increased risk of thromboembolism (110), one of the leading causes of maternal mortality. The theoretical increased risk of stroke in pregnancy has been largely unsubstantiated by data (111,112). A recent population-based study found an incidence of stroke during pregnancy and the puerperium of 1 in 7,500 pregnancies (112). Kittner et al. showed that the relative risk (RR) for ischemic stroke was not increased during pregnancy (RR, 0.7) but was significantly elevated in the puerperium (RR, 5.4), especially during the first postpartum days. For hemorrhagic stroke, the relative risk was 2.5 during pregnancy and 28.3 during the puerperium. The causes of ischemic strokes and hemorrhages were heterogeneous, although preeclampsia-eclampsia was present in 24% of cases. Other identified causes included vasculopathy, dissection, thrombotic thrombocytopenic purpura (TTP), and CVT.

Stroke during pregnancy and the puerperium has been attributed to pregnancy-related hypertensive diseases and to cesarean delivery (113). Preeclampsia affects 3 to 8% of all pregnant women (114). It is described as an endothelial disorder (115) with decreased venous distensibility and altered cerebral blood flow velocity (116,117), which may, therefore, influence the pregnancy-related incidence of stroke. Multiple pregnancy is associated with an increased risk of preeclampsia, higher circulating levels of estrogens, and a greater rise in cardiac output, all of which may affect the risk of stroke (114,118,119). (See also Chapter 16 on preeclampsia-eclampsia). Cesarean delivery is more commonly performed for women with preeclampsia-eclampsia or with multiple pregnancy; it is also associated with an increased risk of thromboembolism, increased platelet counts, and fluctuations in blood pressure due to general or regional anesthesia (120). A recent large, population-based cohort study in Sweden revealed a three- to twelvefold increased risk of stroke during late pregnancy, at delivery, and in the puerperium for women with preeclampsia, multiple gestation, and cesarean delivery (121). These conditions do not fully explain the inherent pregnancy-related risk of stroke, however, and do not account for the majority of this excess risk. The actual contribution of stroke to maternal mortality may be underestimated because proven risk factors for stroke, such as systemic embolism (including intracranial embolism) and hypertensive disease of pregnancy, are often identified as the cause of death, even when they have resulted in stroke.

Numerous other etiologies and risk factors for ischemic stroke are present during pregnancy and puerperium. Cardioembolism is extremely common in young stroke patients (122) and may be due to peripartum cardiomyopathy (123,124) or amniotic fluid embolism (125,126) during this time. Large-artery atherosclerosis is a common cause of stroke in the general population, but it is a relatively uncommon cause of stroke in women of childbearing age. Arterial dissection may lead to ischemic stroke, but no data linking pregnancy or labor with an increased risk of dissection have been found. SLE is the most frequent type of symptomatic vasculitis during pregnancy (127), and there are reported cases of stroke during pregnancy in a patient with lupus (128,129). Pregnancy may increase the risk of stroke in patients with hematologic abnormalities such as sickle cell anemia, APLA syndrome, other hypercoagulable states, and inherited thrombophilias such as antithrombin deficiency, protein C deficiency, protein S deficiency, and activated protein C (APC) resistance (112,113,130–133). TTP occurs with an increased incidence in pregnancy and may cause multiple small infarctions (134,135). Gestational thrombocytopenia, also called benign or essential thrombocytopenia of pregnancy, is the most common cause of thrombocytopenia during pregnancy, but does not increase the risk for maternal hemorrhage or bleeding complications (136).

CVT and Pregnancy

The incidence of CVT is approximately 1 in 11,000 deliveries (137). CVT usually occurs during the postpartum period, particularly during the first week (138–140). The cause of CVT has been attributed to factors such as infection, a hypercoagulable state during pregnancy, a relative dehydration during the puerperium, and the unique anatomy of cerebral venous drainage (141). The pregnant or postpartum patient with CVT tends to differ from other patients with CVT; patients with CVT associated with pregnancy tend to be younger, the disease onset is more acute, the resolution is faster, and the prognosis is better (140). The mortality rate varies between 0% (29) and 50% (142), depending on the study; recovery tends to be almost complete in those who survive.

Arteriovenous Malformation and Aneurysm in Pregnancy

The incidence of nontraumatic intracerebral hemorrhage (ICH) in pregnancy is about 1 in 10,000. Arteriovenous malformation (AVM) and preeclampsia-eclampsia are the most common causes when an etiology can be determined (112). SAH can be caused by ruptured aneurysms or the extension of ICH into the subarachnoid space, which commonly occurs with AVMs. The most frequent cause for SAH during pregnancy is ruptured aneurysm, followed by AVM (112). SAH leads to most intracranial hemorrhages during pregnancy. Although symptomatic aneurysms and AVMs during pregnancy are rare, the mortality rate ranges from 40 to 80% (143). The rate of asymptomatic aneurysmal rupture appears higher during pregnancy, especially in the second and third trimester and the puerperium, compared with the general population (143). After surgical clipping of an aneurysm, mode of delivery proceeds according to obstetrical indications (143). The mode of delivery remains controversial if the aneurysm has been managed conservatively and still has the potential to rupture; many authors recommend an operative vaginal delivery using forceps or a vacuum under epidural anesthesia to shorten the second stage of labor (143–146). The management of aneurysmal SAH in the pregnant patient is based on neurosurgical principles (143–145); in the postpartum patient, management is the same as in the nonpregnant patient. The risk of bleeding from AVMs during pregnancy is thought to be increased (143), with most cases occurring late in pregnancy and during labor and delivery (146,147). AVMs present with hemorrhage about three times more often in pregnant women compared with nonpregnant women (146,148,149). AVMs also result in a larger proportion of SAH during pregnancy—up to 50%—(146,148) compared with about 10% in nonpregnant women and 6% in the general population. The reason for the relatively higher incidence of AVM-associated hemorrhage compared with aneurysm-associated hemorrhage in pregnancy is not known. Neurosurgical criteria are used in the decision to operate on ruptured and unruptured AVMs (141,143), and the optimal mode of delivery in patients with unoperated AVMs is unclear. Women with successfully corrected AVMs are delivered according to obstetrical indications (143).

Management of Stroke in Pregnant Women

In the acute stoke, the use of thrombolytic agents including rt-PA, streptokinase, and urokinase may be used if the mother's condition warrants therapy (144). None of these therapies represents a major risk to the fetus or newborn and may be used safely during pregnancy and lactation (145). Anticoagulants such as aspirin, ticlopidine, heparin, and warfarin are the standard treatments for acute stroke. Low-dose aspirin (less than 150 mg daily) can be used for primary and secondary stroke prevention during pregnancy; it selectively inhibits maternal cyclooxygenase without impairing fetal coagulation (146,147). There is considerable clinical experience with heparin use in pregnancy because it does not cross the placenta and is not excreted in human milk (148). The major concerns with heparin use during pregnancy include maternal heparin-induced osteoporosis and thrombocytopenia. The reversibility of this osteoporosis has not been clearly established, nor does there appear to be a clear dose–response relationship (149). The postpartum evaluation of bone density may have prognostic and therapeutic implications for osteoporosis (151,152). The most common type of heparin-induced thrombocytopenia (HIT) is benign and reversible, occurring within the first few days of therapy, resolving spontaneously, and

not requiring the cessation of heparin therapy. The less common but more severe type is the immune form of HIT, which occurs within 5 to 14 days of full-dose heparin therapy in as many as 3% of patients (9) and may cause widespread thrombosis (153,154). Low molecular weight heparin (LMWH) reduces three of the complications caused by unfractionated heparin: bleeding, osteoporosis, and thrombocytopenia (152,154,155). LMWH does not cross the placenta in pregnancy or appear significantly in breast milk. Additionally, LMWH has improved bioavailability, and dosing may be limited to once or twice daily (156–159). Both standard heparin and LMWH may be discontinued at the onset of labor and resumed after delivery due to their short half-lives. Warfarin crosses the placenta and has been linked to spontaneous abortion, fetal hemorrhage, fetal anomalies and abnormalities, and increased fetal mortality (160–162). Therefore, its use is relatively contraindicated in pregnancy or nursing mothers, because it is also excreted in breast milk (163). It is unknown whether ticlopidine results in maternal, fetal, or neonatal toxicity in humans; use of this agent would require consideration of the relative risks of the drug versus the risk of recurrent stroke.

Limited data exist on the influence of pregnancy on recurrent stroke, making it difficult to counsel women with a history of ischemic stroke on stroke risk in future pregnancies (164,165). A recent large, multicenter series found that young women with a history of ischemic stroke have a low recurrence during subsequent pregnancies (166). The postpartum period, not the pregnancy itself, was associated with an increased relative risk of stroke recurrence, as described above. This suggests a causal role for the large decrease in blood volume or the rapid changes in hormonal status during the puerperium, possibly due to hemodynamic, coagulative, or vessel wall changes (112,166). The outcome of pregnancies in these women was similar to that of the general population and, therefore, a previous ischemic stroke should not be a contraindication to a subsequent pregnancy (166). No data or guidelines are available for the obstetrical management of labor and delivery in women with a history of ischemic stroke.

References

1. American Heart Association. *Stroke statistics*. Dallas: American Heart Association; 2000. Available at: http://www.americanheart.org. Accessed January 2003.
2. Ayala C, Croft J, Greenlund K, et al. Differences in U.S. mortality rates for stroke and stroke subtypes by race/ethnicity and age, 1995–1998. *Stroke* 2002;33: 1197.
3. Holroyd-Leduc JM, Kapral MK, Austin PC, et al. Sex differences and similarities in the management and outcome of stroke patients. *Stroke* 2000;31:1833–1837.

3a. Ridker PM, Cook NR, Lee I, et al. Randomized trial of low-dose aspirin in the primary prevention of cardiovascular disease in women. *N Engl J of Med*, 2005.

4. Barker WH, Mullooly JP. Stroke in a defined elderly population, 1967–1985: a less lethal and disabling but no less common disease. *Stroke* 1997;28: 284–290.

5. Menon SC, Pandey DK, Morgenstern LB. Critical factors determining access to acute stroke care. *Neurology* 1998;51:427–432.

6. Labiche LA, Chan W, Saldin KR, Morgenstern LB. Sex and acute stroke presentation. *Ann Emerg Med* 2002; 40:453–460.

7. Katzan IL, Furlan AJ, et al. Use of tissue-type plasminogen activator for acute ischemic stroke: the Cleveland area experience. *JAMA* 2000;283:1151–1158.

8. Ayanian JZ, Epstein AM. Differences in the use of procedures between women and men for coronary heart disease. *N Engl J Med* 1991;325:221–225.

9. Jaglal SB, Goel V, Naylor CD. Sex differences in the use of invasive coronary procedures in Ontario. *Can J Cardio* 1994;10:239–244.

10. Sivenius J, Laakso M, Penttila IM, et al. The European Stroke Prevention Study: results according to sex. *Neurology* 1991;41:1189–1192.

11. Gent M, Blakely JA, Easton JD, et al. The Canadian American Ticlopidine Study (CATS) in thromboembolic stroke. *Lancet* 1989;1:1215–1220.

12. CAPRIE Steering Committee. *Lancet* 1996;348: 1329–1339.

13. Wolf PA, Abbott RD, Kannel WB. Atrial fibrillation as an independent risk factor for stroke: the Framingham Study. *Stroke* 1991;22:983–988.

14. Norman P.E, Semmens JB, Lawrence-Brown M, et al. The influence of gender on outcome following vascular surgery: a review. *Cardiovasc Surg* 2000;8:111–115.

15. Hertzer NR, O'Hara PJ, Mascha EJ, et al. Early outcome assessment for 2228 consecutive carotid endarterectomy procedures: the Cleveland Clinic experience from 1989 to 1995. *J Vasc Surg* 1997;26:1–10.

16. Schneider J, Drose J, Golan I. Carotid endarterectomy in women versus men; patient characteristics and outcomes. *J Vasc Surg* 1997;25:890–899.

17. Maxwell J, Rutledge R, Covingto D, et al. A statewide hospital-based analysis of frequency and outcomes in carotid endarterectomy. *Am J Surg* 1997;174: 655–661.

18. Ozsvath K, Darling RC, Tabatabi L, et al. Carotid endartectomy in the elderly: does gender effect outcome? *Cardiovasc Surg* 2002;10:534–537.

19. Macko R, Kittner S, Epstein A, et al. Elevated tissue plasminogen activator antigen and stroke risk. The Stroke Prevention in Young Study. *Stroke* 1999;30:7–11.

20. Giles W, Kittner S, Croft J, et al. Distribution and correlates of elevated total homocyst(e)ine: the stroke in young prevention in Young Women Study. *Ann Epidemiol* 1999;9:307–313.

21. Kernan W, Viscoli C, Brass L, et al. Phenylpropanolamine and the risk of hemorrhagic stroke. *N Engl J Med* 2000;343:1826–1832.

22. O'Brien T, Nguyen TT. Lipids and lipoproteins in women. *Mayo Clin Pro* 1997;72:235–244.

23. Voulgari PV, Katsimbri P, Alamanos Y, Drosos AA. Gender and age differences in systemic lupus erythematosus. A study of 489 Greek patients with a review of the literature. *Lupus* 2002;11:722–729.

24. Mitsias P, Levine SR. Large cerebral vessel occlusive disease in systemic lupus erythematosus. *Neurology* 1994;44:385–393

25. Devinsky O, Petito C, Alonso D, et al. Clinical and neuropathological findings in systemic lupus erythematosus: the role of vasculitis, heart emboli, and thrombotic thrombocytopenic purpura. *Ann Neurol* 1988;23: 380–384.

26. Galve E, Candell-Riera J, Pigrau C, et al. Prevalence, morphologic types, and evaluation of cardiac valvular disease in systemic lupus erythematosus. *N Engl J Med* 1988;319:817–823.

27. Provenzale JM, Orel TL, Allen NB. Systemic thrombosis in patients with anti-phospholipid antibodies: lesion distribution and imaging findings. *Am J Roentgenol* 1998;170:285–290.

28. Brey R, Stallworth C, McGlasson D, et al. Antiphospholipid antibodies and stroke in young women. *Stroke* 2002;33:2396–2401.

29. Rand J. The antiphospholipid syndrome. *Annu Rev Med* 2003:54:409–424.

30. Levine S, Salowich-Palm L, Sawaya K, et al. IgG anticardiolipin antibody titer >40 GPL and the risk of subsequent thrombo-occlusive events and death. A prospective cohort study. *Stroke* 1997;28;1660–1665.

31. Caplan LR (ed.) *Caplan's stroke*. 3rd ed. Boston: Butterworth-Heinenmann, 2000;315–317.

32. Moore PM, Richardson B. Neurology of the vasculitides and connective tissue diseases. *J Neurol Neurosurg Psychiatry* 1998;65:10–22.

33. Ford RG, Siekert RG. Central nervous system manifestation of periarteritis nodosa. *Neurology* 1965;15:114–122.

34. Moore PM, Fauci AS. Neurologic manifestations of systemic vasculitis. A retrospective study of the clinicopathologic features and response to therapy in 25 patients. *Am J Med* 1981;71:517–524.

35. Alhalabi M, Moore PM. Serial angiography in isolated angiitis of the central nervous system. *Neurology* 1994;44:1221–1226.

36. Chiche L, Bahnini A, Koskas F, et al. Occlusive fibromuscular disease of arteries supplying the brain: results of surgical treatment. *Ann Vasc Surg* 1997;5:496–504.

37. Caplan LR (ed.) *Caplan's Stroke*. 3rd ed. Boston: Butterworth-Heinenmann, 2000;324–325.

38. Ueki K, Meyer FB, Mellinger JF. Moya-moya disease: the disorder and surgical treatment. *Mayo Clin Proc* 1994:69:749–757.

39. Bruno A, Adams HOP, Bilbe J, et al. Cerebral infarction due to moya-moya disease in young adults. *Stroke* 1988;19:826–833.

40. Wityk RJ, Hillis A, Beauchamp N, et al. Perfusion-weighted magnetic resonance imaging in adult moya-moya syndrome: characteristic patterns and change after surgical intervention: case report. *Neurosurgery* 2002;51:1499–1505.

41. Lipton RB, Stewart WF. Prevalence and impact of migraine. *Neurol Clin* 1997;15(1):1–13.

42. Schwaag S, Nabavi DG, Frese A, et al. The association between migraine and juvenile stroke: a case-control study. *Headache* 2003;43:90–95.

43. Donaghy M, Chang CL, Poulter N. Duration, frequency, recency, and type of migraine and the risk of ischaemic stroke in women of childbearing age. *J Neurol Neurosurg Psychiatry* 2002;73:747–750.

44. Call GK, Fleming MC, Sealfon S. Reversible cerebral segmental vasoconstriction. *Stroke* 1988;19:1159–1170.

45. Caplan LR (ed.) *Caplan's Stroke*. 3rd ed. Boston: Butterworth-Heinenmann, 2000;322–324.

46. Geocadin RG, Razumovsky AY, Wityk RJ, Bhardwaj A, Ulatowski JA. Intracerebral hemorrhage and postpartum cerebral vasculopathy. *Neurol Sci* 2002;205:29–34.

47. Biousse V, Bousser MG. Cerebral venous thrombosis. *Neurologist* 1999;5:326–349.

48. Vidailhet M, Piette JC, Puzio K, et al. Cerebral venous thrombosis in systemic lupus erythematosus. *Stroke* 1990;21:1226–1231.

49. Einhaupl Km, Villringer A, Meister W, et al. Heparin treatment in sinus venous thrombosis. *Lancet* 1991;338: 597–600.

50. De Bruijin SFTM, Stam J, et al. Randomized placebo controlled trial of anticoagulate treatment with low molecular weight heparin for cerebral sinus thrombosis. *Stroke* 1999;30:484–488.

51. Bousser MG. Cerebral venous thrombosis. Nothing, heparin or local thrombolysis? *Stroke* 1999;30:481–483.

52. Breteau G, Mounier-Vehier F, Godefroy O, et al. Cerebral venous thrombosis 3-year clinical outcome in 55 consecutive patients. *J Neurol* 2003;250:29–35.

53. Australasian Cooperative Research on Subarachnoid Hemorrhage Study (ACROSS). Epidemiology of aneurysmal subarachnoid hemorrhage in Australia and New Zealand. *Stroke* 2000;31:1843.

54. Kaminogo M, Yonekura M, Shibata S. Incidence and outcome of multiple intracranial aneurysms in a defined population. *Stroke* 2003;34:16–21.

55. Kongable GL, Lanzino G, Germanson TP. Gender-related differences in aneurysmal subarachnoid hemorrhage. *J Neurosurg* 1996;84:43–48.

56. Masi AT, Dugdale M. Cerebrovascular diseases associated with the use of oral contraceptives. *Ann Intern Med* 1970;72:111–112.

57. Collaborative Group for the Study of Stroke in Young Women. Oral contraceptives and stroke in young women. *JAMA* 1975;231:718–722.

58. Jick H, Porter J, Rothman KJ. Oral contraceptives and non-fatal stroke in healthy young women. *Ann Intern Med* 1978;88:58–60.

59. Stolley PD, Strom BL, Sartwell PK. Oral contraceptives and vascular disease. *Epidemiol Rev* 1989;11:241–243.

60. Stadel BV. Oral contraceptives and cardiovascular disease. *N Engl J Med* 1981;288:871–877.

61. Hannaford PC, Croft PR, Kay CR. Oral contraception and stroke: evidence from the Royal College of General Practitioners' Oral Contraception Study. *Stroke* 1994; 25:935–942.

62. Lindegaard O. Oral conception and risk of a cerebral thromboembolic attack: results of a case-control study. *BMJ* 1993;306:956–963.

63. Burkman RT, Collins JA, Schulman LP, Williams JK. Current perspectives on oral contraceptive use. *Amer J Obstet Gynecol* 2001;185(suppl 2):S4–S12.

64. Burkman RT. Oral contraceptives: current status. *Clin Obstet Gynecol* 2001;44:62–72.

65. Pymar HC, Creinin MD. The risks of oral contraceptive pills. *Semin Repro Med* 2001;19:305–312.

66. World Health Organization. Cardiovascular disease and steroid hormone contraception: report of a WHO Scientific Group. *WHO Technical Report Series* 1998; 877:1–89.

67. World Health Organization. Ischaemic stroke and combined oral contraceptives: results of an international multicentre case-control study: WHO Collaborative Studies of Cardiovascular Disease and Steroid Hormone Contraception. *Lancet* 1996;348:498–505.

68. Schwartz, SM, Siscovick DS, Longstreth WT Jr, et al. Use of low-dose oral contraceptives and stroke in young women. *Ann Intern Med* 1997;127:596–603.

69. Petitti DB, Sidney S, Bernstein A, et al. Stroke in users of low-dose oral contraception. *N Engl J Med* 1996; 335:8–15.

70. Kemmerman J, Tanis B, Van Den Booch MA, et al. Risk of arterial thrombosis in relation to oral contraceptives (RATIO) study: oral contraceptives and the risk of stroke. *Stroke* 2002;33:1202–1208.

71. Schwartz, SM, Petitti DB, Siscovick DS, et al. Stroke and use of low-dose oral contraceptives in young women: a pooled analysis of two U.S. studies. *Stroke* 1998;29: 2277–2284.

72. Heinmann LA, Lewis MA, Thorogood M, et al. Case-control study of oral contraceptives and risk of thromboembolic stroke: results from international study on oral contraceptives and health of young women. *BMJ* 1997;315:1502–1504.

73. Lindegaard O. Oral contraceptives, pregnancy and use of cerebrothromboembolism: the influence of diabetes, hypertension, migraine and previous thrombotic disease. *Br J Obstet Gynecol* 1995;102:153–159.

74. American College of Obstetricians and Gynecologists. The use of hormonal contraception in women with coexisting medical conditions. *ACOG Practice Bulletin No. 18* 2000;18:1–13.

75. Chang CL, Donaghy M, Poulter N. Migraine and stroke in young women: case control study. WHO collaborative study of cardiovascular disease and steroid hormone contraception. *BMJ* 1999;318:13–18.

76. MacGregor EA, Guillebaud J. Combined oral contraceptives, migraine and ischaemic stroke. Clinical and scientific committee of the faculty of family planning and reproductive healthcare and the family planning association. *Br J Fam Plann* 1998;24:53–60.

77. Bruijn de SFTM, Stan J, Koopman MMW, Vandenbroncke JP. Case control study of risk of cerebral sinus thrombosis in oral contraceptive users who are carriers of hereditary prothrombotic conditions. *BJM* 1998; 316:589–593.

78. Martinelli I, Sacchi E, Landi G, et al. High risk of cerebral-vein thrombosis in carriers of a prothrombin-gene mutation and users of oral contraceptives. *N Engl J Med* 1998;338:1793–1797.

79. Martinelli I, Taioli E, Palli D, Mannucci PM. Risk of cerebral vein thrombosis and oral contraceptives. *Lancet* 1998;352:326.

80. Gillum LA, Mauridipudi SK, Johnston SC. Ischemic stroke risk with oral contraceptives: a meta-analysis. *JAMA* 2000;284:72–78.

81. Goldstein LB, Adams R, Becker K, et al. Primary prevention of ischemic stroke: a statement for healthcare professionals from the Stroke Council of the American Heart Association. *Circulation* 2001;103: 163–182.

82. Kaunitz AM. Injectable contraception: new and existing options. *Obstet Gynecol Clin North Am* 2000;27: 741–780.

83. World Health Organization Collaborative Study of Cardiovascular Disease and Steroid Hormone Contraception. Cardiovascular disease and use of oral and injectable progestogen-only contraceptives and combined injectable contraceptives: results of an interna-

tional, multicenter, case-control study. *Contraception* 1998;57:315–324.

84. Bushnell CD, Goldstein LB. Ischemic stroke: recognizing risks unique to women. *Women's Health Primary Care* 1999;2:788–804.

85. Wilson PW, Garrison RJ, Castelli WP. Postmenopausal estrogen use, cigarette smoking, and cardiovascular morbidity in women over 50: the Framingham Study. *N Engl J Med* 1985;313:1038–1043.

86. Lindenstrom E, Boysen G, Nyboe J. Lifestyle factors and risk of cerebrovascular disease in women: the City Heart Study. *Stroke* 1993;24:1468–1472.

87. Boysen G, Nyboe J, Appleyard M, et al. Stroke incidence and risk factors for stroke in Copenhagen, Denmark. *Stroke* 1988;19:1345–1353.

88. Lafferty FW, Fiske ME. Postmenopausal estrogen replacement: a long-term cohort study. *Am J Med* 1994; 97:66–77.

89. Grodstein F, Stamfer MJ, Colditz GA, et al. Postmenopausal hormone therapy and mortality. *N Engl J Med* 1997;336:1769–1775.

90. Finucane FF, Madans JH, Bush TL, et al. Decreased risk of stroke among postmenopausal hormone users. *Arch Intern Med* 1993;153:73–79.

91. Falkeborn M, Persson I, Terent A, et al. Hormone replacement therapy and the risk of stroke: follow-up of a population-based cohort in Sweden. *Arch Intern Med* 1993;153:1201–1209.

92. Petitti DB, Sidney S, Quesenberry CP Jr, et al. Ischemic stroke and use of estrogen and estrogen/progestogen as hormone replacement therapy. *Stroke* 1998;29:23–28.

93. Grodstein F, Manson JE, Colditz GA, et al. A prospective, observational study of postmenopausal hormone therapy and primary prevention of cardiovascular disease. *Ann Intern Med* 2000;133:933–941.

94. Pederson AT, Lindegaard O, Kriener S, et al. Hormone replacement therapy and risk of non-fatal stroke. *Lancet* 1997;350:1277–1283.

95. Paganini-Hill A, Ross PK, Henderson BE. Postmenopausal oestrogen treatment and stroke: a prospective study. *BMJ* 1988;297:519–522.

96. Writing Group for the Women's Health Initiative Investigators. Risks and benefits of estrogen plus progestin in healthy postmenopausal women. Principal results from the Women's Health Initiative randomized controlled trial. *JAMA* 2002;288:321–333.

97. Bush T, Barrett-Conner E, Cowan L, et al. Cardiovascular mortality and noncontraceptive use of estrogen in women: results from the Lipid Research Clinic Program Follow-up Study. *Circulation* 1987;75:1102–1109.

98. Speroff L, Glass RH, Kase NG. In: *Clinical gynecologic endocrinology and infertility.* 6th ed. Baltimore: Lippincott Williams & Wilkins,1999;673.

99. Viscoli CM, Brass LM, Kernan WN, et al. A clinical trial of estrogen-replacement therapy after ischemic stroke. *N Engl J Med* 2001;345:1243–1249.

99a. Wassertheil-Smoller S, Hendrix S, Limacher M, et al. Effect of estrogen plus progestin on stroke in postmenopausal women: the Women's Health Initiative. *JAMA.* 2003;289:2673–2684.

100. Linn FHH, Rinkel GJE, Algra A, van Gijn J. Incidence of subarachnoid hemorrhage: role of region, year, and rate of computed tomography: a meta-analysis. *Stroke* 1996;27:625–629.

101. Stober T, Sen S, Anstatt T, Freier G, Schimrigk K. Direct evidence of hypertension and the possible role of postmenopausal estrogen deficiency in the pathogenesis of berry aneurysms. *J Neurol* 1985;232:67–72.

102. Longstreth WT Jr, Nelson LM, Koepsell TD, van Belle G. Subarachnoid hemorrhage and hormonal factors: a population-based case-control study. *Ann Intern Med* 1994;121:168–173.

103. Stamfer M, Colditz G, Willett W, et al. Postmenopausal estrogen therapy and cardiovascular disease. *N Engl J Med* 1991;325:756–762.

104. Falkeborn M, Persson I, Terent A, et al. Hormone replacement therapy and the risk of stroke: follow-up of a population-based cohort in Sweden. *Arch Intern Med* 1993;153:1201–1209.

105. Mhurchu CN, Anderson C, Jamrozik K, et al. Hormonal factors and risk of aneurysmal subarachnoid hemorrhage: an international population-based, case-control study. *Stroke* 2001;32:606–611.

106. Thorogood M. Stroke and steroid hormonal contraception. *Contraception* 1998;57:157–167.

107. Grodstein F, Stamfer MJ, Manson JE, et al. Postmenopausal estrogen and progestin use and the risk of cardiovascular disease. *N Engl J Med* 1996;335: 453–461.

108. Bamford J, Sandercock P, Dennis M, et al. A prospective study of acute cerebrovascular disease in the community: the Oxfordshire Community Stroke Project-1981-1986, II: incidence, case fatality rates and overall outcome at one year of cerebral infarction, primary intracerebral and subarachnoid hemorrhage. *J Neurol Neurosurg Psych* 1990;53:16–22.

109. Cerneca F, Ricci G, Simone R, et al. Coagulation and fibrinolysis changes in normal pregnancy. Increased levels of procoagulants and reduced levels of inhibitors during pregnancy induce a hypercoagulable state, combined with areactive fibrinolysis. *Eur J Obstet Gynecol Reprod Biol* 1997;73:31–36.

110. Ros Salonen H, Lichtenstein P, Bellocco R, et al. Increased risk of circulatory diseases in late pregnancy and puerperium. *Epidemiology* 2001;12:456–460.

111. Grosset DG, Ebrahim S, Bone I, Warlow C. Stroke in pregnancy and the puerperium: what magnitude of risk? *J Neurol Neurosurg Psych* 1995;58:129–131.

112. Kittner SJ, Stern BJ, Feeser BR, et al. Pregnancy and the risk of stroke. *N Engl J Med* 1996;335:768–774.

113. Lanska D, Kryscio R. Risk factors for peripartum stroke and intracranial venous thrombosis. *Stroke* 2000;31: 1274–1282.

114. Ros Salonen H, Cnattingius S, Lipworth L. Comparison of risk factors for preeclampsia and gestational hypertension in a population-based cohort study. *Am J Epidemiol* 1998;147:1062–1070.

115. Van Wijk M, Kublickiene K, Boer K, Van Bavel E. Vascular function in preeclampsia. *Cardiovasc Res* 2000;47: 38–48.

116. Sakai K, Imazumi T, Maeda H, et al. Venous distensibility during pregnancy. Comparisons between normal pregnancy and preeclampsia. *Hypertension* 1994;24: 461–466.

117. Williams K, McLean C. Peripartum changes in maternal cerebral blood flow velocity in normotensive and preeclamptic patients. *Obstet Gynecol* 1993;82: 334–337.

118. Duff GB, Brown JB. Urinary oestriol excretion in twin pregnancies. *J Obstet Gyn Res* 1974;81:695–700.

119. Robson SC, Hunter S, Boys RJ, Dunlop W. Hemodynamic changes during twin pregnancies. A Doppler and

m-mode echocardiographic study. *Am J Obstet Gyn* 1989;161:1273–1278.

120. Atalla RK, Thompson JR, Oppenheimer CA, et al. Reactive thrombocytosis after cesarean section and vaginal delivery. Implications for maternal thromboembolism and its prevention. *Br J Obstet Gyn* 2000;107:411–414.

121. Ros Salonen H, Lichtenstein P, Belloco R, et al. Pulmonary embolism and stroke in relation to pregnancy: how can high-risk women be identified? *Am J Obstet Gyn* 2002;186:198–203.

122. Kittner SJ, Stern BJ, Wozniak M, et al. Cerebral infarction in young adults: the Baltimore-Washington Cooperative Young Stroke Study. *Neurology* 1998;50:890–894.

123. Ladwig P, Fischer E. Peripartum cardiomyopathy. *Aust NZJ Obstet Gynaecol* 1997;37:156–160.

124. Hodgman MT, Pessin MS, Homans DC, et al. Cerebral embolism as the initial manifestation of peripartum cardiomyopathy. *Neurology* 1982;32:668–671.

125. Martin RW. Amniotic fluid embolism. *Clin Obstet Gynecol* 1996;39:101–106.

126. Clark SL. New concepts of amniotic fluid embolism: a review. *Obstet Gynecol Surv* 1990;45:360–368.

127. Donaldson JO. Cerebrovascular disease. In: *Neurology of pregnancy*. Philadelphia: WB Saunders,1989:347.

128. Suzuki Y, Kitagawa Y, Matsuoka Y, et al. Severe cerebral and systemic necrotizing vasculitis developing during pregnancy in a case of systemic lupus erythematosus. *J Rheumatol* 1990;17:1408–1411.

129. Traboulsi EI, Mansour AM, Aswad MI, et al. Homonymous hemianopia and systemic lupus erythematosus. *J Clin Neuroophthalmol* 1985;5:63–66.

130. Lao T, Lewinsky R, Ohissoin A, Cohen H. Factor XII deficiency and pregnancy. *Obstet Gyn* 1999;78:491–493.

131. Hart R, Kanter M. Hematologic diseases and ischemic stroke: a selective review. *Stroke* 1990;19:1111–1121.

132. Conrad J, Horellon M, Van Dreden P, et al. Thrombosis and pregnancy in congenital deficiencies in AT III, protein C or protein S: study of 78 women. *Throm Haemost* 1990;63:319–320.

133. Linquist P, Daneback B, Marsal K. Thrombotic risk during pregnancy: a population study. *Obstet Gyn* 1999;94:595–599.

134. Wiebers D. Ischemic cerebrovascular complications of pregnancy. *Arch Neurol* 1985;42:1106–1113.

135. Upshaw J, Reidy T, Groshart K. Thrombotic thrombocytopenic purpura in pregnancy: response to plasma manipulations. *South Med J* 1985;78:677–680.

136. Ruggeri M, Schiavotto C, Castaman G, et al. Gestational thrombocytopenia: a prospective study. *Haematologia* 1997;82:341–342.

137. Lanska DJ, Kryscio RJ. Peripartum stroke and intracranial venous thrombosis in the National Hospital Discharge Survey. *Obstet Gynecol* 1997;89:413–418.

138. Amias AG. Cerebral vascular disease in pregnancy. *J Obstet Gynaecol Br Commonw* 1970;77:100–120, 312–315.

139. Biback SM, Franklin A, Sata WK. Puerperal hemiplegia *Am J Obstet Gynecol* 1962;83:45–53.

140. Cantu C, Barinagarvementeria F. Cerebral venous thrombosis associated with pregnancy and puerperium: review of 67 cases. *Stroke* 1993;24:1880–1884.

141. Wiebers DO. Subarachnoid hemorrhage in pregnancy. *Semin Neurol* 1988;8:226-229.

142. Carroll JD, Leak D, Lee HA. Cerebral thrombophlebitis in pregnancy and the puerperium. *QJM* 1966;35:347–368.

143. Dias MS, Sekhar LN. Intracranial hemorrhage from aneurysms and arteriovenous malformations during pregnancy and the puerperium. *Neurosurgery* 1990;27:855–866.

144. Turrentine MA, Braems G, Ramirez MM. Use of thrombolytics: the treatment of thromboembolic disease during pregnancy. *Obstet Gynecol Surv* 1995;50:534–541.

145. Briggs G, Freeman R, Yaffe R. In: *Drugs in pregnancy and lactation*, 5th ed. Baltimore: Williams and Wikins, 31–33, 979–981, 1066–1068.

146. Imperiale TF, Stollenwek-Petrulis A. A meta-analysis of low dose aspirin for the prevention of pregnancy-induced hypertensive disease. *JAMA* 1991;266:260–264.

147. CLASP Collaborative Group. Low dose aspirin in pregnancy and early childhood development: follow up of the collaborative low-dose aspirin study in pregnancy. *Br J Obstet Gynecol* 1995;102:861–868.

148. Ginsberg JS, Kowalchuk G, Hirsh J, et al. Heparin therapy during pregnancy. Risks to the fetus and mother. *Arch Intern Med* 1989;149:2233–2236.

149. Dahlman TC. Osteoporotic fractures and the recurrence of thromboembolism during pregnancy and the puerperium in 184 women undergoing thromboprophylaxis with heparin. *Am J Obstet Gynecol* 1993;168:1265–1270.

150. Barbour LA, Kick SD, Steiner JF, et al. A prospective study of heparin-induced osteoporosis in pregnancy using bone densitometry. *Am J Obstet Gynecol* 1994;170:862–869.

151. Dahlman TC, Sjöberg HE, Ringertz H. Bone mineral density during long-term prophylaxis with heparin in pregnancy. *Am J Obstet Gynecol* 1994;170:1315–1320.

152. Warkentin TE, Levine MN, Hirsh J, et al. Heparin-induced thrombocytopenia in patients treated with low-molecular-weight heparin or unfractionated heparin. *N Engl J Med* 1995;332:1330–1335.

153. Kelton JG. The clinical management of heparin-induced thrombocytopenia. *Semin Hematol* 1999;36(suppl 1):17–21.

154. Hirsh J, Warkentin TE, Raschke R, et al. Heparin and low-molecular-weight heparin: mechanism of action, pharmacokinetics, dosing considerations, monitoring, efficacy and safety. *Chest* 1998;114:489S–510S.

155. Bergqvist D. Low-molecular-weight heparins. *J Intern Med* 1996;240:63–72.

156. Forestier F, Solé Y, Aiach M, et al. Absence of transplacental fragmin (Kabi) during second and third trimesters of pregnancy. *Thromb Haemost* 1992;67:180–181.

157. Nelson-Piercy C, Letsky, deSwiet M. Low-molecular-weight heparin for obstetric thromboprophylaxis: experience of sixty-nine pregnancies in sixty-one women at risk. *Am J Obstet Gynecol* 1997;176:1062–1068.

158. Dulitzki M, Pauzner R, Langevitz P, et al. Low-molecular-weight heparin during pregnancy and delivery: preliminary experience with 41 pregnancies. *Obstet Gynecol* 1996;87:380–383.

159. Rasmussen C, Wadt B, Jacobsen B. Thromboembolic prophylaxis with low molecular weight heparin during pregnancy. *Int J Gynecol Obstet* 1994;47:121–125.

160. Chan WS, Anand S, Ginsberg JS. Anticoagulation of pregnant women with mechanical heart valves. *Arch Intern Med* 2000;160:191–196.

161. Iturbe-Alessio I, Fonseca M, Mutchinik O, et al. Risks of anticoagulant therapy in pregnant women with artificial heart valves. *N Engl J Med* 1986;315:1390–1393.

162. Born D, Martinez EE, Almeida PAM, et al. Pregnancy in patients with prosthetic heart valves: the effects of

anticoagulation on mother, fetus, and neonate. *Am Heart J* 1992;124:413–417.

163. Orme ML, Lewis PJ, deSwiet M, et al. May mothers given warfarin breast-feed their infants? *BMJ* 1987;1: 1564–1565.

164. Grosset DG, Ebrahim S, Bone S, et al. Stroke in pregnancy and puerperium: what magnitude of risk? *J Neurol Neurosurg Psych* 1995;58:129–131.

165. Leys D, Lamy C, Lucas C, et al. Arterial ischemic strokes associated with pregnancy and puerperium. *Acta Neurol Bel* 1997;97:5–16.

166. Lamy C, Hamon JB, Coste J, Mas JL. Ischemic stroke in young women: risk of recurrence during subsequent pregnancies. *Neurology* 2000;55:269–274.

18 Multiple Sclerosis

P.K. Coyle, MD and Mustafa Hamaad, DO

Multiple sclerosis (MS) is one of the major acquired disorders of the central nervous system (CNS) and a leading cause of neurologic disability in young adults (1). It is notable for its strong sex preference, and for the fact that it affects young people in their prime years. MS is more common in women than men, by a ratio of at least 2 to 1 (2,3). The disease involves ongoing CNS lesion formation, with accumulating total disease burden. It is estimated that up to 10% more brain tissue is damaged annually in untreated MS patients (4). The pathologic CNS lesions are called *plaques* and range in size from a millimeter to a centimeter or greater. They may be single or coalesce, and they tend to form close to cerebrospinal fluid (CSF) and around small veins. Plaques involve varying degree of inflammation, demyelination, remyelination, reactive gliosis, axonal loss, and oligodendrocyte and neuronal cell loss (5).

SUBTYPES

MS is probably heterogeneous. Not only does a spectrum of severity exist, but discrete clinical disease types are recognized (Table 18.1) (6). It has been postulated, although not proven, that true biologic differences underlie the various clinical subtypes of MS. The mildest end of the spectrum is subclinical or asymptomatic MS. Autopsy studies indicate that subclinical disease may account for some 20% of all cases. Among symptomatic MS patients, the majority begin with *relapsing disease*, characterized by the acute to subacute onset of neurologic deficits. These episodes are referred to as *relapses*, *attacks*, or *exacerbations*. Most relapsing MS patients have relatively complete recovery from their attacks, at least early in the disease course. Between discrete relapses, they appear clinically stable. A subgroup of relapsing patients, ultimately only 5 to 10%, have a mild (benign) disease that never leads to permanent disability. The remaining relapsing patients ultimately develop disability based on an incomplete recovery from attacks, as well as later entry into a progressive subtype.

In a minority of MS patients, a slow development of neurologic deficits occurs without acute relapses. This form of MS, referred to as *primary progressive disease*, is markedly different from the other subtypes. These patients have an older age onset of their MS, show an equal sex ratio, most often have a clinical course consistent with progressive myelopathy, and show pathologic and neuroimaging features emphasizing tissue or axon damage of the spinal cord, as opposed to contrast enhancing inflammatory lesions in brain (7).

Ultimately, 90% of relapsing MS patients enter a secondary progressive stage of slow worsening. They are then considered to have changed from relapsing to *secondary progressive MS*. Patients may stop having attacks,

TABLE 18.1
Clinical Subtypes of Multiple Sclerosis

Type	Estimated frequency	Characteristics
Subclinical	Up to 20% of all cases	Asymptomatic; diagnosis based on pathologic study
Relapsing	85% at onset and 55% overall	Acute attacks; clinically stable between attacks
Mild relapsing	5–10% of relapsing cases	Few attacks with good recovery; attacks involve optic nerve, sensation, brainstem; minimal impairment despite >20-year history of MS
Primary progressive	10% of symptomatic cases	Slow worsening; never experience acute attacks
Secondary progressive	90% (ultimately) of relapsing cases	After initial relapsing course, patients slowly worsen with or without superimposed attacks
Progressive relapsing	5%	Initial primary progressive course, with subsequent acute attack

or show less frequent attacks superimposed on slow progression. The risk of entering this secondary progressive phase appears to be time locked. It occurs later in early onset relapsing disease and sooner in late onset relapsing disease.

Finally, a few patients begin with a primary progressive course but subsequently experience one or more acute relapses. They are considered to have *progressive relapsing disease.*

In general, the progressive forms of MS are more severe than relapsing disease and associated with greater disability. The clinical subtypes of MS are important to recognize because they have distinct disease courses, prognostic profiles, and therapeutic responses. When therapeutic trials test new drug treatments for MS, they enter patients based on their clinical subtype.

PATHOGENESIS

The etiology of MS is not well understood. Genetic, environmental, and immune factors all appear to be involved in the development of MS. Up to 20% of MS patients report a family member with the disease, and familial clustering of cases can occur. The risk of MS steadily increases when there is a third-, second-, or first-degree relative with MS (8). The risk increases from 0.2% (in the general Caucasian population) to 3 to 5% (9).

Although MS is not an inherited disease, it is genetically heterogeneous, and multiple genes appear to be involved. These genes are associated with disease susceptibility, protection, and severity. Recent multiple stage all-genome screens in multiplex MS families find evidence for multiple interacting susceptibility loci (10). The strongest link thus far is with the human leukocyte antigen (HLA) DRB1*1501 haplotype DQA1* 0102-

DQB1*0602, the DR2 extended haplotype (11). Additional genes have also been implicated. One study reported that combinations of two non-HLA cytokine genes, the interleukin-1 (IL-1) receptor antagonist allele 2+ and the IL-1β allele 2-, was associated with more rapid progression and more severe disease (12). These genes may be MS severity genes, and the IL-1 receptor antagonist allele 2 has been associated with disease severity in a variety of disorders (e.g., alopecia areata, psoriasis, lichen sclerosis, and ulcerative colitis).

Other genes appear to contribute to the development of the MS phenotype. So-called Asian (Japanese, Chinese-Taiwanese, Indian) MS patients show a form of MS with predominant optic nerve and spinal cord involvement, similar to neuromyelitis optica. These patients have an increased frequency of HLA-DPB1*0501 allele (13). Certain women with presumed MS and prominent visual deficit have a pathogenic mitochondrial mutation, consistent with Leber's hereditary optic neuropathy (14–16).

Overall however, it is clear that genetics alone cannot explain MS (17). Twin studies find a higher concordance rate for monozygotic than dizygotic twins with MS, but the maximum genetic loading for monozygotic twins is no greater than 40% (8). Concordance is much higher for female monozygotic twins.

Many studies implicate environmental exposures. The number of MS cases is not uniform worldwide, and zones of high risk, medium risk, and low risk are recognized (18). In many global regions where the disease has been mapped, MS cases are unusual at the Equator but increase as one moves into the northern and southern hemispheres. Migration studies suggest that the lifetime risk of MS is determined by where one spends the first 15 years of life. Epidemics of MS are described, particularly in the Faroe Islands and Iceland, in addition to a number of geographic clusters (19). Although the criti-

---

TABLE 18.2
Infectious Agents Implicated in MS

- Herpes viruses
  - Human herpes virus type 6 (HHV-6)
  - Epstein-Barr virus (EBV)
  - Herpes simplex virus (HSV)
- Retroviruses
  - Human T cell lymphotropic virus type 1 (HTLV-1)
  - Human immunodeficiency virus (HIV)
- Bacteria
  - Chlamydia pneumoniae
  - Borrelia burgdorferi and other spirochetes

---

cal environmental factors are not identified, many believe them to be ubiquitous infectious agents, including viruses and bacteria (Table 18.2). Exposures to common viruses and bacteria relatively early in life, in a way that is not yet understood, set the stage for MS. Infections probably act as disease triggers, although continued active neural or extraneural infection has not been ruled out in selected patients. Molecular mimicry (shared epitope sequences or structurally similar sequences between ubiquitous infectious agents and autoantigens, including CNS antigens) is well documented. It is commonly believed, although not proven, that infection-triggered cross-reactivity to a myelin component initiates MS in genetically vulnerable individuals. Epitope spread occurs when CNS damage releases multiple sequestered antigens to the systemic immune system. The initial attack, even if due to cross-reactivity to a dominant epitope on myelin basic protein, results in subsequent immune responses to multiple cryptic myelin and even nonmyelin epitope targets (20). This expands the immune attack and acts to enhance and perpetuate organ-specific autoimmune disease. Epitope spread occurs in animal models of MS, and preliminary data indicate it is also a factor in MS (21).

The concept of epitope spread carries important therapeutic implications. It argues for starting effective MS treatment at the earliest possible time (ideally, at the first attack of definite MS), to minimize expansion and reinforcement of the damage process. The concept even provides a rationale for considering initial induction therapy (with broad-spectrum immunosuppression), followed by maintenance therapy. Supporting evidence that the early disease process is critical also comes from natural history studies of first-attack, clinically isolated syndrome (CIS) patients (22).

The final factor in the pathogenesis of MS is the host immune system. Although MS does not appear to be an autoimmune disease in the strict sense of the word, it is clearly an immune-mediated disease. Pathologic lesions in this disease involve localized immune responses within the CNS (5). CNS inflammation is most marked in the early

stages of MS, corresponding to the relapsing, reversible phase (23,24). Later, neurodegeneration with axon loss appears to predominate, corresponding to the irreversible progressive phase. A lesion may be initiated when activated T cells from the blood compartment bind, via adhesion molecules, to CNS endothelial cells. Cells then release enzymes, including matrix metalloproteinases, that allow them to pass through the basement membrane and extracellular matrix into CNS parenchyma. This cell penetration is the earliest detectable abnormality; it corresponds to contrast enhancement on magnetic resonance imaging (MRI). Cell entry is followed by the development of an immune cascade of other blood immune system cells, including B cells and antigen presenting cells, the release of cytokines and chemokines, the production of antibodies and enzymes, and the upregulation of immune activation molecules on resident CNS cells, particularly microglia. This localized immune response results in the formation of the plaque, which contributes to an increasing permanent lesion burden.

The new concept in the pathogenesis of MS indicates that both axon density and volume are reduced in MS, not just within the plaque but also in normal-appearing CNS tissue (25,26). The analysis of n-acetyl aspartate (NAA), an axon/neuron marker measured by MR spectroscopy, indicates that whole-brain NAA is reduced even in early MS (27). Loss or shrinkage of axons is a major contributor to brain and spinal cord volume loss (atrophy). In patients with MS, prominent CNS atrophy is present very early, even at the time of the first clinical attack (28,29). On a yearly basis, brain volume loss in MS is accelerated three- to tenfold over that of matched controls.

Recent studies suggest immunopathologic heterogeneity. A multinational consortium of neurologists and neuropathologists has studied acute plaque pathology in MS brain tissue samples obtained at biopsy or autopsy (30). Results of this study reveal four distinct immunopathologies (Table 18.3). These observations await confirmation but, if true, suggest 4 distinct categories of MS based on primary damage mechanisms; this would have profound therapeutic implications.

EPIDEMIOLOGY

Frequency

MS is the most common acquired neurologic disease of young adults. In the United States, it is estimated that up to 400,000 individuals have MS, and these numbers increase with subclinical cases. The frequency of MS varies in different locations. High risk zones (>30/100,000) include the northern United States, northern Europe, Canada, southern Australia, and New Zealand. Medium risk zones (5–30/100,000) include southern parts of the

TABLE 18.3
Heterogeneous MS Immunopathology of Acute Brain Plaques

Pattern	Frequency of patients	Characteristics
I	16%	MO mediated demyelination, oligodendrocytes preserved, remyelination
II	59%	Antibody/complement mediated demyelination, oligodendrocytes preserved, remyelination
III	24%	Distal dying back oligodendrogliopathy and apoptosis (ischemic, toxic, virus-induced, injury)
IV	1–2%	Primary oligodendrocyte degeneration (metabolic injury)

United States and Europe, and northern Australia. Low risk zones (<5/100,000) include Asia and possibly parts of South America. Latitude seems to play some role, since little MS is seen at the Equator but numbers increase as one moves away from the Equator. This observation remains unexplained and has been challenged but not refuted (31). Over 90% of MS patients are Caucasian. MS is rare in Africans. It is unusual in Afro-Americans, who have an incidence that is much less than Caucasian-Americans, but appear to have more severe disease. This likely reflects genetic factors. In certain racial populations MS virtually never occurs, such as the Eskimos and Bantus. There are also restricted populations who experience very little MS despite living in high-risk zones, such as the Lapps in Finland and the Inuit in Canada.

MS may be on the rise. Studies suggest an increase among women and an increase as natural infections in early childhood become less common. MS is now being seen in countries such as China, India, Saudia Arabia, and Egypt, where previously the disease had been rare.

Sex Preference

Over 70% of MS patients are women. This clearcut sex preference is an unexplained but central feature of MS and implicates possible hormonal factors, maternal factors, and X-linked gene factors in the disease (32–35). In general, women predominate in diseases considered to be autoimmune. The immune system is sexually dimorphic, and women as a group show stronger immune responses than men. The nervous system is also sexually dimorphic, with important anatomic, physiologic, hormonal, and circuitry differences based on sex, all of which could also

play a role. The only clinical type of MS where this preference is not seen is in the primary progressive subtype. As noted, these MS patients show a number of differences from the more common relapsing and secondary progressive forms of the disease. Sex impacts on multiple aspects of MS (Table 18.4). This includes such disparate observations as the fact that MRI disease activity may be influenced by sex hormones, sexual dysfunction is a frequent symptom of MS, and symptomatic therapies may have distinct side effects based on sex.

Age of Onset

MS commonly affects young adults within a few years of puberty. Ninety percent of MS patients present between the ages of 15 and 50 years. The mean age of onset is approximately 30 years. Only 0.5% of patients have onset of MS under age 10, or over age 60. Approximately 5% have onset before age 16. Again, the primary progressive form differs from the other clinical MS subtypes in this regard, since the typical onset is 40 years.

Morbidity and Mortality

MS is almost never a primary cause of death, although on occasion, deep brainstem lesions can affect vital cardiovascular and respiratory centers, resulting in mortality. The lifespan of MS patients is minimally shortened (by about 2 years) compared to matched controls. Mortality relates directly to disability. Mortality rates are lowest in ambulatory MS patients, higher in wheelchair-bound

TABLE 18.4
Sex Impact on MS

- Increased disease risk in women
  - 70–75% females
  - Likely to involve genetic, hormonal, and immune factor
- Increasing risk for women postpuberty, declines with perimenopause
  - 90% have onset between ages 15 and 50
  - Average onset age 20 to 30 and peak is early 20s
- Men are more likely to show primary progressive (PP) course, older age at onset
  - No sex preference in PP MS
- PP males have older age onset than PP females
- MS may be increasing (in women only in one study)
- Males have worse prognosis
  - May reflect in part older age onset, but this does not explain the whole picture
- Contrast brain MRI lesion activity may be higher in women
- Polymorphisms in estrogen receptor gene associated with increased disease risk, onset age (Japanese)

patients, and highest in very disabled, bedfast patients. Death in MS patients is generally due to the secondary complications of increased infections, aspirations, and skin breakdown. Death also occurs from suicide. The suicide rate is increased in MS, a reflection of the fact that depression is a common symptom in this disease (36).

The major effect of MS is on morbidity, with impact on the ability to remain mobile, to think, and to hold down a job.

DIAGNOSTIC CRITERIA

Clinical

The basic clinical principles for diagnoses of MS were outlined by Schumacher in 1965 (Table 18.5) (37). The criteria recognized characteristic age, clinical pattern, and objective white matter features, as well as the fact that lesions had to be disseminated in time and space. The criteria also recognized the need to consider other diagnostic possibilities. MS ultimately is a clinical diagnosis, because there are no definitive laboratory tests. It is disturbing, however, that despite modern medical advances, the misdiagnosis rate remains 5 to 10%.

The recently published International Panel (IP) *McDonald criteria* define formal MRI parameters for dissemination in space and time (Table 18.6) (38). They also specify criteria for the diagnosis of primary progressive MS that requires abnormal CSF (Table 18.7). These new criteria emphasize the principles of documenting dissemination in time and space and for relying on objective abnormalities for diagnosis. They specify diagnostic categories of "MS, possible MS, not MS," and endorse as useful supportive laboratory tests MRI, CSF analysis, and visual evoked potentials (VEPs). They do not allow a definite diagnosis on the first attack, because an ongoing disease process is not documented. Documentation of MRI activity, however, now can be used in place of clinical activity. The new diagnostic requirements for relapsing MS, based on initial assessment, are outlined in Table 18.8.

TABLE 18.6

IP McDonald Diagnostic Criteria for MRI-Based Dissemination in Space and Time (38)

- MRI dissemination in space criteria
  - 3 of 4 Criteria:
    - 1Gd+lesion, or 9T2 hyperintense lesions
    - ≥1 infratentorial lesion
    - ≥1 juxtacortical lesion
    - ≥3 periventricular lesions
  - Lesions ordinarily >3 mm
  - 1 spinal cord lesion may substitute for brain lesion
- MRI dissemination in time criteria
  - A. First scan ≥3 months after clinical event
    - 1. Gd+lesion (at independent site) demonstrates dissemination in time
    - 2. Gd-scan: follow-up MRI ≥3 months; new T2 or Gd+ lesion demonstrates dissemination in time
  - B. First scan <3 months after clinical event; on second scan ≥3 months after event
    - 1. Gd+lesion demonstrates dissemination in time
    - 2. Gd-scan: follow-up third MRI ≥3 months after first; new T2 or Gd+lesion disseminated in time

---

TABLE 18.7

IP McDonald Diagnostic Criteria for Primary Progressive MS (38)

1. Abnormal CSF (oligoclonal band positivity or intrathecal IgG production)
2. Any one of the following:
   a. ≥9 T2W brain MRI lesions
   b. ≥2 spinal cord lesions
   c. 4–8 brain + 1 cord lesion(s)
   d. 4–8 brain lesions + abnormal visual evoked potential (VEP)
3. Dissemination in time by MRI criteria or continued progression for 1 year

---

TABLE 18.5

Clinical Criteria for the Diagnosis of Multiple Sclerosis

- Objective CNS abnormalities
- Appropriate age
- CNS white matter disease process
- Lesions disseminated in time and space
- Compatible time course
  - Attacks lasting over 24 hours, spaced 1 month apart
  - Slow or stepwise progression over 6 months
- No better explanation

Clinical features that suggest misdiagnosis of MS are lack of ocular involvement, progressive disease beginning before age 35, localized disease explained by involvement of a single region of the neuraxis, and presence of atypical features (37–41). Atypical features include disease onset before age 10 or over age 65, abrupt onset of hemiparesis, prominent pain syndrome (with the exception of trigeminal neuralgia), associated peripheral neuropathy, nonscotomatous field defect, prominent gray matter disease, complete sparing of sensation and bladder involvement, progressive myelopathy without bladder and bowel involvement, impaired level of consciousness, and very prominent uveitis.

TABLE 18.8
Diagnostic Requirements for Relapsing MS

Clinical presentation	Dissemination in space criteria	Dissemination in time criteria
≥2 attacks; objective clinical evidence of ≥2 lesions	Not needed	Not needed
≥2 attacks; objective clinical evidence of 1 lesion	Abnormal MRI or ≥2 MRI lesions + abnormal CSF or new attack at new site	Not needed
1 attack; objective clinical evidence ≥2 lesions	Not needed	MRI criteria, or second attack
1 attack; objective clinical evidence of 1 lesion (CIS)	MRI criteria, or ≥2 MRI lesions + abnormal CSF	MRI criteria, or second attack

Laboratory Studies

A selective laboratory workup can help to minimize misdiagnosis (Table 18.9). Blood studies are used to exclude other diagnoses or confounding conditions. MRI is used to detect suggestive lesion patterns. Brain MRI is ultimately abnormal in at least 98% of MS patients, but at present lacks the specificity to assure that imaged lesions are due to MS. The value of brain MRI for diagnosis decreases after age 50, when age-related vascular changes become more frequent. Typical abnormalities are scattered white matter lesions, which are hyperintense on T2 and proton density scans. Some are also hypointense on T1 scans. MS MRI lesions have distinctive features (Table 18.10). It is unusual in MS to see basal ganglia (≤25%) or internal capsule (10%) lesions. Spinal cord MRI is particularly valuable in patients over age 50, because there are no age-related changes. Spinal MRI is also helpful with spinal cord presentations and in patients with normal or nonsupportive brain MRI. A minority of MS patients will show MRI lesions confined to the spinal cord.

CSF immune changes that support a diagnosis of MS involve the presence of detectable oligoclonal bands independent of serum bands or the presence of intrathecal IgG production. Bands should be detected through isoelectric focusing followed by immunoblot, and can be done on 100 mcL of unconcentrated CSF. These CSF immune changes become more common over time and, once positive, stay positive. Although not specific for MS, in the setting of a suggestive clinical history, they provide strong supportive data for the diagnosis.

Differential Diagnosis

The differential diagnosis of MS is quite broad (Table 18.11) (42–44). MS should be considered in any young or middle-aged woman with unexplained CNS disease. It is particularly troublesome that women presenting with their first symptoms are often considered to have nonorganic or psychologic diagnoses. In one study of the initial medical assessment of MS patients, 30% of Afro-American and 11% of Caucasian women, but no men, were told that their symptoms were emotional or psychological in origin (45).

TABLE 18.9
Laboratory Diagnostic Workup for MS

- Selective blood work to exclude other conditions:
  - Collagen vascular disease
  - Infections (Lyme, HHV-6, retroviruses, syphilis)
  - Endocrine disease
  - Nutritional deficiency (B12, vitamin E, folate)
  - Vasculitis
  - Adrenoleukodystrophy (very long chain fatty acids)
  - Specific genetic testing (CADISIL, Leber's, familial spastic paraplegia)
  - Antiphospholipid antibodies
  - Angiotensin converting enzyme, quantitative IgG, calcium
  - Antineuronal antibodies
- Magnetic resonance imaging
  - Brain
  - Spinal cord
- Cerebrospinal fluid
  - Oligoclonal bands
  - Intrathecal IgG production
  - Other tests
- Evoked potentials
  - Visual
  - Somatosensory of lower extremities
- Urologic
  - Urodynamics

TABLE 18.10
MRI Features Suggestive of MS

Brain MRI
- Large lesions (≥3 mm in size)
- Multiple lesions
- Lesions in specific locations
  - Predominantly white matter
  - Periventricular
  - Infratentorial/brainstem
  - Juxtacortical
  - Corpus callosum (best seen on sagittal T2 scan, lesions pointing away, moth-eaten appearance, or even frank atrophy)
- Ovoid shape
- Perpendicular orientation to ventricles
- Contrast enhancing lesions
  - Especially open ring

Spinal MRI
- Cervical, thoracic regions
- ≤50% cross-sectional diameter
- <2 segments in length
- Edema unusual
- Lateral, posterior anterior columns
- Asymmetric, multiple scattered lesions

TABLE 18.11
Differential Diagnosis of Multiple Sclerosis

- Variant demyelinating conditions
  - Balo concentric sclerosis
  - Schilder disease/myelinoclastic diffuse sclerosis
  - Infectious/postinfectious encephalomyelitis (acute disseminated encephalomyelitis)
  - Neuromyelitis optica (Devic syndrome)
  - Central pontine myelinolysis
- Collagen vascular disease
- Metabolic/toxic disorders
- Nutritional
- Sarcoidosis
- Uveomeningoencephalitides
- Behçet disease
- Neoplastic
- Structural
- Complicated migraine
- Neurodegenerative diseases
- Psychologic disturbance
- Genetic disorders
  - Hereditary ataxias
  - Mitochondrial cytopathies
  - Adrenoleukodystrophy
  - Metachromatic leukodystrophy
  - Fabry disease
  - Krabbe disease
  - Organic acidemias
  - Hepatolenticular degeneration
  - Adult polyglusan body disease

MANAGEMENT ISSUES IN WOMEN

Symptomatic Therapies

MS produces many symptoms that are bothersome and disruptive. The management of these symptoms is a major component of current MS therapy. Symptoms include fatigue, which is considered to be the single most disabling feature of MS, as well as depression, cognitive difficulties, spasticity, bladder and bowel disturbances, pain, tremor, sexual dysfunction, and impaired mobility. Their treatment is multifactorial. The first step is to identify bothersome symptoms, the extent to which they are disrupting the patient's life, and potential complicating factors (medications, sleep pattern, diet, activity, concurrent problems). This is followed by an individualized therapeutic approach, which may combine changes in lifestyle, physical strategies, surgical therapies, and pharmacologic therapies.

Certain drugs are frequently used for symptom relief (Table 18.12). These drugs can have interactions or potential side effects that women with MS must be aware of, such as the interaction of carbamazepine or phenytoin with estrogen-containing contraceptives. The pregnant or breast-feeding MS patient is at unique risk and must be very familiar with potential drug problems.

Steroids

Glucocorticoids are 21-carbon, four-ringed steroid molecules with potent anti-inflammatory and immunosup-pressive actions (46). They also affect carbohydrate, lipid, and protein metabolism, stimulate neurotransmitter release, enhance conduction and, at high dose, increase neuron excitability. Several synthetic glucocorticoids are used in MS as symptomatic therapy for acute relapses, to hasten recovery (Table 18.13). They temporarily repair the damaged blood–brain barrier, in part through effects on matrix metalloproteinases, and improve acute edema within developing plaques (47–50). They may also influence T cell subsets within the CNS, promote apoptosis in selected cell populations, and have direct physiologic effects on the plaque microenvironment (51). They are not believed to influence the degree of recovery, nor the underlying and ultimate MS disease course. Two recent studies, however, found that steroids at the time of new brain MRI lesion formation led to less permanent tissue damage and that, in a single center phase II trial, regular pulse steroid treatment over 5 years resulted in less disability (52,53).

At present, intravenous methylprednisolone, given as 1 gram over 30 minutes once a day for 3 to 5 days, is the most common steroid treatment regimen. Alternative regimens include dexamethasone 200 mg IV daily, and oral prednisone 1,000 mg daily (give over two

TABLE 18.12
Symptomatic Drugs Used in MS

Drug	Indication	Side effects/problems of specific concern to women
Amantadine	Fatigue	– Livedo reticularis (skin lesions on legs) more common in women – Insomnia (take earlier in day) – Excreted in breast milk – Causes birth defects in some animals; no human data
Modafinil	Fatigue	– May reduce effectiveness of steroid contraception (for up to 1 month after discontinuation)
Fluoxetine	Depression, fatigue	– Can interfere with sleep (AM dose) – Paradoxical suicidal ideation – Excreted in breast milk – May decrease libido, cause menstrual pain
Tricyclics	Depression, pain	– Photosensitivity – Excreted in breast milk – Newborn problems may be noted (muscle, heart, respiratory, urinary) with dose just before delivery – May cause weight gain, increased appetite, decreased sexual performance, enlarged breasts, lactation, hair loss, yellow skin
Carbamazepine	Pain	– Interferes with estrogen contraceptives – Photosensitivity – Potential fetal effects (low birth weight, small head, skull/face defects, undeveloped fingernails, growth delay) – Excreted in breast milk – May cause hair loss
Phenytoin	Pain	– Interferes with estrogen contraceptives – Gingival hyperplasia – Excreted in breast milk – May increase risk of birth defects
Baclofen	Spasticity, trigeminal neuralgia	– Acute withdrawal syndrome – Excreted in breast milk – Animal fetal effects at high dose (hernia, bone, low birth weight)
Tizanidine	Spasticity	– Decreased drug clearance with oral contraceptives – Animal effects at high dose (decreased fertility, fetal loss) – May be excreted in breast milk – Hepatotoxicity
Benzodiazepines (Clonazepam, Diazepam)	Spasticity, tremor	– Excreted in breast milk – Fetus may become dependent – Use prior to delivery may cause newborn problems (weakness, breathing/feeding/temperature problems)
Oxybutynin	Bladder urgency, frequency	May reduce breast milk flow, sexual performance

doses). Steroids have a number of potential side effects. Acute side effects include insomnia, emotional lability, fluid retention, weight gain, and increased appetite. With high-dose intravenous methylprednisolone, cardiac arrhythmias, acute psychosis, and hypotension have been seen. With longer use, glucocorticoids can result in cosmetic side effects such as worsening of acne, cushingoid habitus, prominent stretch marks, and skin atrophy. Other side effects include hypertension, hyperglycemia, increased susceptibility to infection, and gastrointestinal upset. Women must be aware of potential negative effects on bone density. Glucocorticocoids decrease body calcium through several mechanisms,

including inhibition of calcium absorption, increase in calcium excretion, and induction of secondary hyperparathyroidism. Sustained and intense glucocorticoid treatment can result in osteonecrosis, such as aseptic necrosis of the femoral head, while chronic treatment can lead to osteoporosis. MS patients at risk may need to take supplemental calcium and vitamin D. Physical activity is encouraged, and postmenopausal women should be on hormone replacement. Osteoporotic MS patients may need to be monitored with periodic bone density studies and may benefit from bisphosphonates.

Glucocorticoid side effects can be minimized through the use of a single daily dose, preferably in the morning

TABLE 18.13
Synthetic Glucocorticoids Used to Treat MS Relapses

Drug	Biologic half life (hours)	Relative anti-inflammatory potency	Equivalent dose (mg)	Treatment protocol*
Methylprednisolone	8–12	5	4	1,000 mg IV daily 3–5 days (± PO prednisone taper)
Prednisone	8–12	4	5	High dose: 1,000–1,250 mg QD for 3–5 days Low dose: 60–100 mg PO daily (taper over 2–16 weeks)
Dexamethasone	36	30	0.75	PO, IV, or IM in doses equal to above high-dose regimens (200 mg daily for 3–5 days)

*Drug routes include intravenous (IV), oral (PO), and intramuscular (IM); use of oral taper is becoming much less frequent.

TABLE 18.14
DMT for MS

Class	Agent	Recommended dose	FDA pregnancy category
Immunomodulator: antiinflammatory cytokine	Avonex® (IFN-β1a) Rebif® (IFN-β1a) Betaseron® (IFN-β1b)	30 mcg IM once weekly 44 mcg SC three times weekly 875 mcg (28 MIU) SC every week	C
Immunomodulator: random polymers of 4AA (T cell manipulator)	Copaxone® (glatiramer acetate)	20 mg SC once daily	B
Immunosuppressant	Novantrone® (mitoxantrone)	12 mg/m² IV every 3 months (to a lifetime maximum dose of 140 mg/m²)	D

to minimize effects on the hypothalamic pituitary adrenal axis, and by limiting the duration of therapy.

Glucocorticoids are not contraindicated in later pregnancy. Overuse during pregnancy may slow postnatal growth, and in animal studies, birth defects have been noted. As is true for all drugs, with the exception of vitamins (such as folic acid to minimize neural tube defects), one tries to avoid medication use in the early weeks of pregnancy. For the MS patient who is breast-feeding, glucocorticoids are excreted in milk and may affect growth.

Disease-Modifying Agents

Five disease-modifying agents (DMTs) (four immunomodulators and one immunosuppressive) and are currently approved by the Food and Drug Administration (FDA) for the treatment of MS (Table 18.14). The clinical and MRI benefits of these agents are best documented for relapsing forms of MS (Table 18.15), but there is also evidence of benefit for selected first attack high risk and secondary progressive patients.

TABLE 18.15
Documented Benefits of the DMTs in Relapsing Forms of MS

- Clinical benefits
  - ↓ relapse rate and relapse severity
  - ↑ time to next relapse
  - ↑ proportion of relapse-free patients
  - ↑ time to sustained disability/worsening on the neurologic examination
  - ↓ in development of disability
  - ↑ quality of life
- MRI benefits
  - ↓ in lesion (new, contrast) number and size
  - ↓ or stabilize burden of disease

TABLE 18.16

NMSS Disease Management Consensus Statement (46)

- Immunomodulator treatment should be initiated as soon as possible following diagnosis of relapsing MS.
- Immunomodulators should be considered for selected first-attack/high-risk patients.
- Relapse frequency, age, level of disability, or most medical conditions should not limit access to therapy.
- It is permissible to change drugs.
- Immunosuppressant (mitoxantrone) therapy may be considered for selected worsening and/or relapsing patients.
- None of the DMTs are approved for use in women who are pregnant, nursing, or trying to become pregnant.
- Therapy continues indefinitely except in the event of
  - Clear lack of benefit
  - Intolerable side effects
  - New data
  - Better therapy

TABLE 18.17

AAN/MS Council Clinical Practice Guidelines for the Use of DMT (55)

- Type A recommendations (proven)
  - Consider IFNβs in first attack/high risk patients, relapsing MS, SP with relapses
  - Consider GA in relapsing MS

- Type B recommendations (probable)
  - Consider mitoxantrone in relapsing
  - IFNβ dose response curve (may in part reflect dosing frequency)
  - Route of IFNβ administration does not affect efficacy

- Type C recommendations (possible)
  - Consider mitoxantrone in progressive MS

- Type U recommendations (unknown)
  - The benefit of GA in progressive MS is uncertain

The National MS Society has recently updated its consensus guidelines for use of MS DMT (Table 18.16) (38). It endorses the use of an immunomodulator in relapsing forms of MS and selected first-attack/high-risk patients. These agents are not to be used in women who are pregnant, attempting to become pregnant, or are breast-feeding, however. The American Academy of Neurology and the MS Council have provided practice guidelines for the use of the DMTs based on a rigorous evidence-based medicine review of the literature (Table 18.17) (55).

Interferon β

Three recombinant interferon βs are currently available in the United States for the treatment of relapsing MS (Table 18.14) (56–58). Several issues in the use of these agents are especially pertinent to women with MS. In certain animal models, interferon β is an abortifacient, although it is not documented to be a teratogen. Every female MS patient on therapy who is of childbearing age and at risk for pregnancy should use some form of contraceptive. If a woman becomes pregnant, interferon β is usually stopped. The limited group data indicate that babies born to mothers who were taking interferon β have been normal, but the FDA has recently mandated interferon β pregnancy registries (see Pregnancy section).

Interferon β has side effects of particular interest to women. Generally, side effects are dose related and spontaneously remit after several months. Because higher and more frequent doses are more efficacious, for most patients, the goal should be optimal management strategies to maintain patients on treatment at the highest tolerated dose. High-dose interferon β therapy can affect menstruation. The disturbances are mild to moderate rather than severe. In the phase III trial of interferon β 1b, menstrual disorders were noted in 17% of the 124 patients receiving high dose, compared with 8% of the 123 patients receiving placebo (59). When premenopausal women were specifically reviewed, 28% on interferon β had menstrual abnormalities compared with 13% of placebo-treated women. Menstrual problems included intermenstrual bleeding/spotting, intramenstrual clotting/spotting, early or delayed menses, and decreased flow days. Patients who begin therapy must be informed about this particular side effect.

The interferon βs cause a flu-like reaction, characterized by variable combinations of fever, chills, myalgias, fatigue/malaise, and sweats. This is the major side effect of interferon β therapy. Because flu-like symptoms are more likely to occur in young patients and in patients with small body size, young MS women are at increased risk (60). Flu-like reactions are prevented by initial dose escalation (such as 25% dose for 2 weeks, 50% for 2 weeks, 75% for 2 weeks, then full dose), and consistent premedication for the first 4 to 12 weeks of therapy. Premedication can consist of antipyretics (such as acetaminophen), anti-inflammatory agents (such as ibuprofen), low-dose corticosteroids (such as prednisone 30 mg QD), or pentoxifylline (60,61).

When interferon β is injected subcutaneously, it initially causes injection site reactions in up to 85% of patients. This rate falls to 44 to 50% over time. Reactions include redness, inflammation, bruising, pain, hypersensitivity and, very rarely, worsening of psoriasis or subcutaneous atrophy. The most serious reaction, skin necrosis, occurs in less than 1 to 3% of cases and may be more likely to occur when there is intercurrent infection. Necrosis has become quite rare with use of an autoject, which is now standard with SC injections. Management includes changing technique, changing depth of the needle, avoiding problematic body parts, injecting body temperature drug, using ice on the site prior to injection, and using sunscreen to block injection site exposure.

The only significant laboratory effects associated with interferon β therapy are depression of the white blood cell count and elevation in liver transaminases. These usually normalize spontaneously by 3 to 4 months, although lymphopenia may persist. Rare problems involve effects on red blood cells, platelets, and thyroid function. It is uncommon to have to stop interferon β therapy because of an abnormal laboratory test.

Glatiramer Acetate

The fourth immunomodulator is glatiramer acetate (Copaxone®), a synthetic polypeptide consisting of the random polymers of four amino acids (L-alanine, L-glutamic acid, L-lysine, L-tyrosine). It is a biophysical analog of myelin basic protein and disrupts the immune response to this important myelin protein. Glatiramer acetate is given by subcutaneous injection 20 mg daily.

Although it is not known to be an abortifacient, teratogen, or to damage the fetus, pregnancy is still considered a contraindication to treatment with glatiramer acetate and, while on therapy, fertile women must practice contraception. Glatiramer acetate carries a FDA category B pregnancy risk, however, as opposed to the category C of the interferon βs. A recent large registry involving several hundred pregnancies found nothing to indicate any risk from glatiramer acetate use (see Pregnancy section).

This immunomodulator is very well tolerated, with mild injection site reactions. Rare examples occur of lipoatrophy, hard nodules, or urticaria. A small proportion of patients (10 to 15%) experience an immediate postinjection (systemic) reaction. Typically, this is a single self-limited attack that occurs within minutes of injection, lasts 0.5 to 30 minutes, and involves a variable combination of flushing, chest pain, palpitations, anxiety, dyspnea, and throat constriction. No morbidity (in particular cardiac) has been associated with this reaction, although it can be frightening, and no gender preference has been noted in the occurrence of this side effect.

Mitoxantrone is the only FDA-approved immunosuppressant agent for MS. In the pivotal MIMS trial conducted in relapsing and secondary progressive MS patients, mitoxantrone given at 12 mg/m^2 IV every 3 months for 2 years had significant clinical and MRI benefits over placebo (62). Induction strategies with mitoxantrone, given monthly for 6 months, have also been shown to decrease disease activity lasting for up to 4 years (63). The major issue with mitoxantrone is the lifetime maximum of 140 mg/m^2, because of concerns about cardiotoxicity. The majority of premenopausal women treated with mitoxantrone will note menstrual abnormalities. A small risk for permanent sterility exists, especially in women aged 40 or higher.

Immunosuppressives

Immunosuppressive agents have been used to treat the progressive forms of MS as well as severe relapsing disease unresponsive to other therapies (Table 18.18). They include antimetabolites (azathioprine, methotrexate) that are active during the cell cycle S phase (DNA synthesis), and alkylating agents (chlorambucil, cyclophosphamide) that are active throughout the cell cycle (64). These drugs are basically cytotoxic agents that are not only teratogenic, but also carry a risk for late malignancy. Sterility may occur with intensive cyclophosphamide use, and menses may stop or be affected by all these agents. Convincing efficacy data is lacking for any of these agents, although it is clear that individual MS patients may benefit from their use.

A number of therapeutic trials are currently available to MS patients. These range from small single center and relatively brief (weeks to months) phase I studies, to large multicenter phase III studies lasting several years. A great interest exists in assuring that sufficient numbers of women participate in formal studies, particularly in a sex preference disorder such as MS. Pregnancy is a routine exclusion criterion in treatment trials, and women who wish to participate are routinely requested to use contraception to assure that pregnancy does not occur. The rationale is based on avoiding potential risks to a fetus. This is an added responsibility for women who take part in these studies. It is important to emphasize compliance with their chosen birth control method for the required time period.

Hormonal Issues

The increased frequency of MS in women of childbearing age is not unique to this disease. Women are more com-

TABLE 18.18
Immunosuppressive Drugs Used to Treat Multiple Sclerosis

Azathioprine
Chlorambucil
2-Chlorodeoxyadenosine
Cladnibine
Cyclophosphamide
Methotrexate
Mycophenolate mofetil

monly affected in a number of disorders believed to be autoimmune or immune mediated, including systemic lupus erythematosus (SLE), rheumatoid arthritis, Hashimoto's thyroiditis, Sjögren's syndrome, systemic sclerosis, and myathenia gravis. Symptoms in these diseases are often affected by hormonal changes related to pregnancy, menopause, or exogenous hormone use. These diseases likely reflect multiple levels of interaction between the individual's immune system, nervous system, endocrine system, and genetic makeup.

Sex hormones have many nervous system actions including effects on cognitive function, synaptogenesis, coordinated movement, tropic properties (promotion of axon and myelin growth and formation), and modulation of specific neurotransmitter systems (65). Sex hormones affect immune responses (66–69). During pregnancy, for example, a shift occurs in the T helper cell population to favor T helper 2 cells. This subpopulation downregulates cell-mediated responses and promotes antibody responses. Hormonal manipulation can bias towards either a T helper 1 or T helper 2 immune response. In general, women show higher immunoglobulin levels than men but decreased cell-mediated immune responses, consistent with a T helper 2 bias (70). Sex hormone receptors are present on a number of immune system cells, including CD8 T cells and macrophages (antigen presenting cells), thus assuring crosstalk between the endocrine and immune systems. CD4+ T cells respond to estrogens in a dose-related manner, with antigen-stimulated cell cytokine production modulated based on the amount of estrogen present (71). The cytokines involved all have very important roles in controlling immune responses. In animal models of MS, such as the adoptive experimental allergic encephalomyelitis (EAE) model in the SJL strain mouse, gender-related immune differences are clearly demonstrated (35). In fact, multiple sex-specific effects exist in EAE (Table 18.19). It seems likely that sex hormones play some role in MS. Preliminary studies of oral estriol appeared to show MRI and possibly clinical benefits. Ongoing studies are also evaluating testosterone patch therapy in men with MS.

Recent studies suggest that gender impacts on MRI findings in both healthy controls and MS patients. In a 3-year phase III trial of subcutaneous IFNβ1a in secondary progressive MS, men in the placebo arm showed fewer active lesions and less accumulation of T2 lesion burden than women (72). In a cross-sectional study of 413 consecutive patients who underwent MRI at a single outpatient center, male MS patients were found to have fewer contrast-enhancing lesions and active scans, but more T1 hypointense lesions (73). In contrast, women showed fewer T1 hypointense lesions and lower T1:T2 ratios (a lower proportion of their T2 hyperintense lesions were visible on T1 as hypointense), findings consistent with less severe tissue damage. These

---

TABLE 18.19
Sex-Specific Effects in the EAE Animal Model of MS

- Disease course and therapeutic response may differ based on sex
- Female animals are generally more susceptible and show more severe disease
- Pregnancy is protective
- Exogenous estrogen ameliorates disease, whereas removal of ovaries worsens disease
- The disease influencing effects of estrogen are lost in estrogen receptor alpha knockout mice
- Testosterone suppresses or ameliorates disease
- Castration worsens disease and changes a male disease pattern to a female disease pattern
- Combination therapy with estrogen can change a monotherapy nonresponder to a responder.

---

results suggest that men with MS develop less inflammatory but more destructive lesions than women with MS. When analyzed based on relapsing versus secondary progressive MS, a significant sex effect occurred on the T1:T2 lesion ratio: For relapsing MS, the male to female ratio was 0.36 versus 0.27 (p=0.001), whereas for secondary progressive MS it was 0.40 versus 0.33 (p=0.008). A trend was seen in both clinical subtypes for fewer enhancing lesions in men. As expected, the T1:T2 lesion ratio was higher in the secondary progressive group (p=0.003). Studies of primary progressive MS have also noted a higher median T1:T2 lesion ratio in men (74,75).

In another preliminary study, brain water content was measured using MRI T1 mapping on a 4T MRI machine instrument, in 23 healthy adult controls (12 men, 11 women) and 25 MS patients (eight men, 17 women). The MS group (both men and women) shows increased water in brain white matter compared with healthy controls. Among the controls, women had significantly higher white matter water content (76). No significant sex difference was observed in the MS group, although the fact that patients were not well age-matched may have been a possible confounding factor.

In another study, healthy women showed smaller white matter volume fractions and larger gray matter volume fractions than men (77). White matter volume did not change with age, whereas gray matter volume showed significant decrease with age, but only in men. A trend for decreased gray matter with age was observed in women. In men (but not women), CSF volume fraction and white matter water content increased with age. These results give further support for sexual dimorphism in structural and chemical brain parameters.

Pregnancy

Pregnancy is a major issue in MS because the disease affects so many young women. Questions arise not only about the effect of pregnancy on MS disease onset, activity, and prognosis, but whether MS in turn affects the fetus and the birth process. Until 1949, pregnancy was considered to have a negative effect on MS and was discouraged. Over the next few years, several studies were published that failed to confirm this widely held impression (78,79). A number of publications have addressed pregnancy in MS (80–98). Overall, pregnancy does not increase the risk of developing MS. A Scandinavian study found the risk of MS was higher for nulliparous than parous women, and that the risk ratio increased over time (99). Pregnancy does not worsen MS (100). In fact, suggestive data show that pregnancy may improve the disease course and slow time to disability endpoints for relapsing patients (101–103). Anecdotal data suggest this may not be true for secondary progressive MS, however. MS has no significant effects on fertility, conception, fetal viability, and delivery. No increases occur in ectopic pregnancies, spontaneous abortions, stillbirths, or congenital malformations (17,82).

In counseling MS patients on pregnancy, they should be told that there is no negative effect in the short- or long-term. In fact, pregnancy may have a positive effect on their prognosis. A very small but finite increased risk exists for MS in the child. Finally, there is increased risk of relapse in the months following delivery. The extent of physical disability of the MS patient is an obvious factor in deciding on pregnancy. If possible, arrangements should be made to have help available, in the event the mother has an acute relapse.

Pregnancy appears to be protective in MS. Relapses are decreased during the 9 months of gestation, particularly in the latter half. This probably relates to the fact that pregnancy is an immunosuppressive state. Maternal, fetal, and placental factors combine to produce immune suppression by way of pregnancy-associated immunoregulatory proteins; an overall net inhibitory effect of pregnancy-related hormone, prostanglandin, and cytokine changes; maternal–fetal MHC class II disparity; pregnancy-associated inhibition of cell-mediated immune responses; and pregnancy-associated enhancement of immunoglobulin (including blocking antibody and immune complex) responses (93). This pregnancy-associated decrease in disease activity was confirmed by MRI. In two pregnant MS patients scanned serially, the number of new and/or enlarging brain lesions decreased during the second half of pregnancy (104). Of note was the fact that MRI disease activity returned to prepregnancy levels in the first months' postpartum.

Most studies indicate a postpartum rebound in disease activity. A threefold increase in relapses occurs in the 3 to 6 months after giving birth, with 30% of women experiencing clinical attacks. Consistent with findings from this small neuroimaging study, the European study on Pregnancy–related Relapses in MS (PRIMS study), which involved 254 women and 269 pregnancies, documented a 70% decline in the prepregnancy relapse rate during the last trimester (105). A rebound 70% increase also occurred in relapses in the first 3 months postpartum, before the attack rate returned to the prepregnancy baseline level. A recent report provided 2-year postpartum follow-up in the PRIMS cohort. From postpartum month 4, the relapse rate remained at the prepregnancy level. Disability and relapse rate at 2 years were not influenced by pregnancy, type of delivery, use of epidural anesthesia, or decision to breast feed (106). Postpartum relapses should be preventable using available immunotherapies. In one study, nine MS patients who had previously had 12 childbirth-associated relapses received prophylactic intravenous immune globulin postpartum. None went on to have clinical relapses (107).

The mode of delivery, as well as whether the mother breastfeeds, have no adverse effects on MS disease course (98). The only type of anesthesia not recommended for MS patients is spinal anesthesia.

The recently revised National MS Society Disease Management Consensus Statement emphasizes that current DMTs are not approved for use in women who are pregnant (38). These drugs have distinct classifications with regard to their risk. Glatiramer acetate is classified category B (no identified animal/human risk), interferon βs are category C (abortofacients in animal models), and mitoxantrone is category D (cell toxic immunosuppressive agent).

Some data are available on pregnancy outcome in patients exposed to MS DMT. In the United States, normal pregnancy outcome rates are 62% live births, 22% elective abortions, 16% spontaneous abortions, and 0.8% ectopic pregnancies. Congenital anomaly rates are 7 to 10% overall, and 2 to 3% for significant defects. A pregnancy registry for subcutaneous IFNβ1a (Rebif®) cases, collected from clinical trial data (both placebo-controlled and extension studies), examined a range of doses from 22 mcg once a week to 44 mcg three times a week. There were 37 pregnancies among approximately 1,400 women; 30 women were on drug or close to taking drug when they became pregnant. Of these, there were 13 (45%) healthy live births, two (6.9%) premature births, six (21%) elective abortions, and eight (27.6%) spontaneous abortions, including one fetal death. One pregnancy was lost to follow-up (108).

A glatiramer acetate (Copaxone®) pregnancy registry, the largest reported to date, was based on 21 global clinical trials (placebo-controlled and open label), and postmarketing surveillance data from 1996 to September 2002 (109). The clinical trials data involved 2,380 women. There were 40 reported pregnancies. Ten were lost to follow-up. For the 30 with outcome data, there were 18 (60%) elective abortions, five (16.7%) spontaneous abortions, six (20%) healthy live births, and one (3.3%) cleft lip anomaly. In the cleft-lip anomaly, the mother had used carbamazepine during pregnancy, so it was felt that the anomaly was most likely due to the anticonvulsant. In the postmarketing surveillance, 345 pregnancies were reported. The large majority of women discontinued drug once they found they were pregnant. Over 90% had clear DMT exposure in the first trimester. One hundred and thirty women were either lost to follow-up or did not have outcome data because they had not reached their due date. Of the 215 known outcomes, there were 155 healthy live births, 43 spontaneous abortions, 9 elective abortions, 1 ectopic pregnancy, 1 still birth, and 6 congenital anomalies (failure to thrive, finger anomaly, cardiomyopathy, urethrostenosis, anencephaly, adrenal cyst). Overall then, there are 245 pregnancies with outcome data: 66% healthy live births, 20% spontaneous abortions, 11% elective abortions, 2.9% congenital anomalies, 0.4% ectopic pregnancies, and 0.4% still births.

In summary, the DMT immunomodulators and glatiramer acetate in particular do not appear to have significant adverse effects on pregnancy.

Breast-Feeding

Data are conflicting on breast-feeding. Two studies reported no effect, whereas a third found a positive one (110–112). At present, it is not known whether breast-feeding has any real benefit in reducing relapses postpartum. This is an important that needs to be resolved, because breast-feeding is considered a contraindication to use of the DMTs.

Menses

Very little data are available on the menstrual cycle and MS. In one self-report study of 149 women with MS, 70% noted symptom changes associated with their cycle. The majority (60%) noted changes in the week prior to or the week of their menses, while 44% reported relapses at a consistent cycle phase (113). In one study of 30 patients, a single MRI was done in the early follicular (day 1–3), late follicular (days 14–18), or luteal (days 21–23) phase. MRI activity increased when progesterone was low and estradiol was high (114). In another study, eight relapsing patients had two MRI scans during their follicular (days 3–9) and luteal (days 21–28) phases. Although overall MRI activity did not differ between the phases, in the luteal phase, a higher progesterone to estradiol ratio correlated with an increased number and volume of contrast enhancing lesion (115). In a follow-up study of 17 relapsing patients, the association of greater contrast

lesion activity with a higher progesterone to estradiol ratio in the latter half of the menstrual cycle was confirmed. In addition, these MS women showed lower testosterone levels than matched controls. MRI activity was greater in the MS patients with low testosterone levels, whereas the MS patients without any MRI activity had much higher levels (116). These preliminary studies are very intriguing and suggest that sex hormones may affect MRI disease activity markers.

With regard to menopause issues, MS is not a contraindication to hormone replacement therapy (HRT). Menopause is a time of increased bone loss and enhanced risk for osteoporosis, so this should be monitored. Virtually no data are available on whether a relationship of menopause to symptoms, disease activity, or prognosis exists. Anecdotally, symptoms that worsen postmenopause may respond to HRT (40,117). Although historically there has been a sense that the MS disease process lessens with age, this is probably not the case, because ongoing atrophy and axon damage occurs, even though CNS inflammation must be less.

Contraception

The limited data available indicate that the use of oral contraceptives has no effect on the risk of developing MS (118), and no adverse effects on the overall disease course. Data may suggest that young patients on the pill may show less disability and are less likely to experience menstrual worsening of their disease (82). This is another issue that awaits clarification.

PSYCHOSOCIAL ISSUES

MS impacts on virtually all aspects of life, career, and family. Therefore, the woman with MS faces a number of psychosocial issues (Table 18.20). They run the gamut from questions about self image and interpersonal relationships, to economic issues. Women, particularly when there are obvious neurologic deficits, may have a poor self image and feel that they are unattractive and undesirable. They may not be able to apply makeup, fix their hair, or practice appropriate hygiene. Suddenly they are dependent on others to perform very personal tasks. The unpredictable nature of MS and the uncertain prognosis are unsettling. Sexual dysfunction, including decreased sensation, decreased libido, and problems with orgasm, are reported in up to 74% of women with MS (119). This is an extra stress for a marriage, in addition to those stresses caused by the loss of a partner and the need for a spouse or other family member to assume the role of caretaker.

As a whole, MS patients are less likely to be involved in vocational, educational, and homemaking activities. They are more likely to require personal assistance care

TABLE 18.20
*Psychosocial Issues for
Women Multiple Sclerosis Patients*

Issue	Concerns

Self image/
personal life
	Physical attractiveness
	Uncertain future
	Dependency
	Mobility
	Symptom control
	  – Depression
	  – Bladder/bowel
	  – Sexual
	  – Other
	Disruption of lifestyle
	Role playing
	  – Career
	  – Homemaker
	  – Spouse
	  – Parent

Relationships	Marriage
	  – Abandonment/Divorce
	  – Children
	  – Sexuality
	  – Contraception
	  – Caretaker role
	Codependency
	Adjustment/coping
	Abuse
	  – Physical
	  – Mental
	Social isolation

Financial/
economic
	Employment
	Health care
	  – Access
	  – Cost
	  – Long-term care

Some studies suggest that the cost of MS is higher for women (121). Estimated on 1991 dollars, the average lifetime costs of MS were $746,819 for single women, $450,845 for married women, $360,320 for married men, and $332,001 for single men.

Finally, access to health care may be limited for more disabled MS patients. It is important that routine non-neurologic care for female patients, including an annual gynecologic examination, assessment for osteoporosis, and periodic mammography, not be neglected.

SUMMARY

MS is a major neurologic disease of young women. A great deal of accurate information is available on diagnosis, prognosis, and effects of pregnancy in this disease, and expanding options are available to treat both disease activity and symptoms. A well-informed health care team can provide not only useful information to the female MS patient, but can assure that she will receive the optimal management of her neurologic disease.

*R*eferences

1. Noseworthy JH, Lucchinetti C, Rodriguez M, Weinshenker BG. Multiple sclerosis. *N Engl J Med* 2000; 343:938–952.
2. Duquette P, Pleines J, Girard M, Charest L, Senecal-Quevillon M, Masse C. The increased susceptibility of women to multiple sclerosis. *Can J Neurol Sci* 1992; 19:466–471.
3. Minden SL, Marder WD, Harrold LN, Dor A. *Multiple Sclerosis: A statistical portrait*. National MS Society. Cambridge, Mass: Abt Associates 1993.
4. Miller DH, Albert PS, Barkhof F, et al. Guidelines for the use of magnetic resonance techniques in monitoring the treatment of multiple sclerosis. *Ann Neurol* 1996;39: 6–16.
5. Storch M, Lassmann H. Pathology and pathogenesis of demyelinating diseases. *Curr Opinion Neurol* 1997;10: 186–192.
6. Lublin FD, Reingold SC. National Multiple Sclerosis Society (USA). Defining the clinical course of multiple sclerosis: results of an international survey. *Neurology* 1996;46:900–911.
7. McDonnell GV, Hawkins SA. Primary progressive multiple sclerosis: a distinct syndrome? *Multiple Sclerosis* 1996;2:137–141.
8. Sadovnick AD, Ebers GC. Genetics of multiple sclerosis. *Neurol Clin* 1995;13:99–118.
9. Robertson NP, Compston DAS. Prognosis in multiple sclerosis: genetic factors. In: Siva A, Kesselring J, Thompson AJ, (eds.) *Frontiers in multiple sclerosis*. London: Martin Dunitz, 1999;51–61.
10. Oksenberg JR, Hauser SL. New insights into the immunogenetics of multiple sclerosis. *Curr Opinion Neurol* 1997;10:181–185.
11. Dyment DA, Sadovnick AD, Ebers GC. Genetics of multiple sclerosis. *Hum Mol Genet* 1997;6: 1693–1698.

and to use medical services. The entire MS family unit experiences increased stress, with decreased available resources, and decreased satisfaction with life in general.

Psychosocial factors are critical to quality of life. A poor quality of life for MS patients is associated in particular with social isolation, as well as an unstable disease course, denial rather than acceptance of illness, disease symptoms that are moderate to severe, limitations in mobility, and unemployment (117). Women with MS, particularly those who are married, are more likely to be unemployed than men with MS (120). They tend to leave the work force while they are less physically disabled to assume a role in the home. Women tend to feel guilty at perceived failure to meet obligations to their family, whereas men tend to react with anger and frustration at their limited work and other activities.

12. Schrijver HM, Crusius JB, Uitdehaag BM, et al. Association of interleukin-1beta and interleukin-1 receptor antagonist genes with disease severity in MS. *Neurology* 1999;52(3):595–599.

13. Kira J, Kanai T, Nishimura Y, Yamasaki K, et al. Western versus Asian types of multiple sclerosis: immunogenetically and clinically distinct disorders. *Ann Neurol* 1996;40(4):569–574.

14. Harding AE, Sweeney MG, Miller DH, et al. Occurrence of a multiple sclerosis-like illness in women who have a Leber's hereditary optic neuropathy mitochondrial DNA mutation. *Brain* 1992;115(Pt 4):979–989.

15. Kellar-Wood H, Robertson N, Govan GG, Compston DA, Harding AE. Leber's hereditary optic neuropathy mitochondrial DNA mutations in multiple sclerosis. *Ann Neurol* 1994;36(1):109–112.

16. Riordan-Eva P, Sanders MD, Govan GG, Sweeney MG, Da Costa J, Harding AE. The clinical features of Leber's hereditary optic neuropathy defined by the presence of a pathogenic mitochondrial DNA mutation. *Brain* 1995;118(Pt 2):319–337.

17. Sadovnick AD, Baird PA. Reproductive counseling for multiple sclerosis patients. *Amer J Med Gen* 1985;20:349–354.

18. Sadovnick AD, Ebers GC. Epidemiology of multiple sclerosis: a critical overview. *Can J Neurol Sci* 1993;20:17–29.

19. Weinshenker BG. Epidemiology of multiple sclerosis. *Neurol Clin* 1996;14:291–308.

20. Vanderlugt CL, Miller SD. Epitope spreading in immune-mediated disease: implications for immunotherapy. *Nat Rev Immunol* 2002;2:85–95.

21. Tuohy VK, Yu M, Weinstock-Guttman B, Kunkel RP. Diversity and plasticity of self recognition during the development of multiple sclerosis. *J Clin Invest* 1997;99:1682–1690.

22. Brex PA, Ciccarelli O, O'Riordan JI, Sailer M, Thompson AJ, Miller DH. A longitudinal study of abnormalities on MRI and disability from multiple sclerosis. *N Engl J Med* 2002;346:158–164.

23. Cifelli A, Arridge M, Jezzard P, et al. Thalamic neurodegeneration in multiple sclerosis. *Ann Neurol* 2002;52:650–653.

24. Kuhlman T, Lingfeld G, Bitsch A, Schuchardt J, Bruck W. Acute axonal damage in multiple sclerosis is most extensive in early disease stages and decreases over time. *Brain* 2002;125:2202–2212.

25. Trapp BD, Peterson J, Ransohoff RM, Rudick R, Mork S, Bo L. Axonal transection in the lesions of multiple sclerosis. *N Engl J Med* 1998;338:278–285.

26. Ferguson B, Matyszak MK, Esiri MM, Perry VH. Axonal damage in acute multiple sclerosis lesions. *Brain* 1997;120:393–399.

27. Gonen O, Moriarty DM, Li BS, et al. Relapsing-remitting multiple sclerosis and whole-brain N-acetylaspartate measurement: evidence for different clinical cohorts initial observations. *Radiology* 2002;225:261–268.

28. Chard DT, Griffin CM, Parker GJM, et al. Brain atrophy in clinically early relapsing-remitting multiple sclerosis. *Brain* 2002;125:327–337.

29. Dalton CM, Brex PA, Jenkins R, et al. Progressive ventricular enlargement in patients with clinically isolated syndromes is associated with the early development of multiple sclerosis. *J Neurol Neurosurg Psychiatry* 2002;73:141–147.

30. Lucchinetti C, Bruck W, Parisi J, Scheithauer B, Rodriguez M, Lassmann H. Heterogeneity of multiple sclerosis lesions: implications for the pathogenesis of demyelination. *Ann Neurol* 2000;47:707–717.

31. Rosati G. Descriptive epidemiology of multiple sclerosis in Europe in the 1980s: a critical overview. *Ann Neurol* 1994;36:S164–S174.

32. Sadovnick AD, Bulman D, Ebers GC. Parent-child concordance in multiple sclerosis. *Ann Neurol* 1991;29:252–255.

33. Smith R, Studd JWW. A pilot study of the effect upon multiple sclerosis of the menopause, hormone replacement therapy and the menstrual cycle. *J R Soc Med* 1992;85:612–613.

34. Piccinni MP, Giudizi M, Biagiotti R, et al. Progesterone favors the development of human T helper cells producing Th2-type cytokines and promotes both IL-4 production and membrane CD30 expression in established Th1 cell clones. *J Immunol* 1995;155:128–133.

35. Voskuhl RR, Pitchekian-Halabi H, MacKenzie-Graham A, McFarland HF, Raine CS. Gender differences in autoimmune demyelination in the mouse: implications for multiple sclerosis. *Ann Neurol* 1996;39:724–733.

36. Sadovnick AD, Eisen K, Ebers GC, Paty DW. Cause of death in patients attending multiple sclerosis clinics. *Neurology* 1991;41:1193–1196.

37. Schumacher GA, Beebe GW, Kibler RF, et al. Problems of experimental trials of therapy in multiple sclerosis. *Ann NY Acad Sci* 1965;122:552–568.

38. NMSS Expert Opinion Paper. *Disease management consensus paper.* National Multiple Sclerosis Society 2002; http://www.nationalmssociety.org/pdf/forpros/Exp_Consensus.pdf.

39. Herndon RM, Brooks B. Misdiagnosis of multiple sclerosis. *Sem Neurol* 1985;5:94–98.

40. Rudick RA, Schiffer RB, Schwetz KM, Herndon RM. Multipel sclerosis: The problem of incorrect diagnosis. *Arch Neurol* 1986;43:578–583.

41. Rolak LA. The diagnosis of multiple sclerosis. *Neurol Clin* 1996;14:27–43.

42. Murray TJ, Murray SJ. Characteristics of patients found not to have multiple sclerosis. *Can Med Assoc J* 1984;131:336–337.

43. Natowicz MR, Bejjani B. Genetic disorders that masquerade as multiple sclerosis. *Am J Med Gen* 1994;49:149–169.

44. O'Riordan JI. Central nervous system white matter diseases other than multiple sclerosis. *Curr Opinion Neurol* 1994;10:211–214.

45. Kalb RC. *Families affected by multiple sclerosis: disease impacts and coping strategies.* Health Services Research Reports Monograph, National MS Society, 1995.

46. Salman K, LI R. Corticotropin and corticosteroids. In: DiPalma JR, DiGregorio GJ, (eds.) *Basic Pharmacology in Medicine.* 3rd ed. New York: McGraw Hill, 1990;535–546.

47. Troiano R, Hafstein M, Ruderman M, Dowling P, Cook SD. Effect of highdose intravenous sterid administration on contrast-enhancing computed tomographic scan lesion in multiple sclerosis. *Ann Neurol* 1984;15:257–263.

48. Troiano R, Haftein M, Zito G, Ruderman MI, Dowling PC, Cook SD. The effect of oral corticosteroid dosage on CT enhancing multiple sclerosis plaques. *J Neurol Sci* 1985;70:67–72.

49. Kesselring J, Miller DH, Macmanus DG, et al. Quantitative magnetic resonance imaging in multiple sclerosis:

the effect of high dose intravenous methylprednisolone. *J Neurol Neurosurg Psych* 1989;52:14–17.

50. Rosenberg GA, Dencoff JE, Correa N, Reiners M, Ford CC. Effect of steroids on CSF matrix metalloproteinases in multiple sclerosis: relation to blood-brain barrier injury. *Neurology* 1996;46:1626–1632.

51. Durelli L, Poccardi G, Cavallo R. CD8+ high CD11b* low T cells (T suppressor-effectors) in multiple sclerosis cerebrospinal fluid are increased during high dose corticosteroid treatment. *J Neuroimmunol* 1991;31: 221–228.

52. Richert ND, Ostuni JL, Bash CN, et al. Interferon beta-1b and intravenous methylprednisolone promote lesion recovery in multiple sclerosis. *Mult Scler* 2001; 7(1):49–58.

53. Zivadinov R, Rudick RA, De Masi R, et al. Effects of IV methylprednisolone on brain atrophy in relapsing-remitting MS. *Neurology* 2001;57:1239–1247.

54.

55. Goodin DS, Frohman EM, Garmany GP Jr, et al. Disease modifying therapies in multiple sclerosis: Report of the Therapeutics and Technology Assessment Subcommittee of the American Academy of Neurology and the MS Council for Clinical Practice Guidelines. *Neurology* 2002;58:169–178.

56. The IFNB Multiple Sclerosis Study Group: interferon beta-1b is effective in relapsing-remitting multiple sclerosis, I. Clinical results of a multicenter, randomized, double-blind, placebo-controlled trial. *Neurology* 1993;43:655–661.

57. Jacobs LD, Cookfair DL, Rudick RA, et al. Intramuscular interferon beta-1a for disease progression in relapsing multiple sclerosis. The Multiple Sclerosis Collaborative Research Group (MSCRG) *Ann Neurol* 1996; 39:285–294.

58. IFNB Multiple Sclerosis Study Group, University of British Columbia MS/MRI Analysis Group: interferon beta-1b in the treatment of MS: final outcome of the randomized controlled trial. *Neurology* 1995;45: 1277–1285.

59. *Interferon β1b*. Product Monograph, Berlex Laboratories, 1994.

60. Lublin FD, Whitaker JN, Eidelman BH, Miller AE, Arnason BG, Burks JS. Management of patients receiving interferon beta 1b for multiple sclerosis: report of a consensus conference. *Neurology* 1996;46:12–18.

61. Rieckmann R, Weber F, Gunther A, Poster S. The phosphodiesterase inhibitor pentoxifylline reduces early side effects of interferon β-1b treatment in patients with multiple sclerosis. *Neurology* 1997;47:604.

62. Edan G, et al. Therapeutic effect of mitoxantrone combined with methylprednisolone in multiple sclerosis: a randomised multicentre study of active disease using MRI and clinical criteria. *J Neurol Neurosurg Psychiat* 1997;62:112–118.

63. Johnson KP, Brooks BR, Cohen JA, et al. Copolymer 1 reduces relapse rate and improves disability in relapsing-remitting multiple sclerosis: results of a phase III multicenter, double-blind placebo-controlled trial. The Copolymer 1 multiple sclerosis Study Group. *Neurology* 1995;45:1268–1276.

64. Brodsky I, Crilley P, Terzian AEL. Cancer chemotherapy. In: DiPalma JR, DiGregorio GJ, (eds.) *Basic pharmacology in medicine*. 3rd ed. New York: McGraw Hill, 1990;549–565.

65. McEwen BS, Alves SE, Bullock K, Weiland NG. Ovarian steroids and the brain: implications for cognition and aging. *Neurology* 1997;48(S7):8–15.

66. Weinstein Y, Ran S, Segal S. Sex-associated differences in the regulation of immune responses controlled by the MHC of the mouse. *J Immunol* 1984;132:656–661.

67. Ahmed SA, Talal N, Christados P. Genetic regulation of testosterone-induced immune suppression. *Cell Immunol* 1987;104:91–98.

68. Grossman C. Possible underlying mechanisms of sexual dimorphism in the immune response, fact and hypothesia. *J Steroid Biochem* 1989;34:241–251.

69. Schuurs A, Verheul H. Effects of gender and sex steroids on the immune response. *J Steroid Biochem* 1990;35: 157–172.

70. Duquette P, Girard M. Hormonal fractors in susceptibility to multiple sclerosis. *Curr Opinion Neurol Neurosurg* 1993;6:195–201.

71. Gilmore W, Weiner LP, Correale J. Effect of estradiol on cytokine secretion by proteolipid protein-specifc T cell clones isolated from multiple sclerosis patient and normal control subjects. *J Immunol* 1997;158:446–451.

72. Li DK, Zhao GJ, Paty DW. Randomized controlled trial of interferon-beta-1a in secondary progressive MS: MRI results. *Neurology* 2001;56:1505–1513.

73. Pozzilli C, Tomassini V, Marinelli F, Paolillo A, Gasperini C, Bastianello S. 'Gender gap' in multiple sclerosis: magnetic resonance imaging evidence. *Eur J Neurol* 2003; 10(1):95–97.

74. Stevenson VL, Miller DH, Leary SM, et al. One year follow up study of primary and transitional progressive multiple sclerosis. *J Neurol Neurosurg Psychiatry* 2000;68:713–718.

75. Van Walderveen MA, Lycklama A Nijeholt GJ, et al. Hypointense lesions on T1-weighted spin-echo magnetic resonance imaging: relation to clinical characteristics in subgroups of patients with multiple sclerosis. *Arch Neurol* 2001;58:76–81.

76. Rooney WD, Coyle PK, Li X, et al. *Sex differences of brain 1H20 T1 values in controls and MS subjects: the role of estradiol*. Submitted, AAN 2003a (abstract).

77. Rooney WD, Li X, Telang,FW, et al. *Age and sex: sex on brain properties by ^1H_2O T1 histogram*. Submitted, AAN 2003b (abstract).

78. Muller R. Studies on disseminated sclerosis. *Acta Med Scand* 1949;S222:1–214.

79. Tillman AJB. The effect of pregnancy on multiple sclerosis and its management. *Res Publ Ass Res Nerv Ment Dis* 1950;28:548–582.

80. Millar JHD. The influence of pregnancy on disseminated sclerosis. *Proc Royal Soc Med* 1961;54:4–7.

81. Leibowitz U, Antonovsky A, Kats R, Alter M. Does pregnancy increase the risk of multiple sclerosis? *J Neurol Neurosurg Psychiat* 1967;30:354–357.

82. Poser S, Raun NE, Wikstrom, Poser W. Pregnancy, oral contraceptives and multiple sclerosis. *Acta Neurol Scandinav* 1979;59:108–118.

83. Ghezzi A, Caputo D. Pregnancy: a factor influencing the course of multiple sclerosis? *Eur Neurol* 1981;20:115–117.

84. Poser S, Poser W. Multiple sclerosis and gestation. *Neurology* 1983;33:1422–1427.

85. Korn-Lubertzki I, Kahana E, Cooper G, Abramsky O. Activity of multiple scleroisis during pregnancy and puerperium. *Ann Neurol* 1984;16:229–231.

86. Birk K, Rudick R. Pregnancy and multiple sclerosis. *Arch Neurol* 1986;43:719–726.

87. Frith JA, McLeod JG. Pregnancy and multiple sclerosis. *J Neurol Neurosurg Psych* 1988;51:495–498.

88. Thompson DS, Nelson LM, Burns A, Burks JS, Franklin GM. The effects of pregnancy in multiple sclerosis: a retrospective study. *Neurology* 1986;36:1097–1099.

89. Nelson LM, Franklin GM, Jones MC, Multiple Sclerosis Study Group. Risk of multiple sclerosis exacerbation during pregnancy and breastfeeding. *JAMA* 1988;259: 3441–3443.

90. Weinshenker BG, Hader W, Carriere W, Baskerville J, Ebers GC. The influence of pregnancy on disability from multiple sclerosis: a population-based study in Middlesex County, Ontario. *Neurology* 1989;39:1438–4440.

91. Bernardi S, Grasso MG, Bertollini R, Orzi F, Fieschi C. The influence of pregnancy on relapses in multiple sclerosis: a cohort study. *Acta Neurol Scand* 1991;84: 403–406.

92. Roullet E, Verdier-Taillefer MH, Amarenco P, Gharbi G, Alperovitch A. Pregnancy and multiple sclerosis: a longitudinal study of 125 remittent patients. *J Neurol Neurosurg Psych* 1993;56:1062–1065.

93. Abramsky O. Pregnancy and multiple sclerosis. *Ann Neurol* 1994;36:S38–S41.

94. Sadovnick AD, Eisen K, Hashimoto SA, et al. Pregnancy and multiple sclerosis. A prospective study. *Arch Neurol* 1994;51:1120–1124.

95. Stenager E, Stenager EN, Jensen K. Effect of pregnancy on the prognosis for multiple sclerosis. A 5-year follow up investigation. *Acta Neurol Scan* 1994;90:305–308.

96. Verdru P, Theys P, D'Hooghe MB, Carton H. Pregnancy and multiple sclerosis: the influence on long term disability. *Clin Neurol Neurosurg* 1994;96:38–41.

97. Worthington J, Jones R, Crawford M, Forti A. Pregnancy and multiple sclerosis—a 3-year prospective study. *J Neurol* 1994;241:228–233.

98. Flachenecker P, Hartung HP. Multiple sclerosis and pregnancy. Overview and status of the European multicenter PRIMS study. *Nervenarzt* 1995;66:97–104.

99. Runmarker B, Andersen O. Pregnancy is associated with a lower risk of onset and a better prognosis in multiple sclerosis. *Brain* 1995;118:253–261.

100. Lorenzi AR, Ford HL. Multiple sclerosis and pregnancy. *Postgrad Med J* 2002;78:460–464.

101. Damek DM, Shuster EA. Pregnancy and multiple sclerosis. *Mayo Clin Proc.* 1997;72:977–989.

102. Verdru P, Theys P, D'Hooghe MB, Carton H. Pregnancy and multiple sclerosis: the influence on long term disability. *Clin Neurol Neurosurg* 1994;96:38–41.

103. Runmarker B, Andersen O. Pregnancy is associated with a lower risk of onset and a better prognosis in multiple sclerosis. *Brain* 1995;118:253–261,285–291.

104. Van Walderveen MA, Tas MW, Barkhof F, et al. Magnetic resonance evaluation of disease activity during pregnancy in multiple sclerosis. *Neurology* 1994;44: 327–329.

105. Confavreux C, Hutchinson M, Hours MM, et al. Rate of pregnancy-related relapses in multiple sclerosis. *N Engl J Med* 1998;339:285–291.

106. Confavreux C, Vukusic S, Adeleine P, et al. Pregnancy and multiple sclerosis (the PRIMS study): two-year results. *Neurology* 2001;56:A197.

107. Achiron A, Rotstein Z, Noy S, Mashiach S, Dulitzky M, Achiron R. Intravenous immunoglobulin treatment in the prevention of childbirth-associated acute exacerbations in multiple sclerosis: a pilot study. *J Neurol* 1996;243:25–28.

108. *Neurology* 2002;58:A455.

109. Coyle PK, Johnson K, Pardo L, Stark Y. *Pregnancy outcomes in patients with multiple sclerosis treated with glatiramer acetate (Copaxone®).* AAN 2003 (abstract).

110. Nelson L, Franklin GM, Jones MC and the Multiple Sclerosis Study Group. Risk of multiple sclerosis exacerbation during pregnancy and breastfeeding. *JAMA* 1988;259:3441–3443.

111. Confavreux C, Hutchinson M, Hours M, et al. Rate of pregnancy related relapses in multiple sclerosis. *N Engl J Med* 1998;339:285–291.

112. Pisacane A, Impagliazzo N, Russo M, Valiani R, et al. Breast feeding and multiple sclerosis. *BMJ* 1994;308: 1411–1412.

113. Giesser BS, Halper J, Cross AH, et al. Multiple sclerosis symptoms fluctuate during menstrual cycle. *MS Exchange* 1991;3:5.

114. Bansil S, Lee HJ, Jindal S, Holtz CR, Cook SD. Correlation between sex hormones and magnetic resonance imaging lesions in multiple sclerosis. *Acta Neurol Scand* 1999;99:91–94.

115. Pozzilli C, Falaschi P, Mainero C, et al. MRI in multiple sclerosis during the menstrual cycle: relationship with sex hormone patterns. *Neurology* 1999;53(3):622–624.

116. Tomassini V, Giugni E, Mainero C, et al. Relationship between sex hormones and MRI activity in relapsing-remitting multiple sclerosis. *Neurology* 2001;56: P04–025.

117. Aronson KJ. Quality of life among persons with multiple sclerosis and their caregivers. *Neurology* 1997;48: 74–80.

118. Villard-Mackintosh L, Vessey MP. Oral contraceptives and reproductive factors in multiple sclerosis incidence. *Contraception* 1993;47:161–168.

119. Minderhoud MJ, Leemhuis JG, Kremer J, Laban E, Smits PML. Sexual disturbances arising from multiple sclerosis. *Acta Neurol Scand* 1984;70:299–306.

120. LaRocca NG. *Employment and multiple sclerosis. Health Services Research Reports Monograph*, National MS Society, 1995.

121. Harvey C. *Economic costs of multiple sclerosis: how much and who pays?* Health Services Research Reports Monograph, National MS Society, 1995.

19 Optic Neuritis

Neil R. Miller, MD

O ptic neuritis is the most common optic nerve-related cause of visual loss in young women of childbearing age. It is important not only with respect to visual function in affected patients but also to their neurologic prognosis.

The term *optic neuritis* means inflammation of the optic nerve. When optic neuritis occurs with a swollen optic disc, it is called *papillitis* or *anterior optic neuritis*. When the optic disc appears normal, the terms *retrobulbar optic neuritis* or *retrobulbar neuritis* are used.

The pathogenesis of most cases of isolated optic neuritis is presumed to be demyelination, similar to that seen in multiple sclerosis (MS). In the absence of signs of MS or other systemic disease, however, optic neuritis is referred to as isolated, monosymptomatic, or idiopathic.

Optic neuritis does not always present as an acute loss of vision. It may develop as insidious progressive or nonprogressive visual dysfunction, and it may even be asymptomatic. Patients with asymptomatic optic neuritis have laboratory evidence of optic nerve dysfunction and may also have subtle clinical evidence of optic nerve damage if appropriate studies are performed.

Because this book is about those neurologic diseases that occur mainly in women, this chapter deals exclusively with acute, chronic, and subclinical demyelinating or idiopathic optic neuritis. For a discussion of optic neuritis caused by processes other than MS, the reader is referred to the chapter entitled "Optic Neuritis" by Smith (1).

IDIOPATHIC AND PRIMARY DEMYELINATING OPTIC NEURITIS

Optic neuritis almost always occurs as an isolated phenomenon without any neurologic or systemic accompaniments or sequelae or as a demyelinating process that precedes the development of MS. There are three forms of optic neuritis: (i) acute, (ii) chronic, and (iii) subclinical.

Acute Idiopathic or Demyelinating Optic Neuritis

Acute idiopathic or demyelinating optic neuritis is by far the most common type of optic neuritis that occurs throughout the world and is the most frequent cause of optic nerve dysfunction in the young adult population (2). Much of our knowledge regarding this form of optic neuritis was obtained from a study, begun in 1988, called the Optic Neuritis Treatment Trial (ONTT) and continued throughout the 1990s as the Longitudinal Optic Neuritis Study (LONS) (3–18). The ONTT was a multicenter controlled clinical trial that was funded by the National Eye Institute of the National Institutes of Health

(NIH) in the United States. The investigators in this trial enrolled 455 patients with acute unilateral optic neuritis. A similar study was performed in Japan (18). Although the primary objective of these studies was the assessment of the efficacy of corticosteroids in the treatment of optic neuritis, the ONTT and LONS, as well as the Japanese Optic Neuritis Study have also provided invaluable information about the clinical profile of optic neuritis, its natural history, and its relationship to MS.

The entry criteria for patients who were entered into the ONTT were a clinical syndrome consistent with unilateral optic neuritis, including a relative afferent pupillary defect and a visual field defect in the affected eye. Visual symptoms had to have begun within 8 days of randomization. The patient could have no history of a previous episode of optic neuritis in the affected eye, no previous corticosteroid treatment for optic neuritis or MS, and no evidence of a systemic disease other than MS as a cause for the optic neuritis. The Japanese trial had similar criteria for entry.

Demographics

The annual incidence of acute optic neuritis is estimated in population-based studies to be between 1 and 5 per 100,000 (19–25). The majority of patients are between the ages of 20 and 50 years, with a mean age of 30–35 years. Nevertheless, optic neuritis can occur at any age, including children in the first and second decades of life and adults in their sixth to eighth decades. Women are much more commonly affected than men, at a ratio of approximately 4:1. Caucasians are affected much more often than are African-Americans, Africans, or Hispanics (26,27).

Symptoms

The two major symptoms in patients with acute optic neuritis are loss of central vision and pain in and around the affected eye.

LOSS OF CENTRAL VISION.   Loss of central visual acuity is reported by over 90% of patients (4,19). Vision loss is typically abrupt, occurring over several hours to several days. Progression over a longer period can occur but should make the clinician suspicious of an alternative disorder. The degree of visual loss varies widely from a minimal reduction to complete blindness with no perception of light. The majority of patients describe diffuse blurred vision, although some recognize that the blurring is predominantly central. Occasionally, patients complain of a loss of a portion of peripheral field, such as the inferior or superior region or even the temporal or nasal region.

The visual loss is monocular in most cases in adults, but in children and in a small percentage of adults, both eyes are simultaneously affected.

OCULAR OR ORBITAL PAIN.   Pain in or around the eye is present in more than 90% of patients with acute optic neuritis. It is usually mild, but it may be extremely severe and may be more debilitating to the patient than the loss of vision. It may precede or occur concurrently with visual loss, usually is exacerbated by eye movement, and generally lasts no more than a few days (4,19). The presence of pain is a helpful differentiating feature from anterior ischemic optic neuropathy, particularly when the pain is severe and when it occurs or worsens during movement of the eyes, features uncommon in the 10 to 12% of ischemic optic neuropathy patients who experience pain (28,29).

POSITIVE VISUAL PHENOMENA.   Up to 30% of patients with optic neuritis experience positive visual phenomena, called *photopsias*, both at the onset of their visual symptoms and during the course of the disorder. These phenomena consist of spontaneous flashing black squares, flashes of light, or showers of sparks, sometimes precipitated by eye movement or certain sounds (30–33).

Signs

An examination of a patient with acute optic neuritis reveals evidence of optic nerve dysfunction (Table 19.1). Visual acuity is almost always decreased, but varies from a mild reduction (e.g., 20/15 to 20/20) to no light perception.

Contrast sensitivity and color vision also are impaired in almost all cases. The reduction in contrast sensitivity often parallels the reduction in visual acuity (34), although in some cases, it is much worse (3). The reduction in color vision is often much worse than would be expected from the level of visual acuity (35,36). Standard color vision testing with the Ishihara or Hardy-Rand-Rittler pseudoisochromatic plates commonly reveals abnormalities in the affected eye, whereas the

---

TABLE 19.1
Features of Typical Optic Neuritis in Adults

- Acute unilateral loss of visual acuity and color vision
- Periocular pain, often exacerbated with eye movement
- Visual field defect, usually central
- Ipsilateral relative afferent pupillary defect
- Absence of anterior or posterior segment inflammation
- Normal or swollen optic disc
- Spontaneous visual improvement beginning in 2 to 4 weeks
- Strong relationship with multiple sclerosis

more sensitive Farnsworth-Munsell 100-Hue test can reveal more subtle defects. Even when the patient can detect all the pseudoisochromatic figures correctly, a careful comparison of the appearance of a single plate by each eye may reveal a striking difference in color and brightness between the two eyes.

Like visual acuity, visual field loss can vary from mild to severe, may be diffuse or focal, and can involve the central or peripheral field (37–39). Indeed, although the classic visual field defect in acute optic neuritis is the central scotoma, almost any type of field defect can occur in the affected eye (39).

A relative afferent pupillary defect (RAPD) is demonstrable with the swinging flashlight test in all unilateral cases of optic neuritis and in cases with bilateral but asymmetric neuritis (40–43). When such a defect is not present, either there is a coexisting optic neuropathy in the fellow eye (e.g., from previous or concurrent asymptomatic optic neuritis) or the visual loss in the affected eye is not caused by optic neuritis or by any other form of optic neuropathy.

The use of a neutral density filter may help uncover a subtle relative afferent pupillary defect in patients with suspected optic neuritis (44). In this test, a 0.3 log-unit neutral density filter is placed in front of one eye and a swinging flashlight test is performed. The filter is then placed in front of the other eye and the swinging flashlight test is again performed. If there is no RAPD, the result of the swinging flashlight test should be the same regardless of which eye is behind the neutral density filter; that is, there should be a mild observable RAPD. On the other hand, if a minimal RAPD is already present, then placing the filter in front of the eye with the RAPD should make it more obvious, whereas placing the filter in front of the opposite eye should result in normal pupillary responses (44).

Patients with optic neuritis also can be shown to have a reduced sensation of brightness in the affected eye by asking them to compare the brightness of a light shone in one eye and then the other (1). This test is simple to perform and extremely helpful in the patient with a questionable RAPD.

About one-third of patients with acute optic neuritis have some degree of disc swelling (4,19) (Figure 19.1). In most cases, the degree of swelling is quite mild; however, in some cases, the swelling is so severe that it mimics the "choked disc" seen in patients with papilledema (Figure 19.2). The degree of disc swelling usually does not correlate with the severity of either visual acuity or visual field loss (4,19,45). Disc or peripapillary hemorrhages and segmental disc swelling are less common in eyes with acute optic neuritis than in eyes with anterior ischemic optic neuropathy (4,46).

The majority of patients with acute idiopathic or demyelinating optic neuritis have a normal optic disc in the affected eye, unless they have had a previous attack

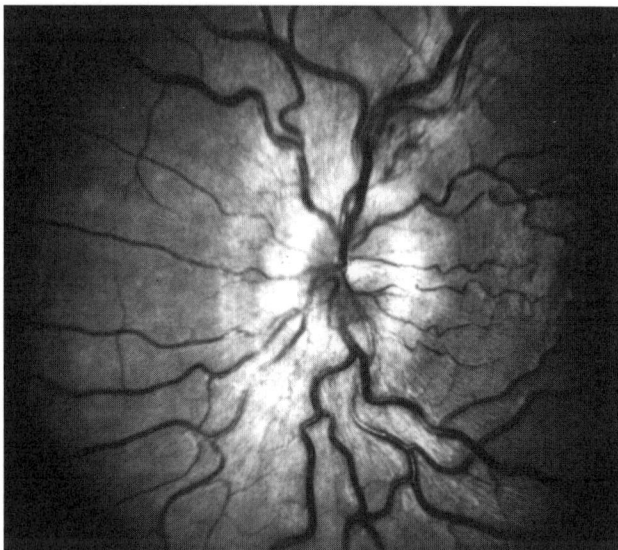

FIGURE 19.1

Mild optic disc swelling in a patient with acute anterior optic neuritis (papillitis).

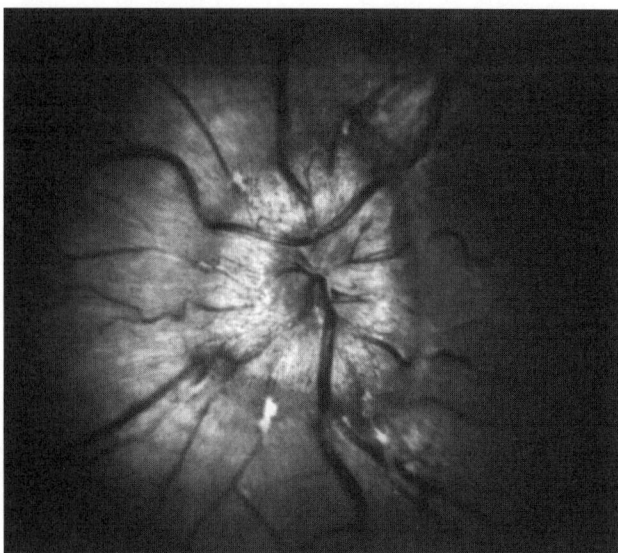

FIGURE 19.2

Severe optic disc swelling in a patient with acute anterior optic neuritis (papillitis). Note resemblance to papilledema.

of acute or asymptomatic optic neuritis or have ongoing chronic optic neuritis (4,19). With time, however, the optic disc usually becomes pale, even as visual acuity, color vision, visual field, and other aspects of visual sensory function improve. The pallor may be diffuse or localized to a particular portion of the optic disc, most often the temporal portion (Figure 19.3).

Slit lamp biomicroscopy in eyes with demyelinating optic neuritis is almost always normal. In some patients

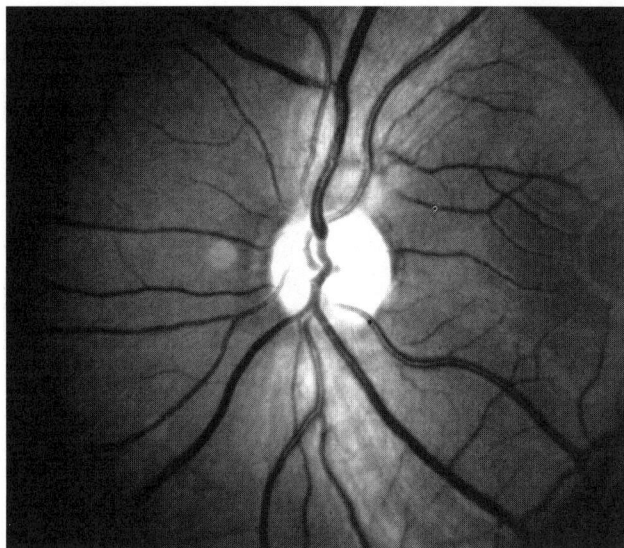

FIGURE 19.3

Diffuse optic disc pallor after an attack of acute retrobulbar optic neuritis. Despite appearance of disc, the patient had 20/20 vision in this eye.

with anterior optic neuritis, a few vitreous cells may be observed, particularly in the vitreous overlying the optic disc. In such cases, sheathing of retinal veins also may be present, especially in patients with MS. Indeed, patients with acute optic neuritis and mild uveitis or retinal phlebitis have an increased risk of developing MS compared with patients with isolated optic neuritis (47,48). When the cellular reaction is extensive, however, etiologies other than demyelination should be considered, including sarcoidosis, syphilis, cat scratch disease, and Lyme disease.

Visual Function in the Fellow Eye

Although bilateral, simultaneous acute optic neuritis is uncommon in adults, a relatively high percentage of patients with acute unilateral optic neuritis have abnormal visual function in their asymptomatic fellow eye, including decreased visual acuity, disturbances of color vision, and visual field defects (4,8). The majority of these deficits resolve over several months, suggesting that such abnormalities are caused by subclinical but concurrent acute inflammation.

Diagnostic, Etiologic, and Prognostic Studies

Studies in patients with presumed acute optic neuritis are usually performed for one of three reasons: (i) to determine if the cause of the optic neuropathy is something other than inflammation, particularly a compressive lesion; (ii) to determine if a cause other than demyelina-

tion is responsible for inflammation of the optic nerve; or (iii) to determine the visual and neurologic prognosis of optic neuritis.

DIAGNOSTIC STUDIES. The major concern of a physician evaluating a patient with sudden visual loss associated with evidence of an optic neuropathy is whether the optic neuropathy is truly optic neuritis or is an acute manifestation of compression from an orbital, canalicular, or intracranial mass. Magnetic resonance imaging (MRI) is the neuroimaging technique of choice in the setting of presumed optic neuritis. It can identify with a high degree of sensitivity mass lesions such as aneurysms that can cause an acute optic neuropathy, and it also can detect evidence of demyelination in the optic nerve, including foci of T2-bright signal, areas of enhancement, and/or enlargement of all or a portion of the nerve (49–54) (Figure 19.4). These abnormalities are much less likely to be seen in patients with other forms of acute optic neuropathy, such as anterior ischemic optic neuropathy (54).

ETIOLOGIC STUDIES. Although systemic and local infectious and inflammatory disorders can cause acute optic neuritis, the majority of such rare cases can be identified by a thorough history and confirmed by appropriate laboratory studies. Thus, in patients without a history of (or suggestive of) sexually transmitted disease, sarcoidosis, cat scratch disease, Lyme disease, systemic lupus erythematosus, or similar disorders, the likelihood of such a condition being responsible for acute optic neuritis is exceptionally low (4,5,55). Serologic tests, chest radiographs, and cerebrospinal fluid (CSF) analysis are unwarranted in such cases unless the patient's course does not follow that of typical optic neuritis.

The most important application of MRI in acute optic neuritis is the identification of signal abnormalities consistent with demyelination in the white matter of the brain, usually in the periventricular region (Figure 19.5) (9,19,56,57). The presence of such lesions suggests not only that the diagnosis of optic neuritis is correct but that the cause of the optic neuritis is demyelination.

Another application of MR in patients with acute optic neuritis is MR spectroscopy. This technique can be used to determine changes in the concentration of N-acetyl-aspartate, a neuronal marker, which may reflect axon dysfunction or loss in normal-appearing white matter and may predict those patients who are at increased risk to develop MS (58).

PROGNOSTIC STUDIES. A substantial percentage of patients with isolated optic neuritis develop MS within months to years after the onset of optic neuritis. It would be helpful if there were certain studies that

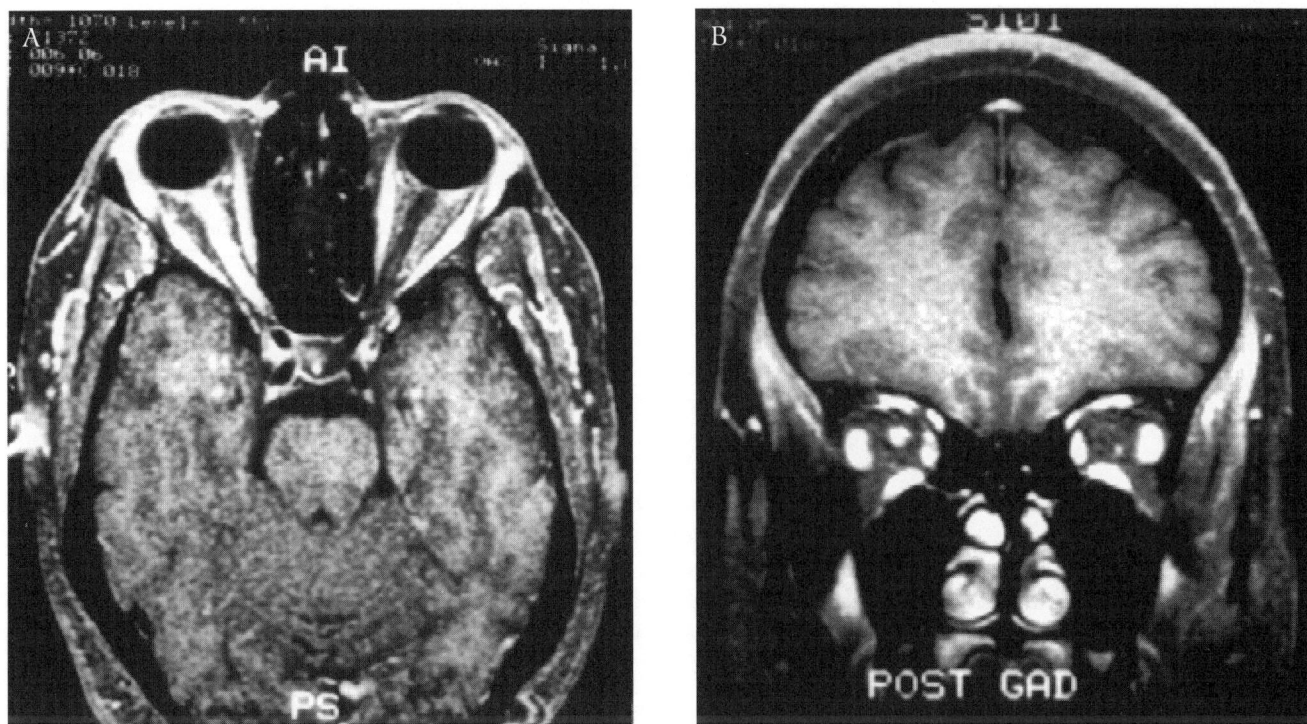

FIGURE 19.4

Magnetic resonance imaging (MRI) of the optic nerve in a young woman with acute optic neuritis affecting the right eye. A. Enhanced T1-weighted axial image shows extensive enhancement and diffuse enlargement of the right optic nerve from the back of the eye to the optic canal. B. Enhanced T1-weighted coronal image shows enhancing right optic nerve in cross section.

could be performed in a patient with isolated optic neuritis that would allow the accurate prediction of the odds of subsequent development of MS. In fact, multiple studies indicate that the results of MRI in the patient with isolated acute optic neuritis correlate with the eventual development of MS (59–61). The more white-matter lesions that are present in the brain of a patient with acute optic neuritis, the greater the risk of MS over the subsequent 10 years (Figure 19.6) (61). Among patients with isolated optic neuritis in the ONTT, the cumulative percentage developing MS within 10 years of the onset of the optic neuritis was 39%; however, among patients with normal MRI, 24% developed MS compared with 64% of patients with more than three lesions (61).

As noted above, MR spectroscopy may one day be useful in predicting which patients with optic neuritis are at increased risk to develop MS; however, there is at present insufficient information to determine if this is the case or if the technique could ever be cost-effective.

Just as patients with acute optic neuritis and multiple white-matter lesions in the brain have a high risk of developing MS, certain patients with acute optic neuritis have a very low risk of developing MS. Patients with acute, painless anterior optic neuritis associated with a normal MRI scan have a probability similar to that of a normal age- and sex-matched population of developing optic neuritis over the succeeding 10 years (61).

SEROLOGIC AND CEREBROSPINAL FLUID STUDIES. Immunologic abnormalities in the CSF are common in patients with optic neuritis, occurring in up to 79% of cases (55,57,62,63). As in patients with MS, CSF pleocytosis, elevated protein concentration, elevated levels of myelin basic protein, increased IgG ratio and IgG synthesis, oligoclonal bands, kappa-light chains, and increased concentrations of cytokines may be detected. Although the predictive value of these CSF findings for the development of MS is somewhat controversial, there appear to be certain CSF and even serologic risk factors that increase the likelihood that a patient with isolated optic neuritis will eventually develop MS. These include oligoclonal banding and elevated levels of myelin basic protein, CSF and serum elevations of cytokines, and positivity for certain HLA types (55,57,64–66). However, the robust predictive value of baseline MRI diminishes the relative usefulness of these other studies in the individual patient with acute optic neuritis who wishes to have some idea of prognosis for the development of MS.

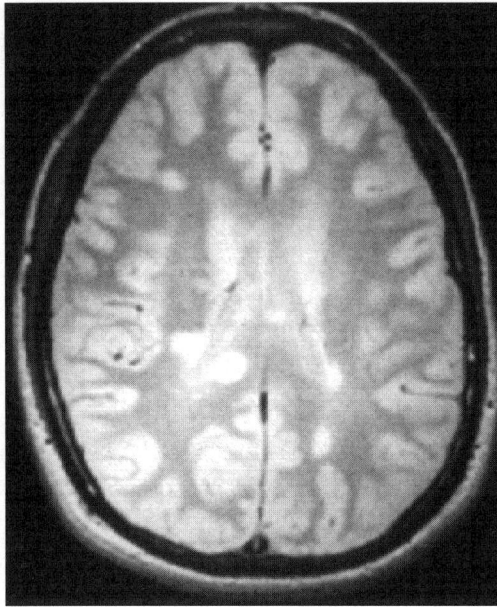

FIGURE 19.5

Magnetic resonance image (MRI) of the brain in a young woman at the time of an attack of acute retrobulbar optic neuritis. The patient had no history of previous neurologic symptoms and had no neurologic signs on examination. T1-weighted axial image shows multiple ovoid lesions in the periventricular white matter of both cerebral hemispheres.

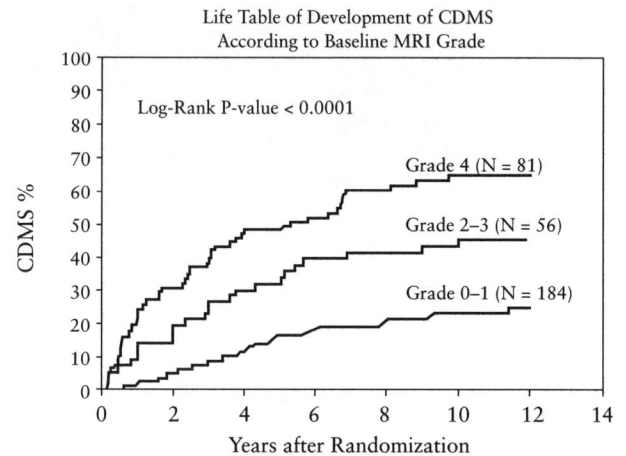

FIGURE 19.6

Graph showing relationship of risk of developing multiple sclerosis (MS) after an attack of acute optic neuritis and initial appearance of brain magnetic resonance imaging (MRI) in patients enrolled in Optic Neuritis Treatment Trial and followed for at least 10 years since the attack. Grade 0–1 indicates normal MR scan, whereas grades 2–4 indicate increasing numbers of white-matter lesions in the periventricular region. Note that the more lesions present at the time of an attack of acute optic neuritis, the higher the likelihood of developing MS over the subsequent 10 years.

Natural History

The natural history of acute demyelinating optic neuritis is to worsen over several days to 2 weeks, and then to improve. The improvement initially is fairly rapid. It then levels off, but further improvement can continue to occur 1 year after the onset of visual symptoms (11,15,67). Among patients in the ONTT who received placebo, visual acuity began to improve within 3 weeks of onset in 79% and within 5 weeks in 93%. For most patients in this study, the recovery of visual acuity was nearly complete by 5 weeks after onset. The mean visual acuity 1 year after an attack of otherwise uncomplicated optic neuritis, is 20/15, and this level of vision remains for up to 10 years following the attack, unless the patient develops another process (61). Indeed, even patients who have recurrences of optic neuritis tend to experience a return of visual acuity to near normal levels, and fewer than 10% of patients have permanent visual acuity less than 20/40 10 years after an attack (61). Other parameters of visual function, including contrast sensitivity, color perception, and visual field, improve in conjunction with the improvement in visual acuity and also tend to remain stable over the subsequent decade (61).

The visual improvement that occurs with acute optic neuritis tends to do so regardless of the degree of visual loss, although some correlation exists between the severity of visual loss and the degree of eventual recovery (5,12,68). In the ONTT, of the 167 eyes in which the baseline visual acuity was 20/200 or worse, only 10 (6%) had this level of vision 6 months later. Of 28 patients whose initial visual acuity in the affected eye was light perception or no light perception, 18 (64%) recovered to 20/40 or better (5,12). Factors such as age, gender, optic disc appearance, and pattern of the initial visual field defect do not appear to have any appreciable effect on the visual outcome (15). Race does seem to be a factor, however, with Africans and African-Americans tending to have a poorer outcome than Caucasians (26,27).

Even though the overall prognosis for visual acuity after an attack of acute optic neuritis is extremely good, some patients have persistent severe visual loss after a single episode (4,5,19,69). Furthermore, patients with recovered optic neuritis frequently complain that their vision in the affected eye is "not right," "remains fuzzy," or that colors are "washed out" (70). One cause of these symptoms is probably a subtle abnormality in the visual field, in which patients experience an abnormally rapid disappearance of focal visual stimuli and abnormally rapid fatigue in sensitivity. These patients typically complain that when they look at something, it appears as if they have "holes" in their vision, some of which fill in while other new ones appear: the so-called "Swiss cheese" visual field

(71). This phenomenon is not limited to optic neuritis, however; it can occur in other optic neuropathies.

Following an episode of acute optic neuritis, some patients describe transient visual blurring during exercise, during a hot bath or shower, or during emotional stress (72,73). This phenomenon, called *Uhthoff's symptom*, also may occur with chronic or subclinical optic neuritis, with Leber hereditary optic neuropathy, and with optic neuropathies from other causes (74,75). Nevertheless, it occurs in about 10% of patients after an attack of demyelinating optic neuritis and, when present, may be a marker for abnormal brain MRI and for the subsequent development of MS (76). Some patients with Uhthoff's symptom note that their visual symptoms improve in colder temperatures or when drinking cold beverages. Two major hypotheses regarding Uhthoff's symptom are that (i) the elevation of body temperature interferes directly with axon conduction and (ii) exercise or a rise in body temperature changes the metabolic environment of the axon which, in turn, interferes with conduction (77–79).

Patients who experience an attack of acute optic neuritis have an increased risk of developing a recurrent attack in the same eye or an acute optic neuritis in the fellow eye (5,80). The risk of a recurrent or new attack of optic neuritis in patients enrolled in the ONTT over 10 years was 35%, with most of the patients experiencing recurrent or new events in the first 5 years after the initial attack (5,61,80). Patients who experience one or two recurrent attacks of acute optic neuritis usually experience substantial improvement in vision, often to normal; however, after multiple attacks of optic neuritis, visual function may improve little or not at all (81,82).

Neurologic Prognosis

Optic neuritis is the initial manifestation of MS in about 20% of patients (83). Several prospective studies have been performed to determine the potential for the development of MS in patients who experience an attack of acute optic neuritis. Although retrospective studies provide figures ranging from 11.5% to 85% (20,24,81,82,84), a study from Germany reported that the risk of developing MS after an attack of acute optic neuritis was 54% over the subsequent 8 years (85). The LONS found that the overall risk of developing MS was almost 40% in patients followed 10 years after an attack of acute optic neuritis (61), and an Australian group of investigators reported a 52% risk of MS after acute optic neuritis in a 13-year prospective study (86). Other prospective studies indicate that the risk of MS eventually increases to about 75% in women and 34% in men with 15 to 20 years of follow-up (87–89). Among 95 incident cases of acute optic neuritis in Olmstead County, Minnesota, the estimated risk of MS was 39% by 10 years, 49% by 20 years, 54% by 30 years, and 60% by 40 years (25). The average time interval from an initial attack of optic neuritis until other symptoms and signs of MS develop varies considerably; however, most studies indicate that the majority of persons who develop MS after optic neuritis do so within 7 years of the onset of visual symptoms (83,61). It therefore seems appropriate to consider most cases of acute optic neuritis a limited form of MS and to counsel patients appropriately (90). We believe that most patients should be told about the relationship between optic neuritis and MS and that this conversation should include a frank discussion of MS and its prognosis. Most patients appreciate this approach and handle this information much better than most physicians anticipate. Indeed, if the physician does not discuss the association of optic neuritis and MS with his or her patient, the patient will almost certainly find out about it from a friend, acquaintance, another physician, or the Internet.

Certain risk factors increase the likelihood that a patient with acute optic neuritis will eventually develop MS. As noted above, the most highly predictive baseline factor is multiple lesions in the periventricular white matter on MRI (60). Gender also appears to be a risk factor, but only in patients with a normal MRI. Among patients in the ONTT who had a normal MRI at the time of their attack of acute optic neuritis, 8% of men and 28% of women have developed evidence of MS (61). Other risk factors for the development of MS in both men and women are Caucasian race, a family history of MS, a history of previous ill-defined neurologic complaints, a previous episode of acute optic neuritis, and winter onset of optic neuritis (10,17). None of these factors predicts the development of MS as much as the results of MRI, however (60).

Although the evidence of immunologic dysfunction (especially oligoclonal banding) in the CSF is common in patients with acute optic neuritis, whether or not their presence in patients with clinically isolated optic neuritis increases the risk for the subsequent development of MS remains controversial. Studies indicate that 25 to 50% of patients with isolated acute optic neuritis and abnormal CSF remain free of neurologic manifestations of MS for many years (if not for life), whereas 10 to 50% of patients with acute optic neuritis and normal CSF develop other manifestations of MS during the same period (55,91). In view of these findings, it seems that CSF abnormalities alone are not a primary risk factor in determining whether a patient with acute optic neuritis eventually develops clinical evidence of disseminated demyelination.

Considerable evidence suggests that genetic factors play a role in the development of MS (92–95). This is based on the familial incidence of the disease, twin studies, and HLA typing patterns. The major predisposing genes in MS are the HLA class II molecules, in particular the haplotype HLA-DR2, which is especially common among MS patients of Northern and Western European ancestry. This haplotype represents a susceptibility locus in specific populations, but a direct contribution to the pathogenesis of the disease is likely small, and presence of the haplotype is not necessary for disease expression in all patients. Indeed, patient groups with MS in different ethnic populations are immunogenetically distinct and thus have HLA polymorphisms that are common within each population but that are different from other populations. HLA type does not seem to strongly influence the subsequent risk for MS in patients with isolated optic neuritis, however. Although the combination of HLA typing and MRI may slightly increase predictive ability, MRI is a much stronger and reliable indicator of risk.

Most studies suggest that patients in whom acute optic neuritis is the initial manifestation of MS tend to have a more benign course than patients in whom MS presents with nonvisual symptoms and signs. Other studies, however, report no difference in the eventual outcome of the disease.

Treatment

Several theoretical reasons exist to consider treating patients with acute optic neuritis: i) to improve visual outcome, ii) to speed visual recovery, and iii) to protect the patient against the development of MS (96,97).

No drugs have been shown to improve the ultimate visual prognosis after an attack of acute optic neuritis compared with the natural history of the disorder. Specifically, the ONTT, the LONS, and similar studies performed in Japan and Europe indicate that the treatment of acute optic neuritis with a 2-week course of low-dose prednisone (1 mg/kg/day) does not improve short- or long-term visual outcome and does *not* speed visual recovery (5,19,61,98). In addition, this treatment is associated with a higher incidence of recurrent and new attacks of optic neuritis (5,61). Thus, it is inappropriate to treat any patient with acute, presumed demyelinating optic neuritis with this regimen.

Treatment with 1 gram of methylprednisolone sodium succinate for 3 days, in either divided doses or a single daily dose, followed by a 2-week course of lower-dose prednisone (1 mg/kg/day) speeds recovery of visual function by 3 to 6 weeks, although it does not affect visual outcome (5).

As noted earlier, a substantial percentage of patients who experience an attack of acute optic neuritis subsequently develop MS. In addition, MS may present as a solitary nonvisual manifestation, such as an episode of weakness or numbness of an extremity or double vision from an oculomotor nerve paresis or internuclear ophthalmoplegia. The Controlled High-Risk Subjects Avonex® Multiple Sclerosis (CHAMPS) study was designed to determine

if interferon beta-1a has any effect on the development of MS in patients who experience an initial acute demyelinating episode (99). The CHAMPS study followed a randomized, double-blind, placebo-controlled design with a total of 383 patients enrolled between 1996 and 2000. All subjects had experienced an initial, acute demyelinating event, 50% of whom had acute optic neuritis and had at least two white-matter lesions consistent with prior subclinical demyelination in the brain by MRI. All patients were first treated according to the ONTT protocol within 14 days of symptom onset with IV methylprednisolone (1 gm/day) for 3 days, followed by oral prednisone (1 mg/kg/day) for 11 days, followed by a rapid taper. During the second week of steroid therapy, about 50% of the patients began receiving weekly intramuscular injections of Avonex® (30 mcg), whereas the remaining 50% began receiving weekly IM placebo injections. The primary outcome measure chosen for the CHAMPS study was the rate of development of clinically definite MS defined as a new neurologic lesion in a different central nervous system (CNS) location lasting more than 48 hours, progressive neurologic disease following 1 month of stable or improved symptoms, or an increase in Kurtzke Expanded Disability Status Scale (EDSS) of 1.5 points without relapse. The secondary outcome measure of the study was the effect of Avonex® on objective MRI findings.

The CHAMPS study was terminated early when an interim preplanned review of the data showed that Avonex® had a beneficial effect in slowing the rate of development to clinically definite MS (CDMS). Most patients had been enrolled in the study for 24 months, and the positive effect of interferon beta-1a had been noted at each 6-month follow-up visit. Kaplan-Meier analysis revealed that Avonex® reduced the development to CDMS in these patients by 43% compared with placebo (p=0.002). The cumulative probability of developing CDMS after 3 years demonstrated a rate ratio of .56 (p=0.002) and an adjusted rate of .49 (p<0.001), with a 35% chance of developing MS on the drug versus a 50% chance on placebo. Flu-like symptoms were seen in the Avonex®-treated group, but the safety and tolerability of Avonex® was comparable to placebo (99).

With regard to the second outcome measure, Avonex® was associated with a 1% increase in the volume of lesions seen on MRI versus a 16% increased volume seen with placebo after 18 months. There were also fewer new and enlarging lesions and 67% fewer enhancing lesions in the treated group compared with the placebo group.

The results of the CHAMPS study indicate that treatment with Avonex® shortly after an initial demyelinating event in patients with white-matter brain lesions on MRI substantially reduces the risk of the development of CDMS in such patients (99,100).

Another clinical trial in Europe, PRISMS (Prevention of Relapses and Disability by Interferon beta-1a Subcutaneously in Multiple Sclerosis), was a double-blind, placebo-controlled study of 560 patients with EDSS scores of 0 to 50, from 22 centers in nine countries (101). These patients were randomly assigned to receive subcutaneous recombinant interferon beta-1a (Rebif®) in a dose of 22 mcg (n=189), the same drug but in a dose of 44 mcg (n=184), or placebo (n=187) 3 times a week for 2 years. Neurologic examinations were performed on all patients every 3 months. All patients had MRI twice yearly, and 205 patients had monthly scans during the first 9 months of treatment.

It was found that the relapse rate was significantly lower at 1 and 2 years with both doses of Rebif® compared with placebo. In addition, time to first relapse was prolonged to 3 and 5 months in the 22 mcg and 44 mcg groups, respectively, and the proportion of relapse-free patients was significantly increased ($p<0.05$). Rebif® also delayed the progression in disability and decreased accumulated disability compared with placebo; the accumulation of burden of disease and number of active lesions on MRI was lower in both treated groups than in the placebo group (101).

PRISMS 4 reported the 3- and 4-year follow-up of patients in the original study (102). This report also included 172 randomized patients who initially received placebo but who were subsequently placed on Rebif® in a dose of 22 or 44 mcg 3 times a week. The investigators concluded that clinical and MRI benefit continued for both doses up to 4 years, with evidence of a dose response; however, outcomes were consistently better for patients treated all 4 years with Rebif® than for patients in the crossover groups (102).

Trials with a third form of interferon beta—Betaseron®—have shown results similar to those of the PRISMS and CHAMPS studies (103).

Several therapies other than interferon beta have been or are currently being evaluated in patients with optic neuritis. For example, Noseworthy et al. (104) found that the administration of intravenous immunoglobulin (IVIg) to patients with persistent visual loss after an attack of acute optic neuritis did not improve vision to a degree that merited general use.

Management Recommendations

In a patient with the typical features of optic neuritis, a clinical diagnosis can be made with a high degree of certainty without the need for ancillary testing. (See Table 19.2). Brain MRI is a powerful predictor of the short-term probability of MS (for at least the first 10 years) and should be considered for all patients with acute optic neuritis. We would avoid the use of low-dose oral prednisone alone to reduce the risk of recurrent or new attacks of optic neuritis, but we would consider treating patients with abnormal MRIs and patients with normal MRIs

---

TABLE 19.2
Management of Acute Optic Neuritis in an Adult

- Avoid low-dose oral steroids
- Obtain a brain MRI before and immediately after IV injection of a paramagnetic contrast agent
- Use high-dose IV/low-dose oral steroid regimen in patients with an abnormal MRI or those in need of rapid visual recovery, such as monocular patients or those with occupational requirements
- Consider treatment with interferon beta-1a for patients with abnormal MRI scan to reduce the risk of developing clinically definite MS

---

who wish to experience a greater speed of recovery with 1 g of methylprednisolone per day for 3 days, followed by a 2-week course of oral prednisone in a dose of 1 mg/kg/day (105,106). We and others also recommend referral of all patients with white-matter lesions on MRI to a neurologist for the consideration of treatment with interferon beta-1a to reduce the risk of subsequent MS (105-108).

CHRONIC DEMYELINATING OPTIC NEURITIS

It was once stated that, for all intents and purposes, chronic optic neuritis does not occur. The reason for this dogmatic statement was that many patients with mass lesions compressing the intracranial portion of the optic nerve were being diagnosed as having chronic optic neuritis, thus leading to the delayed treatment of the underlying lesion, with resultant permanent visual loss and even death in some cases. Thus, the statement that chronic optic neuritis was never a tenable diagnosis was made in an effort to raise the consciousness of the majority of physicians to look for another potentially treatable cause of unilateral progressive optic neuropathy.

In fact, chronic optic neuritis not only occurs but is not uncommon, occurring in about 10% of patients with MS. There are two types of chronic optic neuritis, both of which occur insidiously. One does not progress, whereas progressive visual loss occurs in the other.

Some patients with chronic MS are aware of their visual disturbance, whereas others are unaware of the problem but can be shown to have an optic neuropathy by clinical testing (e.g., visual acuity, color vision, visual fields, ophthalmoscopy) (109–111).

Most patients with chronic unilateral optic neuritis develop visual symptoms after other signs and symptoms of MS have developed, and it is for this reason that the percentage of patients with MS and evidence of chronic progressive optic neuritis increases the longer patients are followed. Nevertheless, slowly progressive visual loss or complaints of blurred or distorted vision in one or both eyes are the first symptoms of underlying neurologic disease in some patients. We are unaware of any consistent efficacious treatment for chronic progressive demyelinating optic neuritis, although individual case reports detailing improvement after treatment with various immunomodulatory agents have been published (112). As new therapies for other forms of chronic progressive MS become available, it is possible that the symptoms and signs of chronic optic neuritis also may respond to treatment.

SUBCLINICAL OPTIC NEURITIS

A substantial percentage of patients with MS have laboratory evidence of optic nerve dysfunction even though they have a normal clinical examination. This is not surprising given that the anterior visual pathways in patients with MS show damage in up to 100% in autopsy studies.

Visually asymptomatic patients suspected or known to have MS may be demonstrated to have disturbances of the visual sensory pathways by electrophysiologic testing. Visual evoked potentials (VEPs) seem to be a particularly sensitive indicator of optic nerve and other visual sensory pathway disturbances in such patients (37,113–117). In addition, psychophysical tests of visual function, such as contrast sensitivity using a Pelli-Robson chart, Arden gratings, oscilloscope screen projections, or similar techniques, may reveal abnormalities in patients with MS who are visually asymptomatic (37,110,116–118). Some psychophysical tests, such as the measurements of sustained visual resolution and the assessment of chromatic, luminance, spatial, and temporal sensitivity, give similar results (119) but are too complex and time-consuming to be of use in screening patients in clinical practice. Other tests, give little more information that one can obtain by an otherwise complete clinical and electrophysiologic examination. One such test assesses the presence or absence of the Pulfrich phenomenon by having the patient gaze at a pendulum swinging at right angles to the line of sight and determine if the pendulum appears to the patient to be swinging in a elliptical path. In another test, the "light of colors" test, a bright light is aimed directly in one eye at a distance of 2.5 cm for 10 seconds while the other eye is covered; the patient then closes both eyes and reports the sequences of colors and duration of the afterimage.

References

1. Smith CH. Optic neuritis. In: Miller NR, Newman NJ (eds.) *Walsh and Hoyt's Clinical Neuro-Ophthalmology*. 5th ed., vol. 1. Baltimore: Lippincott, Williams & Wilkins. 2005;5283–347.
2. Volpe NJ. Optic neuritis: historical aspects. *J Neuroophthalmol* 2001;21:302–309.
3. Beck RW. Optic Neuritis Study Group. The Optic Neuritis Treatment Trial. *Arch Ophthalmol* 1988;106:1051–1053.
4. Optic Neuritis Study Group. The clinical profile of acute optic neuritis: experience of the Optic Neuritis Treatment Trial. *Arch Ophthalmol* 1991;109:1673–1678.
5. Beck RW, Cleary PA, Anderson MM Jr, et al. A randomized, controlled trial of corticosteroids in the treatment of acute optic neuritis. *N Engl J Med* 1992;326:581–588.
6. Beck RW. Optic Neuritis Study Group. The Optic Neuritis Treatment Trial: implications for clinical practice. *Arch Ophthalmol* 1992;110:331–332.
7. Beck RW. Optic Neuritis Study Group. Corticosteroid treatment of optic neuritis: a need to change treatment practices. *Neurology* 1992;42:1133–1135.
8. Beck RW, Kupersmith MJ, Cleary PA, et al. Fellow eye abnormalities in acute unilateral optic neuritis: experience of the Optic Neuritis Treatment Trial. *Ophthalmology* 1993;100:691–698.
9. Beck RW, Arrington J, Murtagh FR, et al. Brain MRI in acute optic neuritis: experience of The Optic Neuritis Study Group. *Arch Neurol* 1993;8:841–846.
10. Beck RW, Cleary PA, Trobe JD, et al. The effect of corticosteroids for acute optic neuritis on the subsequent development of multiple sclerosis. *N Engl J Med* 1993;329:1764–1769.
11. Beck RW, Cleary PA. Optic Neuritis Study Group: Optic Neuritis Treatment Trial: one-year follow-up results. *Arch Ophthalmol* 1993;111:773–775.
12. Beck RW, Cleary PA. Optic Neuritis Study Group: recovery from severe visual loss in optic neuritis. *Arch Ophthalmol* 1993;111:300.
13. Beck RW, Diehl L, Cleary PA, et al. The Pelli-Robson letter chart: normative data for young adults. *Clin Vis Sci* 1993;8:207–210.
14. Cleary PA, Beck RW, Anderson MM Jr, et al. Design, methods and conduct of the Optic Neuritis Treatment Trial. *Controlled Clin Trials* 1993;14:123–142.
15. Beck RW, Cleary PA, Backlund J-C, et al. The course of visual recovery after optic neuritis: experience of the Optic Neuritis Treatment Trial. *Ophthalmology* 1994;101:1771–1778.
16. Beck RW. The Optic Neuritis Treatment Trial: three-year follow-up results. *Arch Ophthalmol* 1995;113:136–137.
17. Beck RW, Trobe JD. Optic Neuritis Study Group: what have we learned from the Optic Neuritis Treatment Trial? *Ophthalmology* 1995;102:1504–1508.
18. Beck RW, Trobe JD. Optic Neuritis Study Group. The Optic Neuritis Treatment Trial: putting the results in perspective. *J Neuroophthalmol* 1995;15:131–135.
19. Wakakura M, Mashimo K, Oono S. Multicenter clinical trial for evaluating methylprednisolone pulse treatment of idiopathic optic neuritis in Japan: Optic Neuritis Treatment Trial Multicenter Cooperative Research Group (ONMRG). *Jpn J Ophthalmol* 1999;133–138.
20. Percy AK, Nobrega FT, Kurland LT. Optic neuritis and multiple sclerosis: an epidemiologic study. *Arch Ophthalmol* 1972;87:135–139.
21. Wikström J. The epidemiology of optic neuritis in Finland. *Acta Neurol Scand* 1975;52:167–178.
22. Kahana E, Alter M, Feldman S. Optic neuritis in relation to multiple sclerosis. *J Neurol* 1976;213:87–95.
23. Haller P, Patzold U, et al. Optic neuritis in Hanover: an epidemiologic and serogenetic study. In: Bauer JH, Poser S, Ritter G, (eds.) *Progress in multiple sclerosis research*. New York: Springer; 1980;546–548.

24. Kinnunen E. The incidence of optic neuritis and its prognosis for multiple sclerosis. *Acta Neurol Scand* 1983;68:371–377.

25. Rodriguez M, Siva A, Cross SA, et al. Optic neuritis: a population-based study in Olmsted County, Minnesota. *Neurology* 1995;45:244–250.

26. Phillips PH, Newman NJ, Lynn MJ. Optic neuritis in African Americans. *Arch Neurol* 1998;186–192.

27. Pokroy R, Modi G, Saffer D. Optic neuritis in an urban black African community. *Eye* 2001;15:469–473.

28. Swartz NG, Beck RW, Savino PJ, et al. Pain in anterior ischemic optic neuropathy. *J Neuroophthalmol* 1995;15:9–10.

29. Gerling J, Janknecht P, Kommerell G. Orbital pain in optic neuritis and anterior ischemic optic neuropathy. *Neuro-ophthalmology* 1998;19:93–99.

30. McDonald WI, Barnes D. The ocular manifestations of multiple sclerosis. Abnormalities of the afferent visual system. *J Neurol Neurosurg Psychiatry* 1992;55:747–752.

31. Davis FA, Bergen D, Schauf C, et al. Movement phosphenes in optic neuritis: a new clinical sign. *Neurology* 1976;26:1100–1104.

32. Lessell S, Cohen MM. Phosphenes induced by sound. *Neurology* 1979;29:1524–1527.

33. Page NGR, Bolger JP, Sanders MD. Auditory evoked phosphenes in optic nerve disease. *J Neurol Neurosurg Psychiatry* 1982;45:7–12.

34. Sanders EA, Volkers AC, Van der Poel JC, et al. Spatial contrast sensitivity function in optic neuritis. *Neuro-ophthalmology* 1984;4:255–259.

35. Tsukamoto M, Adachi-Usami E. Color vision in multiple sclerosis with optic neuritis. *Acta Soc Ophthalmol Jpn* 1987; 91:613–621.

36. Menage MJ, Papakostopoulos D, Hart JCD, et al. The Farnsworth-Munsell 100 hue test in the first episode of demyelinating optic neuritis. *Br J Ophthalmol* 1993;77:68–74.

37. Kupersmith MJ, Nelson JI, Seiple WH, et al. The 20/20 eye in multiple sclerosis. *Neurology* 1983;33:1015–1020.

38. Vighetto A, Grochowicki M, Aimard, G. Altitudinal hemianopia in multiple sclerosis. *Neuro-ophthalmology* 1991;11:25–27.

39. Keltner JL, Johnson CA, Spurr JO, et al. Baseline visual field profile of optic neuritis: the experience of the Optic Neuritis Treatment Trial. *Arch Ophthalmol* 1993;111:231–234.

40. Stanley JA, Baise, G. The swinging flashlight test to detect minimal optic neuropathy. *Arch Ophthalmol* 1968;80:769–771.

41. Thompson HS. Pupillary signs in the diagnosis of optic nerve disease. *Trans Ophthalmol Soc UK* 1976;96:377–381.

42. Ellis CK. The afferent pupillary defect in acute optic neuritis. *J Neurol Neurosurg Psychiatry* 1979;42:1008–1017.

43. Cox TA, Thompson HS, Corbett JJ. Relative afferent pupillary defects in optic neuritis. *Am J Ophthalmol* 1981;92:685–690.

44. Digre KB. Principles and techniques of examination of the pupils, accommodation, and the lacrimal system. In: Miller NR, Newman NJ, (eds.) *Walsh and Hoyt's clinical neuro-ophthalmology*, 5th ed., vol. 1. Baltimore: Williams & Wilkins, 1998;933-960.

45. Perkin GD, Rose FC. *Optic neuritis and its differential diagnosis.* Oxford: Oxford Medical Press, 1979.

46. Warner JEA, Lessell S, Rizzo JF III, et al. Does optic disc appearance distinguish ischemic optic neuropathy from optic neuritis? *Arch Ophthalmol* 1997;115:1408–1410.

47. Lightman S, McDonald WI, Bird AC, et al. Retinal venous sheathing in optic neuritis: its significance for the pathogenesis of multiple sclerosis. *Brain* 1987;110:405–414.

48. Birch MK, Barbosa S, Blumhardt LD, et al. Retinal venous sheathing and the blood-retinal barrier in multiple sclerosis. *Arch Ophthalmol* 1966;114:34–39.

49. Miller DH, Ormerod IEC, McDonald WI, et al. The early risk of multiple sclerosis after optic neuritis. *J Neurol Neurosurg Psychiatry* 1988;51:1569–1571.

50. Youl BD, Turano G, Miller DH, et al. The pathophysiology of acute optic neuritis: an association of gadolinium leakage with clinical and electrophysiological deficits. *Brain* 1991;114:2437–2450.

51. Guy J, Mao J, Bidgood WD Jr, et al. Enhancement and demyelination of the intraorbital optic nerve: fat suppression magnetic resonance imaging. *Ophthalmology* 1992;99:713–719.

52. Vaphiades MS. Disk edema and cranial MRI optic nerve enhancement: how long is too long? *Surv Ophthalmol* 2001;46:56–58.

53. Yieh F-S, Chou P-I. Bilateral optic nerve enlargement in optic neuritis. *Ann Ophthalmol* 2001;33:76–78.

54. Rizzo JF III, Andreoli CM, Rabinov JD. Use of magnetic resonance imaging to differentiate optic neuritis and nonarteritic anterior ischemic optic neuropathy. *Ophthalmology* 2002;109:1679–1684.

55. Rolak LA, Beck RB, Paty DW, et al. Cerebrospinal fluid in acute optic neuritis: experience of the Optic Neuritis Study Group. *Neurology* 1996;46:368–372.

56. Jacobs L, Kinkel PR, Kinkel WR. Silent brain lesions in patients with isolated idiopathic optic neuritis: a clinical and nuclear magnetic resonance imaging study. *Arch Neurol* 1986;43:452–455.

57. Frederiksen JL. A prospective study of acute optic neuritis: clinical, MRI, CSF, neurophysiological, and HLA findings. *Acta Ophthalmol Scand* 2000;78:490–491.

58. Tourbah A, Stievenart J-L, Abanou A, et al. Normal-appearing white matter in optic neuritis and multiple sclerosis: a comparative proton spectroscopy study. *Neuroradiology* 1999;41:738–743.

59. Frederiksen J, Larsson HBW, Olesen J, et al. MRI, VEP, SEP and biothesiometry suggest monosymptomatic acute optic neuritis to be a first manifestation of multiple sclerosis. *Acta Neurol Scand* 1991;83:343–350.

60. Optic Neuritis Study Group. The 5-year risk of MS after optic neuritis. *Neurology* 1997;49:1404–1413.

61. Beck RW, Probe JD, Moke PS, et al. High- and low-risk profiles for the development of multiple sclerosis within ten years after optic neuritis: experience of the optic neuritis trial. *Arch Othmalol* 2003;121:944–949.

62. Frederiksen JL, Larsson HBW, Oleson J. Correlation of magnetic resonance imaging and CSF findings in patients with acute monosymptomatic optic neuritis. *Acta Neurol Scand* 1992;86:317–322.

63. Söderström M, Lindqvist M, Hiller J, et al. Optic neuritis: findings on MRI, CSF examination and HLA class II typing in 60 patients and results of a short-term follow-up. *J Neurol* 1994;241:391–397.

64. Deckert-Schlüter M, Schlüter D, Schwendemann G. Evaluation of IL-2, sIL2R, IL-6, TNF-a, and IL-1b in serum and CSF of patients with optic neuritis. *J Neurol Sci* 1992;113:50–54.

65. Söderström M, Link H, Xu Z, et al. Optic neuritis and multiple sclerosis: anti-MBP and anti-MBP peptide antibody-secreting cells are accumulated in CSF. *Neurology* 1993;43:1215–1222.

66. Link J, Söderström M, Kostulas V, et al. Optic neuritis is associated with myelin basic protein and proteolipid protein reactive cells producing interferon-gamma, interleukin-4, and transforming growth factor-b. *J Neuroimmunol* 1994;49:9–18.

67. Keltner JL, Johnson CA, Spurr JO, et al. Visual field profile of optic neuritis: one-year follow-up in the Optic Neuritis Treatment Trial. *Arch Ophthalmol* 1994;112:946–953.

68. Slamovits TL, Rosen CE, Cheng KP, et al. Visual recovery in patients with optic neuritis and visual loss to no light perception. *Am J Ophthalmol* 1991;111:209–214.

69. Saraux H, Nordmann JPH, Denis PH. Les formes atypiques des nevrites optiques de la sclerose en plaques. *J Fr Ophtalmol* 1991;14:235–244.

70. Cleary PA, Beck RW, Bourque LB, et al. Visual symptoms after optic neuritis: results from the Optic Neuritis Treatment Trial. *J Neuroophthalmol* 1997;17:18–23.

71. Ellenberger C Jr, Ziegler T. The Swiss cheese visual field or time-varying abnormalities of vision after "recovery" from optic neuritis. In: Smith JL, (ed.) *Neuro-ophthalmology focus 1980*. New York: Masson, 1979;175–179.

72. Uhthoff W. Untersuchungen uber die bei der multiplen herdsklerose vorkommenden augenstorungen. *Arch Psychiatr Nervenkr* 1890;21:55–116, 303–410.

73. Goldstein JE, Cogan DG. Exercise and the optic neuropathy of multiple sclerosis. *Arch Ophthalmol* 1964;72:168–170.

74. Smith JL, Hoyt WF, Susac JO. Ocular fundus in acute Leber optic neuropathy. *Arch Ophthalmol* 1973;90:349–354.

75. Nelson D, Jeffreys WH, McDowell F. Effect of induced hyperthermia on some neurological diseases. *Arch Neurol Psychiatr* 1958;79:31–39.

76. Scholl GB, Song H-S, Wray SH. Uhthoff's symptom in optic neuritis: relationship to magnetic resonance imaging and development of multiple sclerosis. *Ann Neurol* 1991;30:180–184.

77. Rasminsky M. The effects of temperature on conduction in demyelinated single nerve fibers. *Arch Neurol* 1973;28:287–292.

78. Bode DD. The Uhthoff phenomenon. *Am J Ophthalmol* 1978;85:721–722.

79. Selhorst JB, Saul RF, Waybright EA. Optic nerve conduction: opposing effects of exercise and hyperventilation. *Trans Am Neurol Assoc* 1981;106:101–105.

80. The Optic Neuritis Study Group. Visual function 5 years after optic neuritis: experience of The Optic Neuritis Treatment Trial. *Arch Ophthalmol* 1997;115:1545–1552.

81. Lynn BH. Retrobulbar neuritis: a survey of the present condition of cases occurring over the last fifty-six years. *Trans Ophthalmol Soc UK* 1959;79:701–716.

82. Hutchinson WM. Acute optic neuritis and the prognosis for multiple sclerosis. *J Neurol Neurosurg Psychiatry* 1976;39:283–289.

83. Sorensen TL, Frederiksen JL, Bronnum-Hansen H, et al. Optic neuritis as onset manifestation of multiple sclerosis: a nationwide, long-term survey. *Neurology* 1999;53:473–478.

84. Anmarkrud N, Slettnes ON. Uncomplicated retrobulbar neuritis and the development of multiple sclerosis. *Acta Ophthalmol* 1989;67:306–309.

85. Druschky A, Heckmann JG, Claus D, et al. Progression of optic neuritis to multiple sclerosis: an 8-year follow-up study. *Clin Neurol Neurosurg* 1999;101:189–192.

86. Frith JA, McLeod JG, Hely M. Acute optic neuritis in Australia: a 13-year prospective study. *J Neurol Neurosurg Psychiatry* 2000;68:246.

87. Francis DA, Compston DAS, Batchelor JR, et al. A reassessment of the risk of multiple sclerosis developing in patients with optic neuritis after extended follow up. *J Neurol Neurosurg Psychiatry* 1987;50:758–765.

88. Rizzo JF, Lessell S. Risk of developing multiple sclerosis after uncomplicated optic neuritis: a long-term prospective study. *Neurology* 1988;38:185–190.

89. Sandberg-Wollheim M, Bynke H, Cronqvist S, et al. A long-term prospective study of optic neuritis: evaluation of risk factors. *Ann Neurol* 1990;27:386–393.

90. Ghosh A, Kelly SP, Mathews J, et al. Evaluation of the management of optic neuritis: audit on the neurological and ophthalmological practice in the north west of England. *J Neurol Neurosurg Psychiatry* 2002;72:119–121.

91. Cole SR, Beck RW, Moke PS, et al. The predictive value of CSF oligoclonal banding for MS 5 years after optic neuritis. *Neurology* 1998;51:885–887.

92. Chataway J, Feakes R, Coraddu F, et al. The genetics of multiple sclerosis: principles, background and updated results of the United Kingdom systematic genome screen. *Brain* 1998;121:1869–1887.

93. Ebers GC, Dyment DA. Genetics of multiple sclerosis. *Semin Neurol* 1998;18:295–299.

94. Oksenberg JR, Barcellos LF, Hauser SL. Genetic aspects of multiple sclerosis. *Semin Neurol* 1999;19:281–288.

95. de Jong BA, Huizinga TWJ, Zanelli E, et al. Evidence for additional genetic risk indicators of relapse-onset MS within the HLA region. *Neurology* 2002;59:549–555.

96. Frohman EM, Racke M, van den Noort S. To treat, or not to treat. The therapeutic dilemma of idiopathic monsymptomatic demyelinating syndromes. *Arch Neurol* 2000;57:930–932.

97. Kaufman DI, Trobe JD, Eggenberger ER, et al. Practice parameter: the role of corticosteroids in the management of acute monosymptomatic optic neuritis. *Neurology* 2000;54:2039–2044.

98. Sellebjerg F, Schaldemose Nielsen H, Frederiksen JL, et al. A randomized, controlled trial of oral high-dose methylprednisone in acute optic neuritis. *Neurology* 1999;52:1479–1484.

99. Jacobs LD, Beck RW, Simon JH, et al. Intramuscular interferon beta-1a therapy initiated during a first demyelinating event in multiple sclerosis. *N Engl J Med* 2000;343:898–904.

100. CHAMPS Study Group. Interferon β-1a for optic neuritis patients at high risk for multiple sclerosis. *Am J Ophthalmol* 2001;132:463–471.

101. Comi G, Filippi M, Barkhof F, et al. Effect of early interferon treatment on conversion to definitive multiple sclerosis: a randomised study. *Lancet* 2001;357:1576–1582.

102. The PRISMS Study Group and The University of British Columbia MS/MRI Analysis Group. PRISMS-4: long-term efficacy of interferon beta-1a in relapsing MS. *Neurology* 2001;56:1628–1636.

103. The IFNB Multiple Sclerosis Study Group and the University of British Columbia MS/MRI Analysis Group. Interferon beta-1b in the treatment of multiple sclerosis: final outcome of the randomized controlled trial. *Neurology* 1995;45:1277–1285.

104. Noseworthy JH, O'Brien PC, Petterson TM, et al. A randomized trial of intravenous immunoglobulin in inflammatory demyelinating optic neuritis. *Neurology* 2001;56:1514–1522.

105. Lee AG, Galetta SL. Update on therapeutics in multiple sclerosis for ophthalmologists. *Compr Ophthalmol Update* 2000;1:349–356.

106. Balcer LJ, Galetta SL. Treatment of acute demyelinating optic neuritis. *Semin Ophthalmol* 2002;17:4–10.

107. Soderstrom M. Optic neuritis and multiple sclerosis. *Acta Ophthalmol Scand* 2001;79:223–227.

108. Van Stavern GP. Management of optic neuritis and multiple sclerosis. *Curr Opin Ophthalmol* 2001;12: 400–407.

109. Kahana E, Leibowitz U, Fishback N, et al. Slowly progressive and acute visual impairment in multiple sclerosis. *Neurology* 1973;23:729–733.

110. Regan D, Bartol S, Murray TJ, et al. Spatial frequency discrimination in normal vision and in patients with multiple sclerosis. *Brain* 1982;105:735–754.

111. Ashworth B. Chronic demyelinating optic neuritis: a reappraisal. *Neuro-ophthalmology* 1987;7:75–79.

112. Milder DG. Partial and significant reversal of progressive visual and neurological deficits in multiple sclerosis: a possible therapeutic effect. *Clin Exp Ophthalmol* 2002;30:363–366.

113. Della Sala S, Comi G, Martinelli V, et al. The rapid assessment of visual dysfunction in multiple sclerosis. *J Neurol Neurosurg Psychiatry* 1987;50:840–846.

114. Engell T, Trojaborg W, Raun NE. Subclinical optic neuropathy in multiple sclerosis: a neuro-ophthalmological investigation by means of visually evoked response, Farnsworth-Munsell 100 hue test and Ishihara test and their diagnostic value. *Acta Ophthalmol* 1987;65: 735–740.

115. Ashworth B, Aspinall PA, Mitchell JD. Visual function in multiple sclerosis. *Doc Ophthalmol* 1990;73:209–224.

116. Pinckers A, Cruysberg JRM. Colour vision, visually evoked potentials, and lightness discrimination in patients with multiple sclerosis. *Neuro-ophthalmology* 1992;12:251–256.

117. Van Diemen HAM, Lanting P, Loetsier JC, et al. Evaluation of the visual system in multiple sclerosis: a comparative study of diagnostic tests. *Clin Neurol Neurosurg* 1992;94:191–195.

118. Nordmann J-P, Saraux H, Roullet E. Contrast sensitivity in multiple sclerosis: a study of 35 patients with and without optic neuritis. *Ophthalmologica* 1987;195: 199–204.

119. Dain SJ, Rammahan KW, Benes SC, et al. Chromatic, spatial, and temporal losses of sensitivity in multiple sclerosis. *Invest Ophthalmol Vis Sci* 1990;31:548–558.

20 Peripheral Nerve Disease in Women

Alan R. Moore, MD, E. Wayne Massey, MD, and Janice M. Massey, MD

A t different stages of life, women are uniquely predisposed to injury or disease of the peripheral nervous system (PNS). Symptoms involving the PNS are perhaps some of the more common neurologic complaints during pregnancy. Although many complaints are of minor significance, severe peripheral nerve dysfunction may threaten the mother and fetus, and this deserves immediate recognition and treatment. An awareness of the structural, immunologic, and metabolic contributions to peripheral nerve disease in pregnancy assists in its appropriate diagnosis and management. Other rheumatologic, neoplastic, and environmental conditions that also exist in the nonpregnant state often have deleterious consequences to the PNS. The special circumstances surrounding these frequently encountered conditions call for a closer evaluation of the diagnosis and management of peripheral nerve disease in women.

PREGNANCY-RELATED DISORDERS DURING PREGNANCY

Mononeuropathies of Pregnancy

Cranial Nerves

FACIAL NERVE. Idiopathic facial nerve palsy has a slightly higher incidence in women, particularly in women of childbearing age (1). The risk for developing Bell's palsy during pregnancy or early puerperium is reported to be three times greater than in nonpregnant women (2). Several case series have demonstrated the increased risk to occur during the third trimester and first 2 weeks postpartum (2,3). Hypercoagulopathy, hypertension, edema, and a propensity for viral infections have all been proposed etiologies, though none proven. Hypertensive disorders of pregnancy occur five to six times more often in patients with Bell's palsy (3,4).

The clinical course of the facial palsy is similar to that in the nonpregnant state. Abrupt upper and lower unilateral facial weakness without objective sensory loss may follow a recent viral syndrome. Bilateral involvement is rare. Ear pain, absence of taste, and hyperacusis may be reported on the affected side. Maximal weakness occurs within the first few days, with the preservation of some degree of motor function is a good prognostic sign for recovery. Electrophysiologic studies are useful in predicting recovery. Complete or near complete recovery of facial weakness occurs in the vast majority of cases. The recurrence of Bell's palsy during subsequent pregnancies has been reported (5).

Treatment with any agent in pregnant patients has not been systematically studied. The early use of prednisone therapy in the nonpregnant patient with Bell's palsy is probably helpful, whereas the role of acyclovir is less clear (6). Patients with complete motor loss should receive stronger consideration for steroid treatment. Close blood pressure monitoring is recommended due to the possible exacerbation of hypertension that may occur with steroid treatment, especially in patients with increased risk for hypertensive disorders of pregnancy. Maintaining adequate lubrication of the eye and protecting the cornea from abrasions remain the mainstay of treatment.

NERVES OF OCULAR MOTILITY. Diplopia from isolated muscle paresis is distinctly rare in pregnant patients. An abducens nerve palsy may occur as a consequence of elevated intracranial pressure in idiopathic intracranial hypertension. Similarly, abrupt hypertension has caused increased intracranial pressure and subsequent abduction palsies in cases of preeclampsia (7). More commonly, transient abnormalities of ocular conversion lasting weeks may occur during labor or the days following delivery. Persistent isolated paresis should prompt a search for causes occurring in the nonpregnant patient, such as aneurysm and nerve infarction. Myasthenia gravis often presents with external ocular muscle dysfunction and may mimic an isolated muscle paresis.

OPTIC NERVE. Visual loss secondary to lesions of the optic nerve is infrequent in pregnancy. Idiopathic intracranial hypertension causing visual loss and headache is an uncommon complication of pregnancy that is important to recognize and manage. The shunting of cerebrospinal fluid by an optic nerve sheath fenestration may be needed to preserve vision, because weight loss and acetazolamide are suboptimal alternatives.

Retrobulbar neuritis has been reported in the second trimester, sometimes producing optic atrophy. This may be bilateral and severe. A detailed clinical neuro-ophthomologic evaluation is useful to clarify this etiology.

Neuroimaging is recommended to pursue other causes of visual loss, including multiple sclerosis or structural lesions such as meningioma, optic nerve glioma, and aneurysmal compression, which may enlarge during pregnancy.

Trunk Intercostal Nerves

Chest or abdominal pain may be attributable to intercostal neuralgia (Figure 20.1) in the last trimester of pregnancy (8). Stretch injury to the intercostal nerve or root from a large fetus or other mechanical factors is the suspected cause. Mild to severe pain follows the distribution of one or two thoracic roots and typically subsides after delivery. Epidural anesthesia has successfully treated disabling cases (9). Examining the skin to exclude herpes zoster is essential. Diabetes mellitus may also cause a thoracolumbar radiculopathy with similar symptoms.

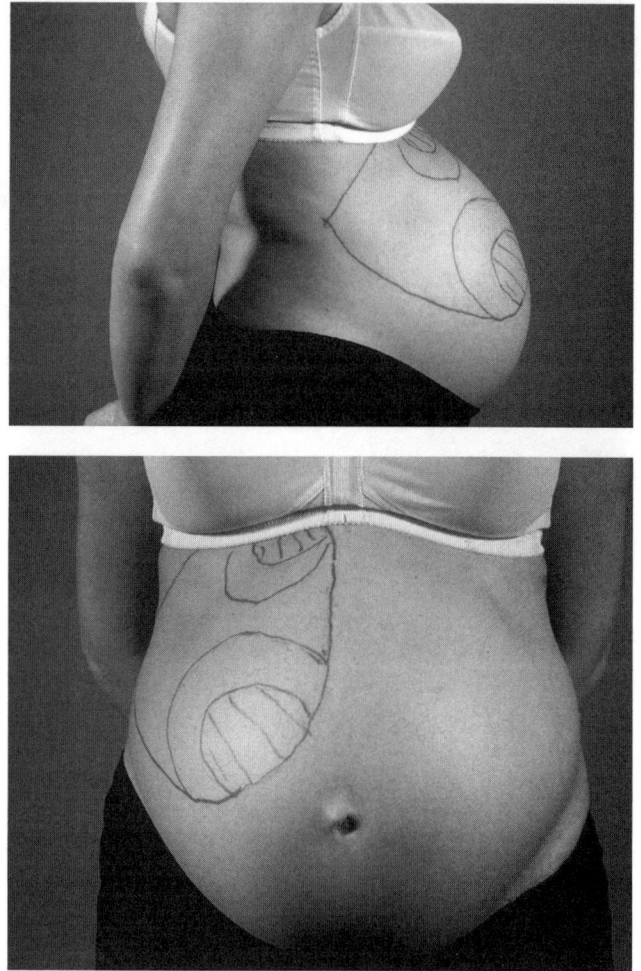

FIGURE 20.1

Sensory loss from stretch injury to the intercostal nerves, intercostal neuralgia, anterior and lateral views.

Upper Extremities

MEDIAN NERVE. Hand symptoms of paresthesias and pain are among the most common complaints during pregnancy. They are present in up to one-third of pregnancies (10). Most hand symptoms are attributed to compression of the median nerve in the carpal tunnel. Objective findings of carpal tunnel syndrome (CTS) have been identified in 7 to 10% of pregnancies (11). Symptoms most often begin in the third trimester but can occur at any time. Pregnant and nonpregnant patients often report hand or arm pain that arouses them at night and is relieved by shaking of the affected hand (Flick sign) (12). Interestingly, pregnant patients may experience more pain than nonpregnant patients (13). Paresthesias may occur in the median nerve distribution or the entire palmar hand. Complaints of hand weakness are infrequent early in CTS. Symptoms are usually bilateral and more severe in the dominant hand. Tinel's sign,

Phalen's sign, median nerve distribution sensory loss, thenar atrophy, and weakness of the abductor pollicis brevis and opponens pollicis may be observed on examination.

Nerve conduction studies allow an accurate diagnosis and assessment of the severity of disease. Serial electrical studies are often useful in following the disease course. Conservative therapy using nighttime wrist splints and modification of activities are usually sufficient to relieve pain. Many find injections of steroids into the carpal tunnel helpful if splinting fails. Other conventional therapies, such as diuretics and nonsteroidal anti-inflammatory drugs (NSAIDs), are discouraged during pregnancy.

Symptoms resolve shortly after pregnancy in about half of the patients (14). Patients developing CTS before the third trimester, however, may have a more severe course and are less likely to improve after delivery. Rarely, patients with hand weakness and significant symptoms unresponsive to conservative therapy, especially when occurring in the first two trimesters, may need surgical decompression (15). The short-term inability to use the hand in the postoperative period may have significant consequences to the expectant or recently delivered mother.

The role of pregnancy on CTS has not been elucidated completely. Increased rates of edema have been associated with pregnancy-related CTS (14,16). Hormonal changes may influence the rates of pregnancy-related CTS just as in the nonpregnant patient (17). Alteration in sleep position has been another proposed risk factor. As pregnancy progresses, sleeping on one's side is necessary. This position is often associated with wrist flexion while sleeping, which may lead to increased pressure in the carpal tunnel, ischemia, and nocturnal pain (18).

ULNAR NERVE. Symptoms of sensory dysfunction and pain in the ulnar nerve distribution occur in 2 to 12% (10,19) of pregnancies. The ulnar nerve may be injured near the elbow at the condylar groove or cubital tunnel by a variety of mechanisms. It is often difficult to distinguish from a wrist lesion at Guyon's canal, which usually spares the dorsal and palmar ulnar cutaneous sensory nerves. Weakness of the flexor digitorum profundus of the fourth and fifth digits and flexor carpi ulnaris suggests a proximal lesion, whereas the absence of weakness in these muscles does not help further localization due to the frequent sparing of these fascicles with injury near the elbow. If no obvious trauma has occurred, limiting compression and flexion of the elbow is important until full recovery, which usually occurs following delivery.

BRACHIAL PLEXUS. Idiopathic brachial plexopathy (neuralgic amyotrophy or Parsonage-Turner syndrome) and hereditary brachial plexus neuropathy have similar peaks of occurrence in the postpartum period (see the section Neuropathies in the Puerperium). Their incidence during pregnancy is significantly less frequent, with only two cases of idiopathic brachial plexopathy reported (20,21). Plexopathies can occur at any time during pregnancy and may have recurrence in the puerperium in the current or subsequent pregnancy (21,22). Unilateral pain of the shoulder or upper arm is the initial, primary feature, followed by weakness, atrophy, and sensory loss in a variable distribution. Axonal damage is the predominant feature on electromyography. In nonpregnant patients, nearly 80% of patients completely recover by two years (23).

Lower Extremities

LATERAL FEMORAL CUTANEOUS NERVE OF THE THIGH (FIGURE 20.2). Pain, paresthesias, and numbness may occur in the anterolateral thigh as a result of damage to the lateral femoral cutaneous nerve of the thigh—

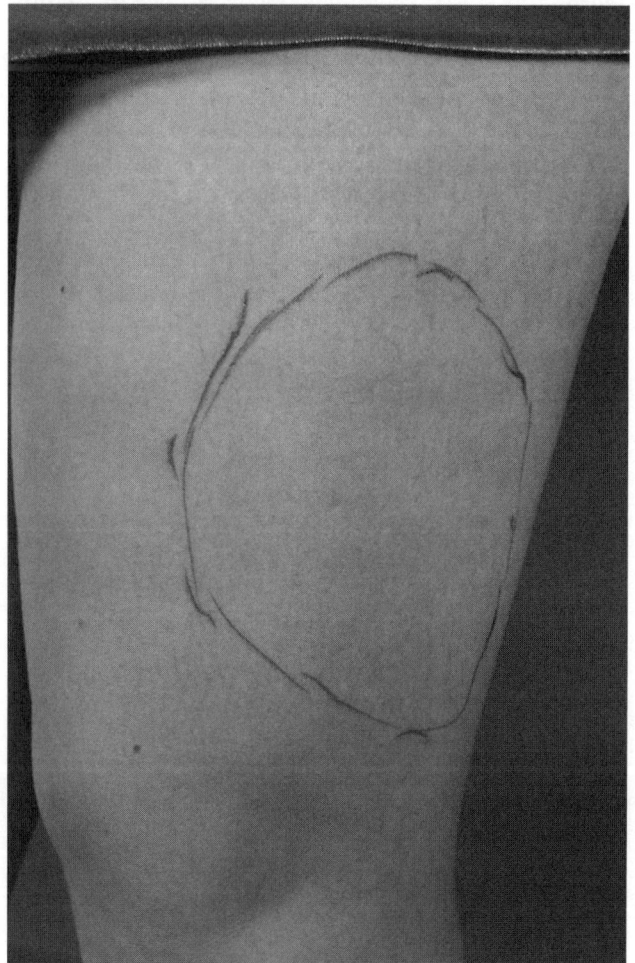

FIGURE 20.2

Characteristic sensory loss with injury of the lateral femoral cutaneous nerve of the thigh, meralgia paresthetica.

meralgia paresthetica. Pregnancy is commonly an inciting factor. Symptoms usually begin in the last trimester of pregnancy (24). Increased abdominal protuberance and weight gain may cause a stretch injury to the nerve, alter the angle of the nerve through the inguinal ligament causing mechanical injury, or entrap the nerve as it penetrates the tensor fascia lata muscle. Reassurance of resolution of symptoms after pregnancy is often all that is required. Local anesthetic injection for disabling cases may be preferred over relatively contraindicated neuropathic pain medications. Lidoderm patches sometimes are benficial.

LUMBOSACRAL PLEXUS.   Uncommonly, pregnancy is complicated by a lumbosacral plexopathy developing during the third trimester (25,26). The proposed etiology is compression of the plexus by the fetus. A large fetal-to-pelvis size ratio and fetal position are presumed factors. Rarely, a lumbosacral plexopathy occurs during pregnancy as part of hereditary brachial plexus neuropathy (22). Complete recovery occurs within months after delivery.

TIBIAL NERVE.   Pregnancy has been implicated in the cause of isolated reports of tarsal tunnel syndrome. Pain at the ankle and/or foot and paresthesias on the sole of the foot are caused by lesions of the tibial nerve in the tarsal tunnel, just inferior to the medial malleolus. The most common etiology in nonpregnant patients is ill-fitting shoes (11), a factor only enhanced by the edema of pregnancy. Symptoms usually abate after delivery and the resolution of pedal edema. Compression of the tibial nerve in the popliteal fossa is easily distinguished from tarsal tunnel syndrome by the presence of plantar flexion weakness and reduced Achilles reflex.

Polyneuropathies of Pregnancy

Autoimmune–Related Polyneuropathies

GUILLAIN-BARRÉ SYNDROME.   Acute inflammatory demyelinating polyradiculoneuropathy or Guillain-Barré syndrome (GBS) is an acute or subacute predominantly motor neuropathy with a monophasic course. Patients generally develop ascending symmetric distal weakness and paresthesias. Weakness may progress for 4 weeks, followed by a gradual return in strength over many weeks or months. Impaired strength, relatively preserved sensation, hyporeflexia, and albuminocytologic dissociation in cerebrospinal fluid are encountered. Electrophysiologic studies may be normal early in the disease but typically show prolonged F-wave latencies, prolonged distal latencies, and slowed conduction velocities later in the disease course.

The incidence of GBS during pregnancy is thought to be similar to that of the nonpregnant state (27). Women may develop rapidly progressive weakness anytime during the course of pregnancy, but more commonly during the third trimester (28). GBS is an immune-mediated illness, although the exact mechanism is unclear. Preceding infection or viral syndrome is present in about two-thirds of patients (29). Associated illnesses may have significant implications for the mother and fetus and warrant screening at the time of diagnosis. Cytomegalovirus has been implicated in a case of CMV placentitis in a patient who developed GBS in the first trimester (30). Epstein-Barr virus, human immunodeficiency virus (HIV), varicella zoster virus, and *Campylobacter jejuni* infections may also have added implications during pregnancy.

Complications of GBS may be more common late in gestation (31). Respiratory decompensation occurs more readily in the third trimester due to diminished lung volumes from an elevated diaphragm, which is restricted by the growing fetus. Serial vital capacities should be performed. Early intubation is indicated when vital capacities are 15mL/kg or less (29). Patients requiring mechanical ventilation may be at a higher risk for premature labor (32), thromboembolic complications, sepsis, and acute respiratory distress syndrome. Care should be taken to ensure adequate nutrition, prevent thromboembolic complications with subcutaneous heparin and sequential compression devices, and prevent aortocaval compression and skin breakdown with frequent turning of the patient. Autonomic dysfunction may be present, and treatment is made difficult by unpredictable responses to even low doses of medications. When possible, fluid management and other conservative measures to treat variations in blood pressure should be initiated.

Treatment with plasmapheresis or intravenous immune globulin (IVIg) is effective in nonpregnant patients (33,34). No consensus on treatment preference exists. Plasmapheresis and IVIg have been used safely and effectively in pregnant patients. (See the section "Immune Modulation Therapy in Pregnancy" for further discussion.) Patients may undergo vaginal delivery, because GBS has no effect on uterine contraction or cervical dilatation. Vacuum extraction may be needed due to an inability to bear down (35), and only rarely is C-section indicated in GBS. Consultation with an experienced anesthesia team may prevent complications of autonomic dysfunction due to inadequate regional pain control or respiratory failure due to a high regional block (36). If general anesthesia is required, succinylcholine should be used with caution because cardiac arrest from succinylcholine-induced hyperkalemia has been reported (37).

The fetal survival rate has been reported to be 96% (31). A case of congenital GBS associated with maternal inflammatory bowel disease has been reported (38), reaffirming the need for adequate pediatric respiratory support at delivery.

CHRONIC INFLAMMATORY DEMYELINATING POLYRADICULONEUROPATHY. Chronic inflammatory demyelinating polyradiculoneuropathy (CIDP) is a motor and sensory autoimmune neuropathy that has features similar to GBS. The time course is much different, however. One-half of the women present with steady or stepwise progressive weakness over many months. The remainder of patients have a chronic relapsing course (39). One case series of nine pregnancies with CIDP noted an increased incidence of relapses during pregnancy, with worsening strength during the third trimester and immediate postpartum period (40). Steroids, plasmapheresis, and IVIg are effective treatments in CIDP (41–43). Indication for treatment and treatment preference is not established in pregnancy. Treatment considerations similar to the pregnant GBS patient should be made. (See the section "Immune Modulation Therapy in Pregnancy" for further discussion.) The patient wanting to become pregnant who is on chronic immunosuppressants for CIDP should be educated about the risks involved for herself and the fetus and switched from potentially harmful agents such as azathioprine, cyclosporine, or cyclophosphamide to the lowest dose of steroids that controls the disease.

MULTIFOCAL MOTOR NEUROPATHY. Pregnancy appears to worsen episodes of weakness in patients with multifocal motor neuropathy (MMN). In one series of three patients, weakness developed in previously affected and unaffected muscles during pregnancy. The patients responded incompletely to IVIg during pregnancy and returned to their prepregnancy state after delivery (44). Several mechanisms for the worsening have been described. Increased maternal steroid production may have similar worsening effects to treatment of MMN with corticosteroids (44). Also, MMN is most likely a humorally mediated disease with antibodies to the gangliosides GM1, GM2, and GD1a. Other humoral disorders are adversely affected by a state of relative cellular immunosuppression and humoral immunostimulation during gestation.

Immune Modulation Therapy in Pregnancy

The improved identification and treatment of autoimmune neuromuscular disease has brought new challenges. Immunosuppressive medications (IS), many of which have significant repercussions on the fetus, are often needed to control the autoimmune neuromuscular disease in pregnancy. Determining a balance between the mother's health and the lowest risk of fetal toxicity can be difficult. Careful medication selection is instrumental

in successfully treating the neuromuscular disease and preventing complications in the mother and child.

Corticosteroids are often used in treating CIDP, myasthenia gravis (MG), and inflammatory muscle disease. Prednisone and prednisolone cross the placental barrier with levels eight- to ten-fold lower than in maternal blood (45). Fluorinated preparations, such as dexamethasone, are less well metabolized by the placenta (46). Congenital malformations are not typically seen with corticosteroid use. However, the incidence of cleft palate may exceed the general population when fetuses are exposed to high doses in the first trimester (47). High doses of the pulsed intravenous preparations frequently used in treating certain neurologic disorders may have more toxicity, given their teratogenicity at extreme doses in animals. The major consequences of corticosteroid therapy include premature rupture of the membranes, intrauterine growth retardation, and maternal complications of steroid use such as diabetes and hypertension (46). After delivery, the newborn is at a theoretic risk for adrenal insufficiency. Steroids are the only IS deemed safe during lactation (48). Low-dose corticosteroid treatment appears to be among the least harmful IS during pregnancy.

Azathioprine is frequently used in the treatment of MG. Epidemiologic data suggest relative safety during pregnancy, despite pregnancy category D status. While there is no definite increased risk of major malformations, a substantial number of pregnancies are premature or small for gestational age (49). Immunologic and hematologic abnormalities have been reported in infants exposed to azathioprine (50,51). Lactation is contraindicated, despite little to no transmission to breast milk (52).

Cyclophosphamide is infrequently used to treat inflammatory and vasculitic neuropathies. No specific malformation has been associated with fetal exposure, although sporadic anomalies have been reported. A case of multiple neoplasms in an offspring exposed to cyclophosphamide has been reported (53). Infertility is the most common adverse effect. Breast-feeding is contraindicated with its use (54).

Mycophenolate mofetil has been gaining acceptance in the treatment of myasthenia gravis and there are anecdotal reports of its use with other immune-mediated disorders. Little data exist regarding its use in pregnancy. Teratogenicity has been established in animals. Two cases of structural malformations have been noted in offspring exposed to mycophenolate mofetil (55). It is not recommended during pregnancy or lactation.

The treatment of refractory neuromuscular diseases with cyclosporine has many of the same effects on pregnancy as azathioprine. There is an increased risk of maternal hypertension, premature labor, spontaneous abortion, and intrauterine growth retardation (56,57). No significant major malformations have been identified. The long-term effects of cyclosporine exposure to the fetus are unknown. A maternal risk of reversible posterior leukoencephalopathy in the third trimester or immediate postpartum period exist (58,59), perhaps as a result of the additive effects of endothelial damage and hypertension, evident in both cyclosporine toxicity and eclampsia. Caution should be used when starting this medication late in pregnancy. Breast-feeding should be avoided.

Methotrexate is a folic acid antagonist infrequently used in the treatment of refractory autoimmune neuropathies, myopathies, and MG. Early fetal exposure to methotrexate may cause fetal demise, whereas exposure later in pregnancy is associated with skeletal abnormalities and cleft palate (60). Lower doses of methotrexate, less than 10 mg per week, taken early in pregnancy may be better tolerated (61). Pregnancy termination should be considered on an individual basis. Patients desiring to become pregnant should discontinue this medication many months before conception. Women of childbearing age taking methotrexate should receive contraceptive counseling. Breast-feeding is not recommended during treatment.

Plasmapheresis and IVIg have been used safely and effectively in pregnant patients with GBS. The complications of plasmapheresis are similar to those of the nonpregnant state. Complications of venous access, hypocalcemia, hypothrombinemia, and hypotension are encountered infrequently with a trained plasmapheresis team. Hypotension may occur less frequently when the procedure is performed in the left lateral decubitus position.

IVIg treatment in pregnancy has been used less often based on the literature (62). Infusion-related reactions including headache, myalgias, chills, and nausea are common and often respond to acetaminophen and diphenhydramine. Hyperviscosity associated with thromboembolic events occurs in up to 5% of nonpregnant patients. This risk may increase in pregnant patients who are already prone to clot formation. Anaphylaxis in IgA deficient patients, aseptic meningitis, renal failure in patients with pre-existing renal insufficiency, and a reversible encephalopathy are reported rare complications (63).

Metabolism-Related Polyneuropathies

DIABETES MELLITUS. Diabetic neuropathy is a heterogenous disorder. Commonly, patients present with a chronic distal sensorimotor neuropathy. Other neuropathic manifestations seen in diabetics at any age or level of glycemic control include acute sensorimotor neuropathy, autonomic neuropathy, diabetic amyotrophy, and thoracolumbar radiculopathy, which may be more frequent in diabetic women during pregnancy. Electrophysiologic abnormalities vary from essentially normal in a patient with a painful small fiber neuropathy to markedly slowed conduction velocities and reduced amplitudes in an asymptomatic patient.

These are just some of the factors that have hindered the accuracy of epidemiologic studies.

Prior pregnancy does not appear to increase the prevalence of diabetic neuropathy in women with insulin-dependent diabetes mellitus (IDDM). The incidence of peripheral neuropathy at postpartum reexamination increased tenfold in one study, however, suggesting neuropathy may progress more rapidly during pregnancy (64). Smaller studies using neurophysiologic testing have failed to demonstrate induction or worsening of sensorimotor or autonomic neuropathies (65–67). A direct correlation between glycemic control and diabetic peripheral neuropathy exists in the nonpregnant patient (68).

Diabetic autonomic neuropathy may have serious consequences in pregnancy. Gastroparesis may worsen during pregnancy, thus significantly jeopardizing the health of the mother and fetus (69). Adequate nutrition and vitamin supplementation should be administered. Gastric motility agents such as erythromycin or metoclopramide may be needed. Also, rapid blood pressure fluctuations and cardiac dysrhythmias may occur during pregnancy and labor, secondary to diabetic autonomic neuropathy; these require close monitoring and therapy.

THIAMINE DEFICIENCY. Pregnant patients with marginal nutritional status or hyperemesis gravidarum may develop thiamine deficiency. A sensorimotor, occasionally asymmetric axonal neuropathy develops with or without signs of Wernicke's encephalopathy. Intravenous thiamine should be administered until the patient tolerates oral medicines and a satisfactory diet. The neuropathy typically improves within weeks to months with proper treatment.

PORPHYRIA. Sensorimotor and autonomic neuropathies are manifestations of the hepatic porphyrias in young to middle-aged women. In acute intermittent porphyria, variegate porphyria, and hereditary coporphyria, enzymatic defects affecting the heme biosynthesis pathway result in excessive production of porphyrins and their precursors. Precipitating factors, such as sex hormones, induce delta-aminolevulinic acid (ALA) synthase, the rate-limiting enzyme in heme biosynthesis, leading to the excessive production of porphobilinogen and delta-ALA. Oral contraceptives and hormonal changes during the menstrual cycle may produce exacerbations of neuropathy, abdominal, or psychiatric disturbance.

Many women experience relapses during pregnancy (70). Proper medication selection during pregnancy and at the time of labor can prevent an attack of porphyria. The treatment of the pregnant patient with a porphyric relapse should be similar to that of the nonpregnant patient. The elimination of exacerbating medications, glucose administration, and high carbohydrate meals should be undertaken. Persistent symptoms should prompt consideration for hematin therapy to prevent permanent neurologic sequella (71).

Toxin-Related Polyneuropathies

NITROFURANTOIN. An acute axonal sensorimotor neuropathy may develop during the treatment of urinary tract disorders with nitrofurantoin, with or without renal failure (72). Symptoms may persist even after discontinuation of this medication. Congenital neuropathies have been proposed to be a consequence of nitrofurantoin therapy during the first trimester (73). Also, due to the possibility of hemolytic anemia due to glutathione instability, this drug is contraindicated near term or delivery, further discouraging its use during pregnancy.

Since the recognition of fetal toxicity associated with use of thalidomide in the 1950s, restricted use of medications during pregnancy has reduced fetal exposure to other toxins.

Hereditary Polyneuropathies

CHARCOT-MARIE-TOOTH (CMT) DISEASE. The hereditary dysmyelinating disorder CMT1 has been associated with exacerbations of weakness during pregnancy. In one review of CMT1 patients (74), 38% of patients reported an exacerbation with at least one pregnancy. Patients who developed symptoms earlier in life appear more prone to these exacerbations. A temporary worsening occurs in one-third of the patients, while deficits persist in the remainder of patients. Improvement after treatment with corticosteroids has been reported in one pregnancy (75), although steroids have not proved to be efficacious in this disorder.

PREGNANCY-RELATED DISORDERS DURING LABOR AND DELIVERY

Acute neuropathies of the lower extremity may develop during labor from injury at the spinal root, lumbosacral plexus, or peripheral nerve. Fortunately, the incidence of intrapartum neuropathies is declining due to modern obstetric practice and awareness of common compression sites.

Lumbosacral Plexopathy

Intrapartum lumbosacral plexopathy occurs during active labor, although cases of lumbosacral plexopathy during the third trimester exist (26). Its estimated incidence is 1:2000 to 1:6400 deliveries (76,77). Patients

may become aware of numbness or pain in the lateral leg during labor or notice foot drop immediately postpartum. Examination typically reveals dysfunction of L4 and L5 innervated muscles. Most patients have an inability to dorsiflex and weakness of foot inversion and eversion. Additional muscles may be involved. Sensory impairment predominates along the L5 dermatome. Achilles reflex is usually preserved. Electrodiagnostic testing is typically consistent with a demyelinating lesion of the lumbosacral trunk.

The lesion is most likely a consequence of compression of the lumbosacral trunk by the fetal head at the pelvic brim where the nerve is unprotected by the psoas muscle (78). Other infrequent causes include lumbar disc herniation, injury from gluteal injection (79), and spinal nerve root damage from epidural anesthesia (80). Neurophysiologic testing may be the only means to distinguish lumbosacral plexopathy from compression of the peroneal nerve at the fibular neck. Risk factors for intrapartum lumbosacral plexopathy include maternal short stature, large gestational weight, cephalopelvic disproportion, and protracted labor (78). Forceps delivery alone is probably not a risk factor. The majority of patients have complete recovery within 6 months. An ankle-foot orthosis is often helpful until strength returns.

Femoral Neuropathy

Femoral mononeuropathy has an estimated incidence of 1.5:1000 deliveries (81). Most women become symptomatic after labor. A few pregnancies may be complicated by unilateral or bilateral femoral neuropathies during the third trimester, however (82). Patients complain of their leg giving away while standing, difficulty climbing stairs, and sensory loss of the anterior and medial thigh. Examination reveals reduced patellar reflex and restricted weakness of the quadriceps femoris or the iliopsoas and the quadriceps femoris. In the former, more common condition, labor and vaginal delivery is in the lithotomy position. Compressive injury of the femoral nerve occurs at the inguinal ligament. Although technically difficult to perform, electrodiagnostic testing is consistent with an area of demyelination at the level of the inguinal ligament (83). Complete recovery occurs within 6 months. Physical therapy may be helpful.

When the iliopsoas is weak, the lesion is likely to be in the pelvis proximal to the inguinal ligament. Fetal compression and stretch injury by excessive hip abduction and external rotation may be the cause. When delivery is by caesarian section, instrumentation may injure the femoral nerve (84). Suspicion for other intrapelvic pathology, such as an iliacus or retroperitoneal hemorrhage should be high when pain is a presenting complaint. Computed tomography (CT) scan or magnetic resonance imaging (MRI) of the pelvis is warranted.

Obturator Neuropathy

Protracted labor may also cause an obturator neuropathy by nerve compression between the fetal head and bony pelvic wall, exacerbated by external rotation and abduction of the thighs. Women report leg weakness while walking, pain in the groin and upper thigh, or paresthesias along the medial thigh. Symptoms may be transient, lasting only days, and the diagnosis is often unrecognized. Weakness of thigh adduction, sensory deficit over the medial thigh, and a circumducting gait are found on evaluation. Normal patellar reflex and quadriceps femoris power help eliminate from suspicion upper plexus lesions or L3 or L4 radiculopathies. Vaginal examination and imaging studies can exclude compression from hematoma or tumor. If pelvic surgery was performed, neurophysiologic testing to assess the continuity of the nerve should be considered. Patients generally recover completely from this compressive neuropathy. Residual neuropathic pain requiring nerve blocks has been reported (85). If symptoms persist, nerve compression from an obturator hernia or endometriosis should be considered.

Peroneal Neuropathy

Foot drop also occurs as result of injury to the peroneal nerve during labor. Patients may report paresthesias along the anterolateral aspect of the leg during labor or foot drop after delivery. Weakness of dorsiflexion, toe extension, and foot eversion are evident on examination. Full foot inversion power can help distinguish a peroneal neuropathy from a lumbosacral plexopathy or L5 radiculopathy, although the tibialis anterior has a minor contribution to foot inversion (Table 20.1). Neurophysiologic testing can readily distinguish the two conditions, because conduction block at the fibular neck or head is common in peroneal neuropathy. Pressure on the peroneal nerve at the fibular head by manual compression during forced knee flexion (86) or by compression against stirrups occurs (85). Mechanical injury to the common peroneal nerve during prolonged squatting or forced abduction of the knees may be other causes (87). The prognosis for recovery is good. Patients should avoid further compromise by abstaining from leg crossing. Many women may need an ankle-foot orthosis until recovery usually within 6 months.

Ilioinguinal, Genitofemoral, and Iliohypogastric Neuropathies

Lesions of the ilioinguinal, genitofemoral, and iliohypogastric nerves may occur during normal pregnancy and delivery from stretch injury or nerve entrapment following Pfannenstiel incision (88). Patients report lower abdominal, inguinal, or upper thigh dysesthesias and pain. Sensory abnormalities from ilioinguinal and genitofemoral lesions occur on the skin overlying the mons pubis, labium majora, inguinal ligament, and upper medial thigh. Iliohypogastric neuropathy may cause sensory dysfunction above the pubis and upper buttocks and a bulging of the lower abdominal muscles. Frequently, the three cannot be differentiated at the bedside or by elec-

---

TABLE 20.1

Localization of Sensory and Motor Complaints in Pregnancy

	Motor findings	Sensory findings	Reflex	Onset	Common causes
Carpal tunnel syndrome	Abductor pollicis brevis	Median distal fingers	None	3rd trimester, postpartum	Possibly edema, wrist flexion in sleep, hand position holding infant
Intercostal neuropathy	None	One or two thoracic nerve roots	None	3rd trimester	Stretch injury from large fetus
Lumbosacral plexopathy	Variable				
Lumbar plexus	Thigh flexion, adduction	Anterior and medial thigh	Patellar	Labor and delivery	Compression by fetal head at pelvic brim, hematoma, gluteal injection, instrumentation
Sacral plexus	Thigh extension, abduction	Posterior thigh	Achilles	Labor and delivery	Compression by fetal head at pelvic brim, hematoma, gluteal injection, instrumentation
Femoral neuropathy	Thigh flexion, leg extension	Anteromedial thigh	Patellar	Labor and delivery	Compression by fetal head, inguinal ligament, hematoma

trodiagnostic testing. Symptoms typically resolve if the etiology is presumed to be a stretch injury. Therapeutic and diagnostic nerve blocks may be needed if neuropathic pain medications fail. Rarely, nerve resection is needed.

Pudendal Neuropathy

The pudendal nerve innervates the muscles of the perineum, external urethral and anal sphincters, and the skin of the perineum, labia majora, and clitoris. Damage to the nerve can occur with large episiotomies and local tissue damage from prolonged fetal compression (89). Numbness and incontinence are the typical sequela.

More commonly, patients develop urinary stress incontinence or fecal incontinence later in life. The role of pudenal neuropathy in incontinence is less clear. Sphincter injury, pelvic floor descent, and cumulative nerve damage from stretch injury during prolonged labor may all have a role (90,91). Neuropathic changes of the anal sphincter by EMG, temporary prolongation of pudendal nerve latencies, and fiber type grouping can be seen in women with fecal incontinence after vaginal delivery (92–94). Continence is poorly achieved by surgical repair of the anal sphincter muscles or Burch colposuspension if pudendal neuropathy is present (95,96). Caesarean section should be offered to patients with incontinence, as progression with subsequent vaginal deliveries is the rule (97).

Anesthesia-Related Neuropathies and Myelopathy

The incidence of neurologic complications from regional anesthesia may be as high as 1:1000 (98). Spinal anesthesia appears to carry a higher risk of neurologic complications than does epidural anesthesia (99). Lumbosacral radiculopathy, polyradiculopathy, thoracic myelopathy, and cauda equina syndrome may result from direct trauma, neurotoxic medications, epidural hematoma, and epidural abscess. Complications are more common with lumbar stenosis, prolonged medication use, and the inadvertent administration of high volumes into subarachnoid (98) space. Neuroimaging should be considered to rule out treatable causes of major neurologic deficits, especially when back pain is a primary complaint. Fortunately, neurologic deficits typically seen with labor and delivery are mild and reversible.

PREGNANCY-RELATED DISORDERS OF THE PUERPERIUM

Carpal Tunnel Syndrome

A small percentage of women develop CTS in the puerperium. Women are typically older and primiparous, have no evidence of peripheral edema, and are breast-feeding (100). Hand positioning during breast-feeding may be a significant contributing factor. Symptoms persist for months and subside with the discontinuation of lactation. Reassurance, proper positioning, and nocturnal splinting are often the only therapy needed.

Guillain-Barré Syndrome

GBS has an increased incidence in the 2 weeks following delivery (27). Possible explanations include exposure to certain risk factors at the end of pregnancy and an increased cell-mediated immunity that is relatively suppressed during pregnancy. Other cell-mediated autoimmune diseases, such as multiple sclerosis, have an increased risk of relapse during the puerperium (see Chapter 18). This supporting evidence of the cell-mediated contribution to GBS is not necessarily contradictory to the presence of anti-ganglioside antibodies found in a variety of GBS subtypes, as a synergistic role of T-cell autoimmunity and humoral response is most likely (101,102). An overview of treatment considerations is discussed in the section under Autoimmune-Related Polyneuropathies.

Brachial Plexus Neuropathy

Hereditary and idiopathic brachial plexus neuropathies develop hours to weeks following delivery (103,104). Patients initially develop pain, more commonly in the dominant extremity, followed by weakness days to weeks later. Clinical weakness varies from single nerves to bilateral plexus lesions. The pathogenesis is believed to be autoimmune in both hereditary and idiopathic conditions. Upper extremity nerve biopsies have revealed inflammatory infiltrates associated with epineural microvessels in patients with hereditary and idiopathic brachial plexus neuropathies (103). Treatment in the hereditary form with high-dose intravenous steroids has proved beneficial in relieving pain in some patients. Other analgesics and narcotics are potentially safer alternatives. Prognosis is good in the nonhereditary form. Relapses, without predictability, do occur in some patients with subsequent deliveries.

NON–PREGNANCY-RELATED POLYNEUROPATHIES

Systemic Diseases Common in Women

Connective Tissue Diseases

SJÖGREN'S SYNDROME. Sjögren's syndrome (SS) is a poorly recognized cause of peripheral neuropathy in women. Several forms of peripheral neuropathy exist

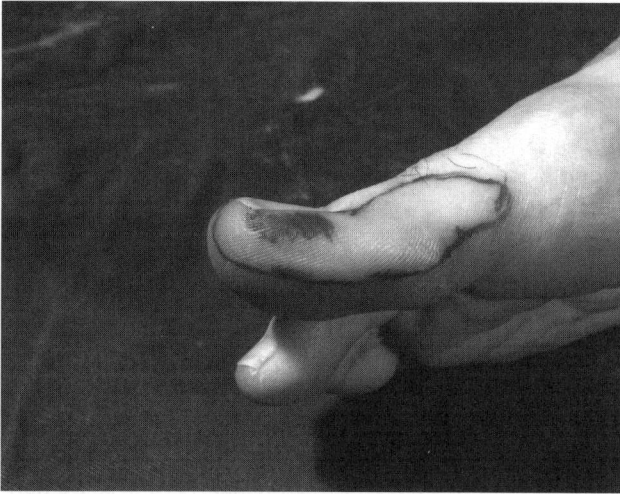

FIGURE 20.3

Digital sensory neuropathy of the great toe.

with this disorder including pure sensory neuronopathy, distal sensory or sensorimotor neuropathy, digital sensory neuropathy (Figure 20.3), trigeminal sensory neuropathy, autonomic neuropathy, and mononeuritis multiplex (105,106). Frequently, patients present with neuropathic complaints of sensory dysfunction without a diagnosis of SS. On further questioning, symptoms of the sicca complex, xerophthalmia, and xerostomia, are elicitable. Schirmer's test of lacrimal secretion, slit lamp examination for filamentary keratitis, and salivary gland biopsy are abnormal. Prominent extraglandular involvement and one of the serologic studies needed for definite SS [rheumatoid factor, anti-Ro(SSA), anti-La(SSB), or ANA] are not necessary for neuropathy to coexist (107). Neuropathies are typically sensory, involving large fibers secondary to lymphocytic infiltration of the dorsal roots and ganglia (106,107). Antineuronal antibodies to the dorsal root ganglia and other neural tissues suggest immunotherapy may benefit patients with early presentation (108,109). Case reports of improvement using plasmapheresis, IVIg, D-penicillamine, and infliximab exist in patients with a sensory neuronopathy, as do reports of spontaneous recovery (110,113). Typically, mild sensory or sensorimotor neuropathies require no further treatment. Rarely, a vasculitic neuropathy as a result of SS can present with mononeuritis multiplex, suggesting the need for advanced immunotherapy. Pain can be prominent and require intervention.

RHEUMATOID ARTHRITIS. A variety of neuropathies can be associated with rheumatoid arthritis (RA). The most common presentation is a symmetric sensory or sensorimotor polyneuropathy. Frequently,

patients have no symptoms (114). A mild reduction in vibration and pinprick may be the only signs. Neurophysiologic testing demonstrates a predominantly axonal sensorimotor neuropathy. RA patients treated with steroids may have a lower occurrence of this form of neuropathy (114). A superimposed CTS is often evident, and successful treatment of the underlying disease can relieve CTSs (115). Rheumatoid vasculitis can occur in longstanding RA, presenting with multiple mononeuropathies or, less commonly, a distal symmetrical sensory or sensorimotor axonal polyneuropathy (116). Despite improvement of the vasculitic neuropathy in the majority of cases, long-term prognosis for these patients is poor (117). Symptoms mimicking polyneuropathy may rarely occur as a result of a myelopathy secondary to high cervical spine dislocation.

SYSTEMIC LUPUS ERYTHEMATOSUS. Systemic lupus erythematosus (SLE) is a multisystem inflammatory autoimmune disease frequently affecting young women. Although central nervous system manifestations are most common, clinical evidence of neuropathy is found relatively infrequently. Electrophysiologic testing can detect a distal symmetric axonal sensorimotor neuropathy in up to one-quarter of SLE patients (118). Neuropathy may be more prevalent with active disease. Rarely, a severe form of neuropathy causes significant weakness. Other neuropathies associated with SLE include acute demyelinating, autonomic, mononeuritis multiplex, and compressive neuropathies (119–121). A vasculitic neuropathy is rare, despite evidence of epineural vasculitis on sural nerve biopsy in some cases (122,123).

THYROID DISEASE. A large number of patients with hypothyroidism have neuromuscular complaints. Compressive neuropathies, especially CTS, can occur in up to 25% of patients (124). The etiology is likely related to an accumulation of myxedematous tissue in the carpal tunnel. Less commonly, a mild distal sensorimotor neuropathy is evident. Both segmental demyelination and axonal loss of predominantly large myelinated fibers have been described on sural nerve biopsy (125–127). Frequently, CTS and sensorimotor neuropathies improve with thyroid replacement therapy. Hyperthyroidism is less commonly associated with compressive and sensorimotor neuropathies (124).

PORPHYRIA. The porphyrias are discussed in the earlier section, Metabolism-Related Polyneuropathies.

Neuropathies Associated with Malignancy

The development of a neuropathy in a patient with malignancy is not an uncommon occurrence. Neuropathies may be caused by direct invasion of the tumor, remote effects of the cancer, or as a consequence of the cancer treatment.

Neoplastic Infiltration

Neoplastic invasion of the PNS can occur at any location. Peripheral nerve involvement is less common than nerve root or plexus involvement. Isolated neuropathy of the mental nerve may be the presenting complaint of patients with breast cancer or lymphoproliferative diseases (128,129). Patients with known cancer and radicular symptoms should have an MRI of the spine with gadolinium, to exclude epidural metastasis, followed by a lumbar puncture to evaluate for the presence of leptomeningeal spread of the disease. Leptomeningeal spread most commonly occurs in breast cancer, lung cancer, melanoma, and nonsolid tumors (130,131).

Differentiation between neoplastic invasion of the brachial plexus (NBP) and radiation-induced brachial plexopathy (RBP) can be difficult in patients with breast or apical lung cancers. NBPs usually present with moderate to severe pain in the affected limb, whereas RBPs present more commonly with paresthesias and dysesthesias. Weakness predominantly affects the lower trunk of the plexus in NBP. Although similar findings can be seen in RBP (132), the entire plexus is usually involved. Horner's syndrome and a rapid progression are more commonly associated with a neoplastic spread of disease. Myokymic discharges can be identified using EMG in many muscles in 63 to 78% of patients with RBP, while occurring in only a few muscles, if at all, in NBP (132,133). MRI and CT have been useful in demonstrating tumor recurrence (134). If suspicion of tumor recurrence still exists, biopsy is indicated. Persistent pain is often difficult to treat. Neuropathic pain medications, steroids, and NSAIDs may not sufficiently treat the pain. Narcotic analgesics or a variety of interventional procedures may be required.

Paraneoplastic Neuropathies

Neuropathies can present as remote manifestations of cancer. In theory, tumor cells express an antigen, which is antigenically similar to molecules expressed by cells in the nervous system. An autoimmune reaction ensues, and neurologic symptoms are manifested. Autoantibodies often serve as a marker for a paraneoplastic process and may appear before the diagnosis of cancer is made. Because autoantibodies are not 100% sensitive for a paraneoplastic process, further cancer evaluation should be routinely performed if suspicion remains high (135).

Neuropathies are just one aspect of the paraneoplastic spectrum. In paraneoplastic neuropathies, typical findings include prominent neuropathic pain, symptoms outside of the peripheral sensory system, and cere-

brospinal fluid abnormalities such as increased protein, mild pleocytosis, elevated IgG index, or oligoclonal bands (136,137). Progression may be subacute, and there may be unusual clinical or electrophysiologic characteristics of the neuropathy. The most common paraneoplastic neuropathy is a multifocal encephalomyelitis with sensory neuronopathy, which seems to occur more often in women. Asymmetric numbness and paresthesias involving the proximal extremities or face is often the presenting symptom (138). Severe sensory ataxia, impaired proprioception, and hyporeflexia reflect dysfunction of the dorsal root ganglia. Most cases have anti-Hu autoantibodies and small cell lung cancer, although either anti-Hu or anti-amphiphysin antibodies in breast cancer can have similar presentations (139).

Breast cancer is associated with other paraneoplastic neuromuscular syndromes. Motor neuron disease presenting with pure upper or lower motor neuron dysfunction has been reported (140,141). Antibodies to amphiphysin and GAD in breast cancer patients have been implicated in cases of stiff-person syndrome (138,142).

Although the treatment of paraneoplastic neuropathies using various forms of immunosuppression and cancer treatment has shown infrequent benefit (136,143), patients with early presentation or less severe neuropathies deserve further consideration for immunotherapy.

Treatment-Related Neuropathies

Radiation therapy and chemotherapy for malignancy are necessary insults to the PNS. In the past, radiation treatment for breast cancer caused a brachial plexopathy in up to 50% of patients, many of whom had a disabling plexopathy (144). Sensory loss and hyporeflexia typically occur more than a year after radiation therapy. Weakness may follow months later. Progressive neuronal damage can occur in cancer survivors (145). Short courses of large fraction size and concomitant chemotherapy increase the risk for developing radiation-induced plexopathies (146). Differentiating radiation-induced plexopathies from tumor invasion is paramount. Their diagnostic evaluation and pain treatment are outlined above.

Chemotherapy-induced neuropathy is a common problem in patients with breast and gynecologic cancers. Cisplatin, commonly used for ovarian cancer, primarily affects the dorsal root ganglion, where its dose-related accumulation is greatest (147). Dysesthesias and paresthesias are reported in up to 90% of patients (148). Marked sensory ataxia, proprioceptive loss, and hyporeflexia are prominent features on exam. Nerve conduction studies (NCS) reveals a purely sensory neuropathy. Nerve biopsy demonstrates predominant loss of the large diameter fibers (148).

Paclitaxel is often used to treat both breast and ovarian cancer. The majority of women treated with high-dose paclitaxel develop a sensorimotor axonal neuropathy shortly after infusion (149). Paresthesias in the distal extremities are a common presentation. Uniform sensory loss, mild weakness, and hyporeflexia are identified on examination. Weakness develops at higher doses. The neurotoxic effects appear dose related. Symptoms and nerve conduction studies can normalize after 3 to 6 months, without further treatment (149).

Concomitant exposure to cisplatin appears to increase the severity of the neuropathy (150). Vincristine causes a similar neuropathy, often with a burning pain in the distal extremities secondary to small fiber dysfunction.

Nutritional Deficiencies

Chronic malnutrition associated with anorexia nervosa and bulimia nervosa is associated with a sensorimotor neuropathy and, more commonly, a metabolic myopathy. One prospective study of anorexic patients demonstrated an 8% incidence of a distal symmetric neuropathy. Neuropathy was more common in patients with chronic malnutrition. A 6% incidence of peroneal palsy also occurred, presumably due to the lack of adipose causing an increased risk for compressive neuropathies (151). Bulimics using ipecac are at a significant risk of a toxic myopathy with or without cardiomyopathy (152,153). Myopathies and neuropathies induced by malnutrition are reversible within months with adequate nutrition and discontinuation of ipecac.

NON–PREGNANCY-RELATED MONONEUROPATHIES

Carpal Tunnel Syndrome

Compressive median neuropathy at the carpal tunnel has a fourfold higher incidence in women than men (154). Smaller carpal canal size, occupational ergonomic risks, hormonal factors, and increased prevalence of diseases known to contribute to CTS are some of the factors that predispose women to CTS (155,156). Diagnosis and management is outlined previously in the section on Mononeuropathies of Pregnancy.

Neuropathies Associated with Endometriosis

Normal endometrial tissue abnormally located outside of the uterus is a common cause of abdominal pain and infertility. Pelvic endometriosis without actual nerve involvement may be the most common cause of cyclic radiating leg pain (157). Pain usually starts shortly before menses and ends after cessation of flow (158). When neurologic signs such as weakness or sensory dysfunction develop,

nerve compression by an endometrioma or nerve sheath infiltration by endometrial tissue at any location in the lumbosacral nerves may be the cause. Lesions of the sciatic nerve (11) at the sciatic notch and the lateral femoral cutaneous nerve of the thigh (meralgia paresthetica) occur most commonly (Figure 20.2). Lower abdominal tenderness particularly after pelvic examination often accompanies neuropathic findings. Electrodiagnostic studies and imaging of the pelvis and lumbosacral plexus using MRI may be useful in the diagnosis (159). Pathologic confirmation is needed. A trial of conservative treatment with hormonal therapy is reasonable for patients without neurologic signs or obvious nerve compression. When nerve dysfunction is present, surgical excision of the lesion may prevent further scarring and accelerate recovery of weakness, which often persists (158,160).

Iatrogenic Mononeuropathies

Ruptured breast implants and subdermal contraceptive implants have been implicated in isolated reports of local nerve injury (161,162). Remote neurologic deficits associated with breast implants have yet to be proved despite an increased incidence of neurologic symptoms in women with breast implants (163). Epidemiologic studies have found no association with breast implants and neurologic or rheumatologic disease (164,165). Variable pathologic changes are seen in a minority of patients with neuropathic complaints and implants (166). Other etiologies should be sought in women with neuropathy.

Domestic Violence and Nerve Injury

Nearly one-third of American women report physical or sexual abuse at some time in their lives (167). Peripheral nerve injury from abuse should be treated similarly to other traumatic nerve lesions. Early electrodiagnostic evaluation is helpful in assessing the extent of nerve injury and identifying patients who may need surgical repair. Chronic pain syndromes may mimic peripheral neuropathy and should alert the clinician to address the possibility of victimization (168). Inquiries concerning victim support options and statutes regarding reporting domestic violence should be sought.

References

1. Katusic SK, Beard CM, Wiederholt WC, Bergstrahl EJ, Kurland LT. Incidence, clinical features, and prognosis in Bell's palsy, Rochester, Minnesota, 1968–1982. *Ann Neurol* 1986;20:622–627.
2. Hilsinger RL, Abdour KK, Doty HE. Idiopathic facial paralysis, pregnancy, and the menstrual cycle. *Ann Otol Rhinol Laryngol* 1975;84:433–442.
3. Falco NA, Eriksson E. Idiopathic facial palsy in pregnancy and the puerperium. *Surg Gynecol Obstet* 1989; 337–340.

4. Shmorgun D, Chan WS, Ray JG. Association of Bell's palsy in pregnancy and pre-eclampsia. *QJM* 2002; 95:359–362.

5. McGregor JA, Guberman A, Amer J, Goodlin R. Idiopathic facial nerve paralysis (Bell's palsy) in late pregnancy and the early puerperium. *Obstet Gynecol* 1987; 69:435–438.

6. Grogan PM, Gronseth PM. Practice parameter: steroids, acyclovir, and surgery for Bell's palsy (an evidence based medicine review): report on the Quality Standards Subcommittee of the American Academy of Neurology. *Neurology* 2001;56:830–836.

7. Barry-Kinsella C, Milner M, McCarthy N, Walsh J. Sixth nerve palsy: an unusual manifestation of preeclampsia. *Obstet & Gynecol* 1994;83:849–851.

8. Pleet AB, Massey EW. Intercostal neuralgia of pregnancy. *JAMA* 1980;243:770.

9. Samlaska S, Dews TE. Long-term epidural analgesia for pregnancy-induced intercostals neuralgia. *Pain* 1995;62: 245–248.

10. Voitk AJ, Mueller JC, Farlinger DE, Johnston RU. Carpal tunnel syndrome in pregnancy. *Can Med Assoc J* 1983;128:277–281.

11. Stewart JD. *Focal Peripheral Neuropathies*, 3rd ed. Philadelphia: Lippincott Williams and Wilkins; 2000.

12. Pryse-Phillips WE. Validation of a diagnostic sign in carpal tunnel syndrome. *J Neurol Neurosurg Psychiatry* 1984;47:870–872.

13. Seror P. Pregnancy-related carpal tunnel syndrome. *J Hand Surg* 1998;23:98–101.

14. Padua L, Aprile I, Caliandro P, et al. The Italian Carpal Tunnel Study Group. Symptoms and neurophysiological picture of carpal tunnel syndrome in pregnancy. *Clinical Neurophys* 2001;112:1946–1951.

15. Stahl S, Blumenfeld Z, Yarnitsky D. Carpal tunnel syndrome in pregnancy: indications for early surgery. *J Neurol Sci* 1996;136:182–184.

16. Ekman-Orderberg G, Salgeback S, Orderberg G. Carpal tunnel syndrome in pregnancy. A prospective study. *Acta Obstet Gynecol Scan* 1987;66:233–235.

17. Stevens JC, Beard CM, O'Fallon WM, Kurland LT. Conditions associated with carpal tunnel syndrome. *Mayo Clin Proc* 1992;67:541–548.

18. Stolp-Smith KA. Carpal tunnel syndrome related to pregnancy. Course G: Neuromuscular Medicine in Pregnancy. 22nd Annual Electrodiagnostic Medicine Courses and Workshops. Vancouver, October 1999.

19. McLennan HG, Oats JN, Walstab JE. Survey of hand symptoms in pregnancy. *Med J Aust* 1987;147:542–544.

20. Rossi M, Morena M, Zanardi M. Neuropathy of the brachial plexus associated with pregnancy. Report of a case. *Recenti Progressi in Medicina* 1993;84:768–771.

21. Redmond JMT, Cros D, Martin JB, Shahani BT. Relapsing brachial plexopathy during pregnancy. Report of a case. *Arch Neurol* 1989;46:462–464.

22. Taylor RA. Heredofamilial mononeuritis multiplex with brachial predilection. *Brain* 1960;83:113–137.

23. Tsairis P, Dyck PJ, Mulder DW. Natural history of brachial plexus neuropathy: report on 99 patients. *Arch Neurol* 1972;27:109–117.

24. Rhodes P. Meralgia paresthetica in pregnancy. *Lancet* 1957;2:831.

25. Turget F, Turget M, Mentes E. Lumbosacral plexus compression by fetus: an unusual cause of radiculopathy during teenage pregnancy. *Eur J Obstet Gynecol Reprod Biol* 1997;73:203–204.

26. Delarue MW, Vles JS, Hassaart TH. Lumbosacral plexopathy in the third trimester of pregnancy: a report of three cases. *Eur J Obstet Gynecol Reprod Biol* 1994;53: 67–68.

27. Jiang GX, de Pedro-Cuesta J, Strigard K, Olsson T, Link H. Pregnancy and Guillian-Barre syndrome: a nationwide register cohort study. *Neuroepidemiology* 1996;15:192–200.

28. Parry GJ, Heiman-Patterson TD. Pregnancy and autoimmune neuromuscular disease. *Sem Neurol* 1988;8: 197–204.

29. Ropper AR, Wijdicks EFM, Traux BT. *Guillain-Barre Syndrome*. Philadelphia: FA Davis, 1991.

30. Mendizabal JE, Bassam BA. Guillain-Barre syndrome and cytomegalovirus infection during pregnancy. *South Med Assoc J* 1997;90:63–64.

31. Nelson LH, Maclean WT. Management of Landry-Guillain-Barre syndrome in pregnancy. *Obstet Gynecol* 1985;65:S25–S29.

32. Gautier PE, Hantson P, Vekemans MC, et al. Intensive care management of Guillain-Barre syndrome during pregnancy. *Intensive Care Med* 1990;16:460–462.

33. van der Meche FGA, Scmitz PIM, and the Dutch Guillain-Barre Syndrome Study Group. A randomized trial comparing intravenous immune globulin and plasma exchange in Guillain-Barre syndrome. *N Engl J Med* 1992;326:1123–1129.

34. Plasma Exchange/Sandoglobulin Guillain-Barre Syndrome Study Group. Comparison of plasma exchange, intravenous gammaglobulin, and plasma exchange followed by intravenous gammaglobulin in the treatment of Guillain-Barre syndrome. *Lancet* 1997;349: 225–230.

35. Rockel A, Wissel J, Rolfs A. GBS in pregnancy—an indication for Caesarian section? *J Perinat Med* 1994;22: 393–398.

36. Brooks H, Christian AS, May AE. Pregnancy anaesthesia and Guillain-Barre syndrome. *Anaesthesia* 2000;55: 894–898.

37. Feldman JM. Cardiac arrest after succinylcholine administration in a pregnant patient recovered from GBS. *Anesthesiology* 1990;72:942–944.

38. Bamford NS, Trojaborg W, Sherbany AA, De Vivo DC. Congenital Guillain-Barre syndrome associated with maternal inflammatory bowel disease is responsive to intravenous immunoglobulin. *Europ J Paediatr Neurol* 2002;6:115–119.

39. Barohn RJ, Kissel JT, Warmolts JR, Mendell JR. Chronic inflammatory demyelinating polyradiculoneuropathy. Clinical characteristics, course, and recommendations for diagnostic criteria. *Arch Neurol* 1989;46:878–884.

40. McCombe PA, McMannis PG, Frith JA, Pollard JD, McLeod JG. Chronic inflammatory demyelinating polyradiculoneuropathy associated with pregnancy. *Ann Neurol* 1987;21:102–104.

41. Dyck PJ, Lais AC, Ohta M, Bastron JA, Okazaki H, Groover RV. Chronic inflammatory polyradiculoneuropathy. *Mayo Clin Proc* 1975;50:621–637.

42. Dyck PJ, Daube J, O'Brien P, et al. Plasma exchange in chronic inflammatory demyelinating polyneuropathy. *N Engl J Med* 1986;314:461–465.

43. Hahn AF, Bolton CF, Zochodne D, Feasby TE. Intravenous immunoglobulin treatment in chronic inflammatory demyelinating polyneuropathy. A double-blind, placebo-controlled, cross-over study. *Brain* 1996;119: 1067–1077.

44. Chaudry V, Escolar DM, Cornblath DR. Worsening of multifocal motor neuropathy during pregnancy. *Neurology* 2002;59:139–141.

45. Beitns IZ, Bayard F, Ances IG, Kowarski A, Migeon CJ. The transplacental passage of prednisone and prednisolone in pregnancy near term. *J Pediatr* 1972;81:936–945.

46. Bermas BL, Hill JA. Effects of immunosuppressive drugs during pregnancy. *Arthritis Rheum* 1995;38:1722–1732.

47. Harris JWS, Ross IP. Cortisone therapy in early pregnancy: relation to cleft palate. *Lancet* 1956;1:1045–1047.

48. Committee on drugs, American Academy of Pediatrics. The transfer of drugs and other chemicals into human breast milk. *Pediatrics* 1994;93:137–150.

49. Pirson Y, van Lierde M, Ghysen J, Squifflet JP, Alexandre GPJ, van Ypersele de Strihou C. Retardation of fetal growth in patients receiving immunosuppressive therapy. *N Engl J Med* 1985:313:328.

50. Cote CJ, Meuwissen HJ, Pickering RJ. Effects on the neonate of prednisone and azathioprine administration to the mother during pregnancy. *J Pediatr* 1974;85:324–328.

51. Cederqvist LL, Merkatz IR, Litwin SD. Fetal immunoglobulin synthesis following maternal immunosuppression. *Am J Obstet Gynecol* 1977;129:687–690.

52. Lawson DH, Lovatt GE, Gurton CS, Hennings RC. Adverse effects of azathioprine. *Adverse Drug React Acute Poisoning Rev* 1984;3:161–171.

53. Zemlickis D, Lishner M, Erlich R, Koren G. Teratogenicity and carcinogenicity in a twin exposed in utero to cyclophosphamide. *Teratog Carcinog Mutagen* 1993;13:139–143.

54. Wiernik PH, Duncan JH. Cyclophosphamide in human milk. *Lancet* 1971;1:912.

55. Amenti VT, Radomski JS, Moritz MJ, et al. Report for the national transplantation pregnancy registry (NTPR): outcomes of pregnancy after transplant. *Clin Transpl* 2001;97–105.

56. Armenti VT, Ahlswede KM, Ahlswede BA, Jarrell BE, Moritz MJ, Burke JF. National transplant pregnancy registry: outcomes of 154 pregnancies in cyclosporine-treated female kidney transplant recipients. *Transplantation* 1994;57:502–506.

57. Haugen G, Fauchald P, Sodal G, Leivestad T, Moe N. Pregnancy outcome in renal allograft recipients in Norway: the importance of immunosuppressive drug regimen and health status before pregnancy. *Acta Obstet Gynecol Scand* 1994;73:541–546.

58. Dor R, Blanshard C. Caution with use of cyclosporine in pregnancy. *Gut* 2003;52:1070.

59. Bung P, Molitor D. Pregnancy and postpartum after kidney transplantation and cyclosporine therapy: a review of the literature adding a new case. *J Perinat Med* 1991;19:397–401.

60. Salko RG, Gold MP. Teratogenicity of methotrexate in mice. *Teratology* 1974;9:159–163.

61. Feldkamp M, Carey JC. Clinical teratology counseling and consultation case report: low-dose methotrexate exposure in the early weeks of pregnancy. *Teratology* 1993;47:533–539.

62. Yamada H, Noro N, Kato EH, Ebina Y, Cho K, Fujimoto S. Massive intravenous immunoglobulin treatment in pregnancy complicated by Guillain-Barre syndrome. *Eur J Obstet Gynecol Reprod Biol* 2001;97:101–104.

63. Brannagan, TH. Intravenous gammaglobulin (IVIg) for treatment of CIDP and related immune-mediated neuropathies. *Neurology* 2002;59:S33–S40.

64. Hemachandra A, Ellis D, Lloyd CE, Orchard TJ. The influence of pregnancy on IDDM complications. *Diabetes Care* 1995;18:950–954.

65. Lapolla A, Cardone C, Negrin P, et al. Pregnancy does not induce or worsen retinal or peripheral nerve dysfunction in insulin-dependent diabetic women. *J Diabetes Complications* 1998;12:74–80.

66. Nylund L, Brismar T, Lunell NO, Persson A, Persson B, Stangenberg M. Nerve conduction in diabetic pregnancy. A prospective study. *Diabetes Res Clin Pract* 1985;1:121–123.

67. Airaksinen KE, Salmela PI. Pregnancy is not a risk factor for a deterioration of autonomic nervous function in diabetic women. *Diabet Med* 1993;10:540–542.

68. Diabetes Control and Complications Trial Research Group. The effect of intensive diabetes therapy on the development and progression of neuropathy. *Ann Intern Med* 1995;122:561–568.

69. Macleod AF, Smith SA, Sonksen PH, Lowy C. The problem of autonomic neuropathy in diabetic pregnancy. *Diabet Med* 1990;7:80–82.

70. Vine S, Shaffer HM, Pauley G, Margolis EJ. A review of the relationship between pregnancy and porphyria and presentation of a case. *Ann Intern Med* 1957;47:834–840.

71. Bosch EP, Mitsumoto H. Disorders of Peripheral Nerves. In: Bradley WG, et al. (ed.) *Neurology in clinical practice: the neurological disorders*, 2nd ed. Boston: Butterworth-Heinemann, 1996.

72. Yiannikas C, Pollard JD, McLeod JG. Nitrofurantoin neuropathy. *Aust N Z J Med* 1981;11:400–405.

73. Philpot J, Muntoni F, Skellet S, Dubowitz V. Congenital symmetrical weakness of the upper limbs resembling brachial plexus palsy: a possible sequel of drug toxicity in the first trimester of pregnancy? *Neuromuscul Disord* 1995;5:67–69.

74. Rudnik-Schoneborn S, Rohrig D, Nicholson G, Zerres K. Pregnancy and delivery in Charcot-Marie-Tooth disease type 1. *Neurology* 1993;43:2011–2016.

75. Gastaut, JL, Benaim J, Livet MO, Philip N. Charcot Marie Tooth disease: exacerbation in pregnancy. *Revue Neurol* 2000;156:778–779.

76. Cole JT. Maternal obstetrical paralysis. *Am J Obstet Gynecol* 1946;52:372–385.

77. Hill EC. Maternal obstetrical paralysis. *Am J Obstet Gynecol* 1962;83:1452–1460.

78. Katirji B, Wilbourn AJ, Scarberry SL, Preston DC. Intrapartum maternal lumbosacral plexopathy. *Muscle Nerve* 2002;26:340–347.

79. Stohr M, Dichagans J, Dorstelmann D. Ischemic neuropathy of the lumbosacral plexus following intragluteal injection. *J Neurol Neurosurg Psychiatry* 1980;43:489–494.

80. Kane RE. Neurologic deficits following epidural anesthesia. *Anesth Analg* 1981;60:150–161.

81. Dar AQ, Robinson A, Lyons G. Postpartum femoral neuropathy: more common than you think. *Anesthesia* 1999;54:512.

82. Kofler M, Kronenberg MF. Bilateral femoral neuropathy during pregnancy. *Muscle Nerve* 1998;21:1106.

83. Hakim MA, Katirji B. Femoral mononeuropathy induced by the lithotomy position: a report of 5 cases with a review of the literature. *Muscle Nerve* 1993;16:891–895.

84. Massey EW. Mononeuropathies in pregnancy. *Semin Neurol* 1988;8:193–196.

85. Warfield CA. Obturator neuropathy after forceps delivery. *Obstet Gynecol* 1984;64:47S–48S.

86. Adornato BT, Carlini WG. "Pushing palsy:" a case of self-induced bilateral peroneal palsy during natural childbirth. *Neurology* 1992;42:936–937.

87. Reif ME. Bilateral common peroneal nerve palsy secondary to prolonged squatting in natural childbirth. *Birth* 1988;15:100–102.

88. Sippo WC, Burhardt A, Gomez AC. Nerve entrapment following Pfannenstiel incision. *Am J Obstet Gynecol* 1989;161:499–500.

89. Beric A. Peripheral nerve disorders. In: Hainline B, Devinsky O, (ed.) *Neurological complications of pregnancy*, 2nd ed. Philadelphia: Lippincott Williams & Wilkins, 2002.

90. Fitzpatrick M, O'Herlihy C. The effects of labour and delivery on the pelvic floor. *Best Pract Res Clin Obstet Gynaecol* 2001;15: 63–79.

91. Ryhammer AM, Lauberg S, Hermann AP. No correlation between perineal position and pudendal nerve terminal motor latency in healthy perimenopausal women. *Dis Colon Rectum* 1998;41:350–353.

92. Allen RE, Hosker GL, Smith ARB. Pelvic floor damage and childbirth: a neurophysiological study. *Br J Obstet Gynecol* 1990;97:770–779.

93. Tetzschner T, Sorensen M, Lose G, Christiansen J. Pudendal nerve function during pregnancy and after delivery. *Int Urogynecol J Pelvic Floor Dysfunct* 1997;8:66–68.

94. Morley R, Cummings J, Weller R. Morphology and neuropathology of the pelvic floor in patients with stress incontinence. *Int Urogynecol J Pelvic Floor Dysfunct* 1996;7:3–12.

95. Sangwan YP, Coller JA, Barrett RC, et al. Unilateral pudendal neuropathy. Impact on outcome of anal sphincter repair. *Dis Colon Rectum* 1996;39:686–689.

96. Kjolhede P, Lindehammar H. Pelvic floor neuropathy in relation to outcome of Burch colposuspension. *Int Urogynecol J Pelvic Floor Dysfunct* 1997;8:61–65.

97. Willis S, Faridi A, Schelzig S, et al. Childbirth and incontinence: a prospective study on anal sphincter morphology and function before and early after vaginal delivery. *Langenbecks Arch Surg* 2002;387:101–107.

98. Yuen EC, Layzer RB, Weitz SR, Olney RK. Neurologic complications of lumbar epidural anesthesia and analgesia. *Neurology* 1995;45:1795–1801.

99. Auroy Y, Narchi P, Messiah A, Litt L, Rouvier B, Samii K. Serious complications related to regional anesthesia: results of a perspective survey in France. *Anesthesiology* 1997;87:479–486.

100. Wand JS. Carpal tunnel syndrome in pregnancy and lactation. *J Hand Surg* 1990;15:93–95.

101. Hahn AF, Feasby TE, Wilkie L, Lovgren D. Antigalactocerebroside antibody increases demyelination in adoptive transfer experimental allergic neuritis. *Muscle Nerve* 1993;16:1174–1180.

102. Cooper JC, Hughes S, Ben-Smith A, Savage COS, Winer JB. T cell recognition of a non-protein antigen preparation of Campylobacter jejuni in patients with Guillain-Barre syndrome. *J Neurol Neurosurg Psychiatry* 2002; 72:413–414.

103. Klein CJ, Dyck PJB, Friedenberg SM, Burns TM, Windebank AJ, Dyck PJ. Inflammation and neuropathic attacks in hereditary brachial plexus neuropathy. *J Neurol Neurosurg Psychiatry* 2002;73:45–50.

104. Lederman RJ, Wilbourn AJ. Postpartum neuralgic amyotrophy. *Neurology* 1996;47:1213–1219.

105. Kaplan JG, Rosenberg R, Reinitz E, Buchbinder S, Schaumberg HH. Invited review: Peripheral neuropathy in Sjögren's syndrome. *Muscle Nerve* 1990;13:570–579.

106. Griffin JW, Cornblath DR, Alexander E, et al. Ataxic sensory neuropathy and dorsal root ganglionitis associated with Sjögren's syndrome. *Ann Neurol* 1990;27: 304–314.

107. Grant IA, Hunder GG, Homburger HA, Dyck PJ. Peripheral neuropathy associated with sicca complex. *Neurology* 1997;48:855–862.

108. Moll JW, Markusse HM, Pinjnenburg JJ, Vecht CJ, Henzen-Logmans SC. Antineuronal antibodies in patients with neurologic complications of primary Sjögren's syndrome. *Neurology* 1993;43:2574–2581.

109. Satake M, Yoshimura T, Iwaki T, Yamada T, Kabayashi T. Anti-dorsal root ganglion neuron antibody in a case of dorsal root ganglionitis associated with Sjögren's syndrome. *J Neurol Sci* 1995;132:122–125.

110. Chen WH, Yeh JH, Chiu HC. Plasmapheresis in the treatment of ataxic sensory neuropathy associated with Sjögren's syndrome. *Eur Neurol* 2001;45:270–274.

111. Molina JA, Benito-Leon J, Bermejo F. Intravenous immunoglobulin therapy and sensory neuropathy associated with Sjögren's syndrome. *J Neurol Neurosurg Psychiatry* 1996;60:699.

112. Asahina M, Kuwabara S, Asahina M, Nakajima M, Hattori T. D-penicillamine treatment for chronic sensory ataxic neuropathy associated with Sjögren's syndrome. *Neurology* 1998;51:1451–1453.

113. Caroyer JM, Manto MU, Steinfeld SD. Severe sensory neuronopathy responsive to infliximab in primary Sjögren's syndrome. *Neurology* 2002;59:1113–1114.

114. Lanzillo B, Pappone N, Crisci C, Di Girolamo C, Massini R, Caruso G. Subclinical peripheral nerve involvement in patients with rheumatoid arthritis. *Arthritis Rheum* 1998;41:1196–1202.

115. Risenbaum R. Neuromuscular complications of connective tissue diseases. *Muscle Nerve* 2001;24:154–169.

116. Said G. Lacroix-Ciaudo C, Fujimura H, Blas C, Faux N. The peripheral neuropathy of necrotizing arteritis: a clinicopathological study. *Ann Neurol* 1988;23:461–465.

117. Chang RW, Bell CL, Hallet M. Clinical characteristics and prognosis of vasculitic mononeuropathy multiplex. *Arch Neurol* 1984;41:618–621.

118. Huynh C, Ho SL, Fong KY, Cheung RTF, Mok CC, Lau CS. Peripheral neuropathy in systemic lupus erythematosus. *J Clin Neurophysiol* 1999;16:164–168.

119. Stahl HD, Kalischewski P, Orda C, Baum P, Grahmann F, Emmrich F. Filtration of cerebrospinal fluid for acute demyelinating neuropathy in systemic lupus erythematosus. *Clin Rheum* 2000;19:61–63.

120. Gamez-Nava JI, Gonzalez-Lopez L, Ramos-Remus C, Fonsecca-Gomez MM, Cardona-Munoz EG, Suarez-Almazor ME. Autonomic dysfunction in patients with systemic lupus erythematosus. *J Rheum* 1998;25: 1092–1096.

121. Campello I, Almarcegui C, Velilla J, Hortells JL, Oliveros A. Peripheral neuropathy in systemic lupus erythematosus. *Rev Neurol* 2001;33:27–30.

122. McCombe PA, McLeod JG, Pollard JD, Guo YP, Ingall TJ. Peripheral sensorimotor and autonomic neuropathy associated with systemic lupus erythematosus. Clinical, pathological and immunological features. *Brain* 1987; 110:533–549.

123. Olney RK. Neuropathies in connective tissue disease. *Muscle Nerve* 1992;15:531–542.

124. Duyff, RF, Van den Bosch J, Laman DM, Potter van Loon BJ, Lnssen WHJP. Neuromuscular findings in thyroid dysfunction: a prospective clinical and electrodiagnostic study. *J Neurol Neurosurg Psychiatry* 2000;68:750–755.

125. Dyck PJ, Lambert EH. Polyneuropathy associated with hypothyroidism. *J Neuropathol Exp Neurol* 1970;29:631–658.

126. Shirabe T, Tawara S, Terao A, Araki S. Myxodematous polyneuropathy: a light and electron microscopic study of the peripheral nerve and muscle. *J Neurol Neurosurg Psychiatry* 1975;38:241–247.

127. Pollard JD, McLeod JG, Honnibal TG, Verheijden MA. Hypothyroid polyneuropathy. Clinical, electrophysiological and nerve biopsy findings in two cases. *J Neurol Sci* 1982;53:461–471.

128. Laurencet FM, Anchiisi S, Tullen E, Dietrich PY. Mental neuropathy: report of five cases and review of the literature. *Crit Rev Oncol Hematol* 2000;34:71–79.

129. Massey EW, Moore J, Schold SC Jr. Mental neuropathy from systemic cancer. *Neurology* 1981;31:1277–1281.

130. Clouston PD, Davies L. Neuropathies in malignant disease. In: Cros D, (ed.) *Peripheral neuropathy: a practical approach to diagnosis and management*. Philadelphia: Lippincott Williams & Wilkins, 2000.

131. Clouston PD, DeAngelis L, Posner JB. The spectrum of neurologic disease in systemic cancer. *Ann Neurol* 1992;31:268–273.

132. Harper CM, Juergen ET, Cascino TL, Litchy WJ. Distinction between neoplastic and radiation-induced brachial plexopathy, with emphasis on the role of the EMG. *Neurology* 1989;39:502–506.

133. Esteban A, Traba A. Fasciculation-myokymic activity and prolonged nerve conduction block. A physiopathological relationship in radiation-induced brachial plexopathy. *Electroencephalogr Clin Neurophysiol* 1993;89:382–391.

134. Qayyum A, MacVicar AD, Padhani AR, Revell P, Husband JE. Symptomatic brachial plexopathy following treatment for breast cancer: utility of MR imaging with surface-coil techniques. *Radiology* 2000;214:837–842.

135. Molinnuevo JL, Graus F, Serrano C, Rene R, Guerrero A, Illa I. Utility of anti-Hu antibodies in the diagnosis of paraneoplastic sensory neuropathy. *Ann Neurol* 1998;44:976–980.

136. Chalk CH, Windebank AJ, Kimmel DW, McManis PG. The distinctive clinical features of paraneoplastic sensory neuropathy. *Can J Neurol Sci* 1992;19:346–351.

137. Dalmau J, Graus F, Rosenblum MK, Posner JB. Anti-Hu–associated paraneoplastic encephalomyelitis/sensory neuronopathy. A clinical study of 71 patients. *Medicine* 1992;71:59–72.

138. Dropcho EJ. Remote neurologic manifestations of cancer. *Neurol Clin* 2002;20:85–122.

139. Bechich S, Graus F, Arboix A, Isiadro A, Marti M, Rosell F. Anti-Hu associated paraneoplastic sensory neuropathy and breast cancer. *J Neurol* 2000;247:552–553.

140. Forsyth PA, Dalmau J, Graus F, Cwik V, Rosenblum MK, Posner JB. Motor neuron syndromes in cancer patients. *Ann Neurol* 1997;41:722–730.

141. Ferracci F, Fassetta G, Butler MH, Floyd S, Solimena M, De Camillo P. A novel antineuronal antibody in a motor neuron syndrome associated with breast cancer. *Neurology* 1999;53:852–855.

142. Folli F, Solimena M, Cofiell R, et al. Autoantibodies to a 128-kd synaptic protein in the women with the stiff-man syndrome and breast cancer. *N Engl J Med* 1993;328:546–551.

143. Keime-Guibert F, Graus F, Fleury A, et al. Treatment of paraneoplastic neurological syndromes with antineuronal antibodies (Anti-Hu, anti-Ro) with a combination of immunoglobulins, cyclophosphamide, and methylprednisolone. *J Neurol Neurosurg Psychiatry* 2000;64:479–482.

144. Olsen NK, Pfeiffer P, Mondrup K, Rose C. Radiation-induced brachial plexus neuropathy in breast cancer patients. *Acta Oncol* 1990;29:885–890.

145. Johansson S, Svensson H, Denekamp J. Timescale of evolution of late radiation injury after postoperative radiotherapy of breast cancer. *Int J Radiat Oncol Biol Phys* 2000;48:745–750.

146. Olsen NK, Pfeiffer P, Johannsen L, Schroder H, Rose C. Radiation-induced brachial plexopathy: neurological follow-up in 161 recurrence-free breast cancer patients. *Int J Radiat Oncol Biol Phys* 1993;26:43–49.

147. Gregg RW, Molepo JM, Monpetit VJ, et al. Cisplatin neurotoxicity: the relationship between dosage, time, and platinum concentration in neurologic tissues, and morphologic evidence of toxicity. *J Clin Oncol* 1992;10:795–803.

148. Roelofs RI, Hrushesky W, Rogin J, Rosenberg L. Peripheral sensory neuropathy and cisplatin chemotherapy. *Neurology* 1984;34:934–938.

149. Iniguez C, Larrode P, Mayordomo JI, et al. Reversible peripheral neuropathy induced by a single administration of high-dose paclitaxel. *Neurology* 1998;51:868–870.

150. Pace A, Bove L, Aloe A, et al. Paclitaxel neurotoxicity: clinical and neurophysiological study of 23 patients. *Ital J Neurol Sci* 1997;18:73–79.

151. MacKenzie JR, LaBan MM, Sackeyfio AH. The prevalence of peripheral neuropathy in patients with anorexia nervosa. *Ach Phys Med Rehab* 1989;70:827–830.

152. Palmer EP, Guay AT. Reversible myopathy secondary to ipecac in patients with major eating disorders. *N Engl J Med* 1985;313:1457–1459.

153. Dresser LP, Massey EW, Johnson EE, Bossen E. Ipecac myopathy and cardiomyopathy. *J Neurol Neurosurg Psychiatry* 1993;56:560–562.

154. Mondelli M, Giannini F, Giacchi M. Carpal tunnel syndrome incidence in a general population. *Neurology* 2002;58:289–294.

155. Dekel S, Papaioannou T, Rushworth G, Coates R. Idiopathic carpal tunnel syndrome caused by carpal stenosis. *Br Med J* 1980;280:1297–1299.

156. Ferry S, Hannaford P, Warskyj M, Lewis M, Croft P. Carpal tunnel syndrome: a nested case-control study of risk factors in women. *Am J Epidemiol* 2000;151:566–574.

157. Vilos GA, Vilos AW, Haebe JJ. Laparoscopic findings, management, histopathology, and outcome of 25 women with cyclic leg pain. *J Am Assoc Gynecol Laparsc* 2002;9:145–151.

158. Dhote R, Tudoret L, Bachmeyer C, Legmann P, Christoforov B. Cyclic sciatica: a manifestation of compression of the sciatic nerve by endometriosis: a case report. *Spine* 1996;21:2277–2279.

159. Torkelson SJ, Lee RA, Hildahl DB. Endometriosis of the sciatic nerve: a report of two cases and review of the literature. *Obstet Gynecol* 1988;71:473–477.

160. Zager EL, Pfeifer SM, Brown MJ, Torosian MH, Hackney DB. Catamenial mononeuropathy and radiculopa-

thy: a treatable neuropathic disorder. *J Neurosurg* 1999;90:374.

161. Sanger JR, Matloub HS, Yousif NJ, Komorowski R. Silicone gel infiltration of a peripheral nerve and constrictive neuropathy following rupture of breast prosthesis. *Plast Reconstr Surg* 1992;89:949–952.

162. Hueston WJ, Locke KT. Norplant neuropathy: peripheral neurologic symptoms associated with subdermal contraceptive implants. *J Fam Pract* 1995;40:184–186.

163. Nyren O, McLaughlin JK, Yin L, et al. Breast implants and risk of neurologic disease: a population-based cohort study in Sweden. *Neurology* 1998;50:956–961.

164. Gabriel SE, O'Fallon WM, Kurland LT, Beard CM, Woods JE, Melton LJ. Risk of connective-tissue diseases and other disorders after breast implantation. *N Engl J Med* 1994;330:1697–1702.

165. Winther JF, Friis S, Bach FW, et al. Neurological disease among women with silicone breast implants in Denmark. *Acta Neurol Scand* 2001;103:93–96.

166. Vogel H. Pathologic findings in nerve and muscle biopsies from 47 women with silicone breast implants. *Neurology* 1999;53:293–297.

167. The Commonwealth Fund 1998 Survey of Women's Health. *Women's Health Issues* 2000;10:35–38.

168. Massey JM. Domestic violence in neurologic practice. *Arch Neurol* 1999;56:659–660.

21 Muscle Disease in Women

James M. Gilchrist, MD

A ny discussion of muscle disease in women is dominated by the effects of pregnancy and the puerperium. These considerations aside, men and women have similar disease presentations, prognoses, responses to treatment, and demographic risks. Scant literature exists on the effects of puberty, menarche, or menopause on muscle disease. My own clinical experience has been that these otherwise resounding events in the lives of every woman have little effect on diseases of muscle. This chapter includes a discussion of prenatal genetic counseling and testing where important, a brief explanation of maternal inheritance (Figure 21.1) as it pertains to mitochondrial encephalomyopathies and a summary of those diseases that have different expressions depending on gender (Table 21.1).

MUSCULAR DYSTROPHY

Muscular dystrophy (MD) has several forms, such as oculopharyngeal MD and facioscapulohumeral MD, without differences in women. Emery-Dreifuss MD is an X-linked recessive trait, affecting only males, and is not addressed.

Duchenne and Becker Muscular Dystrophy

Duchenne muscular dystrophy (DMD) and Becker muscular dystrophy (BMD) are allelic X-linked recessive dis-

orders that arise from defects in a gene situated in the Xp21 region of the X-chromosome, coding for a large structural protein called dystrophin (1). Boys become symptomatic for Duchenne dystrophy at approximately 5 years of age, become wheelchair bound at approximately 10 to 12 years of age, and die by their early 20s. Becker dystrophy is milder and the symptoms, although similar, reach the same milestones a decade or so later (2). By nature of the chromosomal location, females are at risk for being carriers but not for the dystrophy (infrequently, carrier females can manifest a milder form of the disease) (3,4) except for rare cases of Turner's syndrome (XO), X; autosome translocation (5,6), and uniparental disomy of the female X chromosome (7). Female carriers have an increased incidence of breech deliveries, regardless of the genetic status of the neonate, indicating a maternal factor such as subtle uterine or pelvic floor muscle weakness (8).

Manifesting Carriers

Uncommonly (5 to 10%) (9), a female carrier of an altered dystrophin gene will develop myopathic features similar to but milder than those of Duchenne or Becker dystrophy (3). These women have muscle fibers containing either normal or abnormal dystrophin, or none (10), which in many cases may be related to a skewed (i.e., dysproportionate) inactivation of the X-chromosome carry-

TABLE 21.1
A summary of disorders discussed in this chapter.

Disease	Onset	Clinical Features	Unique Features	Diagnostic Test	Treatment	Prognosis
Manifesting DMD carrier	1st–3rd decade	Proximal weakness, contractures	Asymmetry, cardiomyopathy	DNA deletion	None	Slow progression
X; autosome translocation DMD	1st decade	Proximal weakness	Looks like DMD in a girl	Muscle dystrophin	Consider prednisone	Poor
Limb-girdle muscular dystrophy	1st–3rd decade	Proximal weakness		Muscle biopsy	None	Slow progression
FSH dystrophy	1st–3rd decade	Proximal weakness	Facial, scapular, humeral weakness	DNA test	None	Slow progression
Congenital muscular dystrophy	Birth-childhood	Hypotonia, weakness, retardation	Early onset, progression	CK, muscle biopsy	None	Poor
Myotonic dystrophy type 1	2nd–6th decade	Distal weakness	Myotonia, cataracts, cardiomyopathy	EMG, DNA triplet repeat	None	Variable
Congenital myotonic dystrophy	Birth-childhood	Hypotonia, respiratory distress	Mental retardation	DNA triplet repeat	None	Poor
Myasthenia Gravis	2nd–7th decade	Ptosis, diplopia, weakness	Fatigable weakness	AchR antibody, EMG	Antichol-inesterases, immuno-suppression	Good
Neanatal myasthenia gravis	Birth	Hypotonia, poor suck & cry	Lasts days to weeks	Neostigmine test	Antichol-inesterases	Excellent
Polymyositis	Childhood, 5th–6th decade	Proximal weakness	Myalgias	CPK, EMG, muscle biopsy	Immuno-suppression	Fair
Periodic paralysis	1st–3rd decade	Intermittent paralysis	Transient weakness, myotonia	Serum potassium	Potassium replacement or lowering	Good
Myotonia Congenita	1st–3rd decade	Myotonia	Muscle hypertrophy	EMG	Mexilitine, etc	Good
Metabolic myopathies	2nd–3rd decade	Myalgia	Myoglobinuria	Muscle enzyme assay	Dietary	Fair
Mitochondrial myopathy	1st–6th decade	Proximal weakness	Opthalmoplegia, lactic acidosis	Muscle biopsy, genetic test	None	Poor
Carnitine deficiency	1st–5th decade	Proximal weakness		Carnitine assay	Carnitine	Good
Thyroid myopathy	3rd-5th decade	Proximal weakness	Other signs of dysthyroidism	Thyroid tests	Treat thyroid disease	Good
Congenital Myopathy	Birth	Weakness, hypotonia	Skeletal abnormalities	Muscle biopsy	None	Stable
Toxic Myopathy	3rd–7th decade	Weakness	Cardiomyopathy	History	Abstinence	Fair
Fibromyalgia	3rd–5th decade	Myalgia	Trigger points	None	Tricyclics	Fair

ing the normal dystrophin gene (11,12). Such nonrandom inactivation would explain the occasional discordance for myopathic disease in monozygotic female twins carrying the gene defect (13).

The age of onset may be during childhood, but more commonly is in the second and third decades, with more severe disease following earlier onset. Proximal weakness, which affects the legs first and then the arms, is often asymmetric. Calf hypertrophy is very common but contractures are not, except in the more severely affected and wheelchair-bound, and unassisted ambulation commonly persists for decades after onset. Unlike males with dystrophinopathy, carrier females with dystrophy may derive significant and prolonged improvement in function from exercise training, presumably via hypertrophy of normal muscle fibers. The similarity of the clinical picture to that of limb girdle muscular dystrophy (LGMD) has led to speculation that females with sporadic LGMD may be manifesting carriers of DMD or BMD (4). This has important genetic implications, and a thorough evaluation, including muscle biopsy with dystrophin analysis and dystrophin deletion studies, should be done in appropriate females with LGMD (sporadic cases, or with no affected males in the family).

Cardiomyopathy is a frequent occurrence in DMD and BMD and can also be seen in symptomatic carriers, occasionally as the only manifestation (14,15). A recent study (16) found 84% of female carriers had preclinical or clinical myocardial involvement, with incidence increasing with age, from 55% of patients under 16 years of age, to 90% of those over 16 years old. Myocardial hypertrophy, dysrhythmias, and dilated cardiomyopathy were found in clinically affected patients, a pattern similar to males with DMD and BMD.

X; Autosome Translocations

Rarely, DMD can be found in females due to de novo translocations involving the Xp21 region. Twenty-four such cases have been described, with the breakpoint within the dystrophin gene, which is then disabled (17). Skewed X-inactivation of the normal chromosome leads to clinical manifestations of a severe myopathy beginning in childhood and progressing to nonambulation by the second decade. It is clinically indistinguishable from boys with DMD.

Prenatal Diagnosis and Counseling

Because of the devastating effect on parent and child and the lack of a cure, it is important to provide prepregnancy genetic counseling regarding risk to women with affected offspring, siblings, or other relatives. Unfortunately, the dystrophin gene region is quite large, and up to one-third of cases of Duchenne and Becker muscular dystrophy are

new mutations (2). Carrier detection and prenatal diagnosis of affected fetuses is available in families with known dystrophinopathies, however (18). The calculated risk of being a carrier depends on the pedigree; that is, the number of affected males and their relationship to the female patient. Bayesian analysis enables a calculation of the genetic risk for being a carrier (2). For a known carrier, each of her offspring, male or female, carries a 50% chance of inheriting the abnormal gene. The situation is often more complex (2), and the calculation of risk may be improved through DNA analysis (18).

Abnormal dystrophin quantity and quality are the sine qua non of Duchenne and Becker muscular dystrophy, and this can be determined through muscle assay (19). Female carriers are not reliably diagnosed by quantitation of dystrophin, however (4). Immunostaining of muscle for dystrophin may be useful (4), but a normal examination does not exclude being a carrier and DNA analysis is essential. Approximately 60% of Duchenne cases arise from a deletion of the dystrophin gene, whereas another 7% arise from duplications (20). If either is present in the affected male(s) of a family, the presence or absence of the deletion or duplication can be easily and quickly determined in at-risk females by a blood test for DNA. Absence of the DNA abnormality can exclude the risk, although germline mosaicism must also be considered. The presence of the DNA defect indicates the female is a carrier. If a large deletion or duplication is not found in the affected male, then a search for small mutations [detection of virtually all mutations-single strand conformational polymorphism (SSCP); (DOVAMS-S)] can detect mutations in 78.5% of patients with previously unidentified mutations (21). This blood-based method improves the overall success rate in finding the genetic defect in DMD and BMD to 93%. In the remaining 7% of families, DNA linkage analysis is indicated (18). This necessitates obtaining blood from members of the family, especially affected males, if alive. Prenatal testing can be used to identify affected fetuses in families known to be at risk. If the fetus is male, DNA linkage using polymerase chain reaction (PCR) techniques can be done to determine if the fetus carries the defective gene. This may be done by chorionic villus sampling or amniocentesis. Other methods include fetal muscle biopsy for dystrophin analysis (22), cleavage cell embryo biopsy (23), and dystrophin delection analysis of nucleated maternal erythrocytes (24). At least one report documents maternal contamination of a fetal muscle biopsy (25). These tests are only helpful if therapeutic abortion is being considered (see also Chapter 5).

Limb-Girdle Muscular Dystrophy

A diagnosis of LGMD has long been a respository for patients who have muscle disease that is not otherwise explained. Typically, it appears in the second and third decades of life, with proximal legs and then arms affected over a prolonged course. Ambulation may be lost, but not until 20 years or so after onset. LGMD is sporadic or inherited as a autosomal recessive trait in 95% of patients, with the remaining cases inherited in an autosomal dominant pattern.

A severe childhood form of the disease is seen less commonly. This form looks very much like DMD but is distinguishable from it by an autosomal recessive pattern of inheritance (severe childhood autosomal recessive muscular dystrophy; SCARMD).

The molecular genetics of LGMD have been clarified to a great extent in the past 10 years, with localization of 10 autosomal recessive forms and five autosomal dominant forms (26,27). Several of the genes code for proteins of the dystrophin-associated glycoprotein complex, which, with dystrophin, comprise the major underlying structural support of the muscle fiber membrane (28).

LGMD and Pregnancy

The incidence and severity of LGMD does not vary between the sexes, so it does not convey a special risk or benefit to females. There may well be an effect of the disease upon pregnancy and vice versa, however. In an unpublished study, Lauren Donald and I did a retrospective survey of 38 women with autosomal recessive LGMD from 31 families. There were 59 pregnancies in 22 women with 38 children, and a known spontaneous abortion rate of 31%, with one perinatal death. Difficulty with labor and delivery was reported in 29% of births without other complications. Seven women suffered significant and permanent decline in function while pregnant, usually in the first two trimesters, and most frequently in more severely affected women. Similar findings were reported from a retrospective review of nine LGMD women with 15 pregnancies (29). Therapeutic abortion occurred in three (20%), with no miscarriages noted. Operative delivery was necessary in five of the remaining 12 pregnancies, of which two were emergencies. Five of the nine women experienced worsening weakness during pregnancy, one of whom improved after delivery. Five of the women required assistance in child care after delivery because of physical limitations. Women with LGMD should therefore be counseled that pregnancy may increase spontaneous abortion and may significantly and permanently increase weakness, the risk being greater with increasing disease severity.

LGMD Genetic Counseling

The majority of LGMD patients have an autosomal recessively inherited trait. Therefore, the risk of their offspring inheriting the disease is increased only marginally over the general population, as long as the mat-

ing is not consanguinous. The challenge, then, is in families who already have one child with SCARMD and wish to have another child. The risk of any further children having the disease is 25% if there is no consanguinity. Prenatal screening is possible, but requires linkage analysis, mutation analysis, or fetal muscle biopsy at a center able to do the testing, which is not widely available (30–32).

Facioscapulohumeral Dystrophy

Facioscapulohumeral dystrophy (FSHD) is inherited as an autosomal dominant trait. Approximately 95% of families have been linked to chromosome 4q35, near the telomere (33). FSHD is an MD of characteristic and defining weakness involving the face and scapular muscles. The age of onset is variable, from childhood (these patients are frequently more severely affected) to the early third decade. The weakness is slowly progressive and may arrest for several years or more. The disease also may progress in sudden accelerations, however.

Despite the relative frequency of FSHD, there is only one report of 26 pregnancies in 11 patients (29). Three miscarriages (12%), two preterm births, and six operative deliveries occurred. Three women had symptomatic worsening during gestation, but all recovered after delivery and there were no long-term sequelae.

FSHD Genetic Counseling

As with any autosomal dominant inherited trait, the risk of intergenerational transmission is 50% for each child. The gene for FSHD has not been found nor is the gene product known. More than 90% of FSHD patients have a deletion on chromosome 4q35, however, which results in a small EcoR1 restriction fragment that can be used to confirm the disease and for prenatal diagnosis (34). For further information on the genetics of other neuromuscular diseases, please see Chapter 7.

Myotonic Dystrophy

Myotonic dystrophy (also known as dystrophica myotonica, myotonia atrophica, and Steinert's disease) is a multisystem disorder affecting both sexes equally. It is characterized by the variable expression of progressive, predominantly distal, skeletal muscle weakness, cataracts, frontal balding, cardiac conduction defects, clinical and electrical myotonia, smooth muscle weakness of the esophagus, stomach, bowel, and uterus, and endocrine disturbances (35). Onset is usually in the second to third decade but can be much later (35) or as early as birth (36,37).

Myotonic dystrophy is inherited as an autosomal dominant trait. The abnormal gene has been localized to chromosome 19 and cloned (38–40). It encodes for myotonin, a member of the protein kinase family (38), whose function is poorly understood. The disease is correlated to the presence of triplet repeats (CTG) inserted in the gene, which then increase in size in succeeding generations, explaining the clinical phenomenon of "anticipation," in which subsequent generations manifest the disease more severely and at an earlier age (41). The triplet repeat expansion is present in essentially all patients who have myotonic dystrophy (41). The transgenerational expansion of the triplet repeat sequence is greater when the transmitting parent is male (42).

Congenital Myotonic Dystrophy

Myotonic dystrophy can present in the fetus during pregnancy, at birth, or in early childhood. For reasons still unexplained (43,44), this congenital myotonic dystrophy occurs only when the mother is the affected parent (45). The risk of an affected woman having a congenitally affected child is 10%, but increases to almost 40% if she has already had congenitally affected offspring (43). Women who have multisystem disease at the time of pregnancy and delivery are at the highest risk for a child with congenital myotonic dystrophy (43), but even asymptomatic women have borne congenitally affected children (46). The mother's age at birth may have an effect on the severity of her offspring's disease, with the children of older women being more severely affected (47).

The disease can manifest in utero as polyhydramnios and reduced fetal movements, resulting in arthrogryposis multiplex congenita at birth (48–52). Vanier described congenital myotonic dystrophy in 1960 (53). Dyken and Harper subsequently reported 38 patients from 24 families who had symptoms referable to myotonic dystrophy from birth (37). Symptoms vary from severe respiratory involvement at birth to clumsiness and mental retardation becoming evident in early childhood. The neonatal onset of myotonic dystrophy is frequently fatal, with a 25% mortality rate before age 18 months (52), often due to respiratory failure (50–52). Survivors are very impaired, with hypotonia, diffuse weakness, developmental delay, poor feeding, mental retardation, talipes, and arthrogryposis (51,52). In these cases, fetal muscle exhibits maturational arrest, principally involving the limb, pharyngeal, and diaphragmatic muscles (54). Rutherford and co-workers reported that respiratory function at birth determined survival in congenital myotonic dystrophy, with the duration of mechanical ventilation providing the best guide to prognosis (55). Electrodiagnostic studies may confirm the diagnosis (56), but they often do not show myotonia and may be more informative when they are performed on the mother rather than on the infant. In the infant with respiratory failure and failure to feed, a high index of suspicion for congenital myotonic dystrophy is important because the mother often has not been diagnosed. Affected children without fetal or neonatal presentation exhibit talipes, facial diplegia, mental retardation, developmental delay, weakness, clumsiness, strabismus, and dysarthria (36,37).

Pregnancy and Myotonic Dystrophy

Large sibships are not uncommon in families with myotonic dystrophy, and fertility is not drastically reduced. Women appear to have few clinical or hormonal gonadal abnormalities (57,58) and, in two studies of six women, no abnormalities of estrogen, gonadotrophin, or testosterone were apparent (57,59). In a group of 33 women followed by Thomasen "menstrual irregularities [were] more frequently found in women with severe degrees of muscle dystrophy" (60) although others are not sure this is significant (58). Harper studied 44 affected females and compared them to 25 unaffected siblings and spouses. He found a tendency towards irregular and painful menses, and an earlier onset of menopause (58). A case of amenorrhea with hypothalamic hypogonadism reported normal gonadal hormone levels (61). Fertility seems to be reduced to 75% of normal in both sexes. Because this number includes severely affected members who are unlikely to conceive, however, the fertility of less affected women may well be normal or even increased (62).

The Effect of Pregnancy on Myotonic Dystrophy

Pregnancy rarely has an adverse affect on the course of myotonic dystrophy (63). No evidence suggests that pregnancy has a beneficial effect upon the disease. Several case reports indicate myotonia, muscle wasting, and weakness can first become symptomatic or significantly worsen during pregnancy (64–68). This usually occurs during the third trimester (48,65), corresponding to the time of maximal progesterone levels, and leading some investigators to implicate progesterone in the temporary worsening of the disease (65). Because progressive loss of muscle function in the mother is expected regardless of pregnancy, the question of whether pregnancy accelerates permanent disability is difficult to answer but may rarely occur (63). A single report documents a pregnant woman with recurrent myotonic spasms affecting distal limbs beginning in the second trimester and continuing until delivery (69).

Fall and co-workers (70) described a pregnant myotonic woman who developed heart failure at 32 weeks gestation, with an endomyocardial biopsy suggestive of myotonic dystrophy. She improved after delivery but died suddenly from a cardiac arrhythmia 8 weeks later.

The Effect of Myotonic Dystrophy on Pregnancy

Myotonic dystrophy may have a devastating effect during pregnancy (Table 21.2) due to the mother's disease (48,50,63,64,67,71–74) and the disease of the fetus (48–50,63,71,75). Postpartum hemorrhage from a failure of uterine contraction may occur (71,73). The first (65) and second stages of labor can be prolonged because of poor uterine contraction from myometrial involvement (48,64) and the inability to "bear down" because of voluntary muscle weakness (66,68). Despite this, most women do not have prolonged labor (63). Women should avoid prolonged bed rest leading to disuse of muscles, which further weakens patients with myotonic dystrophy.

Special risks accrue to anesthesia and surgery. Depolarizing neuromuscular blockade with succinylcholine may cause *myotonic spasm* (76,77), in which muscles diffusely contract and cannot relax, thus preventing ventilation of the patient. Nondepolarizing agents (e.g., curare) may safely be used. Myotonic dystrophy does not place patients at higher risk for malignant hyperthermia (78). Thiopental may cause marked respiratory depression in patients with myotonic dystrophy (74). All things considered, local anesthesia is preferable (74).

Genetic Counseling

In the absence of a foreseeable cure for myotonic dystrophy, genetic counseling offers an opportunity to help develop a patient's understanding of the disease, establish individual risk for symptoms, determine the risk for myotonic dystrophy, and offer advice for dealing with these risks. Carrier and prenatal detection can be done with almost 100% accuracy (79,80), thus allowing better genetic counseling and the option of elective abortion of affected fetuses. For prenatal detection, chorionic villus sampling circa 10 weeks, or amniocentesis circa 16 weeks, is needed to establish fetal genotype. Trophoblast cells from endocervical canal flushing between 7 and 9 weeks gestation can also provide fetal DNA (81). The expansion of the trinucleotide repeat in fetal tissue compared to maternal tissue does not reliably predict congenital myotonic dystrophy (82). Contraction of the trinucleotide repeat expansion from parent to child may complicate the determination of fetal status (83).

Proximal Myotonic Myopathy, Myotonic Dystrophy Type 2

Accurate genetic testing for myotonic dystrophy has revealed families without either a triplet repeat expansion or linkage to DNA markers on chromosome 19. These patients were clinically similar to those having myotonic dystrophy except for proximal rather than distal weakness, thus the newly coined diagnosis of proximal myotonic myopathy (PROMM) (84). PROMM has been linked to a locus on chromosome 3q, as have two other myotonic entities—proximal myotonic dystrophy and myotonic dystrophic type 2 (85). Whether the three diseases are allelic or represent phenotypic variation of single genetic mutation is unknown (85). A new classification proposes calling myotonic dystrophy linked to chromosme 19q *myotonic dystrophy type 1* and the entities linked to chromosome 3q *myotonic dystrophy type 2* (85). Newman and associates report three sisters with PROMM who had myotonic dystrophy present during pregnancy but the disease disappeared after delivery (86). One report documents a congenital hypotonic infant with PROMM, born to an asymptomatic mother (87). PROMM, or myotonic dystrophy type 2, affects genetic counseling because patients without clinical signs but with a family history of myotonic dystrophy and normal triplet repeat numbers cannot be definitely excluded as carriers until an affected family member has been shown to have an expanded triplet repeat region (see also Chapter 7).

Congenital Muscular Dystrophy

Congenital muscular dystrophy (CMD) comprises a group of inherited disorders with progressive muscular weakness and variable amounts of CNS involvement. CMD has been classified into the classic form without CNS involvement, and Fukuyama muscular dystrophy. The classic form has been further divided by the presence or absence of merosin, a protein that connects the dystrophin-associated glycoprotein complex to the extracellular matrix. Merosin-deficient CMD has been linked to the locus of the laminin alpha2 chain of merosin on chromosome 6q2 (88). Merosin-deficient and merosin-positive CMD share similar characteristics of hypotonia, muscle weakness, and developmental delay with onset in early infancy (89). Imaging studies of the brain reveal white matter changes but no malformations. Mental retardation occurs in a minority of patients with classical CMD.

TABLE 21.2

The Effects of Myotonic Dystrophy on the Pregnant Mother and Her Fetus

Maternal effects	Fetal effects
Prolonged labor	Hydramnios
Premature labor	Increased neonatal mortality
Uterine atony	Reduced fetal movements
Retained placenta	
Placenta previa	
Spontaneous abortion	
Postpartum hemorrhage	
Variable response to oxytocin	

The progressive weakness and the mental retardation may be milder in the merosin-positive patients (89). Fukuyama CMD has early infantile onset of severe weakness, brain malformation, severe mental retardation, and early death. It has been linked to a locus on chromosome 9q31 (90).

The finding of a genetic locus for merosin-negative CMD and for Fukuyama CMD has made prenatal genetic determination possible in families at risk. Trophoblast tissue immunocytochemistry and DNA linkage analysis have been used to determine affected and unaffected merosin-negative CMD fetuses (91,92). Linkage analysis using PCR markers has been used in Fukuyama CMD for the same purpose (93,94).

MYASTHENIA GRAVIS

Myasthenia gravis (MG) is an autoimmune disorder in which polyclonal antibodies are directed against the nicotinic acetylcholine receptor (AchR) of skeletal muscle (95). This results in a degradation of the neuromuscular junction and failure of neuromuscular transmission (95). The clinical hallmark of the disease is fatiguable weakness, causing intermittent symptoms (usually following repetitive action) such as ptosis, diplopia, dysphagia, dysarthria, and facial and limb muscle weakness. Respiratory compromise can occur in severe cases.

MG has a bimodal peak incidence, affecting older men and young women of childbearing age (96). Sex hormones may play an important role in juvenile MG (disease onset before 20 years of age). Female predominance is slight before puberty but becomes marked during and after puberty (female:male incidence = 14:1) (97), as does disease severity (more severe and persistent disease and fewer spontaneous remissions in females with pubertal onset than in males or prepubertal females) (98).

Although the clinical history and examination are often typical and highly suggestive, confirmation of the diagnosis rests on pharmacologic, immunologic, and electrodiagnostic grounds. Tensilon® (edrophonium chloride), in doses from 1 to 10 mg given intravenously, will quickly but briefly reverse the signs of myasthenia gravis and thus serves as a good bedside test (99). Assay for the presence of serum acetylcholine receptor antibodies is very specific for MG, and is abnormal in 70 to 90 % of cases (100). Sensitivity is lower in patients who have only ocular signs. Electrodiagnostic tests of neuromuscular transmission include repetitive nerve stimulation (abnormal in 50 to 75% of cases) (101) and single fiber EMG (abnormal in 98%) (102).

Treatment can be symptomatic or curative. Anticholinesterases can be used to briefly improve the symptoms attributable to MG, but they do not affect the underlying immunologic dysfunction. These drugs work by inhibiting the breakdown of acetylcholine, the neuro-transmitter released by terminal motor nerve fibers. Edrophonium (Tensilon®), neostigmine, and pyridostigmine (Mestinon®) are all anticholinesterases, the latter being the most commonly used because of its longer duration of action (2–4 hours) and lesser muscarinic side effects. A time-release form of Mestinon® is also available, usually for overnight use. Pyridostigmine is commonly used alone in mild cases and in conjunction with immunosuppression in more severe cases. Side effects include diaphoresis, hypersalivation, diarrhea, nausea, abdominal cramping, bradycardia, and fasciculations. Pyridostigmine can enter the fetal circulation, at 85 to 90% of maternal levels (103). Despite this, only one case of disputed possible fetal teratogenicity has been reported in the 50 years it has been available, and that was in a woman taking four to eight times (1,500 to 3,000 mg daily), the recommended dose (104–106). At recommended doses (less than 600 mg daily) pyridostigmine is safe to use during pregnancy. Parenteral formulations of neostigmine and pyridostigmine are available when needed before or after surgery, during labor, or early in pregnancy if emesis gravidarum is severe. Intravenous dosages are 1/30 the oral dose for both drugs.

A suppression of the immune system attack on the acetylcholine receptor is indicated when the disease is generalized, involves vital functions such as breathing or swallowing, or is not satisfactorily responsive to anticholinesterase drugs. Various treatments can be used including corticosteroids; immunosuppressants such as azathioprine, cyclosporine, and mycophenylate mofetil; plasmapheresis; intravenous human immunoglobulin; and thymectomy. In the pregnant patient, corticosteroids are preferred over the other immunosuppressants. Corticosteroids can cause a dramatic worsening of symptoms at the initiation of therapy, and patients must be carefully monitored, preferably as inpatients (107–108). Deterioration can be limited by starting at very low doses with a gradual increase in dose, although this delays the clinical benefit (109). Plasmapheresis is indicated in the severely compromised patient, in the patient who is refractory to other treatments, and in the patient in whom an immediate response is desired. Plasmapheresis rapidly lowers AchR antibody titers and may be indicated when high maternal AchR titers threaten fetal development (110) or when the possibility of neonatal myasthenia exists. Plasmapheresis has been used to successfully treat fulminant MG in a pregnant patient (111) without increase in risk (112).

Thymomas are present in 10 to 15% of patients with MG, and MG occurs in 30% of patients with thymomas (113). Thymic hyperplasia is present in another 70% of patients with MG (113). Malignant thymoma is uncommon in the pregnant patient but appears to carry a poor prognosis when it does occur (114). The thymus gland is the likely site for initial sensitization to the acetylcholine receptor (115). Removal of thymic tissue increases remission rate from 15 to 30% and results in significant clinical improvement in two-thirds of patients, although the improvement may take up to 5 years (116). Thymectomy has been noted to decrease the incidence of neonatal MG (discussed in a later section) (117). Thymectomy has been performed in pregnant women with refractory disease (118) and, when it is done before pregnancy, it can decrease disease exacerbation during pregnancy (119). If possible, it is advisable for a woman with generalized MG who is considering pregnancy to have thymectomy before becoming pregnant (120). I generally recommend thymectomy in all patients between 18 and 55 years of age who have generalized MG.

Menstruation

Menstruation exacerbates MG in approximately 40% of women (121), particularly just before menses. After thymectomy, this effect disappears in 50% of patients. Pregnanediol, a measure of progesterone metabolism, is at or below normal in the luteal stage of the menstrual cycle in women with MG, increases dramatically within weeks of thymectomy, and remains high for up to 2 years (122). Birth control pills are not reported to affect myasthenia gravis, although progesterone, 50 mg daily, exacerbated one woman's symptoms (123) and levonorgestrol implants have been associated with MG in at least 35 women (124).

Effects of Pregnancy on Myasthenia Gravis

A review of the literature revealed 31% of pregnancies in myasthenic women did not affect the disease, 28% improved, and 40% worsened, usually in the puerperium (125). Maternal mortality was 10%, most commonly from myasthenic crisis, but also from cholinergic crisis and postpartum hemorrhage (125). These numbers reflect a reporting bias towards more severe disease, but indicate that pregnancy frequently has an adverse effect on the myasthenic patient. A study of 47 myasthenic women with 64 pregnancies from a single institution (126) showed that, during pregnancy, 39% improved, 42% remained unchanged, and 19% deteriorated or relapsed. After delivery, however, 28% had worsening of symptoms. Exacerbations tend to be most sudden and dangerous in the postpartum period and are frequently accompanied by respiratory failure (125). Physiologic worsening of neuromuscular transmission has been confirmed by single-fiber EMG (126). Therapeutic abortion is of little benefit in the treatment of MG (127,128).

Alpha-fetoprotein (AFP) very effectively inhibits the binding of AchR antibodies (129). The presence of AFP may explain the oft-seen symptomatic improvement in the third trimester (117), and its absence may account for the frequent postpartum exacerbation of MG, when AFP levels precipitously fall.

Effects of Myasthenia Gravis on Pregnancy

MG slightly increases the risk of premature delivery (114,130) but does not affect the incidence of preeclampsia (130,131). Magnesium sulfate is contraindicated in the myasthenic patient because it interferes with neuromuscular transmission and muscle fiber excitability (132), thus leading to the onset or deterioration of myasthenic symptoms and signs.

MG does not affect smooth muscle but may weaken the voluntary muscles used during the second stage of labor; parenteral anticholinesterases (e.g., pyridostigmine 2 mg IV) may be useful at this point. Care must be taken not to push the myasthenic patient beyond her physical capabilities during labor, and the criteria for caesarean section should be relaxed (117). MG does not prolong the overall length of labor (123,133). Women on corticosteroids during pregnancy should have stress doses of steroids given during labor and delivery.

Regional anesthesia is preferred over other anesthetic methods. Myasthenic patients are particularly sensitive to even small doses of neuromuscular blocking agents, especially of the nondepolarizing type such as curare, and these drugs should be avoided. Lidocaine is the recommended local anesthetic because it is not affected by the decreased cholinesterase activity seen in patients who are receiving anticholinesterase drugs (134,135). Combined spinal and epidural anesthesia using intrathecal opioids can provide analgesia without inhibiting muscular strength (136).

Perinatal infant death rates are increased in babies with antenatal and neonatal MG (123). Both conditions are presumed to be due to the transplacental transfer of maternal AchR antibodies (137), which affects fetal acetylcholine receptors much more so than adult receptors (138,139). Antenatal problems occur because skeletal muscle movement and development are inhibited, resulting in pulmonary hypoplasia, arthrogryposis multiplex, and polyhydramnios (110), consistent with the fetal akinesia deformation sequence (140). Mothers with previously affected infants or very high titers of AchR antibodies are at higher risk. Ultrasound monitoring of total fetal and diaphragmatic movement, and an assessment of AchR antibody titers—particularly determining the antifetal/antiadult receptor antibody titer ratio (141)—may identify those women at risk in whom an aggressive lowering of the antibody load to the placenta (such as with plasmapheresis) might prevent congenital anomalies (110,142). The syndrome may occur in asymptomatic women (143).

Neonatal Myasthenia Gravis

A less severe but more common occurrence is neonatal MG, which is characterized by transient weakness in the newborn infant (144). Affecting up to 19% of children born to mothers who have myasthenia gravis, the disease becomes symptomatic within the first 3 days of life and can persist for weeks before improving (144). Symptoms include poor feeding, weak suck, feeble cry, floppiness, generalized weakness, and respiratory distress. Treatment is supportive but can be supplemented by cholinesterase inhibitors. Neostigmine 0.1 mg intramuscularly (IM) or subcutaneously, or pyridostigmine 0.15 mg IM, are effective (103) but must be sparingly used because they may increase oral secretions. Further therapeutic interventions, such as plasmapheresis, are rarely needed. The disease is self-limited and does not represent a risk to the infant for later MG (145). Subsequent infants are at higher risk for neonatal MG (144).

The etiology of neonatal MG is not entirely clear. Nearly all infants born to myasthenic mothers are exposed to intrauterine maternal AchR antibodies (146) yet only a minority develop symptoms. The acetylcholine receptor consists of five subunits, with the fetal and adult forms differing by an ϵ subunit instead of a γ subunit in the adult. An increased ratio of antibodies against the fetal form of the receptor predisposes to antenatal and neonatal MG and may explain why both conditions have occurred in infants born to mothers in remission (147). A positive correlation exists between maternal AchR antibody titers and neonatal MG (146). Because AFP binds AchR antibody (129), its decline after birth may result in the emergence of symptoms (125,130). See also Chapter 11.

POLYMYOSITIS AND DERMATOMYOSITIS

Polymyositis and dermatomyositis are inflammatory disorders that affect striated and cardiac muscle. Dermatomyositis differs from polymyositis primarily by the presence of skin involvement and is thought to be a vasculopathy. The etiology of polymyositis/dermatomyositis is unknown. Both diseases can occur in isolation or in conjunction with connective tissue diseases. Both are characterized by proximal weakness, elevated creatine kinase (CK) levels, myopathic changes on electromyography, and inflammatory myonecrosis on muscle biopsy. Dermatomyositis in childhood affects girls (70%) much more frequently than boys, and this female preponderance persists into adulthood (55% female incidence) (148).

Dermatomyositis, and to a lesser extent, polymyositis (149) carry an increased risk of cancer, which can occur before, at the time of, or years after the diagnosis is made, particularly when the onset of dermatomyositis is after the age of 40 years (150). Women with dermatomyositis have a particular risk of gynecologic malignancies, including vaginal (151) and most particularly, ovarian carcinoma (152–154), which usually appear within months to years after the diagnosis of dermatomyositis. One study cited the incidence as high as 13% compared with 1% in the general female population, with the risk rising to 21% in women over 40 years of age (154). A thorough and continuing search for cancer, especially ovarian, is indicated in all women with dermatomyositis, in an attempt to catch the disease at an early stage. One study found that despite repeated cancer screenings, several women still presented with advanced stages of ovarian cancer (153). Indications of susceptibility to ovarian cancer include severe, skin disease (153), and vesicle formation, a rare complication in dermatomyositis (152).

Polymyositis and dermatomyositis rarely occur in pregnancy. Although females are affected twice as often as men, the bimodal age of onset largely spares the child-bearing years, and the average age of onset of the inflammatory myopathies is 47 years (155). A review of the literature reveals 34 patients with 48 examined pregnancies, approximately evenly split between polymyositis/dermatomyositis antedating pregnancy or starting during pregnancy (156–181). Preexisting inflammatory myopathy does not result for the most part in gestational exacerbation but when it does, it occurs in later pregnancy (156,181). This is in contrast with de novo disease, which usually occurs during the first trimester (156), but can appear postpartum (162). In preexisting polymyositis/dermatomyositis, the inflammatory myopathy is rarely fulminant or difficult to control. De novo inflammatory myopathy is often active throughout gestation, even with treatment, but with remission following close on the heels of delivery (156,181).

Several complications of pregnancy have been reported in patients with polymyositis/dermatomyositis, including postpartum microangiopathic hemolytic anemia (160), placental abruption, uterine atony, and postpartum maternal death (166, 175). More frequently encountered are intrauterine growth retardation, spontaneous abortion, and preterm labor, the latter being quite common (156). There are no reports of newborns of mothers with myositis having myositis themselves, but CK levels can be elevated dramatically in the newborn for several weeks (177).

Fetal wastage is increased in pregnancies complicated by inflammatory myopathies, with a rate of 50 to 60% found by Gutierrez and co-workers (162). My review of the literature is not so gloomy: In de novo disease, 40% fetal deaths occurred; and in preexisting disease, the rate was 21%.

The treatment of gestational polymyositis/dermatomyositis is predicated by the clinical condition of the patient and the length of gestation. Mild disease may not warrant treatment. For those patients who need treatment, corticosteroids are the drugs of choice, in doses approximating 1 mg prednisone/kg/day. Although the effect of corticosteroids on fetal development is not clear, they are a much better choice than the antimetabolites, which in the first trimester almost invariably result in spontaneous abortion or fetal malformation (182) (see also Chapter 4). Unfortunately, even with corticosteroids, no controlled studies of efficacy are available.

In general, women with either mildly active inflammatory myopathy or women in remission should have an uneventful pregnancy, while using corticosteroids to manage exacerbations. Pregnancy should be avoided in patients who have severe disease or in patients requiring antimetabolite therapy. In patients who have onset in pregnancy, corticosteroid therapy should be tried but, if ineffective, should lead to consideration of therapeutic abortion (183). Postpartum corticosteroid taper should be done slowly to avoid severe exacerbations.

Myositis in pregnancy also occurs in systemic connective tissue disorders, such as mixed connective tissue disease (184), systemic lupus erythematosis (SLE), scleroderma (185), and interstitial lung disease (172). Interstitial pneumonitis with myositis is more frequent in women (55%) (186). See also Chapter 22.

CHANNELOPATHIES (MYOTONIA CONGENITA AND PERIODIC PARALYSIS)

Channelopathy refers to a group of inherited muscle disorders that are caused by genetic defects of the muscle membrane channels. These include the SCN4A gene on chromosome 17q23, coding for the adult sodium channel α-subunit (187); the CLCN1 gene on chromosome 7q35, encoding the chloride channel (187); the CACNL1A3 gene on 1q31-32, coding for the dihydropyridine receptor of the calcium channel (187); and the RYR1 gene on 19q, coding for the ryanodine receptor of the calcium release channel (27). Mutations of the SCN4A gene result in several autosomal dominant phenotypes, including hyperkalemic periodic paralysis, normokalemic periodic paralysis, and paramyotonia congenita (187). These diseases cause a transient paralysis of muscles, beginning in legs and progressing to involve arm and even facial muscles, and rarely, the muscles of respiration. Each attack lasts hours to days, and onset is in childhood. All have electrical, and to a lesser extent, clinical myotonia. A form of hypokalemic periodic paralysis has also been localized to a mutation of the SCN4A gene (27). Mutations of the CLCN1 gene cause either autosomal dominant (Thomsen disease) or autosomal recessive (Becker-type myotonia) myotonia congenita (187); the former is the more common. Both are characterized by electrical and clinical myotonia of skeletal muscles, with normal muscle strength. Patients complain of stiffness, which abates with continued use of the muscle, after "warming up." Sudden movement, however, may result in such stiffness as to cause falls. The multisystem involvement of myotonic dystrophy is not present in any of the channelopathies. Mutations of the calcium chan-

nel gene result in a hypokalemic periodic paralysis in which patients suffer a transient weakness of limbs, as in the hyperkalemic form, but have no myotonia. This weakness is associated with low serum potassium. Mutations of the RYR1 gene result in malignant hyperthermia.

In a multigeneration family with hyperkalemic periodic paralysis that I follow, affected males suffer early, frequent, and severe attacks, whereas affected women have infrequent attacks that abate by the third decade.

The effect of pregnancy on myotonia congenita in two women was a temporary worsening in the second half of the pregnancy (188–190). As with myotonic dystrophy, increased symptoms in the pregnant mother occur but are probably uncommon. Obstetric problems have not been described. Exceptionally, patients with autosomal dominant myotonia congenita may develop weakness and fluctuating symptoms only during pregnancy (191).

Anesthetics pose some risks to the pregnant woman with myotonia congenita. *Myotonic spasms* may occur with the use of depolarizing neuromuscular blockers such as succinylcholine (76). Malignant hyperthermia has been reported in two cases of myotonia congenita (192,193), although a connection between the two disorders remains doubtful (78).

There are no reports of problems with pregnancy in periodic paralysis. The women that I follow who have hyperkalemic periodic paralysis have had multiple uneventful pregnancies. It is uncertain whether certain anesthetics precipitate attacks of paralysis (194). Paralytic attacks with surgery may be related more to the stress of the operation, long periods of fasting, or overeating the night before surgery than to any anesthetic agent.

METABOLIC MYOPATHIES

Myophosphorylase Deficiency

Metabolic myopathies are inborn errors of metabolism affecting muscle. Several glycogen storage disorders involve muscle, and all of them are rare. A gender effect on expression would not be expected, although nine of ten patients with phosphorylase β kinase deficiency were males (195). Little is known of the effect of glycogen storage deficiency upon pregnancy. McArdle disease, or myophosphorylase deficiency, which is another enzyme in the glycolytic pathway, manifests as exercise-induced muscle contractures and myoglobinuria. One report documents an uneventful pregnancy and delivery in McArdle disease (196). Dawson and associates (197) mention one multiparous woman with McArdle disease who had leg cramps and myoglobinuria after her last delivery. Smooth muscle phosphorylase is normal in McArdle patients (198), and uterine activity should be unimpaired. Neither deterioration nor exacerbation is expected during pregnancy.

Myoglobinuria

Myoglobinuria is a sign of rhabdomyolysis, not a specific disease. Markedly elevated serum CPK and the presence of myoglobin in the urine are the biochemical hallmarks of the syndrome. Idiopathic and polymyositis-associated myoglobinuria have been reported during pregnancy (157,199). Extreme unaccustomed exertion also can be associated with rhabdomyolysis, as illustrated by a woman with severe hyperemesis gravidarum (200).

Malignant Hyperthermia

Malignant hyperthermia is a potentially fatal syndrome that includes hyperpyrexia, muscle rigidity, and rhabdomyolysis. It may be triggered by certain anesthetic agents (e.g., depolarizing muscle relaxants, inhalation anesthetics). It is inherited as an autosomal dominant trait, and six chromosomal locations have been identified (27). In susceptible patients, hyperpyrexia can be triggered by stress and infection. The incidence in adults is 1:50,000 operative cases, which raises the question of why malignant hyperthermia is not encountered more frequently in pregnancy and delivery (201). Females may be less susceptible (202), because only three cases have been reported during pregnancy, all during cesarean section (203–205). In susceptible patients, prophylactic dantrolene may permit uneventful labor and delivery, including cesarean section (206–208). Dantrolene crosses the placenta (208) and has unknown effects upon the newborn, but one study of 20 pregnancies found no adverse effect upon fetus or newborn (207). Careful monitoring and avoiding provocative anesthetics may obviate the need for dantrolene (201,209).

MITOCHONDRIAL ENCEPHALOMYOPATHIES

Mitochondrial myopathies are a heterogenous group of diseases in which mitochondrial metabolism is defective. The disorders have been defined by morphologic, genetic, and biochemical means but, at present, are best grouped into four categories (210): (i) defects of mitochondrial substrate transport, (ii) defects of the respiratory chain, (iii) defects of substrate utilization, (iv) and defects of energy conservation and transduction. In the context of the pregnant woman, I discuss the first three categories.

Intramitochondrial fatty acid oxidation is largely dependent upon the transport of long-chain fatty acids across the mitochondrial membrane by attachment to carnitine. Deficiency of carnitine can be purely myopathic, which will not effect pregnancy, or systemic. Primary systemic carnitine deficiency is rare, and most deficiencies are secondary to other metabolic disorders (210). Weakness, predominantly of proximal muscles, is fre-

quent, and muscle biopsy shows abnormal lipid storage. A rapid progression of weakness has been reported during pregnancy (211) and in the postpartum period in three cases (212,213), two of which were fatal (211,213). The only patient who was treated with 2 g daily carnitine replacement improved (212). A fourth patient with systemic carnitine deficiency and a defect in the respiratory chain had rapidly progressive worsening of her weakness in the last trimester of her pregnancy. She improved following treatment with 6 g carnitine daily (210). Worsening is probably related to the low carnitine stores in pregnant women (214), which are further depleted by lactation (212) and increased fetal demand. Carnitine is actively transported to the fetus via the placenta (215), which produces little carnitine (216). Untreated systemic carnitine deficiency in pregnancy can be fatal: Treated patients do well.

A rare disease but a common cause of myoglobinuria, carnitine palmitoyltransferase deficiency (CPT) prevents linkage of long chain fatty acids to carnitine for transport across the mitochondrial membrane, where they will undergo oxidation. This provides a major source of muscle energy, especially during aerobic exercise lasting more than 20 minutes. The prolonged exertion of labor would seem to make patients with CPT deficiency quite susceptible to severe rhabdomyolysis and myoglobinuria, but pregnancy and delivery are uneventful (217). The disease is inherited as an autosomal recessive trait, but only 20% of documented cases are women (218). A hormonal protective effect has been postulated (218).

Many defects of the respiratory chain are possible, and several syndromes have been described, some associated with particular mutations of the mitochondrial genome. As recognition of the syndromes and the ability to test the mitochondrial genome improve, more case reports of pregnancy in patients with defects of the respiratory chain appear. A frequent feature of mitochondrial syndromes is small stature, which by itself may explain an association with hypertension and preterm labor in several patients (219, 220). Commonly, pregnancy proceeds normally or with mild exercise intolerance (221–224), although rarely it may progress to complete immobility (225).

Two women had initial presentation of mitochondrial encephalopathy, lactic acidosis, and stroke-like episodes (MELAS) during pregnancy. Both women had a spontaneous improvement of symptoms as the pregnancy progressed and normal deliveries (226, 227). Another woman had preterm labor, gestational diabetes, and a postpartum cardiomyopathy (228).

The deficiencies of numerous enzymes involved in mitochondrial substrate utilization have been reported, and a discussion of each is not relevant. At least one, long-chain 3-hydroxyacyl-CoA dehydrogenase deficiency, predisposes female carriers to preeclamptic complications of pregnancy. In Finland, carrier frequency has been reported to be 1:240 (229).

Mitochondrial Maternal Inheritance

The oxidative metabolism of fatty acids is an important source of energy in muscle. It takes place in the mitochondrial electron transport chain (respiratory chain). Approximately 85% of the proteins comprising the respiratory chain are encoded by nuclear DNA, with 15% (in total, 13 proteins) encoded on DNA within the mitochondria itself (210). No mitochondria are found in spermatozoa, but they are found in ova. Therefore, all human mitochondria arise from maternal sources, thus causing the maternal (nonmendelian) inheritance of mitochondrial encephalomyopathies. These disorders do not follow the rules for nuclear DNA inheritance (230). Mitochondrial diseases do not all arise from mitochondrial genomic defects; some follow mendelian inheritance patterns. Because mitochondria replicate autonomously, a range of mitochondrial genomes exists in any ovum. The presence and percentage of mutated mitochondria determine the expression of a particular mitochondrial defect, which explains the variable expression of mitochondrial encephalomyopathies (231). Figure 21.1 illustrates maternal inheritance in one family. The disease is passed between generations by females only, although all offspring of a carrier mother may carry the genetic defect (see also Chapter 7). The higher the load of maternal mutant mitochondrial DNA, the higher the chance of affected offspring (231).

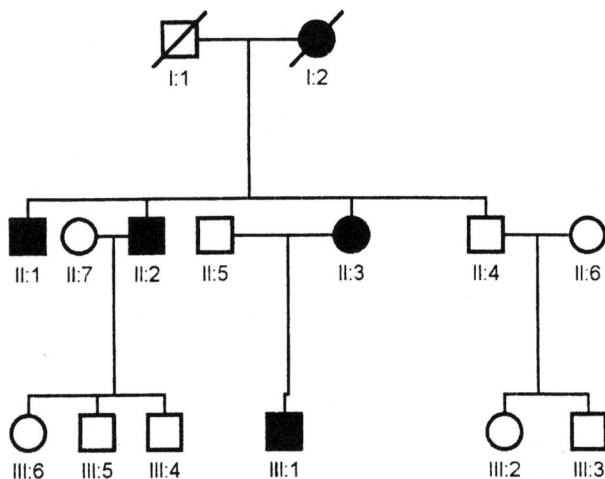

FIGURE 21.1

This family pedigree demonstrates maternal inheritance. Women are affected and can transmit the mitochondrial trait; men can manifest the trait but not transmit it.

Genetic Counseling

Antenatal diagnosis of mitochondrial disease is complicated by both maternal and autosomal patterns of inheritance. For those mitochondrial diseases with mendelian inheritance, or syndromes caused by mutations at base pair 8993 of the mitochondrial genome [Leigh's syndrome, or neuropathy ataxia and retinitis pigmentose (NARP)], prenatal diagnosis can be done using chorionic villus sampling (232). Beyond that, prenatal diagnosis becomes markedly less reliable because it is not possible to predict how heteroplasmic mitochondrial DNA will behave (233). Successful prenatal diagnosis has been accomplished by direct mutation screening of the fetus using chorionic villus sampling at 10 weeks (234) but with less success utilizing the determination of respiratory chain enzyme activity in the fetus, which can give false negative results (235). See also Chapter 7.

ENDOCRINE MYOPATHIES

Many endocrine abnormalities may affect muscle function, including Cushing syndrome, iatrogenic steroid myopathy, hypothyroidism, hyperthyroidism and rarely, Addison disease. The mechanisms that produce myopathy differ and, for the most part, remain poorly understood. Treatment is aimed at the endocrine dysfunction rather than the muscle disease.

Thyroid-Related Myopathy

Both hyperthyroidism and hypothyroidism can cause myopathy, manifesting as proximal painless weakness and fatigue. Beyond the known female preponderance of cases (5:1 for Graves disease, and 20:1 for Hashimoto thyroiditis), however, there is no predilection for muscle disease attributable to gender. Weakness is infrequently the sole presenting complaint, but it is often a presenting symptom. Propanolol does not improve weakness in hyperthyroidism, but the myopathy quickly improves with thyroid suppression.

CONGENITAL MYOPATHY

A number of congenital myopathies exist, and these often require muscle biopsy for diagnosis. These disorders reflect a developmental arrest of muscle, with the pathologic and clinical manifestations dependent on the timing of insult or the nature of the genetic defect. These diseases do not progress, although the patient may be severely affected and may die. Myotubular myopathy has been linked to the X-chromosome, and prenatal diagnosis is possible by mutation testing of the MTM1 gene

(236) and by linkage analysis of DNA markers in the Xq28 region (237,238). Severe X-linked myotubular myopathy has been reported in one girl with extremely skewed x-inactivation (239).

Congenital nemaline myopathy is a static muscle disease of variable severity, usually diagnosed in childhood. Antenatal onset may occur, with consequences characteristic of the fetal akinesia sequence (140,240), including arthrogryposis, polyhydramnios, lung hypoplasia, and neonatal demise (240). Hypotonia, weakness, jaw and palatal abnormalities, and scoliosis are frequent findings. It is inherited as either an autosomal dominant or recessive trait. Four cases of congenital nemaline myopathy were reported in pregnant women: Pregnancy was uneventful in all, and vaginal or cesarean deliveries were normal, except when micrognathia, prognathia, and high arched palate made intubation difficult, and scoliosis inhibited epidural anesthesia (241,242). All infants were unaffected.

A retrospective report (29) detailed the 12 pregnancies of five women with central core congenital myopathy and the two pregnancies of a woman with cytoplasmic body congenital myopathy. For the most part, the women had mild weakness that was not progressive prior to pregnancy. Three of the patients with central core myopathy had worsening of weakness during pregnancy, with no improvement after delivery. There were no miscarriages, three preterm, and two assisted deliveries (prolonged labor in one, and threatened fetal asphyxia in another), and no adverse fetal outcomes. Two of the children inherited central core myopathy. The chromosomal locus for central core myopathy is 19q13.1, and the gene product is the ryanodine receptor, the same as for one of the familial malignant hyperthermia types (243).

TOXIC MYOPATHY

A plethora of substances are capable of harming muscle at physiologic and supraphysiologic doses. Few have any particular tendency to affect women more than men, or vice versa. I will discuss two substances, emetine and ethanol, and then discuss the possible effects of antiretroviral therapy for HIV infection on the fetus.

Emetine is a major component of syrup of ipecac and is not specifically toxic for females. It is commonly abused as an aid to weight loss, however, by inducing postprandial vomiting. As such, the common victim of emetine myopathy is a young woman who has an eating disorder (244,245). Women present with diffuse weakness, and studies show a necrotizing vacuolar myopathy; cardiomyopathy may also occur. Emetine is slowly excreted, so large doses and chronic intake conspire to accumulate emetine, thus producing toxic levels. The myopathic syndrome slowly improves over months following cessation of intake.

Abuse of ethanol is certainly not limited to either sex, and acute and chronic skeletal and cardiomyopathies can be seen in men and women. It appears, however, that women are differentially prone to myopathic toxicity from alcohol (246). The sum total of lifetime alcohol intake necessary to cause myopathy is less in women, and there is an enhanced deleterious effect on female cardiac muscle (246).

In 1999, Blanche and others reported eight children with mitochondrial dysfunction who had been exposed to zidovudine, or zidovudine and lamivudine in utero. All had neurologic symptoms or abnormalities. An analysis of respiratory chain enzymes was abnormal in all, but none had mitochondrial mutations known to cause disease and none were HIV-infected (247). This remains controversial: a retrospective review of 35 non-HIV infected children who had died after exposure to nucleoside reverse transcriptase inhibitors showed none were related to mitochondrial dysfunction. Of 1,954 uninfected living children exposed to perinatal antiretroviral agents, no evidence suggested mitochondrial disease (248).

CRAMPS AND MYALGIA

The question of muscle cramps frequently occurs in discussions I have with other physicians. They are usually surprised when told cramps are rarely a sign of muscle disease, but rather are a sign of neuronal or metabolic disturbance, if not simply a normal response. Additionally, the word "cramp" is often misused to cover any type of muscle pain or myalgia. In fact, a muscle cramp is a specific clinical and electrophysiologic syndrome that must be differentiated from muscle contracture, myalgia, tetany, stiffness, spasticity, myotonia, neuromyotonia, and dystonia.

A cramp is a "sudden, forceful, painful, involuntary contraction of one muscle or part of a muscle, lasting anywhere from a few seconds to several minutes" (249). Electromyography during a cramp reveals a full interference pattern that is indistinguishable from a maximal voluntary contraction of the muscle. Cramps often begin and end with fasciculations. This is in contrast with muscle contractures, as in McArdle disease, which are electrically silent.

Cramps are seen in normal individuals at night or related to exercise. Several metabolic disorders can also cause cramps, including uremia, hypothyroidism, and hypoadrenalism. Acute extracellular volume depletion (perspiration, diarrhea, vomiting, diuresis, hemodialysis) is also associated with cramps (249). Pregnant women suffer an increased frequency of cramping, probably secondary to changes in metabolic and extracellular volume parameters. Cramps are more sinister as part of disorders of the motor neuron, in diseases such as amyotrophic lateral sclerosis, radiculopathy, neuropathy, and remote poliomyelitis. Stretching the affected muscle is the best immediate treatment for cramping. Active exercise during pregnancy, especially the last trimester, may result in less cramping. If no correctable cause is present, recurrent cramps can be treated with quinine (250), oral magnesium (251), phenytoin, or carbamazepine for prophylaxis, although the latter two drugs carry some risk for teratogenesis.

HYPERCKEMIA

Increased estrogens decrease muscle enzyme efflux and are thought to have some stabilizing effect upon muscle (252), including lowering baseline CK levels during pregnancy. The normalization of idiopathic hyperCKemia has been reported during pregnancy, with a recrudescence of elevated CK levels after delivery (253). Menarchial women have lower CK levels at rest than premenarchial or menopausal women, and have a higher efflux of CK after exercise than either of the other two groups (254). Women tend to have less of a rise in CK after exercise than men, and even though estrogen levels inversely correlate with resting CK level, no correlation exists between estrogen and postexercise CK levels (254). Oral contraceptives have no effect upon serum levels of CK (255). In general, men have higher resting CK levels than women, and blacks have higher levels than whites, with Hispanics having intermediate levels (256). Because most laboratories use normal ranges based on the prevailing racial profile, which is largely white, African-American men and women may have falsely abnormal CK values. Teenage girls, particularly if premenarcheal, have higher levels than adult women, and CK is higher in the postpartum than in pregnancy due to the involution of myometrium (257). These circumstances are particularly important if the CK is being used to determine carrier status, such as in X-linked Duchenne dystrophy.

FIBROMYALGIA

Fibromyalgia is a common diagnosis whose features are nonspecific. It is characterized by chronic, multifocal pain, arthralgias, and myalgias, with focal tender points and subjectively poor sleep. Laboratory and pathologic evaluation is usually normal. Women are affected much more frequently than men, and 80% of cases are women between the ages of 20 and 50 years (258). One possible mechanism is a disturbed sleep cycle, and alpha-wave intrusion in delta sleep has been described (259). This may explain the efficacy of tricyclic compounds such as amitriptyline in reducing pain. Nonsteroidal anti-inflammatory drugs, exercise, selective serotonin reuptake inhibitors, and physical therapy may also help (259).

References

1. Hoffman EP, Brown RH, Kunkel LM. Dystrophin: the protein product of the Duchenne muscular dystrophy locus. *Cell* 1987;51:919–928.
2. Emery AEH. *Duchenne muscular dystrophy*. New York: Oxford Press, 1987.
3. Barkhaus PB, Gilchrist JM. Duchenne muscular dystrophy manifesting carriers. *Arch Neurol* 1989;46:673–675.
4. Hoffman EP, Arahata K, Minetti C, et al. Dystrophinopathy in isolated cases of myopathy in females. *Neurology* 1992;42:967–975.
5. van Bakel I, Holt S, Craig I, Boyd Y. Sequence analysis of the breakpoint regions of a x;5 translocation in a female with Duchenne muscular dystrophy. *Am J Hum Genet* 1995;57:329–336.
6. Nevin NC, Hughes AE, Calwell M, Lim JHK. Duchenne muscular dystrophy in a female with a translocation involving Xp21. *J Med Genet* 1986;23:171–187.
7. Quan F, Janas J, Toth-Fejel S, Johnson DB, Wolford JK, Popovich BW. Uniparental disomy of the entire X chromosome in a female with Duchenne muscular dystrophy. *Am J Hum Gen* 1997;60:160–165.
8. Geifman-Holtzman O, Bernstein IM, Capeless EL, Hawley P, Specht LA, Bianchi DW. Increase in fetal breech presentation in female carriers of Duchenne muscular dystrophy. *Am J Med Genet* 1997;73:276–278.
9. Moser H. Duchenne muscular dystrophy: pathogenetic aspects and genetic prevention. *Hum Genet* 1984;66:17.
10. Hoshino S, Ohkoshi N, Watanabe M, Shoji S. Immunohistological staining of dystrophin on formalin-fixed paraffin-embedded sections in Duchenne/Becker muscular dystrophy and manifesting carriers of Duchenne dystrophy. *Neuromuscul Disord* 2000;10:425–429.
11. Matthews PM, Benjamin D, van Bakel I, et al. Muscle X-inactivation patterns and dystrophin expression in Duchenne muscular dystrophy carriers. *Neuromuscul Disord* 1995;5:209–220.
12. Pegoraro E, Schimke RN, Garcia C, et al. Genetic and biochemical normalization in female carriers of Duchenne muscular dystrophy: evidence for failure of dystrophin production in dystrophin-competent myonuclei. *Neurology* 1995;45:677–690.
13. Abbadi N, Phillipe C, Chery M, et al. Additional case of female monozygotic twins discordant for the clinical manifestations of Duchenne muscular dystrophy due to opposite X-chromosome inactivation. *Am J Med Genet* 1994;52:198–206.
14. Kinoshita H, Goto Y, Ishikawa M, et al. A carrier of Duchenne muscular dystrophy with dilated cardiomyopathy but no skeletal muscle symptoms. *Brain Dev* 1995;17:202–205.
15. Davies JE, Winokor TS, Aaron MF, Benza RL, Foley BA, Holman WL. Cardiomyopathy in a carrier of Duchenne's muscular dystrophy. *J Heart Lung Transplant* 2001;20:781–784.
16. Politano L, Nigro V, Nigro G, et al. Development of cardiomyopathy in female carriers of Duchenne and Becker muscular dystrophies. *JAMA* 1996;275:1335–1338.
17. Cockburn DJ, Munro E, Craig IW, Boyd Y. Mapping of x;autosome translocation breakpoints in females with Duchenne muscular dystrophy with respect to exons of the dystrophin gene. *Hum Genet* 1992;90:407–412.
18. Clemens PR, Fenwick RG, Chamberlain JS, et al. Carrier detection and prenatal diagnosis in Duchenne and

Becker muscular dystrophy families, using dinucleotide repeat polymorphisms. *Am J Hum Gen* 1991;49: 951–960.

19. Hoffman EP, Fischbeck KH, Brown RH, et al. Characterization of dystrophin in muscle-biopsy specimens from patients with Duchenne's or Becker's muscular dystrophy. *N Engl J Med* 1988;318:1363–1368.

20. Den Duneen JT, Grootscholten PM, Bakker E, et al. Topography of the Duchenne muscular dystrophy (DMD) gene: FIGE and cDNA analysis of 194 cases reveals 115 deletions and 13 duplications. *Am J Hum Gen* 1989;45:835–847.

21. Mendell JR, Buzin CH, Feng J, et al. Diagnosis of Duchenne dystrophy by enhanced detection of small mutations. *Neurology* 2001;57:645–650.

22. Heckel S, Favre R, Flori J, et al. In utero fetal muscle biopsy: a precious aid for the prenatal diagnosis of Duchenne muscular dystrophy. *Fetal Diagn Ther* 1999;14:127–132.

23. Liu J, Lissens W, Devroey P, Liebaers I, Van Steirteghem A. Cystic fibrosis, Duchenne muscular dystrophy and preimplantation genetic diagnosis. *Hum Reprod Update* 1996;2:531–539.

24. Sekizawa A, Kimura T, Sasaki M, Nakamura S, Kobayashi R, Sato T. Prenatal diagnosis of Duchenne muscular dystrophy using a single fetal nucleated erythrocyte in maternal blood. *Neurology* 1996;46: 1350–1353.

25. Overton TG, Smith RP, Sewry CA, Holder SE, Fisk NM. Maternal contamination at fetal muscle biopsy. *Fetal Diagn Ther* 2000;15:118–121.

26. Bushby K. Towards the classification of the autosomal recessive limb-girdle muscular dystrophies. *Neuromuscul Disord* 1996;6:439–441.

27. Neuromuscular disorders: gene location. *Neuromuscul Disord* 2003;13:97–108.

28. Cohn RD, Campbell KP. Molecular basis of muscular dystrophies. *Muscle Nerve* 2000;23:1456–1471.

29. Rudnick-Schoneborn S, Glauner B, Rohrig D, Zerres K. Obstetric aspects in women with facioscapulohumeral muscular dystrophy, limb-girdle muscular dystrophy, and congenital myopathies. *Arch Neurol* 1997;54: 888–894.

30. Restagno G, Romero N, Richard I, et al. Prenatal diagnosis of limb-girdle muscular dystrophy type 2A. *Neuromuscul Disord* 1996;6:173–176.

31. Dincer P, Piccolo F, Leturcq F, Kaplan JC, Jeanpierre M, Topaloglu H. Prenatal diagnosis of limb-girdle muscular dystrophy type 2C. *Prenat Diagn* 1998;18:1300–1303.

32. Pegoraro E, Fanin M, Angelini C, Hoffman EP. Prenatal diagnosis in a family affected with beta-sarcoglycan muscular dystrophy. *Neuromuscul Disord* 1999;9: 323–325.

33. Fisher J, Upadhyaya M. Molecular genetics of facioscapulohumeral muscular dystrophy (FSH). *Neuromuscul Disord* 1997;7:55–62.

34. Galluzzi G, Deidda G, Cacurri S, et al. Molecular analysis of 4q35 rearrangements in facioscapulohumeral muscular dystrophy (FSHD): application to family studies for correct genetic advice and a reliable prenatal diagnosis of the disease. *Neuromuscul Disord* 1999;9: 190–198.

35. Harper PS. *Myotonic dystrophy*, 3rd ed. Philadelphia: WB Saunders, 2001;17–45.

36. Ibid, 223–252.

37. Dyken PR, Harper PS. Congenital dystrophica myotonica. *Neurology* 1973;23:465–473.

38. Brook JD, McCurrach ME, Harley HG, et al. Molecular basis of myotonic dystrophy: expansion of a trinucleotide (CTG) repeat at the 3' end of a transcript encoding a protein kinase family member. *Cell* 1992;68: 799–808.

39. Fu Y-H, Pizzuti A, Fenwick RG, et al. An unstable triplet repeat in a gene related to myotonic muscular dystrophy. *Science* 1992;255:1256–1258.

40. Mahadevan M, Tsilfidis C, Sabourin L, et al. Myotonic dystrophy mutation: an unstable CTG repeat in the 3' untranslated region of the gene. *Science* 1992;255: 1253–1255.

41. Redman JB, Fenwick RG, Fu Y-H, Pizzuti A, Caskey CT. Relationship between parental trinucleotide GCT repeat length and severity of myotonic dystrophy in offspring. *JAMA* 1993;269:1960–1965.

42. Brunner HG, Bruggewirth HT, Nillesen W, et al. Influence of sex of the transmitting parent as well as of parental allele size on the CTG expansion in myotonic dystrophy. *Am J Hum Gen* 1993;53:1016–1023.

43. Koch MC, Grimm T, Harley HG, Harper PS. Genetic risks for children of women with myotonic dystrophy. *Am J Hum Gen* 1991;48:1084–1091.

44. Poulton J. Congenital myotonic dystrophy and mtDNA. *Am J Hum Gen* 1992;50:651–652.

45. Harper PS, Dyken PR. Early onset dystrophica myotonica: evidence supporting a maternal environmental factor. *Lancet* 1972;2:53–55.

46. Howeler CJ, Bush HTM. An asymptomatic mother of children with congenital myotonic dystrophy. *J Neurol Sci* 1990;98(suppl):197.

47. Andrews PI, Wilson J. Relative disease severity in siblings with myotonic dystrophy. *J Child Neurol* 1992;7:161–167.

48. Shore RN, MacLachlan TB. Pregnancy with myotonic dystrophy: course, complications and management. *Obstet Gynecol* 1971;38:448–454.

49. Sarnat HB, O'Connor T, Byrne PA. Clinical effects of myotonic dystrophy on pregnancy and the neonate. *Arch Neurol* 1976;33:459–465.

50. Broekhuizen FF, Elejalde de M, Elejalde R, Hamilton PR. Neonatal myotonic dystrophy as a cause of hydramnios and neonatal death. *J Reprod Med* 1983;28:595–599.

51. Pearse RG, Howeler CJ. Neonatal form of dystrophica myotonica. *Arch Dis Child* 1979;54:331–338.

52. Reardon W, Newcombe R, Fenton I, Sibert J, Harper PS. The natural history of congenital myotonic dystrophy: mortality and long term clinical aspects. *Arch Dis Child* 1993;68:177–181.

53. Vanier TM. Dystrophica myotonica in childhood. *Br Med J* 1960;2:1284–1288.

54. Sarnat HB, Silbert SW. Maturational arrest of fetal muscle in neonatal myotonic dystrophy. *Arch Neurol* 1976;33:466–474.

55. Rutherford MA, Heckmatt JZ, Dubowitz V. Congenital myotonic dystrophy: respiratory function at birth determines survival. *Arch Dis Child* 1989;64: 191–195.

56. Swift TR, Ignacio OJ, Dyken PR. Neonatal dystrophica myotonica: electrophysiological studies. *Am J Dis Child* 1975;29:734–737.

57. Sagel J, Distiller LA, Morley JE, Issacs H. Myotonia dystrophica: studies on gonadal function using luteinizing hormone-releasing hormone. *J Clin Endo Metab* 1975; 40:1110–1113.

58. Harper PS. *Myotonic dystrophy*, 3rd ed. Philadelphia: WB Saunders; 2001;169–178.

59. Marshall J. Observations on endocrine function in dystrophica myotonica. *Brain* 1959;82:221–231.

60. Thomasen E. *Myotonia: Thomsen's disease (Myotonic congenita), paramyotonia, and dystrophica myotonica: a clinical and heredobiologic investigation.* London: MK Lewis, 1948.

61. Febres F, Scaglia H, Lisker R, et al. Hypothalamic-pituitary-gonadal function in patients with myotonic dystrophy. *J Clin Endocrinol* 1975;41:833–840.

62. Harper PS. *Myotonic dystrophy*, 3rd ed. Philadelphia: WB Saunders, 2001:345–346.

63. O'Brien TA, Harper PS. Reproductive problems and neonatal loss in women with myotonic dystrophy. *J Obstet Gynecol* 1984;4:170–173.

64. Sciarra JJ, Steer CM. Uterine contractions during labor in myotonic muscular dystrophy. *Am J Obstet Gynecol* 1961;82:612–615.

65. Hopkins A, Wray S. The effect of pregnancy on dystrophica myotonica. *Neurology* 1967;17:166–168.

66. Gardy HH. Dystrophica myotonica in pregnancy. *Obstet Gynecol* 1963;21:441–445.

67. Jaffe R, Mock M, Abramowitz J, Ben-Aderet N. Myotonic dystrophy and pregnancy: a review. *Obstet Gynecol Surv* 1986;41:272–278.

68. Davis HA. Pregnancy in myotonia dystrophica. *J Obstet Gynecol Brit Empire* 1958;65:479–480.

69. Benito-Leon J, Aguilar-Galan EV. Recurrent myotonic crisis in a pregnant woman with myotonic dystrophy. *Eur J Obstet Gynecol Reprod Biol* 2001;95:181.

70. Fall LH, Young WW, Power JA, Faulkner CS, Hettleman BD. Severe congestive heart failure and cardiomyopathy as a complication of myotonic dystrophy in pregnancy. *Obstet Gynecol* 1990;76:481–485.

71. Webb D, Muir I, Faulker J, Johnson G. Myotonia dystrophica: obstetric complications. *Am J Obstet Gynecol* 1978;132:265–270.

72. Maas O. Observations on dystrophica myotonica. *Brain* 1937;60:498–524.

73. Watters GV, Williams TV. Early onset myotonic dystrophy. Clinical and laboratory findings in five families and a review of the literature. *Arch Neurol* 1967;17:137–152.

74. Hook R, Anderson EF, Noto P. Anesthetic management of a parturient with myotonia atrophia. *Anesthiol* 1975;43:689–692.

75. Esplin MS, Hallam S, Farrington PF, Nelson L, Byrne J, Ward K. Myotonic dystrophy is a significant cause of idiopathic polyhydramnios. *Am J Obstet Gynecol* 1998;179:974–977.

76. Thiel RE. The myotonic response to suxamethonium. *Brit J Anaesth* 1967;39:815–820.

77. Mitchell MM, Ali HH, Savarese JJ. Myotonia and neuromuscular blocking agents. *Anesthiol* 1978;49:44–48.

78. Harper PS. *Myotonic dystrophy*, 3rd ed. Philadelphia: WB Saunders, 2001:132.

79. Norman AM, Floyd JL, Meredith AL, Harper PS. Presymptomatic detection and prenatal diagnosis for myotonic dystrophy by means of linked DNA markers. *J Med Gen* 1989;26:750–754.

80. Fokstuen S, Myring J, Evans C, Harpte PS. Presymptomatic testing in myotonic dystrophy: genetic counseling approaches. *J Med Genet* 2001;35:846–850.

81. Massari A, Novelli G, Colosimo A, et al. Non-invasive early prenatal molecular diagnosis using retrieved transcervical trophoblast cells. *Hum Genet* 1996;97:150–155.

82. Geifman-Holtzman O, Fay K. Prenatal diagnosis of congenital myotonic dystrophy and counseling of the pregnant mother: case report and literature review. *Am J Med Gen* 1998;78:250–253.

83. Amiel J, Raclin V, Jouannic J-M, et al. Trinucleotide repeat contraction: a pitfall in prenatal diagnosis of myotonic dystrophy. *J Med Genet* 2001;35:850–852.

84. Moxley RT. Proximal myotonic myopathy: mini-review of a recently delineated clinical disorder. *Neuromuscul Disord* 1996;6:87–93.

85. The International Myotonic Dystrophy Consortium. New nomenclature and DNA testing guidelines for myotonic dystrophy type 1 (DM1). *Neurology* 2000;54:1218–1221.

86. Newman B, Meola G, O'Donovan DG, Schapira AH, Kingston H. Proximal myotonic myopathy (PROMM) presenting as myotonia during pregnancy. *Neuromuscul Disord* 1999;9:144–149.

87. Khwaja S, Sripathi N, Shmad BK, et al. Proximal myotonic myopathy presenting a congenital hypotonia with asymptomatic mother. *Muscle Nerve* 1998;21:1598.

88. Helbling Leclerc A, Zhang X, Topaloglu H, et al. Mutation sin the laminin alpha 2-chain gene (LAMA 2) cause merosin-deficient congenital muscular dystrophy. *Nature Genet* 1995;11:216–218.

89. Kobayashi O, Hayashi Y, Arahata K, Ozawa E, Nonaka I. Congenital muscular dystrophy: clinical and pathologic study of 50 patients with classical (Occidental) merosin-positive form. *Neurology* 1996;46:815–818.

90. Toda T, Segawa M, Nomura Y, et al. Localization of a gene for Fukuyama type congenital muscular dystrophy to chromosome 9q31-33. *Nature Genet* 1993;5:283–286.

91. Naom I, Sewry C, D'Alessandro M, et al. Prenatal diagnosis of merosin-deficient congenital muscular dystrophy. *Neuromuscul Disord* 1997;7:176–179.

92. Nass D, Goldberg I, Sadeh M. Laminin alpha2 deficient congenital muscular dystrophy: prenatal diagnosis. *Early Hum Dev* 1999;55:19–24.

93. Kondo E, Saito K, Toda T, et al. Prenatal diagnosis of Fukuyama type congenital muscular dystrophy by polymorphism analysis. *Am J Med Genet* 1996;66:169–174.

94. Takai Y, Tsutsumi O, Harada I, et al. Prenatal diagnosis of Fukuyama-type congenital muscular dystrophy by microsatellite analysis. *Hum Reprod* 1998;13:320–323.

95. Lindstrom JM. Acetylcholine receptors and myasthenia. *Muscle Nerve* 2000;23:453–477.

96. Schwab RS, Leland CC. Sex and age in myasthenia gravis as critical factors in incidence and remission. *JAMA* 1953;153:1270–1273.

97. Andrews PI, Massey JM, Sandres DB. Acetylcholine receptor antibodies in juvenile myasthenia gravis. *Neurology* 1993;43:977–982.

98. Andrews PI, Massey JM, Howard JF, Sanders DB. Race, Sex and puberty influence onset, severity, and outcome in juvenile myasthenia gravis. *Neurology* 1994;44:1208–1214.

99. Daroff RB. The office Tensilon test for ocular myasthenia gravis. *Arch Neurol* 1986;43:843–844.

100. Lindstrom J, Shelton D, Fujii Y. Myasthenia gravis. *Adv Immunol* 1988;42:233–284.

101. Oh SJ, Eslami N, Nishihira T, et al. Electrophysiological and clinical correlation in myasthenia gravis. *Ann Neurol* 1982;12:348–354.

102. Sanders DB, Stalberg EV. Single fiber electromyography. *Muscle Nerve* 1996;19:1069–1083.

103. Lefvert AK, Osterman PO. Newborn infants to myasthenic mothers: a clinical study and an investigation of acetylcholine receptor antibodies in 17 children. *Neurology* 1983;33:133–138.

104. Niesen CE, Shah NS. Pyridostigmine-induced microcephaly. *Neurology* 1999;54:1873–1874.

105. Shekhlee A, Robin N, Kaminski H. Pyridostigmine-induced microcephaly (Comment). *Neurology* 2001;56:1606.

106. Polizzi A, Ruggieri M, Vincent A. Pyridostigmine-induced microcephaly (Comment). *Neurology* 2001;56:1606–1607.

107. Pascuzzi RM, Coslett HB, Johns TR. Long-term corticosteroid treatment of myasthenia gravis: report of 116 patients. *Ann Neurol* 1984;15:291–298.

108. Miller RG, Milner-Brown HS, Mirka A. Prednisone-induced worsening of neuromuscular function in myasthenia gravis. *Neurology* 1986;36:729–732.

109. Seybold ME, Drachman DB. Gradually increasing doses of prednisone in myasthenia gravis. *N Engl J Med* 1974;290:81–84.

110. Carr SC, Gilchrist JM, Abuelo D, Clark D. Antenatal treatment of myasthenia gravis. *Obstet Gynecol* 1991;78:485–489.

111. Levine SE, Keesey JC. Successful plasmapheresis for fulminant myasthenia gravis during pregnancy. *Arch Neurol* 1986;43:197–198.

112. Watson WJ, Katz VL, Bowes WA. Plasmapheresis during pregnancy. *Obstet Gynecol* 1990;76:451–457.

113. Castleman B. The pathology of the thymus gland in myasthenia gravis. *Ann NY Acad Sci* 1966;135:496–503.

114. Goldman KP. Malignant thymomas in pregnancy. *Brit J Dis Chest* 1974;68:279–283.

115. Hohlfeld R, Wekerle H. The immunopathogenesis of myasthenia gravis. In: Engel AG, (ed.) *Myasthenia gravis and myasthenic disorders.* New York: Oxford University Press, 1999;87–110.

116. Perlo VP, Arnason B, Poskanzer D, et al. The role of thymectomy in treatment of myasthenia gravis. *Ann NY Acad Sci* 1971;183:308–315.

117. Genkins G, Kornfeld P, Papatestas AE, Bender AN, Matta RJ. Clinical experience in more than 2000 patients with myasthenia gravis. *Ann NY Acad Sci* 1987;505:500–513.

118. Ip MSM, So SY, Lam WK, Tang LCH, Mok CK. Thymectomy in myasthenia gravis during pregnancy. *Postgrad Med J* 1986;62:473–474.

119. Eden RD, Gall SA. Myasthenia gravis and pregnancy: a reappraisal of thymectomy. *Obstet Gynecol* 1983;62:328.

120. Donaldson JO. Neurologic emergencies in pregnancy. *Obstet Gynecol Clin N Am* 1991;18:199–212.

121. Keynes G. Obstetrics and gynaecology in relation to thyrotoxicosis and myasthenia gravis. *J Obstet Gynecol Brit Commonweal* 1952;59:173–182.

122. Schrire I. Progesterone metabolism in myasthenia gravis. *Quart J Med* 1959;28:59–75.

123. Frenkel M, Ehrlich EN. The influence of progesterone and mineralcorticoids upon myasthenia gravis. *Ann Intern Med* 1964;60:971–981.

124. Brittain J, Lange LS. Myasthenia gravis and levonorgestrol implant. *Lancet* 1995;346:1556.

125. Plauche WC. Myasthenia gravis in mothers and their newborn. *Clin Obstet Gynecol* 1991;34:82–99.

126. Batocchi AP, Majolini L, Evoli A, Lino MM, Minisci C, Tonali P. Course and treatment of myasthenia gravis during pregnancy. *Neurology* 1999;52:447–452.

127. Massey JM, Sanders DB. Single fiber electromyography in myasthenia gravis during pregnancy. *Muscle Nerve* 1993;6:458–460.

128. Hay DM. Myasthenia gravis and pregnancy. *J Obstet Gynecol Brit Commonweal* 1969;76:323–329.

129. Brenner T, Beyth Y, Abramsky O. Inhibitory effect of alpha fetoprotein on the binding of myasthenia gravis antibody to acetylcholine receptor. *Proc Natl Acad Sci USA* 1980;77:3635–3639.

130. Fennell DF, Ringel SP. Myasthenia gravis and pregnancy. *Obstet Gynecol Surv* 1987;41:414–421.

131. Duff GB. Preeclampsia and the patient with myasthenia gravis. *Obstet Gynecol* 1979;54:355–358.

132. Bashuk RG, Krendel DA. Myasthenia gravis presenting as weakness after magnesium administration. *Muscle Nerve* 1990;13:708–712.

133. Giwa-Osagie OF, Newton JR, Larcher V. Obstetric performance of patients with myasthenia gravis. *Int J Gynecol Obstet* 1981;19:267.

134. Kalow W. Hydrolysis of local anesthetics by human serum cholinesterase. *J Pharm Exper Therap* 1952;104:122–134.

135. Rolbin SH, Levinson G, Shnider SM, et al. Anesthetic consideration for myasthenia gravis and pregnancy. *Anesth Analg* 1978;57:441.

136. D'Angelo R, Gerancher JC. Combined spinal and epidural analgesics in a parturient with severe myasthenia gravis. *Reg Anesth Pain Med* 1998;23:201–203.

137. Keesey J, Lindstrom J, Cokely H. Anti-acetylcholine receptor antibody in neonatal myasthenia gravis. *N Engl J Med* 1977;296:55.

138. Vincent A, Newland C, Brueton L, et al. Arthrogryposis multiplex congenita with maternal autoantibodies specific for a fetal antigen. *Lancet* 1995;346:24–25.

139. Riemersma S, Vincent A, Beeson D, et al. Association of arthrogryposis multiplex congenita with maternal antibodies inhibiting fetal acetylcholine receptor function. *J Clin Invest* 1996;98:2358–2363.

140. Moessinger AC. Fetal akinesia deformation sequence: an animal model. *Pediatrics* 1983;72:857–863.

141. Gardnerova M, Eymard B, Morel F, et al. The fetal/adult acetylcholine receptor antibody ratio in mothers with myasthenia gravis as a marker for transfer of the disease to the newborn. *Neurology* 1997;48:50–54.

142. Stoll C, Ehret-Mentre MC, Treisser A, Tranchant C. Prenatal diagnosis of congenital myasthenia with arthrogryposis in a myasthenic mother. *Prenat Diag* 1991;11:17–22.

143. Brueton LA, Huson SM, Cox PM, et al. Asymptomatic maternal myasthenic as a cause of the Pena-Shokeir phenotype. *Am J Med Genet* 2000;92:1–6.

144. Namba T, Brown SB, Grob D. Neonatal myasthenia gravis: report of two cases and review of the literature. *Pediatrics* 1970;45:488–504.

145. Ahlsten G, Lefvert AK, Osterman PO, Stalberg E, Safwenberg J. Follow-up study of muscle function in children of mothers with myasthenia gravis during pregnancy. *J Child Neuro* 1992;7:264–269.

146. Eymard B, Morel E, Dulac O, et al. Myasthenia and pregnancy: a clinical and immunologic study of 42 cases (21 neonatal myasthenia gravis). *Rev Neurol* 1989;145:696–701.

147. Elias SB, Butler I, Appel S. Neonatal myasthenia gravis in an infant of a myasthenic mother in remission. *Ann Neurol* 1979;6:72.

148. Beeson PB. Age and sex associations of 40 autoimmune diseases. *Am J Med* 1994;96:457–462.

149. Buchbinder R, Hill CL. Malignancy in patients with inflammatory myopathy. *Curr Rheum Rep* 2002;4: 415–426.

150. Callen JP. Relationship of cancer to inflammatory muscle diseases. Dermatomyositis, polymyositis, and inclusion body myositis. *Rheum Dis Clin North Am* 1994;20: 943–953.

151. Cormio G, DiVagno G, Loverro G, Selvaggi L. Polymyositis and vaginal carcinoma. *Arch Gynecol Obstet* 1993;253:145–147.

152. Kubo M, Sato S, Kitahara H, Tsuchida T, Tamaki K. Vesicle formation in dermatomyositis associated with gynecologic malignancies. *J Am Acad Dermatol* 1996; 34:391–394.

153. Whitmore SE, Rosenshein NB, Provost TT. Ovarian cancer in patients with dermatomyositis. *Medicine (Baltimore)* 1994;73:153–160.

154. Cherin R, Piette JC, Herson S, et al. Dermatomyositis and ovarian cancer: a report of 7 cases and literature review. *J Rheumatol* 1993;20:1897–1899.

155. Bohan AJ, Peter JB, Pearson CM. A computer-assisted analysis of 150 patients with polymyositis and dermatomyositis. *Medicine* 1977;56:255.

156. Rosenzweig BA, Rotmensch S, Binnette SP, Phillippe M. Primary idiopathic polymyositis and dermatomyositis complicating pregnancy: diagnosis and management. *Obstet Gynecol Surv* 1989;44:162–170.

157. Ditzian-Kadanoff R, Reinhard JD, Thomas C, Segal AS. Polymyositis with myoglobinuria in pregnancy: a report and review of the literature. *J Rheum* 1988;15:513–514.

158. Ishii N, Ono H, Kawaguchi T, Nakajima H. Dermatomyositis and pregnancy. Case report and review of the literature. *Dermatologica* 1991;183:146–149.

159. Glickman FS. Dermatomyositis associated with pregnancy. *US Armed Forces Med J* 1958;9:417–425.

160. Tsai A, Lindheimer MD, Lamberg SI. Dermatomyositis complicating pregnancy. *Obstet Gynecol* 1973;41: 570–573.

161. Katz AL. Another case of polymyositis in pregnancy. *Arch Intern Med* 1980;140:1123.

162. Gutierrez G, Dagnino R, Mintz G. Polymyositis/dermatomyositis and pregnancy. *Arthr Rheum* 1984;27: 291–294.

163. Barnes AB, Lisak DA. Childhood dermatomyositis and pregnancy. *Am J Obstet Gynecol* 1983;146:335–336.

164. Bauer KA, Siegler M, Lindheimer MA. Polymyositis complicating pregnancy. *Arch Intern Med* 1979;139: 449.

165. Houck W, Melnyk C, Gast MJ. Polymyositis in pregnancy. *J Reprod Med* 1987;32:208–210.

166. England MJ, Perlmann T, Veriava Y. Dermatomyositis in pregnancy. *J Reprod Med* 1986;31:633–636.

167. King CR, Chow S. Dermatomyositis and pregnancy. *Obstet Gynecol* 1985;66:589–592.

168. Emy PH, Lenormand V, Maitre F, et al. Polymyosite, dermatomyosite et grossesse: grossesse a haut risk, nouvelle observation et revue de la literature. *J Gynecol Obstet Biol Reprod* 1986;15:785.

169. Masse MR. Grossesses et dermatomyosite. *Bull Soc Franc Derm Syph* 1962;69:921.

170. Satoh M, Ajmani AK, Hirakata M, Suwa A, Winfield JB, Reeves WH. Onset of polymyositis with autoantibodies to threonyl-tRNA synthetase during pregnancy. *J Rheumatol* 1994;21:1564–1566.

171. Harria A, Webley M, Usherwood M, Burge S. Dermatomyositis presenting in pregnancy. *Br J Dermatol* 1995;133:783–785.

172. Boggess KA, Easterling TR, Raghu G. Management and outcome of pregnant women with interstitial and restrictive lung disease. *Am J Obstet Gynecol* 1995;173: 1007–1014.

173. Kofteridis DP, Malliotakis PI, Sotsiou F, Vardakis NK, Vamvakas LN, Emmanouel DS. Acute onset of dermatomyositis presenting in pregnancy with rhabdomyolysis and fetal loss. *Scand J Rheumatol* 1999;28:192–194.

174. Papapetropoulos T, Kanellakopoulou N, Tsibri E, Paschalis C. Polymyositis and pregnancy: report of a case with three pregnancies. *J Neurol Neurosurg Psychiat* 1998;64:406.

175. Case Records of the Massachusetts General Hospital. *N Engl J Med* 1999;340:455–464.

176. Takei R, Suzuki S, Kijima K, et al. First presentation of polymyositis postpartum following intrauterine fetal death. *Arch Gynecol Obstet* 2000;264:47–48.

177. Messina S, Fagiolari G, Lamperti C, et al. Women with pregnancy-related polymyositis and high serum CK levels in the newborn. *Neurology* 2002;58:482–484.

178. Tojyo K, Sekiyima Y, Hattori T, et al. A patient who developed dermatomyositis during the 1st trimester of gestation and improved after abortion. *Rinsho Shinkeigaku* 2001;41:635–638.

179. Ishikawa S, Takei Y, Maruyama T, Koyama S, Hanyu N. A case of polymyositis presenting pregnancy with acute respiratory failure. *Rinsho Shinkeigaku* 2000;40:140–144.

180. Hepburn A, Damani N, Sandison A, Pandit N. Idiopathic focal myositis in pregnancy. *Rheumatology (Oxford)* 2001;40:704–706.

181. Kanoh H, Izumi T, Seishma M, Nojiri M, Ichiki Y, Kitajima Y. A case of dermatomyositis that developed after delivery: the involvement of pregnancy in the induction of dermatomyositis. *Br J Dermatol* 1999;141:897–900.

182. Nicholson HO. Cytotoxic drugs in pregnancy. *J Obstet Gynecol Brit Commonweal* 1968;75:307–312.

183. Mintz G. Dermatomyositis. *Rheum Dis Clin N Am* 1989;15:375–382.

184. Kaufman RL, Kitridou RC. Pregnancy in mixed connective tissue disease: comparison with systemic lupus erythematosus. *J Rheum* 1982;9:549–555.

185. Spellacy WN. Scleroderma and pregnancy. *Obstet Gynecol* 1964;23:297–300.

186. Nambu Y, Mouri M, Toga H, Ohya N, Iwata T, Kobashi Y. Gender and underlying diseases affect the frequency of the concurrence of adult polymyositis/dermatomyositis and interstitial pneumonia. *Chest* 1994;106: 1931–1932.

187. Lehmann-Horn F, Rudel R. Hereditary nondystrophic myotonias and periodic paralyses. *Curr Opin Neurol* 1995;8:402–410.

188. Gardiner CF. A case of myotonia congenita. *Arch Ped* 1901;18:925–928.

189. Hakim CA, Thomlinson J. Myotonia congenita in pregnancy. *J Obstet Gynecol Brit Commonweal* 1969;76: 561–562.

190. Rana SS, Kunschner L, Small G. Pregnancy induced worsening of symptoms in a patient with myotonia congenita. *Muscle Nerve* 2002;26:587–588.

191. Lacomis D, Gonzales JT, Guiliani MJ. Fluctuating clinical myotonia and weakness from Thomsen's disease occurring only during pregnancies. *Clin Neurol Neurosurg* 1999;101:133–136.

192. Morley JB, Lambert TF, Kakulas BA. *Excerpta Medica International Congress Series* 1973;295:543.

193. Saidman LJ, Havard ES, Eger EI. Hyperthermia during anesthesia. *JAMA* 1964;190:1029–1032.

194. Miller JD, Lee C. Muscle diseases. In: Katz J, Benumof JL, Kadis LB, (eds.) *Anesthesia and uncommon diseases*, 3rd ed. Philadelphia: WB Saunders, 1990;622–626.

195. Wilkinson DA, Tonin P, Shanske S, Lombes A, Carlson GM, DiMauro S. Clinical and biochemical features of 10 adult patients with muscle phosphorylase kinase deficiency. *Neurology* 1994;44:461–466.

196. Cochrane P, Alderman B. Normal pregnancy and successful delivery in myophosphorylase deficiency (McArdle's disease). *J Neurol Neurosurg Psychiatry* 1973;36:225–227.

197. Dawson DM, Spong FL, Harrington JF. McArdle's disease: lack of muscle phosphorylase. *Ann Intern Med* 1968;69:229–235.

198. Engel WK, Eyerman EL, Williams HE. Late-onset type of skeletal-muscle phosphorylase deficiency: a new familial variety with completely and partially affected members. *N Engl J Med* 1962;268:135–137.

199. Owens OJ, Macdonald R. Idiopathic myoglobinuria in the early puerperium. *Scott Med J* 1989;34:564–565.

200. Fukada Y, Ohta S, Mizuno K, Hoshi K. Rhabdomyolysis secondary to hyperemesis gravidarum. *Acta Obstet Gynecol Scand* 1999;78:71–73.

201. Kaplan RF, Kellner KR. More on malignant hyperthermia during delivery. *Am J Obstet Gynecol* 1985;152:608–609.

202. Strazis KP, Fox AW. Malignant hyperthermia: a review of published cases. *Anesth Analg* 1993;77:297–304.

203. Liebenschutz F, Mai C, Pickerodt VWA. Increased carbon dioxide production in two patients with malignant hyperthermia and its control by dantrolene. *Br J Anaesth* 1979;51:899–903.

204. Lips FJ, Newland M, Dutton G. Malignant hyperthermia triggered by cyclopropane during cesarean section. *Anesthesiol* 1982;56:144–146.

205. Cupryn JP, Kennedy A, Byrick RJ. Malignant hyperthermia in pregnancy. *Am J Obstet Gynecol* 1984;150:327–328.

206. Sorosky JI, Ingardia CJ, Botti JJ. Diagnosis and management of susceptibility to malignant hyperthermia in pregnancy. *Am J Perinatol* 1989;6:46–48.

207. Shime J, Gare D, Andrews J, Britt B. Dantrolene in pregnancy: lack of adverse effects on the fetus and newborn infant. *Am J Obstet Gynecol* 1988;159:831–834.

208. Morison DH. Placental transfer of dantrolene. *Anesthesiol* 1983;59:265.

209. Lucy SJ. Anaesthesia for caesarean delivery of a malignant hyperthermia susceptible parturient. *Can J Anaesth* 1994;41:1220–1226.

210. Morgan-Hughes JA. Mitochondrial Disease. In: Engel AG, Franzini-Armstrong C, (eds.) *Myology*, 2nd ed. New York: McGraw-Hill, 1994;1610–1660.

211. Cornelio F, DiDonato S, Peluchetti D, et al. Fatal cases of lipid storage myopathy with carnitine deficiency. *J Neurol Neurosurg Psychiat* 1977;40:170–178.

212. Angelini C, Govoni E, Bragaglia M, Vergani L. Carnitine deficiency: acute postpartum crisis. *Ann Neurol* 1978;4:558–561.

213. Boudin G, Mikol J, Guillard A, Engel AG. Fatal systemic carnitine deficiency with lipid storage in skeletal muscle, heart, liver and kidney. *J Neurol Sci* 1976;30:313–325.

214. Marzo A, Cardace G, Corbellata C, et al. Plasma concentration, urinary excretion and renal clearance of L-carnitine during pregnancy: a reversible secondary L-carnitine deficiency. *Gynecol Endocrinol* 1994;8:115–120.

215. Hahn P, Skala JP, Secombe DW, et al. Carnitine content of blood and amniotic fluid. *Pediatr Res* 1977;11:878–880.

216. Warshaw JB, Terry ML. Cellular energy metabolism during fetal development, Part 2. *J Cell Biol* 1970;44:354–360.

217. Dreval D, Bernstein D, Zakut H. Carnitine palmitoyl transferase deviciency in pregnancy-a case report. *Am J Obstet Gynecol* 1994;170:1309–1392.

218. Zierz S. Carnitine palmitoyltransferase deficiency. In: Engel AG, Franzini-Armstrong C, (eds.) *Myology*, 2nd ed. New York: McGraw Hill, 1994;1577–1586.

219. Ewart RM, Burrows RF. Pregnancy in chronic progressive external opthalmoplegia: a case report. *Am J Perinatol* 1997;14:293–295.

220. Torbergsen T, Oian P, Mathiesen E, Borud O. Preeclampsia—a mitochondrial disease? *Acta Obstet Gynecol Scand* 1989;68:145–148.

221. Berkowitz K, Monteagudo A, Marks F, Jackson U, Baxi L. Mitochondrial myopathy and preeclampsia associated with pregnancy. *Am J Obstet Gynecol* 1990;162:146–147.

222. Rosaeg OP, Morrison S, MacLeod JP. Anaesthetic management of labour and delivery in the parturient with mitochondrial myopathy. *Can J Anaesth* 1996;43:403–407.

223. Larsson N-G, Eiken HG, Boman H, Holme E, Oldfors A, Tulinius MH. Lack of transmission of deleted mtDNA from a woman with Kearns-Sayre syndrome to her child. *Am J Hum Gen* 1992;50:360–363.

224. Blake LL, Shaw RW. Mitochondrial myopathy in a primigravid pregnancy. *Br J Obstet Gynecol* 1999;106:871–873.

225. Soccio PS, Phillips WP, Bonisteel P, Bennett KA. Pregnancy with cytochrome oxidase-deficient mitochondrial myopathy. *Obstet Gynecol* 2001;97:815–816.

226. Yanagawa T, Sakaguchi H, Nakao T, et al. Mitochondrial myopathy, encephalopathy, lactic acidosis, and stroke-like episodes with deterioration during pregnancy. *Intern Med* 1998;37:780–783.

227. Kokawa N, Ishii Y, Yamoto M, Nakano R. Pregnancy and delivery complicated by mitochondrial myopathy, encephalopathy, lactic acidosis, and stroke-like episodes. *Obstet Gynecol* 1998;91:865.

228. Kovilam OPO, Cahill W, Siddiqi TA. Pregnancy with mitochondrial encephalopathy, lactic acidosis, and strokelike episodes syndrome. *Obstet Gynecol* 1999;93:853.

229. Tyni T, Pihko H. Long-chain 3-hydroxyacyl-CoA dehydrogenase deficiency. *Acta Paediatr* 1999;88:237–245.

230. Giles RE, Blanc H, Cann HM, Wallace DC. Maternal inheritance of human mitochondrial DNA. *Proc Natl Acad Sci USA* 1980;77:6715.

231. Chinnery PF, Howell N, Lithowlers RN, Turnbull DM. MELAS and MERRF. The relationship between maternal mutation load and the frequency of clinically affected offspring. *Brain* 1998;121:1889–1894.

232. White SL, Shanske S, Biros I, et al. Two cases of prenatal analysis for the pathogenic T to G substitution at nucleotide 8993 in mitochondrial DNA. *Prenat Diagn* 1999;19:1165–1168.

233. Poulton J, Marchington DR. Progress in genetic counseling and prenatal diagnosis of maternally inherited

mtDNA diseases. *Neuromuscul Disord* 2000;10: 484–487.

234. Amiel J, Pigarel N, Benacki A, et al. Prenatal diagnosis of respiratory chain deficiency by direct mutation screening. *Prenat Diagn* 2001;21:602–604.

235. Faivre L, Cormier-Daire V, Chretien D, et al. Determination of enzyme activities for prenatal diagnosis of respiratory chain deficiency. *Prenat Diagn* 2000;20: 732–737.

236. Tanner SM, Laporte J, Guirad-Chaumeil C, Liechti-Gallati S. Confirmation of prenatal diagnosis results of X-linked recessive myotubular myopathy by mutational screening, and description of three new mutations in the MTM1 gene. *Hum Mutat* 1998;11:62–68.

237. Hu LJ, Laporte J, Kress W, Dahl N. Prenatal diagnosis of X-linked myotubular myopathy: strategies using new and tightly linked DNA markers. *Prenat Diagn* 1996;16:231–237.

238. Liechti-Gallati S, Wolff G, Ketelsen UP, Braga S. Prenatal diagnosis of X-linked centronuclear myopathy by linkage analysis. *Pediatr Res* 1993;33:201–204.

239. Jungbluth H, Sewry CA, Buj-Bello A, et al. Early and severe presentation of X-linked myotubular myopathy in a girl with skewed X-inactivation. *Neuromuscul Disord* 2003;13:55–59.

240. Lammens M, Moerman P, Fryns JP, et al. Fetal akinesia sequence caused by nemaline myopathy. *Neuropediatrics* 1997;28:116–119.

241. Stackhouse R, Chwlmow D, Dattel BJ. Anesthetic complications in a pregnant patient with nemaline myopathy. *Anesth Analg* 1994;79:1195–1197.

242. Wallgren-Pettersson C, Hilesmaa VK, Paatero H. Pregnancy and delivery in congenital nemaline myopathy. *Acta Obstet Gynecol Scand* 1995;74:659–661.

243. Quane KA, Healey JMS, Keating KE, et al. Mutations in the ryanodine receptor gene in central core disease and malignant hyperthermia. *Nature Genet* 1993;5:51–55.

244. Dresser LP, Massey EW, Johnson EE, Bossen E. Ipecac myopathy and cardiomyopathy. *J Neurol Neurosurg Psychiatry* 1993;56:560–562.

245. Thyagarajan D, Day BJ, Wodak J, Gilligan B, Dennett X. Emetine myopathy in a patient with an eating disorder. *Med J Aust* 1993;159:757–760.

246. Urbano-Marquez A, Estruch R, Fernandez-Sola J, Nicolas JM, Pare JC, Rubin E. The greater risk of alcoholic cardiomyopathy and myopathy in women compared with men. *JAMA* 1995;274:149–154.

247. Blanche S, Tardieu M, Rustin P, et al. Persistent mitochondrial dysfunction and perinatal exposure to antiretroviral nucleoside analogues. *Lancet* 1999;354:1084–1089.

248. Bulterys M, Nesheim S, et al. Perinatal Safety Review Working Group. Lack of evidence of mitochondrial dysfunction in the offspring of HIV-infected women. *Ann NY Acad Sci* 2000;918:212–221.

249. Layzer RB. Diagnosis of Neuromuscular Disorders. *Neuromuscular manifestations of systemic disease*. Philadelphia: FA Davis, 1985;19–22.

250. Man-Son-Hing M, Wells G. Meta-analysis of efficacy of quinine for treatment of nocturnal leg cramps in elderly people. *BMJ* 1995;310:13–17.

251. Young GL, Jewell D. Interventions for leg cramps in pregnancy. *Cochrane Database Syst Rev* 2002;l: CD000121.

252. Thomsen WHS, Smith I. Effects of oestrogen on erythrocyte enzyme efflux in normal men and women. *Clin Chim Acta* 1980;103:203–208.

253. Fukutake T, Hattori T. Normalization of creatine kinase level during pregnancy in idiopathic hyperCKemia. *Clin Neurol Neurosurg* 2001;103:168–170.

254. Arnett MG, Hyslop R, Dennehy CA, Schneider CM. Age-related variations of serum CK and CK MB response in females. *Can J Appl Physiol* 2000;25:419–429.

255. Simpson J, Zellweger H, Burmeister LF, Christee R, Nielsen MK. Effect of oral contraceptive pills on the level of creatine phosphokinase with regard to carrier detection in Duchenne muscular dystrophy. *Clin Chim Acta* 1974;52:219–223.

256. Black HR, Quallich H, Gareleck CB. Racial differences in serum creatine kinase levels. *Am J Med* 1986;81: 479–487.

257. Emery AEH. Prevention. In: *Duchenne muscular dystrophy*. Oxford: Oxford University Press. 1987; 181–211.

258. Kelley W, Harris E, Ruddy S, Sledge C. The fibromyalgia syndrome: myofascial pain and the chronic fatigue syndrome. In: Bennett R, (ed.) *Textbook of rheumatology*, 4th ed. Philadelphia: WB Saunders, 1993;471–483.

259. Moldofsky H, Scarisbrick P. Induction of neurasthenic musculoskeletal pain syndrome by selective sleep stage deprivation. *Psychosom Med* 1976;38:35–41.

22 Neurologic Presentations of Autoimmune Disorders in Women

Michelle Petri, MD, MPH

Connective tissue diseases and some types of vasculitis disproportionately affect women. The rheumatologic diseases in women that most frequently have neurologic manifestations are Takayasu arteritis, giant cell arteritis, systemic lupus erythematosus (SLE), Sjögren's syndrome, rheumatoid arthritis (RA), and scleroderma. Medium-vessel vasculitides, including Wegener granulomatosis and polyarteritis nodosa, do not have a special female predominance and are not covered in this chapter. The neurologic manifestations of rheumatic diseases often require long-term corticosteroid therapy, leading to corticosteroid complications (such as cataracts and osteoporosis) in many patients.

The treatment of women during pregnancy presents particular problems in management, both because the diseases (and their activity) can be difficult to diagnose and follow and because many of the effective medications are either contraindicated during pregnancy or, as is the case with corticosteroids, aggravate hyperglycemia, osteoporosis, and preeclampsia.

Antiphospholipid antibody syndrome (APS) is a hypercoagulable state that occurs equally in patients with connective tissue diseases, usually lupus, and in a primary form, without known autoimmune disease. Many of these patients are women. APS has many neurologic presentations, including transient ischemic attack (TIA), stroke, chorea, and transverse myelopathy (see also Chapters 17 and 24). The neurologic manifestations of connective tissue diseases, vasculitis, and APS are reviewed in this chapter.

TAKAYASU ARTERITIS

Takayasu arteritis is a large-vessel vasculitis that predominantly affects young women, with a sex ratio of 9:1. Most patients present between 15 and 25 years of age. In the United States, the incidence is very low, at 2.6 per million per year (1); it is more common in Asia (2,3). It is a vasculitis of the aorta and major branches, typically presenting as a two-stage illness. In the first stage, systemic phase ("pre-pulseless"), symptoms include fever, malaise, night sweats, arthralgias, myalgias, and tender arteries (4). In the late "pulseless" phase, there are symptoms of ischemia, with claudication, headache, syncope, paresthesia, and visual disturbance (5,6). Many patients do not follow the two-stage pattern, however.

On physical examination, the classic findings are those of decreased pulses (especially carotid, radial, ulnar, and brachial), blood pressure differential between the arms, and bruits over vessels, especially the subclavian arteries or aorta. Laboratory abnormalities include an elevated erythrocyte sedimentation rate (ESR) in most patients. Arteriography is the usual mode of diagnosis,

---

TABLE 22.1
Presentations of Takayasu Arteritis

Typical Presentation
- Female patient under 40 years of age
- Clinical features include systemic symptoms (malaise, fever) followed by symptoms due to vascular occlusion (arterial bruits and absent pulses)

Neurologic Presentations
- Brain
- Dizziness
- Syncope
- Stroke/transient ischemic attack
- Headache
- Ocular
- Difficulty with upward gaze
- Visual impairment
- Hypertensive retinopathy
- Limb weakness

TABLE 22.2
Presentations of Giant Cell Arteritis

Typical Presentation
- Patient over 50 years of age
- Clinical features include malaise, headache, jaw claudication, visual disturbance, scalp tenderness, and/or polymyalgia rheumatica
- Laboratory features include a greatly elevated ESR, anemia, and/or elevated liver function tests (alkaline phosphatase)

Neurologic Presentations
- Brain
- Headache
- Amaurosis fugax
- Blindness
- Diplopia
- Focal cerebral ischemia (transient ischemic attacks, strokes)
- Peripheral neuropathy

---

revealing one of three patterns: type I, with aortic arch and branch involvement; type II, with involvement of the descending thoracic and abdominal aorta; and type III, a combination of type I and type II (7,8).

Neurologic presentations include syncope, stroke, or TIA; limb weakness from vascular insufficiency; dizziness; and multiple ocular manifestations (diplopia, amaurosis, and retinal changes) (Table 22.1) (1,3,9,10).

Treatment is often delayed because most patients are not diagnosed in the early phase, in which most symptoms are systemic (fever, malaise). Treatment with corticosteroids is helpful in improving these systemic symptoms and slowing, progression of vascular occlusion (1,11,12). Some patients require additional immunosuppression, using azathioprine, cyclophosphamide, or methotrexate (13). Those patients who have fixed claudication or major vascular insufficiency may require angioplasty (13–15) or bypass procedures (16).

GIANT CELL ARTERITIS

Giant cell arteritis (GCA), or temporal arteritis, is more common in women than in men, with similar clinical presentations in both sexes. Most affected patients are over the age of 50. In the United States, it is more common in people of Scandinavian extraction. Giant cell arteritis is one of the most frequent types of vasculitis, with an incidence of 20 to 30 per 100,000 (17). Typical presentations include headache, amaurosis fugax, muscle and joint aches and pains (with a shoulder-hip girdle predominance and morning accentuation, i.e., polymyalgia rheumatica), jaw claudication, scalp tenderness, fever, and sometimes cough or sore throat (Table

22.2). Physical examination may reveal enlargement, beading (alternating enlargement and narrowing), and tenderness of the temporal arteries. The laboratory examination may show the classic triad of a greatly elevated ESR, anemia, and elevated alkaline phosphatase. Diagnosis is based on the characteristic large-vessel vasculitis with giant cells on temporal artery biopsy. Because the vasculitis may skip certain regions, a large segment is obtained and bilateral biopsies should be done if the first one is negative. It is extremely unusual to have biopsy-negative GCA or to have a normal ESR before treatment.

Treatment is initially high-dose corticosteroids (usually 40 to 60 mg of prednisone daily). The ESR usually falls promptly, with relief of symptoms following shortly thereafter. The high doses of corticosteroids are usually reduced gradually after the first 4 to 6 weeks, with maintenance therapy often required for a year or longer. It is not necessary to normalize the ESR; it is more important to follow the important symptoms and signs of disease, including headache and visual disturbance. Both sexes are at risk for corticosteroid complications, including diabetes mellitus; infections; increase in cardiovascular risk factors such as weight, hypertension, and hyperlipidemia; and osteoporosis. Because nearly all women who have this disease are postmenopausal, it is extremely important to treat presumptively for corticosteroid-induced osteoporosis using calcium, vitamin D, and bisphosphonates (either daily or weekly alendronate). Because the Women's Health Initiative study showed an increase in cardiovascular events in women randomized to hormone replacement therapy (HRT), it is no longer recommended for osteoporosis.

SYSTEMIC LUPUS ERYTHEMATOSUS

Systemic lupus erythematosus (SLE) is the classic example of an autoimmune disease, with a 9:1 female-male ratio and a disproportionate predilection for African-Americans. It usually has its clinical onset post puberty; the sex ratio is equal before puberty. Although the cause is unknown, several predisposing factors have been identified. Genetic factors include HLA-D alleles and null (lack of the gene product for C4 or C3, due to either deletion or mutation) complement alleles. Environmental factors include exposure to ultraviolet light and sulfa antibiotics (18). Hormonal factors include oral contraceptive pills (although this may have been more true for pills in the past that contained more estrogen) and pregnancy (19).

The diagnosis of SLE is made by history, physical examination, and confirmatory laboratory tests. The history reveals symptoms or signs in multiple organ systems. Frequent presenting symptoms and signs include malar (erythematous rash on the cheeks) or discoid (deeper, inflammatory rash healing with scarring, often hyper- or hypopigmentation) rash, photosensitivity, oral ulcers, alopecia, polyarthritis, and fever. Physical examination will confirm the presence of lupus rashes, reveal whether there is serositis (pleural rub or effusion and/or pericardial rub), and demonstrate polyarthritis, characteristically involving the proximal interphalangeal (PIP), metacarpophalangeal (MCP), and wrist joints of both hands. Some manifestations of SLE are only apparent through laboratory testing, including, in some but not all patients, hemolytic anemia, leukopenia, lymphopenia, thrombocytopenia, elevated ESR, elevated creatinine, hematuria and red blood cell casts, and proteinuria. Serologic tests can be helpful in the diagnosis: A positive antinuclear antibody (ANA) is found in 95% of patients with SLE, but a positive ANA is also found in up to 20% of normal young women. Therefore, a diagnosis of lupus can never be based on a positive ANA alone; evidence of a multiorgan (some combination of dermatologic, musculoskeletal, renal, serositis, hematologic, and neurologic manifestations) systemic disease should exist. Other serologic tests are more specific but are not found in all patients. The autoantibodies anti-dsDNA and anti-Smith (anti-Sm) are found only in SLE. Other autoantibodies, including anti-Ro, anti-La, and anti-RNP, can be found in other connective tissue diseases as well as in SLE. Many patients with SLE will also have evidence of complement consumption, with decreased levels of serum complement (C3, C4, or both). Other connective tissue diseases, vasculitis, and cryoglobulinemia can also cause complement consumption.

Two neurologic events (seizures—due to lupus, not due to a prior stroke—and psychosis) are part of the neurologic criterion for SLE (four of eleven American College of Rheumatology criteria must be present to classify patients as having SLE for research purposes) (20). The eleven criteria include malar rash, discoid rash, photosensitivity, oral ulcers, arthritis, serositis, renal disorder, neurologic disorder, hematologic disorder, immunologic disorder, and positive ANA. The neurologic criterion consists of seizures and psychosis. In the Hopkins Lupus Cohort, our longitudinal study of SLE, only 11% of the cohort have had seizures or psychosis due to SLE. Other neurologic events are actually more common (Table 22.3), including other brain involvement and cranial nerve, cord, and peripheral nervous system manifestations.

Brain involvement in SLE includes stroke, meningitis, seizure, organic brain syndrome, coma, cognitive function abnormalities, chorea, psychosis, and lupus

---

TABLE 22.3
Presentations of Systemic Lupus Erythematosus

Typical Presentations
- Female patient, post puberty, and premenopausal
- Clinical features include fever, fatigue, photosensitivity, malar rash, discoid lupus, aphthous ulcers, polyarthritis, lupus nephritis (hematuria and proteinuria), serositis (pericarditis and pleurisy), hemolytic anemia, leukopenia, thrombocytopenia, seizures, and/or psychosis
- Laboratory features include hematologic abnormalities, renal abnormalities, positive ANA, multiple organ autoantibodies, and/or low serum complement (C3, C4)

Neurologic Presentations
- Brain
- Stroke
- Meningitis
- Organic brain syndrome/delirium
- Coma
- Cognitive function deficits
- Chorea
- Psychosis
- Headache
- Pseudotumor cerebri (see APS)
- Cranial neuropathy
- Spinal cord
- Transverse myelopathy
- Peripheral nerve
- Entrapment neuropathy, especially carpal tunnel syndrome
- Peripheral neuropathy
- Mononeuritis multiplex
- Demyelinating neuropathy
- Autonomic neuropathy (rare)
- Muscle
- Polymyositis
- Steroid myopathy
- Myasthenia gravis

headache (21). The American College of Rheumatology has recently codified neuropsychiatric manifestations of SLE (22). Some strokes are not due to active SLE but to other disease processes or to comorbid conditions, including hypertension. For example, some SLE patients have a hypercoagulable state APS, which can present as a TIA or stroke. This syndrome is discussed in detail later in this chapter. Additionally, SLE patients who have been receiving maintenance corticosteroids are at risk for premature atherosclerosis. Brain magnetic resonance imaging (MRI) is a more sensitive test than a computed tomographic (CT) scan to detect infarcts and other lesions from SLE (23). Strokes due to active SLE often do not have demonstrable vasculitis on angiogram, although there are exceptions (24). The vessel pathology is usually a small-vessel vasculopathy (25,26).

Organic brain syndrome (encephalopathy) and coma are frightening manifestations of SLE that can sometimes occur very acutely, over days or a few weeks. As with other manifestations of CNS-SLE, other diagnoses need to be considered. Infections, multiple cerebral infarcts, tumor, intracranial bleeding, status epilepticus, metabolic states [syndrome of inappropriate secretion of antidiuretic hormone (SIADH), hepatic encephalopathy, uremia, myxedema], and drug toxicity may be mistaken for SLE flare and must be excluded. Nearly all patients will require a brain MRI scan and lumbar puncture. It is also important to perform an electroencephalogram to rule out the possibility of status epilepticus. Other diseases that can mimic SLE in this situation are thrombotic thrombocytopenic purpura (TTP) and the catastrophic (i.e., life-threatening multiorgan vasculopathy and/or infarcts) presentation of APS. In TTP, fever, thrombocytopenia, and renal involvement would be additional clues leading to the diagnosis (discussed later in this chapter). An examination of the blood smear for schistocytes is crucial. Treatment with plasmapheresis is indicated for TTP and may be helpful in the catastrophic form of APS, when multiple organs fail due to vasculopathy and/or thrombosis.

If the organic brain syndrome or coma is due to SLE, it is important to treat early (often while the patient is still in the emergency room) and effectively. Most patients are given intravenous "pulse" methylprednisolone, 1,000 mg daily over 90 minutes, for 3 days. This is the same dosage that is used for the treatment of renal transplant rejection. Many patients begin to show improvement within hours or a day of receiving the methylprednisolone. A patient who is slow to respond, or who is critically ill, may require additional treatment. Several studies have proven the efficacy of intravenous cyclophosphamide for severe CNS-SLE. It is usually given in doses between 750 and 1,000 mg/m^2 body surface area, initially once monthly for up to 6 months, provided that there are no concerns about bone marrow suppression (27,28). Because most SLE patients are young women, it is important that they be protected against some of the major complications of cyclophosphamide, such as hemorrhagic cystitis and bladder carcinoma. For that reason, we and others recommend that cyclophosphamide be preceded by prehydration and that it be given with mesna, which binds toxic metabolites.

A lupus patient who presents with symptoms or signs of meningitis must have a lumbar puncture. Patients with SLE, especially those who are receiving treatment with prednisone or immunosuppressive drugs, are at risk for both typical (i.e., pneumococcal) and opportunistic infections, including tuberculosis, cryptococcus, and candidemia, all of which can be complicated by meningitis. Patients who have SLE may be more susceptible to infection by some viruses, such as herpes zoster, that can cause meningitis. Additionally, certain drugs, such as nonsteroidal anti-inflammatory drugs (NSAIDs), especially ibuprofen, can rarely cause a drug meningitis in SLE patients (29).

Lumbar puncture may show a number of different abnormalities in lupus meningitis, or in CNS-SLE in general, none of which are specific for SLE. These abnormalities include elevated protein, decreased glucose, pleocytosis, oligoclonal bands, and elevated IgG index. The measure of autoantibodies or complement in the cerebral spinal fluid (CSF) is not helpful diagnostically. If infection is ruled out, lupus meningitis is treated initially with high-dose corticosteroids.

Seizures are less common in SLE patients today than they were decades ago, perhaps reflecting earlier diagnosis and treatment. In most series, SLE seizures are more common early in the disease course (21,30,31). Most seizures due to SLE are generalized tonic-clonic seizures (32–34). SLE seizures can occur as part of a systemic flare (i.e., activity outside the neurologic system) or can be isolated, without non–CNS-SLE activity. The etiology of SLE seizures is not understood. Antiphospholipid and/or antineuronal antibodies may, through direct binding to neural tissue, lead to a metabolic change that lowers the seizure threshold.

An SLE patient with new-onset seizures needs a complete evaluation for CNS-SLE and non-SLE causes of seizures (35). The first question is whether the patient is having true seizures or pseudoseizures, such as syncope, movement disorders, narcolepsy, or psychogenic seizures (36). Second, potentially reversible conditions that cause seizures should be investigated. These include infections, metabolic derangements, medication toxicity (including phenothiazines, clozapine, radiographic contrast agents, and some SLE medications, such as antimalarial drugs, that are very rarely associated with seizures) and CNS-SLE. SLE patients with renal failure are at risk for seizure if they are given meperidine hydrochloride; we have seen this problem several times in postoperative patients. Third, it is important to ascertain whether a new focal cause of chronic epilepsy exists, such as a stroke or tumor.

The evaluation of an SLE patient with new-onset seizure includes a search for infection, laboratory testing (complete blood count, electrolytes, BUN, creatinine, liver enzymes), medication review, and a search for activity of SLE outside the neurologic system. Lumbar puncture, EEG, and brain MRI with gadolinium are usually performed.

If the seizures are due to active SLE, initial treatment consists of both corticosteroids and antiepileptic drugs (AEDs). Most seizures in SLE patients are tonic-clonic seizures, which can be successfully treated with phenytoin. Phenytoin can affect the metabolism of corticosteroids and, on rare occasions, causes a drug fever in SLE patients. Patients whose seizure was due to a reversible precipitant, such as infection or lupus flare (reactive seizures), may not need long-term AEDs.

Cognitive function deficits, including problems with memory, concentration, and judgment, are probably the most common manifestations of CNS-SLE (37). They are also, unfortunately, one of the more nonspecific manifestations and are consequently very difficult to attribute to SLE alone (38). SLE, corticosteroids, other drugs (including tricyclic antidepressants and NSAIDs), and comorbid processes such as APS, dementia, and depression can also contribute to cognitive function abnormalities (39). Formal cognitive function tests are important in localizing the deficits, establishing a baseline, and can often suggest processes such as anxiety and/or depression as possible contributing causes. Patients with major cognitive function deficits should have a brain MRI with gadolinium as part of their evaluation. The role of brain single photon emission computerized tomography (SPECT) scan or brain positron emission tomography (PET) is limited because scans can be abnormal in patients without neurologic symptoms or signs (40,41). Treatment with corticosteroids is used if there is evidence of progression and if SLE is thought to be the primary cause (39). Most SLE patients have mild, stable deficits that may not require treatment with corticosteroids or alkylating drugs.

Chorea is a very unusual presentation of CNS-SLE (42). Its presence should always mandate evaluation for APS, especially if infarcts are found in the basal ganglia on brain MRI scan.

Psychosis is an unusual manifestation of CNS-SLE. It may be associated with antiribosomal P antibody (43–45). Antiribosomal P does not have sufficient predictive value to warrant testing for it in all SLE patients, however. Psychosis can also occur from steroid psychosis, infection, and very rarely, drugs such as antimalarials (including hydroxychloroquine and chloroquine). Psychosis, if due to active SLE, is treated with corticosteroids and major tranquilizers (such as haloperidol).

Severe unremitting headache, unresponsive to narcotics and other general headache remedies, can occur as a result of SLE, but is unusual. Headache can be the first presenting sign of other SLE neurologic syndromes, including lupus meningitis, organic brain syndrome, pseudotumor cerebri, and stroke, but it can also represent an infection, tumor, or drug toxicity. Thus, a new severe headache, especially with neurologic symptoms or signs, should be evaluated with brain MRI and lumbar puncture to look for evidence of an opportunistic infection. Chronic recurrent headache is usually not due to lupus and should lead to an evaluation for the common causes of headache, especially migraine. SLE patients with antiphospholipid antibodies should be checked for dural sinus thrombosis.

Cranial neuropathies, including Bell's palsy, are rare in SLE, occurring in only 1 to 2% of patients. Some cases of trigeminal sensory neuropathy do not correspond to trigeminal branches and may be caused by medulla oblongata lesions (46). Most cranial neuropathies in SLE are due to vasculitis or infarction (47–49), although facial nerve palsy has been reported due to angioedema (50). The presence of a new cranial neuropathy, especially Bell's palsy, should lead to an evaluation of other causes, including Lyme disease in endemic areas and space-occupying lesions. Cranial neuropathies due to SLE are treated with corticosteroids.

Transverse myelitis can occur both from SLE (51) and from the APS (52,53). The differential diagnosis includes vertebral compression fractures (54), cord lipomas, infections (herpes zoster) (55), tuberculosis (56), and polyoma JC virus (57). In the case of SLE, lumbar puncture often shows elevated CSF protein, pleocytosis, and/or decreased CSF glucose (58,59). MRI of the cord may show increased signal intensity, edema, or infarct (60). Because of poor long-term function in many cases (61), if infection and compression fracture can be quickly ruled out with an MRI of the affected cord segment, it is important to institute effective treatment, such as intravenous pulse methylprednisolone, within hours of presentation (62). Those patients with relapsing or nonimproving courses can benefit from the addition of "pulse" intravenous cyclophosphamide.

SLE is one of the more common causes of mononeuritis multiplex (63,64). Patients usually first present with pain, hypesthesia, and dysesthesia, followed by motor signs (including weakness). Nerve conduction studies confirm mononeuritis multiplex. If nerve-muscle biopsy is performed, vasculitis is usually demonstrated. Corticosteroids in high doses are the initial therapy, but often it is necessary to add a second drug, such as azathioprine, to allow eventual reduction of the corticosteroid dose. Patients with SLE can also develop peripheral neuropathy (65), entrapment neuropathies (especially carpal tunnel syndrome), demyelinating neuropathy, and autoimmune neuropathy (66,67).

Muscle weakness in an SLE patient can be due to polymyositis, typically with proximal accentuation, and with elevated creatinine phosphokinase (CPK) and/or aldolase. The diagnosis can be confirmed through EMG and muscle biopsy. In a corticosteroid-treated patient, the possibility of steroid myopathy must be considered. Electromyography and muscle biopsy are helpful to rule out inflammatory myopathy, but improvement with corticosteroid reduction is the sine qua non. An occasional patient with SLE may also develop myasthenia gravis (68). All SLE patients with muscle weakness and/or elevated CPK should be checked for hypothyroidism.

SJÖGREN'S SYNDROME

Sjögren's syndrome is predominantly a disease of middle-aged women, affecting between 2 and 5% of adults over 55 years of age (69–71). The usual presenting symptoms and signs are dry eyes and mouth, with keratoconjunctivitis sicca and decreased salivary pool. Some patients have parotid enlargement or hepatosplenomegaly. The diagnosis can be confirmed by an abnormal Schirmer test or rose bengal staining in the case of keratoconjunctivitis sicca, or minor salivary gland biopsy (showing inflammation and/or fibrosis) in the case of dry mouth. Many patients have anti-Ro (also called anti-SSA) and anti-La (also called anti-SSB) autoantibodies in the serum.

The prevalence of severe neurologic disease in Sjögren's syndrome is controversial. Alexander and colleagues reported neurologic complications in as many as 20% of patients (72). Other centers have reported mostly mild neurologic symptoms, which are often explained by the primary autoimmune disease in patients with secondary Sjögren's syndrome (73,74). Most centers report predominantly cranial (especially trigeminal) neuropathy (75) and mild sensory or mixed peripheral neuropathies (76).

Severe CNS-Sjögren's disease is not common, except perhaps in referral centers where there is likely to be a selection bias (77). Clinically, it can resemble multiple sclerosis, with multifocal events occurring over months to years. Presentations include CNS involvement (spasticity, visual loss, ataxia, hemiparesis, cranial neuropathy, dysarthria, nystagmus, and internuclear ophthalmoplegia) and cord involvement (transverse myelopathy and neurogenic bladder) (Table 22.4). Evoked potential and CSF abnormalities are frequently found. In the series of Alexander and colleagues, 16 of 18 patients had one or more oligoclonal bands, and 10 patients had an elevated IgG index (77). CNS-Sjögren's disease is treated in a similar fashion to CNS-SLE, using high-dose corticosteroids and the addition of cyclophosphamide in severe or refractory cases.

The most common neurologic presentation is peripheral neuropathy (72,73,77–81). Mononeuritis multiplex can also occur (82). A pure sensory neuropathy caused by a lymphocytic infiltration of the dorsal root

---

TABLE 22.4
Presentations of Sjögren's Syndrome

Typical Presentation
- Female patient, postmenopausal
- Clinical features include keratoconjunctivitis sicca and dry mouth

Neurologic Presentations
- Brain
- Stroke (72)
- Nystagmus
- Cerebellar ataxia
- Seizures
- Hemianopsia
- Unilateral internuclear ophthalmoplegia
- Optic neuropathy (78)
- Vasculitis (79)
- Multiple sclerosis–like (77)
- Meningitis (80)
- Cognitive function deficits (81)
- Migraine headache (156)
- Cranial neuropathy
- Spinal cord
- Transverse myelitis/myelopathy (157)
- Spinal subarachnoid hemorrhage
- Peripheral nerve
- Entrapment neuropathy, especially carpal tunnel syndrome
- Peripheral neuropathy
- Sensory (75,158–160)
- Motor
- Mononeuritis multiplex (82)
- Muscle
- Polymyositis

---

ganglia has been reported, sometimes preceding the diagnosis of Sjögren's disease itself. Patients who have this disorder present with an asymmetric sensory deficit, initially in the hands, often in association with Adie's pupil or trigeminal sensory neuropathy (76,83). Progressive major peripheral neuropathy is treated with corticosteroids.

RHEUMATOID ARTHRITIS

Rheumatoid arthritis (RA) preferentially affects females, with a ratio of 4:1. It is one of the most common autoimmune diseases, affecting 1% of postmenopausal women. The disease may present in the late twenties or thirties, but many patients present in the peri- or postmenopausal years. Although the cause is unknown, genetic factors are important. One of the most important is the "shared epitope," an HLA sequence that confers susceptibility (84). Hormonal factors play a role in the pathogenesis of the disease. Epidemiologic evidence exists that oral contraceptive use may be protective, and the disease often remits during pregnancy (85). Remissions during pregnancy are due to HLA mismatch between the woman and her partner (86). There is great interest in the role of the nervous system in the pathophysiology of RA, especially in terms of the symmetric nature of the polyarthritis and the preference for distal joints (87). For example, substance P is able to activate rheumatoid synoviocytes (88).

RA presents as a symmetric arthritis of the joints of the hand (MCP and PIP joints) and wrist (carpal joints) (Table 22.5). Pronounced morning stiffness occurs. Eventually, many joints may be involved, including elbows, shoulders, knees, ankles, and tarsal joints. Severe disease results in joint erosions and deformities. Laboratory abnormalities include anemia (usually the anemia of chronic disease, although an anemia that is responsive to erythropoietin is also found), elevated ESR, thrombocytosis, and hypergammaglobulinemia. Some patients have rheumatoid factor, an IgM autoantibody that is directed against IgG.

The treatment of RA consists of drugs that help to suppress acute inflammation, such as NSAIDs and prednisone, and drugs that are "disease-modifying," slowing the progression of erosive changes and deformities. The major oral disease-modifying drugs that are used in the United States are methotrexate and leflunamide (in Europe, azulfidine is also widely used). Neither are allowed during pregnancy. Other disease-modifying drugs

that are used include hydroxychloroquine, azathioprine, and cyclosporine. These are continued during pregnancy only if absolutely required for the health of the mother. Because RA often improves during pregnancy, it is usually possible to stop disease-modifying drugs. Gold and penicillamine have fallen into disfavor because of lower efficacy and greater toxicity. They are not used during pregnancy. Over the past few years, biologic agents that block tumor necrosis factor (etanercept, infliximab, adalimunab) have been shown to be very effective for both the symptoms and signs of RA. These biologics are associated with an increase in extrapulmonary tuberculosis and may cause anti-dsDNA, anticardiolipin, or a drug-induced lupus; they worsen multiple sclerosis and congestive heart failure. They are not approved for use in pregnancy.

Rheumatoid involvement of the CNS is very rare (89,90). Intracranial lesions include vasculitis (91,92), meningitis (93), and rheumatoid nodules (90,94). Seizures can be due to rheumatoid nodules (95) or to leptomeningitis (96). Rheumatoid pachymeningitis can be localized to a discrete location, such as the lumbar cord (97). Finally, normal pressure hydrocephalus has been reported in RA (98).

Several of the neurologic complications of RA are directly related to joint swelling and deformity. Carpal tunnel syndrome is the most common nerve entrapment in rheumatoid patients and usually improves as the joint synovitis is controlled. Cock-up wrist splints and carpal tunnel corticosteroid injections are also beneficial treatments. Tarsal tunnel syndrome may occur in the foot. Other entrapment neuropathies found in RA include the posterior interosseous nerve, the femoral nerve, the peroneal nerve, and the interdigital nerve (at the metatarsophalangeal joint) (99,100).

Life-threatening problems can arise from myelopathies due to cervical spine instability (101). C1–2 subluxation, due to destruction of the transverse ligament of C1 or erosion of the odontoid peg, can occur. Atlantoaxial impaction (pseudobasilar invagination or cranial settling) has occurred in 5 to 32% of patients in two series (102,103). Patients present with pain in the occipital area of the neck, retro-orbital area, or temporal area (101). Additionally, there may be upper and lower motor neuron signs, pathologic reflexes, vertebrobasilar insufficiency, and urinary and fecal incontinence (101). Lateral spine films taken in extension and flexion can help to confirm the diagnosis (104), but MRI and somatosensory evoked potentials may be needed (105). Neurosurgical procedures to stabilize the cervical spine are necessary (106). Subluxation of the thoracic or lumbar spine has been reported with RA but is rare (107).

Extra-articular neurologic manifestations of RA include mononeuritis multiplex and peripheral neuropathy. Mononeuritis multiplex is caused by rheumatoid vas-

---

TABLE 22.5
Presentations of Rheumatoid Arthritis

Typical Presentation
- Female patient, peri- or postmenopausal
- Clinical features include malaise, symmetric bilateral polyarthritis, especially of the joints of the hands and wrists, and/or rheumatoid arthritis

Neurologic Presentations
Brain
- Meningitis
- Vasculitis
- Intracranial rheumatoid nodules
- Normal-pressure hydrocephalus
- Optic atrophy
Spinal Cord
- Pachymeningitis
Cervical Myelopathy
- C1–2 subluxation
Peripheral Nerve
- Entrapment neuropathy
- Carpal tunnel syndrome
- Tarsal tunnel syndrome
- Peripheral neuropathy
- Mononeuritis multiplex

culitis. Patients present with onset of sensory or motor loss in a single nerve distribution, often followed by additional nerve lesions. Nerve conduction studies may demonstrate axonal involvement. The diagnosis may be confirmed with a nerve (usually sural)/muscle biopsy showing vasculitis.

SCLERODERMA

Progressive systemic sclerosis (PSS), or scleroderma, is a rare autoimmune disorder. It is much more common in females, with a gender ratio of 15:1, and is particularly common in African-Americans. Epidemiologic studies differ widely in prevalence estimates, with earlier studies finding 0.1 to 13.8 cases per 100,000 (108) and a recent study finding 19 to 75 cases per 100,000 (109). Although certain toxins, such as toxic oil, can cause a syndrome that mimics scleroderma (110), there is little evidence that silicone breast implants are associated with scleroderma (111). The early pathology of scleroderma includes an inflammatory infiltrate in the dermis, but the primary pathology is one of widespread vascular damage and fibrosis.

The clinical presentation of scleroderma includes Raynaud phenomenon, with nailfold capillary changes in most patients (Table 22.6). Patients can be characterized into two groups: in the first, diffuse type, patients have diffuse cutaneous involvement, with rapidly progressive, widespread thickened skin that affects the distal and proximal extremities and trunk. In the second type, there may be limited cutaneous involvement, with calcinosis, Raynaud phenomenon, esophageal dysmotility, sclerodactyly, and telangiectasias (CREST) usually affecting the fingers and face. Patients who have diffuse cutaneous involvement are more likely to develop interstitial pulmonary fibrosis and other systemic complications of scleroderma.

The diagnosis of scleroderma is usually suspected in patients with severe Raynaud phenomenon and the characteristic thickened skin. Other edematous, indurative, and atrophic conditions may mimic scleroderma, and a skin biopsy may be necessary to confirm the diagnosis. Esophageal dysmotility, abnormal pulmonary function tests, calcinosis, and telangiectasias may also help in the diagnosis. Helpful laboratory tests, in addition to antinuclear antibody (which is present in 95% of patients), are anti-centromere antibody (which is positive in 50% of patients who have limited cutaneous involvement), and anti-topoisomerase I antibody, or anti-Scl 70 (which is positive in 40% of patients who have diffuse cutaneous disease).

Current therapy for scleroderma is unsatisfactory. Symptoms of Raynaud phenomenon can be managed with calcium channel blockers, especially nifedipine, diltiazem, and amlodipine. Penicillamine is frequently used

---

TABLE 22.6
Presentations of Progressive Systemic Sclerosis (Scleroderma)

Typical Presentation
- Female patient
- Clinical features include Raynaud's syndrome, tight thick skin and internal involvement, including lung, kidney, and gastrointestinal tract
- Laboratory features include anticentromere in the limited form and antitopoisomerase (anti-Scl 70) in the diffuse form

Neurologic Presentation
- Cranial neuropathy
- Trigeminal sensory neuropathy
- Peripheral
- Entrapment neuropathy
- Carpal tunnel syndrome
- Peripheral neuropathy
- Mononeuritis multiplex
- Muscle
- Myopathy

---

for skin manifestations, in the hope that it will retard pulmonary and renal scleroderma, but a clinical trial comparing low versus high dose showed no benefit of the latter (112). The hypertensive crises in patients with renal involvement can be treated and possibly prevented by ACE inhibitors. No effective therapy exists for the relentless fibrosis. Pulmonary hypertension is treated with calcium channel blockers, intravenous prostacyclin, and an endothelin-receptor antagonist, bosentan.

Neurologic presentations of scleroderma are uncommon (113), found in only 6% of patients (114). Trigeminal neuropathy (115) and other cranial neuropathies (including vocal cord palsy, facial, chorda tympani, and auditory, glossopharyngeal, and hypoglossal neuropathy) (114–120) can occur, more often in the limited form of the disease. Entrapment neuropathy resulting from carpal tunnel syndrome can be due to active arthritis or edematous hands (114). Trigeminal neuropathy (121–123) and carpal tunnel syndrome usually occur early in the course of disease, with mononeuritis multiplex and peripheral neuropathy (124) occurring as late manifestations (114). Autonomic neuropathy has been reported, with or without evidence of peripheral neuropathy (125–127). Both parasympathetic and sympathetic dysfunction can occur.

Most women with scleroderma will either be beyond menopause or too ill with cardiac, pulmonary, or renal manifestations to contemplate pregnancy. ACE inhibitors are normally stopped before pregnancy because of the risk of fetal renal agenesis. Penicillamine is also stopped before pregnancy.

ANTIPHOSPHOLIPID ANTIBODY SYNDROME

Antiphospholipid antibody syndrome (APS) is one of the more common acquired causes of a hypercoagulable state (128). It occurs equally in patients with SLE (the secondary form) and in patients with no known connective tissue disease (the primary form). The secondary form is much more common in women; the gender ratio for the primary form is equal.

APS usually presents as thrombosis (venous or arterial), pregnancy loss (recurrent first trimester loss or late pregnancy loss), and/or thrombocytopenia. It is an unusual hypercoagulable state in that it affects both the arterial and the venous sides of the circulation. Antiphospholipid antibodies consist of a family of autoantibodies. The first one to be discovered, the false-positive test for syphilis, is not highly associated with APS. It still has clinical importance, however, because as many as 20% of young women who have a biologic false-positive for syphilis (VDRL or RPR) go on to develop lupus or a related connective tissue disease.

The three antiphospholipid antibodies that are clinically important are the lupus anticoagulant, anticardiolipin antibody, and anti-β2 glycoprotein I. The lupus anticoagulant is a double misnomer because most of the patients with the autoantibody do not have lupus and because it is a procoagulant. In vitro, however, it does prolong clotting times—hence its name.

The results of lupus anticoagulant assays, because they are clotting assays, are not reliable in patients who are receiving heparin or warfarin. Lupus anticoagulant assays do not measure the amount of autoantibody; rather they measure its action in interfering with the prothrombin activator complex. The lupus anticoagulant is a heterogeneous antibody, so that no single assay can identify more than 90 to 95%. Among the sensitive screening assays in wide use are the modified Russell viper venom time (129), the kaolin clotting time, and the sensitive partial thromboplastin time (PTT). The usual PTT performed in hospital laboratories is an unreliable screening assay. In one study, it missed 50% of SLE patients who had a lupus anticoagulant that was demonstrable using more sensitive tests (130).

Anticardiolipin antibody (aCL) is an assay for antiphospholipid antibody performed in solid phase, providing measures of IgG, IgM, and IgA isotypes. High-titer IgG is most closely associated with the manifestations of APS, although there are patients with only IgM who have thrombosis and/or pregnancy loss. Anticardiolipin antibody can be measured in serum or plasma and is not affected by the presence of heparin or warfarin. Patients with APS may make lupus anticoagulant or anticardiolipin alone. Beta-2 glycoprotein I is the target of anticardiolipin antibodies. It is a plasma protein involved in the control of coagulation. ELISA assays have been developed that measure antibodies to beta-2 glycoprotein I.

Classification criteria have been developed for APS (131). The criteria are the presence of a lupus anticoagulant or moderate to high titer anticardiolipin of IgG or IgM isotype, and the presence of one of the following: venous thrombosis or arterial thrombosis; or pregnancy morbidity including multiple first trimester losses, one or more late fetal losses, or placental insufficiency (132).

The approaches to treatment of APS depend on the clinical manifestations. Thrombosis is treated with long-term high-intensity warfarin, aiming for an international normalized ratio (INR) of 3.0 to 4.0. These recommendations are based on three retrospective series that showed a high frequency of recurrent thrombosis in patients who were not anticoagulated to this degree (133–135). Prospective clinical trials are lacking, however.

Immunosuppression with corticosteroids to decrease the titer of the antiphospholipid antibodies is not sufficient therapy and exposes patients to the long-term risks of corticosteroids. The preferred regimen during pregnancy is heparin and low-dose aspirin (136). Warfarin cannot be given during pregnancy because of its teratogenic potential. This treatment should be extended for 6 to 8 weeks post partum because that is the time of greatest risk for thrombosis (137).

APS has multiple neurologic manifestations (Table 22.7). Thrombosis frequently affects the brain, resulting

---

TABLE 22.7
Presentations of Antiphospholipid Antibody Syndrome

Typical Presentation
- The primary form is equally prevalent in women and men; the secondary form (usually due to SLE) occurs predominantly in women
- Clinical features include venous or arterial thrombosis, recurrent pregnancy loss, and/or thrombocytopenia
- Laboratory features include the lupus anticoagulant (prolonged PTT or other more sensitive clotting assay) and/or anticardiolipin antibody

Neurologic Presentations
- Brain
- Stroke (and multi-infarct dementia)
- Transient ischemic attack
- Encephalopathy
- Pseudotumor cerebri (venous sinus thrombosis)
- Migraine-associated focal neurologic events
- Ocular
- Ischemic optic neuropathy
- Amaurosis fugax
- Retinal vessel occlusion
- Spinal cord
- Transverse myelopathy

in strokes. Embolic strokes arise largely from vegetations on the mitral or aortic valves (138,139) and are more easily demonstrated on transesophageal rather than transthoracic Doppler studies. TIAs are another typical manifestation of APS.

Some of the neurologic manifestations of APS are referred to as vasculopathic rather than thrombotic. Some patients present with encephalopathy, sometimes without frank infarcts. Vasculopathic changes may be found postmortem.

Some CNS manifestations of APS are due to venous rather than arterial thrombosis. Pseudotumor cerebri may occur following cerebral venous sinus thrombosis (140) and may also occur in SLE without thrombosis in association with corticosteroid treatment. Although a rare presentation, the presence of pseudotumor cerebri in a patient with SLE or in any young person should warrant a search for APS (see also Chapter 22).

A few patients with classic presentations of APS had migraine headache as their initial complaint. Uncomplicated migraine headaches are not associated with APS (141,142). Antiphospholipid antibodies were found to be more frequent in young patients with migraine-associated focal neurologic events however, (143). (See also Chapter 17 on cerebrovascular disease).

Chorea, whose pathophysiology is not completely understood, is a manifestation of APS. Chorea appears to be more frequent in the primary form of APS than in SLE, although it can occur in SLE patients (even without antiphospholipid antibodies) (144–146). Chorea is more common in children and frequently is associated with additional precipitants, including pregnancy and oral contraceptive medication (see also Chapter 24). Many case reports exist of antiphospholipid antibodies in patients who developed chorea while receiving oral contraceptives (147,148). Although it is usually bilateral, chorea can be unilateral. Chorea often responds to corticosteroids, aspirin, and/or haloperidol, suggesting that it represents reversible binding of antiphospholipid antibodies rather than a fixed ischemic lesion.

Transverse myelopathy is another hallmark of APS. As with chorea, not all patients have demonstrable infarcts, and many improve rapidly with corticosteroid therapy (149). Many patients termed "lupoid sclerosis" patients because of overlapping features of multiple sclerosis and SLE (often optic neuritis and transverse myelitis) probably had APS (52,150,151).

Ocular manifestations of APS are frequently seen. In a series of patients with cerebrovascular disease, ischemic optic neuropathy, amaurosis fugax, and retinal artery or vein occlusion are frequently found (152–154). A characteristic severe retinal vaso-occlusive disease should suggest APS (155).

CONCLUSION

Because the connective tissue diseases, vasculitides, and APS are systemic diseases, it is not surprising that they frequently involve the nervous system. In a young woman presenting with neurologic involvement, connective tissue disease (lupus or rheumatoid arthritis), vasculitis (Takayasu), or APS would be in the differential diagnosis. Future pregnancy is often an issue in these women, requiring consideration of the safety of medications, and usually, the consultation of maternal-fetal medicine. In a middle-aged woman, a connective tissue disease (RA, Sjögren's syndrome), vasculitis (GCA or medium vessel vasculitis), and APS remain an essential part of the differential diagnosis. A suspicion of a rheumatologic disease will always be based on a thorough history and physical examination, with appropriate laboratory and serologic testing.

References

1. Hall S, Barr W, Lie JT, et al. Takayasu's arteritis: a study of 32 North American patients. *Medicine* 1985;64:89–99.
2. Shimizu K, Sano K. Pulseless disease. *J Neuropathol Clin Neurol* 1951;1:37–47.
3. Ishikawa K, Uyama M, Asayama K. Occlusive thrombo-aortopathy (Takayasu's disease): cervical arterial stenosis, retinal arterial pressure, retinal microaneurysms and prognosis. *Stroke* 1983;14:730–735.
4. Ask-Upmark E. On the "pulseless disease" outside of Japan. *Acta Med Scand* 1954;149:161–178.
5. Lande A, Bard R, Rossi P, Passariello R, Castrucci A. Takayasu's arteritis. A worldwide entity. *NY State J Med* 1976;76:1477–1482.
6. Sano K, Aiba T. Pulseless disease. Summary of our 62 cases. *Jpn Circ J* 1966;30:63–71.
7. Lande A, Rossi P. The value of total aortography in the diagnosis of Takayasu's arteritis. *Radiology* 1975;114:287–297.
8. Lupi-Herrera E, Sanchez-Torres G, Marcushamer J, et al. Takayasu's arteritis. Clinical study of 107 cases. *Am Heart J* 1977;93:94–103.
9. Shelhamer JH, Volkman DJ, Parrilo JE, et al. Takayasu's arteritis and therapy. *Ann Intern Med* 1985;103:121–126.
10. Edwards KK, Lindsley HB, Lai C-W, van Veldhuizen PJ. Takayasu arteritis presenting as retinal and vertebrobasilar ischemia. *J Rheumatol* 1989;16:1000–1002.
11. Fraga A, Mintz G, Valle L, Flores-Izquierdo G. Takayasu's arteritis: frequency of systemic manifestations (study of 22 patients) and favorable response to maintenance steroid therapy with a-adrenocorticosteroids (12 patients). *Arthritis Rheum* 1972;15:617–624.
12. Gardner JD, Lee KR, Abdou NI. Takayasu's arteritis: reversal of pulse deficits after early treatment with corticosteroids. *J Rheumatol* 1984;11:92–93.
13. Liang GC, Nemickas R, Madayag M. Multiple percutaneous transluminal angioplasties and low-dose pulse methotrexate for Takayasu's arteritis. *J Rheumatol* 1989;16:1370–1373.
14. Park JH, Han MC, Kim SH, et al. Takayasu arteritis: angiographic findings and results of angioplasty. *AJR* 1989;153:1069–1074.

15. Yagura M, Sano I, Akioka H, Hayashi M, Uchida H. Usefulness of percutaneous transluminal angioplasty for aortitis syndrome. *Arch Intern Med* 1984;144:1465–1468.

16. Takagi A, Tada Y, Sato O, Miyata T. Surgical treatment for Takayasu's arteritis. A long-term follow-up study. *J Cardiovasc Surg* 1989;30:553–558.

17. Machado EBV, Michet CJ, Ballard DJ, et al. Trends in incidence and clinical presentation of temporal arteritis in Olmsted County, Minnestoa, 1950–1985. *Arthritis Rheum* 1988;31:745–749.

18. Petri M, Allbritton J. Antibiotic allergy in SLE: a case-control study. *J Rheumatol* 1992;19:265–269.

19. Petri M. Systemic lupus erythematosus. In: Rich RR, Fleisher TA, Schwartz BD, Shearer WT, Strober W, (eds.) *Clinical immunology: principles and practice*. St. Louis: Mosby, 1995;1072–1092.

20. Tan EM, Cohen AS, Fries JF, et al. The 1982 revised criteria for the classification of systemic lupus erythematosus. *Arthritis Rheum* 1982;25:1271–1277.

21. Feinglass EJ, Arnett FC, Dorsch CA, Zizic TM, Stevens MB. Neuropsychiatric manifestations of systemic lupus erythematosus: diagnosis, clinical spectrum, and relationships to other features of the disease. *Medicine* 1976;55:323–329.

22. The American College of Rheumatology nomenclature and case definitions for neuropsychiatric lupus syndromes. *Arthritis Rheum* 1999;42:599–608.

23. McCune WJ, MacGuire A, Aisen AM, Gebarski S. Identification of brain lesions in neuropsychiatric systemic lupus erythematosus by magnetic resonance scanning. *Arthritis Rheum* 1988;31:159–166.

24. Scharre D, Petri M, Engman E, DeArmond S. Large cell arteritis with giant cells in systemic lupus erythematosus. *Ann Intern Med* 1986;104:661.

25. Johnson RT, Richardson EP. The neurologic manifestations of systemic lupus erythematosus. A clinical-pathological study of 24 cases and review of the literature. *Medicine* 1968;47:337–369.

26. Ellis SG, Verity MA. Central nervous system involvement in systemic lupus erythematosus: a reviw of neuropathologic findings in 57 cases. 1955–1977. *Sem Arthritis Rheum* 1979;8:212–221.

27. McCune WJ, Golbus J, Zeldes W, et al. Clinical and immunologic effects of monthly administration of intravenous cyclophosphamide in severe systemic lupus erythematosus. *N Engl J Med* 1988;318:1423–1431.

28. Boumpas DT, Yamada H, Patronas NJ, et al. Pulse cyclophosphamide severe neuropsychiatric lupus. *Q J Med* 1991;296:975–984.

29. Agus B, Nelson J, Kramer N, Mahal SS, Rosenstein ED. Acute central nervous system symptoms caused by ibuprofen in connective tissue disease. *J Rheumatol* 1990;17:1094–1096.

30. Mackworth-Young CG, Hughes GRV. Epilepsy: an early symptom of systemic lupus erythematosus. *J Neurol Neurosurg Psychiatry* 1985; 48:185–192.

31. McCure WJ, Globus J. Neuropsychiatric lupus. *Rheum Dis Clin North Am* 1988;14:149–167.

32. Wong KL, Woo EKW, Wong YL. Neurological manifestations of systemic lupus erythematosus: a prospective study. *Q J Med* 1991;294:857–870.

33. Sibley JT, Olszynski WP, Decoteau, Sundaram MB. The incidence and prognosis of central nervous system disease in systemic lupus erythematosus. *J Rheumatol* 1992;19:47–52.

34. Futrell N, Schultz LR, Millikan C. Central nervous system disease in patients with systemic lupus erythematosus. *Neurology* 1992;42:1649–1657.

35. Mayes B, Brey RL. Evaluation and treatment of seizures in patients with systemic lupus erythematosus. *J Clin Rheumatol* 1996;2:336–345.

36. Scheuer ML, Pedley TA. The evaluation and treatment of seizures. *N Engl J Med* 1990;323:1468–1474.

37. Ginsburg KS, Wright EA, Larson MG, et al. A controlled study of the prevalence of cognitive dysfunction in randomly selected patients with systemic lupus erythematosus. *Arthritis Rheum* 1992;35:776–782.

38. Hanly JG, Fisk JD, Sherwood G, Eastwood B. Clinical course of cognitive dysfunction in systemic lupus erythematosus. *J Rheumatol* 1994;21:1825–1831.

39. Denburg SD, Carbotte RM, Denburg JA. Corticosteroids and neuropsychological functioning in patients with systemic lupus erythematosus. *Arthritis Rheum* 1994;37:1311–1320.

40. Rubbert A, Marienhagen J, Pirner K, et al. Single-photon-emission computed tomography analysis of cerebral blood flow in the evaluation of central nervous system involvement in patients with systemic lupus erythematosus. *Arthritis Rheum* 1993;36:1253–1262.

41. Rogers MP, Waterhouse E, Nagel JS, et al. I-123 iofetamine SPECT scan in systemic lupus erythematosus patients with cognitive and other minor neuropsychiatric symptoms: A pilot study. *Lupus* 1992;1:215–219.

42. Bruyn GW, Padberg G. Chorea and lupus erythematosus: a critical review. *Eur Neurol* 1984;23:435–448.

43. Teh LS, Hay EM, Amos N, et al. Anti-P antibodies are associated with psychiatric and focal cerebral disorders in patients with systemic lupus erythematosus. *Br J Rheumatol* 1993;32:287–290.

44. Schneebaum AB, Singleton JD, West SG, et al. Association of psychiatric manifestations with antibodies to ribosomal-P proteins in systemic lupus erythematosus. *Am J Med* 1991;90:54–62.

45. Ahearn JM, Provost TT, Dorsch CA, et al. Interrelationships of HLA-DR, MB and MT phenotypes, autoantibody expression, and clinical features in systemic lupus erythematosus. *Arthritis Rheum* 1982;55:313–322.

46. Lundberg PO, Werner I. Trigeminal sensory neuropathy in systemic lupus erythematosus. *Acta Neurol Scand* 1972;48:330–340.

47. Aragon Diez A, Garcia-Consuegra Sanchez-Camacho G, Hernandez Rodriguez I, Morillas Lopez L. Blepharoptosis and systemic lupus erythematosus. *Rev Clin Exp* 1987;181:173.

48. Ribaute E, Weill B, Ing H, Badelon I, Menkes CJ. Occulomotor paralysis in disseminated lupus erythematosus [Eng. abstr.]. *Ophthalmologie* 1989;3:125–128.

49. Rosenstein ED, Sobelman J, Kramer N. Isolated, pupil-sparing third nerve palsy as initial manifestation of systemic lupus erythematosus. *J Clin Neuro Ophthalmol* 1989;9:285–288.

50. Cuenca R, Simeon CP, Montablan J, Bosch JA, Vilardell M. Facial nerve palsy due to angioedema in systemic lupus erythematosus. *Clin Exp Rheumatol* 1991;9:89–97.

51. Andrianakos AA, Duffy J, Suzuki M, Sharp JT. Transverse myelopathy in systemic lupus erythematosus. Report of three cases and review of the literature. *Ann Intern Med* 1975;83:616–624.

52. Harris EN, Gharavi AE, Mackworth-Young CG, et al. Lupoid sclerosis: a possible pathogenetic role for

antiphospholipid antibodies. *Ann Rheum Dis* 1985; 44:281–283.

53. Lavalle C, Loyo E, Paniagua R, et al. Correlation study between prolactin and androgens in male patients with systemic lupus erythematosus. *J Rheumatol* 1987;14: 268–272.

54. Henry AK, Brunner CM. Relapse of lupus transverse myelitis mimicked by vertebral fractures and spinal cord compression. *Arthritis Rheum* 1985;28:1307–1311.

55. Baethge BA, Lidsky MD. Intractable hiccups associated with high dose intravenous methylprednisolone therapy. *Ann Intern Med* 1986;104:58–59.

56. Drosos AA, Constantopoulos SH, Moutsopoulos HM. Tuberculosis spondylitis: a cause for paraplegia in lupus. *Rheumatol Int* 1985;5:185–186.

57. Stoner GL, Best PV, Mazio M, et al. Progressive multifocal leukoencephalopathy complicating systemic lupus erythematosus: distribution of JC virus in chronically demyelinated cerebellar lesions. *J Neuropath Exp Neurol* 1988;47:307.

58. Warren RW, Kredich DW. Transverse myelitis and acute central nervous system manifestations of systemic lupus erythematosus. *Arthritis Rheum* 1984;27:1058–1060.

59. Al-Husaini A, Jamal GA. Myelopathy as the main presenting feature of systemic lupus erythematosus. *Eur Neurol* 1985;24:94–105.

60. Sills EM. Systemic lupus erythematosus in a patient previously diagnosed as having Shulman disease [letter]. *Arthritis Rheum* 1988;31:694–695.

61. Chang R, Quismorio Jr. P. Transverse myelopathy in systemic lupus erythematosus (SLE) [abstract]. *Arthritis Rheum* 1990;33:S102.

62. Barile L, LaValle C. Transverse myelitis in systemic lupus erythematosus: the effect of IV pulse methylprednisolone and cyclophosphamide. *J Rheumatol* 1992;19:370–372.

63. Hellmann DB, Laing TJ, Petri M, Whiting-O'Keefe Q, Parry GJ. Mononeuritis multiplex: the yield of evaluations for occult rheumatic diseases. *Medicine* 1988;67: 145–153.

64. Bergemer AM, Fouquet B, Goupille P, Valat JP. Peripheral neuropathy as the initial manifestation of systemic lupus erythematosus. Report of a case. *Sem Hop Paris* 1987;63:1979–1982.

65. Estes D, Christian CL. The natural history of systemic lupus erythematosus by prospective analysis. *Medicine* 1971;50:85–95.

66. Hoyle C, Ewing DJ, Parker AC. Acute autonomic neuropathy in association with systemic lupus erythematosus. *Ann Rheum Dis* 1985;44:420–424.

67. Tooke AF, Stuart RA, Maddison PJ. The prevalence of autonomic neuropathy in systemic lupus erythematosus. *Br J Rheumatol* 1990;30:22.

68. Vaiopoulos G, Sfikakis PP, Kapsimali V, et al. The association of systemic lupus erythematosus and myasthenia gravis. *Postgrad Med J* 1994;70:741–745.

69. Hochberg MC. Adult and juvenile rheumatoid arthritis: Current epidemiologic concepts. *Epidemiol Rev* 1981;3:27–44.

70. Reveille JD, Hochberg MC, Bias WB, Arnett FC. Rheumatic disease and autoantibodies in the old order Amish: prevalence and HLA associations [abstract]. *Arthritis Rheum* 1983;26:S40.

71. Strickland RW, Tesar JT, Berne BH, et al. The prevalence of Sjögren's syndrome and associated rheumatic diseases in an elderly population [abstract]. *Arthritis Rheum* 1984;27:S45.

72. Alexander EL, Provost TT, Stevens MB, Alexander GE. Neurologic complications of primary Sjögren's syndrome. *Medicine* 1982;61:247–257.

73. Andonopoulos AP, Lagos G, Drosos AA, Moutsopoulos HM. The spectrum of neurological involvement in Sjögren's syndrome. *Br J Rheumatol* 1990;29:21–23.

74. Binder A, Snaith ML, Isenberg D. Sjögren's syndrome: a study of its neurological complications. *Br J Rheumatol* 1988;27:275–280.

75. Kaltreider HB, Talal N. The neuropathy of Sjögren's syndrome: trigeminal nerve involvement. *Ann Intern Med* 1969;70:751–762.

76. Font J, Valls J, Cervera R, et al. Pure sensory neuropathy in patients with primary Sjögren's syndrome: clinical, immunological, and electromyographic findings. *Ann Rheum Dis* 1990;49:775–778.

77. Alexander EL, Malinow K, Lejewski JE, et al. Primary Sjögren's syndrome with central nervous system disease mimicking multiple sclerosis. *Ann Intern Med* 1986; 104:323–330.

78. Wise CM, Agudelo CA. Optic neuropathy as an initial manifestation of Sjögren's syndrome. *J Rheumatol* 1988;15:799–802.

79. Ferreiro JE, Robalino BD, Saldana MJ. Primary Sjögren's syndrome with diffuse cerebral vasculitis and lymphocytic interstitial pneumonitis. *Am J Med* 1987;82: 1227–1232.

80. de la Monte SM, Hutchins GM, Gupta PK. Polymorphous meningitis with atypical mononuclear cells in Sjögren's syndrome. *Ann Neurol* 1983;14:455–461.

81. Sato K, Miyasaka N, Nishioka K, et al. Primary Sjögren's syndrome associated with systemic necrotizing vasculitis: a fatal case. *Arthritis Rheum* 1987;30:717–718.

82. Massey EW. Sjögren's syndrome and mononeuritis multiplex [letter]. *Ann Intern Med* 1980;92:130.

83. Molina R, Provost TT, Alexander EL. Two types of inflammatory vascular disease in Sjögren's syndrome. Differential association with seroreactivity to rheumatoid factor and antibodies to Ro (SSA) and with hypocomplementemia. *Arthritis Rheum* 1985;28:1251–1258.

84. Gregersen PK, Silver J, Winchester RJ. The shared epitope hypothesis: an approach to understanding the molecular genetics of susceptibility to rheumatoid arthritis. *Arthritis Rheum* 1987;30:1205–1213.

85. Spector TD, Da Silva JA. Pregnancy and rheumatoid arthritis: an overview. *Am J Reprod Immunol* 1992;28:222–225.

86. Nelson JL, Hughes KA, Smith AG, et al. Maternal-fetal disparity in HLA class II alloantigens and the pregnancy-induced amelioration of rheumatoid arthritis. *New Engl J Med* 1993;329:466–471.

87. Levine JD, Collier DH, Basbaum AI, Moskowitz MA, Helms CA. Hypothesis: the nervous system may contribute to the pathophysiology of rheumatoid arthritis. *J Rheumatol* 1985;12:406–411.

88. Lotz M, Carson DA, Vaughan JH. Substance P activation of rheumatoid synoviocytes: neural pathway in pathogenesis of arthritis. *Science* 1987;235:893–895.

89. Bathon JM, Moreland LW, DiBartolomeo AG. Inflammatory central nervous system involvement in rheumatoid arthritis. *Sem Arthritis Rheum* 1989; 18:258–266.

90. Ouyang R, Mitchell DM, Rozdilsky B. Central nervous system involvement in rheumatoid disease. *Neurology* 1967;17:1099–1105.

91. Steiner JW, Gelbloom AJ. Intracranial manifestations in two cases of systemic rheumatoid disease. *Arthritis Rheum* 1959;2:537–545.

92. Watson P, Fekete J, Deck J. Central nervous system vasculitis in rheumatoid arthritis. *Can J Neurol Sci* 1977; 4:269–272.

93. Spurlock RG, Richman AV. Rheumatoid meningitis: a case report and review of the literature. *Arch Pathol Lab Med* 1983;107:129–131.

94. Jackson CG, Chess RL, Ward JR. A case of rheumatoid nodule formation within the central nervous system and review of the literature. *J Rheumatol* 1984;11: 237–240.

95. Ellman P, Cudkowicz L, Elwood J. Widespread serous membrane involvement by rheumatoid nodules. *J Clin Pathol* 1954;7:239–244.

96. Sunter JP. Rheumatoid disease with involvement of the leptomeninges presenting as symptomatic epilepsy. *Beirtr Pathol* 1977;161:194–202.

97. Markenson JA, McDougal JS, Tsairis P, Lockshin MD, Christian CL. Rheumatoid meningitis: a localized immune process. *Ann Intern Med* 1979;90:786–789.

98. Rasker JJ, Jansen ENH, Haan J, Oostrom J. Normal-pressure hydrocephalus in rheumatic patients. A diagnostic pitfall. *N Engl J Med* 1985;312:1239–1241.

99. Grabois M, Puentes J, Lidsky M. Tarsal tunnel syndrome in rheumatoid arthritis. *Arch Phys Med Rehabil* 1981; 62:401–403.

100. Chamberlain MA, Corbett M. Carpal tunnel syndrome in early rheumatoid arthritis. *Ann Rheum Dis* 1970;29: 149–152.

101. Bland JH. Rheumatoid subluxation of the cervical spine. *J Rheumatol* 1990;17:134–137.

102. Dirheimer Y. *The cranio-vertebral region in chronic inflammatory rheumatoid diseases*. Berlin: Springer-Verlag, 1977.

103. Rasker JJ, Cash JA. Radiologic study of cervical spine and hand in patients with rheumatoid arthritis of 15 years duration: an assessment of the effects of corticosteroid treatment. *Ann Rheum Dis* 1978;37:529–537.

104. Halla JT, Hardin Jr. JG. The spectrum of atlanto-axial facet joint involvement in rheumatoid arthritis. *Arthritis Rheum* 1990;33:325–328.

105. Watt I, Cummins B. Management of rheumatoid neck. *Ann Rheum Dis* 1990;49:805–807.

106. Crockard HA, Essigman WK, Stevens JM, et al. Surgical treatment of cervical cord compression in rheumatoid arthritis. *Ann Rheum Dis* 1985;44:809–816.

107. van der Horst-Bruinsma IE, Markusse HM, MacFarlane JD, Vielvoye CJ. Rheumatoid discitis with cord compression at the thoracic level. *Br J Rheumatol* 1990;29:65–68.

108. Tamaki T, Mori S, Takehara K. Epidemiological study of patients with systemic sclerosis in Tokyo. *Arch Dermatol Res* 1991;283:366–371.

109. Maricq HR, Weinrich MC, Keil JE, et al. Prevalence of scleroderma spectrum disorders in the general population of South Carolina. *Arthritis Rheum* 1989;32: 998–1006.

110. Toxic epidemic syndrome study group. Toxic epidemic syndrome, Spain, 1981. *Lancet* 1982;2:697–702.

111. Angell M. Evaluating the health risks of breast implants: the interplay of medical science, the law, and public opinion. *N Engl J Med* 1996;334:1513–1518.

112. Clements PJ, Furst DE, Wong WK, et al. High-dose versus low-dose D-penicillamine in early diffuse systemic sclerosis: analysis of a two-year, double-blind, randomized, controlled clinical trial. *Arthritis Rheum.* 1999;42:1194–1203.

113. Gordon RM, Silverstein A. Neurologic manifestations in progressive systemic sclerosis. *Arch Neurol* 1970;22: 126–134.

114. Lee P, Bruni J, Sukenik S. Neurological manifestations in systemic sclerosis (scleroderma). *J Rheumatol* 1984;11: 480–483.

115. Teasdall RD, Frayha RA, Shulman LE. Cranial nerve involvement in systemic sclerosis (scleroderma): a report of 10 cases. *Medicine* 1980;59:149–159.

116. Singh RR, Malaviya AN, Kumar A, Kacker SK. Vocal cord palsy in a patient with progressive systemic sclerosis. *J Rheumatol* 1988;15:882–883.

117. Beighton P, Gumpel JM, Cornes NGM. Prodromal trigeminal sensory neuropathy in progressive systemic sclerosis. *Ann Rheum Dis* 1968;27:367–369.

118. Ashworth B, Tait GBW. Trigeminal neuropathy in connective tissue disease. *Neurology* 1971;21:609–614.

119. Kabadi UM, Sinkoff MW. Trigeminal neuralgia in progressive systemic sclerosis. *Postgrad Med J* 1977; 61:176–177.

120. Kumar A, Malaviya AN, Tiwari SC, et al. Clinical and laboratory profile of systemic sclerosis in Northern India. *J Assoc Physicians India* 1990;38:765–768.

121. Burke MJ, Carty JE. Trigeminal neuropathy as the presenting symptom of systemic sclerosis. *Postgrad Med J* 1979;55:423–425.

122. Casey EB, Lawton NF. Progressive systemic sclerosis presenting with Raynaud's phenomenon in the tongue and sensory trigeminal neuropathy. *Rheum Phys Med* 1971;11:131–133.

123. Thompson PD, Robertson GJ. Trigeminal neuropathy heralding scleroderma. *J Maine Med Assoc* 1973;64: 123–124.

124. Dierckx RA, Aichner F, Gerstenbrand F, Fritsch P. Progressive systemic sclerosis and nervous system involvement. *Eur Neurol* 1987;26:134–140.

125. Sonnex C, Paice E, White AG. Autonomic neuropathy in systemic sclerosis: a case report and evaluation of six patients. *Ann Rheum Dis* 1986;45:957–960.

126. Klimiuk PS, Taylor L, Baker RD, Jayson MIV. Autonomic neuropathy in systemic sclerosis. *Ann Rheum Dis* 1988;47:542–545.

127. Dessein PHMC, Gledhill RF. Autonomic dysfunction in systemic sclerosis: the site of damage [letter]. *Ann Rheum Dis* 1989;48:877–888.

128. Petri M. Clinical and management aspects of the antiphospholipid syndrome. In: Wallace DJ, Hahn BH, (eds.) *Dubois' lupus erythematosus*, 5th ed. Baltimore: Williams & Wilkins, 1997:57.

129. Thiagarajan P, Pengo V, Shapiro SS. The use of the dilute Russell viper venom time for the diagnosis of lupus anticoagulants. *Blood* 1986;68:869–874.

130. Petri M, Rheinschmidt M, Whiting-O'Keefe Q, Hellmann D, Corash L. The frequency of lupus anticoagulant in systemic lupus erythematosus: a study of 60 consecutive patients by activated partial thromboplastin time, Russell viper venom time, and anticardiolipin antibody. *Ann Intern Med* 1987;106:524–531.

131. Asherson RA, Cervera R. Anticardiolipin antibodies, chronic biologic false positive tests for syphilis and other antiphospholipid antibodies. In: Wallace DJ, Hahn BH, (eds.) *Dubois' lupus erythematosus*, 4th ed. Philadelphia: Lea & Febiger, 1993.

132. Wilson WA, Gharavi AE, Koike T, Lockshin MD, et al. International consensus statement on preliminary classification criteria for definite antiphospholipid syn-

drome: report of an international workshop. *Arthritis Rheum* 1999;42:1309–1311.

133. Rosove MH, Brewer PMC. Antiphospholipid thrombosis: clinical course after the first thrombotic event in 70 patients. *Ann Intern Med* 1992;117:303–308.

134. Derksen RHWM, de Groot PG, Kater L, Nieuwenhuis HK. Patients with antiphospholipid antibodies and venous thrombosis should receive long term anticoagulant treatment. *Ann Rheum Dis* 1993;52:689–692.

135. Khamashta MA, Cuadrado MJ, Mujic F, et al. The management of thrombosis in the antiphospholipid antibody syndrome. *N Engl J Med* 1995;332:993–997.

136. Cowchock FS, Reece EA, Balaban D, Branch DW, Plouffe L. Repeated fetal losses associated with antiphospholipid antibodies: a collaborative randomized trial comparing prednisone with low-dose heparin treatment. *Am J Obstet Gynecol* 1992;166:1318–1323.

137. Kittner SJ, Stern BJ, Feeser BR, et al. Pregnancy and the risk of stroke. *N Engl J Med* 1996;335:768–74.

138. Leung W-H, Wong K-L, Lau C-P, Wong C-K, Liu H-W. Association between antiphospholipid antibodies and cardiac abnormalities in patients with systemic lupus erythematosus. *Am J Med* 1990;89:411–419.

139. Chartash EK, Lans DM, Paget SA, Qamar T, Lockshin MD. Aortic insufficiency and mitral regurgitation in patients with systemic lupus erythematosus and the antiphospholipid syndrome. *Am J Med* 1989;86:407–412.

140. Kaplan RE, Spirngate JE, Feld LG, Cohen ME. Pseudotumor cerebri associated with cerebral venous sinus thrombosis, internal jugular vein thrombosis, and systemic lupus erythematosus. *J Pediatr* 1985;107:266–268.

141. Montalban J, Cervera R, Font J, et al. Lack of association between anticardiolipin antibodies and migraine in systemic lupus erythematosus. *Neurology* 1992;42:681–686.

142. Hering R, Couturier EGM, Asherson RA, Steiner TJ. Antiphospholipid antibodies in migraine. *Cephalalgia* 1991;11:19–20.

143. Tietjen GE, Levine SR, Brown E, Mascha E, Welch KMA. Factors that predict antiphospholipid immunoreactivity in young people with transient focal neurological events. *Arch Neurol* 1993;50:833–836.

144. Bouchez B, Arnott G, Hatron PV. Choré et lupus erythemateux disséminé avec anticoagulant circulant. Trois cas. *Rev Neurol (Paris)* 1985;141:571–577.

145. Asherson RA, Derksen RHWM, Harris EN, et al. Chorea in systemic lupus erythematosus and "lupus-Like" disease: association with antiphospholipid antibodies. *Sem Arthritis Rheum* 1987;16:253–259.

146. Asherson RA, Hughes GRV. Antiphospholipid antibodies in chorea. *J Rheumatol* 1988;15:377–379.

147. Asherson RA, Harris NE, Gharavi AE, Hughes GR. Systemic lupus erythematosus, antiphospholipid antibodies, chorea, and oral contraceptives [letter]. *Arthritis Rheum* 1986;29:1535–1536.

148. Asherson RA, Harris EN, Hughes GRV. Complications of oral contraceptives and antiphospholipid antibodies [letter]. *Arthritis Rheum* 1988;31:575–576.

149. Propper DJ, Bucknall RC. Acute transverse myelopathy complicating systemic lupus erythematosus. *Ann Rheum Dis* 1989;48:512–515.

150. Oppenheimer S, Hoffbrand BI. Optic neuritis and myelopathy in systemic lupus erythematosus. *Can J Neurol Sci* 1986;13:129–132.

151. Fulford KWM, Catterall RD, Delhanty JJ, Doniach D, Kremer H. A collagen disorder of the nervous system presenting as multiple sclerosis. *Brain* 1972;95:373–386.

152. Bacharach JM, Lie JT, Homburger HA. The prevalence of vascular occlusive disease associated with antiphospholipid syndromes. *Int Angiol* 1992;11:51–56.

153. Hughes GRV. The antiphospholipid syndrome: Ten years on. *Lancet* 1993;342:341–344.

154. Montalban J, Codina A, Ordi J, et al. Antiphospholipid antibodies in cerebral ischemia. *Stroke* 1991;22:750–753.

155. Dunn JP, Noorily SW, Petri M, et al. Antiphospholipid antibodies and retinal vascular disease. *Lupus* 1996;5:313–322.

156. Pal B, Gibson C, Passmore J, Griffiths ID, Dick WC. A study of headaches and migraine in Sjögren's syndrome and other rheumatic disorders. *Ann Rheum Dis* 1989;48:312–316.

157. Konttinen Y, Kinnuner E, von Bonsdorff M, et al. Acute transverse myelopathy successfully treated with plasmapheresis and prednisone in a patient with primary Sjögren's syndrome. *Arthritis Rheum* 1987;30:339–344.

158. Alexander GE, Provost TT, Stevens MB, Alexander EL. Sjögren's syndrome: Central nervous system manifestations. *Neurology* 1981;31:1391–1396.

159. Spillane JD, Wells CEC. Isolated trigeminal neuropathy: a report of sixteen cases. *Brain* 1959;82:391–416.

160. Attwood W, Poser C. Neurologic complications of Sjögren's syndrome. *Neurology* 1961;11:1034–1041.

23 Gender Differences in Movement Disorders

Yvette M. Bordelon, MD, PhD and Stanley Fahn, MD

M ovement disorders are commonly encountered in general neurology practice, and in many academic institutions, a separate division is dedicated to the treatment of this subspecialty. Despite the large number of patients with movement disorders, there is a relative paucity of epidemiologic data. In particular, little information is available on the influence of gender on the occurrence and even less on the clinical manifestations of these disorders. This chapter reviews the gender differences that have been identified in the more common movement disorders, and the influence of hormonal states on disease expression.

The etiology for most movement disorders remains unknown, with the majority being idiopathic in nature. Although some gene mutations have been defined (e.g., DYT1 gene mutation in early-onset generalized dystonia), the genetic contributions for the majority of movement disorders remain under investigation (1). Consequently, the impact of gender on these factors is still not clear.

Disorders of movement are broadly categorized into those of predominantly decreased movement, or hypokinetic, and those of primarily excessive movement, or hyperkinetic. Parkinsonism makes up the bulk of hypokinetic movement disorders. Hyperkinesias are comprised of a variety of disease states with tremor, dystonia, chorea, myoclonus, or tics as manifestations. Basal ganglia pathology (including alterations in the connectivity of this group of subcortical nuclei) is responsible for the expression of most but not all movement disorders.

HYPOKINETIC DISORDERS

Parkinson's Disease

Parkinson's disease (PD) is a neurodegenerative disorder with characteristic motor manifestations of rest tremor, rigidity, and bradykinesia. It is typically accompanied by gait and postural instability. The degeneration of dopamine-containing pigmented neurons in the substantia nigra pars compacta and the presence of Lewy bodies are the pathologic hallmarks of the disease. Most cases of Parkinson disease are idiopathic, but heritable forms of PD have also been found and linked to specific gene mutations, including parkin, alpha-synuclein, DJ-1, PINK1 and LRRK2 (2,3). Onset is typically in the sixth to seventh decades of life.

Male predominance of idiopathic PD has been found in most population- and clinic-based studies. Male to female ratios of disease prevalence range from 1.2:1.0 to 1.7:1.0 (4). Incidence data for PD are scanty, but the few studies to date have supported the finding of higher rates in males (5). PD estimates in populations in Rochester, Minnesota, and northern California found a higher incidence of PD in men than women, with 13.0

and 19.0 per 100,000 in men, compared with 8.8 and 9.9 per 100,000 in women, respectively (6,7). A 2 to 1 ratio of men to women with PD was found in Italy (8). The male predominance of PD remains controversial, however, as some studies have found either no difference in prevalence of PD between men and women or a higher prevalence in women (9,10). Several studies in Japan have confirmed a higher prevalence of PD in women (11–14).

Estrogen and PD

Gender differences in the clinical aspects of PD onset and progression have been found. Comparisons of Mini-Mental State Examinations (MMSE) and Unified Parkinson's Disease Rating Scale (UPDRS) motor scores were made between men and women in the Kansas Medical Center's PD Registry (15). Lyons et al. found that women had more dyskinesias than men and slightly better MMSE scores. Men had more motor disability on UPDRS and required higher doses of levodopa, thus suggesting a more severe disease progression overall. This, in addition to the higher incidence of PD in men discussed earlier, has led to investigations into the possible protective effects of estrogen and how hormonal states may influence the disease.

Animal studies have documented that estrogen increases dopamine concentrations in the brain by increasing tyrosine hydroxylase activity, enhancing dopamine release and inhibiting dopamine reuptake (16–19). Estrogen also exerts postsynaptic effects by modulating dopamine D2 receptors, thus increasing receptor density and sensitivity (20–22). Neuroprotection by estrogen may be accomplished through this modulation of the dopaminergic system, antioxidant effects, and inhibition of neurotoxin uptake through the dopamine transporter (23).

The role that estrogen plays in modulating dopaminergic function is not firmly established, however. Indeed, studies have shown the opposite effects, with a decrease in dopamine D2 receptors with estrogen treatment and increases in dopamine transporter density (24–26). It has been suggested that these conflicting results are due to the biphasic effects of estrogen on dopamine modulation, but this has not been resolved (27). See also Chapter 12.

Similar controversy exists in human studies of estrogen effects on nigrostriatal function, particularly in patients with PD. It has been demonstrated that PD symptoms are influenced by the menstrual cycle, in which estrogen levels are lowest just before the onset of menses and peak at the time of ovulation. Studies have shown that parkinsonism worsens premenstrually and dyskinesias increase during ovulation, supporting a dopaminergic effect of estrogen (27–29). In addition, Saunders-Pullman et al. (30) found that women already diagnosed with PD who were on hormone replacement therapy (HRT) had milder symptoms of disease than those who were not. Also, nursing home residents with PD demonstrated bet-

ter ADL scores in women on HRT (31). Supporting the hypothesis of the beneficial effects of estrogen, treatment with estrogen versus placebo led to improvement in UPDRS motor scores (32) and a lower required dose of levodopa to treat symptoms (33). Yet, conflicting data suggest that estrogen does not influence the expression of PD. No difference in the risk of PD was found between women who were taking HRT and those who were not (34,35). Ascherio et al. also found that women taking HRT and large amounts of caffeine had a fourfold higher risk of developing PD. No correlation was found between estrogen level changes through the menstrual cycle and worsening of parkinsonism (36). Another study showed no change in UPDRS motor scores with estrogen use versus placebo (37). Thus, the full story of estrogen effects on dopaminergic function remains to be elucidated.

Gender Differences in Disease Manifestation and Treatment

Initial motor manifestations are similar in men and women, as documented in a study by Scott et al. who obtained data via a mailed questionnaire to members of a Swedish Parkinson organization (38). They described that the symptom profile at onset of disease was the same between sexes except that women more commonly reported neck and low back pain. Later in disease progression, both men and women reported tremor, rigidity, and fatigue as the most common disease manifestations.

Gender differences have been found in the nonmotor symptoms of PD as well. In a nursing home population, women with PD were found to be depressed slightly more often than men, whereas men exhibited behavioral disturbances, including verbal and physical abusiveness and wandering, more commonly than women (39).

One study has documented that the response to surgical treatment of PD varies between men and women. Women who underwent either thalamotomy, pallidotomy, or deep brain stimulation of the thalamus, globus pallidus, or subthalamic nucleus had greater improvement on scores measuring dyskinesias, activities of daily living, emotions, and social life than men (40). Both men and women had significantly improved motor scores in this study.

Menarche, Menses, Pregnancy, and Menopause

The effects of pregnancy on PD are not well documented, as the occurrence is relatively uncommon. However, Golbe (41) described that eight of 14 women he interviewed reported worsening of their parkinsonism during pregnancy, and the PD did not fully return to baseline after delivery. Two recent studies have also found that there was a worsening of parkinsonism during pregnancy (42,43). All three reports documented the safety of levodopa use during pregnancy. Complications occurred in association with amantadine use. Therefore, monotherapy with levodopa during pregnancy is recommended, if necessary, although data are still insufficient to clearly establish its safety in pregnancy.

Women with PD were found to have an older age at menarche and fewer children when compared to controls (44). Women having PD onset prior to menopause had longer disease duration, with more dysmenorrhea and premenstrual worsening of motor symptoms compared with women having disease onset after menopause. In contrast, a separate study by Benedetti et al. found that women with PD had earlier onset of menopause than controls (45).

Parkinson-Plus Syndromes

Parkinsonism occurs as part of a number of Parkinson-plus syndromes, which are much less common in the population than idiopathic PD. Progressive supranuclear palsy (PSP) is manifested by parkinsonism with prominent axial rigidity, postural instability, and supranuclear gaze palsy. Multiple epidemiologic studies have shown a male preponderance of PSP similar to PD (46,47). Multiple system atrophy (MSA), characterized by varying contributions of parkinsonism and autonomic and cerebellar dysfunction, has been found with equal frequency in both sexes (48). Parkinsonism associated with asymmetric dystonia, rigidity, myoclonus, and cortical sensory loss is known as corticobasal ganglionic degeneration (CBGD). No clear gender predominance occurs in CBGD (49,50). Given the lower incidence of these atypical parkinsonian syndromes, there are no detailed studies of the influence of hormonal states on disease manifestations in women.

HYPERKINETIC DISORDERS

Dystonia

Dystonia is defined as the sustained contraction of agonist and antagonist muscles resulting in abnormal movements or postures. Dystonia can be classified by: (i) etiology (primary, secondary, dystonia-plus, or heredodegenerative); (ii) location (generalized, focal, or segmental); and (iii) age at onset (childhood, adolescent, or adult). Among the primary or idiopathic forms of dystonia, several causative gene mutations have been identified, although the majority of cases are sporadic. Secondary and heredodegenerative dystonias result from central nervous system injury or progressive neurodegenerative processes associated with other systemic and neurologic abnormalities.

Women are affected by primary focal dystonia more often than men, as documented by several epidemiologic studies (51–53). Duffey et al. reported a prevalence of primary dystonia in North England of 14.28 per 100,000, with 1.42 per 100,000 generalized and 12.86 per 100,000 focal (54). Overall, women had a relative risk of having dystonia of 2:1 versus men. They also found a higher prevalence of cervical dystonia and blepharospasm among women compared with men. The Epidemiological Study of Dystonia in Europe (ESDE) reported prevalence data from eight European countries. The overall prevalence of primary dystonia was 152 per million, with 117 per million being affected by focal dystonia (55). A higher prevalence of blepharospasm, cervical, focal, and segmental dystonia occurred among women than men, whereas men were affected with writer's cramp more often than women.

Dopa-responsive dystonia (DRD) is a dystonia-plus syndrome characterized by childhood onset, typically starting in the lower extremities and diurnal variation in symptoms. It is easily treated with levodopa. Mutations in the gene encoding GTP-cyclohydrolase I cause this autosomal dominant disorder (56). Women are affected more often than men (4:1 ratio) and also have a higher penetrance of disease (57,58).

A common form of generalized dystonia, Oppenheim's dystonia, is inherited in an autosomal dominant fashion and has been linked to a mutation in the torsinA gene, DYT1, which has variable penetrance (59). Both sexes are affected equally.

Little is known about hormonal influences on dystonic symptoms. Gwinn-Hardy et al. (60) found that 38.7% of premenopausal women with dystonia (both focal and generalized) had worsening of symptoms prior to or during menses. They found no change in symptoms surrounding menopause, pregnancy, or associated with HRT.

Chorea

Chorea is defined as continuous, quick movements that flow from one muscle group to another. The list of potential causes of chorea is extensive. Heritable forms of chorea, such as Huntington's disease, are autosomal dominant disorders, and secondary forms of chorea resulting from CNS injury, metabolic perturbations, or autoimmune processes are also described.

Conditions particularly relevant for women include chorea associated with pregnancy (chorea gravidarum), which is discussed in detail in Chapter 24, and oral contraceptive use. Sydenham's chorea is a syndrome of chorea, ataxia, and cognitive and behavioral changes that can occur in children following infection with group A beta hemolytic streptococcus (61). It is twice as common in females as in males, and women who had Sydenham's chorea as children seem to be predisposed to chorea gravidarum.

Chorea is also seen in systemic lupus erythematosus (SLE), although the mechanisms responsible have not been completely elucidated. A higher incidence of SLE occurs among women, and the presence of antiphospholipid antibodies seems to correlate with the presence of chorea seen in 2% of patients at times occurring before diagnosis (62).

Essential Tremor

Essential tremor (ET) is the most common movement disorder and is characterized by kinetic tremor typically affecting the hands but also at times involving the head, voice, and lower extremities. It is inherited in an autosomal dominant fashion typically, but the causative gene mutations have not been identified. ET occurs at approximately the same frequency in men and women. It has been found that women are affected by head tremor 2 to 6 times more often than men, however (63,64).

Restless Leg Syndrome

Restless leg syndrome (RLS) is characterized by uncomfortable sensations in the lower extremities at rest, resulting in the need to move about for relief. This motor restlessness is sometimes accompanied by sleep disturbance and limb movements in sleep. It is likely the most common movement disorder that occurs during pregnancy. Ten to twenty percent of pregnant women are affected by RLS (41). Symptoms typically emerge in the second or third trimester and resolve after delivery.

Tardive Dyskinesia

Movement disorders resulting from exposure to dopamine receptor antagonists are referred to as tardive syndromes, with tardive dyskinesia (TD) of the oral-buccal-lingual region being a common manifestation. TD is characterized by repetitive, choreic-like movements of the face and mouth to a greater extent than limbs and trunk. The movements appear typically after prolonged use of dopamine receptor blockers, which include most neuroleptics and certain gastrointestinal medications. The syndrome is difficult to treat and can be persistent and disabling.

Women develop TD more often than men, with more severe clinical manifestations. Frequency increases in older postmenopausal women (65). More recent data have not fully supported this finding, however, and report no gender difference in the risk for developing TD (66). Therefore, the influence of gender on the development and expression of TD requires further investigation.

Tic Disorders

Tics are defined as sudden brief movements that are typically associated with a premonitory sensation that is only relieved by completion of the movement. Tics are classified as motor or vocal (phonic), and both must be present for a diagnosis of Tourette's syndrome (TS). The etiology of TS is unknown but is believed to be heritable; the search for gene mutations is ongoing (67). Males are more often affected than females, but the reason for this gender dissociation is not yet clear.

Tics are known to fluctuate in frequency and intensity over time in individuals. Studies have investigated whether women have fluctuations correlating with different hormonal states. Schwabe et al. (68) found that 26% of women reported an increase in tic frequency in the premenstrual cycle, but no consistent changes were associated with pregnancy, oral contraceptive use, or menopause.

Psychogenic Movement Disorders

Movement disorders with no definable organic basis are currently referred to as psychogenic movement disorders. Depending on the root psychologic cause, they are classified as conversion disorders, somatization disorders, factitious disorders, or malingering. The possible clinical manifestations span the spectrum of movement disorders itself with tremor, dystonia, parkinsonism, chorea, and myoclonus as possible expressions.

A great disparity exists in the prevalence of psychogenic movement disorders between genders, with a definite female preponderance. A detailed review by Williams et al. (69) discusses the clinical presentation. In their cohort of psychogenic movement disorder patients, 109 of the 131 patients were female (83%), a ratio that is similar to that seen in other somatoform disorders.

Treatment is very difficult and necessitates the close cooperation of psychiatrists, neurologists, and physiatrists. Treatment success rates are not well documented and, if relapses occur, it may be with a different somatization. This may result in consultation with different medical specialties and loss to further neurologic follow-up.

CONCLUSION

In conclusion, much is still to be learned about the impact of gender on the incidence and expression of movement disorders. Although there is clearly a female predominance in a number of these disorders, including focal dystonia, dopa-responsive dystonia, Sydenham's chorea, and psychogenic movement disorders, the role of gender in the majority of movement disorders must be further defined. Further investigation must be conducted to determine the influence of hormonal states such as pregnancy, menses, menopause, and medication taken specifically by women on the expression and treatment of these diseases. We anticipate that, as the genetic bases for multiple movement disorders are identified in the future, some insight will be gained into pathophysiology and gender influences.

References

1. Harris J, Fahn S. Genetics of movement disorders. In: Rosenberg R, Prusiner S, DiMauro S, Barchi R, Nestler E, (eds.) *The molecular and genetic basis of neurologic and psychiatric disease*, 3rd ed. Philadelphia: Butterworth-Heinemann, 2003;351–368.
2. Dauer W, Przedborski S. Parkinson's disease: mechanisms and models. *Neuron* 2003;39(6):889–909.
3. Paisan-Ruiz C, Jain S, Evans EW, et al. Cloning of the gene containing mutations that cause PARK8-linked Parkinson's disease. *Neuron* 2004;44:595–600.
4. Swerdlow RH, Parker WD, Currie LJ, et al. Gender ratio differences between Parkinson's disease patients and their affected relatives. *Parkinsonism and Related Disorders* 2001;7(2):129–133.
5. Mayeux R, Marder K, Cote LJ, et al. The frequency of idiopathic Parkinson's disease by age, ethnic group, and sex in northern Manhattan, 1988–1993. *Am J Epidemiol* 1995;142(8):820–827.
6. Bower JH, Maraganore DM, McDonnell SK, Rocca WA. Incidence and distribution of parkinsonism in Olmsted County, Minnesota, 1976–1990. *Neurology* 1999;52(6):1214–1220.
7. Van Den Eeden SK, Tanner CM, Bernstein AL, et al. Incidence of Parkinson's disease: variation by age, gender, and race/ethnicity. *Am J Epidemiol* 2003;157(11):1015–1022.
8. Baldereschi M, Di Carlo A, Rocca WA, et al. Parkinson's disease and parkinsonism in a longitudinal study: twofold higher incidence in men. ILSA Working Group. Italian Longitudinal Study on Aging. *Neurology* 2000;55(9):1358–1363.
9. Zhang ZX, Roman GC. Worldwide occurrence of Parkinson's disease: an updated review. *Neuroepidemiology* 1993;12(4):195–208.
10. de Rijk MC, Launer LJ, Berger K, et al. Prevalence of Parkinson's disease in Europe: a collaborative study of population-based cohorts. Neurologic Diseases in the Elderly Research Group. *Neurology* 2000;54(11 suppl 5):S21–23.
11. Okada K, Kobayashi S, Tsunematsu T. Prevalence of Parkinson's disease in Izumo City, Japan. *Gerontology* 1990;36(5-6):340–344.
12. Kusumi M, Nakashima K, Harada H, Nakayama H, Takahashi K. Epidemiology of Parkinson's disease in Yonago City, Japan: comparison with a study carried out 12 years ago. *Neuroepidemiology* 1996;15(4):201–207.
13. Moriwaka F, Tashiro K, Itoh K, et al. Prevalence of Parkinson's disease in Hokkaido, the northernmost island of Japan. *Intern Med* 1996;35(4):276–279.
14. Kimura H, Kurimura M, Wada M, et al. Female preponderance of Parkinson's disease in Japan. *Neuroepidemiology* 2002;21(6):292–296.
15. Lyons KE, Hubble JP, Troster AI, Pahwa R, Koller WC. Gender differences in Parkinson's disease. *Clin Neuropharmacol* 1998;21(2):118–121.
16. Pasqualini C, Olivier V, Guibert B, Frain O, Leviel V. Acute stimulatory effect of estradiol on striatal dopamine synthesis. *J Neurochem* 1995;65(4):1651–1657.
17. Xiao L, Becker JB. Effects of estrogen agonists on amphetamine-stimulated striatal dopamine release. *Synapse* 1998;29(4):379–391.
18. Disshon KA, Boja JW, Dluzen DE. Inhibition of striatal dopamine transporter activity by 17beta-estradiol. *Eur J Pharmacol* 1998;345(2):207–211.
19. Disshon KA, Dluzen DE. Use of in vitro superfusion to assess the dynamics of striatal dopamine clearance: influence of estrogen. *Brain Res* 1999;842(2):399–407.
20. Levesque D, Di Paolo T. Modulation by estradiol and progesterone of the GTP effect on striatal D-2 dopamine receptors. *Biochem Pharmacol* 1993;45(3):723–733.
21. Roy EJ, Buyer DR, Licari VA. Estradiol in the striatum: effects on behavior and dopamine receptors but no evidence for membrane steroid receptors. *Brain Res Bull* 1990;25(2):221–227.
22. Hruska RE, Ludmer LM, Pitman KT, De Ryck M, Silbergeld EK. Effects of Estrogen on striatal dopamine receptor function in male and female rats. *Pharmacol Biochem Behav* 1982;16(2):285–291.
23. Dluzen DE. Neuroprotective effects of estrogen upon the nigrostriatal dopaminergic system. *J Neurocytol* 2000;29(5-6):387–399.
24. Morissette M, Di Paolo T. Effect of chronic estradiol and progesterone treatments of ovariectomized rats on brain dopamine uptake sites. *J Neurochem* 1993;60(5):1876–1883.
25. Bazzett TJ, Becker JB. Sex differences in the rapid and acute effects of estrogen on striatal D2 dopamine receptor binding. *Brain Res* 1994;637(1-2):163–172.
26. Lammers CH, D'Souza U, Qin ZH, Lee SH, Yajima S, Mouradian MM. Regulation of striatal dopamine receptors by estrogen. *Synapse* 1999;34(3):222–227.
27. Horstink MW, Strijks E, Dluzen DE. Estrogen and Parkinson's disease. *Adv Neurol* 2003;91:107–114.
28. Quinn NP, Marsden CD. Menstrual-related fluctuations in Parkinson's disease. *Mov Disord* 1986;1(1):85–87.
29. Sandyk R. Estrogens and the pathophysiology of Parkinson's disease. *Int J Neurosci* 1989;45(1-2):119–122.
30. Saunders-Pullman R, Gordon-Elliott J, Parides M, Fahn S, Saunders HR, Bressman S. The effect of estrogen replacement on early Parkinson's disease. *Neurology* 1999;52(7):1417–1421.
31. Fernandez HH, Lapane KL. Estrogen use among nursing home residents with a diagnosis of Parkinson's disease. *Mov Disord* 2000;15(6):1119–1124.
32. Tsang KL, Ho SL, Lo SK. Estrogen improves motor disability in parkinsonian postmenopausal women with motor fluctuations. *Neurology* 2000;54(12):2292–2298.
33. Blanchet PJ, Fang J, Hyland K, Arnold LA, Mouradian MM, Chase TN. Short-term effects of high-dose 17beta-estradiol in postmenopausal PD patients: a crossover study. *Neurology* 1999;53(1):91–95.
34. Marder K, Tang MX, Alfaro B, et al. Postmenopausal estrogen use and Parkinson's disease with and without dementia. *Neurology* 1998;50(4):1141–1143.
35. Ascherio A, Chen H, Schwarzschild MA, Zhang SM, Colditz GA, Speizer FE. Caffeine, postmenopausal estrogen, and risk of Parkinson's disease. *Neurology* 2003;60(5):790–795.
36. Kompoliti K, Comella CL, Jaglin JA, Leurgans S, Raman R, Goetz CG. Menstrual-related changes in motoric function in women with Parkinson's disease. *Neurology* 2000;55(10):1572–1575.
37. Strijks E, Kremer JA, Horstink MW. Effects of female sex steroids on Parkinson's disease in postmenopausal women. *Clin Neuropharmacol* 1999;22(2):93–97.
38. Scott B, Borgman A, Engler H, Johnels B, Aquilonius SM. Gender differences in Parkinson's disease symptom profile. *Acta Neurol Scand* 2000;102(1):37–43.
39. Fernandez HH, Lapane KL, Ott BR, Friedman JH. Gender differences in the frequency and treatment of behav-

ior problems in Parkinson's disease. SAGE Study Group. Systematic Assessment and Geriatric drug use via Epidemiology. *Mov Disord* 2000;15(3):490–496.

40. Hariz GM, Lindberg M, Hariz MI, Bergenheim AT. Gender differences in disability and health-related quality of life in patients with Parkinson's disease treated with stereotactic surgery. *Acta Neurol Scand* 2003;108(1):28–37.

41. Golbe LI. Pregnancy and movement disorders. *Neurol Clin* 1994;12(3):497–508.

42. Hagell P, Odin P, Vinge E. Pregnancy in Parkinson's disease: a review of the literature and a case report. *Mov Disord* 1998;13(1):34–38.

43. Shulman LM, Minagar A, Weiner WJ. The effect of pregnancy in Parkinson's disease. *Mov Disord* 2000; 15(1):132–135.

44. Martignoni E, Nappi RE, Citterio A, et al. Parkinson's disease and reproductive life events. *Neurol Sci* 2002; 23(suppl 2):S85–86.

45. Benedetti MD, Maraganore DM, Bower JH, et al. Hysterectomy, menopause, and estrogen use preceding Parkinson's disease: an exploratory case-control study. *Mov Disord* 2001;16(5):830–837.

46. Golbe LI. The epidemiology of progressive supranuclear palsy. *Adv Neurol* 1996;69:25–31.

47. Bower JH, Maraganore DM, McDonnell SK, Rocca WA. Incidence of progressive supranuclear palsy and multiple system atrophy in Olmsted County, Minnesota, 1976 to 1990. *Neurology* 1997;49(5):1284–1288.

48. Wenning GK, Ben Shlomo Y, Magalhaes M, Daniel SE, Quinn NP. Clinical features and natural history of multiple system atrophy. An analysis of 100 cases. *Brain* 1994;117(pt 4):835–845.

49. Riley DE, Lang AE, Lewis A, et al. Cortical-basal ganglionic degeneration. *Neurology* 1990;40(8):1203–1212.

50. Rinne JO, Lee MS, Thompson PD, Marsden CD. Corticobasal degeneration. A clinical study of 36 cases. *Brain* 1994;117(pt 5):1183–1196.

51. Nutt JG, Muenter MD, Aronson A, Kurland LT, Melton LJ 3rd. Epidemiology of focal and generalized dystonia in Rochester, Minnesota. *Mov Disord* 1988;3(3):188–194.

52. Claypool DW, Duane DD, Ilstrup DM, Melton LJ 3rd. Epidemiology and outcome of cervical dystonia (spasmodic torticollis) in Rochester, Minnesota. *Mov Disord* 1995;10(5):608–614.

53. Soland VL, Bhatia KP, Marsden CD. Sex prevalence of focal dystonias. *J Neurol Neurosurg Psychiatry* 1996; 60(2):204–205.

54. Duffey PO, Butler AG, Hawthorne MR, Barnes MP. The epidemiology of the primary dystonias in the north of England. *Adv Neurol* 1998;78:121–125.

55. A prevalence study of primary dystonia in eight European countries. *J Neurol* 2000;247(10):787–792.

56. Ichinose H, Ohye T, Takahashi E, et al. Hereditary progressive dystonia with marked diurnal fluctuation caused by mutations in the GTP cyclohydrolase I gene. *Nat Genet* 1994;8(3):236–242.

57. Nagatsu T, Ichinose H. GTP cyclohydrolase I gene, dystonia, juvenile parkinsonism, and Parkinson's disease. *J Neural Transm Suppl* 1997;49:203–209.

58. Furukawa Y, Lang AE, Trugman JM, et al. Gender-related penetrance and de novo GTP-cyclohydrolase I gene mutations in dopa-responsive dystonia. *Neurology* 1998;50(4):1015–1020.

59. Bressman SB. Dystonia genotypes, phenotypes, and classification. *Adv Neurol* 2004;94:101–107.

60. Gwinn-Hardy KA, Adler CH, Weaver AL, Fish NM, Newman SJ. Effect of hormone variations and other factors on symptom severity in women with dystonia. *Mayo Clin Proc* 2000;75(3):235–240.

61. Chuang C, Ford B. Sydenham Chorea. In: Noseworth JH, (ed.) *Neurological therapeutics: principles and practice.* London: Martin Dunitz, 2003;2569–2572.

62. Khamashta MA, Gil A, Anciones B, et al. Chorea in systemic lupus erythematosus: association with antiphospholipid antibodies. *Ann Rheum Dis* 1988;47(8):681–683.

63. Hubble JP, Busenbark KL, Pahwa R, Lyons K, Koller WC. Clinical expression of essential tremor: effects of gender and age. *Mov Disord* 1997;12(6):969–972.

64. Hardesty DE, Maraganore DM, Matsumoto JY, Louis ED. Increased risk of head tremor in women with essential tremor: longitudinal data from the Rochester Epidemiology Project. *Mov Disord* 2004;19(5):529–533.

65. Yassa R, Jeste DV. Gender differences in tardive dyskinesia: a critical review of the literature. *Schizophr Bull* 1992;18(4):701–715.

66. van Os J, Walsh E, van Horn E, Tattan T, Bale R, Thompson SG. Tardive dyskinesia in psychosis: are women really more at risk? UK700 Group. *Acta Psychiatr Scand* 1999;99(4):288–293.

67. Pauls DL. An update on the genetics of Gilles de la Tourette syndrome. *J Psychosom Res* 2003;55(1):7–12.

68. Schwabe MJ, Konkol RJ. Menstrual cycle-related fluctuations of tics in Tourette syndrome. *Pediatr Neurol* 1992;8(1):43–46.

69. Williams DT, Ford B, Fahn S. Phenomenology and psychopathology related to psychogenic movement disorders. *Adv Neurol* 1995;65:231–257.

24 Chorea Gravidarum

Gretchen L. Birbeck, MD MPH

As early as 1817, published accounts noted the occurrence of chorea during pregnancy and, by 1932, Wilson and Preece had published a review of 951 cases of chorea gravidarum (1). The disease was thought to be rare, occurring in 1:2,000 to 3,000 pregnancies, generally in primiparous women, but prognosis was grim, with 18 to 33% maternal and 50% fetal mortality rates.

Wilson and Preece believed the etiology to be an autoimmune phenomenon related to acute rheumatic heart disease presenting in pregnancy. Their assumption was supported by the 86% incidence rate of rheumatic heart disease noted among the patients they reviewed. The etiology previously had been attributed to a variety of problems, including psychic conflict, illegitimacy, hysteria, epidemic encephalitis, allergic reaction, and a "cervical reflex" phenomenon. Elaborate treatment schemes existed, many of which undoubtedly contributed to the high fetal and maternal mortality rates (Table 24.1). Medical student relays were used for the continuous administration of chloroform, and "therapeutic" abortions (with a 34% mortality rate) were advocated in florid cases (1–3).

In 1956, serendipity led to one of the more useful therapies (3). A patient with chorea gravidarum who was receiving morphine and sodium amytal developed severe nausea and vomiting. A physician noted that the chorea abruptly ceased after the administration of 25 mg of intramuscular chlorpromazine given for the gastrointestinal complaints.

PRESENTATION, COURSE, AND TREATMENT

Chorea gravidarum falls into the category of rare neurologic entities. It is not a disease, but rather a symptom of underlying central nervous system (CNS) pathology. Chorea consists of rapid, usually distal, nonrhythmic, nonstereotyped movements that may coexist with the slower, writhing movements termed athetosis. Women typically present with the abrupt onset of chorea during an otherwise uneventful pregnancy. The trimester during which onset most frequently occurs is unclear but may depend on the etiology. Symptoms include choreiform movements of the face, arm, and leg, which are often unilateral. Even without obvious facial involvement, there may be slurred speech. Psychiatric symptoms may precede the chorea and range from emotional lability with subtle mental status changes to flagrant psychosis mimicking schizophrenia. The patient initially may appear restless, assuming postures with crossed legs and clasped hands in order to suppress the movements. Intermittent hemiplegia has been noted. The movements may progress to hemiballismus, and severe cases can result in self-injury, rhabdomyolysis, and hyperthermia. Even relatively mild cases can result in the inability to walk, eat, and perform

TABLE 24.1
*Previously Used Therapies for
Chorea Gravidarum (1–3,16,20,24–26)*

Paraldehyde
Barbiturates
Salicylates
Chloroform
Chloral hydrate
Magnesium sulfate
Arsenic compounds
Potassium bromide
Parenteral horse serum
Extract of thymus gland
Morphine (frequently complicated by fatal overdose)
Colonics
Tonsillectomy
Restrictive diets
Blood transfusions
Isolation and restraints
Extraction of septic teeth
Cervical iodine applications
Hysterectomy (with abortion)

TABLE 24.2
*Etiologies of Chorea Gravidarum
(5,14,17,19,27,28)*

Lupus anticoagulant
Anticardiolipin antibody
Systemic lupus erythematosus
Rheumatic disease (similar to Sydenham's chorea)
Vascular malformation (basal ganglia region)
Cerebrovascular accident (basal ganglia region)
Thyrotoxicosis
Wilson's disease
Huntington's disease
Neuroacanthocytosis

routine activities of daily living. The movements subside with sleep. The course and prognosis depend on the etiology, but an overall mortality rate is estimated at less than 1%. The chorea generally abates hours after delivery of the baby (4).

Rheumatic Disease and Chorea Gravidarum

Although there have been several cited causes of chorea gravidarum (Table 24.2), the vast majority are due to rheumatic and autoimmune disease. Most early reports of chorea gravidarum were probably cases due to rheumatic disease, but since the advent of antibiotics, the sequelae of rheumatic disease have declined. These patients had a history of rheumatic heart disease, recurrent tonsillitis, or Sydenham's chorea (1,2). The symptoms typically presented in the first trimester and often subsided in the mid to late second trimester. Imaging studies are usually normal, but an underlying pathology is presumed (5). Antistreptolysin antibodies are elevated and may continue to rise throughout the pregnancy. Cardiac valvular disease is often evident, but patients usually do well with supportive care, reassurance, and medical intervention. In the first trimester, phenothiazines are the drug of choice for chorea gravidarum. All phenothiazines are class C drugs during pregnancy (6), but obstetricians have much experience using chlorpromazine in *hyperemesis gravidarum*. If treatment is needed in the second trimester, haloperidol is favored because it is less sedating (7,8). Reports of limb deformities prohibit the use of haloperidol during the first

trimester (9) (see also Chapter 4). Prophylactic antibiotics should be given during delivery (10), and although patients usually do well, there is a 25% recurrence rate with subsequent pregnancies (1).

Systemic lupus erythematosus (SLE), anticardiolipin antibody, and lupus anticoagulant are the predominant causes of chorea gravidarum in industrialized nations today (11–15). Patients present with symptoms in the second or third trimester, particularly with mental status changes such as agitation and confusion. These patients are more likely to develop rhabdomyolysis, seizures, hemiplegia, and coma, with hyperthermia being a particularly poor prognostic factor (1,4,12,16). The patient may have no history of autoimmune disease, so a full evaluation, particularly if there is a history of previous fetal loss, is indicated. Imaging studies may be normal or may reveal focal abnormalities in the basal ganglia and caudate nucleus. Cerebrospinal fluid may be normal, may show a mild pleocytosis, or may reveal elevated protein. Postmortem studies have shown diffuse foci of small hemorrhages present throughout the brain, most evident in the basal ganglia and caudate nucleus (15). A widespread vasculitis has also been reported (12). Neuroleptics may also be useful, but the mainstay of treatment is immunosuppression using steroids (11,15,17). In patients with lupus anticoagulant, aspirin therapy may also be indicated (14). If gross structural damage occurs, the chorea may persist after delivery. Recurrence with subsequent pregnancies has been reported, sometimes with fatal results (1,10).

In a well-described series of 50 patients with antiphospholipid antibodies, 12% developed chorea after starting estrogen-containing oral contraceptives and 6% developed chorea gravidarum. Among those with chorea, 55% had bilateral symptoms, and imaging revealed frank infarcts in 35%. Notably, 34% experienced recurrent symptoms when challenged with high estrogen states (18).

ETIOLOGY

In 1950, Beresford and Graham speculated, "it may be that pregnancy lowers the resistance of a patient who is inherently susceptible to chorea" (16). Sydenham's chorea was known to affect males and females equally before puberty, after which a 2:1 female predominance appears (1), but it was not until oral contraceptive agents became widely used that an epidemic of chorea in young women pointed to estrogen as a cause (19). For some time, it has been assumed that a modification of the postsynaptic dopamine receptor produces dopamine hypersensitivity in high estrogen states (20). More recent data indicate that estrogen augments neuronal function by increasing the expression of the active D5 receptor (21). Furthermore, estradiol acts as a DA agonist on the striatal D2 receptor, particularly in the medial part of the striatum (22). Estrogens do not appear to have a net effect on the striatal dopamine receptor expression (23). Presumably, a previously asymptomatic injury to the inhibitory striatopallidal pathways becomes manifest during high estrogen states, including pregnancy.

EVALUATION

A history, physical examination, and pertinent investigations enable a diagnosis in most cases (Table 24.3). Given the high rates of reported, otherwise asymptomatic strokes, an imaging study is warranted. In choosing treatments, the teratogenic risks to the fetus must be weighed against the benefit to the mother. Most case reports suggest that haloperidol offers the most effective symptomatic relief. Recent studies of the use of phenothiazines

---

TABLE 24.3
Evaluation of Chorea Gravidarum

Brain MRI
Toxicology screen
Antistreptolysin antibody (ASO)
Sedimentation rate
Blood cultures
Antinuclear antibody (ANA)
Echocardiography
Coagulation times (PT and APTT)
Anticardiolipin antibody
Lupus anticoagulant
Complete blood count
Liver function tests
Electrolytes
Slit lamp examination of eyes
Peripheral RBC smear for acanthocytes

---

for antiemetic effects in pregnancy have confirmed their relative safety.

CONCLUSION

Chorea gravidarum is a rare entity today. In industrialized nations, the etiology is probably autoimmune in nature, whereas in developing nations rheumatic heart disease is the likely cause. Although historically chorea gravidarum is a highly morbid or even fatal condition, pregnancy in these patients can usually proceed to term following a careful assessment and management of the chorea.

References

1. Wilson P, Preece A. Chorea gravidarum. *Arch Intern Med* 1932;471(49):671–697.
2. Zegart KN, Schwarz RH. Chorea gravidarum. *Obstet Gynecol* 1968;32(1):24–27.
3. Winkelbauer R, Kimsly L. Chorea gravidarum treated with chlorpromazine. *Am J Obstet Gyn* 1956: 1353–1354.
4. Lewis BV, Parsons M. Chorea gravidarum. *Lancet* 1966;1(7432):284–286.
5. Ginnetti RA, Bredfeldt RC, Pegg EW 3rd. Chorea gravidarum. A case report including magnetic resonance imaging results. *J Fam Pract* 1989;29(1):87–89.
6. McEvay R. Drug Information; 1996.
7. Donaldson JO. Control of chorea gravidarum with haloperidol. *Obstet Gynecol* 1982;59(3):381–382.
8. Patterson JF. Treatment of chorea gravidarum with haloperidol. *S Med J* 1979;72(9):1220–1221.
9. Kopelman A, McCullan F, Heggness L. Limb malformation following maternal use of haloperidol. *JAMA* 1975;231:62–64.
10. Ghanem Q. Recurrent chorea gravidarum in four pregnancies. *Can J Neurol Sci* 1985;12(2):136–138.
11. Donaldson IM, Espiner EA. Disseminated lupus erythematosus presenting as chorea gravidarum. *Arch Neurol* 1971;25(3):240–244.
12. Ichikawa K, Kim RC, Givelber H, Collins GH. Chorea gravidarum. Report of a fatal case with neuropathological observations. *Arch Neurol* 1980;37(7):429–432.
13. Lubbe WF, Butler WS, Palmer SJ, Liggins GC. Lupus anticoagulant in pregnancy. *Br J Obstet Gynecol* 1984; 91(4):357–363.
14. Lubbe WF, Walker EB. Chorea gravidarum associated with circulating lupus anticoagulant: successful outcome of pregnancy with prednisone and aspirin therapy. Case report. *Br J Obstet Gynecol* 1983;90(5):487–490.
15. Johnson R, Richardson E. The neurological manifestations of systemic lupus erythematosus. *Medicine* 1968;47(4):337–369.
16. Beresford O, Graham A. Chorea gravidarum. *J Obstet Gyn* 1950;57:616–625.
17. Agrawal BL, Foa RP. Collagen vascular disease appearing as chorea gravidarum. *Arch Neurol* 1982;39(3): 192–193.
18. Cervera R, Asherson RA, Font J, et al. Chorea in the antiphospholipid syndrome. Clinical, radiologic, and immunologic characteristics of 50 patients from our clin-

ics and the recent literature. *Medicine* 1997;76(3): 203–212.

19. Beicherstaff E. *Neurological complications of oral contraceptives*. Oxford: Clarendon Press, 1975.

20. Nausuda P, Koller W, Weiner W, Klawans H. Modification of post-synaptic dopaminergic sensitivity by female sex hormones. *Life Sci* 1979;25:521–526.

21. Lee D, Dong P, Copolov D, Lim AT. D5 dopamine receptors mediate estrogen-induced stimulation of hypothalamic atrial natriuretic factor neurons. *Mol Endocrinol* 1999;13(2):344–352.

22. Levesque D, Di Paolo T. Modulation by estradiol and progesterone of the GTP effect on striatal D-2 dopamine receptors. *Biochem Pharmacol* 1993;45(3):723–733.

23. Lammers CH, D'Souza U, Qin ZH, Lee SH, Yajima S, Mouradian MM. Regulation of striatal dopamine receptors by estrogen. *Synapse* 1999;34(3):222–227.

24. Magee LA, Mazzotta P, Koren G. Evidence-based view of safety and effectiveness of pharmacologic therapy for nausea and vomiting of pregnancy (NVP). *Am J Obstet Gynecol* 2002;185(5 Suppl Understanding):S256–261.

25. Greenhill J. *Obstetrics*. Philadelphia: WB Saunders, 1965.

26. King A. Neurological conditions occurring as complications of pregnancy. *Arch Neurol Psych* 1950;63:471.

27. Barber P, Arnold A, Evans G. Recurrent hormone dependent chorea: effect of oestrogens and progesterones. *Clin Endocrinol* 1976;5:291–293.

28. Korenyi C, Whittier JR, Conchado D. Stress in Huntington's disease (chorea). (Review of the literature and personal observations.) *Dis Nervous Sys* 1972;33(5): 339–344.

25 Giant Cell Arteritis

David B. Hellmann, MD, Mary Betty Stevens, Professor of Medicine

G iant cell arteritis (GCA) is a systemic vasculitis of unknown cause that chiefly occurs in a person more than 60 years old and preferentially affects the extracranial branches of the carotid artery. The most feared complication of GCA—irreversible blindness—usually can be prevented by early diagnosis and treatment. Diagnosis is not always straightforward, however, because GCA often presents with a wide variety of symptoms, including many neurological ones, that can camouflage their vasculitic origins. A detailed knowledge of the clinical presentation of GCA helps neurologists determine which patients with headache, transient ischemic attack (TIA), or amaurosis fugax have underlying GCA.

The terms "giant cell arteritis," "temporal arteritis," or "cranial arteritis" have all been used to designate the same disease process. Each designation captures some characteristic features of the disease and each has its faults (e.g., not all patients have giant cells in the biopsy and not all patients have involvement of the temporal or other cranial arteries). In this chapter, giant cell arteritis and temporal arteritis are used interchangeably.

EPIDEMIOLOGY

GCA is the most common systemic vasculitis in adults, and its incidence is profoundly influenced by age (1–5). The overall yearly incidence is 3 per 100,000 persons, but rises to 17 per 100,000 after the age of 50, and to 56 per 100,000 after age 80 (1). Indeed, GCA very rarely occurs before age 50, and the average age at onset is 72 (7). Women are affected 2 to 3 times as often as men (1,6). In addition, the prevalence varies among racial and ethnic groups, with the highest prevalence in persons of northern European ancestry (4). Latitude also appears to be important, because GCA is twice as common in Sweden as it is in Italy or Spain (8,9). GCA occurs more commonly in people who have specific HLA-DR4 haplotypes (10,11). The infrequency of these haplotypes in African Americans may explain the rarity of GCA in that population (12).

PATHOLOGY, PATHOGENESIS, AND ETIOLOGY

GCA produces an inflammatory reaction that affects all layers of large- and medium-sized arteries (9,13,14). The infiltrate is chiefly mononuclear, consisting largely of CD4+ T cells and macrophages. The classic multinuclear giant cells are found in only 50% of affected arteries. B cells are noticeably absent. The inflammatory infiltrate characteristically causes a marked disruption of the internal elastic lamina and occlusive internal hyperplasia (9,13).

Immunohistologic and immunochemical studies have demonstrated a striking layer-specific expansion of inflammatory cells and cytokines (15–20). For example, gamma interferon secreting T cells are almost exclusively localized to the adventitia. Although macrophages are found throughout the vessel wall, distinct subsets of macrophages producing different cytokines are found in each layer (15–19).

Although the etiology of GCA is unknown, the layer-specific pathology and cytokine pattern suggest that the disease begins in the adventitia and is antigen- and T cell driven (13,18). Speculation about the provocative antigen has centered on viruses, intracellular bacteria, and neoantigens created by degenerating arterial structures (13).

DISTRIBUTION OF AFFECTED VESSELS

Although GCA is a systemic disease that can affect virtually any artery, GCA most frequently affects the superficial temporal, ophthalmic, posterior ciliary, and vertebral arteries (21,22). The proximal central retinal and the cavernous portions of the internal and external carotids arteries are also commonly affected (17). Intracranial arteritis is very rare, perhaps because intracranial arteries lose the internal elastic lamina 5 mm beyond penetration of the dura (22). GCA also commonly affects the aorta (22–24). Subclavian, axillary, and brachial artery disease can result in claudication, local bruits, and produce a characteristic angiographic appearance (22). The descending aorta, mesenteric, coronary, renal, and femoral arteries are infrequently involved.

CLINICAL PRESENTATIONS

Classical Presentation

Headache

The most common presenting symptoms are headache, polymyalgia rheumatica, jaw-claudication, and visual abnormalities (Tables 25.1 and 25.2) (1–5,9). Many patients also experience nonspecific symptoms of malaise, fatigue, depression, and weight loss (1–5,9). Headache is the commonest symptom, occurring at some point in 90% of patients (2). The most remarkable aspect of the headache is that the patient perceives it as new. Whether the patient has rarely had headaches or frequently had headaches, the headaches of GCA are usually perceived as new and different. No other characteristic holds up so well. Although the headache most often occurs temporally, it may be felt in the frontal or occipital areas. Although in the majority of patients the headache is not severe and does not limit activities, in some, the headache is so severe the patient is forced to lie quietly in a darkened room. Frequently, patients note associated tenderness of the scalp (e.g., hurts to comb the hair), and some of the tender areas may feel nodular (3).

Jaw Claudication

Jaw claudication is pain in the masseter muscles occurring with chewing and caused by ischemia of the facial arteries. Jaw claudication is nearly pathognomonic for GCA (1), although it does rarely occur in Wegener's granulomatosis and in systemic amyloidosis (25). Jaw claudication usually commences only after protracted chewing, as with meat from the hospital cafeteria. Unlike temporal mandibular joint disease, claudication is not influenced merely by maximally opening the mouth. Some patients, however, do not explicitly relate this pain to eating. Rather, some simply have a vague sense of jaw discomfort that can

TABLE 25.1
Classical Symptoms and Findings in Giant Cell Arteritis

Symptoms	Initial (%)	Ever (%)
Headache	86	90
Jaw claudication	64	67
Polymyalgia	21	50
Visual symptoms	35	40
Findings		
Fever	19	21
Abnormal physical exam of temporal artery	40	50

Modified and reproduced with permission from Huston KA, Hunder GG, Lie JT, Kennedy RH, Elveback LR. Temporal arteritis. A 25-year epidemiologic, clinical, and pathologic study. *Ann Intern Med* 1978;88:162-167.

TABLE 24.2
Laboratory Abnormalities in Giant Cell Arteritis

Test (Normal Values)	% Abnormal	Median	Range
ESR (1–15 mm/h)	100	72	42–136
Hemoglobin (7–10.4 mmol/L)	57	7.1	47.8.8
Platelets (140–400x10⁹/L)	47	374	164–766
Alkaline phosphatase (50–155 u/L)	24	192	95–1,160

Modified and reproduced with permission from Boesen P, Sørensen SF. Giant cell arteritis, temporal arteritis, and polymyalgia rheumatica in a Danish country. A prospective investigation, 1982-1985. *Arthritis Rheum* 1987;30:294-299.

confuse the patient and doctor. One patient, for example, initially attributed her pterygoid area pain to a face lift, though the surgical scar had been painless for months after the surgery. More commonly, the jaw discomfort may be attributed to occult dental problems. Thus, the doctor should inquire about all types of new jaw discomfort and not just classical jaw claudication.

Polymyalgia Rheumatica

Polymyalgia rheumatica (PMR) is pain and stiffness in the shoulder and hip areas that develops in half of the patients who have GCA (1,3,9,26–28). PMR tends to be worse in the morning. Patients may complain of both pain and weakness, but (in contrast to polymyositis) the pain predominates. PMR occurs about twice as often alone as it does with GCA (26). PMR by itself is associated with a low risk of blindness and requires treatment with smaller doses of prednisone.

Visual Abnormalities

Approximately 30% of patients with GCA experience neurologic symptoms outside of headache (Table 25.3), with visual abnormalities being most common (Tables 25.4, 25.5, 25.6) (9,22,29–32). Permanent vision loss develops in about 5 to 10% and frequently renders the patient legally blind (some may be able to perceive light) (9,32). The types of visual loss in GCA are detailed in Table 25.4. Most patients sustain vision loss as a result of ischemia of

TABLE 25.4
Neuro-Ophthalmologic Syndromes in Giant Cell Arteritis

Syndrome	Frequency
Vision loss	5–17%
Ophthalmoparesis	3–15%
Autonomic dysfunction – Horner's syndrome – Parasympathetic pupillary light dysfunction	Rare
Hallucinations	Rare

Modified and reproduced with permission from Mehler MF, Rabinowich L. The clinical neuro-ophthalmologic spectrum of temporal arteritis. *Am J Med* 1988;85:839–844.

TABLE 25.5
Types of Vision Loss in GCA

Pathogenesis	Signs	Prevalence
Anterior ischemic optic neuropathy	Total visual loss, normal (acute) or pale, swollen disk retinal edema	Common
Central retinal artery occlusion	Pale, swollen disk macula—cherry red spot	Rare
Retrobulbar optic neuritis	Optic pallor	Rare
Anterior segment ischemia	Chemosis, corneal edema	Rare
Cortical or chiasmal ischemia	Bitemporal or hemianopic field defects	Rare

Modified and reproduced with permission from Mehler MF, Rabinowich L. The clinical neuro-ophthalmologic spectrum of temporal arteritis. *Am J Med* 1988;85:839–844.

TABLE 25.3
Neurologic Manifestations in Giant Cell Arteritis

Finding	Frequency (%)*
Any neurologic abnormality	31
Neuropathies	14
– Mononeuropathies (esp. optic nerve)	7
– Peripheral neuropathy	7
TIA/stroke	7
Neuro-otologic	7
– Isolated vertigo	6
Tremor	4
Neuropsychiatric	3
– Organic brain syndrome	2
– Dementia	1
Tongue numbness	2
Transverse myelopathy	1

*n=166 patients
Modified and reproduced with permission from Caselli RJ, Hunder GG, Whisnant JP. Neurologic disease in biopsy-proven giant cell (temporal) arteritis. *Neurology* 1988;38:352–359.

the anterior ischemic optic nerve, which in turn is caused by infarction of the posterior ciliary artery (a branch of the ophthalmic artery) (9,22,30,32). The risk of losing vision appears lowest in those patients who have striking signs of systemic inflammation [e.g., fever, high erythrocyte sedimentation rate (ESR)] (9,13). Other causes of vision loss are less common (Table 25.5). In the first few hours of anterior ischemic optic neuritis, the fundoscopic exam may be normal. Within 24 to 36 hours, the disk will become pale and edematous (29,32). Edema resolves within 10 days and is later replaced by optic atrophy (29,32).

Amaurosis fugax occurs in about 10% of patients, and is monocular in two-thirds (29) (Table 25.6). The great majority of patients who sustain permanent vision

TABLE 25.6
Ophthalmologic Signs in Giant Cell Arteritis

Visual Abnormality	Frequency (%)*
Any abnormality	21
Amaurosis fugax	10
– Mono	7
– Binocular	3
Permanent vision loss	8
Permanent vision loss without amaurosis fugax	7
Scintillating scotoma	5
Diplopia	2

*n=166 patients
Modified and reproduced with permission from Caselli RJ, Hunder GG, Whisnant JP. Neurologic disease in biopsy-proven giant cell (temporal) arteritis. *Neurology* 1988;38:352–359.

TABLE 25.7
Stroke and TIA in Giant Cell Arteritis

Prevalence: (12/166) 7%

Location:	All events	Carotid:vestibular = 2:1
	Stroke	Carotid:vestibular = 3:2

Timing: Mean 1 month after temporal artery biopsy

Pathophysiology: Vasculitis of extracranial arteritis; atherosclerosis?

Modified and reproduced with permission from Caselli RJ, Hunder GG, Whisnant JP. Neurologic disease in biopsy-proven giant cell (temporal) arteritis. *Neurology* 1988;38:352–359.

loss do not experience amaurosis fugax (29). Still, vision loss is rarely the first symptom of GCA. On average, vision loss develops 5 months after other symptoms of GCA have been present.

Ophthalmoparesis resulting in diplopia—the second most common ophthalmologic sign of GCA after visial loss—occurs in 3 to 15% of patients (30,32). Defects in vertical gaze caused by ischemia of the third cranial nerve is most common. GCA may also cause abducens or trochlear nerve palsies (30,32). Ophthalmoparesis has a good prognosis, because it usually responds to corticosteroid treatment. Although ophthalmoparesis has been attributed to vasculitis affecting the cranial nerves, myositis of the extraocular muscles has also been described (30,32).

Nonclassical Presentations

Stroke or TIAs have been reported in 7% of patients with GCA (22,29,31) (Table 25.7). Whether stroke occurs more commonly in GCA than in any other population of older individuals has not been firmly established. However, a causal link of GCA and stroke is suggested by the relative frequency of posterior circulation strokes. That is, the ratio of carotid to vestibular strokes is 3:2 compared to the 5:1 ratio seen in the normal population. The mean time of onset of strokes is 1 month after temporal artery biopsy (31). The few angiograms and autopsies performed suggest that intracranial vessels are almost always spared; strokes appear to result from thrombosis of, or platelet embolization from extracranial vessels (31).

Peripheral nervous system involvement in GCA occurs in 1 to 14% of patients (Table 25.8) (22,29,31,33–37). GCA differs from all other forms of systemic vasculitis in preferentially involving the brachial

plexus to produce a lesion that mimics a C5 radiculopathy (33). Patients experience the sudden onset of pain and inability to abduct the shoulder on the affected side. Mononeuropathies involving the hands or feet—common in polyarteritis, Wegener's granulomatosis, and other forms of systemic vasculitis—occur less frequently in GCA. Other uncommon neurologic abnormalities reported in GCA include syndrome of inappropriate antidiuretic hormone (SIADH) secretion, coma, multi-infarct dementia, aseptic meningitis, seizures, anosmia, and spinal cord infarction (38–49).

Other symptoms may be present in GCA. Up to 40% of patients do not present with headache, visual abnormalities, and polymyalgia rheumatica, but instead present with nonclassical symptoms (Table 25.9) (9,13,50–52). Almost half of patients with GCA develop fever, and 15% of patients present as fever of unknown origin (FUO) (53). Indeed, GCA accounts for 15% of all FUOs seen in patients over the age of 65 (53). The fever

TABLE 25.8
Peripheral Nervous System Involvement in Giant Cell Arteritis

Frequency   1–14%

Types (in 24 cases)
- Mononeuropathy
  especially brachial plexopathy, C5 radiculopathy
- Polyneuropathy

Clinical picture: Neuropathy was chief symptom in 13/23

Prognosis: 16/18 improved with prednisone

Summary: GCA causes picture of C5 radiculopathy

Reproduced with permission using data from Nesher G, Rosenberg P, Shorer Z, Gilai A, Solomonovich A, Sonnenblick M. Involvement of the peripheral nervous system in temporal arteritis-polymyalgia rheumatica. Report of 3 cases and review of the literature. *J Rheumatol* 1987;14:358–360.

TABLE 25.9
Manifestations of Occult GCA

Fever of unknown origin
Respiratory tract symptoms (especially cough)
Otologic manifestations
   – Glossitis
   – Lingual infarction
   – Tongue ulceration
   – Throat pain
Large artery disease
   – Limb claudication
   – Aortic dissection
   – Raynaud's disease
Neurologic manifestations (see Table 25.3 and text)
Myocardial infarction
Microangiopathic hemolytic anemia
Glomerulonephritis
Liver disease
Breast mass (arteritis)
Uterine and ovarian mass (arteritis)

can reach 40°C and, in two-thirds of patients, is associated with rigors and drenching sweats (53). Almost all patients with FUO from GCA have a normal white blood cell count (before corticosteroids) (53). Most also have other manifestations of GCA, but in a few patients FUO may be the only symptom.

Respiratory symptoms occur in 9%, and most commonly consist of a dry cough (54). The cause of the cough is not known; the chest x-ray is invariably normal. Tongue pain with or without glossitis, ulcerations, and throat pain are other manifestations of GCA in the respiratory tract (3,54).

Large vessel disease occurs in 3 to 10% of patients presenting as Raynaud's phenomenon, loss of pulses (upper extremities are most common), arm claudication, or unequal limb pressures (9,13,23,55–57). Aortic involvement—causing thoracic aortic dissection, aortic regurgitation, or sudden death—develops in at least 3% of patients with GCA (13,23). Aortic disease may occur early, but most typically develops 7 years after the diagnosis of GCA, emphasizing the need for long-term follow-up (55,57).

Other uncommon manifestations of GCA are listed in Table 25.9. GCA presenting as breast, uterine, or ovarian masses has been described (50,58,59).

SIGNS AND LABORATORY FINDINGS

Physical examination is normal in many patients. The temporal arteries are normal to palpation in 50% of cases (1–5). Thus, the absence of temporal artery abnormali-

ties on physical examination does not exclude the diagnosis of GCA. Abnormalities of the temporal arteries can include nodularity, tenderness, enlargement, and loss of pulse. Occult large artery involvement may be reflected by unequal arm pressures, aortic murmurs, or bruits over the supraclavicular or infraclavicular areas or over the carotids or axillary arteries. The ophthalmologic findings already have been described.

The laboratory findings seen in most patients are a markedly elevated Westergren ESR (averaging 88) and a modest normochromic, normocytic anemia (60) (Table 25.2). More modest elevations of the ESR occur (61–65): One study of 167 patients with GCA showed that at the time of presentation, 10.8% had an ESR <50, 5.4% <40, and 3.6% <30 (61). The platelet count—"a poor person's ESR"—is also frequently elevated (2,4,28). Many patients also develop a mildly elevated alkaline phosphatase, attributed to otherwise occult liver involvement (2,4,19).

DIAGNOSIS

The diagnosis of GCA should be considered nearly certain in patients who have classic symptoms of headache, PMR, jaw claudication, and visual abnormality associated with a high ESR (9,60). When the patient's chief complaint is not one of the classic symptoms, then the probability of GCA depends on whether the review of symptoms reveals other typical (though less prominent) symptoms of GCA and whether the patient has the characteristic laboratory abnormalities (anemia and elevated ESR). Thus, the 78-year-old woman who develops a TIA in the absence of other symptoms with a normal ESR should not be suspected of having GCA, whereas a similarly aged woman with a TIA, 2 months of malaise and fatigue, a 5-pound weight loss, and subtle but definite new headaches and jaw pain associated with a hematocrit of 32 and an ESR of 110 should be suspected of having GCA.

Diagnosis usually rests on finding pathologic changes in the temporal artery biopsy. Unilateral biopsies are approximately 85 to 90% sensitive (65,66). About 4% of patients with a negative unilateral biopsy are found to have GCA when the contralateral temporal artery is biopsied (66). Because GCA does not involve the artery continuously but in a skip fashion, 3 to 5 cm of artery should be removed and multiple sections examined pathologically (66). In some patients, the diagnosis of GCA is established by autopsy, by pathologic examinations of an aortic aneurysm, by angiography showing typical large vessel changes of GCA, or by biopsy of another extracranial artery, such as the occipital artery (65,67). Color duplex ultrasonography of the temporal arteries has been reported to be sensitive (68), but its specificity and usefulness remain debatable (69). Magnetic resonance angiography (MRA) may be useful in patients with involvement of the aorta or subclavian arteries (70,71).

There are many reasons to recommend temporal artery biopsy (65). First, biopsy has virtually no morbidity. Second, rarely, other diseases—polyarteritis, Wegener's granulomatosis, systemic amyloidosis, and thyroiditis—can mimic GCA (9,25,65). Third, even when the initial symptoms appear classical, in the absence of biopsy confirmation, doubt may arise later when the patient develops symptoms that could be attributed to either corticosteroid toxicity (e.g., weakness, fatigue) or be signs of another condition.

TREATMENT

Initial Therapy

Because the goal of treatment is to prevent blindness and because blindness is usually irreversible, corticosteroid therapy should be started as soon as the diagnosis of GCA is thought to be likely. Temporal artery biopsies appear to remain reliable for at least the first 2 weeks after treatment has been initiated (7). The initial dose is 60 to 80 mg of prednisone per day orally. Small series of patients suggest that those who experience sudden recent visual change should be admitted and given high-dose intravenous methylprednisone (500 to 1,000 mg per day in divided doses). Unfortunately, vision loss is almost invariably irreversible (72,73). After 3 to 5 days, the oral regimen (again in divided doses, e.g., 30 mg po bid) may be started. Once treatment has begun, subsequent vision loss is rare (74,75).

Patients with GCA respond dramatically to corticosteroids. Most feel "miraculously" improved within 48 hours, and some feel better within hours of the first dose (1–5,9). PMR, headache, and fever respond especially rapidly. Jaw claudication may take weeks to resolve. Virtually all patients will be symptom free and have a normal ESR 1 month after starting treatment (1).

Every effort should be made at the onset to limit the toxicity of corticosteroids. Placing the patient on a diet and exercise program and prescribing an appropriate therapy of osteoporosis prophylaxis should be done early.

Late Treatment

After the first month, prednisone can be tapered slowly, for example, by 5 mg/wk. The patient is followed carefully for any symptoms or signs of reoccurrences. Most authorities do monitor the ESR, but base treatment changes on the complete clinical picture (history, examination, and laboratory studies) (4). Treatment of the ESR alone should be avoided. Once the patient achieves a prednisone dose in the range of 20 mg/d, small decrements (by 1 to 2.5 mg) become better tolerated. Flares can usually be treated by raising the prednisone dose to 10 mg above the dose at which the patient was last asymptomatic. Many but not all patients will be able to be tapered off prednisone within 2 years (4). Alternate day dose prednisone does not work in the first month, but some have reported successful use thereafter (4,76). The effectiveness of methotrexate as a steroid-sparing agent is controversial since placebo-controlled trials have reached opposing conclusions (77,78). No other drugs have proved to be successful, but cyclophosphamide, azathioprine, and cyclosporine have been used in the rare patient who could not be managed with prednisone alone (79).

Most studies show that GCA does not decrease survival (80). Patients whose disease remits should be warned, however, that the disease may reoccur and be advised to always mention their history of GCA to any new physician. Involvement of the thoracic aorta with dissection, or congestive heart failure from aortic regurgitation, is an increasingly noted late complication of GCA (9,13,57).

*R*eferences

1. Goodman BW Jr. Temporal arteritis. *Am J Med* 1979;67: 839–852.
2. Huston KA, Hunder GG, Lie JT, Kennedy RH, Elveback LR. Temporal arteritis. A 25-year epidemiologic, clinical, and pathologic study. *Ann Intern Med* 1978;88:162–167.
3. Hamilton CR Jr, Shelley WM, Tumulty PA. Giant cell arteritis: Including temporal arteritis and polymyalgia rheumatica. *Medicine* 1971;50:1–27.
4. Huston KA, Hunder GG. Giant cell (cranial) arteritis: a clinical review. *Am Heart J* 1980:99–107.
5. Hunder GG, Bloch DA, Michel BA, et al. The American College of Rheumatology 1990 criteria for the classification of giant cell arteritis. *Arthritis Rheum* 1990;33: 1122–1128.
6. Machado EBV, Michet CJ, Ballard DJ, et al. Trends in incidence and clinical presentation of temporal arteritis in Olmsted County, Minnesota, 1950–1985. *Arthritis Rheum* 1988;31:745–749.
7. Achkar AA, Lie JT, Hunder GG, O'Fallon M, Gabriel SE. How does previous corticosteroid treatment affect the biopsy findings in giant cell (temporal) arteritis? *Ann Intern Med* 1994;120:987–992.
8. González-Gay MA, Garcia-Porrua C, Rivas MJ, et al. Epidemiology of biopsy proven giant cell arteritis in northwestern Spain: trend over an 18-year period. *Ann Rheum Dis* 2001;60:367–371.
9. Salvarani C, Cantini F, Boiardi L, Hunder GG. Polymyalgia rheumatica and giant-cell arteritis. *N Engl J Med* 2002;347:261–271.
10. Wilke WS, Hoffman GS. Treatment of corticosteroid-resistant giant cell arteritis. *Rheum Dis Clin North Am* 1995;21:59–71.
11. Weyand CM, Hunder NNH, Hicok KC, Hunder GG, Goronzy JJ. HLA-DRB1 alleles in polymyalgia rheumatica, giant cell arteritis, and rheumatoid arthritis. *Arthritis Rheum* 1994;37:514–520.
12. Bielory L, Ogunkoya A, Frohman LP. Temporal arteritis in blacks. *Am J Med* 1989;86:707–708.

13. Levine SM, Hellmann DB. Giant cell arteritis. *Curr Opin Rheumatol* 2002;14:3–10.

14. McDonnell PJ, Moore GW, Miller NR, Hutchins GM, Green WR. Temporal arteritis. A clinicopathologic study. *Ophthalmology* 1986;93:518–530.

15. Weyand CM, Hicok KC, Hunder GG, Goronzy JJ. Tissue cytokine patterns in patients with polymyalgia rheumatica and giant cell arteritis. *Ann Intern Med* 1994;121:484–491.

16. Wagner AD, Goronzy JJ, Weyand CM. Functional profile of tissue-infiltrating and circulating CD68+ Cells in giant cell arteritis. Evidence of two components of the disease. *J Clin Invest* 1994;94:1134–1140.

17. Hunder GG, Lie JT, Goronzy JJ, Weyand CM. Pathogenesis of giant cell arteritis. *Arthritis Rheum* 1993;36:757–761.

18. Weyand CM, Goronzy JJ. Arterial wall injury in giant cell arteritis. *Arthritis Rheum* 1999;42:844–853.

19. Weyand CM, Wagner AD, Bjornsson J, et al. Correlation of the topographical arrangement and the functional pattern of tissue-infiltrating macrophages in giant cell arteritis. *J Clin Invest* 1996;98:1642–1649.

20. Weyand CM, Tetzlaff N, Bjornsson J, et al. Disease patterns and tissue cytokine profiles in giant cell arteritis. *Arthritis Rheum* 1997;40:19–26.

21. Reich KA, Giansiracusa DF, Strongwater SL. Neurologic manifestations of giant cell arteritis. *Am J Med* 1990;89:67–72.

22. Caselli RJ, Hunder GG. Neurologic complications of giant cell (temporal) arteritis. *Rheum Dis Clin North Am* 1994;14:349–353.

23. Evans JM, O'Fallon M, Hunder GG. Increased incidence of aortic aneurysm and dissection in giant cell (temporal) arteritis: a population-based study. *Ann Intern Med* 1995;122:502–507.

24. Blockmans D, Stroobants S, Maes A, et al. Positron emission tomography in giant cell arteritis and polymyalgia rheumatica: evidence for inflammation of the aortic arch. *Am J Med* 2000;15;108:246–249.

25. Rao JK, Allen NB. Primary systemic amyloidosis masquerading as giant cell arteritis. Case report and review of the literature. *Arthritis Rheum* 1993;36:422–425.

26. Chuang T-Y, Hunder GG, Ilstrup DM, Kurland LT. Polymyalgia rheumatica. A 10-year epidemiologic and clinical study. *Ann Intern Med* 1982;97:672–680.

27. Healey LA, Wilske KR. Polymyalgia rheumatica and giant cell arteritis. *West J Med* 1984;141:64–67.

28. Boesen P, Sørensen SF. Giant cell arteritis, temporal arteritis, and polymyalgia rheumatica in a Danish country. A prospective investigation, 1982–1985. *Arthritis Rheum* 1987;30:294–299.

29. Caselli RJ, Hunder GG, Whisnant JP. Neurologic disease in biopsy-proven giant cell (temporal) arteritis. *Neurology* 1988;38:352–359.

30. Mehler MF, Rabinowich L. The clinical neuro-ophthalmologic spectrum of temporal arteritis. *Am J Med* 1988;85:839–844.

31. Caselli RJ, Hunder GG. Neurologic aspects of giant cell (temporal) arteritis. *Rheum Dis Clin N Am* 1993;19:941–953.

32. Miller NR. Visual manifestations of temporal arteritis. In: Rheumatic Disease Clinics of North America. Stone J, Hellmann DB, (eds). New York: WB Saunders, 2001:781–797.

33. Golbus J, McCune WJ. Giant cell arteritis and peripheral neuropathy: a report of 2 cases and review of the literature. *J Rheumatol* 1987;14:129–134.

34. Small P. Giant cell arteritis presenting as a bilateral stroke. *Arthritis Rheum* 1984;27:819–821.

35. Shapiro L, Medsger TA Jr, Nicholas JJ. Brachial plexitis mimicking C5 radiculopathy—A presentation of giant cell arteritis. *J Rheumatol* 1983;10:670–671.

36. Nesher G, Rosenberg P, Shorer Z, Gilai A, Solomonovich A, Sonnenblick M. Involvement of the peripheral nervous system in temporal arteritis-polymyalgia rheumatica. Report of 3 cases and review of the literature. *J Rheumatol* 1987;14:358–360.

37. Sánchez MC, Arenillas JIC, Gutierrez DA, Alonso JLG, Alvarez JDP. Cervical radiculopathy: a rare symptom of giant cell arteritis. *Arthritis Rheum* 1983;26:207–209.

38. Wolfovitz E, Levy Y, Brook JG. Sudden deafness in a patient with temporal arteritis. *J Rheumatol* 1987;14:384–385.

39. Sheehan MM, Keohane C, Twomey C. Fatal vertebral giant cell arteritis. *J Clin Pathol* 1993;46:1129–1131.

40. Luzar MJ, Whisler RL, Hunder GG. Syndrome of inappropriate antidiuretic hormone secretion in association with temporal arteritis. *J Rheumatol* 1982;9:957–960.

41. Dautzenberg PL, Leijtens JP. Reversible perfusion disorder on brain SPECT after treatment with prednisone in temporal arteritis. *Clin Nucl Med* 1995;20:463–464.

42. Lie JT, Tokugawa DA. Bilateral lower limb gangrene and stroke as initial manifestations of systemic giant cell arteritis in an African-American. *J Rheumatol* 1995;22:363–366.

43. Tomer Y, Neufeld MY, Shoenfeld Y. Coma with triphasic wave pattern in EEG as a complication of temporal arteritis. *Neurology* 1992;42:439–440.

44. Pascuzzi RM, Roos KL, Davis TE Jr. Mental status abnormalities in temporal arteritis: a treatable cause of dementia in the elderly. *Arthritis Rheum* 1989;32:1308–1311.

45. Caselli RJ. Giant cell (temporal) arteritis: a treatable cause of multi-infarct dementia. *Neurology* 1990;40:753–755.

46. Thomson GTD, Johnston JL, Sharpe JA, Inman RD. Internuclear ophthalmoplegia in giant cell arteritis. *J Rheumatol* 1989;16:693–695.

47. Dashefsky SM, Cooperberg PL, Harrison PB, Reid JDS, Araki DN. Total occlusion of the common carotid artery with patent internal carotid artery. Identification with color flow Doppler imaging. *J Ultrasound Med* 1991;10:417–421.

48. Büttner T, Heye N, Przuntek H. Temporal arteritis with cerebral complications: report of four cases. *Eur Neurol* 1994;34:162–167.

49. Fruchter O, Ben-Ami H, Schapira D, Gallimidi Z, Gaitini D, Goldsher D. Giant cell arteritis complicated by spinal cord infarction: a therapeutic dilemma. *J Rheumatol* 2002;29:1556–1558.

50. Hellmann DB. Occult manifestations of giant cell arteritis. *Med Rounds* 1989;2:296–301.

51. Fitzcharles M-A, Esdaile JM. Atypical presentations of polymyalgia rheumatica. *Arthritis Rheum* 1990;33:403–406.

52. Healey LA, Wilske KR. Presentation of occult giant cell arteritis. *Arthritis Rheum* 1980;23:641–643.

53. Calamia KT, Hunder GG. Giant cell arteritis (temporal arteritis) presenting as fever of undetermined origin. *Arthritis Rheum* 1981;24:1414–1418.

54. Larson TS, Hall S, Hepper NGG, Hunder GG. Respiratory tract symptoms as a clue to giant cell arteritis. *Ann Intern Med* 1984;101:594–597.

55. Klein RG, Hunder GG, Stanson AW, Sheps SG. Large artery involvement in giant cell (temporal) arteritis. *Ann Intern Med* 1975;83:806–812.

56. Ninet JP, Bachet P, Dumontet CM, Du Colombier PBD, Stewart MD, Pasquier JH. Subclavian and axillary involvement in temporal arteritis and polymyalgia rheumatica. *Am J Med* 1990;88:13–20.

57. Evans JM, O'Fallon WM, Hunder GG. Increased evidence of aortic aneurysm and dissection in giant cell (temporal) arteritis. A population-based study. *Ann Intern Med* 1995;122:502–507.

58. Kohn NN. Giant cell arteritis of the female productive tract associated with temporal arteritis. *J Rheumatol* 1989;16:832–833.

59. Kariv R, Sidi Y, Gur H. Systemic vasculitis presenting as a tumorlike lesion. Four case reports and an analysis of 79 reported cases. *Medicine* 2000;79:349–359.

60. Smetana GW, Shmerling RH. Does this patient have temporal arteritis? *JAMA* 2002;287:92–101.

61. Salvarani C, Hunder GG. Giant cell arteritis with low erythrocyte sedimentation rate: frequency of occurrence in a population-based study. *Arthritis Care Res* 2001;45:140–145.

62. Wong RL, Korn JH. Temporal arteritis without an elevated erythrocyte sedimentation rate. Case report and review of the literature. *Am J Med* 1986;80:959–964.

63. Jundt JW, Mock D. Temporal arteritis with normal erythrocyte sedimentation rates presenting as occipital neuralgia. *Arthritis Rheum* 1991;34:217–223.

64. Wise CM, Agudelo CA, Chmelewski WL, McKnight KM. Temporal arteritis with low erythrocyte sedimentation rate: a review of five cases. *Arthritis Rheum* 1991;34:1571–1574.

65. Hall S, Lie JT, Kurland LT, Persellin S, O'Brien PC, Hunder GG. The therapeutic impact of temporal artery biopsy. *Lancet* 1983;26:1217–1220.

66. Klein RG, Campbell RJ, Hunder GG, Carney JA. Skip lesions in temporal arteritis. *Mayo Clin Proc* 1976;51:504–510.

67. Kattah JC, Cupps T, Manz HJ, Khodary AE, Caputy A. Occipital artery biopsy: a diagnostic alternative in giant cell arteritis. *Neurology* 1991;41:949–950.

68. Schmidt WA, Kraft HE, Vorpahl K, et al. Color duplex ultrasonography in the diagnosis of temporal arteritis. *N Engl J Med* 1997;6:337:1336–1342.

69. Salvarani C, Silingardi M, Ghirarduzzi A, et al. Is duplex ultrasonography useful for the diagnosis of giant cell arteritis? *Ann Intern Med* 2002;137:232–238.

70. Atalay MK, Bluemke DA. Magnetic resonance imaging of large vessel vasculitis. *Curr Opin Rheumatol* 2001;13:41–47.

71. Mitomo T, Funyu T, Takahashi Y, et al. Giant cell arteritis and magnetic resonance angiography. *Arthritis Rheum* 1998;41:1702.

72. Liu GT, Glaser JS, Schatz NJ, Smith JL. Visual morbidity in giant cell arteritis. Clinical characteristics and prognosis for vision. *Ophthalmology* 1994;101:1779–1785.

73. Hayreh SS. Steroid therapy for visual loss in patients with giant-cell arteritis. *Lancet* 2000;355:1572–1573.

74. Myles AB, Perera T, Ridley MG. Prevention of blindness in giant cell arteritis by corticosteroid treatment. *Br J Rheumatol* 1992;31:103–105.

75. Aiello PD, Trautmann JC, McPhee TJ, Kunselman AR, Hunder GG. Visual prognosis in giant cell arteritis. *Ophthalmology* 1993;100:550–555.

76. Bengtsson B-Å, Malmvall B-E. An alternate-day corticosteroid regimen in maintenance therapy of giant cell arteritis. *Acta Med Scand* 1981;209:347–350.

77. Jover JA, Hernández-Garcia C, Morado IC, et al. Combined therapy of giant-cell arteritis with methotrexate and prednisone. *Ann Intern Med* 2001;134:106–114.

78. Hoffman GS, Cid MC, Hellmann DB, et al. A multicenter randomized, double-blind, placebo controlled trial of adjuvant methotrexate for giant cell arteritis. *Arthrit Rheum* 2002;46:1309–1318.

79. Silva MD, Hazleman BL. Azathioprine in giant cell arteritis/polymyalgia rheumatica: a double-blind study. *Ann Rheum Dis* 1986;45:136–138.

80. Matteson EL, Gold KN, Bloch DA, Hunder GG. Long-term survival of patients with giant cell arteritis in the American College of Rheumatology Giant Cell Arteritis Classification Criteria Cohort. *Am J Med* 1996;100:193–196.

26 Neurologic Basis of Common Pelvic Floor Disorders

Linda Brubaker, MD, FACOG, FACS and J. Thomas Benson, MD

The neural regulation of pelvic viscera is critical to normal bowel and bladder control as well as to anatomic support of the pelvic viscera. In the presence of local or systemic neural disorders, pelvic floor problems may become clinically apparent. Thus, the clinical neurologist should have a working knowledge of the neural contribution to common pelvic floor disorders in women. Such pelvic floor problems include abnormal bowel and bladder control, as well as pelvic organ prolapse.

The neurologist and urogynecologist contribute special expertise in the treatment of two groups of patients: patients with established neurologic disease and coexisting bowel or bladder dysfunction, and patients with diagnosed pelvic dysfunction and suspected but undiagnosed neurologic problems. The significance of neuropathy as an element in urinary and fecal incontinence is well recognized (1,2). The chief cause of this neuropathy is vaginal delivery. In normal vaginal deliveries, the perineal pressure may reach 240 mm Hg (3), and it is known that 80 mm Hg is sufficient to stop axonal blood flow, causing ischemic nerve damage. Likewise, nerve stretch over 15% of the original length can induce neuropathy. The pudendal nerve, in particular, is anatomically vulnerable to the stretch and compressive forces during vaginal delivery. Clinical studies have demonstrated that 80% of women have measurable pudendal neuropathy following a single vaginal delivery (4). This damage persists for at least 5 years in one-third of women (5).

This chapter focuses on the specific entities of urinary incontinence, urinary retention, and fecal incontinence, as well as those known neurologic entities that have pelvic floor manifestations.

INCIDENCE OF PELVIC FLOOR DISORDERS

It is well recognized that patients with congenital or acquired spinal cord injury are likely to have abnormalities in bowel and/or bladder control. Furthermore, these disorders are quite common in the ambulatory population. Urinary incontinence, which is a social and hygienic problem, is estimated to affect at least 10 million American women throughout the age span, with an increasing incidence and prevalence with aging (6). Approximately 11% of American women will undergo surgery for urinary incontinence and/or pelvic organ prolapse (7). Many more women will either receive medical treatment or suffer in silence. Urinary retention, although less common than urinary incontinence, poses a significant risk to affected women. Ineffective bladder emptying increases the risk of urinary tract infection, and in an important subset of patients, it increases the risk of renal damage. A paucity of information exists about the incidence and

367

prevalence of fecal incontinence; however, conservative estimates suggest that one in every five patients who has urinary incontinence also suffers from some degree of fecal incontinence (8). An additional patient group has primary fecal incontinence with concomitant disturbance of the lower urinary tract. The physician's level of understanding regarding these disorders greatly enhances the patient's opportunity for appropriate evaluation, treatment, and alleviation of some of the more socially disabling conditions.

ANATOMY

The following section focuses on the neuromuscular regulation that is critical for normal bowel and bladder control. In the healthy adult, the neural pathway is complete and appropriately myelinated, which allows the lower urinary tract and the anorectum to be under central nervous system (CNS) control.

The lower bowel and bladder are supported primarily by the levator ani muscle. This large pelvic muscle provides visceral support and an important sling-like function that is critical for fecal continence. This muscle is innervated by a direct sacral branch (nerve to the levator ani). Recent anatomic dissections have demonstrated that no pudendal nerve innervation of the levator ani is present (9). Loss of muscular function (through denervation or severe disuse atrophy) frequently results in loss of normal visceral support and function. Connective tissue supports exist in the pelvis (endopelvic fascia), but they are secondary support structures. It is important to realize that with significant anatomic support abnormalities, visceral function may become abnormal despite a normal or near-normal neural system.

NORMAL VOIDING AND DEFECATION

Normal voiding and defecation are under voluntary cortical control. Discrete areas within the brain provide for the upper motor neuron control of the urinary and anal sphincters, as well as the detrusor muscle. In particular, the precentral gyrus, lateral prefrontal cortex (especially the right side), anterior cingulate gyrus of the cortex, basal ganglia, brainstem raphe nuclei, locus ceruleus, hypothalamus, midbrain aqueductal gray, and medial and lateral pons are areas of involvement of reflex pathways for the lower urinary tract (10).

The muscular components of the urinary and anal sphincters include both smooth and skeletal muscle. The skeletal muscle is supplied primarily by the somatic branches of the peripheral pudendal nerve, originating from S3 and S4, with occasional S2 contributions. These cell bodies reside within Onuf's nucleus (Figure 26.1).

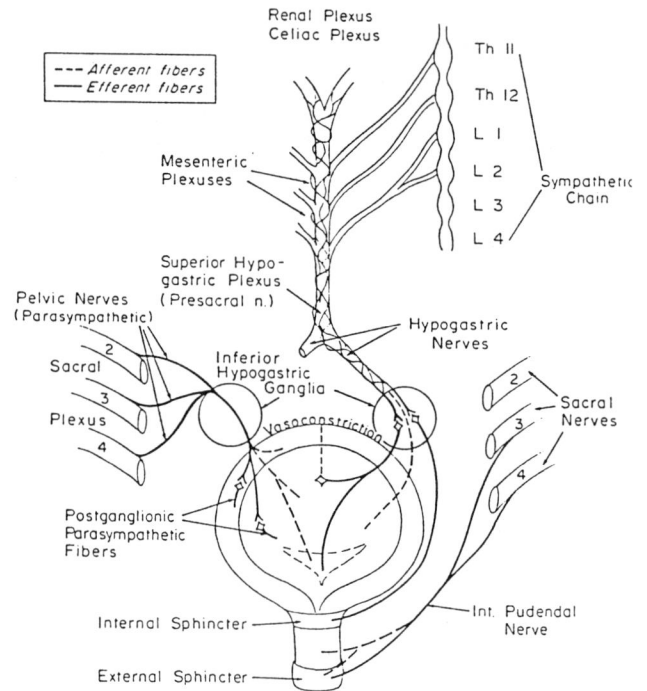

FIGURE 26.1

Innervation of the urinary bladder and its sphincters.

The normal female urethra is approximately 4 cm in length. The muscular composition of the urinary sphincter includes both smooth and skeletal muscle, but the precise ratios are not known. The smooth muscle is present throughout almost the entire urethral length, whereas the circumferential band of skeletal muscle is located predominantly in the central portion. The skeletal muscle consists entirely of type I fibers.

The anal sphincter is approximately 3 to 5 cm in length, and the smooth muscle component accounts for 80% of the total anal pressure. The skeletal muscle component is composed primarily of slow, type I fibers with relatively rare fast-twitch fibers. These discrete sphincteric fibers also receive contributions from the puborectalis portion of the levator ani muscle, a critically important structure for fecal continence. These muscles also receive a dual nerve supply: The puborectalis is innervated through the pelvic plexus, primarily from above, whereas the sphincter musculature, which is an embryologic cloacal structure, receives innervation from the pudendal nerve below (Table 26.1).

Autonomic innervation to the smooth musculature of the colon and anal canal has similarities to the lower urinary tract in that, generally speaking, the parasympathetic system modulates smooth muscle contraction in the gut for elimination (peristalsis), and stimulation of the sympathetic nerves favors storage. At the internal anal sphincter, the alpha sympathetic stimulation causes con-

TABLE 26.1
Mechanisms of Sphincter Function

	Anatomic Length	Muscle Components	Somatic Nerve Supply	Intrinsic Reflexes
Urethral	4 cm	Smooth and skeletal	Pudendal (perineal branch)	None described
Anal	3–4 cm	Smooth and skeletal	Pudendal (inferior hemorrhoidal branch)	Anorectal inhibitory reflex

traction and the parasympathetics promote relaxation of the smooth muscle.

An important difference between the colon and urinary innervation is that the colon sympathetic inhibition is not a supraspinal or spinal afferent reflex but consists of lumbar cord endogenous circuits. The colon and bladder neurons have different locations in the sacral parasympathetics. Defecation is triggered by C-fiber, unmyelinated afferents, whereas micturition is triggered by a-delta myelinated afferents, which become replaced by C-fiber activity after spinal section, urethral obstruction or bladder irritation. Thus, C-fiber afferentation is developed as a common response of the lower urinary tract to various insults. This response is indicative of neuronal plasticity and is abolished if nerve growth factor is not present (11).

Normal bowel and bladder control relies on the appropriate sensation of visceral filling and the intact motor response of the sphincters. Visceral afferent pathways are involved in remarkable abilities—anorectal sensation that can distinguish among features of gas, liquid, or solid stool; and in the urinary tract, perception of discrete, subtle differences in sensation involved in filling, fullness, desire to micturate, urgency, and pain. Afferents from pelvic viscera go through pelvic and hypogastric pathways to the afferent nerve cell bodies which, similar to the somatic sensory neurons, are located in the dorsal root ganglia. Spinal cord transmission is complex, with involvement of the dorsal, lateral, and ventral columns.

The smooth muscle (detrusor) of the bladder is innervated autonomically and functions as a compliant reservoir (increasing volume with low pressure) for the storage of urine. During storage, the detrusor muscle is under the inhibitory influence of the sympathetic system. Parasympathetic stimulation causes detrusor contraction. The sensation of bladder filling is perceived primarily by stretch receptors in the smooth muscle of the detrusor. In the healthy adult, the perceived urge to urinate may be effectively delayed. The urinary sphincter promotes urinary storage by actively contracting and maintaining a higher pressure in the urethra than in the bladder.

For normal voiding, the urinary sphincter relaxes and a detrusor contraction of sufficient strength and dura-

tion occurs, effectively emptying the bladder. After voiding, the urethral sphincter regains its activity and the detrusor returns to its low-pressure reservoir state. This coordination between the urethral sphincter and the detrusor muscle is critical for normal voiding and is neurally regulated in the pons. The area of the pons exerting such regulation is called the "M" region, the pontine micturition center (PMC), or the "Barrington's nucleus" and leads to the coordination of sacral cord parasympathetic preganglionic neurons and the nucleus of Onuf motor neurons to the sphincter. The PMC neurons are glutaminergic, excitatory to sacral parasympathetic neurons that produce bladder contraction; PMC terminals on the sacral dorsal commissural gray contact are inhibitory gamma-aminobutyric acid (GABA) neurons that inhibit Onuf neurons to the sphincter. The "on-off" glutaminergic and GABA activities are modulated by norepinephrine and serotonin. Contraction of the pelvic floor musculature is controlled by another group of neurons in the pons, the "L" region.

The autonomic nervous system is also involved in sphincteric function, with sympathetic stimulation (alpha receptors) increasing urethral sphincter smooth muscle closure and facilitating urinary storage by inhibiting parasympathetic bladder detrusor muscle contraction. A malfunction in these systems can lead to urinary incontinence and/or retention.

Lower bowel function has many similarities to lower urinary tract function, but there are some important differences. Anal continence is maintained through an elaborate neuromuscular interaction with visceral function. Like the bladder, the rectum acts as a compliant reservoir. With distention of the rectum, the rectal anal inhibitory reflex decreases the resting pressure of the anal canal. This rectal anal inhibitory reflex is intrinsic in the bowel wall and is absent in localized failure of myenteric plexus development (Hirschsprung disease). The contents of the rectum then enter the anal canal, wherein an elaborate sensory nerve plexus, together with sensors in the levator ani musculature, provide "sampling" of the rectal contents in order to distinguish gas, liquid, and solid. After sampling, if voluntary assessment is made that it is an inopportune time for emptying, external anal sphincter contraction, including the puborectalis muscle, again places the contents into the rectum for further storage. The puborectalis muscle helps in the formation of the anorectal angle with an anterior/posterior "kink," and the intra-abdominal downward pressure maintains this angle. The puborectalis muscle and external anal sphincter are in a state of tonic contraction.

To allow defecation, relaxation of the puborectalis and external anal sphincter occurs, followed by straightening of the anorectal angle, and with an associated Valsalva maneuver, increases in intra-abdominal pressure, and some involuntary smooth muscle activity in the bowel wall, evacuation may proceed.

SPECIFIC DISORDERS

Urinary Incontinence

Urinary incontinence is a symptom, not a diagnosis. The evaluation should follow a systematic approach to achieve a clinically appropriate understanding of the etiology (Figure 26.2). Given the complex neural control of normal urine storage and voiding, it is not unusual that patients who have local or systemic neurologic disease may present with urinary incontinence. Urinary incontinence may occur from a variety of causes.

It is essential that clinicians use accurate terminology for the diagnosis of urinary incontinence. Previously used terms, such as "neurogenic bladder," do not meet the current internationally accepted terminology and should be discarded (12). Simplistically, loss of urinary

control can occur from bladder muscle disorders, loss of urethral sphincteric integrity, or neural control of the continence systems, or a combination of these mechanisms. There are unusual causes for urinary incontinence, such as extraurethral incontinence (fistulas) and urethral diverticulum, which are not reviewed in this chapter.

A normal bladder muscle is characterized as "normoactive," that is, it maintains a low pressure during bladder filling and voids with a contraction of appropriate strength and duration to completely empty the bladder. Abnormalities in the detrusor muscle can cause uninhibited, inappropriate bladder contractions, which result in urinary leakage. This abnormality, which is called detrusor overactivity, can be documented by cystometrogram testing (Figure 26.3). Patients typically report symptoms of urinary urgency, urge incontinence, frequency, and nocturia. In the presence of a pertinent neurologic disorder, the diagnosis of "neurogenic detrusor overactivity" can be made. In the absence of any relevant neurologic disease, the clinician can make a diagnosis of detrusor overactivity. Older terminology, such as detrusor dyssynergia and neurogenic bladder, should be replaced with this current nomenclature.

It is important that the urethral sphincter response to a bladder contraction be characterized. During normal voiding, the urethral sphincter relaxes under the influence of the pons. A loss of "coordinated" voiding (urethral contraction during detrusor contraction) is termed detrusor-sphincter dyssynergia and is pathognomonic for a lesion between the pons and the bladder. Thus, the diagnosis of detrusor-sphincter dyssynergia is important for the detection of previously undiscovered neurologic disease. This

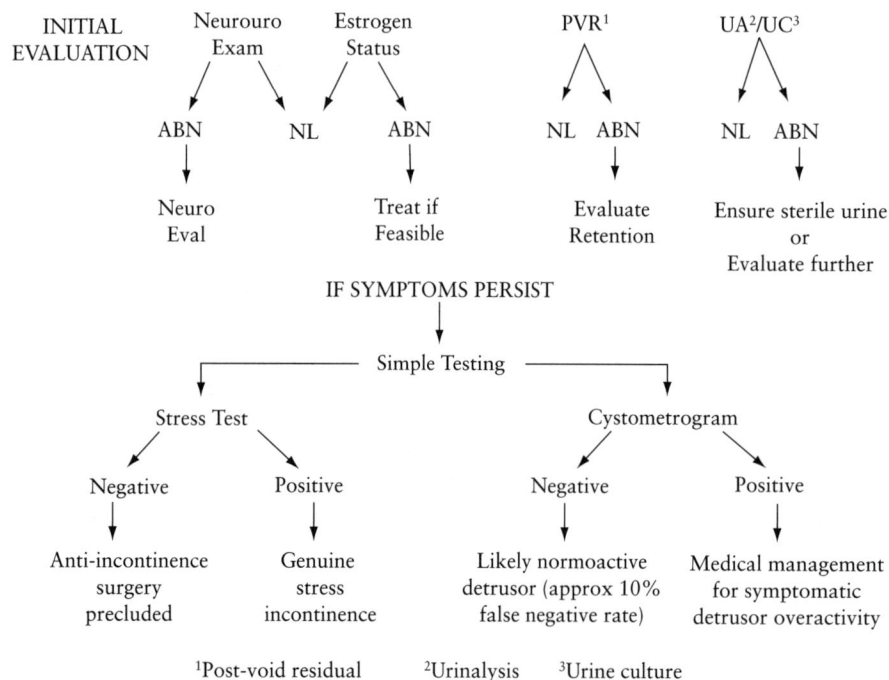

FIGURE 26.2

Flow diagram of initial testing for urinary incontinence.

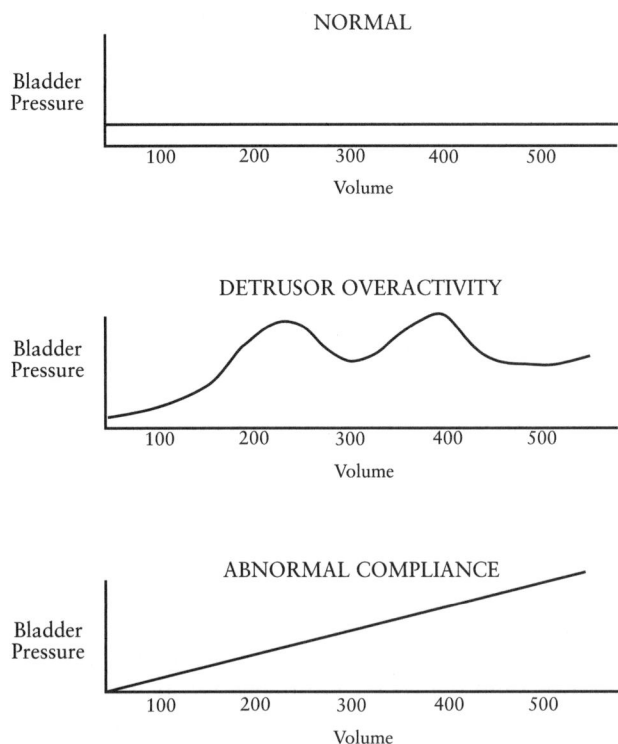

NORMAL

Bladder Pressure

100   200   300   400   500

Volume

DETRUSOR OVERACTIVITY

Bladder Pressure

100   200   300   400   500

Volume

ABNORMAL COMPLIANCE

Bladder Pressure

100   200   300   400   500

Volume

FIGURE 26.3

Normal and abnormal cystometrogram tracings.

can be clearly confirmed or refuted with needle electromyography (EMG) of the urethra during voiding.

Abnormalities in visceral sensation may contribute to incontinence by allowing filling to nonphysiologic bladder volumes. Patients may describe a loss of sensation during filling or insensible urinary loss. This also can be assessed objectively during some forms of urodynamic testing, as well as by neurophysiologic tests, which are described later in this chapter.

A second form of urinary incontinence is stress incontinence. Patients who have this disorder typically present with the symptom of loss of urine during moments of increased abdominal pressure (cough, sneeze). In patients with stress incontinence, the urethral sphincter does not perform its function of holding back urine that is in the bladder. This may occur because the sphincter is at an anatomic disadvantage (urethral hypermobility) or because the intrinsic neuromuscular components of the sphincter are abnormal. Not uncommonly, elements of neuromuscular abnormalities may be combined with anatomic support deficits. The internationally recommended term "urodynamic stress incontinence" indicates stress-induced, transurethral urine loss that occurs in the absence of a bladder contraction. Assessment of the sphincteric function is an important area of active neurophysiologic investigation. Urodynamic studies using concentric needle EMG of the urethra demonstrate a difference between stress incontinent women and those who are stress continent (13).

Urinary Retention

Urinary retention is a symptom of an underlying abnormality that causes the incomplete expulsion of urine. The abnormality may lie in the detrusor muscle itself. This is relatively common in older patients who have detrusor insufficiency; that is, the smooth muscle of the detrusor does not contract with adequate force or duration to completely empty the bladder. Neural control mechanisms influence the efficacy of the detrusor contraction, however. When these mechanisms are destroyed, the term detrusor areflexia is used. This is also known as an acontractile bladder. To demonstrate an acontractile bladder, there must be no detrusor activity whatsoever under any circumstance. Bethanecol denervation testing is appropriate when this diagnosis is entertained.

A second important form of urinary retention occurs in patients who have spinal cord disease or involvement of the pontine area of the brain stem that is responsible for coordinating active urination. Patients with detrusor-sphincter dyssynergia have detrusor contractions that are met with inappropriate urethral contraction, which leads to ineffective voiding and urinary retention. The diagnosis of detrusor-sphincter dyssynergia requires a demonstration of simultaneous detrusor contraction and urethral activation.

Fecal Incontinence

Fecal incontinence has many etiologies. Problems that result in loss of liquid stool may be produced by infection or inflammatory bowel disease, irritable bowel, rapid colon transit, or small bowel dysfunction, such as lactase deficiency. A rectum that has an inadequate reservoir is present in inflammatory bowel disease, cancer, pelvic masses, pelvic adhesions, and scleroderma. Inadequate rectal sensation may result from neurologic injury that leads to a sensory deficit with improper interpretation of the sensations, or fecal impaction, which is one of the leading causes of anal incontinence in nursing homes. Fecal incontinence may be associated with defects in neuromuscular function. Childbirth causes direct injury to the sphincter muscles, but also causes direct and indirect injury to the pelvic and/or pudendal nerves. Surgical sphincter injury following fistula repair is common, and traumatic sphincteric injury is also seen.

The neuropathy associated with fecal incontinence is most commonly a mononeuropathy involving the pudendal nerve and/or pelvic plexus as a result of mechanical injury. Other types of neuropathic processes, however, are associated with anorectal dysfunction. These are reviewed in the following section.

INITIAL EVALUATION

Patients who present with pelvic floor complaints have directed neurologic examinations for mental status, tremor, posterior column deficits (vibration and position senses), peripheral sensation, and gait (including postural reflexes). Pelvic neurologic clinical examination includes evaluating the sacral 2, 3, and 4 dermatomes, knee and ankle reflexes, bulbocavernosus reflex, and tone of pelvic floor sphincter musculature.

Clinical Neurophysiologic Studies

A function of the World Health Organization, the 2nd International Consultation on Incontinence, was held in Paris, France, July 1–3, 2001. A subcommittee of this was the Clinical Neurophysiology Committee (14), which attempted to determine current clinical and research applications of the various techniques for pelvic floor neurophysiologic investigation.

The committee opinion included the following: "The information gained by clinical examination and urodynamic testing may be enhanced by uroneurophysiological tests in selected patient groups. It seems that tests have often been performed by non-neurophysiologists in research but for routine diagnostics, an established service would seem necessary, and the physicians performing the tests should be appropriately trained, as required by national policies. As a rule, the service should be in liaison with general clinical neurophysiology. It seems optimal to create interdisciplinary programs between urology, urogynecology, and neurology departments. Eventually, 'neurourology' or 'uroneurology' sections should provide the appropriate setting for testing of the individual patient to be performed within a wider scope of clinical evaluation, and treatment. Such specialized teams, sections, or even departments within larger institutions are as yet few, but the organization of such teams in tertiary medical centres should be encouraged."

Appropriate clinical neurophysiologic studies are indicated when sensory or reflex abnormalities are noted in the clinical examination. Such neurophysiologic studies are performed to clarify the neurologic diagnosis and to determine the need for anatomic studies such as magnetic resonance imaging (MRI). Abnormalities on urodynamic study that can lead to clinical neurophysiologic studies include storage abnormalities with accommodation loss or sensory abnormality, and voiding disorders, particularly detrusor-sphincter dyssynergia, detrusor areflexia, or overflow incontinence. The clinical neurophysiologic studies help document the degree of sphincter neuropathy in order to select an appropriate surgical intervention. The preoperative degree of anal sphincter neuropathy is also related to the outcome of sphincteroplasty surgery.

SPECIFIC NEUROLOGIC DISORDERS

The neurologist may consider the pathophysiologic processes relating to pelvic floor dysfunction as processes that involve somatic motor or sensory nerves or visceral nerves. Somatic motor nerve pathology may include nerve damage occurring at any point from the anterior horn cell via the nerve root, the plexus, the peripheral nerves, or the neuromuscular junction and muscle fibers.

Lumbosacral radiculopathies commonly involve bladder and bowel dysfunction. In fact, bladder and bowel involvement is a clinical marker that distinguishes radiculopathy from anterior horn cell disease. The S2–S4 nerve roots going to the pelvis originate in the small terminal portion of the spinal cord (conus medularis) and constitute the central portion of the cauda equina (Table 26.2).

Cauda equina lesions are very common, with central disc protrusion affecting nerve roots to the bladder and bowel. Many clinicians consider this to be a major indication for disc surgery. Cauda equina lesions are seen with congenital caudal aplasia (in children of diabetic mothers) and congenital and acquired spinal stenosis (pseudoclaudication syndrome). Ankylosing spondylitis, schwannomas, primary and metastatic malignancies, lymphomas, meningiomas, neural fibromas, chordomas, acquired immunodeficiency syndrome (AIDS), and cytomegalovirus (CMV) infection are other causes of cauda equina disease.

Conus medularis lesions may be produced by ankylosing spondylitis, epidendymomas, lipomas, dermoid cysts, transverse myelitis, arteriovenous malformations, and congenital meningomyelocele with cord tethering. It is a fairly common complication of abdominal aortic aneurysm surgery secondary to prolonged aortic clamping.

Transverse myelitis with neurologic features, including progressive areflexic paraplegia with loss of bowel and bladder function being a typical finding, is often of unknown and presumed inflammatory etiology, but it can also exist in mixed connective disease (15). Patients with tethered cord syndrome typically have dermatologic changes in the lumbosacral region, neurogenic foot deformities, and disturbed bladder function. Surgery in children before the onset of symptoms does have a place. (16) (11).

Bladder dysfunction is typically present in sacral agenesis, even if it is only unilateral, with absent detrusor contractility being the most common abnormality. Although surgery does not usually restore lost bladder function, surgery is indicated in the presence of deterioration of bladder or lower limb function to stop further deterioration (12).

Lumbosacral plexus lesions are most commonly associated with malignancies (uterine cervical cancer or rectal lymphoma), surgical or radiation damage, or hematomas. Mononeuropathies occur frequently in pelvic nerves secondary to injury that may be mechanical, thermal, elec-

TABLE 26.2
Neurologic Entities Causing Pelvic Dysfunction

Category	Causes	Clinical Features (may be variable)
Lumbosacral Radiculopathy	Disc protrusion Benign tumors Malignant tumors	Incontinence Unilateral sensory deficits
Cauda equina lesions	Disc protrusion Sacral agenesis Spinal stenosis Ankylosing spondylitis Schwannomas Malignancy Benign tumor Viral infection (HIV, CMV)	Sacral sensory deficits Patellar reflex loss—higher lesion Loss of Achilles tendon reflex—lower lesion Hypocontractile detrusor Asymmetric motor deficit with atrophy
Conus medullaris lesions	Disc protrusion Ankylosing spondylitis Epidendymomas Lipomas Dermoid cysts Transverse myelitis Arteriovenous malformation Congenital meningomyelocele with cord tethering Postoperative (aortic aneurysm surgery)	Loss of sacral reflexes Loss of Achilles tendon reflex Detrusor areflexia Sensory dissociation Symmetric, milder motor deficits More severe sphincter dysfunction

trical, radiation-related, vascular, granulomatous, or the result of primary or metastatic neoplastic lesions. The leading cause of pelvic mononeuropathy is the mechanical effect (compression and stretching) of vaginal delivery.

Pelvic nerve damage that is diffuse and bilaterally symmetric suggests possible polyneuropathy. Any of the established causes of polyneuropathy may equally affect the pelvic floor nerves. Generally, relatively little is known about the pathology of the effects of peripheral neuropathy on the autonomic nerves innervating the viscera because of the difficulties inherent in the histologic examination of the peripheral autonomic nerves. Recently, changes have been observed in fine axons in the bladder wall in diabetic subjects. Pathologic changes have also been observed in ganglia and in the nerve trunks, all of which may be important in the development of urinary bladder dysfunction (18). With distal autonomic neuropathy, the innervation of the striated muscle of the urethra is apparently unaffected, even when there is almost total loss of nerves in the bladder muscularis. The subepithelial plexus of nerve tends to be preserved (19). Neurologic disease is frequently found in studies of voiding difficulties in human females (20).

Typically, the anterior horn cell diseases do not significantly involve Onuf's nucleus, reflecting the unique properties of these neurons. Single-fiber EMG comparisons of sphincter muscles with semimembranosus-semitendi-nosus muscles revealed that neurogenic change was more marked in the latter than in the external anal sphincter. The external anal sphincter is not normal in amyotrophic lateral sclerosis. However, there is a relative resistance of the external anal sphincter to amyotrophic lateral sclerosis that is sufficient to prevent incontinence, even in older patients who survive longer (21) (see also Chapter 20).

In most myopathies, sphincter muscles tend to be clinically spared. Incontinence is occasionally reported in Duchenne muscular dystrophy, although no patient demonstrates myopathic motor units in the sphincters. Urinary incontinence in Duchenne muscular dystrophy is most often due to upper motor neuron dysfunction, most likely caused by severe scoliosis or a complication of spinal fusion surgery (22) (see also Chapter 21).

Neuromuscular junction disorders, such as myasthenia gravis or myasthenic syndrome, typically have minor effects on sphincters. Myasthenia gravis has been known to present with uncontrollable flatus and fecal incontinence, albeit rarely (23).

Upper motor neuron lesions have a profound effect on motor nerves to the sphincters as well as on motor neurons to the bladder and bowel. Detrusor hyperreflexia is common after cerebrovascular accidents, particularly those involving the right side of the cortex, occurring in slightly less than 50% of patients (24). It is frequently asymptomatic.

Patients with Parkinson's disease frequently have detrusor hyperreflexia. Inadequate detrusor contractility has also been reported (25). A subset of patients with parkinsonism are those who have progressive autonomic failure and multiple system atrophy. These patients typically have incompetent bladder necks, and the striated muscle of the urethra is uniformly affected by marked denervation and reinnervation. These findings help distinguish patients with autonomic failure from those who have idiopathic Parkinson's disease (26).

In Parkinson's disease, the abnormalities of detrusor function are ascribed to abnormalities in the basal ganglia (27). Urodynamically, increased urethral sphincter activity with loss of coordination with the detrusor activity is typically seen with lesions below the pontine micturition center (Table 26.3).

Spinal cord disorders markedly affect pelvic floor function, as already outlined. In a series of patients with malignant extradural tumors of the spine who were operated on for decompression or back pain, approximately one-third of patients treated surgically had improved bladder function, but no patient with complete paraplegia gained useful neurologic recovery (28). Putty and coworkers report a series of spinal cord injury patients who had dorsal longitudinal myelotomy to treat spasticity. Although successful in providing relief of painful spasms, the procedure had no effect on bladder function (29).

In general, conus medullaris lesions have more symmetric bilateral loss of clitoral anal reflex along with S2–S4 dermatomal changes. Cauda equina lesions demonstrate varying symmetry with deficits in dermatome testing. Reflex changes may also occur. Typically, higher lesions result in absent knee reflexes, whereas a loss of Achilles tendon reflexes occurs with lower lesions.

Sensory nerve involvement also impacts pelvic floor function. The anatomic separation of the sensory nerve axon into proximal and distal segments is used during electrodiagnostic tests to localize disease processes. The peripheral sensory nerve has a greater capacity for repair and remyelination than does the proximal portion of the nerve, which lies within the CNS. Certain processes have a predilection for sensory nerves and even particular sensory nerve fiber sizes. Fecal or urinary incontinence due

TABLE 26.3
Specific Disorders of Micturition Control

Terminology	Definition	Symptom	Causes	Investigations	Treatment
Detrusor instability	Inappropriate phasic detrusor contractions (no known neurologic disorder)	Nocturia Urgency Frequency Urge incontinence	Idiopathic	Cystometrogram	Behavioral Electrical stimulation Pharmacotherapy
Detrusor hyperreflexia	Inappropriate phasic detrusor contractions with known, relevant neurologic disorder	Nocturia Urgency Frequency Urge incontinence	Pertinent neurologic disorder (e.g., stroke)	Cystometrogram Electrodiagnostic testing	Behavioral Electrical stimulation Pharmacotherapy
Detrusor-sphincter dyssynergia	Simultaneous detrusor contraction with urethral sphincter activation during voiding effort	Urinary retention Post-void fullness	Spinal cord or brain stem lesions involving CNS below pontine micturition center	Urethral needle EMG during urodynamic study	Pharmacotherapy (a-blocker, small muscle relaxant) Self-catheterization Other drainage techniques
Urodynamic stress incontinence	Transurethral loss of urine during increase in abdominal pressure in absence of detrusor contraction	Stress incontinence		Anatomic displacement of urethral sphincter Intrinsic neuromuscular dysfunction of urethral sphincter	Urodynamics Pharmacotherapy Surgery

to sensory loss is difficult to treat, and surgery has disappointing results. Friedreich's ataxia, vitamin B12 deficiency, and occasionally subacute sensory neuropathies tend to produce large fiber loss, whereas predominantly small fiber loss is seen in hereditary sensory neuropathy (type I), diabetes, leprosy, amyloidosis, Tangier's disease, Fabry's disease, and congenital insensitivity to pain. Visceral motor dysfunction occurs most commonly secondary to diabetic neuropathy. Generalized autonomic syndromes involve bladder and bowel dysfunction. The syndromes are "pure cholinergic dysfunction," characterized by bladder atony, Adie's pupil, alacrima, constipation, dry mouth, hyperpyrexia; cardiovagal failure, and impotence. Etiologies include Lambert-Eaton (myasthenia) syndrome and neuromuscular junction toxicity from organic phosphates in insecticides or botulinum toxin in improperly canned food.

In acute inflammatory demyelinating polyradiculoneuropathy (Guillain-Barré syndrome), urinary retention early in the course of the disease is a predictor of disease severity; more than 80% of patients with early urinary retention later require ventilatory assistance (30). Acute intermittent porphyria is an autosomal dominant disease that generally presents in the third or fourth decade with premenstrual abdominal pain, constipation, voiding dysfunction, quadriparesis, and "bathing trunk" dysesthesia. Generalized sympathetic disorders tend to be length-dependent and are characterized by early postural hypotension and overactivity, with cold, sweaty feet, and later loss of activity, with red, swollen, anhidrotic distal extremities.

Disease processes that affect small sensory nerves and autonomic nerves can similarly affect visceral afferent nerves. Clinical manifestations include overflow incontinence or megacolon with loss of the visceral reflexes necessary for proper function.

TESTS

Normative Values

One of the difficulties in electrodiagnostic testing in pelvic floor disorders is the paucity of normative values. Collection of such data requires dichotomous definitions—normal versus abnormal. Vaginally parous women typically have some birth-induced alterations, but may be entirely asymptomatic. Table 26.4 displays the known data sets for normative data in the pelvic floor.

Table 26.5 demonstrates anal sphincter data obtained with three different techniques of motor unit action potential (MUAP) analysis. Although the data obtained by Podnar et al. differ slightly from that of Weidner et al. it may be important to weigh these differences against the pragmatic approach of data acquisition using multi-MUAP technology.

TABLE 26.4
Motor Unit Action Potential Analysis (31)

Test	Value
EMG (Quant) External Anal Sphincter	
Amplitude (mV)	0.37 + 0.13
Duration (ms)	8.27 + 2.5
Phases (No.)	3.77 + 0.9
Turns (No.)	2.28 + 0.4
Area (mV/ms)	0.36 + 0.2
Amplitude-area ratio (ms)	0.91 + 0.4
Polyphasic motor units (%)	21.6 + 17.1
EMG (Quant) Levator Ani Muscle	
Amplitude (mV)	0.48 + 0.2
Duration (ms)	10.40 + 2.2
Phases (No.)	3.70 + 1.0
Turns (No.)	2.80 + 0.8
Area (mV/ms)	0.65 + 0.3
Amplitude-area ratio (ms)	1.4 + 0.3
Polyphasic motor units (%)	29.8 + 17.7
Interference Pattern Analysis	
External Sphincter	
Turns per sec (No.)	183.9 + 90
Amplitude (μV)	225.3 + 39.4
Activity	61.2 + 39.4
Envelope size (μV)	567.6 + 185.7
Small segments (No.)	81.4 + 51.8
Levator Ani	
Turns per sec (No.)	241.6 + 68.9
Amplitude (μV)	302.7 + 46.9
Activity	95.6 + 43.9
Envelope size (μV)	861.1 + 194
Small segments (No.)	105.8 + 55

Electromyography

Surface electrodes are used to monitor voluntary muscle contraction during kinesiologic studies such as in urodynamic testing or anal manometry. Surface electrodes may be applied to a Foley catheter to record or stimulate from the bladder base or proximal urethra. Various types of surface electrodes can be mounted on anal plugs or vaginal sponges.

Needle Electromyography

Needle EMG can give information concerning denervation, reinnervation, upper and lower motor neuron function, and the activity and time course of neurologic disease. In most skeletal muscles at rest, there is no electrical activity except for "spontaneous" activity. The constant firing of activity in the sphincters makes spontaneous activity assessment more difficult.

TABLE 26.5
Comparison of Methods for External Anal Sphincter MUAP Assessment (Podnar et al.) (32)

	Single MUAP	Manual MUAP	Multi-MUAP
MUAP parameter	Mean + SD	Mean + SD	Mean + SD
Amplitude (µV)	609 + 193	358 + 89	405 + 128
Log (amplitude)	2.77 + 0.13	2.54 + 0.11	2.59 + 0.14
Duration (ms)	7.0 + 1.4	6.6 + 1.0	5.5 + 1.1
Area (µV)	572 + 188	362 + 106	356 + 135
Thickness (ms)	0.95 + 0.14	1.03 + 0.16	0.85 + 0.14
Size index	0.28 + 0.31	−0.09 + 0.25	−0.20 + 0.3
Phases	3.4 + 0.5	3.2 + 0.4	3.0 + 0.4
Turns	3.4 + 0.6	3.0 + 0.5	2.9 + 0.5
Rise-time (ms)	0.79 + 0.24	0.80 + 0.21	0.53 + 0.05
Spike duration (ms)	3.5 + 0.9	5.6 +1.5	2.9 + 0.55

The number of fibers and fiber distribution of nerves innervating the urinary bladder and urethra in humans has been estimated by quantitative nerve analysis (33). The numbers are small, leading to the clinical implication that one intercostal nerve (containing 9,000 afferent nerves and 1,000 efferent nerves), with its dissectable skin, muscle, and mixed branches, contains enough myelinated fibers for a reinnervation of the detrusor (with 3,200 afferent nerves and 800 efferent nerves), the external anal and bladder sphincters (with 30 afferent nerves and 30 efferent nerves), the mucosa of the urethra, trigone, and anal canal (with 200 afferent nerves), and the lower sacral skin (with 6,000 afferent nerves).

The sacral roots to the urethra fire rhythmically. Alpha 3 motor neurons innervating slow fatigue-resistant muscle fibers fire at approximately 0.7 Hz, with impulse trains of 11 to 60 action potentials. Alpha 1 motor neurons are not observed. The alpha 2 motor neurons increase the mean activity from 0.5 to 18 Hz during filling by changing the firing pattern from the occasional spike mode to the continuous oscillatory mode. The activity decreases and overflow incontinence occurs at 800 cc (34).

Nerve Conduction Studies

Nerve conduction studies most commonly involve pudendal motor conduction. Pudendal studies are performed using a pudendal nerve stimulator mounted over a gloved hand. The electrode over the tip of the index finger is passed vaginally or rectally to lie at the level of the ischial spine. Electrodes at the base of the finger record the muscle action potential of the external anal sphincter. The pudendal motor nerve distal latency and amplitude of the compound muscle action potential can be checked for reproducibility.

The sacral reflexes that are used most often in our laboratory are the clitoral anal reflexes and urethral anal reflexes. Clinically, the clitoral anal reflex is obtained by touching the clitoral region with a cotton swab and observing contraction in the external anal sphincter. Ten percent of neurologically normal females do not have this reflex on physical examination, although it is present with electrodiagnostic testing. The reflex tests the afferent and efferent pudendal nerve pathways, hence the roots of the cauda equina and conus medullaris. It has two components, the first of which occurs at 30 to 50 msec latency, the second at 60 to 70 msec. The response may be selectively recorded on the left and right sides, and stimulation may likewise be done selectively on the left or right side. Localized lesions may be indicated as being either afferent or efferent and right or left. The reflex is suppressed during voiding, and failure of such suppression has been found to be highly sensitive in detecting spinal cord lesions above the sacral level (35). The intensity of stimulation used for the response is generally three to four times the intensity at perception threshold, which is normally less than 9 mA of constant current stimulation.

Urethral Anal Reflex

Using a catheter-mounted ring electrode for stimulation, a reflex response may be obtained at the right and left external anal sphincters. This has been termed urethral electromyelography by Bradley (36). The reflex has a long latency of approximately 60 msec because the very proximal urethral response is carried by small myelinated or unmyelinated pelvic and hypogastric nerves, and the pathway is multisynaptic. The sensory threshold is generally less than 13 mA, and the reflex requires a stimulus intensity of three times the sensory threshold. This reflex is suppressed during voiding. The test may also be performed by stimulating in the bladder to obtain a bladder-anal reflex. The reflex pathway duplicates the urethral-anal reflex but with separate afferent initiating sites.

Cortical Evoked Potentials

Recording electrodes are best placed in the midline, with the reference electrode midway between Fpz and Fz (Fpz') and one just posterior to the scalp vertex (Cpz). Recording is done over the spinal column, with one electrode over T12–L1 and the second over the iliac crest, or alternatively over the L5 vertebra. The initial component of this potential represents the afferent volley to the cauda equina, and the subsequent component represents the root entry zone/dorsal horns of the lower spinal cord; these allow calculation of the "peripheral" component of the evoked potential tests. The "central" component, then, is represented in the impulse transmission from the cord to the cortex. Peripherally, either tibial or pudendal stimulation can be used.

Pudendal Nerve Somatosensory Evoked Potentials

The stimulus may be applied to either the right or left clitoral region, with the anode lateral to the clitoris and the cathode adjacent to it. Cortical responses are reliably obtained in women, with the first positive peak between 35 and 43 msec, a latency very similar to that obtained in tibial nerve somatosensory evoked potentials when the posterior tibial at the ankle is stimulated. Recording over the spinal column is technically difficult in women.

Proximal Urethral Evoked Potential

By stimulating with a ring electrode on a Foley catheter, this produces waveforms with longer latencies (approximately 50 msec to the first positive peak). The responses are very small, and absence may be due to technical factors. Obtaining a response with normal latency is very valuable in excluding a subpontine neurogenic bladder disorder, however (30).

Autonomic Tests

Autonomic tests include quantitative sudomotor axon reflex test (QSART), sympathetic skin response, orthostatic blood pressure and heart rate responses to tilt, heart rate responses to deep breathing, and beat-to-beat blood pressure responses to Valsalva maneuver, tilt, and deep breathing.

Bethanechol Test for Vesical Denervation

A cystometrogram is recorded as a baseline control, recording bladder pressure to a volume of 100 cc. Bethanechol chloride 0.05 mg per kilogram filling fluid is injected subcutaneously, and postinjection cystometrograms are collected at 10, 20, and 30 minutes, performed in the same manner as the control cystometrogram. A positive test is an intravesical pressure increase of more than 15 cm of water over the control cystometrogram at 100 cc volume.

The Clinical Neurophysiology Committee of the 2nd International Consultation on Incontinence summarized the value of the respective tests, as indicated in Tables 26.6 and 26.7. The tests were judged by difficulty to perform, sensitivity for diagnosis, cost, and current use.

The tests of most clinical use at present are the kinetic and concentric needle EMG and the sacral reflex.

CONCLUSION

Bladder and bowel dysfunction can accompany neuromuscular disease. Clinical neurophysiologic testing provides unique information regarding these functions. Such testing is complementary to imaging and urodynamic studies. Patients who are particularly helped by electrophysiologic testing include those being evaluated for anal sphincter repair; those with voiding disorders, detrusor-sphincter dyssynergia, overflow incontinence, stress incon-

TABLE 26.6
Comparison of Tests Used in Incontinence Analysis (I) Committee Opinion Summary

Test	Difficulty	Sensitive	Cost	Use
kEMG	Low	Fair	$$	Good
CNEMG	High	Good	$$$	Good
SFEMG	High	Good	$$$	Poor
PNTML	Low	Fair	$$	Debated
Sacral stim	Moderate	Unknown	$$$	Research
Mag. stim	Moderate	Unknown	$$$	Poor
Q. sens.	Variable	Fair	$$	Research

kEMG = kinetic EMG
CNEMG = concentric needle EMG
SFEMG = single fiber EMG
PNTML = pudendal nerve terminal motor latency
Mag. = magnetic
Q. sens = quantitative sensory testing

TABLE 26.7
Comparison of Tests Used in Incontinence Analysis (II) Committee Opinion Summary

Test	Difficulty	Cost	Perform	Use
Pud. SEP	Moderate	$$	Good	Poor
Visceral SEP	Difficult	$$	Good	Research
Sacral reflex	Not difficult	$$	Good	Good
Viscero reflex	Moderate	$$$	Unknown	Research
Autonom.	Moderate	$$$	Fair	Research

Pud. SEP = pudendal somatosensory evoked potentials
Viscero reflex = urethral-anal reflex and bladder-anal reflex
Autonom. = autonomic tests

tinence (especially when intrinsic sphincter deficiency is suspected), spinal myelopathies, peripheral or autonomic neuropathies; diabetic patients with bladder or bowel symptoms; those with pelvic floor trauma from childbirth or other sacral injuries; and those with unexplained perineal numbness or pain, or with failure of diagnosis on standard evaluations for bladder or rectal dysfunction.

Neurologists have an important contribution to make to the clinical care of patients with pelvic floor abnormalities, particularly urinary and fecal incontinence. Awareness of the prevalence of these common disorders, as well as an understanding of the methods for evaluation and treatment, will improve patient care and facilitate communication among health care providers.

References

1. Parks AG, Swash M, Urich H. Sphincter denervation in anal rectal incontinence and rectal prolapse. *Gut* 1977; 18:656–665.
2. Beersiek F, Parks AG, Swash M. The pathogenesis of anal rectal incontinence. *J Neurolog Sci* 1974;42:111–127.
3. Rempen A, Kraus M. Measurement of head compression during labor: preliminary results. *J Perinatal Med* 1991;19:115–120.
4. Allen RE, Hosker GL, Smith ARB, et al. Pelvic floor damage in childbirth: a neurophysiologic study. *Brit J Obstet Gynecol* 1990;91:770–779.
5. Snooks SJ, Swash M, Matthews SE, et al. Effect of vaginal delivery on the pelvic floor: a 5-year follow up. *Brit J Surg* 1990;77:1358–1360.
6. Urinary Incontinence Guideline Panel. Urinary incontinence in adults: Clinical practice guidelines, 2nd ed. Rockville, MD: Agency for Health Care Policy and Research, Public Health Service, U.S. Department of Health and Human Services, 1996.
7. Olson AL, Smith VJ, Bergstrom JU, et al. Incidence and clinical characteristics of surgically managed pelvic organ prolapse and urinary incontinence. *Obstet Gynecol* 1997;89:501–506.
8. Haadem K, Dahlstrom JA, Bengtsson M, et al. Sphincter function in the urethra and the anal canal: A comparison in women with manifest urinary incontinence. *Int Urogynecol J* 1991;2:85–89.
9. Barber MD, Bremer RE, Thor KB, et al. Innervation of the female levator ani muscles *Am J Obstet Gynecol* 2002;187(1):64-71.
10. Blok BF, Holstege G. The central nervous system control of micturition in cats and humans. *Behav Brain Res* 1998;92(2):119–125.
11. Steers WD, Creedon D, Tuttle JB. Immunity to NGF prevents afferent plasticity following hypertrophy of the urinary bladder. *J Urol* 1996,155:378–385.
12. Abrams P, Cardozo L, Fall M, et al. Standardisation Sub-Committee of the International Continence Society. The standardisation of terminology in lower urinary tract function: report from the standardisation sub-committee of the International Continence Society.
13. Kenton K, Fitzgerald MP, Shott S, Brubaker L. Role of urethral electromyography in predicting outcome of Burch retropubic urethropexy. *Am J Obstet Gynecol* 2001;185:51–55.
14. Fowler CJ, Benson JT, Craggs MD, Vodusek DB, Yang CC, Podnar S. In: Abrams P, Cardoza L, Khoury K, Wein A, (eds.) *Incontinence*. Plymouth, UK: Health Publication Ltd, 2002.
15. Weiss TD, Nelson JS, Woolsey RM, et al. Transverse myelitis in mixed connective tissue disease. *Arthrit Rheum* 1978;21:982–986.
16. Zumkeller MB, Seifert V, Stolke D. Intraspinal lipoma with tethered cord syndrome in childhood. *Zeitschrift Fur Kinderchirurgie* 1988;43:384–390.
17. Saito M, Kondo A, Kato K. Diagnosis and treatment of neurogenic bladder due to partial sacral agenesis. *Brit J Urol* 1991;67:472–476.
18. Mastri AR. Neuropathology of diabetic neurogenic bladder. *Ann Intern Med* 1980;92:316–318.
19. Kirby RS. Studies of the neurogenic bladder. *Ann Royal Coll Surg Eng* 1988;70:285–288.
20. Stanton SL, Ozsoy C, Hilton P. Voiding difficulties in the female: Prevalence, clinical and urodynamic review. *Obstet Gynecol* 1983;61:144–147.
21. Arvalho M, Schwartz MS, Swash M. Involvement of the external anal sphincter in amyotrophic lateral sclerosis. *Muscle Nerve* 1995;18:848–853.
22. Caress JB, Kothari MJ, Bauer SB, et al. Urinary dysfunction in Duchenne muscular dystrophy. *Muscle Nerve* 1996;19:819–822.
23. Berger AR, Swerdlow M, Herskovitz S. Myasthenia gravis presenting as uncontrollable flatus and urinary/fecal incontinence. *Muscle Nerve* 1996;19:113–114.
24. Kong KH, Chan KF, Lim AC, et al. Detrusor hyperreflexia in strokes. *Ann Acad Med Sing* 1994;23:319–321.
25. Anderson JT, Hepjorn S, Frimodt-Moller C, et al. Disturbances of micturition in Parkinson's disease. *Acta Neurol Scand* 1976;53:161–170.
26. Kirby RS. Studies of the neurogenic bladder. *Ann Royal Coll Surg Engl* 1988;79:285–288.
27. Andersen JT, Bradley WE. Cystometric, sphincter and electromyelographic abnormalities in Parkinson's disease. *J Urol* 1976;116:75–78.
28. Turner PL, Prince HG, Webb JK, et al. Surgery for malignant extradural tumors of the spine. *J Bone Joint Surg Brit* 1988;70:451–455.
29. Putty TK, Shapiro SA. Efficacy of dorsilongitudinal myelotomy in treating spinal spasticity: A review of 20 cases. *J Neurosurg* 1991;75:397–401.
30. Ropper AH, Wijdicks EFM, Truaz BT. *Guillain-Barre syndrome. Contemporary neurology sciences*. Philadelphia: FA Davis, 1991.
31. Weidner AC, Sanders DB, Nandedkar SD, Bump RC. Quantitative electromyographic analysis of levator ani and external anal sphincter muscles of nulliparous women. *Am J Obstet Gynecol* 2000;183: 1249–1256.
32. Podner S, Vodusek DB, Stalberg E. Comparison of quantitative techniques in anal sphincter electromyography. *Muscle Nerve* 2002;25:83–92.
33. Schalow G. Number of fibers in fiber diameter distributions of nerves innervating the urinary bladder in humans. *Electromyography Clin Neurophysiol* 1992;32:187–196.
34. Schalow G. Oscillatory firing of single human sphincteric motor neurons. *Electromyography Clin Neurophysiol* 1991;31:323–355.
35. Dyro FM, Yalla SV. Refractoriness of urethral striated sphincter during voiding: studies with afferent pudendal reflex arc stimulation. *J Urol* 1986;135:732–736.
36. Bradley WE. Urethral electromyelography. *J Urol* 1972; 108:563–564.

27 Infections of the Nervous System in Women

David N. Irani, MD

The incidence, severity, and clinical manifestations of many diseases can vary between men and women. With regard to infections of the central nervous system (CNS), some diseases display a predilection for women, particularly during pregnancy, whereas others are less common in women than in men. Although incompletely understood, these differences may in part relate to the complex effects that female sex hormones exert on the cells of the immune system. This chapter updates the clinically relevant aspects of neurologic infections affecting women, including differences in the frequency, manifestations, prognosis, and management of these disorders. Consideration of the diagnosis and treatment of neurologic infections during pregnancy are addressed in particular detail.

THE FEMALE IMMUNE SYSTEM

Differences in the immune responses mounted by men and women against similar antigens have long been recognized. In general, cell-mediated immunity is relatively enhanced in men, whereas humoral or antibody-mediated immune responses are more easily elicited in women (1–7). Based on our current understanding of how these two types of immune responses are generated, this immunologic variability between the sexes is hypothesized to result from the differential activation of regulatory T lymphocytes. Studies in animals now confirm this hypothesis (8), and multiple lines of evidence suggest that estrogens in particular are responsible for the variability in immune responses between the sexes in humans (1–7). These differences may help account for the predominance of antibody-mediated autoimmune diseases such as rheumatoid arthritis (RA) and systemic lupus erythematosus (SLE) in females (3,6). They may also explain why women show particular clinical responses to certain infections that involve the CNS. Despite recent progress, however, a more complete understanding of the specific immunologic differences between the sexes remains to be achieved.

During pregnancy, the cellular immune responses important in graft rejection must be suppressed in order to prevent the maternal immune system from reacting to the many foreign antigens presented by the fetus and placenta (9,10). This immune tolerance is achieved through both a physical separation of the maternal and fetal circulations, as well as by the production of factors that exert modulatory effects on the maternal immune system. Placental syncytial trophoblasts produce a variety of hormones including progesterone, estrogen, chorionic gonadotropin, and cortisol-binding globulin that can cause immunosuppression (11). Cytokines derived from fetal lymphocytes and alpha-fetoprotein can also cross the placenta and alter maternal immune responses (12). Collectively, these factors suppress maternal cell-mediated immunity to a degree that protects the fetus. However, they also increase the maternal risk of infection particularly by intracellular pathogens that are eradicated via these same cell-mediated immune responses.

SUSCEPTIBILITY TO INFECTION DURING THE MENSTRUAL CYCLE

The rapid hormonal changes that occur during the menstrual cycle do not cause lasting effects on the immune system, and an increased susceptibility to CNS infection during any stage of the menstrual cycle remains unproven. The particular conditions of menstruation can result in toxic shock syndrome (TSS), however, a disorder characterized by high fever, profound hypotension, a diffuse erythematous rash, and varying degrees of vomiting, diarrhea, myalgias, and mental confusion without focal neurologic signs (13). Epidemiologic studies have linked the disease to the use of hyperabsorbable tampons; accordingly, it is rare in the pediatric population, in males, and in nonmenstruating females (14). TSS has recently been shown to be mediated by toxins released from strains of *Staphylococcus aureus* that can normally colonize the vagina but which proliferate under conditions promoted by the presence of these tampons (14).

Although it is not known whether TSS toxins have any direct effects on the CNS, the muscle pain and weakness that can accompany this disorder probably represent a toxin-mediated myositis (15). The cerebrospinal fluid (CSF) is abnormal in many TSS patients who show evidence of confusion or an altered sensorium; a pleocytosis of up to 100 cells per cubic millimeter and a protein elevation up to 75 milligrams per deciliter can occur (15). Although the glucose is usually normal and cultures are typically negative, these CSF abnormalities suggest that the CNS manifestations of TSS represent an encephalitis rather than simply a direct effect of bacterial toxins on the brain. Neuropsychologic sequelae, including memory and behavioral abnormalities, can persist for as long as a year following the acute illness, and electroencephalographic findings such as diffuse slowing and even epileptiform discharges may accompany these chronic disease manifestations (15). The acute management of TSS patients frequently necessitates their treatment in an intensive care unit, with prompt correction of hypotension and metabolic abnormalities as well as the administration of antistaphylococcal antibiotics. With appropriate management, mortality is less than 5% (14).

NEUROLOGIC INFECTIONS DURING PREGNANCY

As noted previously, the susceptibility of women to infection by certain intracellular pathogens increases during

pregnancy as cell-mediated immunity wanes. This may alter the frequency, severity, or clinical presentation of these illnesses. In addition, it must be remembered that certain antimicrobial drugs are relatively contraindicated during pregnancy, and the drugs of first choice for various CNS infections may need to be adjusted during this interval. Chloramphenicol and the tetracyclines, in particular, can adversely affect the fetus and should be avoided if possible. The problems associated with common antimicrobial drugs during pregnancy are summarized in Table 27.1, while treatment considerations are outlined in Table 27.2, and proposed treatment regimens for common CNS infections during pregnancy are listed in Table 27.3. Although the potential teratogenic and embryotoxic effects of all medications should be thoroughly investigated in prescription drug references, and their risks discussed with the patient before being administered, many of these infections are life-threatening events that often justify the risks associated with their use. The most important examples of these neurologic infections during pregnancy are considered individually below.

Tuberculosis (TB)

Although pregnancy itself does not alter the rate at which dormant *Mycobacterium tuberculosis* infections are reactivated, pulmonary TB is generally more severe during pregnancy (16). Furthermore, women with tuberculous meningitis during pregnancy have a higher morbidity and mortality than nonpregnant patients (17,18). Because the presenting signs and symptoms of TB meningitis are not themselves different in pregnancy, some have suggested that the worse outcome in pregnant patients is due to a delay in diagnosis rather than a more fulminant infection (17). Therapeutic regimens for TB meningitis in pregnant patients uphold the concept that multiple antimycobacterial drugs should be given in combination for prolonged intervals (Table 27.2). Isoniazid more frequently produces hepatitis during pregnancy, and while not absolutely contraindicated, liver function tests should be closely monitored when this drug is being given (16). Streptomycin should be avoided because of its potential to cause vestibulocochlear nerve toxicity in the fetus.

Listeriosis

Infection with *Listeria monocytogenes* presents either as a bacteremia or a meningitis, usually in patients with underlying disorders that cause immunodeficiency (19). In one large series of 722 cases, 34% of infections occurred during pregnancy, making it the most common single condition predisposing to infection (20). Listeriosis may occur at any time, but is most common during the third trimester of pregnancy. Patients usually present with fever, chills, and back pain. These symptoms can resolve

TABLE 27.1

*Adverse Effects of Common Antimicrobial Drugs during
Pregnancy Used in Various Neurologic Infections*

Drug	FDA Category*	Experience in Experimental Animals or in Pregnant Women
Antibacterials		
Gentamicin	C	No studies in pregnant women
Other aminoglycosides	D	Reports of congenital deafness with streptomycin
Chloramphenicol	D	"Gray syndrome" when given late in pregnancy or during labor
Sulfonamides	C	Small risk of kernicterus when used in last trimester
Tetracyclines	D	Retardation of bone growth, dental discoloration, or hypoplasia
Antifungals		
Amphotericin B	B	Harmless in animals; no studies in pregnant women
Fluconazole	C	Embryotoxic in animals; no studies in pregnant women
Antimycobacterials		
Rifampicin	C	Teratogenic in animals; may cause a postnatal coagulopathy when used in the last trimester that is sensitive to vitamin K
Streptomycin	D	Congenital deafness due to cochlear toxicity
Antiparasitics		
Quinine	X	Congenital malformations after large doses; sometimes used to induce abortion
Antivirals		
Acyclovir	B	Chromosomal damage in animals at high doses
Zidovudine	C	Teratogenic in animals, but no adverse effects reported in humans

*FDA Pregnancy Categories
A: Controlled studies in women fail to show fetal risk in the first trimester, there is no evidence of risk in later trimesters, and the possibility of fetal harm appears remote.
B: Animal studies fail to show fetal risk, plus no studies in pregnant women, *or* animal studies show an adverse effect that is not confirmed in controlled studies in pregnant women in first trimester, and there is no evidence of risk in later trimesters.
C: Studies in animals show adverse effects, and there are no studies in women, *or* there are no studies in women or animals. Drugs in this category should be given only if the need justifies the risk.
D: There is evidence of human fetal risk, but the need for the drug may still sometimes justify the risk.
X: Studies in animals or patients have demonstrated fetal abnormalities *or* there is evidence of fetal risk based on patient experience; the risk of the drug clearly outweighs the potential benefit.

spontaneously, and a positive blood culture may provide the only clue to the diagnosis. If cultures are not obtained, the infection may go completely undetected. In some cases, however, bacterial transmission across the placenta can result in premature labor or fetal death. Pregnant mothers may also present with a meningoencephalitis that varies in severity from mild headache and confusion to fulminant meningitis with decreased consciousness, elevated intracranial pressure, and a CSF pleocytosis of up to several hundred cells per cubic millimeter. In these more severe infections, the brain parenchyma itself can become involved, resulting in focal neurologic deficits and seizures (19). Although the organism can be missed on gram stain because of its intracellular life cycle, it is usually grown from the CSF without difficulty under standard laboratory conditions. Treatment of the infection with ampicillin should be initiated promptly (Table 27.2).

Coccidioidomycosis

Coccidioidomycosis is a fungal infection endemic to the southwest United States. It can become symptomatic during pregnancy and commonly disseminates to the CNS (21). Nearly one-third of the population become infected in endemic areas by inhaling airborne spores that are released from the soil (22). Symptomatic disease, however, occurs in less than 0.5% of infected individuals and most commonly presents as a pulmonary illness. Disseminated coccidioidomycosis is an infrequent complication of symptomatic disease with the skin, bones, and meninges being the usual sites of extrapulmonary involvement (21). Although males are more likely to develop severe disease, pregnancy clearly predisposes to fungal dissemination in women (21). It has been postulated that the effects of female sex hormones on both the immune

TABLE 27.2

Treatment Considerations for Common Neurologic Infections during and Immediately after Pregnancy

Disease	Drug of Choice	Teratogenicity*	Breast-feeding Ok?†	Recommendations
Tuberculous meningitis	Isoniazid	+	No	Treat with multidrug regimen at all stages of pregnancy
	Rifampicin	+	No	
	Pyrazinamide and/or	+	No	
	Ethambutol	+	No	
Listerial meningitis	Ampicillin	–	Yes	Treat with standard antibiotic doses as soon as possible
Coccidioidal meningitis	Amphotericin B	–	Unknown	Begin antifungal therapy as soon as pathogen is identified
Cerebral malaria	Quinidine gluconate	–	Yes	Treat as indicated as soon as possible
Disseminated HSV	Acyclovir	–	Yes	Use IV dosing for all forms of disseminated infection (including encephalitis)

* – = No adverse effects demonstrated or no adverse effects known (Class A or B), + = adverse effects in animals and no studies in women (Class C), ++ = significant fetal risk (Class D or X).

† Yes = absent or low concentrations of the drug excreted into breast milk, No = systemic or concentrated levels found in milk, proceed with caution, or avoid breast-feeding altogether.

system and the pathogen itself are responsible for the spread of infection during pregnancy (1–7,23). Coccidioidal meningitis is subtle in its presentation with lethargy, confusion, headache, low-grade fever, and generalized weight loss developing gradually. Diagnosis may be further delayed when meningitis occurs without any apparent pulmonary disease, a pattern of presentation that occurs in almost two-thirds of cases involving the CNS (24). The CSF is always abnormal in patients with coccidioidal meningitis, and the diagnosis is made either by detecting anticoccidioidal complement fixing (CF) antibodies or by growing *C. immitis* from the CSF. Because it is invariably fatal when left untreated, aggressive therapy for all patients is indicated (Table 27.2). The main therapeutic regimen requires intravenous followed by intraventricular amphotericin B at least until the CSF anticoccidioidal CF antibody titers remain negative for 6 to 12 months, and sometimes for life (Table 27.3) (25). Although pregnant mothers usually survive, the fetus often succumbs (21,25).

Malaria

Only one of the four species of plasmodia that infect humans, *Plasmodium falciparum*, is capable of causing severe cerebral disease. Falciparum malaria is especially common in pregnancy during which the level of parasitemia is increased and both fetal and maternal morbidity are high. In Thailand, malaria is the most common cause of mortality during pregnancy (26). Patients with

cerebral malaria present with headache, increasing drowsiness, confusion, delirium, seizures, and finally coma; the fever, anemia, and jaundice that accompany these findings serve as clues to the diagnosis. An important feature of falciparum malaria in pregnancy is the frequent development of hypoglycemia that becomes particularly severe during the intravenous administration of quinine (27). This derangement, along with a high sequestration of parasites in the placenta, thereby impeding oxygen and nutrient supply to the fetus, are believed to result in the fetal mortality (27,28). Serum glucoses should therefore be carefully monitored and hypoglycemia managed aggressively. Because untreated cerebral malaria is commonly fatal, it requires prompt intervention. Many strains of *P. falciparum* in Africa, Asia, and South America are now chloroquine-resistant, and because high doses of quinine may rarely cause stillbirths and fetal anomalies (28), it is now advisable to treat pregnant patients with intravenous quinidine gluconate (Table 27.2) (29). The combination of artesunate and mefloquine has also recently been tested in pregnancy and shown to have comparable efficacy to quinine in a small study (30). Antimalarial drugs can appear in breast milk, but not in quantities that can treat infant malaria (31). The use of antimalarials is not a contraindication to breast-feeding (31).

Viruses

Despite the fact that cell-mediated immunity is suppressed during pregnancy, viral meningitis and viral encephalitis

TABLE 27.3
Antimicrobial Regimens Commonly Used to Treat Neurologic Infections during Pregnancy

Drug	Dose	Frequency	Duration
Antimycobacterials			
Isoniazid	5 mg/kg PO	Daily	9 mo. to 1 yr.
Rifampin	10 mg/kg PO	Daily	9 mo. to 1 yr.
Pyrazinamide	15–30 mg/kg PO	Daily	2 months
Ethambutol	15–25 mg/kg PO	Daily	2 months
Antibacterials			
Ampicillin	2 g IV	Every 4 hours	2–3 weeks
Antifungals			
Amphotericin B*	0.5 mg/kg IV	Daily	Total dose of 30–40 mg/kg, plus:
	0.2–0.5 mg intraventricular**	Every other day	at least until CSF titer (–) for 6–12 mo.
Antimalarials			
Quinidine gluconate***	10 mg base/kg IV load, then 0.02 mg/kg/h	TID	Until oral Rx can be started, then: 7 days plus:
	648 mg PO		
Sulfadoxine-pyrimethamine			3 tablets all at once at the end of quinidine therapy
Antivirals			
Acyclovir	10 mg/kg IV	Every 8 hours	2–3 weeks

  * Adverse effects are common; requires an initial test dose of 1 mg under close observation (see reference 25).
  ** Duration of therapy typically necessitates the placement of an intraventricular reservoir.
*** Cardiac monitoring is indicated during infusion. Slow or stop if QRS lengthens >25% of baseline or if QTc interval >500 msec.

are not increased in frequency or severity during pregnancy (32). Paralytic poliomyelitis is slightly more common in pregnant women (33), and some nonneurologic viral infections, including smallpox, influenza, and varicella-zoster, can be more severe in these patients (32). Herpes simplex virus (HSV) infections of the genital tract can lead to intrauterine fetal infection or neonatal disease when contracted during vaginal birth (34,35). Although these may have devastating effects on the infant, no data show that pregnancy itself increases the rate with which latent genital HSV infections reactivate. Likewise, whereas reactivated genital HSV infections can rarely disseminate to the CNS, this does not occur more commonly in pregnant women (35,36). In a small number of cases, however, disseminated HSV infection during pregnancy (either with or without obvious CNS involvement) was associated with a maternal mortality of greater than 50% (35). As a result, despite its potential for causing chromosome breaks at very high concentrations (37), acyclovir should be given to all pregnant women with disseminated HSV infection in doses that are standard for the treatment of encephalitis (Table 27.3). Isolated genital HSV infections typically should not be treated since acyclovir simply decreases the duration of viral shedding and has no beneficial effect on preventing subsequent

reactivations (36). Active genital HSV infection during labor, however, may be considered an indication to deliver the baby by caesarean section to prevent neonatal infection (35).

VACCINATION DURING PREGNANCY

Because of the theoretical risk of transplacental transmission, immunizing pregnant women with live virus vaccines is generally avoided. The Centers for Disease Control (CDC) have stated that inactivated vaccines are officially safe during pregnancy, however (38). Circumstances can arise during pregnancy when there is a need to immunize a woman against an infection that might potentially involve the nervous system. For example, it is important to ensure that pregnant women are immunized against tetanus because the transplacental transfer of maternal antibodies is important in preventing this disease in neonates. Pregnant women can safely be given a combination of tetanus and diphtheria toxoids (38). Similarly, in pregnant women potentially exposed to rabies virus, post-exposure rabies vaccine can be given (38). The live vaccine of greatest concern is the attenuated oral polio vaccine (OPV), because recently immunized children can spread these fecally excreted viruses to pregnant mothers through close household contact. OPV was recently given to pregnant women during a poliomyelitis outbreak in Finland. No vaccine-related cases of paralysis occurred, and no harmful effects on fetal development were noted (39). Nevertheless, the CDC does not recommend its routine use in the United States during pregnancy (38).

GENDER-BASED DIFFERENCES IN THE FREQUENCY, MANIFESTATIONS, AND OUTCOMES OF SPECIFIC NEUROLOGIC INFECTIONS

In a few examples, apart from pregnancy, neurologic infections differ in their frequency, manifestations, and/or clinical outcomes between men and women. Sex differences in the susceptibility to viral infection of the CNS have also been documented in experimental animals (40,41). These animal studies are helpful because they begin to address the mechanisms underlying gender-based differences in outcome. In these reports, both groups of investigators showed that female animals generated more robust immune responses to infection than males (40,41). This led to an improved overall outcome for females with one infection (40). In the other case, however, where symptoms of the infection were predominantly immune-mediated, the enhanced immune response in female animals resulted in more severe disease and greater mortality (41). In humans, examples in which differences between the sexes have been identified typically show that women either do better or less commonly have the disease than men.

Mumps

Mumps is a systemic infection caused by a paramyxovirus. Although salivary gland enlargement, especially parotitis, is the most easily recognized clinical manifestation of mumps, CNS involvement frequently occurs (42). This ranges from a mild aseptic meningitis to a fulminant and potentially fatal encephalitis. The disease has largely been controlled by vaccination over the last three decades, but cases in unvaccinated individuals still occur (42). This is most common in urban populations, where school-aged children are typically affected. Although boys and girls have the same incidence of mumps parotitis (43), a distinct male predominance (up to 80%) of CNS disease exists. In most series, the ratio of males to females is between 3:1 and 4:1 (42,44–46). The peak incidence of CNS involvement in mumps occurs at about age 7 in both sexes (44–46).

Brain Abscess

Brain abscesses are focal areas of infection within the brain parenchyma itself. They occur as single or multiple lesions, commonly in association with three clinical situations: (i) a contiguous focus of infection such as a sinusitis or otitis media, (ii) hematogenous spread from a distant source, such as pneumonia or bacterial endocarditis, or (iii) following cranial trauma. Several large series report a male predominance among patients with brain abscesses, as high as 3:1 (47–50). The reason for this difference between men and women is unknown, and the disease is otherwise the same for both sexes.

Subdural Empyema

A subdural empyema is an infection that occupies the space between the dura mater and the arachnoid mater. It is most often a complication of ear, nose, and throat infection, but may also occur following head trauma, neurosurgery, osteomyelitis of the skull, bacteremic spread from a distant source, or leptomeningitis in infants (51). As with brain abscesses, males with subdural empyemas outnumber females by 3:1 (52). Nearly 70% are in their second or third decade of life (52), and the growing posterior wall of the frontal sinus in boys between the ages of 9 and 20 has been offered as a possible explanation for this striking sex and age susceptibility (53).

HORMONAL THERAPY AND NEUROLOGIC INFECTIONS IN WOMEN

Exogenous female sex hormones are used therapeutically for a number of purposes. Some examples include progesterone, either alone or with estrogen, in contraceptive pills and conjugated estrogens that are used to treat the vasomotor symptoms associated with menopause ("hot flashes") and to prevent postmenopausal osteoporosis. Although these treatments may increase the susceptibility of women to both cardiovascular and cerebrovascular disease, they have never been directly linked to an increased risk of infection. Some drug interactions, however, may occur between contraceptive pills and certain antibiotics including rifampin, tetracycline, and ampicillin (54). These drugs all decrease the effectiveness of contraceptive pills (54). This effect may be particularly enhanced by the concurrent administration of anticonvulsants such as phenytoin and carbamazepine.

CONCLUSION

Infections of the CNS in women present a number of unique situations and challenges that are not applicable to men. Conditions present during menses may predispose women to develop TSS, which can involve the CNS. This uncommon disorder requires prompt recognition and appropriate antibiotic therapy. Immune suppression during pregnancy increases the susceptibility of women to certain neurologic infections, and the adverse effects of particular antimicrobial drugs on the fetus may complicate the treatment of these disorders. Particular care is likewise required in determining the appropriateness of vaccines against neurologic infections during pregnancy. Women taking contraceptive pills or hormone supplements during menopause may find that the effectiveness of these drugs decreases in the presence of certain antibiotics that are used to treat neurologic infections. In contrast to their striking susceptibility during pregnancy, however, women also resist certain neurologic infections such as mumps and brain abscesses compared to men. Whereas studies in experimental animals have begun to elucidate the immunologic underpinnings for these differences in susceptibility to CNS infections, only the in vitro effects of estrogens on cells of the immune system have begun to be delineated. Pregnancy is a critical period during which neurologic infections require prompt identification and careful management, because of the often subtle presenting features, changes in antibiotic metabolism, and potentially damaging effects of both infection and treatment on the fetus.

References

1. Grossman CJ. Regulation of the immune system by sex steroids. *Endocrine Rev* 1984;5:435–451.
2. Paavonen T. Hormonal regulation of lymphocyte functions. *Med Biol* 1987;65:229–236.
3. Sarvetnick N, Fox HS. Interferon-gamma and the sexual dimorphism of autoimmunity. *Mol Biol Med* 1990;7:323–330.
4. Styrt B, Sugarman B. Estrogens and infection. *Rev Infect Dis* 1991;13:1139–1151.
5. Bhalla AK. Hormones and the immune response. *Ann Rheum Dis* 1989;48:1–6.
6. Ansar-Ahmed S, Penhale WJ, Talal N. Sex hormones, immune responses, and autoimmune diseases. *Am J Path* 1985;121:531–551.
7. Paavonen T, Anderson LC, Adlercreutz H. Sex hormone regulation of in vitro immune response. *J Exp Med* 1981;154:1935–1945.
8. Huber SA, Pfaeffle B. Differential Th1 and Th2 cell responses in male and female BALB/c mice infected with coxsackievirus group B type 3. *J Virol* 1994;68:5126–5132.
9. Wegmann TG, Lin H, Guilbert L, Mosmann TR. Bidirectional cytokine interactions in the maternal-fetal relationship: is successful pregnancy a Th2 phenomenon? *Immunol Today* 1993;14:353–356.
10. Siiteri PK, Stites DP. Immunologic and endocrine interrelationships in pregnancy. *Bil Reprod* 1982;26:1–14.
11. Johnson PM. Immunobiology of the human placental trophoblast. *Exp Clin Immunogenetics* 1993;10:118–122.
12. Robertson SA, Seamark RF, Guilbert LJ, Wegmann TG. The role of cytokines in gestation. *Crit Rev Immunol* 1994;14:239–292.
13. Davis JP, Chesney PJ, Wand PJ, La Venture M. Toxic shock syndrome: epidemiologic features, recurrence, risk factors, and prevention. *N Engl J Med* 1980;303:1429–1435.
14. Waldvogel FA. Staphylococcus aureus (including toxic shock syndrome). In: Mandell GL, Bennett JE, Dolin R, (eds.) *Principles and practice of infectious diseases.* New York: Churchill Livingstone, 1995;1754–1777.
15. Bharucha NE, Bhabha SK, Bharucha EP. Bacterial infections of the nervous system. In: Bradley WG, Daroff RB, Fenichel GM, Marsden CD, (eds.) *Neurology in clinical practice.* Boston: Butterworth-Heinemann, 1991;1049–1084.
16. Hamadeh MA, Glassroth J. Tuberculosis and pregnancy. *Chest* 1992;101:1114–1120.
17. Kingdom JCP, Kennedy DH. Tuberculous meningitis in pregnancy. *Br J Obstet Gynecol* 1989;96:233–235.
18. D'Cruz IA, Dandeker AC. Tuberculous meningitis in pregnant and puerperal women. *Obstet Gynecol* 1968;31:775–779.
19. Armstrong D. Listeria monocytogenes. In: Mandell GL, Bennett JE, Dolin R, (eds.) *Principles and practice of infectious diseases.* New York: Churchill Livingstone, 1995;1880–1885.
20. McLauchlin J. Human listeriosis in Britain 1967–1985, a summary of 722 cases. 1. Listeriosis during pregnancy and in the newborn. *Epidemiol Infect* 1990;104:181–190.
21. Ampel NM, Wieden MA, Galgiani JN. Coccidioidomycosis: clinical update. *Rev Infect Dis* 1989;11:897–911.
22. Dodge RR, Lebowitz MD, Barbee R, Burrows B. Estimates of *Coccidioides immitis* infection by skin test reactivity in an endemic community. *Am J Public Health* 1985;75:863–865.
23. Drutz DJ, Huppert M. Coccidioidomycosis: factors affecting the host-parasite interaction. *J Infect Dis* 1983;147:372–390.
24. Bouza E, Dreyer JS, Hewitt WL, Meyer RD. Coccidioidal meningitis. An analysis of thirty-one cases and review of the literature. *Medicine (Baltimore)* 1981;60:139–172.
25. Dal Pan GJ. Fungal infections of the central nervous system. In: Johnson RT, Griffin JW, (eds.) *Current therapy in neurologic disease.* St. Louis: Mosby-Year Book, 1997;146–151.
26. Khanavongs M. Maternal mortality rate at Phaholpolpayuhasena from 1977–1979. *Thai Med Council Bull* 1980;9:877–881.
27. Looareesuwan S, White NJ, Karbwang J, et al. Quinine and severe falciparum malaria in late pregnancy. *Lancet* 1985;2:4–8.
28. Dilling WJ, Gemmell AA. A preliminary investigation of of fetal deaths following quinine induction. *J Obst Gyn* 1929;36:352–366.
29. Miller KD, Greenberg AE, Campbell CC. Treatment of severe malaria in the United States with a continuous infusion of quinidine gluconate and exchange transfusion. *N Engl J Med* 1989;321:66–70.
30. Bounyasong S. Randomized trial of artesunate and mefloquine in comparison with quinine sulfate to treat P. falciparum malaria in pregnant women. *J Med Assoc Thai* 2001;84:1289–1299.
31. Murphy GS, Oldfield EC. Falciparum malaria. In: Lutwick LI, (ed.) *Infectious disease clinics of North America.* Philadelphia: WB Saunders, 1996;10(4):747–775.
32. Johnson RT. Infections during pregnancy. In: Devinsky O, Feldmann E, Hainline B, (eds.) *Neurological complications of pregnancy.* New York: Raven Press, 1994;153–162.

33. Weinstein L, Aycock WL, Feemster RF. The relation of sex, pregnancy, and menstruation to susceptibility in poliomyelitis. *N Engl J Med* 1951;245:54-58.

34. Whitley RJ, Schlitt M. Encephalitis caused by herpesviruses, including B virus. In: Scheld WM, Whitley RJ, Durack DT, (eds.) *Infections of the central nervous system.* New York: Raven Press, 1991;41–86.

35. Whitley RJ, Stagno S. Perinatal viral infections. In: Scheld WM, Whitley RJ, Durack DT, (eds.) *Infections of the central nervous system.* New York: Raven Press, 1991; 167–200.

36. Corey L, Adams HG, Brown ZA, Holmes KK. Genital herpes simplex virus infections: clinical manifestations, course, and complications. *Ann Intern Med* 1983;98: 958–972.

37. Stahlmann R, Klug S, Lewandowski C. Teratogenicity of acyclovir in rats. *Infection* 1987;15:261–262.

38. Centers for Disease Control and Prevention. Recommendation of the Immunization Practices Advisory Committee (ACIP): general recommendations on immunization. *MMWR* 1994;43 (RR-1).

39. Harjulehto T, Hovi T, Aro T, Saxen L. Congenital malformations and oral poliovirus vaccination during pregnancy. *Lancet* 1989;1:771–772.

40. Barna M, Komatsu T, Bi Z, Reiss CS. Sex differences in susceptibility to viral infection of the central nervous system. *J Neuroimmunol* 1996;67:31–39.

41. Muller D, Chen M, Vikingsson A, Hildeman D, Pederson K. Estrogen influences CD4+ T lymphocyte activity in vivo and in vitro in ß2-microglobulin-deficient mice. *Immunology* 1995;86:162–167.

42. Gnann JW. Meningitis and encephalitis caused by mumps virus. In: Scheld WM, Whitley RJ, Durack DT, (eds.) *Infections of the central nervous system.* New York: Raven Press, 1991;113–125.

43. Levitt LP, Mahoney DH, Casey HL, Bond JO. Mumps in a general population: a sero-epidemiologic study. *Am J Dis Child* 1970;120:134–138.

44. Levitt LP, Rich TA, Kinde SW, Lewis AL, Gates EH, Bond JO. Central nervous system mumps. *Neurology* 1970;20: 829–834.

45. Ritter BS. Mumps meningoencephalitis in children. *J Pediatr* 1958;52:424–432.

46. Murray HGS, Field CMB, McLeod WJ. Mumps meningo-encephalitis. *Br Med J* 1960;1:1850–1853.

47. Morgan H, Wood M, Murphy F. Experience with 88 consecutive cases of brain abscess. *J Neurosurg* 1973;38: 698–704.

48. Chun CH, Johnson JD, Hofstetter M, Raff MJ. Brain abscess. A study of 45 cases. *Medicine (Baltimore)* 1986;65:415–431.

49. Samson DS, Clark K. A current review of brain abscess. *Am J Med* 1973;54:201–210.

50. Spires JR, Smith RJH, Catlin FI. Brain abscesses in the young. *Otolaryngol Head Neck Surg* 1985;93:468–474.

51. Helfgott DC, Weingarten K, Hartman BJ. Subdural empyema. In: Scheld WM, Whitley RJ, Durack DT, (eds.) *Infections of the central nervous system.* New York: Raven Press, 1991;487–498.

52. Luken MG, Whelan MA. Recent diagnostic experience with subdural empyema. *J Neurosurg* 1980;52:764–771.

53. Kaufman DM, Litman N, Miller MM. Sinusitis-induced subdural empyema. *Neurology* 1983;33:123–132.

54. Bartlett JG. *Pocket book of infectious disease therapy.* Baltimore, Md: Williams & Wilkins; 1998.

28 Neuro-oncologic Diseases in Women

Alessandro Olivi, MD and John J. Laterra, MD, PhD

T he goal of this chapter is to provide an overview of the more common intracranial tumors and neurologic complications of cancer that are unique to women, with particular emphasis on the possible relationship between certain conditions and female sex hormones or oral contraceptives, female-specific cancers, and on the special therapeutic considerations regarding women affected by brain tumors during their childbearing years or during pregnancy.

In general, females are not more frequently affected by intracranial tumors than are males (1). The sex ratio (SR) for all histologic types as a group is 1:2 (2). The incidence rate per 100,000 population for primary brain tumors is 9.2 for males and 8.7 for females. Some histologic subtypes such as meningioma and pituitary adenoma are more frequently observed in women of childbearing age, however (3). This observation has led to the hypothesis of a link between the female sex hormones and these tumors. Indeed, research studies have shown the presence of estrogen and progesterone receptors in meningioma cells (4).

This chapter also describes the most recent diagnostic modalities that enable us to obtain more accurate and timely diagnoses in women affected by brain tumors for establishing appropriately individualized treatment plans.

GLIAL TUMORS

Glial tumors are the most common primary brain tumors of adults, comprising half of all diagnosed brain tumors. The average adult incidence rate is 5.2 per 100,000, and the most common histologic type is the asytrocytoma (5). Among asytrocytomas, glioblastoma multiforme is the most common and the most malignant histologic variant. Other histologic types include oligodendroglioma and ependymoma. The presenting symptoms can be divided into nonfocal, typically the result of increased intracranial pressure, and focal, as the consequence of direct destructive or irritative involvement of the surrounding nervous tissue. Nonfocal symptoms include headache, drowsiness, nausea, and vomiting. When these symptoms appear without any other accompanying symptom or sign, they can be difficult to distinguish from the common disturbances of pregnancy. Conversely, focal symptoms such as motor or sensory deficits, cranial nerve dysfunctions, or seizure can be more promptly related to a new pathologic process in the central nervous system (CNS).

A direct influence on tumor growth by hormonal changes has been hypothesized for glial tumors, but little experimental evidence has been demonstrated (6).

Glial tumors are often surrounded by brain edema, which is thought to be the result of incompetent neoplastic vessels that lack mature tight junctions between endothelial cells and thus allow extracellular fluid to accumulate in the vicinity of the brain tumor. The tendency to retain extra- and intracellular fluid during pregnancy is considered a predisposing factor for the development of more extensive perineoplastic edema and, subsequently, more severe symptoms (7).

Diagnosis

When an intracranial lesion is suspected, the standard diagnostic test is a high-resolution computed tomographic (CT) scan or magnetic resonance imaging (MRI) performed with and without intravenous contrast. The MRI remains the imaging test of choice because it can provide precise information about the configuration of the lesion, its relative vascularity, the presence of a cystic component or obstructive hydrocephalus, and the extent of mass effect on the surrounding structures. It is also a test that does not expose the pregnant woman to ionizing radiation. Rarely, an angiogram is needed to complete the assessment. Special sequences on the MRI or a magnetic resonance angiogram (MRA) can provide enough information about the vascular component of the brain tumor.

Treatment

When a glial tumor is accessible, and removal does not involve unacceptable loss of essential brain function, a surgical resection is recommended. This treatment allows tissue sampling for accurate diagnosis and a longer survival both in highly malignant and less aggressive glial tumors (8).

For deep-seated lesions or tumors in direct proximity to eloquent portions of the brain, stereotactic biopsies are performed. These procedures allow the clinician to obtain the initial diagnosis of the tumor with a very low rate of morbidity.

Conventional external beam radiotherapy plays a very important role in the treatment of aggressive glial tumors as an adjuvant measure after surgery. In addition, chemotherapeutic regimens in selected patients may play a role in prolonging survival in patients affected with malignant gliomas (9). More recently, stereotactic radiosurgery using precisely converging radiation beams (gamma knife and linear accelerators) has been used as an alternative to surgery for the treatment of small, deep-seated lesions (10).

In pregnant women with glial tumors, the treatment plan must be individualized. Surgery is usually indicated when the tumor is causing progressive symptoms or considerable mass effect and increased intracranial pressure. If the increase in intracranial pressure is the result of obstructive hydrocephalus, a shunting procedure should be performed. Conversely, if the tumor is not producing significant mass effect and the clinical condition is stable, the option to postpone any kind of invasive procedure until

after delivery is available. In this situation, however, the patient should be followed up closely with frequent neurologic examinations and neuroimaging studies and, if necessary, with medical therapy (e.g., steroids, antiepileptic drugs [AEDs]) throughout the pregnancy.

The most common medical therapy for these lesions consists of synthetic corticosteroids, which are very effective in reducing perineoplastic brain edema, and AEDs for seizure control. Both these treatment modalities should be used very cautiously in pregnant women because of their possible consequences to the fetus (see Chapter 4). In particular, the use of prolonged doses of corticosteroids can cause hypoadrenalism in infants, and teratogenicity has been reported with the use of AEDs (11). Therefore, the use of AEDs should be limited to pregnant women with generalized tonic-clonic seizures or multiple seizures that would jeopardize the health of mother and fetus.

Special recommendations should be given to women receiving radiotherapy and chemotherapy during childbearing years. In view of the possible effects on the embryo and the fetus, it is recommended that these women adhere to a strict birth control regimen or practice sexual abstinence during the entire time of treatment. As to pregnant women, in most instances, these therapies can be postponed until after delivery. However, if the treatment is required during gestation, some important safety precautions should be taken to protect the fetus.

Acute radiation of 100 rads or more through the 15th week of gestation represents a substantial risk for either abortion or mental retardation and congenital defects to the surviving embryo (12). Given the relatively long distance from the maternal brain to the developing fetus, however, and the limited scattering of the ionizing radiation through the body, the use of appropriate lead shielding can reduce radiation diffusion and adequately protect the fetus from dangerous radiation levels. Except in extenuating circumstances, chemotherapeutic agents should be avoided during pregnancy (13). Animal studies have identified the teratogenic effects of carmustine (BCNU), the most widely used agent for malignant gliomas, when it is given early in pregnancy (14). Although there is no evidence of increased risk of teratogenicity associated with the administration of cytotoxic drugs in the second and third trimesters (15,16), the general recommendation is to postpone systemic chemotherapy until after delivery, if possible. Interstitial chemotherapy consisting of BCNU-impregnated polymers placed directly into the tumor bed at the time of surgical resection has recently been approved by the Food and Drug Administration (FDA) in the form of Gliadel®. Although this ideal administration of BCNU dramatically reduces drug delivery to system organs, information regarding its safety during pregnancy is lacking. Finally, because of the likelihood for chemotherapeutic agents to be secreted in human milk, breast-feeding is not advised while receiving chemotherapy.

PITUITARY TUMORS

Pituitary adenomas are the most common intrasellar lesions, comprising 5 to 8% of all intracranial tumors. They have a peak incidence in women of childbearing age (17). They manifest with an endocrinopathy and local mass effect. Functional adenomas produce excessive quantities of pituitary hormones, causing characteristic symptoms. Prolactin-secreting tumors cause the amenorrhea-galactorrhea syndrome; growth hormone–secreting adenomas may produce acromegaly; and ACTH-secreting tumors may cause Cushing's syndrome. Because of these hormonal symptoms, functional adenomas often can be diagnosed while they are still small.

Nonfunctional adenomas are usually manifested by direct compression of the surrounding structures. This can result in pituitary stalk compression and subsequent pituitary insufficiency, optic chiasm compression causing bitemporal hemianopsia, and cavernous sinus compression causing oculomotor problems. Headaches usually are associated with pituitary adenomas and probably are caused by stretching of the surrounding sensory innervated dural membranes.

Because of the frequent infertility associated with this tumor, it is rare to find them in pregnancy. In those cases in which the reproductive cycle is not affected, however, or when medical treatment such as bromocriptine has restored normal ovulatory function, this association can occur. The well-documented increase in size of the normal pituitary gland during pregnancy, plus the reported observation that pituitary adenomas may expand more rapidly in pregnant women (18), warrant close clinical monitoring of this particular population. The effect of pregnancy on the size of pituitary adenomas is reported more frequently in patients with macroadenoma than in those with microadenoma and usually is more accentuated in the second and third trimesters. Thus, such patients should be followed up closely with ophthalmologic testing and laboratory and imaging studies to monitor disease progression.

Pituitary adenomas can rarely present with "pituitary apoplexy." This event is caused by acute hemorrhage within the pituitary adenoma that causes a rapid increase of the intrasellar pressure. Violent headaches, rapid deterioration of vision, nausea, and vomiting are the common presenting symptoms. Pituitary apoplexy is a condition that requires emergency surgical treatment to avoid progression of the deficit and possible death.

Diagnosis

Endocrinologic and neuro-ophthalmologic evaluation should be performed in any patient with a suspected pituitary tumor. A general baseline determination of anterior and posterior pituitary function should be completed with the measurements of serum prolactin, early morning cortisol, serum gonadotropins, urine volume, serum electrolytes and osmolarity, and a thyroid profile. A formal neuro-ophthalmologic evaluation including visual field assessment should be completed. A high-resolution CT scan or MRI remains the test of choice. In particular, MRI scans can allow the detection of even small tumors using special coronal sections following intravenous injection of paramagnetic contrast agents, such as gadolinium. MRI scans also enable the visualization of the details of the vascular structures and may eliminate the need for angiography in the evaluation of these patients. High-resolution CT scans provide detailed definition of the sella and surrounding bony structures. This information is particularly valuable in the preoperative evaluation of the sphenoidal bones when a transsphenoidal resection is planned.

Treatment

Medical treatment involves controlling the growth of functional adenomas such as prolactin-secreting adenomas. Bromocriptine is particularly effective. Patients with prolactinomas presenting with a classic amenorrhea-galactorrhea syndrome and placed on bromocriptine may resume regular ovulatory cycles and subsequently become pregnant. To minimize any possible effects of bromocriptine on the developing fetus, it is recommended that women discontinue the medication while trying to conceive (19). Other medical therapies for less frequent hyperfunctional pituitary adenomas include a somatostatin analog (SMS-201–995) for acromegaly and cyproheptadine and ketoconazole for Cushing's disease. A transsphenoidal resection of the tumor is indicated when patients do not respond to the medical therapy, if there is clear progression of the disease with compression of surrounding structures (i.e., optic chiasm causing visual field loss), and if pituitary apoplexy occurs. Radiotherapy can be used as an adjunctive measure after surgery if the residual tumor is particularly large. In rare cases, radiotherapy is the initial form of treatment.

Generally, pregnant women affected by pituitary adenomas can be safely followed up clinically with frequent ophthalmologic evaluations and MRI scans. Medical management can be quite effective even in pregnant patients. Only a small portion of these patients require further surgical treatment before parturition.

MENINGIOMA

Meningiomas are tumors that clearly appear more frequently (20) in females than in males, with a ratio of 2:1 to 3:1. Meningiomas originate from the meninges and generally are slow growing. The expression of hormonal receptors in these tumors has been of particular interest. Progesterone receptors are commonly found in these tumors and estrogen receptors occur, although at much lower frequency (4). The clinical presentation of meningioma is determined by their location. Presenting symptoms can include mental status changes, lethargy, and apathy. In tumors that become large enough to increase intracranial pressure, headaches and visual symptoms can occur. Focal irritative signs such as focal motor or complex-partial seizures can occur in tumors located next to the motor strip or other areas of the sensitive cortex. Motor or sensory loss also can be the initial manifestation of these tumors. Pregnant women may have a more rapid increase in size of these tumors, presumably because of rapid vascular engorgement as a result of the generalized increase in blood volume during pregnancy (21). There also may be a direct hormonal effect on the rate of tumor growth, presumably via progesterone and estrogen receptor stimulation. The appropriate diagnosis of these tumors is based on CT and MRI studies. An MRA or traditional angiography can be useful in determining the vascularization of these tumors.

Treatment

Whenever possible, surgical resection remains the only definitive treatment for these benign tumors. Pregnant women affected by meningioma can be followed up very closely in view of the usually slow-growing characteristics. It is therefore generally safe to defer surgery until after pregnancy, unless progression of the disease becomes significant. Repeat surgical resection may be an option in the setting of local recurrence. Radiosurgery or external beam radiotherapy also can be effective therapies following biopsy of a meningioma that is believed to be unresectable due to location or after tumor recurrence.

OTHER TUMORS

A number of less frequently encountered tumors can occur in women. Acoustic neuroma, ependymoma, hemangioblastoma, medulloblastoma, and choroid plexus papilloma are among them. Again, in general, the incidence of these tumors is not higher in women than in men, and the therapeutic recommendations are similar. Special consideration should be paid to metastatic tumors in general and metastatic choriocarcinoma and breast cancer in particular. The treatment of these tumors is largely palliative and varies according to the nature of the primary tumor and the extent of the systemic and CNS dissemination. Choriocarcinoma can occur during pregnancy and can also metastasize to the brain. This tumor originates from the trophoblast that produces human chorionic gonadotropin and has a known tendency to hemorrhage spontaneously. This can cause rapid deterioration of the neurologic condition, and urgent surgical resection is indicated. In general, when dealing with a solitary brain metastasis, surgical resection followed by whole brain radiotherapy is the treatment of choice (22). More recently, surgical treatment in selected cases has been recommended even in cases in which two or three metastases are present, with the aim of providing the patient with an improved quality of life (23).

The radiosensitivity of these tumors and response to radiotherapy should be considered. In women, breast cancer is the most common tumor to metastasize to the brain, followed by lung cancer. This differs from men, in whom the most common metastases to the brain are from primary lung carcinoma. Metastatic breast cancer to the brain usually is approached in the same fashion with surgery, radiotherapy, and in selected cases, chemotherapy.

Radiosurgery recently has been used as an alternative or as an adjunctive treatment for metastatic tumors to the brain. The advantages are that it can be given on an outpatient basis, and it is readily applied to deep-seated brain metastases or multiple inoperable tumors. However, it is still unclear whether radiosurgery is more advantageous than traditional surgical intervention in prolonging survival.

PARANEOPLASTIC SYNDROMES

Structures within the central or peripheral nervous systems can be injured as a result of the paraneoplastic effects of cancers that do not directly involve the nervous system. Some of the best-characterized paraneoplastic neurologic syndromes result from cancers that occur exclusively in women. Most if not all paraneoplastic neurologic disorders are believed to be immune-mediated by the systemic cancer initiating an anticancer immune response that causes autoimmune neuronal injury (24). This mechanism is supported by the strong association between specific paraneoplastic neurologic syndromes and specific diagnostic antibodies directed against tumor-associated antigens sharing epitopes with macromolecules expressed by the affected neurons. Paraneoplastic neurologic disorders are relatively rare, appearing in approximately 1 in 10,000 patients with systemic cancer. Paraneoplastic syndromes typically develop as the initial sign of underlying cancer (25). Recognizing these unusual syndromes is essential to their rapid diagnosis and treatment.

Specific paraneoplastic neuronal syndromes including their most commonly associated malignancies and

TABLE 28.1
Paraneoplastic Neurologic Disorders

Syndrome	Antibody	Tissue Target	Malignancy
Cerebellar degeneration	Anti-Yo	Purkinje cell	Ovarian, breast, lung
Ataxia ± opsoclonus-myoclonus	Anti-Ri	CNS neurons	Breast, gynecologic, bladder
Stiff-man syndrome, encephalomyelitis	Anti-amphiphysin	Presynaptic terminals	Breast, lung
Retinopathy	Anti-retinal	Ganglia, photoreceptors	Gynecologic, lung, melanoma
Lambert-Eaton	Anti-voltage-gated K+ channel	Presynaptic neuromuscular junction	Small cell lung
Encephalomyelitis, sensory Neuronopathy, cerebellar degeneration	Anti-Hu	Neurons	Lung, prostate
Encephalitis, cerebellar degeneration	Anti-MA1/2	Neurons	Lung, testes
Peripheral neuropathy	Anti-MAG	Peripheral nerve	Waldenströms macroglobulinemia

antibodies are listed in Table 28.1. The paraneoplastic syndromes specific to women are those associated with gynecologic and mammary cancers. These include anti-Yo+ cerebellar degeneration (25,26), anti-Ri+ opsoclonus-myoclonus (27), anti-amphihysin+ stiff-man syndrome (28,29), and cancer-associated retinopathy (30). The relative incidence of the other syndromes in men versus women is in general determined by the relative incidence of their underlying associated malignancies. Essentially, any part of the nervous system can be affected by paraneoplastic autoimmune mechanisms. The neurologic deficits of paraneoplastic neuronal injury reflect the specific neuronal sites of injury and typically develop subacutely over the course of a few weeks followed by symptom stabilization. Spontaneous improvement in the absence of therapy directed at either the neurologic disorder or underlying cancer points strongly to an alternate diagnosis.

Diagnosis

Because these syndromes develop most commonly in otherwise healthy individuals, a meticulous search for the underlying cancer is mandatory. Evaluations should include CT of the chest, abdomen and pelvis, mammography, and whole body glucose positron emission tomography (PET) to locate any occult malignancy. Electromyography and nerve conduction studies should be performed in the setting of neuropathy or suspected neuromuscular junction defect. Cerebrospinal fluid analysis frequently reveals nonspecific abnormalities such as mild pleiocytosis, mildly elevated protein, elevated IgG/albumin ratio, and the presence of oligoclonal bands. The identification of specific paraneoplastic antibodies in blood can help make a specific diagnosis and can guide the search for occult malignancy (i.e., anti-Yo antibodies and ovarian carcinoma).

Treatment

Therapy focuses on treating the underlying malignancy. Immune-specific approaches to inhibit humoral and cellular autoimmune mechanisms should also be initiated in patients displaying an objective progression of neurologic deficits. The benefits of immune-based therapies remain unpredictable and controversial. Initiating treatment early is critical to preserving neurologic function. Therapy may minimize progression of neurologic deficits but typically will not reverse deficits resulting from paraneoplastic autoimmune neuronal death (e.g., anti-Yo paraneoplastic cerebellar degeneration). In contrast, deficits due to ion channel dysfunction (e.g., Lambert-Eaton syndrome) may improve with treatments that target the blood-borne pathogenic antibodies (31,32). Increasing evidence suggests that cytotoxic T-cell responses play a fundamental role in the pathogenesis of these disorders (33). Patients presenting with paraneoplastic neurologic syndromes tend to have more favorable cancer outcomes than others with the same malignancy. This is likely due to the combination of early cancer diagnosis and the antineoplastic effects of the immune response to tumor-associated antigens. For the majority of the syndromes, generally a small temporal window exists for impacting positively upon neurologic outcome.

CONCLUSION

Neuro-oncological problems in women are diagnosed and treated by balancing the health risks from the tumor against temporary health issues such as pregnancy. In general, the incidence of CNS tumors and neurologic complications of systemic cancer in women during pregnancy is not higher than in the rest of the population. Special therapeutic considerations should be given to women during pregnancy and the childbearing years, however. The influences of female sex hormones and their effect on brain tumors should be considered. The availability of sophisticated diagnostic tools can enable the early diagnosis of these lesions and appropriate treatment plans. Recent advances in the techniques for surgical resection and the delivery of adjuvant therapy have provided improved survival for these patients. Certain rare neurologic complications of systemic cancer, in particular types of paraneoplastic syndromes, are associated with systemic cancers unique to women. Recognizing these early tumor-specific signs of cancer can expedite diagnoses and the initiation of appropriate treatments.

References

1. Walker AE, Robins M, Weinfeld FD. Epidemiology of brain tumors: the national survey of intracranial neoplasms. *Neurology* 1985;35:219–226.

2. Radhakreshnan K, Bohmen NI, Kurland LT. Brain tumors. In: Morantz RA, Walsh JM, (eds.) *Epidemiology of brain tumors*. New York: Marcel Dekker, 1994;1–8.

3. Robinson N, Beral V, Ashley JSA. Incidence of pituitary adenoma in women (letter). *Lancet* 1879;2:630.

4. Martuza RL, McLaughlin DT, Ojemann RG. Specific estradiol binding in schwannomas, meningiomas and neurofibromas. *Neurosurgery* 1981;9:665.

5. Kurland LT, Schoenberg BS, Annegers JF, Okazaki H, Molgaard CA. The incidence of primary intracranial neoplasms in Rochester, Minnesota, 1935–1977. *Ann NY Acad Sci* 1982;381:6–16.

6. Roelvink NCA, Kamphorst W, Van Alpen HAM, et al. Pregnancy-related primary brain and spinal tumors. *Arch Neurol* 1987;44:209–215.

7. Kemper MD. Management of pregnancy associated with brain tumors. *Am J Obstet Gynecol* 1963;87:858–864.

8. Wood JR, Green SB, Shapiro WR. The prognostic importance of tumor size in malignant gliomas: a computed tomographic scan study by the Brain Tumor Cooperative Group. *J Clin Oncol* 1988;6:338–343.

9. Shapiro WR, Green SB, Burger PC, et al. Randomized trial of three chemotherapy regimens and two radiotherapy regimens in postoperative treatment of malignant glioma. *J Neurosurg* 1989;71:1–9.

10. Lundsgotf LD, Flickinger J, Coffey RJ. Stereotactic gamma knife radiosurgery: initial North American experience in 207 patients. *Arch Neurol* 1990;47:169–175.

11. Dalessio DJ. Seizure disorders and pregnancy. *N Engl J Med* 1985;312:559.

12. Otake M, Schull WJ. In utero exposure to A-bomb radiation and mental retardation: A reassessment. *Br J Radiol* 1984;57:409–414.

13. Doll DC, Ringenberg QS, Yarbro JW. Antineoplastic agents and pregnancy. *Semin Oncol* 1989;16:337–346.

14. Briggs GC, Bodendorfer TQ, Freeman RK, et al. *Drugs in pregnancy and lactation*. Baltimore: Williams & Wilkins, 1983.

15. Lowenthal RM, Marsden KA, Newman NM. Normal infant after treatment of acute myeloid leukemia in pregnancy with daunorubicin. *Aust NZ J Med* 1978;8:431–432.

16. Brem H, Plantadosi S, Burger PC, et al. Placebo-controlled trial of safety and efficacy of intraoperative controlled delivery by biodegradable polymers of chemotherapy for recurrent gliomas. *Lancet* 1995;345:1008–1012.

17. Gold EB. Epidemiology of pituitary adenomas. *Epidemiol Rev* 1981;3:163–183.

18. Scheithauser BW, Sano T, Kovacs KT, et al. The pituitary gland in pregnancy: a clinicopathologic and immunohistochemical study of 69 cases. *Mayo Clin Proc* 1990;65:461–474.

19. Evans WS, Thorner MO. Bromocriptine. In: Wilkins RN, Rengachary SS, (eds.) *Neurosurgery*. New York: McGraw-Hill, 1985;873–878.

20. Rohringer M, Sutherland GR, Louw DF, Sima AAF. Incidence and clinicopathological features of meningioma. *J Neurosurg* 1989;71:665–672.

21. Fox MW, Harms RW, Davis DH. Selected neurologic complications of pregnancy. *Mayo Clin Proc* 1990;65:1595–1618.

22. Patchell RA, Tibbs PA, Walsh JW, et al. A randomized trial of surgery in the treatment of single metastases to the brain. *N Engl J Med* 1990;322:494–500.

23. Sawaya R, Ligon BL, Bindal RK. Management of metastatic brain tumors. *Ann Surg Oncol* 1994;1:169–178.

24. Darnell RB, Posner JB. Paraneoplastic syndromes involving the nervous system. *N Engl J Med* 2003;47:1543–1554.

25. Peterson K, Rosenblum MD, Kotanides H, Posner JB. Paraneoplastic cerebellar degeneration. I. A clinical analysis of 55 anti-Y0 antibody positive patients. *Neurology* 1992;42:1931–1937.

26. Fathallah-Shaykh H, Wolf S, Wong E, Posner JB, Furneaux HM. Cloning of a leucine-zipper protein recognized by the sera of patients with antibody-associated paraneoplastic cerebellar degeneration. *Proc Natl Acad Sci USA* 1991;88:3451–3454.

27. Luque FA, Furneaux HM, Ferziger R, et al. Anti-Ri: an antibody associated with paraneoplastic opsoclonus and breast cancer. *Ann Neurol* 1991;29:241–251.

28. DeCamilli P, Thomas A, Cofiell R, et al. The synaptic vesicle-associated protein amphiphysin is the 128 kD autoantigen of stiff-man syndrome with breast cancer. *J Exp Med* 1993;178:2219–2223.

29. Folli F, Solimensa M, Cofiell R, et al. Autoantibodies to a 128-kd synaptic protein in three women with the stiff-man syndrome and breast cancer. *N Engl J Med* 1993;328:546–551.

30. Maeda T, Maeda A, Maruyama I, et al. Mechanisms of photoreceptor cell death in cancer-associated retinopathy. *Invest Ophthalmol Vis Sci* 2000;42:705–712.

31. Bain PG, Motomura M, Newsom-Davis J, et al. Effects of intravenous immunoglobulin on muscle weakness and calcium-channel autoantibodies in the Lambert-Eaton myasthenic syndrome. *Neurology* 1996;47:678–683.

32. Das A, Hochberg FH, McNelis S. A review of the therapy of paraneoplastic neurologic syndromes. *J Neurooncol* 1999;41:181–194.

33. Albert ML, Austin LM, Darnell RB. Detection and treatment of activated T cells in the cerebrospinal fluid of patients with paraneoplastic cerebeller degeneration. *Ann Neurol* 2000;9–17.

29

Pseudotumor Cerebri

Neil R. Miller, MD

Pseudotumor cerebri (PTC) is the term used to describe a syndrome that occurs mainly in young women of child-bearing age. It is characterized by five features: (i) increased intracranial pressure (ICP), (ii) normal or small sized ventricles by neuroimaging, (iii) no evidence of an intracranial mass, (iv) normal cerebrospinal fluid (CSF) composition, and (v) papilledema (1).

The disorder was first recognized by Quincke in 1897 (2), but it was Warrington (3) who first called it "pseudotumor cerebri." Foley (4) introduced the term "benign intracranial hypertension" in 1955. The use of the prefix "benign" was challenged by Bucheit et al. (5), who emphasized that the visual outcome of this syndrome is not always "benign." These authors also suggested that the term idiopathic intracranial hypertension (IIH) be used for those cases of PTC for which no cause could be identified, and we agree. Readers interested in a history of PTC should consult the short but excellent monograph written by Bandyopadhyay (6).

EPIDEMIOLOGY

The incidence of PTC varies throughout the world. It is almost unknown in countries in which the incidence of obesity is low; obesityis a significant factor in the idio-

pathic form of the condition. Correspondingly, it is common in countries with an increased incidence of obesity. Durcan et al. (7) calculated the incidence of PTC in Iowa and Louisiana. In Iowa, the incidence was 0.9 per 100,000 in the general population, 3.5 per 100,000 in women aged 20 to 44 years, 13 per 100,000 in women who were 10% over ideal weight, and 19 per 100,000 in women who were 20% over ideal weight. Durcan et al. (7) found a similar incidence in Louisiana. Radhakrishnan et al. (8) reported an incidence of PTC in Rochester, Minnesota, of 1 per 100,000 in the general population, 1.6 in the female population, and 7.9 per 100,000 in obese women [defined as body mass index (BMI) greater than 26]. Radhakrishnan et al. (9) also reported that the annual incidence of PTC in Benghazi, Libya, was 2.2 per 100,000 in the general population, 4.3 per 100,000 in women, and 21.4 per 100,000 in women aged 15 to 44 years who were 20% over ideal weight.

The age range in patients with PTC is broad. Children and even infants are not infrequently affected (10–13), and older adults may also develop the condition (14). The peak incidence of the disease, however, seems to occur in the third decade. As noted, a female preponderance occurs that ranges from 2:1 in some studies to 8:1 in others (15,16). Men who develop PTC have clinical features identical with those of affected women; however, most men who develop PTC are not overweight (17).

CLINICAL MANIFESTATIONS

The most common presenting symptom in patients with PTC is headache, which occurs in more than 90% of cases (15,16,18–20). The headache is usually generalized, worse in the morning, and aggravated when cerebral venous pressure is increased by some type of Valsalva maneuver (coughing, sneezing, etc.). When caused by venous sinus thrombosis, it may be described as the "worst headache of my life," similar to that caused by subarachnoid hemorrhage (21). Other common nonvisual manifestations of PTC include nausea, vomiting, dizziness, and pulsatile tinnitus (18,20). Focal neurologic deficits in patients with PTC are extremely uncommon, and their occurrence should make one consider alterna-

tive diagnoses. Nevertheless, isolated unilateral and bilateral facial pareses, hemifacial spasm, trigeminal sensory neuropathy, hearing loss, hemiparesis, ataxia, paresthesias, mononeuritis multiplex, arthralgias, and both spinal and radicular pain have been reported in patients with PTC (19,22–31). Patients with chronic PTC can also develop persistent disturbances in cognition (32). In addition, a substantial percentage of patients with PTC, particularly young obese women, have evidence of clinical depression and anxiety (33–37).

The visual manifestations of PTC are usually preceded by headache and occur in 35 to 70% of patients. These symptoms are identical with those described by patients with increased ICP from other causes and include: (i) transient visual obscurations; (ii) loss of vision

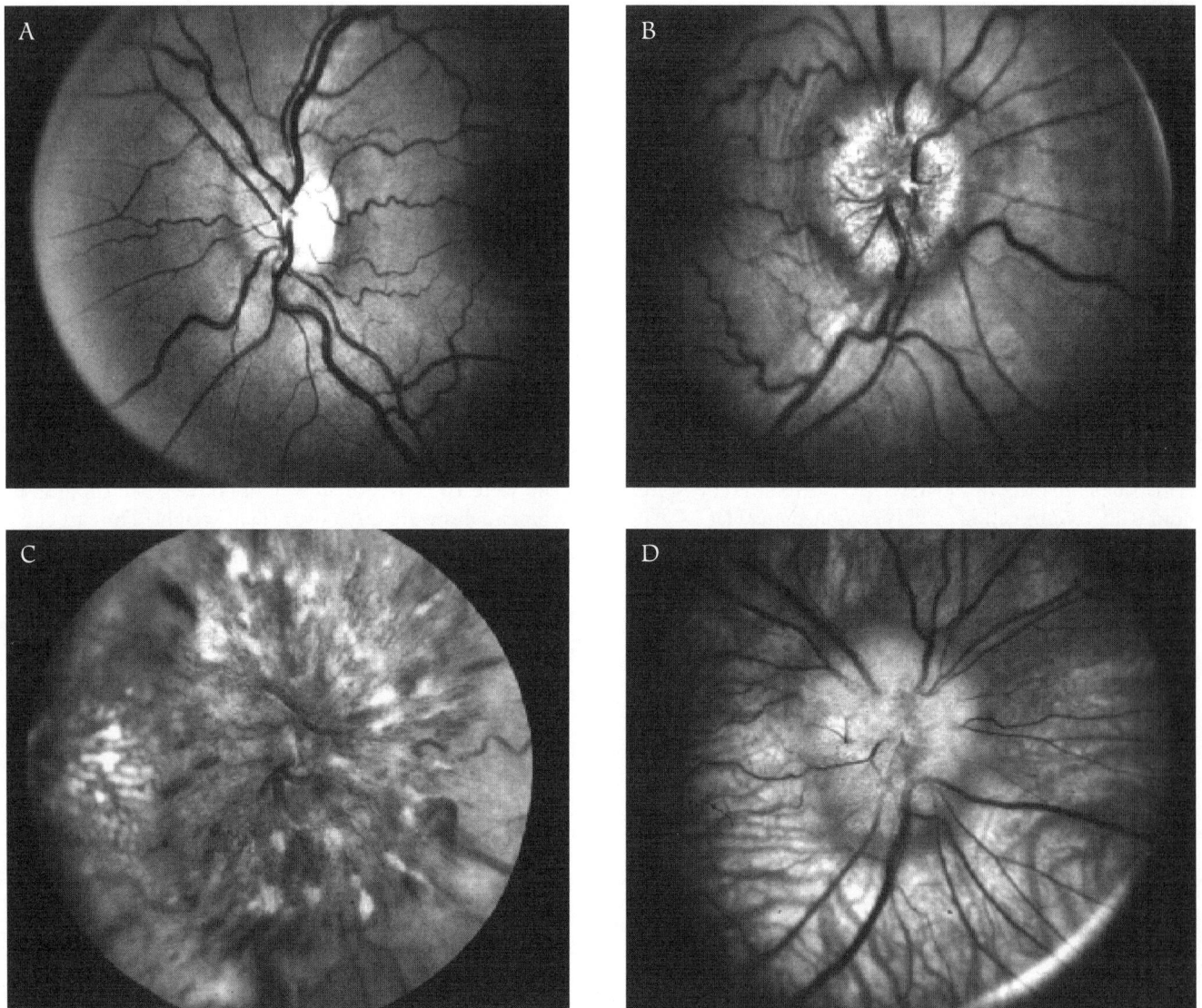

FIGURE 29.1

Papilledema in pseudotumor cerebri. (A) Mild; (B) moderate; (C) severe; (D) chronic.

from macular hemorrhages, exudates, pigment epithelial changes, retinal striae, choroidal folds, subretinal fluid or neovascularization, or optic atrophy; (iii) horizontal diplopia from unilateral or bilateral abducens nerve paresis; and, rarely, (iv) vertical or oblique diplopia from trochlear nerve paresis, oculomotor nerve paresis, or skew deviation (18,19,38–41). Among 110 patients with PTC examined by Johnston and Paterson (15,16), 57% had disturbances of visual acuity and 36% complained of diplopia.

The papilledema that occurs in patients with PTC is identical with that which occurs in patients with other causes of increased ICP. It may be mild, moderate, or severe (Figure 29.1). There is no correlation between

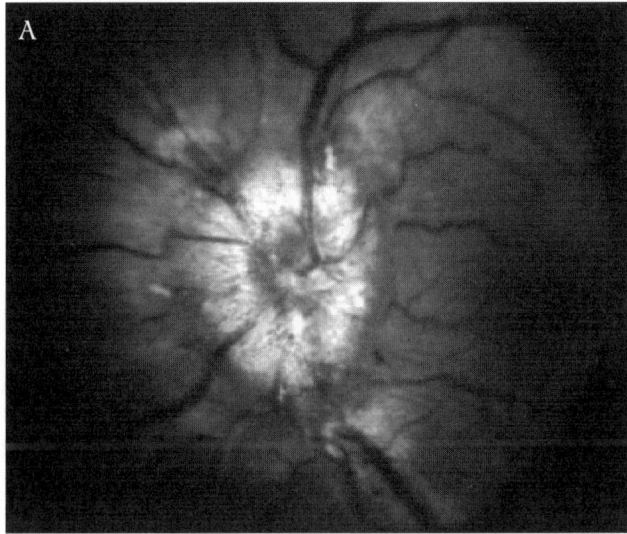

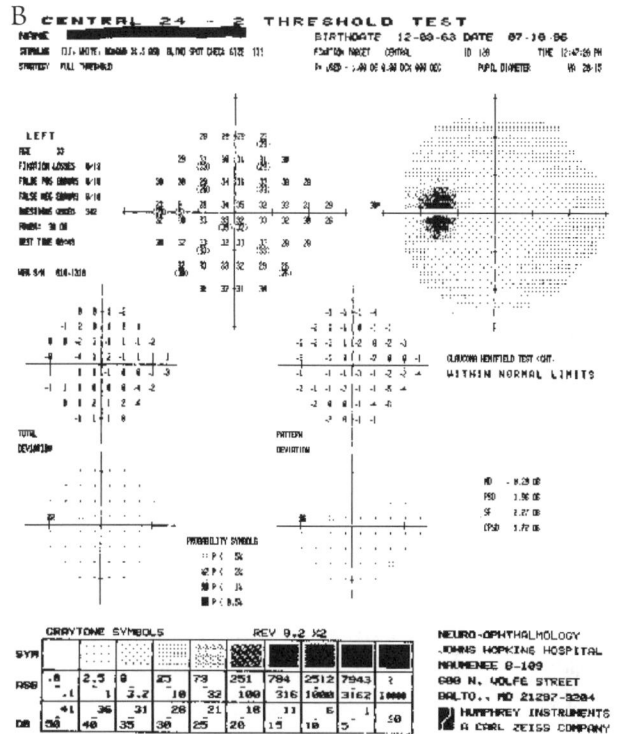

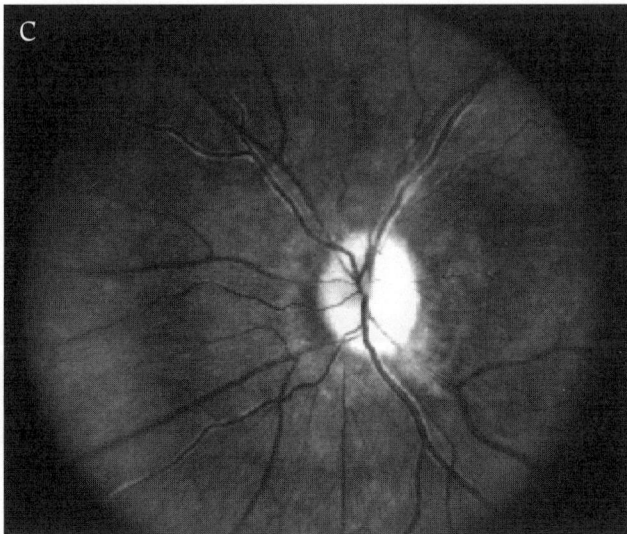

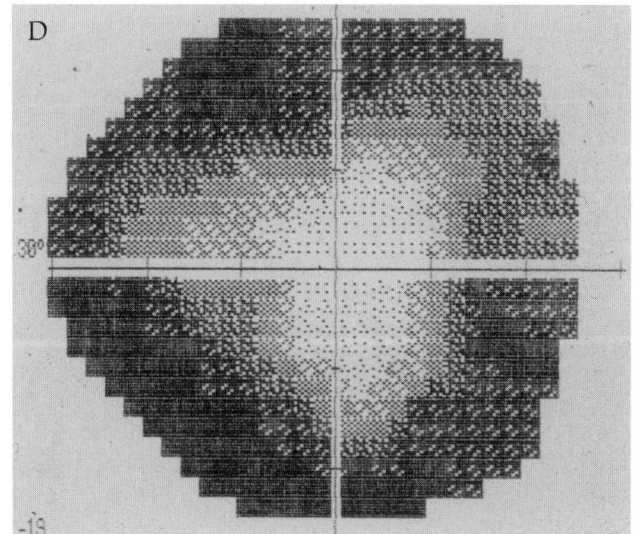

FIGURE 29.2

Comparison of visual fields and optic disc appearance in a patient with pseudotumor cerebri. (A) Left optic disc shows moderate papilledema. (B) Static perimetry shows enlargement of blind spot. (C) Postpapilledema optic atrophy. (D) Static perimetry shows generalized reduction in sensitivity and marked field constriction.

severity of optic disc swelling and age, race, or body weight in patients with PTC (42). Postpapilledema optic atrophy occurs in untreated or inadequately treated patients after a variable period of time, usually over several months, but occasionally within weeks of the onset of symptoms (Figure 29.2). Some patients have persistent chronic papilledema without the development of atrophy. Postpapilledema optic atrophy in patients with PTC usually develops symmetrically, but just as papilledema may be asymmetric (Figure 29.3), so postpapilledema optic atrophy can be asymmetric, and some patients develop a pseudo-Foster Kennedy syndrome characterized by postpapilledema optic atrophy on one side and papilledema on the other (43).

ETIOLOGY

Over 90% of cases of PTC occur in young obese women with no evidence of any underlying disease (15,16,18,19). In such cases, the condition is called "idiopathic pseudotumor cerebri" or idiopathic intracranial hypertension (1). In about 10% of patients, however, particularly young men, young nonobese women, and middle-aged adults of both genders, the condition occurs in a number of different settings, including: (i) obstruction or impairment of cerebral venous drainage, (ii) endocrine and metabolic dysfunction, (iii) exposure to exogenous drugs and other substances, (iv) withdrawal of certain drugs, (v) systemic illnesses, and (vi) as an idiopathic phenomenon (5,14,44,45).

Obstruction or Impairment of Intracranial Venous Drainage

The uncompensated obstruction of cerebral venous drainage may result in increased ICP and papilledema without enlargement of the ventricles and with otherwise normal cerebrospinal fluid (CSF) (21,45-49) (Table 29.1). The obstruction is most often caused by compression or thrombosis, with the vessels most often affected being the superior sagittal and transverse (lateral) sinuses (see also Chapter 28 on brain tumors in women). Tumors that obstruct the superior sagittal sinus are usually extra-axial lesions such as meningiomas (50), which are much more common in women than in men. The transverse sinus can also become occluded by meningiomas, vestibular schwannomas, and metastatic tumors (50-52), particularly carcinomas of the breast and lung. All these tumors, except for carcinoma of the lung, are more frequent in women than in men.

Septic thrombosis of the transverse sinus tends to occur in the setting of acute or chronic otitis media, in which there is an extension of the infection to the mastoid air cells and then to the adjacent lateral sinus (53,54). In such cases, papilledema usually occurs early and tends to be bilateral and symmetric (55,56). A similar appearance occurs with septic thrombosis of the superior sagittal sinus, a much less common condition. Septic thrombosis of the cavernous sinus may also be associated with papilledema, although it develops late.

Aseptic thrombosis usually occurs in the nonpaired sinuses of both adults and children, with the superior sagittal sinus most frequently affected (48,49). In such cases, a

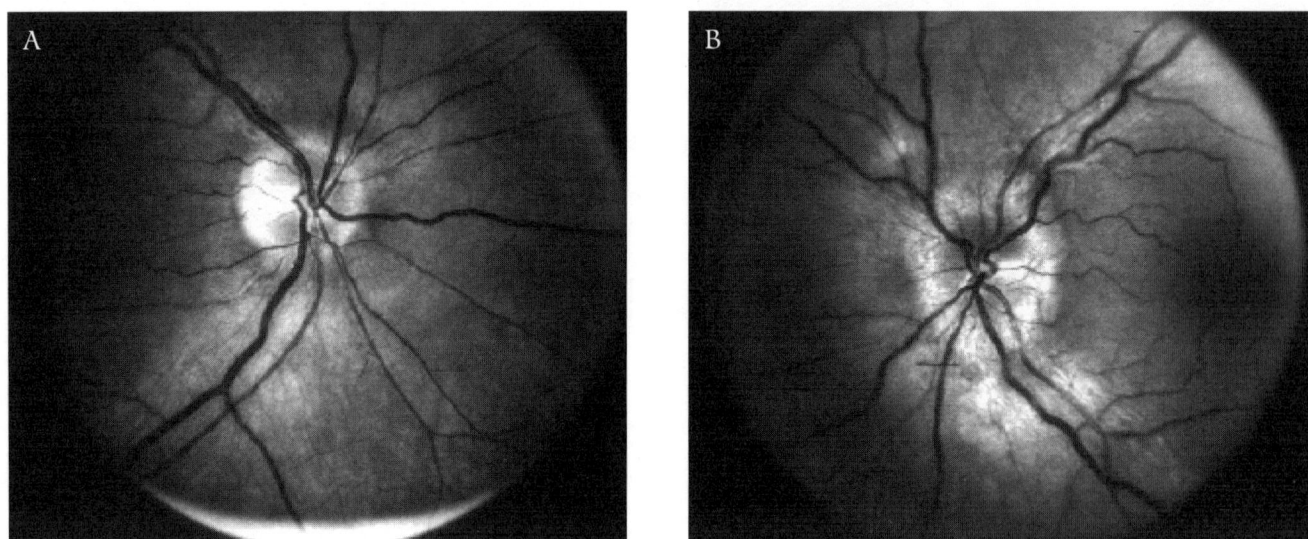

FIGURE 29.3

Asymmetric papilledema in pseudotumor cerebri. (A) Right optic disc is markedly swollen. Note folds in peripapillary retina. (B) Left optic disc is mildly swollen.

TABLE 29.1
*Etiologies of Obstruction/Impairment
of Cerebral Venous Drainage Associated
with Pseudotumor Cerebri*

Obstruction of Superior Sagittal Sinus
  Primary hematologic
    Antiphospholipid antibody syndrome
    Antithrombin III deficiency
    Essential thrombocythemia
    Protein S deficiency
    Protein C deficiency
  Systemic conditions associated with coagulopathy
    Behçet's disease
    Cancer
    Neurosarcoidosis
    Pregnancy
    Renal disease
    Systemic lupus erythematosus
    Trichinosis
  Traumatic
  Tumors
    Extravascular
    Intravascular
Obstruction of Transverse Sinus
  Dural arteriovenous fistula
  Hematologic (see above)
  Infection (mastoiditis)
  Tumors (extravascular)
Occlusion of Internal Jugular Vein
  Iatrogenic
  Indwelling catheter
  Surgery
  Traumatic
  Tumors (extravascular)

Dural or pial arteriovenous fistulae may reduce venous outflow sufficiently to produce PTC (58-61). In some of these cases, an associated venous sinus thrombosis is present, whereas in others, the flow through the cerebral venous sinuses is simply reduced. In all cases, the successful treatment of the fistula usually results in a resolution of the symptoms and signs of increased ICP.

Ligation of one jugular vein (if it is the principal vein draining the intracranial area) or both jugular veins may produce papilledema. In most instances, the occlusion of the jugular veins occurs during radical neck dissection for regional tumors; in other cases, the veins become thrombosed from the effects of indwelling catheters (57). The papilledema in such cases usually does not appear for a week or two. It is virtually always bilateral and severe; however, it typically resolves in 2 to 3 months, as collateral venous drainage from the head develops to meet the demands of cerebral blood flow.

Endocrine and Metabolic Dysfunctions

Patients with endocrine and metabolic dysfunction can develop pseudotumor cerebri (Table 29.2). As noted earlier, obesity is the most common finding in patients with PTC (1,15,17–19). In many of these patients, a history of menstrual irregularity is also present (62,63). Greer (64) described a self-limited PTC syndrome in 10 pubertal females at the time of menarche. He related this syndrome to the direct or indirect effects of ovarian hormones on the intracranial contents. This theory is based on experimental evidence obtained by other investigators indicating a mild increase in brain water content in the immature female rat given estrogen injections. Tessler et al. (65) reported a similar case. These reports, as well as the observation that idiopathic PTC almost never occurs in postmenopausal women, suggest that the ovarian hormones

pronounced engorgement may occur in the vessels of the scalp, retina, and conjunctiva, in addition to papilledema. Many of these patients have no underlying condition that can be linked to the thrombosis; however, in some, a coagulopathy from a primary hematologic disorder (e.g., protein C or S deficiency, antiphospholipid antibody syndrome, essential thrombocythemia) is found, whereas in others, a systemic process (e.g., cancer, pregnancy, recent delivery of a child, recent abortion) is identified. Still other patients with aseptic cerebral venous sinus thrombosis and PTC have a systemic inflammatory or infectious disease that affects venous coagulation (e.g., systemic lupus erythematosus, Behçet syndrome, trichinosis, sarcoidosis). Lam et al. (57) reported a patient who developed PTC after surgical ligation of the dominant sigmoid sinus to treat longstanding pulsatile tinnitus. Patients who develop PTC from a cerebral venous sinus thrombosis may experience complete resolution of their signs and symptoms if the obstructed sinus can be opened (48,49).

TABLE 29.2
*Endocrine and Metabolic Disorders,
and Physiologic Changes Associated
with Pseudotumor Cerebri*

Addison's disease
Hypoparathyroidism
    Primary
    Secondary
Hyperthyroidism
Hypothyroidism
Menarche
Menopause
Obesity (idiopathic)
Pregnancy
Turner syndrome

are indeed important in the genesis of this condition.

Donaldson and Binstock (66) studied extraovarian estrogen production in an obese young woman with pathologically confirmed mosaic Turner syndrome and PTC. Because such patients have no functional ovarian tissue, all estrogen production occurs through the action of the adrenal gland. These investigators found that diet plus enough dexamethasone to suppress adrenal steroidogenesis promptly lowered CSF pressure and serum concentrations of androstenedione, estrone, and testosterone. Estrone was detected in CSF before and after, but not during, dexamethasone administration. The findings of this study suggest that extraovarian estrogen may produce the menstrual irregularities in some obese young women with PTC.

The findings of Donaldson and Binstock (66) notwithstanding, most attempts made to detect specific endocrinologic disturbances in patients with the pseudotumor syndrome have been unsuccessful. For example, Greer (67) studied 20 obese women with classic PTC and could not obtain laboratory evidence of endocrine abnormality. Johnston and Paterson (15,16) measured plasma and urinary adrenal steroids in eight patients and found no consistent abnormality. They also estimated urinary gonadotrophins in three male patients. The values were normal in each case.

PTC not infrequently occurs during pregnancy. Greer (68) described eight patients who developed PTC during pregnancy. In all cases, the time of diagnosis was between the second and fifth months of gestation and coincided with the expected normal decline in levels of adrenal corticoids and the expected increase in estrogen concentration. In addition, the brief duration of the illness in each case corresponded to the time when a second rise in glucocorticoids normally occurs.

Permanent vision loss occurs with the same frequency in pregnant women who develop PTC as in nonpregnant women who develop the condition (69). Thus, although patients who develop PTC during pregnancy generally have good maternal and neonatal outcomes, we agree with those who recommend that nonpregnant women with active PTC be encouraged to delay pregnancy until the disease is under control. Such patients should also be monitored carefully throughout the pregnancy and should be instructed to contact their primary care physician, neurologist, or ophthalmologist should they develop any recurrent symptoms suggesting increased ICP (see "Clinical Manifestations" section).

Papilledema occurs in patients with both primary and secondary hypoparathyroidism, both of which are more common in women than in men. Sambrook and Hill (70) studied CSF absorption in a patient with primary hypoparathyroidism, papilledema, and seizures using I-131 RISA scanning. They found a marked reduction of CSF absorption that returned to normal after correction of the patient's hypocalcemia. It has been postulated that the hypocalcemia that occurs in patients with hypoparathyroidism leads to an increase in intracellular sodium and water that, in turn, interferes with the transport of CSF through the arachnoid granulations.

Exogenous Substances

Patients who are exposed to, or ingest, a variety of substances can develop PTC (Table 29.3). For some of these substances, the association between exposure or ingestion and the development of PTC is well-documented in numerous reports and investigations; for others, however, a causative relationship is supported by only a single case report and is tenuous at best.

Systemic corticosteroid therapy has been recognized as a cause of PTC since the report by Dees and McKay in 1959 (71). Steroid-induced PTC can occur in both adults and children, with the primary disease for which the steroids are administered not being a significant factor. In most cases, ICP returns to normal and papilledema and headache resolve as soon as steroids are discontinued (72–75).

PTC may occur in women taking oral contraceptives (76–78) or estrogen replacement after hysterectomy (79);

TABLE 29.3

Exogenous Substances Whose Exposure or Ingestion Is Associated with Pseudotumor Cerebri

Amiodarone
Antibiotics
    Nalidixic acid
    Penicillin
    Tetracyclines
Carbidopa/Levodopa (Sinemet®)
Chlordecone (Kepone®)
Corticosteroids
    Systemic
    Topical
Cyclosporine
Danazol
Growth hormone
Indomethecin
Ketoprofen
Lead
Leuprolide acetate (Lupron®)
Levonorgesterol implants (Norplant®)
Lithium carbonate
Oral contraceptives
Oxytocin (intranasal)
Perhexiline maleate
Phenytoin
Thyreostimulin suppression hormonotherapy
Vitamin A

however, a causal relationship between drug intake and increased ICP has not yet been established.

Several antibiotics may be associated with the development of PTC. The most common are the tetracyclines, which can produce the syndrome in infants, children, and both young and older adults (80,81). In infants, the condition manifests itself as a bulging of the fontanelles and occasionally by spreading of sutures. Irritability, drowsiness, feeding disturbances, and vomiting are common symptoms, although some infants are asymptomatic. The mechanism of the reaction is obscure. No correlation exists between the onset of the syndrome and either the dosage of the drug or the length of therapy. Cessation of tetracycline administration causes prompt regression of symptoms. Older children and adults have manifestations more consistent with typical PTC. Gardner et al. (80) described teenage fraternal twin sisters who developed PTC while taking tetracycline for acne. Both children had a rapid resolution of papilledema and headaches after stopping the drug. This report suggests that tetracycline-induced PTC may have a genetic predisposition.

The development of apparent PTC in a patient taking tetracycline or one of its derivatives does not necessarily indicate that the patient truly has PTC or that the drug is causing the illness. Aroichane et al. (82) described a young woman who developed headaches and papilledema while taking minocycline for acne. Magnetic resonance imaging (MRI) revealed some fullness of the basal ganglia; however, the ventricular system was not dilated, and there were no intracranial masses. Two lumbar punctures revealed increased ICP with normal CSF content. Specifically, cytopathologic examination revealed no malignant cells. A diagnosis of minocycline-induced PTC was made. The patient was taken off the antibiotic and treated with acetazolamide. She did not improve, however, and several weeks after the onset of symptoms, she experienced acute loss of vision. Neuroimaging now showed a mass in the region of the chiasm that was biopsied and found to be a glioblastoma multiforme.

Other substances associated with the development of PTC include amiodarone (83–85), cyclosporine (86), danazol (87,88), growth hormone (89,90), indomethacin (91), ketoprofen (92), leuprolide acetate (Lupron®—a gonadotropin-releasing hormone) (93,94), levonorgestrel implants (Norplant®) (95,96), lithium carbonate (97,98), various psychotherapeutic drugs (99), oxytocin (taken nasally) (100), phenytoin (101), and thyreostimulin suppression hormonotherapy (102).

It must be emphasized that when a patient develops PTC while taking a drug that is known or thought to cause the condition, one should not necessarily assume that the drug really is the cause. We examined a somewhat obese young woman who was taking lithium carbonate for a psychiatric disorder when she developed headaches and was found to have bilateral optic disc swelling. Neuroimaging and lumbar puncture established a diagnosis of PTC, which was assumed to have been caused by the lithium, a well-documented association. The patient was taken off lithium and treated with acetazolamide. Her headaches immediately disappeared, and her papilledema resolved. The acetazolamide was stopped, and the patient was free of symptoms for several months. However, 6 months later, while taking no psychotropic drugs, the patient's papilledema recurred. A diagnosis of idiopathic PTC was made, and acetazolamide was resumed, again with resolution of papilledema and normalization of ICP.

Daily ingestion of 100,000 or more units of vitamin A may, within a few months, produce increased ICP. In infants and small children, the condition is characterized by anorexia, lethargy, and an increasing head circumference (103). Older children and adults develop PTC (104,105). Some of these patients exhibit other manifestations of hypervitaminosis A, including fissuring of the angles of the lips, loss of hair, migratory bone pain, hypomenorrhea, hepatosplenomegaly, and dryness, roughness, and desquamation of the skin; however, most do not.

The diagnosis of PTC caused by hypervitaminosis A is usually simple, providing the physician knows that the patient is ingesting excessive amounts of vitamin A, either as the vitamin itself or in calf, bear, chicken, or shark liver (106–108). In some cases, however, the physician may not be aware that the patient is eating something high in vitamin A content. For example, Donahue (109) described a remarkable patient with resolved idiopathic PTC whose condition recurred after she began to eat 2 to 3 pounds of raw baby carrots per week as part of her weight-loss program. The patient's serum retinol level was markedly elevated. The condition resolved again after the patient discontinued her intake of carrots, which Donahue emphasized contain extremely large quantities of retinol. As emphasized by the case described by Donahue, reduction of the excessive vitamin A intake is invariably associated with resolution of all symptoms and signs, although Morrice et al. emphasized that resolution of disc swelling may take 4 to 6 months (110).

PTC can also occur after *withdrawal* or *deficiency* of certain substances and has been reported within several weeks after reduction or withdrawal of: (i) steroids following chronic use for a variety of disorders (111); (ii) danazol being used to treat endometriosis (112); (iii) a nonergot dopamine antagonist being used in two women for hyperprolactinemia (113); and (iv) beta-human chorionic gonadotropin (β-HCG) (114,115).

A deficiency of vitamin A can produce PTC (116), as can a deficiency of vitamin D (117), particularly in infants. According to Lessell (10), the child at special risk is an exclusively breast-fed child of a strict vegan mother. This form of PTC resolves slowly.

Systemic Illnesses

Increased ICP with papilledema can occur in patients with meningitis and encephalitis. In many of these cases, the ventricular system is blocked in some location and is thus dilated, and the CSF contains white blood cells or an elevated protein content. Such cases are not, by definition, examples of PTC. In other cases, such as Whipple disease, neuroborreliosis, and neurosarcoidosis, the ventricular system appears normal, although the CSF contains white blood cells, malignant cells, an increased protein content, or a combination of these. Such cases are considered examples not of PTC but of the "pseudotumor cerebri syndrome," as are cases of meningeal lymphomatosis and carcinomatosis. In such cases, it is the CSF and not neuroimaging that indicates that the clinical manifestations are not caused by PTC. Nevertheless, some systemic inflammatory, infectious, and noninfectious disorders rarely may be associated with increased ICP, papilledema, normal-sized ventricles, and normal CSF content (Table 29.4). In such cases, treatment of the underlying condition commonly results in a normalization of ICP and resolution of papilledema (118).

Papilledema is a rare finding in patients with various types of anemia, including microcytic, iron-deficiency, megaloblastic, and hemolytic anemia (119–122). The mechanism of increased ICP in patients with anemia is unknown and may be multifactoral; however, it is most likely that in most cases, low hemoglobin levels result in compensatory changes in cerebral blood volume, leading to increased ICP. In any event, in cases of PTC associated with anemia, correction of the hematologic disorder is associated with normalization of ICP and resolution of papilledema (121,122).

TABLE 29.4
Systemic Illnesses Associated with Pseudotumor Cerebri

Anemia
Brucellosis
Chronic respiratory insufficiency
    Pickwickian syndrome
    Obstructive sleep apnea
Familial Mediterranean fever
Hypertension
Multiple sclerosis
Polyangiitis overlap syndrome
Psittacosis
Renal disease
Reye syndrome
Sarcoidosis
Systemic lupus erythematosus
Thrombocytopenic purpura

Chronic respiratory insufficiency may be associated with increased ICP and papilledema (123). Affected patients have chronic hypercapnia, with retention of carbon dioxide (CO_2), reduced blood oxygen (O_2) levels, polycythemia, increased venous pressure, and increased ICP. Respiratory acidosis in such cases causes an accumulation of CO_2 in brain tissue, reflected by an inversion of the normal CO_2 tension ratio between CSF and arterial blood. This, in turn, causes dilation of cerebral capillaries and increases intracranial blood volume.

In most cases of increased ICP related to pulmonary insufficiency, the pulmonary dysfunction is caused by primary pulmonary disease. In other patients, however, respiratory insufficiency is caused by a systemic myopathy, such as muscular dystrophy. In still others, hypoventilation from extreme obesity causes a typical cardiopulmonary syndrome—the Pickwickian syndrome—a condition that is more common in women than in men. The obesity in these patients causes diminished vital capacity, polycythemia, and cyanosis. Severe drowsiness is common, and many patients have obstructive sleep apnea (124–126). The disc swelling and fundus abnormalities usually resolve rapidly once respiratory acidosis and sleep apnea, if present, are treated. Not all patients with obstructive sleep apnea are markedly obese, however. Thus, if a patient with presumed PTC has a history of insomnia or snoring, obstructive sleep apnea should be considered, and an evaluation for a sleep disorder obtained. If sleep apnea is found, treatment with continuous positive airway pressure (CPAP) may be beneficial.

The neurologic manifestations of respiratory failure include somnolence, asterixis, other movement disorders, and in severe cases, coma (127). It was once thought that papilledema in association with other neurologic symptoms in patients with chronic respiratory failure was indicative of impending death; however, this is not the case. Supportive respiratory therapy and prompt treatment of the acute physiologic, metabolic, and electrolyte abnormalities can significantly prolong survival and improve the quality of survival time (128).

PTC can occur in patients with systemic lupus erythematosus (129), a disease that is more frequent in women than in men. In some of these cases, the pathogenesis is occlusion of one of the dural venous sinuses, usually the superior sagittal sinus (130,131). In other cases, the pathogenesis is unclear (132). Because the condition usually resolves when the patients are treated with systemic corticosteroids, however, it is possible that inflammation and tissue necrosis in the region of the arachnoid villi interfere with CSF absorption, thereby raising ICP without causing a generalized inflammatory response in the CSF (133).

Thrombocytopenic purpura can be caused by a number of mechanisms, including decreased platelet production and decreased platelet survival. PTC occurs in association with two forms of this condition, both of which are associated with decreased platelet survival: immune idiopathic thromocytopenic purpura (ITP) and nonimmune thrombotic thrombocytopenic purpura (TTP).

ITP occurs in two forms, acute and chronic. Acute ITP occurs most often in children, usually after an upper respiratory tract infection, whereas chronic ITP occurs most often in women between 20 and 45 years of age. The etiology of this condition is a spontaneously appearing antibody that damages the platelets, causing them to be removed from the circulation by the reticuloendothelial system. Furuta et al. (134) described a 53-year-old woman with ITP who developed PTC from thrombosis of the superior sagittal sinus.

TTP is characterized by severe thrombocytopenia, hemolytic anemia, fever, renal dysfunction, and CNS disturbances (135). Patients with this condition occasionally develop PTC, presumably from an obstruction of the cerebral venous sinuses.

FAMILIAL PSEUDOTUMOR CEREBRI

The occurrence of PTC in family members is well recognized. Bucheit et al. (5) first described two sisters with this syndrome, and numerous other examples have been reported (80,136). We have seen it in a father and his daughter.

COMPLICATIONS OF PSEUDOTUMOR CEREBRI

PTC is a self-limited condition in some cases. In most cases, however, the ICP remains elevated for many years, even if systemic and visual symptoms resolve. Corbett et al. (137) followed a group of 57 patients with a diagnosis of PTC for 5-41 years. These investigators performed complete neuro-ophthalmologic examinations, including fundus photographs, on all patients. In over 80% of the patients studied by these investigators, CSF pressure remained elevated, regardless of the treatment the patients had received. The chronic nature of PTC has been substantiated by reports of patients who have developed recurrent headaches and papilledema after either removal (138) or blockage (139) of their lumboperitoneal shunts. Some of these patients have experienced permanent loss of vision from the rapid increase in ICP in these settings.

The effects of even self-limited PTC on the visual system may be catastrophic. In the study by Corbett et al. (137), severe visual impairment occurred in one or both eyes in 26% of patients, several of whom experienced visual loss months to years after initial symptoms appeared. In this study, systemic hypertension was a statistically significant risk factor for visual loss. Other investigators have reported similar results (140–146).

PATHOPHYSIOLOGY OF IDIOPATHIC PSEUDOTUMOR CEREBRI

As noted earlier, the etiology of the increased ICP in about 10% of patients with PTC can be determined. For example, patients with occlusion of the superior sagittal sinus develop raised venous pressure that reduces the absorption of CSF across the arachnoid villi. A similar mechanism is responsible for the PTC that occurs in some patients after ligation of the internal jugular vein. The pathogenesis of increased ICP in 90% of patients with idiopathic PTC is unclear, however (147), although numerous studies have suggested potential mechanisms. For example, it is well known that vitamin A ingestion can produce PTC. Jacobson et al. (148) prospectively determined serum retinol and retinyl ester concentration in 16 women with the idiopathic form of PTC and compared the results with those from 70 healthy women. These investigators found that the serum retinol concentration was significantly higher in the patient group compared with controls, even after adjusting for age and body mass index (p<0.001), even though there was no significant difference in the amounts of vitamin A ingested by the patients or the controls. A similar study was performed by Selhorst et al. (149), who measured serum retinol and retinol binding protein. These investigators also found that mean retinol values were higher in patients than in controls, although the values did not reach a significant level. In addition, 7 of 30 patients with IIH had elevated retinol binding protein levels, whereas none of the 40 control subjects did. These findings may indicate that the abnormal metabolism of vitamin A is responsible for some cases of so-called idiopathic PTC (150).

Another hypothesis is that the elevation of intracranial venous pressure is responsible for idiopathic PTC (151); however, King et al. found, in patients with IIH, that when transducer-measured intracranial venous pressure is high, reduction of CSF pressure by removal of CSF predictably lowers the venous sinus pressure (152). The results of this study indicate that increased venous pressure is caused by elevated ICP and not the other way around (153). Thus, elevated venous pressure is *not* the primary event in the elevation of CSF pressure with IIH.

Despite the investigations described above, we still do not know what initiates the chain of events leading to increased CSF pressure (152), and we continue to agree with Fishman (154) that despite the numerous investigations into the pathophysiology of PTC, "there are more speculations than data available."

DIAGNOSIS

The diagnosis of PTC is based on three crucial findings (1,155,156) (Figure 29.4). First, the patient must have normal or small ventricles and no intracranial mass lesion. Second, the ICP must be increased. Third, the CSF must have no cells and a normal protein and glucose concentration. It is inappropriate to diagnose PTC in a patient with a "slightly elevated" concentration of protein or a pleocytosis in the CSF. Such patients do not have PTC but rather the "pseudotumor cerebri syndrome;" that is, they satisfy all the criteria required to diagnose PTC except that the CSF does not have a normal content (157). Such patients must undergo further evaluation for possible carcinomatous, lymphomatous, or aseptic meningitis.

In order to satisfy the criteria required to diagnose PTC, a patient *must* undergo some type of neuroimaging study followed by a lumbar puncture (1,158,159). Computed tomography (CT) scanning usually is adequate to detect any intracranial mass lesion that could produce

increased ICP and to determine the size of the ventricles, but it is not as sensitive as MRI in detecting cerebral venous thrombosis unless CT venography is performed at the same time (160). We thus prefer to obtain MRI, including MR venography, whenever possible. Lumbar puncture should then be performed in the lateral decubitus position. The opening pressure should be measured with a manometer, and adequate CSF should be obtained for the assessment of cellular content, concentrations of protein and glucose, and any other tests deemed appropriate by the treating physician. We find that the easiest method of performing a lumbar puncture in obese patients is with fluoroscopic guidance. If a lumbar puncture cannot be performed using fluoroscopy, the patient can undergo a lumbar puncture in the sitting position. Once the subarachnoid space is entered, as evidenced by flow of CSF through the hollow needle, the patient can be carefully placed in decubitus position and the CSF pressure obtained.

It is inappropriate and dangerous to make a diagnosis of PTC without both neuroimaging studies and lumbar puncture, even if the clinical setting appears straightforward. We have examined several obese patients in whom a diagnosis of PTC was suspected after they developed headaches and papilledema and were found to have normal results on neuroimaging studies but in whom the increased ICP was found to have been caused by septic or aseptic meningitis, gliomatosis cerebri, or leptomeningeal carcinoma or lymphoma. In addition, not all optic disc swelling in an obese young woman is caused by increased ICP. We recently evaluated a 34-year-old obese woman complaining of blurred vision in both eyes associated with pain behind the eyes. She had been examined by an ophthalmologist who found visual acuity of 20/25 in both eyes associated with severe bilateral optic disc swelling. Because of her appearance and the bilateral disc swelling, he referred her immediately to a neurologist, who obtained MRI that was normal. He made a diagnosis of PTC without performing a lumbar puncture and placed the patient on acetazolamide. When she progressively lost vision in both eyes over the next several days, he referred the patient for emergency optic nerve sheath fenestration (see "Treatment" section). It was our opinion that the loss of vision was out of proportion to the severity of optic disc swelling. We therefore obtained an emergency lumbar puncture, which gave normal results. We stopped the patient's acetazolamide and performed a second lumbar puncture 48 hours later, again with normal results. We thus concluded that the patient had bilateral anterior optic neuritis and treated her with intravenous high-dose corticosteroids. She subsequently made a complete recovery. Other physicians have reported similar cases (161). We even have seen obese patients with brain tumors in whom an initial

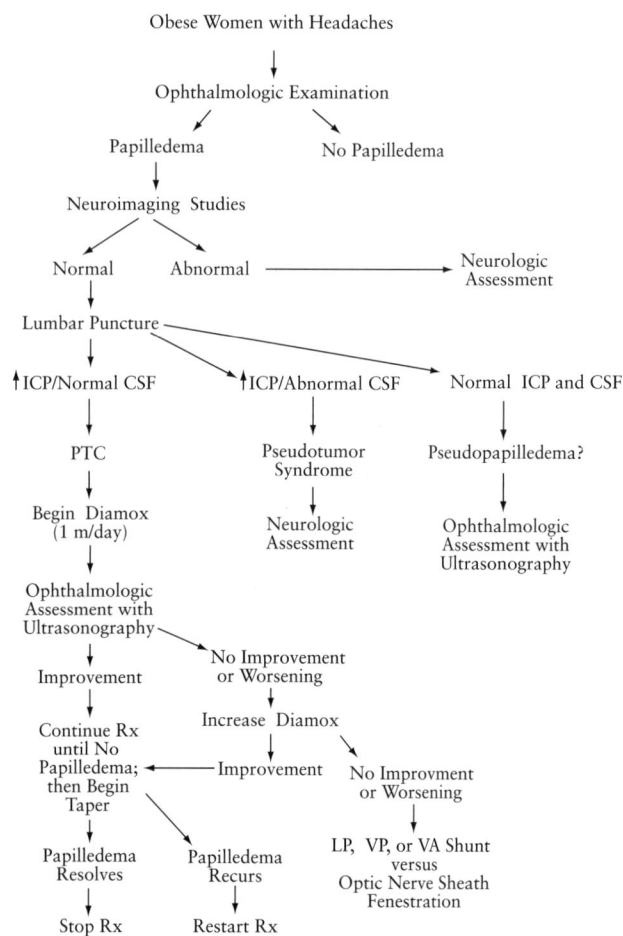

FIGURE 29.4

Decision pathway for the diagnosis and management of pseudotumor cerebri.

diagnosis of PTC was made on the basis of headaches and papilledema without either neuroimaging or a lumbar puncture.

Once a diagnosis of PTC is made by neuroimaging followed by lumbar puncture, the physician should attempt to determine if an etiology can be found. This is particularly important in young nonobese women, in older women, and in men, regardless of age or body habitus, because such patients are much less likely to develop the idiopathic form of PTC (7-9,19,145,146). In addition, we have examined several obese women—one after a spontaneous abortion—in whom a diagnosis of presumed idiopathic PTC was found to be incorrect after neuroimaging revealed evidence of cerebral venous sinus thrombosis. We therefore recommend that all patients, not just nonobese women and men, undergo MRI before it is concluded that they have idiopathic PTC. Such an assessment is best performed using a combination of standard MRI and MR venography or CT scanning and venography (160,162). Catheter angiography is rarely required in such cases.

MONITORING

Patients with papilledema can develop progressive loss of visual function in a manner similar to that which occurs in patients with chronic open-angle glaucoma. Visual field defects, usually arcuate scotomas and nasal steps, are an early finding, whereas loss of central vision is usually a very late phenomenon. Thus, it is inappropriate to monitor patients with PTC by simply measuring visual acuity. Such patients should not only undergo testing of best-corrected visual acuity at distance and near, but also color vision testing using pseudoisochromatic plates or a similar method, visual field testing, and ophthalmoscopic examination of the optic discs (163,164).

Although all patients with papilledema should be tested to determine if a relative afferent pupillary defect is present, papilledema tends to be a bilateral symmetric condition. Thus, when present in a patient with papilledema, a relative afferent pupillary defect generally indicates damage to the retina or optic nerve of the eye with the defect. The absence of a relative afferent pupillary defect, however, cannot be taken as evidence of no optic nerve damage from increased ICP (165).

We believe that, in addition to standard clinical testing, stereo color photographs of the optic discs should be obtained on a regular basis on any patient with papilledema to provide the examiner with objective evidence of the appearance of the optic discs. We do not routinely perform other tests of visual sensory function, such as contrast sensitivity testing, motion perimetry, or visual evoked potentials, but these tests may be useful in individual patients in whom issues of management develop (166).

The intervals between the clinical assessments of patients with papilledema must be individualized. We examine some patients every 1 to 2 weeks until we have a sense of the progression or stability of their condition. Other patients are examined every 1 to 3 months, and patients with stable papilledema may only be examined every 4 to 12 months.

The importance of monitoring visual function in patients with papilledema associated with PTC cannot be overemphasized, because most visual defects associated with papilledema are reversible if ICP is lowered before there is severe vision loss, chronic papilledema, or optic atrophy (167,168).

Patients with papilledema should be monitored not only with respect to their clinical manifestations, but also with respect to their increased ICP. In most patients, simple assessment of the optic discs is sufficient. In other patients, however, repeat lumbar puncture is needed. As noted above, we find that performing a lumbar puncture in patients with PTC is straightforward when the procedure is performed under fluoroscopy.

Although both CT scanning and MRI can be used to visualize papilledema and its resolution (12,169–171), we do not believe that these techniques are useful in the diagnosis and management of a patient with papilledema compared with the information gained from a combination of clinical assessment and a lumbar puncture.

TREATMENT

The treatment of PTC depends on whether an underlying etiology can be identified and treated. If so, treatment of the causative process should result in a normalization of ICP and resolution of papilledema (48,49). Conversely, if no etiology can be identified; that is, if the patient has idiopathic PTC, then treatment is directed at lowering ICP (1,144,145) (Figure 29.4).

There are generally only two reasons to treat patients with idiopathic PTC: severe intractable headache that is clearly related to increased ICP, and evidence of progressive visual field and/or visual acuity loss from optic neuropathy. Methods of treatment include weight loss, medical therapy, serial lumbar punctures, and surgery. No single procedure is completely effective in this regard (19,20,144,172).

The optimum treatment for obese patients with idiopathic PTC is weight loss. It has been shown that as little as a 7 to 10% drop in weight may be associated with a rapid resolution of papilledema and the symptoms of PTC (173–175). Thus, a patient may be given a target weight to achieve, making the weight loss perhaps a bit easier. In general, weight loss in patients with idiopathic PTC should be achieved through a combination of diet and exercise prescribed by a registered dietitian or nutritionist. It must be remembered that these patients often have attempted to lose weight in the past without success and may therefore need special assistance.

When standard weight loss methods fail, as they often do (176,177) or when the patient is morbidly obese, gastric-bypass surgery can be performed. Such surgery is generally followed by reduction in weight, normalization of ICP, and resolution of papilledema (178–180), although it has significant potential complications, including anastomotic leaks, small bowel obstruction, and gastrointestinal bleeding. One of our patients had a fatal pulmonary embolism following otherwise successful gastric-bypass surgery for morbid obesity.

As noted above, patients with PTC in the setting of morbid obesity who have sleep apnea (i.e., the Pickwickian syndrome) may respond not only to weight loss, but also to low-flow oxygen and positive airway ventilation using either CPAP or bilevel positive airway pressure (bi-PAP) (125,128,181–183).

Although weight loss is, in our opinion, the optimum way to treat PTC, it is often difficult to achieve. Indeed, we find that even though patients understand the need to lose weight and the consequences of not doing so, they simply cannot lose weight or if they do, they subsequently gain it back. Thus, other methods of treatment must be considered.

A number of medical substances can be used to lower ICP. The most effective is acetazolamide (11,184,185). This drug decreases the production of CSF by an inhibition of carbonic anhydrase, resulting in decreased sodium ion transport across the choroidal epithelium (186-189). Güçer and Viernstein (190) found that patients with idiopathic PTC who were treated with acetazolamide often responded within several hours. Acetazolamide should be started at a dose of 1 g per day, given in divided doses of either 250 mg qid or 500 mg sequels bid. Theoretically, the dose can be increased up to a maximum of 4 g per day, but we have never found anyone who could tolerate this dosage because of the side effects, which include paresthesias of the extremities, lethargy, decreased libido, and a metallic or dry taste in the mouth. These side effects can be reduced but not eliminated by using sequels (191).

Jefferson and Clark (192) used a variety of dehydrating agents to treat PTC with excellent results. Guy et al. (193) reported improvement in three patients with uremia and PTC who responded to furosemide, and Schoeman (11) found the combination of acetazolamide and furosemide to be helpful in several children with PTC. Despite these reports, we find that most dehydrating drugs are not particularly efficacious in lowering ICP in patients with PTC.

Although systemic corticosteroids are clearly beneficial in the treatment of PTC associated with various systemic inflammatory disorders, such as sarcoidosis and systemic lupus erythematosus, they are not generally recommended for use in idiopathic PTC. Nevertheless, Liu et al. (194) reported that the use of high-dose intravenous methylprednisolone (250 mg four times per day) combined with oral acetazolamide resulted in a lowering of ICP and marked improvement in visual function in four patients with PTC who had severe papilledema and vision loss.

Although a single case report suggests that indomethacin can cause PTC (91), this drug may reduce ICP in selected patients with the idiopathic form of PTC. Forderreuther and Straube injected seven patients with IIH and ICPs between 350 and 500 mm H_2O (mean, 400 mm H_2O) with indomethacin while monitoring their ICP (195). During administration of indomethacin, all seven patients showed a marked reduction of CSF pressure within 1 minute (mean, 139 mm H_2O; range, 80 to 200 mm H_2O). Five patients were subsequently treated with oral indomethacin (75 mg per day) and all reported improvement of headache. In addition, ophthalmologic follow-up in these patients revealed improvement in papilledema. These findings have yet to be corroborated by other investigators.

Multiple lumbar punctures are advocated as a nonmedical, nonsurgical method of relieving the increased ICP of idiopathic PTC. We have found this treatment to be effective in a few children with the condition but not in the majority of adults. The theory behind this treatment is that the needle used for the lumbar puncture creates an opening in the dura through which CSF leaks. With several lumbar punctures, one creates a "sieve" that allows sufficient egress of CSF and ICP is normalized.

Surgical decompression procedures are generally used only when patients initially present with severe optic neuropathy or when other forms of treatment have failed, and the patients are incapacitated by headache or have begun to develop evidence of progressive optic neuropathy (146). Subtemporal decompression was advocated in the past and occasionally is still performed in select cases (196), but most neurosurgeons favor some form of shunting procedure. Ventriculoperitoneal or ventriculoatrial shunting is quite effective in lowering intracranial pressure in patients with PTC (197), but this procedure can be difficult unless some type of stereotactic method is used, because the ventricles in patients with PTC are normal in size rather than being enlarged. Thus, in many institutions, the preferred technique is the lumboperitoneal shunt, in which a silicone tube is placed percutaneously between the lumbar subarachnoid space and the peritoneal cavity. Complications of the shunt procedure are minimal and usually benign but include spontaneous obstruction of the shunt, usually at the peritoneal end, excessive low pressure, infection, radiculopathy, and migration of the tube, resulting in abdominal pain (198,199). Some patients also develop a Chiari malformation that may or may not be symptomatic (198,200).

Nevertheless, most patients treated with a lumboperitoneal shunt experience a rapid return of ICP to normal and resolution of papilledema, often with improvement in visual function (200,201). Shunts that fail usually do so within the first 2 years after initial placement (200).

Optic nerve sheath fenestration has been advocated for the treatment of patients with severe papilledema, particularly that which occurs in intractable PTC. A successful optic nerve sheath fenestration results in resolution of papilledema on that side and, occasionally, on the other, with improvement in visual function in many cases (202–206). Regardless of the technique used, the procedure immediately reduces pressure on the nerve by creating a filtration apparatus that controls the intravaginal pressure surrounding the orbital segment of the optic nerve (207,208); however, it may not reduce ICP. Kaye et al. (209) monitored ICP before and after bilateral optic nerve decompression in a patient with PTC. These investigators found no postoperative changes in ICP and concluded that the decrease in papilledema and the visual improvement after optic nerve sheath surgery occurred from a local decrease in optic nerve sheath pressure rather than from a generalized decrease in ICP. Similar results were reported by Jacobson et al. (210). These investigators reported six patients who had ICP, CSF resistance, or both measured both before and after optic nerve sheath fenestration. Pressure was elevated in five of six patients preoperatively. It decreased in all six patients after optic nerve sheath fenestration, but not to normal. In addition, four of the six patients still had high CSF resistance after the surgery.

The risks of optic nerve sheath fenestration, although low, are nevertheless significant. They include loss of vision from vascular occlusion, diplopia, and infection (202–206,211). Because of these potential complications, the low permanent success rate of the procedure of about 16% within 6 years of the procedure (212), and the difficulty in performing repeat optic nerve sheath fenestration in patients whose initial procedure has failed (202), we favor ventricular or lumboperitoneal shunts as the surgical treatments of choice in most patients with PTC in whom medical therapy has failed or cannot be tolerated. Nevertheless, long-term benefit from optic nerve sheath fenestration is well-documented (205,206,213), and the procedure may be appropriate for patients with PTC who refuse, cannot undergo, or do not respond to shunting. It may also be the treatment of choice for patients with severe papilledema caused by a malignant brain tumor in whom a long-term solution is not required, and for patients with severe vision loss on presentation in whom immediate decompression of the optic nerve is mandatory. These latter patients may benefit from a combined shunt and an optic nerve sheath fenestration.

The major difficulty in assessing surgical results in patients with PTC is that generally these procedures are not used until evidence of optic neuropathy is already present. In such patients, it is impossible to know at what stage irreversible visual acuity or field loss has occurred. For this reason, a "successful" procedure may still be followed by optic atrophy, with diminished visual acuity or reduced visual field. The continuous monitoring of ICP and the use of more sophisticated testing of optic nerve function may ultimately enable physicians to decide whether to use medical or surgical therapy to reduce ICP and at what stage a change in therapy must be considered.

It is important to recognize that a substantial percentage of patients with PTC have headaches that are unrelated to increased ICP (214). Indeed, some of these patients have tension headaches, whereas others have migraines. Correctly identifying the nature of these headaches will prevent inappropriate treatment in such patients.

Women who develop PTC during pregnancy can be treated in much the same way as nonpregnant women except that caloric restriction and the use of diuretics are contraindicated (69,215,216). Specifically, lumboperitoneal shunting can be performed with little or no maternal or fetal risk (216), and this treatment should not be withheld simply because the patient is pregnant.

References

1. Friedman DI, Jacobson DM. Diagnostic criteria for idiopathic intracranial hypertension. *Neurology* 2002;59: 1492–1495.
2. Quincke H. Ueber Meningitis Serosa und verwandte Zustande. *Dtsch Z Nervenheilkd* 1897;9:149–218.
3. Warrington WB. Intracranial serous effusions of inflammatory origin: meningitis or ependymitis serosa—meningism—with note on "pseudo-tumors" of the brain. *Q J Med* 1914;7:93–118.
4. Foley J. Benign forms of intracranial hypertension—"toxic" and "otitic hydrocephalus." *Brain* 1955;78:1–41.
5. Bucheit WA, Burton D, Haag B, et al. Papilledema and idiopathic intracranial hypertension. *N Engl J Med* 1969; 280:938–942.
6. Bandyopadhyay S. Pseudotumor cerebri. *Arch Neurol* 2001;58:1699–1701.
7. Durcan FJ, Corbett JJ, Wall M. The incidence of pseudotumor cerebri: population studies in Iowa and Louisiana. *Arch Neurol* 1988;45:875–877.
8. Radhakrishnan K, Ahlskog JE, Cross SA, et al. Idiopathic intracranial hypertension (pseudotumor cerebri): Descriptive epidemiology in Rochester, Minn, 1976 to 1990. *Arch Neurol* 1993;50:78–80.
9. Radhakrishnan L, Thacker AK, Bohlaga NH, et al. Epidemiology of idiopathic intracranial hypertension: a prospective and case-control study. *J Neurol Sci* 1993; 116:18–28.
10. Lessell S. Pediatric pseudotumor cerebri (idiopathic intracranial hypertension. *Surv Ophthalmol* 1992;37: 155–166.
11. Schoeman JF. Childhood pseudotumor cerebri: clinical and intracranial pressure response to acetazolamide and furosemide treatment in a case series. *J Child Neurol* 1994;9:130–134.

12. Brodsky MC, Glasier CM. Magnetic resonance visualization of the swollen optic disc in papilledema. *J Neuroophthalmol* 1995;15:122–124.

13. Youroukos S, Psychou F, Fryssiras S, et al. Idiopathic intracranial hypertension in children. *J Child Neurol* 2000;15:453–457.

14. Bandyopadhyay S, Jacobson DM. Clinical features of late-onset pseudotumor cerebri fulfilling the modified Dandy criteria. *J Neuroophthalmol* 2002;22:9–11.

15. Johnston L, Paterson A. Benign intracranial hypertension: I. Diagnosis and prognosis. *Brain* 1974;97:289–300.

16. Johnston I, Paterson A. Benign intracranial hypertension: II. Cerebrospinal fluid pressure and circulation. *Brain* 1974;97:301–312.

17. Kesler A, Goldhammer Y, Gadoth N. Do men with pseudotumor cerebri share the same characteristics as women? A retrospective review of 141 cases. *J Neuroophthalmol* 2001;21:15–17.

18. Giuseffi V, Wall M, Siegel PZ, et al. Symptoms and disease associated in idiopathic intracranial hypertension (pseudotumor cerebri): a case-control study. *Neurology* 1991;41:239–244.

19. Biousse V, Bousser MG. L'hypertension intracranienne benigne. *Rev Neurol* 2001;157:21–34.

20. Salman MS, Kirkham FJ, MacGregor DL. Idiopathic "benign" intracranial hypertension: case series and review. *J Child Neurol* 2001;16:465–470.

21. Purvin VA, Trobe JD, Kosmorsky G. Neuro-ophthalmic features of venous sinus thrombosis. *Arch Neurol* 1995;52:880–885.

22. Zachariah SB, Jimenez L, Zachariah B, et al. Pseudotumor cerebri with focal neurological defect. *J Neurol Neurosurg Psychiatry* 1990;53:360–361.

23. Davie C, Kennedy P, Katifi HA. Seventh nerve palsy as a false localising sign. *J Neurol Neurosurg Psychiatry* 1992;55:510–511.

24. Davenport RJ, Will RG, Galloway PJ. Isolated intracranial hypertension presenting with trigeminal neuropathy. *J Neurol Neurosurg Psychiatry* 1994;57:381–386.

25. Selky AK, Purvin VA. Hemifacial spasm: an unusual manifestation of idiopathic intracranial hypertension. *J Neuroophthalmol* 1994;14:196–198.

26. Selky AK, Dobyns WB, Yee RD. Idiopathic intracranial hypertension and facial diplegia. *Neurology* 1994;44:357.

27. Bortoluzzi M, Di Lauro L, Marini G. Benign intracranial hypertension with spinal and radicular pain: case report. *J Neurosurg* 1995;57:833–705.

28. Dorman PJ, Campbell MJ, Maw AR. Hearing loss as a false localising sign in raised intracranial pressure. *J Neurol Neurosurg Psychiatry* 1995;58:516.

29. Benegas NM, Volpe NJ, Liu GT, et al. Hemifacial spasm and idiopathic intracranial hypertension. *J Neuroophthalmol* 1996;16:70.

30. Jobges EM, Johannes S, Schubert M, et al. Mononeuropathia multiplex and idiopathic intracranial hypertension. *Clin Neurol Neurosurg* 1996;98:37–39.

31. Rowe FJ. The symptoms of raised intracranial pressure in idiopathic intracranial hypertension. *Br Orthopt J* 2000;57:15–18.

32. Soelberg Serensen P, Gjerris F, Svenstrup B. Endocrine studies in patients with pseudotumor cerebri: estrogen levels in blood and cerebrospinal fluid. *Arch Neurol* 1986;43:902–906.

33. Coffey CE, Ross DR, Massey EW, et al. Familial benign intracranial hypertension and depression. *Can J Neurol Sci* 1982;9:45–47.

34. Coffey CE, Massey EW, Ross DR, et al. Benign intracranial hypertension and depression. *Neurology* 1983;33 (suppl 2):223.

35. Coffey CE. Idiopathic intracranial hypertension. *Neurology* 2000;55:901.

36. Digre KB, Kleinschmidt JJ. Idiopathic intracranial hypertension. *Neurology* 2000;55:901.

37. Kleinschmidt JJ, Digre KB, Hanover R. Idiopathic intracranial hypertension. *Neurology* 2000;54:319–324.

38. Akova YA, Kansu T, Yazar Z, et al. Macular subretinal neovascular membrane associated with pseudotumor cerebri. *J Neuroophthalmol* 1994;14:193–195.

39. Carter SR, Seiff SR. Macular changes in pseudotumor cerebri before and after optic nerve sheath fenestration. *Ophthalmology* 1995;102:937–941.

40. Lee AG. Fourth nerve palsy in pseudotumor cerebri. *Strabismus* 1995;3:57–59.

41. Rowe FJ. Acquired ocular motility disorders in idiopathic intracranial hypertension. *Neuro-ophthalmology* 2000;24:445–453.

42. Mansour AM, Zatorski J. Analysis of variables for papilledema in pseudotumor cerebri. *Ann Ophthalmol* 1994;26:172–174.

43. Torun N, Sharpe JA. Pseudotumor cerebri mimicking Foster Kennedy syndrome. *Neuro-ophthalmology* 1996;16:55–57.

44. Digre KB, Corbett JJ. Pseudotumor cerebri in men. *Arch Neurol* 1988;45:866–872.

45. Biousse V, Ameri A, Bousser MG. Isolated intracranial hypertension as the only sign of cerebral venous thrombosis. *Neurology* 1999;53:1537–1542.

46. Purvin VA, Dunn DW, Edwards M. MRI and cerebral venous thrombosis. *Comput Radiol* 1987;22:75–79.

47. Horton JC, Seiff SR, Pitts LH, et al. Decompression of the optic nerve sheath for vision-threatening papilledema caused by dural sinus occlusion. *Neurosurgery* 1992;31:302–312.

48. Kollar C, Parker G, Johnston I. Endovascular treatment of cranial venous sinus obstruction resulting in pseudotumor syndrome. *J Neurosurg* 2001;94:646–651.

49. Higgins JNP, Owler BK, Cousins C, et al. Venous sinus stenting for refractory benign intracranial hypertension. *Lancet* 2002;359:228–230.

50. Repka MX, Miller NR. Papilledema and dural sinus obstruction. *J Clin Neuroophthalmol* 1984;4:247–250.

51. Graus F, Slatkin NE. Papilledema in the metastatic jugular foramen syndrome. *Arch Neurol* 1983;40:816–818.

52. Truong DD, Holgate RC, Hsu CY, et al. Occlusion of the transverse sinus by meningioma simulating pseudotumor cerebri. *Neuro-ophthalmology* 1987;7:113–117.

53. Lenz RP, McDonald GA. Otitic hydrocephalus. *Laryngoscope* 1984;94:1451–1454.

54. Rosa A, Mizon JP. Benign intracranial hypertension: follow-up of seven cases. *Neuro-ophthalmology* 1984;3:171–174.

55. Dill JL, Crowe SJ. Thrombosis of the sygmoid or lateral sinus: report of thirty cases. *Arch Surg* 1934;29:705–722.

56. Kanai H, Takahashi Y, Shindo Y, et al. A case of lateral and sigmoid sinus thrombosis with bilateral severe papilledema. *Folia Ophthalmol Jpn* 2002;53:60–65.

57. Lam BL, Schatz NJ, Glaser JS, et al. Pseudotumor cerebri from cranial venous obstruction. *Ophthalmology* 1992;99:706–712.

58. Barrow DL. Unruptured cerebral venous malformation presenting with intracranial hypertension. *Neurosurgery* 1988;23:484–490.

59. Rosenfeld JV, Widaa HA, Adams CBT. Cerebral arteriovenous malformation causing benign intracranial hypertension: case report. *Neurol Med Chir* 1991;31:523–525.

60. Kamite Y, Akimithu T, Ohta K, et al. A case of intracranial arteriovenous malformation presenting with intracranial hypertension. *No Shinkei Geka* 1994;22:485–489.

61. Vorstman EBA, Niemann DB, Molyneux AJ, et al. Benign intracranial hypertension associated with arteriovenous malformation. *Dev Med Child Neurol* 2002;44:133–135.

62. McCullagh EP. Menstrual edema with intracranial hypertension (pseudotumor cerebri): report of a case. *Cleve Clin Q* 1941;8:202–212.

63. Greer M. Benign intracranial hypertension: V. Menstrual dysfunction. *Neurology* 1964;14:668–673.

64. Greer M. Benign intracranial hypertension: IV. Menarche. *Neurology* 1964;14:569–573b.

65. Tessler Z, Biender B, Yassur Y. Papilloedema: benign intracranial hypertension in menarche. *Ann Ophthalmol* 1985;17:76–77.

66. Donaldson JO, Binstock ML. Pseudotumor cerebri in an obese woman with Turner syndrome. *Neurology* 1981;31:758–760.

67. Greer M. Benign intracranial hypertension: VI. Obesity. *Neurology* 1965;15:382–388.

68. Greer M. Benign intracranial hypertension: III. Pregnancy. *Neurology* 1963;13:670–672.

69. Digre KB, Varner MW, Corbett JJ. Pseudotumor cerebri and pregnancy. *Neurology* 1984;34:721–729.

70. Sambrook MA, Hill LF. Cerebrospinal fluid absorption in primary hypoparathyroidism. *J Neurol Neurosurg Psychiatry* 1977;40:1015–1017.

71. Dees SC, McKay HW Jr. Occurrrence of pseudotumor cerebri during treatment of children with asthma by adrenal steroids. *Pediatrics* 1959;23:1143–1151.

72. Cohn GA. Pseudotumor cerebri in children secondary to administration of adrenal steroids. *J Neurosurg* 1963;20:784–786.

73. Greer M. Benign intracranial hypertension: II. Following corticosteroid therapy. *Neurology* 1963;13:439–441.

74. Walker AE, Adamkiewicz JJ. Pseudotumor cerebri associated with prolonged corticosteroid therapy. *JAMA* 1964;188:779–784.

75. Levine A, Watemberg N, Hager H, et al. Benign intracranial hypertension associated with budesonide treatment in children with Crohn's disease. *J Child Neurol* 2001;16:458–461.

76. Arbenz JP, Wormser P. Pseudotumor cerebri by sex hormones. *Schweiz Med Wochenschr* 1965;95:1654–1656.

77. Cogan DG. Oral contraceptives having neuro-ophthalmologic complications. *Arch Ophthalmol* 1965;73:461–462.

78. Walsh FB, Clark DB, Thompson RS, et al. Oral contraceptives and neuro-ophthalmologic interest. *Arch Ophthalmol* 1965;74:628–640.

79. Longueville E, Dautheribes M, Williamson W, et al. L'hypertension intra-cranienne dite aigue benigne iatrogene: a propos d'un cas. *Bull Soc Ophtalmol Fr* 1990;90:1009–1012.

80. Gardner K, Cox T, Digre KB. Idiopathic intracranial hypertension associated with tetracycline use in fraternal twins: case reports and review. *Neurology* 1995;45:6–10.

81. Xenard L, George J-L, Maalouf T, et al. Les effets indesirables potentiels des tetracyclines: a propos de deux observations. *Bull Soc Ophtalmol Fr* 1996;96:154–157.

82. Aroichane M, Miller NR, Eggenberger ER. Glioblastoma multiforme masquerading as pseudotumor cerebri: case report. *J Clin Neuroophthalmol* 1993;13:105–112.

83. Fikkerrs BG, Bogousslavsky J, Regli F, et al. Pseudotumor cerebri with amiodarone. *J Neurol Neurosurg Psychiatry* 1986;49:606.

84. Van Sandijcke M, Dewachter A. Pseudotumor cerebri with amiodarone. *J Neurol Neurosurg Psychiatry* 1986;49:1463–1464.

85. Grogan WA, Narkun DM. Pseudotumor cerebri with amiodarone. *J Neuro Neurosurg Psychiatry* 1987;50:651.

86. Cruz OA, Fogg SG, Roper-Hall G. Pseudotumor cerebri associated with cyclosporine use. *Am J Ophthalmol* 1996;122:436–437.

87. Hamed LM, Glaser JS, Schatz NJ, et al. Pseudotumor cerebri induced by danazol. *Am J Ophthalmol* 1989;107:105–110.

88. Shah A, Roberts R, McQueen IN, et al. Danazol and benign intracranial hypertension. *BMJ* 1989;294:1323.

89. Malozowski S, Tanner LA, Wysowski D, et al. Growth hormone, insulin-like growth factor 1, and benign intracranial hypertensiion. *N Engl J Med* 1994;329:665–666.

90. Price DA, Clayton PE, Lloyd IC. Benign intracranial hypertension induced by growth hormone treatment. *Lancet* 1995;345:458–459.

91. Konomi H, Imai M, Nihel K, et al. Indomethacin causing pseudotumor cerebri in Bartter's syndrome. *N Engl J Med* 1978;298:855.

92. Larizza D, Colombo A, Lorini R, et al. Ketoprofen causing pseudotumor cerebri in Bartter's syndrome. *N Engl J Med* 1979;300:796.

93. Arber N, Shirin H, Fadila R, et al. Pseudotumor cerebri associated with leuprorelin acetate. *Lancet* 1990;335:668.

94. Fraunfelder FT, Edwards R. Possible ocular adverse effects associated with leuprolide injections. *JAMA* 1995;273:773–774.

95. Sunku AJ, O'Duffy AE, Swanson JW. Benign intracranial hypertension associated with levonorgestrel implants. *Ann Neurol* 1993;34:299.

96. Alder JB, Fraunfelder FT, Edwards R. Levonorgestrel implants and intracranial hypertension. *N Engl J Med* 1995;332:1720–1721.

97. Lobo A, Pilek E, Stokes PE. Papilledema following therapeutic dosages of lithium carbonate. *J Nerv Ment Dis* 1978;16:526–529.

98. Saul RF, Hamburger HA, Selhorst JB. Pseudotumor cerebri secondary to lithium carbonate. *JAMA* 1985;253:2869–2870.

99. Blumberg AG, Klein DF. Severe papilledema associated with drug therapy. *Am J Psychiatr* 1961;118:168–170.

100. Mayer-Hubner B. Pseudotumor cerebri from intranasal oxytocin and excessive fluid intake. *Lancet* 1996;347:623.

101. Kalanie H, Niakan E, Harati Y, et al. Phenytoin-induced benign intracranial hypertension. *Neurology* 1986;36:443.

102. Serratrice J, Granel B, Conrath J, et al. Benign intracranial hypertension and thyreostimulin suppression hormonotherapy. *Am J Ophthalmol* 2002;134:910–911.

103. Gangemi M, di Martino L, Maiuri F, et al. Intracranial hypertension due to acute vitamin A intoxication. *Acta Neurol* 1985;7:27–31.

104. Fraunfelder FT, LaBraico JM, Meyer SM. Adverse ocular reactions possibly associated with isotretinoin. *Am J Ophthalmol* 1985;100:534–537.

105. Marcus DF, Turgeon P, Aaberg TM, et al. Optic disk findings in hypervitaminosis. *Ann Ophthalmol* 1985;17: 397–402.

106. Misbah SA, Peiris JB, Atukorala TM. Ingestion of shark liver associated with pseudotumor cerebri due to acute hypervitaminosis A. *J Neurol Neurosurg Psychiatry* 1984;47:216.

107. Selhorst JB, Waybright EA, Jennings S, et al. Liver lover's headache: pseudotumor cerebri and vitamin A intoxication. *JAMA* 1984;252:3364.

108. Sirdofsky M, Kattah J, Macedo P. Intracranial hypertension in a dieting patient. *J Neuroophthalmol* 1994; 14:9–11.

109. Donahue SP. Recurrence of idiopathic intracranial hypertension after weight loss: the carrot craver. *Am J Ophthalmol* 2000;130:850–851.

110. Morrice G Jr, Havener WH, Kapetansky F. Vitamin A intoxication as a cause of pseudotumor cerebri. *JAMA* 1960;173:1802–1805.

111. Fukuda S, Kogure M, Ohsawa M. A case of pseudotumor cerebri after renal transplantation. *Folia Ophthalmol Jpn* 1990;41:1850–1857.

112. Fanous M, Hamed LM, Margo CE. Pseudotumor cerebri associated with danazol withdrawal. *JAMA* 1991;266:1218–1219.

113. Atkins SL, Masson EA, Blumhardt LD, et al. Benign intracranial hypertension associated with the withdrawal of a non-ergot dopamine agonist. *J Neurol Neurosurg Psychiatry* 1994;54:371–372.

114. March LF, Morgan DAL, Jefferson D. Benign intracranial hypertension during chemotherapy for testicular teratoma. *Br J Radiol* 1988;61:692.

115. Haller JS, Meyer DR, Cromie W, et al. Pseudotumor cerebri following beta-human chorionic gonadotropin hormone treatment for undescended testicles. *Neurology* 1981;43:448–456.

116. Kasarskis EJ, Bass NH. Benign intracranial hypertension induced by deficiency of vitamin A during infancy. *Neurology* 1982;32:1292–1295.

117. DeJong AR, Callahan CA, Weiss JL. Pseudotumor cerebri and nutritional rickets. *Eur J Pediatr* 1985;143: 219–220.

118. Gungor K, Bekir NA, Namiduru M. Pseudotumor cerebri complicating brucellosis. *Ann Ophthalmol* 2002; 34:67–69.

119. Ikkala E, Laitinen L. Papilloedema due to iron deficiency anemia. *Acta Haematol* 1963;29:368–370.

120. van Gelder T, van Gemert HMA, Tjiong HL. A patient with megaloblastic anaemia and idiopathic intracranial hypertension: Case history. *Clin Neurol Neurosurg* 1991;93:321–322.

121. Taylor JP, Galetta SL, Asbury AK, et al. Hemolytic anemia presenting as idiopathic intracranial hypertension. *Neurology* 2002;59:960–961.

122. Biousse V, Newman NJ. Anemia and patilledema. *MJ Opthamol* 2003;135:437–446.

123. Cameron AJ. Marked papilledema in pulmonary emphysema. *Br J Ophthalmol* 1993;17:167–169.

124. Sharp JT, Barrocas M, Chokroverty S. The cardio-respiratory effects of obesity. *Clin Chest Med* 1980;1:103–118.

125. Purvin VA, Kawasaki A, Yee RD. Papilledema and obstructive sleep apnea syndrome. *Arch Ophthalmol* 2000;118:1626–1630.

126. Marcus DM, Lynn J, Miller JJ, et al. Sleep disorders: a risk factor for pseudotumor cerebri? *J Neuroophthalmol* 2001;21:121–123.

127. Kilburn KH. Neurologic manifestations of respiratory failure. *Arch Intern Med* 1965;116:409–415.

128. Strollo PJ Jr, Rogers RM. Obstructive sleep apnea. *N Engl J Med* 1996;334:99–104.

129. Carlow TJ, Glaser JS. Pseudotumor cerebri syndrome in systemic lupus erythematosus. *JAMA* 1974;228:197–200.

130. Kaplan RE, Springate JE, Feld LG, et al. Pseudotumor cerebri associated with cerebral venous sinus thrombosis, internal jugular vein thrombosis, and systemic lupus erythematosus. *J Pediatr* 1985;107:266–268.

131. Shiozawa Z, Yoshida M, Kobayashi K, et al. Superior sagittal sinus thrombosis and systemic lupus erythematosus. *Ann Neurol* 1986;20:272.

132. Li EK, Ho PCP. Pseudotumor cerebri in systemic lupus erythematosus. *J Rheumatol* 1989;16:113–116.

133. Frohman LP, Joshi VV, Wagner RS, et al. Pseudotumor cerebri as a cardinal sign of the polyangitis overlap syndrome. *Neuro-ophthalmology* 1991;11:337–345.

134. Furuta M, Satoh S, Toriumi T, et al. An autopsy case of cerebral sinus thrombosis which showed papilledema and was accompanied by idiopathic thrombocytopenic purpura. *Acta Soc Ophthalmol Jpn* 1991;95:199–203.

135. Ridolfi RL, Bell WR. Thrombotic thrombocytopenic purpura: report of 25 cases and review of the literature. *Medicine* 1981;60:413–428.

136. Bynke G, Bynke H, Ljunggren B. Familial idiopathic intracranial hypertension and variegate porphyria: is there any connection? *Neuro-ophthalmology* 1994;14: 153–165.

137. Corbett JJ, Savino PJ, Thompson HS, et al. Visual loss in pseudotumor cerebri: follow-up of 57 patients from five to 41 years and a profile of 14 patients with permanent severe visual loss. *Arch Neurol* 1982;39: 461–474.

138. Repka MX, Miller NR, Savino PJ. Pseudotumor cerebri. *Am J Ophthalmol* 1984;98:741–746.

139. Liu GT, Volpe NJ, Schatz NJ, et al. Severe sudden visual loss caused by pseudotumor cerebri and lumboperitoneal shunt failure. *Am J Ophthalmol* 1996;122:129–131.

140. Sorensen PS, Krogsaa B, Gjerris F. Clinical course and prognosis of pseudotumor cerebri: a prospective study of 24 patients. *Acta Neurol Scan* 1988;77:164–172.

141. Wall M, George D. Idiopathic intracranial hypertension: a prospective study. *Brain* 1991;114:155–180.

142. Rowe FJ, Sarkies NJ. Assessment of visual function in idiopathic intracranial hypertension: a prospective study. *Eye* 1998;12:111–118.

143. Golnik KC, Devoto M, Kersten RC, et al. Visual loss in idiopathic intracranial hypertension after resolution of papilledema. *Ophthalmic Plast Reconstr Surg* 1999;15: 442–444.

144. Rowe FJ, Sarkies NJ. Visual outcome in a prospective study of idiopathic intracranial hypertension. *Arch Ophthalmol* 117:1571.

145. Wall M. Idiopathic intracranial hypertension: mechanisms of visual loss and disease management. *Semin Neurol* 2000;20:89–95.

146. Merle H, Smadja D, Cabre P, et al. Idiopathic intracranial hypertension: a retrospective study of 20 cases. *Ann Ophthalmol* 2001;33:21–26.

147. Walker RWH. Idiopathic intracranial hypertension: any light on the mechanism of the raised pressure? *J Neurol Neurosurg Psychiatry* 2001;71:1–7.

148. Jacobson DM, Berg R, Wall M, et al. Serum vitamin A concentration is elevated in idiopathic intracranial hypertension. *Neurology* 1999;53:1114–1118.

149. Selhorst JB, Kulkantrakorn K, Corbett JJ, et al. Retinol-binding protein in idiopathic intracranial hypertension (IIH). *J Neuroophthalmol* 2000;20:250–252.

150. Sass JO, Arnold T, Tzimas G. Serum vitamin A is elevated in idiopathic intracranial hypertension. *Neurology* 2000;54:2192–2193.

151. Karahalios DG, Rekate HL, Khayata MH, et al. Elevated intracranial venous pressure as a universal mechanism in pseudotumor of varying etiologies. *Neurology* 1996;46:198–202.

152. King JO, Mitchell PJ, Thomson KR, et al. Manometry combined with cervical puncture in idiopathic intracranial hypertension. *Neurology* 2002;58:26–30.

153. Corbett JJ, Digre K. Idiopathic intracranial hypertension. An answer to, "the chicken or the egg?" *Neurology* 2002;58:5–6.

154. Fishman RA. The pathophysiology of pseudotumor cerebri: An unsolved puzzle. *Arch Neurol* 1984;41:257–258.

155. Silberstein SD, Marcelis J. Headache associated with changes in intracranial pressure. *Headache* 1992;32:84–94.

156. Miller NR. Papilledema. In: Miller NR, Newman NJ, (eds.) *Walsh and Hoyt's clinical neuro-ophthalmology*, 5th ed, vol 1. Baltimore: Williams & Wilkins, 1997;487–548.

157. Johnston I, Hawke S, Halmagyi M, Teo C. The pseudotumor syndrome. *Arch Neurol* 1991;48:740–747.

158. Frisch E, Hamard H, Cabanis E-A, et al. Hypertension intracranienne dite benigne: a propos de huit observations. *Bull Soc Ophtalmol Fr* 1991;91:371–374.

159. Gibby WA, Cohen MS, Goldberg HI, et al. Pseudotumor cerebri: CT findings and correlation with visual loss. *AJR* 1993;160:143–146.

160. Connor SE, Jarosz JM. Magnetic resonance imaging of cerebral venous sinus thrombosis. *Clin Radiol* 2002;57:449–461.

161. Del Brutto OH, Sotelo J. Neurocysticercosis simulating pseudotumor cerebri (pseudopseudotumor). *J Clin Neuroophthalmol* 1988;8:87–91.

162. Lee AG. Letter to the editor. *Arch Neurol* 1996;53:401.

163. Wall M. Sensory visual testing in idiopathic intracranial hypertension: Measures sensitive to change. *Neurology* 1990;40:1859–1864.

164. Wall M, Conway MD, House PH, et al. Evaluation of sensitivity and specificity of spatial resolution and Humphrey automated perimetry in pseudotumor cerebri patients and normal subjects. *Invest Ophthalmol Vis Sci* 1991;32:3306–3312.

165. Frenkel REP. Evaluation of the relative afferent pupillary defect in pseudotumor cerebri in regard to surgical intervention. *Arch Ophthalmol* 1991;107:634–635.

166. Wall M, Montgomery EB. Using motion perimetry to detect visual field defects in patients with idiopathic intracranial hypertension: a comparison with conventional automated perimetry. *Neurology* 1995;45:1169–1175.

167. Wall M, Hart WM Jr, Burde RM. Visual field defects in idiopathic intracranial hypertension (pseudotumor cerebri). *Am J Ophthalmol* 1983;96:654–669.

168. Orcutt JC, Page NGR, Sanders MD. Factors affecting visual loss in benign intracranial hypertension. *Ophthalmology* 1984;91:1303–1312.

169. Manfre L, Lagalla R, Mangioameli A, et al. Idiopathic intracranial hypertension: orbital MRI. *Neuroradiology* 1995;37:459–461.

170. Gass A, Barker GJ, Riordan-Eva P, et al. MRI of the optic nerve in benign intracranial hypertension. *Neuroradiology* 1996;38:769–773.

171. Jinkins JR, Athale S, Xiong L, et al. MR of optic papilla protrusion in patients with high intracranial pressure. *AJNR* 1996;17:665–668.

172. Sedwick L, Boghen D, Moster M. How to handle the pressure or too much of a good thing. *Surv Ophthalmol* 1996;40:307–311.

173. Newberg B. Pseudotumor cerebri treated by rice/reduction diet. *Arch Intern Med* 1974;133:802–807.

174. Johnson LN, Krohel GB, Madsen RW, et al. The role of weight loss and acetazolamide in the treatment of idiopathic intracranial hypertension (pseudotumor cerebri. *Ophthalmology* 1998;105:2313–2317.

175. Kupersmith MJ, Gamell L, Turbin R, et al. Effects of weight loss on the course of idiopathic intracranial hypertension in women. *Neurology* 1998;50:1094–1098.

176. Johnson D, Drenick EJ. Therapeutic fasting in morbid obesity: long-term follow-up. *Arch Intern Med* 1977;137:1381–1382.

177. Wing RR. Behavorial treatment of severe obesity. *Am J Clin Nutr* 1992;55:545S–551S.

178. Noggle JD, Rodning CB. Rapidly advancing pseudotumor cerebri associated with morbid obesity: an indication for gastric exclusion. *South Med J* 1986;79:761–763.

179. Amaral JF, Tsiaris W, Morgan T, et al. Reversal of benign intracranial hypertension by surgically induced weight loss. *Arch Surg* 1987;122:946–949.

180. Sugerman HJ, Felton WL 3rd, Salvant JB Jr, et al. Effects of surgically induced weight loss on idiopathic intracranial hypertension in morbid obesity. *Neurology* 1995;45:1655–1659.

181. Alpert MA, Hashimi MW. Obesity and the heart. *Am J Med Sci* 1993;207:117–123.

182. Reeves-Hoche MK, Hudgel DW, Meck R, et al. Continuous versus bilevel positive airway pressure for obstructive sleep apnea. *Am J Resp Crit Care Med* 1995;151:443–449.

183. Wolin MJ, Brannon SL, Kay MD, et al. Disk edema in an overweight woman. *Surv Ophthalmol* 1995;39:307–314.

184. Tomsak RL, Niffenegger AS, Remler BF. Treatment of pseudotumor cerebri with Diamox (acetazolamide). *J Clin Neuroophthalmol* 1988;8:93–98.

185. Killer HE, Blumer B, Burde RM. Pseudotumor cerebri, Verlaufsparameter und Therapiemodalitaten. *Klin Monatsbl Augenheilkd* 1992;200:562–563.

186. Tschirgi RD, Frost RW, Taylor JL. Inhibitions of cerebrospinal fluid formation by a carbonic anhydrase inhibitor, 2-acetyl-1,3,4-thiadiazole-t-sulfonamide (Diamox). *Proc Soc Exp Biol Med* 1954;87:373–376.

187. Davison H, Luck CP. The effect of acetazolamide on the chemical composition of the aqueous humor and cerebrospinal fluid of some mammalian species and on the rate of turnover of 24Na in these fluids. *J Physiol* 1957;137:279–283.

188. Maren TH, Robinson B. The pharmacology of acetazolamide as related to cerebrospinal fluid and the treatment of hydrocephalus. *Johns Hopkins Hosp Bull* 1960;106:1–24.

189. Maren TH. Carbonic anhydrase: chemistry, physiology and inhibition. *Physiol Rev* 1967;47:595.

190. Gücer G, Viernstein L. Long-term intracranial pressure recording in the management of pseudotumor cerebri. *J Neurosurg* 1978;49:256–263.

191. Lichter PR. Reducing side effects of carbonic anhydrase inhibitors. *Ophthalmology* 1981;88:266–269.

192. Jefferson A, Clark J. Treatment of benign intracranial hypertension by dehydrating agents with particular reference to the measurement of the blindspot area as a means of recording improvement. *J Neurol Neurosurg Psychiatry* 1976;39:627–639.

193. Guy J, Johnston PK, Corbett JJ, et al. Treatment of visual loss in pseudotumor cerebri associated with uremia. *Neurology* 1990;40:28–32.

194. Liu GT, Glaser JS, Schatz NJ. High-dose methylprednisolone and acetazolamide for visual loss in pseudotumor cerebri. *Am J Ophthalmol* 1996;122:129–131.

195. Forderreuther S, Straube A. Indomethacin reduces CSF pressure in intracranial hypertension. *Neurology* 2000;55:1043–1045.

196. Kessler LA, Novelli PM, Reigel DH. Surgical treatment of benign intracranial hypertension—subtemporal decompression revisted. *Surg Neurol* 1998;50:73–76.

197. McGirt MJ, Woodworth G, Thomas G, et al. Cerebrospinal fluid shunt placement for psuedotumor cerebri associated with intractible headache: predictors of treatment response and an analysis of long-term outcomes. J Neurosurg 2004;101:627–632.

198. Chumas PD, Kulkarni AV, Drake JM, et al. Lumboperitoneal shunting: a retrospective study in the pediatric population. *Neurosurgery* 1993;32:376–383.

199. Rosenberg ML, Corbett JJ, Smith C, et al. Cerebrospinal fluid diversion procedures in pseudotumor cerebri. *Neurology* 1993;43:1071–2072.

200. Eggenberger ER, Miller NR, Vitale S. Lumboperitoneal shunt for the treatment of pseudotumor cerebri. *Neurology* 1996;46:1524–1530.

201. Burgett RA, Purvin VA, Kawasaki A. Lumboperitonal shunting for pseudotumor cerebri. *Neurology* 1997;49: 734–739.

202. Spoor TC, Ramocki JM, Madison MP, et al. Treatment of pseudotumor cerebri with primary and secondary optic nerve sheath decompression. *Am J Ophthalmol* 1991;112:177–185.

203. Kelman SE, Heaps R, Wolfe A, et al. Optic nerve decompression improves visual function in patients with pseudotumor cerebri. *Neurosurgery* 1992;3:391–395.

204. Acheson JF, Green WT, Sanders MD. Optic nerve sheath decompression for the treatment of visual failure in chronic raised intracranial pressure. *J Neurol Neurosurg Psychiatry* 1994;57:1426–1429.

205. Herzau V, Baykal HE. Langzeitergebnisse nach Optikusscheidenfensterung bei Pseudotumor cerebri. *Klin Monatsbl Augenheilkd* 1998;213:154–160.

206. Banta JT, Farris BK. Pseudotumor cerebri and optic nerve sheath decompression. *Ophthalmology* 2000; 107:1907–1912.

207. Keltner JL, Albert DM, Lubow M, et al. Optic nerve decompression: a clinical pathologic study. *Arch Ophthalmol* 1977;95:97–104.

208. Hamed LM, Tse DT, Glaser JS, et al. Neuroimaging of the optic nerve after fenestration for management of pseudotumor cerebri. *Arch Ophthalmol* 1992;110: 636–639.

209. Kaye AH, Galbraith JEK, King L. Intracranial pressure following optic nerve decompression for benign intracranial hypertension. *J Neurosurg* 1981;55:453–456.

210. Jacobson EE, Johnston IH, McCluskey P. The effects of optic nerve sheath decompression on cerebrospinal fluid dynamics. *Neuro-ophthalmology* 1996;16(suppl):290.

211. Mauriello JA Jr, Shaderowfsky P, Gizzi M, et al. Management of visual loss after optic nerve sheath decompression in patients with pseudotumor cerebri. *Ophthalmology* 1995;102:441–445.

212. Spoor TC, McHenry JG. Long-term effectiveness of optic sheath decompression for pseudotumor cerebri. *Arch Ophthalmol* 1993;111:632–635.

213. Kellen RI, Burde RM. Optic nerve decompression. *Arch Ophthalmol* 1987;105:889.

214. Friedman DI, Rausch EA. Headache diagnoses in patients with treated idiopathic intracranial hypertension. *Neurology* 2002;58:1551–1553.

215. Kassam SH, Hadi HA, Fadel HE, et al. Benign intracranial hypertension in pregnancy: current diagnostic and therapeutic approach. *Obstet Gynecol Surg* 1983;38: 314–321.

216. Shapiro S, Yee R, Brown H. Surgical management of pseudotumor cerebri in pregnancy: case report. *Neurosurgery* 1995;37:839–831.

30 Alzheimer Disease in Women

Julene K. Johnson, PhD and Kristine Yaffe, MD

Alzheimer disease (AD) is among the top ten causes of death in the United States (1) and is one of the most common reasons for the institutionalization of elderly individuals (2). Even after controlling for age, women have a slightly higher risk of developing AD compared with men (3–4). In addition, unique issues exist regarding the clinical presentation and treatment of AD among women. This chapter highlights these issues and addresses more recent advances in the field that focus on the importance of the preclinical stage of AD and dementia in the oldest old.

CLINICAL PRESENTATION AND DIAGNOSIS OF AD

AD is a degenerative brain disorder characterized by a progressive decline in cognition and behavior. It is the most common cause of dementia, accounting for approximately two-thirds of all cases of dementia (5). AD currently affects 4 million individuals in the United States and has an annual cost of $100 billion (6). However, by 2050, the number of individuals affected by AD is projected to increase to 12 million (7). Although memory impairment is the hallmark early symptom of AD, other cognitive domains, such as language, executive function, and visuospatial skills, are also affected. Individuals with

AD also experience progressive difficulty with functional activities, such as cooking, driving, and shopping. The clinical criteria for the diagnosis of AD were published in 1984 (8) (Table 30.1). These criteria require memory impairment and at least one other cognitive domain impairment in the absence of "reversible" conditions. The median length of time from diagnosis to death is approximately 7 to 10 years among individuals diagnosed in their 60s and 70s, and a median of 3 years in individuals diagnosed in their 90s (9). Currently, no cure exists for AD; however, treatment efforts focus on the management of behavioral symptoms and the prevention of further cognitive decline.

Prevalence and Incidence of AD

The prevalence of AD increases dramatically with age. Approximately 10% of persons over 65 years of age and 50% of those over 85 years of age exhibit impairment in cognitive functioning (10–11). Pooled data from four U.S. studies (i.e., Framingham, East Boston, Rochester, and Baltimore) indicate that the age-specific incidence rates rise from 0.2% per year at 65 years of age to 0.7%, 1.0%, and 2.9% per year at 75, 77, and 85 years of age, respectively (12) (Figure 30.1). However, additional studies are needed with individuals over age 85 because much less is known about AD in the oldest old. Women live an average of 2 to 6 years longer than men in the United States, and life

---

TABLE 30.1
NINCDS-ADRDA Criteria for
Probable Alzheimer Disease (8)

- Dementia
- Deficit in two or more areas of cognition (memory required)
- Gradual onset
- Onset after age 40
- Absence of other systemic disorder or brain disease that could account for progressive cognitive decline

---

expectancy is related to both age and ethnicity. In 2000, women had a mean life expectancy of 79.5 years of age, whereas men had a mean lifespan of 74.1 years (1). After controlling for age, women have a slightly higher risk of AD than men (3–4). Women over age 80 also have a slightly higher risk for AD (3,13). This gender difference in the incidence of AD is not seen in other common dementias. The cause of it is unknown but may be linked to differences in sex hormones or in other risk factors.

Risk Factors for AD

The primary risk factors for AD include age, genetic susceptibility from the apolipoprotein epsilon (APOE) 4 allele on chromosome 21, and low education. As discussed above, the risk for AD increases with age. The APOE 4 allele represents a major risk for AD and is evi-

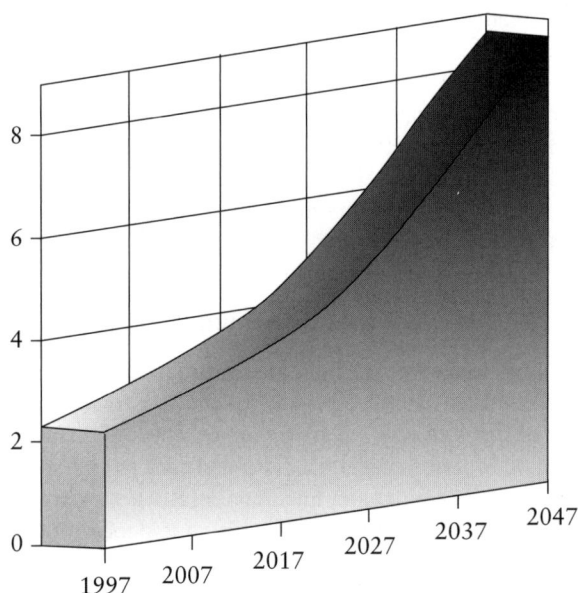

FIGURE 30.1

Projected prevalence (percent of population) in the United States of AD by the year 2050 (12).

dent across all ages (14). Women who are homozygous for APOE 4 allele have a slightly greater risk for developing AD than homozygous men (14). In addition, nondemented women with at least one APOE 4 allele were more likely to exhibit cognitive decline than women without any APOE 4 alleles (15). A low educational level also appears to be a risk for AD and may have a stronger effect in women (16–17). Other possible factors include a family history of AD in a first degree relative (18), a history of head injury (19), and depression (20–21). It may be that the APOE genotype interacts with some of these other risk factors for AD (22).

Comorbidity and Mortality Due to AD

Women with AD are less likely than men to have comorbid medical conditions, and they have a reduced risk for mortality due to AD. One study found that, when compared with men, women with AD had fewer comorbid medical conditions, such as chronic obstructive pulmonary disease, Parkinson's disease, cancer, and arrhythmia (23). In addition, women with AD have a significantly reduced risk of mortality (23–24).

GENDER DIFFERENCES IN COGNITIVE FUNCTION AND BEHAVIOR IN AD

Previous studies suggest that, when compared with men, women with AD exhibit more severe deficits in some cognitive domains. When controlling for dementia severity and demographic variables, women with AD tend to have more difficulty on several tests of language, including confrontational naming (25–28), vocabulary (28), and semantic fluency (e.g., animal naming) (25). In a longitudinal study, Ripich and colleagues (26) also found that the severe impairment on language measures in women with AD persisted throughout the progression of dementia. Other studies, however, have not documented gender-related differences on tests of language (29–30). In other studies, women with AD, compared with men, exhibit more severe deficits on tests of memory, in particular delayed recall of verbal information (25), delayed recall of stories (28), and semantic memory (27). Other studies have not observed this pattern (30), however, and it is not yet clear whether these patterns are gender-specific. The different conclusions may be related to the patient populations, the cognitive tests used, and the analytic methods used. Although some evidence suggests that women with AD may have more severe deficits on language and memory tasks, future studies need to address the lack of consistent results.

In addition to the cognitive symptoms associated with AD, alterations in behavior are also common with patients, especially those in severe stages, exhibiting agitation, psychotic symptoms, and wandering. Cohen and colleagues (31) found that women with AD manifested more psychiatric symptoms than men with AD. In another study, women with AD were more likely to exhibit reclusiveness and emotional lability, whereas men with AD were more likely to have apathy and vegetative signs (32). In a recent study by Sink and colleagues (33), women with AD were more likely to exhibit verbal outbursts, whereas men with AD were more likely to exhibit aggressive physical behaviors (i.e., psychomotor agitation, anger, waking caregiver). It is yet unclear how premorbid personality contributes to these putative gender-related differences in behavior.

MILD COGNITIVE IMPAIRMENT

Although dementia is common in older individuals, the prevalence of *cognitive impairment in the absence of dementia* is even more common. Individuals with cognitive impairment in the absence of dementia exhibit a decline in cognitive ability that does not meet the clinical criteria for dementia. Generally, the cognitive impairment experienced by these individuals falls between healthy aging and dementia. Numerous terms have been proposed to label individuals with isolated cognitive impairment (e.g., age-associated cognitive decline, cognitive impairment no dementia, age-consistent memory decline); however, the term "mild cognitive impairment" (MCI) has become the most widely used term and construct. By definition, individuals with MCI complain of memory problems and exhibit objective memory impairment on standard tests of memory (34). The memory impairment does not significantly impact the ability to perform everyday activities, however (Table 30.2). The identification of individuals with MCI is important because these persons have an increased risk of converting to AD. In a review of several large longitudinal studies, Petersen and colleagues (35) concluded that individuals with MCI convert to dementia with an annual rate between 6 and 25%, which is substantially greater than healthy elderly. Other studies, however, have found that a subset of individuals with MCI revert to normal levels of functioning (36), and some may not convert to dementia for long periods. In terms of the underlying neuropathologic changes, individuals with MCI are also likely to have neuropathologic changes consistent with AD at autopsy, thereby suggesting that MCI represents very early AD and not just a benign state (37). Only a few autopsy studies have been completed, however.

A recent study by Larrieu and colleagues (36) suggests that women may have a higher risk than men for developing MCI. The reasons for the gender difference in MCI are not known, but this finding is consistent with the higher incidence of AD in women. Although there is

TABLE 30.2
Criteria for Mild Cognitive Impairment (34)

- Subjective complaint of memory loss
- Objective impairment on tests of memory
- Preserved functioning on other cognitive domains
- Preserved activities of daily living
- Absence of medical condition causing memory deficit
- Absence of dementia

no currently approved treatment for MCI, these individuals should be closely monitored over time for a possible conversion to dementia and so that any reversible causes of cognitive dysfunction can be identified. The results of ongoing trials for MCI will soon help identify potential therapeutic strategies to prevent the progression to AD.

AD IN THE OLDEST-OLD

Individuals over age 85 are the fastest growing segment of society, and estimates of the prevalence of AD in these individuals range from 13 to 51% (11,32,37–38). The issue of possible gender differences in the oldest-old (e.g., over age 85) has only recently been addressed. Although some studies document a higher incidence of AD in the oldest-old women when compared with men (3,13), other studies do not find gender differences (4,37). A recent study by Miech and colleagues (38) suggested that, whereas the incidence of AD increases dramatically until 85 to 90 years of age, a decline in incidence was observed in men after age 93 and women after age 97. In a large autopsy series of individuals over 85 years of age, 33% of the subjects met the neuropathologic criteria for AD, whereas only 16% met the clinical criteria for AD (39). In this study, a strong relationship also existed between the presence of the apolipoprotein epsilon 4 allele and AD neuropathology, suggesting that the APOE genotype may also modify the expression of AD in the oldest-old. It is likely that many of the factors that influence the expression of AD in younger elderly also affect AD in the oldest-old. Further studies are needed to confirm this, however.

HORMONES AND COGNITIVE AGING

A dramatic decline in estrogen levels occurs in women during menopause, which may be associated with cognitive decline and an increased risk for developing AD. Considerable basic science evidence suggests that estrogen has a protective effect on the brain, particularly in areas that are important for cognition. Mechanisms by which estrogen could improve cognition and prevent decline remain unknown, but several have been suggested. One is the modulation of neurotransmitters, particularly seen with estrogen's enhancement of acetylcholine activity (40–41). Estrogen stimulates axonal sprouting and dendritic spine formation in adult rat CA1 hippocampal pyramidal neurons (42–43), and this may be another mechanism for sex hormone protection, because neuronal loss in the hippocampal CA1 region is found in patients with AD and cognitive decline. In addition, estradiol may be neuroprotective, limiting oxidative stress injury induced by excitotoxins. Estradiol treatment protects neuronal cells from the toxicity of Alzheimer-type β-amyloid (44) and reduces the generation of β-amyloid peptide in neurons (45). Estradiol thus may reduce the risk of cognitive decline through a variety of mechanisms.

Observational studies in women suggest that estrogen therapy may help prevent AD and cognitive decline. There has been tremendous interest in the effect of both exogenous and endogenous hormones on the risk of AD and pre-clinical cognitive decline, especially in women. While several recent trials have failed to show that treatment with estrogen reduced symptoms among women with AD (46,47), there is some observational evidence that estrogen therapy may reduce risk of developing AD. It may be that once the disease is fairly advanced, certain strategies are not efficacious for treatment of symptoms but still may be effective for prevention. In both prospective and case-control studies, women who take estrogen therapy had up to a 50% lower risk of developing AD (48–50). A meta-analysis of most of these observational studies reported a 29% decreased risk of developing AD among estrogen users, supporting the hypothesis that postmenopausal estrogen use protects against the development of AD (51). However, several recently completed randomized trials, such as the Womens Health Initiative Memory Study, reported that conjugated estrogens, either alone or in combination with progestins, did not reduce risk of developing AD. Indeed, women assigned to hormone therapy had an increased risk of developing all-cause dementia and slightly worse performance on a test of global cognitive function (52,53). The current data at this time are insufficient to recommend hormone therapy for the prevention of AD, especially in light of recent findings of increased side effects (54).

Recent studies have begun to investigate the role of sex hormone receptor polymorphisms and cognitive function in older women. Estrogen receptors are located throughout the brain, especially in regions involved in learning and memory such as the hippocampus and amygdala (55). The gene for the estrogen receptor alpha has several single nucleotide polymorphisms (SNPs), the PvuII, XbaI, and B-variants, that may be associated with receptor expression and function (56–57). Recently, several case-controls studies (58–60), but not all (57), have found an increased frequency of the PvuII and XbaI poly-

morphisms (polymorphic sites that are in linkage disequilibrium) in patients with AD compared with controls. One recent prospective study reported that polymorphisms in the estrogen receptor alpha genes PvuII and XbaI are associated with a risk of cognitive decline in older women (61). More research is needed to determine the mechanisms that may explain this association. See also Chapters 6 and 12.

TREATMENT OF AD IN WOMEN

Cholinesterase inhibitors are currently the only FDA-approved treatment for AD. AD is associated with a reduction of acetylcholine, and cholinesterase inhibitors help increase the concentration of acetylcholine in the brain. The major therapeutic effect is the maintenance of cognitive function. Additional effects may include slowing of cognitive decline and improving behavioral symptoms. A recent meta-analysis concluded that cholinesterase inhibitors have a modest beneficial impact on neuropsychiatric symptoms and functional status for patients with AD (62).

The effect of cholinesterase inhibitor treatment may differ between men and women with AD. For example, one study found that after 3 months of cholinesterase inhibitor therapy, men had a 73% greater chance of responding than women (63). APOE genotype may also interact with gender on the effect of cholinesterase inhibitor treatment. Treatment with cholinesterase inhibitors had less of an effect in women with the APOE 4 allele than women with either the epsilon 2 or 3 allele. In contrast, the treatment effect was no different between men with different APOE alleles (64).

CAREGIVING IN AD

Women account for approximately 75% of caregivers for patients with dementia (65). Studies suggest that caregiving may adversely impact the physical and psychologic health of the caregiver. In addition, the caregivers of demented patients tend to experience greater stress and worse mental health than the caregivers of nondemented patients (65). A meta-analysis of 14 studies suggested that female caregivers experience approximately a 20% greater degree of burden than the male caregivers. Yee and Schulz (66) also noted that female caregivers experience more depression than male caregivers. When specifically evaluating possible gender differences in caring for dementia patients, Gallicchio and colleagues (67) found that the burden, and not depression, was higher in female caregivers when compared with male caregivers of dementia patients. Additional research is needed to address the effect of caring for patients with AD, especially among women, because they disproportionately assume the responsibility of caregiving in our society.

CONCLUSION

AD impacts women in several unique ways. First, women have a slightly increased risk for AD and mild cognitive impairment, even possibly in the oldest-old. Second, the clinical presentation of AD may differ in men and women. In addition, treatment approaches in women with AD may be slightly different from men. Finally, women also experience more keenly the impact of caregiving for patients with AD. Current research efforts are attempting to better define normal aging and the earliest transition from healthy aging to dementia. Clearly, a need exists to continue to explore possible gender-related differences in both healthy aging and AD, with a goal of identifying the underlying biological mechanism for these differences.

References

1. Minino AM, Arias E, Kochanek KD, Murphy SL, Smith BL. *Deaths: final data for 2000. National Vital Statistics Reports.* Hyattsville, Md: National Center for Health Statistics, 2002, vol. 50 (15).
2. Agüero-Torres H, von Strauss E, Biitanen M, Winblad B, Fratiglioni L. Institutionalization in the elderly: the role of chronic diseases and dementia. Cross-sectional and longitudinal data from a population-based study. *J Clin Epidemiol* 2001;54(8):795–801.
3. Andersen K, Launer LJ, Dewey ME, et al. Gender differences in the incidence of AD and vascular dementia: the EURODEM studies. *Neurology* 1999;53:1992–1997.
4. Ruitenberg A, Ott A, van Swieten JC, Hofman A, Breteler MM. Incidence of dementia: does gender make a difference? *Neurobio of Aging* 2001;22:575–580.
5. The Canadian Study of Health and Aging. Risk factors for Alzheimer's disease in Canada. *Neurology* 1994;44: 2073–2080.
6. DeKosky ST, Orgogozo JM. Alzheimer disease: diagnosis, costs, and dimensions of treatment. *Alzheimer Dis Assoc Disord* 2001;15(suppl 1):S3–7.
7. Sloane PD, Zimmerman S, Suchindran C, et al. The public health impact of Alzheimer's disease 2000-2050: potential implication of treatment advances. *Annu Rev Public Health* 2002;23:213–231.
8. McKhann G, Drachman D, Folstein M, Katzman R, Price D, Stadlan EM. Clinical diagnosis of Alzheimer's disease: report of the NINCDS-ADRDA Work Group under the auspices of Department of Health and Human Services Task Force on Alzheimer's Disease. *Neurology* 1984; 34(7):939–944.
9. Brookmeyer R, Corrada MM, Curriero FC, Kawas C. Survival following a diagnosis of Alzheimer disease. *Arch Neurol* 2002;59:1764–1767.
10. Evans DA, Funkenstein HH, Albert MS, et al. Prevalence of Alzheimer's disease in a community population of older persons. Higher than previously reported. *JAMA* 1989;262:2551–2556.
11. Andersen-Ranberg K, Schroll M, Jeune B. Healthy centenarians do not exist, but autonomous centenarians do: a population-based study of morbidity among Danish centenarians. *J Am Geriatr Soc* 2001;49:900–908.
12. Brookmeyer R, Gray S, Kawas C. Projections of Alzheimer's disease in the United States and the public health impact of delaying disease onset. *Am J Public Health* 1998;88:1337–1342.
13. Fratiglioni L, Viitanen M, von Strauss E, Tontodonati V, Herlitz A, Winblad B. Very old women at highest risk of dementia and Alzheimer's disease: incidence data from the Kungsholmen Project, Stockholm. *Neurology* 1997; 48:132–138.
14. Farrer LA, Cupples LA, Haines JL, et al. Effects of age, sex, and ethnicity on the association between apolipoprotein E genotype and Alzheimer disease. A meta-analysis. APOE and Alzheimer Disease Meta Analysis Consortium. *JAMA* 1997;278:1349–1356.
15. Yaffe K, Cauley J, Sands L, Browner W. Apolipoprotein E phenotype and cognitive decline in a prospective study of elderly community women. *Arch Neurol* 1997;54: 1110–1114.
16. Launer LJ, Andersen K, Dewey ME, et al. Rates and risk factors for dementia and Alzheimer's disease: results from EURODEM pooled analyses. *Neurology* 1999;52: 78–84.
17. Letenneur L, Launer LJ, Andersen K, et al. Education and risk for Alzheimer's disease: sex makes a difference. EURODEM pooled analyses. EURODEM incidence research group. *Am J Epidemiol* 2000;151:1064–1071.
18. Green RC, Cupples LA, Go R, et al. MIRAGE Study Group. Risk of dementia among white and African American relatives of patients with Alzheimer disease. *JAMA* 2002;287:329–336.
19. Guo Z, Cupples LA, Kurz A, et al. Head injury and risk of AD in the MIRAGE study. *Neurology* 2000;54: 1316–1323.
20. Mehta KM, Yaffe K, Covinsky KE. Cognitive impairment, depressive symptoms, and functional decline in older people. *JAGS* 2002;50:1045–1050.
21. Wilson RS, Barnes LL, Mendes de Leon CF, et al. Depressive symptoms, cognitive decline, and risk of AD in older persons. *Neurology* 2002;59:364–370.
22. Mayeux R, Ottman R, Maestre G, et al. Synergistic effects of traumatic head injury and apolipoprotein-epsilon 4 in patients with Alzheimer's disease. *Neurology* 1995;45:555–557.
23. Gambassi G, Lapane KL, Landi F, Sgadari A, Mor V, Bernabie R. Gender differences in the relation between comorbidity and mortality of patients with Alzheimer's disease. Systematic Assessment of Geriatric drug use via Epidemiology (SAGE) Study Group. *Neurology* 1999;53: 508–516.
24. Lapane KL, Gambassi G, Landi F, Sgadari A, Mor V, Bernabei R. Gender differences in predictors of mortality in nursing home residents with AD. *Neurology* 2001;13:56:650–654.
25. Henderson VW, Buckwalter JG. Cognitive deficits of men and women with Alzheimer's disease. *Neurology* 1994;44:90–96.
26. Ripich DN, Petrill SA, Whitehouse PJ, Ziol EW. Gender differences in language of AD patients: a longitudinal study. *Neurology* 1995;45:299–302.
27. Buckwalter JG, Rizzo AA, McCleary R, Shankle R, Dick M, Henderson VW. Gender comparisons of cognitive performances among vascular dementia, Alzheimer disease,

and older adults without dementia. *Arch Neurol* 1996;53:436–439.

28. McPherson S, Back C, Buckwalter JG, Cummings JL. Gender-related cognitive deficits in Alzheimer's disease. *Int Psychogeriatr* 1999;11:117–122.

29. Bayles KA, Azuma T, Cruz RF, Tomoeda CK, Wood JA, Montgomery EB Jr. Gender differences in language of Alzheimer disease patients revisited. *Alzheimer Dis Assoc Disord* 1999;13:138–146.

30. Hebert LE, Wilson RS, Gilley DW, et al. Decline of language among women and men with Alzheimer's disease. *J Gerontol B Psychol Sci Soc Sci* 2000;55:354–360.

31. Cohen D, Eisdorfer C, Gorelick P, et al. Sex differences in the psychiatric manifestations of Alzheimer's disease. *J Am Geriatr Soc* 1993;41:229–232.

32. Ott BR, Tate CA, Gordon NM, Heindel WC. Gender differences in the behavioral manifestations of Alzheimer's disease. *J Am Geriatr Soc* 1996;44:583–587.

33. Sink K, Covinsky K, Newcomer, Yaffe K. Gender and ethnic differences in dementia-related neuropsychiatric symptoms. *American Geriatrics Society Conference* 2003.

34. Petersen RC, Smith GE, Waring SC, Ivnik RJ, Tangalos EG, Kokmen E. Mild cognitive impairment: clinical characterization and outcome. *Arch Neurol* 1999;56:303–308.

35. Petersen RC, Doody R, Kurz A, et al. Current concepts in mild cognitive impairment. *Arch Neurol* 2001;58: 1985–1992.

36. Larrieu S, Letenneur L, Orgogozo JM, et al. Incidence and outcome of mild cognitive impairment in a population-based prospective cohort. *Neurology* 2002;59: 1594–1599.

37. Morris JC, Storandt M, Miller JP, et al. Mild cognitive impairment represents early-stage Alzheimer disease. *Arch Neurol* 2001;58:397–405.

38. Fratiglioni L, Grut M, Forsell Y, et al. Prevalence of Alzheimer's disease and other dementias in an elderly urban population: relationship with age, sex and education. *Neurology* 1991;41:1886–1892.

39. Polvikoski T, Sulkava R, Myllykangas L, et al. Prevalence of Alzheimer's disease in very elderly people. A prospective neuropathological study. *Neurology* 2001;56: 1690–1696.

40. Gibbs RB. Effects of estrogen on basal forebrain cholinergic neurons vary as a function of dose and duration of treatment. *Brain Res* 1997;757:10–16.

41. Luine VN. Estradiol increases choline acetyltransferase activity in specific basal forebrain nuclei and projection areas of female rats. *Exp Neurol* 1985;89:484–490.

42. McEwen BS. Clinical review 108: the molecular and neuroanatomical basis for estrogen effects in the central nervous system. *J Clin Endocrinol Metab* 1999;84: 1790–1797.

43. Matsumoto A. Synaptogenic action of sex steroids in developing and adult neuroendocrine brain. *Psychoneuroendocrinology* 1991;16:25–40.

44. Behl C, Skutella T, Lezoualc'h F, Post A, Widmann M, Newton CJ, Holsboer F. Neuroprotection against oxidative stress by estrogens: structure-activity relationship. *Mol Pharmacol* 1997;51:535–541.

45. Xu H, Gouras GK, Greenfield JP, et al. Estrogen reduces neuronal generation of Alzheimer beta-amyloid peptides. *Nat Med* 1998;4:447–451.

46. Henderson VW, Paganini-Hill A, Miller BL, et al. Estrogen for Alzheimer's disease in women: randomized, double-blind, placebo-controlled trial. *Neurology* 2000;54: 295–301.

47. Mulnard RA, Cotman CW, Kawas C, et al. Estrogen replacement therapy for treatment of mild to moderate Alzheimer disease: a randomized controlled trial. *JAMA* 2000;283:1007–1015.

48. Kawas C, Resnick S, Morrison A, et al. A prospective study of estrogen replacement therapy and the risk of developing Alzheimer's disease: the Baltimore Longitudinal Study of Aging. *Neurology* 1997;48: 1517–1521.

49. Tang MX, Jacobs D, Stern Y, et al. Effect of oestrogen during menopause on risk and age at onset of Alzheimer's disease. *Lancet* 1996;348:429–432.

50. Henderson VW, Paganini-Hill A, Emanuel CK, Dunn ME, Buckwalter JG. Estrogen replacement therapy in older women. Comparisons between Alzheimer's disease cases and nondemented control subjects. *Arch Neurol* 1994;51:896–900.

51. Yaffe K, Sawaya G, Lieberburg I, Grady D. Estrogen therapy in postmenopausal women: effects on cognitive function and dementia. *JAMA* 1998;279:688–695.

52. Shumaker A, Legault C, Rapp SR, et al., WHIMS investigators. Estrogen plus progestin and the incidence of dementia and mild cognitive impairment in postmenopausal women. The women's health initiative memory study: a randomized controlled trial. *JAMA* 2003; 289:2651–2662.

53. Espeland MA, Rapp SR, Shumaker SA, Brunner R, Manson JE, Sherwin BB, Hsia J, Margolis KL, Hogan PE, Wallace R, Dailey M, Freeman R, Hays J; Women's Health Initiative Memory Study. Conjugated equine estrogens and global cognitive function in postmenopausal women: Women's Health Initiative Memory Study. *JAMA* 2004;291(24):2959–2968.

54. Rossouw JE, Anderson GL, Prentice RL, et al. Writing Group for the Women's Health Initiative Investigators. Risks and benefits of estrogen plus progestin in healthy postmenopausal women: principal results from the Women's Health Initiative randomized controlled trial. *JAMA* 2002;288:321–333.

55. Shughrue PJ, Lane MV, Merchenthaler I. Comparative distribution of estrogen receptor-alpha and -beta mRNA in the rat central nervous system. *J Comp Neurol* 1997; 388:507–525.

56. Albagha OM, McGuigan FE, Reid DM, Ralston SH. Estrogen receptor alpha gene polymorphisms and bone mineral density: haplotype analysis in women from the United Kingdom. *J Bone Miner Res* 2001;16:128–134.

57. Maruyama H, Toji H, Harrington CR, et al. Lack of an association of estrogen receptor alpha gene polymorphisms and transcriptional activity with Alzheimer disease. *Arch Neurol* 2000;57:236–240.

58. Brandi ML, Becherini L, Gennari L, et al. Association of the estrogen receptor alpha gene polymorphisms with sporadic Alzheimer's disease. *Biochem Biophys Res Commun* 1999;265:335–338.

59. Isoe-Wada K, Maeda M, Yong J, et al. Positive association between an estrogen receptor gene polymorphism and Parkinson's disease with dementia. *Eur J Neurol* 1999;6:431–435.

60. Mattila KM, Axelman K, Rinne JO, et al. Interaction between estrogen receptor 1 and the epsilon4 allele of apolipoprotein E increases the risk of familial Alzheimer's disease in women. *Neurosci Lett* 2000;282:45–48.

61. Yaffe K, Lui LY, Grady D, Stone K, Morin P. Estrogen receptor 1 polymorphisms and risk of cognitive impairment in older women. *Biol Psychiatry* 2002;51:677–682.

62. Trinh NH, Hoblyn J, Mohanty S, Yaffe K. Efficacy of cholinesterase inhibitors in the treatment of neuropsychiatric symptoms and functional impairment in Alzheimer disease: a meta-analysis. *JAMA* 2003;289:210–216.

63. MacGowan SH, Wilcock GK, Scott M. Effect of gender and apolipoprotein E genotype on response to anticholinesterase therapy in Alzheimer's disease. *Int J Geriatr Psychiatry* 1998;13:625–630.

64. Farlow MR, Lahiri DK, Poirier J, Davignon J, Schneider L, Hui SL. Treatment outcome of tacrine therapy depends on apolipoprotein genotype and gender of the subjects with Alzheimer's disease. *Neurology* 1998;50:669–677.

65. Ory MG, Hoffman RR 3rd, Yee JL, Tennstedt S, Schulz R. Prevalence and impact of caregiving: a detailed comparison between dementia and nondementia. *Gerontologist* 1999;39:177–185.

66. Yee JL, Schulz R. Gender differences in psychiatric morbidity among family caregivers: a review and analysis. *Gerontologist* 2000;40:147–164.

67. Gallicchio L, Siddiqi N, Langenberg P, Baumgarten M. Gender differences in burden and depression among informal caregivers of demented elders in the community. *Int J Geriatr Psychiatry* 2002;17:154–163.

31 Psychiatric Disorders in Women

Angela S. Guarda, MD and Karen L. Swartz, MD

Psychiatric disorders are extremely common. One-year population prevalence rates of mental or substance abuse disorders in American adults exceeds 15%, whereas lifetime prevalence rates for psychiatric disorders have been estimated at 32% (1). This chapter provides an overview of the psychiatric conditions most common in women, their prevalence, diagnosis, and initial treatment interventions (Table 31.1). Women are more likely than men to develop several psychiatric disorders including major depression, seasonal affective disorder (SAD), rapid cycling bipolar disorder, eating disorders, panic disorder, phobias, generalized anxiety disorder, somatization disorder, pain disorder, and borderline and histrionic personality disorder (2). Women are also more likely to attempt suicide and have higher rates of medical disability (3).

Despite the greater prevalence of many psychiatric conditions in women, etiologic studies, clinical research, drug trials, and outcome studies have usually studied men, and results have been generalized to women without regard for gender variability in phenomenology, drug response, drug metabolism, or side effect profiles. Such generalizations are particularly concerning given that 75% of psychotropic medications are prescribed to women and that drug reaction fatalities are more common in women (4). Lower gastric acidity, body weight, and blood volume, and a higher percentage of body fat

compared with men, affect the absorption and distribution of medications in women. Women also have lower plasma protein binding, slower hepatic glucuronidation and hydroxylation, lower renal clearance, and greater cytochrome P450 3A4 activity than men (5). Furthermore, women's cyclical hormonal fluctuations may interfere significantly with serum levels of a variety of psychotropic drugs over the menstrual cycle.

All physicians should be familiar with the signs and symptoms of psychiatric disorders, first-line interventions, and available referral options for mental health. Unfortunately, many cases of psychiatric illness remain undetected, untreated, or undertreated, and only a small fraction is ever evaluated by psychiatrists. The majority seek care from nonpsychiatric physicians; however, primary care providers have been found to detect only 50% of psychiatric disorders in their practices (6). Many patients present with somatic complaints and do not volunteer emotional symptoms, contributing to these low detection rates in nonpsychiatric settings (7). Affective disorders in particular are extremely common in patients with chronic medical illness (8), and the prevalence of mental illness and substance abuse in patients seen by general medical practitioners is twice that for psychiatric disorders in community samples. The rates of psychiatric illness are even higher for hospitalized severely ill medical patients and high users of medical services. Neurologic disorders, such as stroke, Parkinson's disease, Alzheimer's

TABLE 31.1
Common Psychiatric Disorders in Women

I.   **Eating Disorders**
     Anorexia nervosa
     Bulimia nervosa
     Binge eating disorder
II. **Affective Illnesses**
     Major depression
     Adjustment disorder with depressed mood
     Premenstrual dysphoric disorder
     Postpartum affective illnesses
     Seasonal affective disorder
     Bipolar disorder
     Dysthymia
III. **Alcohol Abuse and Dependence**
IV. **Sexual Disorders**
     Sexual desire disorders
     Sexual arousal disorders
     Orgasmic disorders
     Sexual pain disorders
       Vaginismus
       Dyspareunia
V.   **Anxiety Disorders**
     Phobic disorders
       Specific phobia
       Social phobia
       Agoraphobia
     Panic disorder
     Generalized anxiety disorder
     Obsessive-compulsive disorder
     Post-traumatic stress disorder
VI. **Somatoform Disorders and Factitious Disorders**
     Factitious disorder
       Malingering
     Somatoform disorders
       Somatization disorder
       Conversion disorder
       Hypochondriasis
       Somatoform pain disorder
VII. **Schizophrenic Illnesses**
     Schizophrenia
     Paraphrenia
VIII. **Delirium**

disease and tinnitus are among medical conditions strongly associated with psychiatric illness, most commonly depression (9).

Untreated major depression may worsen the prognosis of medical conditions and increases the use of medical services. Depression can amplify somatic symptoms and lower pain thresholds, thus increasing functional disability. A longitudinal study of high users of ambulatory services revealed that 50% were depressed. Only those with decreased depressive symptoms at a 1-year follow-

up showed an improvement in disability scores (10). The depressive symptoms of decreased mood, concentration, attention, and memory as well as hopelessness, anhedonia, and fatigue often impair the motivation to comply with treatment recommendations. A timely diagnosis and effective treatment of depression in the chronically medically ill helps improve prognosis, lessen disability, and decrease the high use of health services.

The socioeconomic burden of mental illness is very high. Approximately 60% of suicides are attributable to affective disorders alone, and 95% of suicides meet the diagnostic criteria for a psychiatric diagnosis on psychiatric postmortem. Annual U.S. costs for treatment, mortality, and morbidity associated with cases of treated depression have been estimated at over $43 billion (11). Because most individuals with affective illness are either untreated or undertreated, this figure underestimates the total cost of depression to society (12). The mortality and morbidity in the undertreated population, most of which is female, is especially worrisome, because 70 to 90% of depressed patients respond to antidepressant therapy. Given the availability of effective treatment, timely diagnosis and psychiatric care are likely to decrease medical morbidity, mortality, and overall health care expenditure.

PSYCHIATRIC ILLNESSES ACROSS THE FEMALE LIFESPAN

Throughout a woman's life, specific periods occur during which she is at increased risk for developing particular psychiatric disorders. Although the most common psychiatric illnesses—mood and anxiety disorders—may occur at any age, a number of psychiatric conditions are more likely to occur at specific periods of the female lifespan. During these critical periods, the clinician must include appropriate questions in the history and mental status examination to screen for these disorders.

In childhood, young girls are at risk for school phobias, anxiety disorders, attention-deficit hyperactivity disorder (ADHD), and learning disabilities. Adolescence and puberty are accompanied by a marked increase in the incidence of eating disorders. With menarche, 2% of young women develop late luteal premenstrual dysphoria. The premenstrual drop in estrogen and progesterone levels, both of which modulate serotonin, dopamine, norepinephrine, and gamma aminobutyric acid (GABA) function, may explain the monthly fluctuations in psychiatric symptoms observed in several studies and the increase in psychiatric symptoms and hospital admissions associated with the premenstrual and menstrual phases of the female cycle (13). The divergence in risk of depression after puberty, with women developing approximately twice the risk when compared with men of the same age, also suggests a role for the hormonal environment in influencing susceptibility to different psychiatric conditions. In childhood by contrast, girls tend to have lower or equal incidence and prevalence rates for common psychiatric disorders.

During the childbearing years, women are more vulnerable to anxiety and depressive disorders than men but appear to be protected from schizophrenia (14). Women who have a history of psychiatric illness often taper psychiatric medications when planning a pregnancy, resulting in an increased risk of relapse, because pregnancy increases the susceptibility to certain psychiatric disorders. Following delivery, most women experience some change in their mood. The majority has a short-lived, self-limited period of depression or "baby blues," which requires no treatment. Others have severe, disabling symptoms of postpartum depression, and a small number of women develop psychotic symptoms.

The use of psychotropic medication during pregnancy and the postpartum period presents several problems. Physiologic changes associated with pregnancy, including high levels of estrogen, decreased gastrointestinal motility, and increased plasma volume affect pharmacokinetics, and limited data are available on the effect of psychotropic drugs on the developing fetus. Risks from medication during pregnancy and periods of breast-feeding make treatment decisions challenging because each woman's risk–benefit of treatment is greatly influenced by the severity of her symptoms. Besides the teratogenic risks of medication, the offspring of mentally ill women are at higher risk of low birth weight as well as birth and neonatal complications. Psychiatrically ill women are also at higher risk of becoming pregnant without the support of a partner or to have an unplanned pregnancy.

The mid-life period is associated with a continued risk of mood and anxiety disorders as well as other psychiatric illnesses such as schizophrenia. Perimenopause is associated with symptoms of depression, irritability, insomnia, and fatigue, and women may experience changes in sexual function. If treated with antidepressants for affective and anxiety disorders, women are at risk for side effects, including decreased sexual functioning. Although no clear evidence suggests that menopause is associated with an increased risk for depression, most women face many changes during this period, particularly in their roles within the family. Many women exchange their active roles in raising their children for the role of caretaker for their aging parents. Caring for elderly parents on a daily basis is almost exclusively done by women (15). The importance of monitoring the mental state of the caretaker cannot be overstated, given the potential impact on the well-being of the patient. See also Chapter 13.

As women age, they are at increased risk for dementia and the psychiatric complications of medical conditions such as stroke. Because women have a longer lifespan than men, and the risk for dementia increases with age, more women will be affected by dementing illnesses.

Furthermore, Alzheimer's disease disproportionately affects women even after correcting for their longer lifespan. This increase in risk may be related to postmenopausal drops in estrogen levels. Estrogen appears to play a neuromodulatory and neuroprotective role and, as estrogen levels drop during menopause, women lose brain cells at a faster rate than men (14). Randomized controlled trials support a protective effect of estrogen replacement therapy on verbal memory in nondemented postmenopausal women. However, estrogen does not appear to be effective in reversing or slowing cognitive loss in Alzheimer's disease. Whether estrogen replacement delays onset of Alzheimer's remains unanswered and is currently being evaluated in several large prospective, randomized, double-blind, placebo-controlled studies (16).

Older women with multiple medical conditions also face an increased risk for delirium if they are taking multiple medications; decreases in renal and hepatic clearance related to advanced age contribute to an increased risk of toxicity. Women have an elevated risk of paraphrenia, a psychotic disorder with onset typically after the age of 60. Given their longer life expectancy and the fact that they tend to focus more on interpersonal relationships, women are more likely to deal with bereavement, making such losses particularly unsettling.

APPROACH TO THE FEMALE PSYCHIATRIC PATIENT

Psychiatry is the study of affective, cognitive, and behavioral disorders that arise in conscious experience. Psychiatric evaluation and treatment follow the same logic of history taking and examination, differential diagnosis, and treatment planning that is found in other medical conditions. A psychiatric formulation should encompass four perspectives (17): (i) psychiatric diseases, or what the patient has; (ii) disorders of temperament, or what the patient is; (iii) behavioral disorders, or what the patient does; and (iv) disorders that arise from life circumstances and life stressors, or what the patient encounters.

PSYCHIATRIC DISEASES

Schizophrenia and major depression are examples of psychiatric diseases. These conditions are similar to other medical illnesses in that they present with a discrete onset, course, and clinical syndrome of signs and symptoms judged as categorically present or absent in a specific individual. As with other medical diagnoses, they are presumed to be the result of a "broken part," in terms of brain function, resulting in some cases from a genetic or neurodevelopmental abnormality. When symptoms are clearly abnormal and bizarre, as with auditory hallucinations, delusions, or severe obsessions and compulsions, the diagnosis of an abnormal mental state is straightforward. In other cases, distinguishing the pathologic symptoms, such as depressed mood in major depression, from normal feelings of sadness or discouragement arising from life circumstances, can be challenging. The focus should be on eliciting stereotypical patterns of symptoms or symptom complexes that are characteristic of the common psychiatric diseases, combined with knowledge of those diseases that are more common in women.

DISORDERS OF TEMPERAMENT

The second perspective approaches the patient in terms of her personality, or what she is like as a person. Understanding a patient's temperament contributes to an improved therapeutic alliance. Personality traits such as perfectionism, indecisiveness, or impulsiveness exist along a graded continuum normally distributed in the population, much like physiologic traits such as height or weight. Unlike psychiatric diseases, no clear distinction exists between characteristics that are "symptoms of disease" versus healthy variations, and diverseness in personality styles is normal among individuals in a population. Psychopathology or functional impairment in an individual may be evident when traits fall at the extremes of the population distribution. When a woman's temperament leads to serious interference with her professional or interpersonal function, severe enough to qualify as a probable personality disorder, medical care may be impacted and collaboration with a psychiatrist often is helpful.

BEHAVIORAL DISORDERS

Behavioral disorders have an addictive, self-reinforcing quality. They involve goal-directed, compelling behaviors dominant to all other aspects of the behavior of an affected individual. Examples of these disorders include substance abuse disorders and eating disorders. The treatment for these conditions must be staged and should include attention to the behavioral aspects of the condition. The initial goals of treatment are engaging the patient, monitoring and stopping problematic behaviors, and neutralizing sustaining factors. Sustaining factors may include comorbid psychiatric conditions, such as depression or anxiety disorders, or illogical thoughts, such as an anorectic's belief that "if I eat more than 800 calories daily I will get fat." Group therapy is particularly effective in treating behavioral disorders. The final step in treatment is the prevention of relapse. Transient relapse is the norm rather than the exception in the course of behavioral disorders.

THE PATIENT'S LIFE STORY

The fourth perspective is one of narrative. It involves weaving a meaningful story out of a patient's life experiences. Stressors, life circumstances, and social forces are formative factors that can modulate disease expression, personality, and behavior. Developmental life stages, including puberty, pregnancy, and menopause, can be associated with an increased risk for certain disorders. Social conditioning and differences in gender roles may help explain the increased frequency of specific symptom complexes in women. For example, the media's focus on the thinness ideal in Western societies is a likely contributor to the preponderance of women with eating disorders. Such conflicting female roles for contemporary Western women as "devoted wife," "doting mother," and "successful career woman" add to this stress. The perspective of the patient's life story is the approach most closely aligned with methods of insight-oriented psychotherapy, or finding a "meaning to life." The curative power of such therapies does not reside in finding the "right" meaning for a patient's symptoms. Rather, the process enriches the patient's understanding of herself by working with an empathic authority to make sense of her past and to empower her with a feeling of mastery and goal-directedness in the present and for the future (18).

In summary, the formulation of a psychiatric case should include answers to the following four questions:

- Does this patient have an illness with a clear time of onset, probable defined etiology, and likelihood of response to pharmacologic treatment?
- What lifelong personality traits have influenced this woman's interaction with her environment, and how?
- Is there a driven, self-sustained, and pervasive goal-directed behavioral disorder in this individual?
- What events in this woman's life have shaped her as an individual, and what has she learned from them?

EATING DISORDERS

Of all psychiatric conditions, none pertain as exclusively to women as the eating disorders: anorexia nervosa, bulimia nervosa, and binge eating disorder. Ten women are affected with anorexia nervosa or bulimia for every one man, and the overall incidence and prevalence rates of eating disorders are increasing. Young white women and adolescents from the middle and upper classes in Western cultures are at highest risk for anorexia nervosa or bulimia. Prevalence rates in this population are as high as 4%. Rates of eating disorders in other age, racial, and socioeconomic groups are also increasing (19).

As with substance abuse, eating disorders are best formulated as behavioral disorders resulting from a disturbance in hunger, satiety, and the consumption of food. Szmukler and Tantam (20) have described anorexia nervosa as an "addiction to starvation" to illustrate its parallel with substance abuse disorders. Behaviors associated with eating disorders include bingeing or restricting food intake, purging behaviors (vomiting, laxative abuse, and diuretic abuse), excessive exercise, and stimulant abuse. These behaviors develop a driven, compulsive quality fueled by psychologic preoccupations with food and weight. Together, the thoughts and behaviors dominate all aspects of the affected woman's life, developing into a "ruling passion" that impairs physical, psychological, and social function (21). As with substance abuse, conflict over committing to treatment is typical, and treatment must be staged and tailored to the patient's readiness for change.

As defined in the Diagnostic and Statistical Manual of Mental Disorders (DSM-IV), anorexia nervosa includes three criteria: self-starvation, with refusal to maintain weight above 85% of expected; psychologic preoccupation with fear of fatness and body dissatisfaction related to shape and weight; and endocrine disturbance resulting in amenorrhea of 3 months' duration or more (22).

Bulimia nervosa is characterized by the same fear of fatness and body dissatisfaction seen in anorexia nervosa, coupled with binge eating and compensatory behaviors aimed at preventing weight gain from the excess calories ingested. In DSM-IV, anorexia and bulimia are distinguished primarily by whether the patient is significantly underweight and amenorrheic, not by the behaviors that are employed to control weight. Compensatory behaviors in either condition cover a range that includes intermittent fasting, excessive exercise, laxative and diuretic abuse, stimulant abuse, and self-induced vomiting.

Binge eating disorder is distinguished from bulimia nervosa by the absence of compensatory behaviors to prevent or limit weight gain; as a result, binge eaters are generally obese. Most cases of anorexia nervosa, bulimia nervosa, and binge eating disorder are thought to fall along a spectrum of disordered eating pathology. Some patients shift with time from one diagnosis to another, the most common direction being from a restrictive type of anorexia nervosa, in which restriction of food intake and excessive exercise are the predominant behaviors employed to control weight, to bulimia nervosa. No unitary model of causation exists for the eating disorders, and they are best viewed as multifactorial in origin. Identifiable risk factors can be divided into biological, temperamental, and societal predispositions.

Some evidence supports a genetic predisposition to anorexia nervosa. Twin studies of anorexia nervosa (23,24) have shown higher concordance rates for anorexia nervosa in identical versus fraternal twins. One family study yielded a tenfold increased risk of anorexia nervosa in female relatives of anorectic probands (25). Hormonal environment may also play a role in exacerbating eating disorders. For example, binge behavior in both bulimia and binge eating disorder has been observed to increase premenstrually in several small studies.

Temperamental or personality factors that predispose to the development of an eating disorder include introverted, perfectionistic, and self-critical traits. Anorectics who primarily restrict food intake and do not engage in purging behaviors are likely to be anxious persons who tend to avoid harmful and risk-taking behavior, whereas bulimic individuals often have impulsive, novelty-seeking personality traits. Women who binge and purge may exhibit other impulse control behaviors, including substance abuse, sexual promiscuity, shoplifting, and self-harm.

Social forces contribute to the development of eating disorders and stem largely from Western culture's contemporary idealization of thinness and an underweight, androgynous body. The majority of young Western women follow a restrictive diet, a behavior that increases the risk for developing an eating disorder eightfold. Women are conditioned to compare their appearance with one another and to the media's ideal of beauty, and to strive to match the latter. These pressures are felt most strongly in adolescence and young adulthood, a time when pubertal changes increase the distribution of the female body's fat content by 50%, while adolescent girls struggle with the developmental tasks of identity formation, individuation from family, and sexual maturity. The incidence of eating disorders in young women over the past several decades has increased in concert with escalating social conflict over women's roles and the media's increasing emphasis on thinness as a symbol of female success.

Other risk factors or precipitants for the development of an eating disorder include family conflict, loss of or separation from an important attachment figure such as a parent, physical illness, sexual conflict, and trauma. Participation in sports or professions that emphasize thinness such as ballet or modeling, being bullied by peers, or the developmental stressors such as marriage and pregnancy can also be triggers.

Although some may overlap, it is important to distinguish the aforementioned predisposing risk factors from those that maintain the eating disorder once the associated behaviors become entrenched. Eating disorders tend to take on a self-sustaining quality over time, becoming independent of the original precipitating factors. Sustaining factors include the development of pathologic eating habits and the consequences of starvation. The anorectic patient starts starving by dieting. She is often socially reinforced for her initial weight loss by receiving compliments on her appearance and self-discipline. Over time, the behaviors and thoughts associated with the eating disorder develop a sense of primacy and a subjective anxiolytic purpose. The patient uses them with escalating frequency and intensity to self-treat unpleasant thoughts or feelings, much as an alcoholic expands his or her use of alcohol from an initial social situation to a reflexive and learned way of reacting to any emotional stress by reaching for a drink.

Eating disorders are often underdiagnosed. Patients tend not to volunteer signs or symptoms due to feelings of shame, conflict over giving up the associated behaviors, and fears of being judged or stigmatized. The physiologic signs of an eating disorder may be evident on physical examination and are primarily related to starvation or purging behavior. In addition to low body weight, starvation may result in bradycardia, hypotension, chronic constipation, delayed gastric emptying, osteoporosis, and menstrual irregularities. Purging behaviors are associated with electrolyte abnormalities, dental problems, parotid gland hypertrophy, and gastrointestinal symptoms. Seizures may occur due to hyponatremia. The presence of any of these complaints in a young woman should prompt the clinician to ask basic screening questions, including the patient's highest and lowest lifetime weight and a brief history of dieting behaviors such as skipping meals or counting fat grams and calories. Further questioning should explore bingeing behavior, frequency and use of compensatory behaviors to prevent weight gain, preoccupations with food and weight, and whether the patient herself, friends, or family have ever been worried about her having an eating disorder.

Underweight anorectics who purge are at highest risk for serious or life-threatening complications. Anorexia nervosa has one of the highest mortalities of any psychiatric diagnosis, with up to 20% dying over 33 years in one cohort study (26). Death is generally due to the physical complications of starvation or suicide. In bulimia nervosa, deaths are most often the result of hypokalemia-associated arrhythmias or suicide.

The psychologic symptoms of an eating disorder can be classified as secondary to eating disordered behaviors or to a comorbid psychiatric condition. Starvation-induced symptoms include a syndrome of depression and obsessive-compulsive symptoms. In a 1950s study, male subjects who starved to less than 75% of their ideal body weight developed many of the characteristic signs seen in anorexia nervosa (27). Their symptoms included depressed mood, escalating preoccupations with and dreams of food, decreased concentration, ritualistic eating, decreased libido, and social isolation, followed by bingeing when given unlimited access to food. All these behaviors eventually reversed with refeeding. This study highlights the starvation-related, self-sustaining features of an eating disorder and stresses the importance of refeeding and rapid attainment of a normal weight. In bulimia nervosa, feelings of shame and secrecy about bingeing and purging contribute to increased social iso-

lation, self-critical thinking, and demoralization.

Most patients who have an eating disorder are also at risk for comorbid psychiatric conditions. The most common of these are major depression, anxiety disorders, substance abuse, and personality disorders. Comorbid major depression or dysthymia has been reported in 50 to 75% of anorectic patients (19) and 24 to 88% of bulimics (28). A lifetime history of obsessive compulsive disorder was found in 26% of anorectics (29). Failure to recognize and treat these comorbid psychiatric illnesses affects prognosis and interferes with recovery for the individual patient. The social consequences of an eating disorder include increased isolation and avoidance of social situations because these often revolve around food, interpersonal difficulties, problems with sex and intimacy, and academic or occupational impairment.

The treatment of eating disorders must be a staged process, starting with an assessment of the severity of the eating pathology, psychiatric comorbidity, and motivation for change. A referral to a nutritionist or cognitive behavioral therapist who is experienced in the treatment of patients with eating disorders is often necessary. It is important to appreciate that stopping the behaviors involved in these disorders is the primary intervention, and that only after these behaviors are brought under control does more insight-oriented therapy yield progress. A parallel is readily made with the primacy of abstinence in substance abuse treatment, where psychodynamic therapy with an alcoholic who continues drinking is generally accepted to be of little therapeutic use.

When a patient is failing outpatient treatment or is medically compromised, a referral should be made for admission to an eating disorders specialty service having a coordinated treatment team, behavioral protocol, and staff experienced in the treatment of eating disorders. Treatment on a general psychiatric unit is less likely to be effective in motivating the patient to give up her eating disorder, and long-term mortality has been shown to be lower for anorectic patients treated on a specialty unit (30). Group therapy and the close monitoring of meals and bathroom use by nurses on a behavioral unit minimizes manipulative behavior and provides patients with the structure, peer support, and reshaping of their relationship with food necessary for a successful outcome.

Several classes of psychopharmacologic agents have been used to treat patients with eating disorders. Double-blind placebo-controlled trials confirm the efficacy of a wide range of antidepressant drugs in decreasing binge-purge frequency in bulimia nervosa. Imipramine, desipramine, trazodone, and fluoxetine have all been found to decrease the frequency of binge-purge behaviors independent of the presence of comorbid depression. In the case of fluoxetine, higher doses (60 mg) than those commonly used in depression are most effective (31). Monoamine oxidase inhibitors (MAOIs) and buproprion are relatively contraindicated because of the need for dietary restraint with MAOIs and an increased risk of seizures with buproprion in bulimics. First-line intervention for bulimia should include a trial of a tricyclic antidepressant drug or selective serotonergic reuptake inhibitor (SSRI) in conjunction with cognitive-behavioral therapy.

In anorexia nervosa, no medication has been proved effective in increasing weight gain in controlled trials. Except when a patient is severely depressed or has marked obsessive compulsive symptoms, most clinicians recommend monitoring a patient's mental state during refeeding, rather than treating patients with medication while they are still underweight. Most of the depressive symptoms, preoccupations, and rituals around food and weight remit as a patient reaches a healthy weight. When a decision is made to prescribe an antidepressant, a low-dose SSRI is often the safest choice, given the potential risk of a cardiac arrhythmia or hypotension with tricyclic antidepressant drugs and the general risk of increased side effects in this underweight population. A small double-blind controlled trial of fluoxetine in anorexia nervosa indicates that this agent may be useful in preventing weight loss in anorexia after inpatient weight restoration (32).

Studies of neurotransmitters and neuropeptides in ill and recovered patients with eating disorders are limited in number but indicate dysfunction in central nervous system (CNS) serotonergic, noradrenergic, and opiate systems. Feeding behavior studies in animal models implicate the same neurotransmitter systems. The efficacy of serotonergic and noradrenergic antidepressant medications in bulimia nervosa may well relate to the physiology of feeding behavior (33). Data from human studies conflict, and it is unclear whether observed neurotransmitter abnormalities in patients with eating disorders are state-related, arising from dieting and binge-purge behaviors themselves, or trait-related, preceding the onset of the eating disorder behaviors in susceptible individuals and failing to remit with treatment.

Outcome studies for anorexia nervosa show that of hospitalized patients at 4-year follow-up, 44% have a good outcome, with weight restoration and resolution of amenorrhea; 28% have an intermediate outcome; 24% remain chronically underweight and have a poor outcome; and 4% die (19). Poor prognostic factors include binge-purge type anorexia, lower minimum weight, and previous treatment failure. Up to 40% of anorectics develop some bulimic behaviors at follow-up.

The long-term outcome of bulimia nervosa is largely unknown. Abstinence is uncommon, and episodic waxing and waning of symptoms is frequent. Decreased bulimic symptoms are reported by 70% of patients in short-term outcome studies employing combined medication and psychosocial therapies. Controlled treatment studies show better outcomes for cognitive-behavioral or interpersonal therapy than for behavioral therapy alone (34), and the combination of an antidepressant medication and cognitive-behavioral therapy has been shown to be superior to therapy or drug alone (35). As with anorectics, the severity of symptoms in bulimia is related to prognosis. Of patients with severe bulimia requiring inpatient treatment, 33% have a poor outcome at 3 years and engage daily in ongoing bingeing and vomiting behaviors (19).

Eating disorders are complex psychiatric disorders that are primarily found in women. Although frequently undertreated, they are associated with high morbidity and are increasing in prevalence in Western societies. Treatment using psychologic, psychoeducational, and pharmacologic techniques significantly improves prognosis. Although initial intervention may not require specialty care, failure to respond to treatment warrants early referral to a psychiatrist or an eating disorders program. Further research is needed to clarify the reasons for the preponderance of eating disorders in the female population, to identify preventive measures and risk factors, and to develop focused and effective treatments.

AFFECTIVE DISORDERS

Affective disorders are psychiatric illnesses that have a change in mood as their principal feature. Everyone experiences variations in mood, but few know the extreme mood states of the affective disorders. Depression and mania are the two principal mood states seen in the major affective illnesses. Affective disorders include major depression, bipolar disorder, dysthymia, and adjustment disorder with depressed mood. Hormonal status may impact the risk for affective disorders throughout a woman's lifespan, with increased symptoms associated with menstruation and pregnancy.

Depression

Depression is one of the most prevalent psychiatric disorders and occurs more commonly in women (36). Most population-based studies have estimated prevalence rates of depression to be twice as high for women as for men. In a cross-nation study, Weissman demonstrated higher rates of depression in women in 10 countries (37). This finding may be partially influenced by the tendency of women to have better recall of past episodes of depression (38). The range of clinical presentations and lack of specific diagnostic signs or laboratory tests associated with the illness complicate the diagnosis of depression. The experience of feeling depressed is universal. When diagnosing depression, the challenge is to distinguish between short-lived periods of sadness that are related to life circumstances and depression arising from a particular illness. For example, sadness and a lack of enjoyment in activities may be expected during periods of bereavement, making it difficult to distinguish during the initial period of grief between a normal grief reaction and a depressive episode with relatively mild symptoms. The key to the differential diagnosis is recognizing typical symptoms and monitoring their course. A grieving individual usually will not have a change in self-attitude, suicidal thoughts, feelings of hopelessness, or persistent neurovegetative symptoms such as disturbances in sleep, appetite, and energy level lasting continuously for weeks to months.

The diagnosis of major depression is based on clinical history and an examination of mental status. Cardinal symptoms include a sad or depressed mood and anhedonia—a lack of interest in and an inability to enjoy usual activities. At least one of these symptoms is a requirement in the diagnostic criteria of the DSM-IV (22). In addition to depression or anhedonia lasting for at least 2 weeks, a major depressive episode is characterized by a change in vital sense marked by at least four of the following neurovegetative symptoms: significant weight loss or weight gain, insomnia or hypersomnia, psychomotor retardation or agitation, fatigue or loss of energy, diminished ability to concentrate, or indecisiveness. Additionally, most individuals are self-critical, with feelings of worthlessness, hopelessness, excessive guilt, and recurrent thoughts of death or suicidal ideation. This change in self-attitude may also result in patients believing themselves to be a burden to their family and friends. Patients presenting with major depression have a combination of some of these symptoms. The underlying clinical syndrome combines depressed mood, a change in vital sense, and a change in self-attitude.

The continuation of symptoms for periods of at least 2 weeks helps distinguish a major depressive episode from a briefer adjustment disorder with depressed mood. An adjustment disorder is a "reactive" depression in which symptoms are a reaction to a clear stressor and are typically self-limited and responsive to supportive therapy. This does not mean that a major depressive episode cannot be triggered by a stressful life event or should not be treated because the depressive episode appears to be understandable. As with bereavement, it is the severity and course of symptoms that distinguishes an adjustment disorder from an episode of major depressive disorder.

Certain groups, such as the elderly, are less likely to report the classic symptoms of depression, such as low mood and sadness, which probably results in an underestimation of the prevalence of depression in such groups (39). A concern also exists that particular ethnic groups may report somatic symptoms rather than classic depressive symptoms. In older women, symptoms of social withdrawal and a change in the reporting of somatic symptoms should be taken seriously because they are likely to represent a significant change in health status—the emergence of a depressive or other medical illness. Although some laboratory tests, such as the dexamethasone suppression test, have been purported to be diagnostic, they have been shown to be nonspecific. No reliable laboratory diagnostic studies are available for diagnosing depression. The diagnosis of a major depression remains clinical and is made after a careful history and mental status examination.

The incidence of depression during childhood is approximately equal for boys and girls. The divergence in the reported incidence begins around puberty. Angola and Worthman reviewed evidence for a hormonal cause of this disparity and concluded that hormonal developmental changes are likely to be contributing factors in a complex etiologic mechanism (40). With menarche, women are at risk for premenstrual dysphoric disorder (PMDD). This form of mood disorder is characterized by symptoms of major depression, including anxiety and mood lability, which occur during the last week of the luteal phase of the menstrual cycle and remit during the first few days of the follicular phase (41). Although premenstrual mood symptoms affect 20 to 30% of women, severe incapacitating premenstrual mood cycling is less common, with a prevalence of 3 to 8% in the female population (42). Two large, multicenter, randomized, controlled trials have investigated the treatment of PMDD with SSRIs. A randomized, controlled trial of sertraline at doses of 50 to 150 mg versus placebo demonstrated a significant improvement in both symptoms and self-reported disability in women treated with sertraline. Sixty-two percent of sertraline-treated women and 34% of those receiving placebo responded to treatment (43). Fluoxetine at doses of 20 to 60 mg per day has also been shown to decrease premenstrual symptom severity in up to 50% of women tested in a multicenter, placebo-controlled trial (44). In a meta-analysis, Dimmock and colleagues demonstrated the efficacy of fluoxetine, sertraline, paroxetine, and citalopram in treating PMDD (45). Growing evidence suggests that intermittent dosing during the late-luteal phase may be equally effective for a subset of women with PMDD (46,47). In a study comparing the SSRI sertraline to the tricyclic antidepressant (TCA) desipramine, the SSRI was significantly more effective, whereas the TCA was comparable to placebo (48). Aside from the distinct syndrome of PMDD present in a small minority of women, women in the midst of a major depressive episode may also have worsening of symptoms premenstrually. It is unclear whether this is simply the worsening of one condition or the superimposition of two conditions (49). Similarly, in women with bipolar illness, worsening of depressive symptoms or increase in mood cycling may occur in the premenstrual period.

Pregnant women may experience an entire range of affective symptoms either during gestation or postpartum. Population studies have estimated that the prevalence rate of major depression (approximately 10%) is similar to that in nonpregnant women (50,51). Additionally, women may experience less severe depressive symptoms, elated mood, mania, or periods of psychosis with hallucinations and delusions. Special concerns with respect to treatment during pregnancy involve both the onset of new episodes and the continuation of medications as prophylaxis against recurrent episodes. Women with a pre-existing mood disorder such as depression or bipolar illness have been shown to have high relapse rates when medications are discontinued during pregnancy (52–54). The risk of fetal complications from medications used to treat mood disorders must be weighed against the risk to mother and fetus if the mother's mood symptoms worsen.

In a comprehensive review, Altshuler and colleagues (55) outlined treatment guidelines for various psychiatric illnesses during pregnancy. Generally, pharmacologic treatments should be avoided if possible during the first trimester, given the risks of teratogenicity. If the symptoms are severe, however, treatment with an antidepressant medication or mood stabilizer may be necessary. The specific medication should be chosen to minimize risk to the fetus. Wisner and colleagues reviewed the treatment of depression during pregnancy, including recent prospective studies of the TCAs and SSRIs. Exposure to TCAs and SSRIs did not increase the risk for intrauterine or major birth defects (56). See also Chapter 4. Electroconvulsive therapy (ECT) is another relatively safe treatment for severe depression during pregnancy. First-trimester exposure to lithium is associated with congenital cardiovascular malformations. Antiepileptic drugs and benzodiazepines have also been associated with an increased risk of congenital malformations and should be avoided if possible. Each woman's case must be evaluated on an individual basis, with careful consideration of the level of symptom severity. A consultation with a psychiatrist is advisable to assess the risks of untreated illness versus the risk of pharmacologic complications to mother and fetus. Many women experience a mood change after delivery. A wide range exists in the severity of symptoms from the "baby blues" to major depression to psychotic episodes. Most women experience this mood change in the first 6 months following delivery, with a resolution of the symptoms of dysphoria and irritability by the end of this period. The range of mood changes is quite broad, and some women continue to experience depressive symptoms for many months to years, often experiencing several episodes. In a study of 119 women followed up after the birth of their first child, one-half of those receiving psychiatric treatment soon after delivery had a recurrence of psychiatric problems during the following 3 years (57). The early detection of symptoms and prompt treatment is critical for both the mother and the child, because depression may affect a mother's ability to bond with and care for her infant. The management of depression with antidepressants in nursing mothers requires careful consideration of the risks versus benefits of continued breast-feeding, however. Tricyclic antidepressants have been the most studied antidepressants in breast-feeding and are detected in breast milk at concentrations approximating those in maternal plasma. Studies of the effects of tricyclics on infants are very limited, and caution is advisable in prescribing them. To avoid peak plasma levels, it is advisable to prescribe once daily dosing in the evening and have mothers feed with formula overnight and breastfeed only during the day. Of the SSRIs, sertraline and paroxetine are secreted in breast milk at lower concentrations than fluoxetine and are preferable for this reason (58).

Mood changes at the time of menopause have long been noted. Recent studies, however, have not supported a clear association between menopause and affective illness. In a review of this subject, Schmidt and Rubinow (59) outline the major limitations of published studies of this association. One criticism has been the often unclear delineation of affective symptoms from affective disorders, and a specific pattern of mood disturbance or behavior change has not been demonstrated.

Mood symptoms related to the hormonal changes of menopause may be distressing and may warrant a trial of hormone replacement therapy (HRT). The results of the 10th interim analysis of the Women's Health Initiative resulted in a termination of the trial of the combined estrogen/progesterone arm of the trial (60). These results have complicated the risk–benefit analysis for HRT, thus necessitating careful assessment of each individual case. See also Chapter 12. If symptoms are severe, interfere with function, or meet diagnostic criteria for an affective disorder, initial management with an antidepressant medication should be considered.

Given the longer average life expectancy of women, most women in long-term relationships and marriages outlive their spouses. As a result, most elderly women face bereavement and grief. Although empathic support is usually sufficient to deal with the symptoms of grief, older women should be monitored for the emergence of severe depressive symptoms. The history and mental status examination of elderly women should include screening for somatic symptoms and new feelings of "being a burden" to family, because older patients are less likely to report sad, depressed mood as a primary complaint. The treatment of depression in the elderly is often complicated by a poorer tolerance of antidepressant medications, which may necessitate starting with small initial doses and gradually increasing the dose. SSRIs are less likely to cause anticholinergic side effects, such as sedation and orthostasis, which are of particular concern in the elderly. However, SSRIs may interact with other medications metabolized by the cytochrome P450 system, and if a patient is taking several medications, the monitoring of all drug blood levels and potential side effects is essential.

There is no known single cause of depression. The clearest demographic risk factor is female gender. An analysis of population-based data demonstrated an increased risk for major depression in divorced and separated individuals and in the unemployed (61). The role of psychologic causes has been extensively studied without a clear consensus. Family studies have demonstrated an increased prevalence of affective disorders in the first-degree relatives of probands with depression (62). Twin studies have also supported a genetic predisposition in some patients (63). Evidence for a hereditary basis is stronger for bipolar disorder than for major depression (64). Research efforts support probable abnormalities in the functioning of the neurochemical systems involving serotonin and norepinephrine (65–67).

The usual treatment of major depression is the combination of pharmacologic management with an antidepressant and psychological treatment incorporating supportive or cognitive-behavioral psychotherapy. The development of new generations of antidepressants that have relatively few side effects has expanded treatment options for patients with depression. The four major categories of antidepressants are in use: (i) tricyclic antidepressants (TCAs), (ii) selective serotonin reuptake inhibitors (SSRIs), (iii) MAO inhibitors (MAOIs), and (iv) other/atypical antidepressant drugs. Table 32.2 outlines the antidepressant drug classes, drugs within each class, typical starting and maintenance doses, and common side effects.

The key principle in the use of antidepressant medications is completing an adequate trial of at least 6 to 8 weeks for each antidepressant at a therapeutic dose. Unfortunately, patients often have trials of antidepressant drugs discontinued before reaching a therapeutic level or after only a few weeks because there has been no clear benefit. For the TCAs, the monitoring of blood levels is helpful to confirm that the patient's dosage is at a therapeutic level. Blood levels are less helpful with SSRIs, and the therapeutic level may vary significantly. If a patient fails a full trial with an antidepressant medication and continues to have symptoms of a major depressive episode, another trial of antidepressant drugs using a medication from a different class should be initiated. Caution is warranted in generalizing the results of pharmacologic antidepressant treatment studies done on men to women. For example, premenopausal depressed women appear to have better response to serotonergic antidepressants, whereas men tend to respond more favorably to TCAs (9).

All patients being treated with antidepressant medications should be monitored for the emergence of manic symptoms. Although they are a relatively rare complication of antidepressant treatment, manic symptoms including elated or irritable mood, decreased need for sleep, increased energy, and increased agitation may occur, especially in individuals who have a family or personal history of bipolar disorder. All patients should be asked about previous symptoms of mania or hypomania, a mood state with milder symptoms of mania such as decreased need for sleep, increased energy level, and increased self-confidence. For patients who have a personal history of bipolar illness or a strong family history of manic-depressive illness, consultation with a psychiatrist is helpful to plan treatment with a mood stabilizer such as lithium or valproic acid, possibly in combination with antidepressant medications.

Seasonal Affective Disorders

Some persons have a seasonal pattern of depression, with a worsening of symptoms during the winter months. The clinical presentation of this disorder ranges from mild symptoms that do not significantly impair functioning to major depression. If symptoms are mild, management with a full-spectrum nonultraviolet light (10,000 lux) for 15 to 30 minutes each morning during the winter months may be sufficient. These full-spectrum lights are commercially available. If symptoms meet the criteria for major depression, antidepressant medication should be combined with light therapy.

Bipolar Disorder

The essential distinction between major depression, or unipolar depression, and bipolar disorder is the presence of both depressed and manic episodes. The criteria for a depressive episode in bipolar disorder are essentially the same as those for a major depressive episode. A manic episode is characterized by persistently elevated, expansive, or irritable mood lasting for at least 1 week. This mood change is accompanied by several of the following symptoms: elevated self-attitude or grandiosity, decreased need for sleep, loud and rapid speech, racing thoughts, flight of ideas, distractibility, increased activity, or agitation. This general increase in the patient's vital sense often includes overinvolvement in pleasurable activities such as spending more money, substance abuse, increased and often promiscuous sexual activity, and more erratic business investments.

The spectrum of bipolar illness ranges from bipolar type I disorder, the classic form with a history of both depressive and manic episodes, to bipolar type II disorder, which combines depressive episodes and hypomanic periods. Hypomanic episodes are a milder form of typical mania in which similar symptoms occur but do not impair the patient's social and occupational functioning to a marked degree. Other forms of bipolar illness include rapid cycling, in which mood states change rapidly, and mixed states, in which the patient simultaneously experiences the symptoms of both mania and depression. Mixed states are particularly distressing because patients experience both depressive symptoms and an energized, agitated state.

TABLE 31.2
Common Antidepressants

Class of Antidepressants	Starting Dose	Usual Therapeutic Dose	Blood Levels	Common Side Effects
Tricyclics				
Nortriptyline (Pamelor®)	10–25 mg qhs	50–150 mg qhs titrated to level	70–140 ng/mL	Sedation, dry mouth, orthostasis, constipation
Desipramine (Norpramin®)	10–25 mg qhs	50–200 mg qhs titrated to level	>125 ng/mL	Sedation, dry mouth, orthostasis, constipation
Imipramine (Tofranil®)	10–25 mg qhs	100–300 mg qhs	200–250 ng/dL	Sedation, dry mouth, orthostasis, constipation
SSRIs				
Citalopram (Celexa®)	20 mg qd	20–40 mg qd	Unclear	Insomnia, agitation, nausea, anorexia, sexual dysfunction
Escitalopram (Lexapro®)	10 mg qd	10–20 mg qd	Unclear	Insomnia, agitation, nausea, anorexia, sexual dysfunction
Fluoxetine (Prozac®)	10–20 mg qd	20–60 mg qd	Unclear	Insomnia, agitation, nausea, anorexia, sexual dysfunction
Fluvoxamine (Luvox®)	50 mg qd	100–300 mg qd	Unclear	Insomnia, agitation, nausea anorexia, sexual dysfunction
Paroxetine (Paxil®)	10–20 mg qd	20–50 mg qd	Unclear	Insomnia, agitation, nausea, anorexia, sexual dysfunction
Sertraline (Zoloft®)	25–50 mg qd	50–200 mg qd	Unclear	Insomnia, agitation, diarrhea, nausea, anorexia, sexual dysfunction
MAOIs				
Tranylcypromine (Parnate®)	10 mg qd	20–40 mg qd	Unclear	Insomnia, dizziness, dry mouth
Phenelzine (Nardil®)	15 mg qd	45–60 mg qd	Unclear	Dizziness, dry mouth, dyspepsia, sedation
Others				
Buproprion (Wellbutrin®)	75 mg bid	200–450 mg qd in divided doses	Unclear	Agitation, insomnia, anxiety, restlessness
Buproprion, SR (Wellbutrin SR®)	100 mg qd	200–400 mg qd in divided doses (bid)	Unclear	Agitation, insomnia, anxiety, restlessness
Mirtazapine (Remeron®)	15 mg	15–45 mg qd	Unclear	orthostasis, drowsiness, dry mouth, weight gain, sexual dysfunction
Nefazodone (Serzone®)	100 mg bid	300–600 mg qd	Unclear	Nausea, dry mouth, sedation, dizziness, constipation
Trazodone (Desyrel®)	50–100 mg qd	50–100 mg qhs for sleep 200–400 mg qd for depression	Unclear	Sedation, orthostasis, nausea
Venlafaxine (Effexor®)	37.5 mg bid	150–375 mg qd		Anxiety, nausea, insomnia, dizziness, sedation
Venlafaxine, ER (Effexor XR®)	37.5 mg qd	150–375 mg qd		Anxiety, nausea, insomnia, dizziness, sedation

SR = sustained release, ER = extended release

The primary treatment for all forms of bipolar disorder is a mood-stabilizing agent such as lithium, carbamazepine, or valproic acid. Lithium dosage should be initiated at 300 mg once or twice daily and titrated to a blood level between 0.8 and 1.0 mEq/L for bipolar type I disorder. Blood level ranges for valproic acid are not as clearly established for the management of affective disorders, but the levels used for the treatment of epilepsy can be used as a guide, with a target range between 50 and 150 µg/mL. For some patients, a combination of a mood stabilizer and an antidepressant medication is needed to manage persistent depressive symptoms. The combination of a mood stabilizer and a low-dose neuroleptic medication may be needed to control the symptoms of acute mania. Although they have not been as extensively studied, a number of newer antiepileptic medications including gabapentin, lamotrigine, and topiramate are also being prescribed to treat bipolar disorder.

A past history of bipolar disorder in pregnant women who are not currently on medication is associated with a 30 to 50% risk of postpartum psychosis and warrants close monitoring by a psychiatrist (58). During pregnancy, both carbamazepine and valproate are associated with fetal neural tube defects (NTDs) and lithium can cause cardiac anomalies. The risk of NTDs is less than 2% with the mood stabilizers. Although the relative risk for Ebstein's is 10 to 20 times greater than in the general population, the absolute risk of Ebstein's anomaly following first trimester exposure to lithium is only 0.1 to 0.05% (68). In pregnancy, when risk of relapse outweighs the risk of discontinuing the medication, a careful second trimester fetal ultrasound to screen for NTDs or cardiac anomalies is indicated. If lithium is continued during pregnancy, levels should be followed closely. The dose of lithium usually must be increased as the pregnancy progresses due to increased renal clearance (58). The dose then needs to be decreased approximately 2 weeks prior to delivery to decrease the risk of the "floppy baby" syndrome (69). Little is known about the risks associated with the newer antiepileptics during pregnancy and lactation (70). Although most clinicians advise against breast-feeding while on lithium, studies of infant toxicity are lacking.

Dysthymia

Dysthymia is a more chronic depressive state lasting for at least 2 years but with fewer symptoms than major depression. The severity and number of symptoms are not sufficient to meet the criteria for a major depressive episode but they do interfere with work or social functioning. Common symptoms include appetite disturbance, decreased energy, impaired concentration, disturbed sleep, and feelings of hopelessness. Community studies from different countries have consistently reported higher rates of dysthymia in women (71). The National Comorbidity Study estimated the lifetime prevalence of dysthymia to be 8% of women compared with 5% of men (72). Although treatment trials involving dysthymia are limited, some evidence suggests that SSRIs such as fluoxetine and sertraline may have a role in treating this chronic form of depressed mood. In some patients, episodes of major depression may be superimposed on a chronic dysthymic disorder.

Comorbid Affective and Neurologic Disorders

Numerous demonstrated associations exist between neurologic conditions and affective illnesses, with depressive illnesses more commonly associated than bipolar disorder. The occurrence of major depressive episodes requiring treatment is frequently seen in Huntington's disease, Parkinson's disease, and Alzheimer's disease. Approximately 40% of patients with Parkinson's disease have depressive symptoms; on average, half the depressed patients have major depression and half have dysthymia (73). A study of 221 patients with multiple sclerosis (MS) found that approximately 35% had a current or lifetime diagnosis of major depression (74). Bipolar disorder also occurs at higher than expected rates in MS patients (75). Several studies have demonstrated an association between left anterior hemispheric stroke and depression (76). Patients with AIDS may develop both depression and mania as well as the subcortical dementia characteristic of human immunodeficiency virus (HIV) infection. Interestingly, although the prevalence of depression in individuals without neuropathology is twice as high for women as it is for men, focal neurologic illness such as stroke or Parkinson's disease is associated with a 1:1 prevalence ratio between genders. This increased relative vulnerability to depressive illness in men with stroke or Parkinson's may reflect a protective effect of estrogen in women. Because estrogen regulates serotonergic tone, it may counteract the expected effect of focal neurologic damage (9).

In the neurologic patient, the most important diagnostic distinction is differentiating an adjustment disorder from a major depressive episode. Because the symptoms of neurologic conditions can be debilitating, depressive symptoms are often "misunderstood" as a natural reaction to a serious medical condition. Patients who meet the diagnostic criteria for an affective disorder should be treated, because treatment of the comorbid affective illness is likely to impact on the response to medical treatment for their neurologic condition. If the clinical picture does not meet the criteria for an affective disorder, the treatment is usually supportive psychotherapy to help the patient come to terms with the changes and challenges of the neurologic disorder. Peer support groups also may be very helpful. If the patient has a psychiatric disorder such as depression, the treatment is essentially the same as that for someone without a comorbid medical condition. Comorbidity implies a higher likelihood of polypharmacy and sensitivity to medications, increasing the risk of delirium with treatment. For patients receiving multiple medications, antidepressant medications should be started at low doses and carefully increased, with monitoring for symptoms of delirium.

ALCOHOL ABUSE

Alcohol is the most commonly abused substance in the United States, and 6% of the adult female population has a serious alcohol problem. Although the rates of alcohol abuse are lower in women than in men, alcohol dependence and alcohol-related morbidity and mortality are disproportionately higher, and physicians less commonly take a substance abuse history or detect alcoholism in women than in men (77). Studies of alcoholism have focused on male populations, and the extension of their findings to female populations is speculative and of questionable validity. Diagnostic instruments often include questions regarding occupational or legal problems that are less likely to be evident in women, since women who work in the home are unlikely to be exposed to the professional problems that often force men into treatment. Although alcoholic women more commonly drink alone and less often have histories of violent acts when intoxicated, they are more likely to become the victims of sexual and physical violence, often by an intoxicated partner, and to develop post-traumatic stress disorder (PTSD) (78). Indeed, alcoholic women are more likely to have an alcoholic partner than are alcoholic men and are strongly influenced by spouses or partners to use. Substance abusing partners are also less likely to pressure their wives to seek help while non–substance abusing husbands may avoid confronting their wives because women who drink heavily are stigmatized more than male drinkers, contributing to increased denial and under-reporting of alcohol-related problems by both women and their spouses. Taken together, these factors suggest that the reported prevalence rates of alcohol abuse in the female population are probably underestimated

Women develop alcohol-related medical complications faster and at lower levels of absolute alcohol intake than men. Cirrhosis, hypertension, fatty liver, gastrointestinal bleeding, alcohol-related cardiac problems, cognitive impairment, stroke, and malnutrition all occur earlier in women, and mortality rates are higher both due to medical complications and alcohol-related accidents. Women who consume 1.5 drinks daily have an approximately equal risk of alcoholic liver disease as do men who drink four or more drinks a day (79). At-risk drinking for women has been defined by the National Institute on

Alcohol Abuse and Alcoholism as more than seven drinks per week or three drinks per occasion. Women's lower levels of gastric alcohol dehydrogenase and higher ratio of body fat/water volume help to account for the observed discrepancies in levels of first-pass metabolism and absolute blood alcohol between the sexes (80). As with medical complications, alcohol dependence is "telescoped" in women, occurring faster and at lower absolute levels of consumption. A compression of the time frame needed for the development of a withdrawal syndrome in women is also seen with other substances of abuse, including opiates and cocaine (81).

Evidence suggests that the incidence of alcohol abuse and rates of alcohol-related problems are increasing in cohorts of women born after 1950, making the need for studies comparing alcoholic with nonalcoholic women a priority. Physiologic risks related to alcohol abuse vary across the female lifespan. No consistent changes in alcohol metabolism have been found by menstrual phase, but menstrual irregularities, early menopause, and fertility problems are more prevalent in heavy drinkers. Obstetric complication and fetal alcohol syndrome are also common in female alcoholics (79). The incidence of cirrhosis increases precipitously after menopause, and heavy alcohol consumption elevates the risk of invasive breast cancer (82). Elderly women are more likely to use prescription drugs with side effects that are intensified by concomitant alcohol use and are therefore at higher risk of injury due to falls or motor vehicle accidents while intoxicated. Finally, older women are at a higher risk of longer and more severe withdrawal, complicated by related medical problems.

Comorbid psychiatric diagnoses, especially polysubstance abuse, mood disorders, bulimia nervosa, anxiety, and psychosexual disorders, are more common in women who drink heavily compared with nonalcoholic women or alcoholic men. In one study, the prevalence of depression in alcoholic women was 19% compared with 7% in nonalcoholic women (83). Many women report drinking in order to self-medicate mood states including depression, anxiety, or premenstrual dysphoria. Although alcohol use may provide short-term relief, it inevitably exacerbates these conditions and can precipitate substance-induced mood or anxiety disorders in susceptible individuals. It may take several weeks of abstinence for these symptoms to resolve. Women with a family history of paternal-side alcoholism, generalized anxiety disorder, and premenstrual syndrome drink more premenstrually, perhaps in an attempt to self-medicate anxiety or depressive symptoms (84). Suicidality has also been reported to be significantly elevated in alcoholic women.

Women are likely to seek treatment for alcoholism indirectly, presenting to counselors or physicians with complaints of marital or family problems and nonspecific physical or emotional symptoms including nervousness, insomnia, and anxiety. Less than half of these cases are correctly identified as alcohol-related. Women are also more likely to be admitted to non–alcohol-specific treatment, such as general psychiatric units rather than conventional alcohol treatment services (81) and are more likely to drop out of treatment (85). Because female alcoholics often have low self-esteem and feelings of shame and embarrassment, they may balk at confrontational techniques and require more supportive and skill-building approaches. The very serious consequences of alcoholism for women's health make it crucial for physicians to screen for alcohol abuse, to educate female patients on the risks of drinking what are often seen as moderate amounts of alcohol for men, and to refer patients to specialized substance abuse treatment when appropriate. Women of childbearing age should be made aware of the consequences of alcohol abuse as they relate to fertility, as well as to fetal and maternal health.

Although direct questions about the amounts of alcohol consumed tend to be unreliable, screening for alcohol abuse should not be limited to an assessment of laboratory values suggestive of alcoholism, such as anemia, increased red blood cell mean corpuscular volume, or elevated liver function tests and triglycerides. The question "Have you ever had a drinking problem?" and the four-item CAGE questionnaire (Table 31.3) (86) provide an easy two-minute screen for an alcohol use problem. Since the sensitivity of the CAGE is lower for women than for men, a cut off for a positive response of one affirmative response has been suggested.

Faced with the diagnosis of alcohol abuse, initial denial and rationalization are common. Support, education, and discussion of the physical, psychologic, and social costs of drinking on repeat visits will help a patient commit to treatment. Patient fears that they may lose their partner or custody of their children if they enter treatment and child care issues are important obstacles to treatment access for women. Brief physician interventions consisting of two counseling sessions have been found effective in individuals who are heavy drinkers but not alcohol dependent and appear more effective in women than in

men, resulting in a 31% reduction in alcohol consumption (87). Alcoholics Anonymous is the most widely used and effective self-help group for alcoholism, and all-women groups are available in many areas. Encouraging a patient to call and set up a meeting for the same day from the physician's office has been shown to increase compliance with treatment recommendations. In patients at risk for alcohol withdrawal, detoxification as an outpatient can be accomplished by prescribing a starting dose of 10 to 20 mg of diazepam a day and tapering the dose by 5 mg every 3 days. The number of pills prescribed at each visit should be limited to the number needed until the next office visit. The patient should be seen at least twice weekly and should agree to take 250 to 500 mg of disulfiram daily. Signs of withdrawal, including diaphoresis, tachycardia, hypertension, and tremor, should be monitored at each checkup and should be used to pace the taper of diazepam. Inpatient detoxification is indicated for patients who are medically unstable, those who fail outpatient treatment, and for suicidal patients.

Although alcohol abuse is less common in women than in men, the faster progression of physiologic, psychologic, and social effects of alcohol in women implies that its cost in terms of associated morbidity and mortality is considerably higher for the individual female patient. More research is needed to clarify the pathophysiology and psychopathology responsible for this telescoping effect. Additionally, improved screening of women for substance abuse and treatment outcome studies are urgently needed, given the narrower window for intervention before advanced disease progression than in men (78).

SEXUAL DISORDERS

Common sexual dysfunctions are often conceptualized as pertaining to three sexual response stages: disorders of desire, arousal, and orgasm. DSM-IV lists sexual pain disorders as a fourth category of sexual dysfunction. Disorders of desire are further subdivided into hypoactive sexual desire and sexual aversion. Sexual pain disorders include vaginismus and dyspareunia. Clinically, women often present with more than one sexual dysfunction, and population prevalence estimates for all female sexual disorders combined approximate 50%.

The role of reproductive hormones and the female menstrual cycle in sexual function remains unclear. Most research suggests that endogenous variations in estrogen and progesterone do not significantly affect sexual desire in women of reproductive age. Evidence suggests, however, that desire decreases in surgically oophorectomized premenopausal women and can be restored by estradiol or testosterone administration (88). Studies of fluctuations in sexual arousal and orgasm with respect to menstrual cycle–related hormonal variations have been incon-

---

TABLE 31.3
The CAGE Questionnaire

- Have you ever felt you ought to **Cut down** on your drinking?
- Have people **Annoyed** you by criticizing your drinking?
- Have you ever felt bad or **Guilty** about your drinking?
- Have you ever had a drink first thing in the morning to steady your nerves or get rid of a hangover (**Eye-opener**)?

clusive (89). In contrast, oxytocin has been implicated in both arousal and orgasm, and levels of plasma oxytocin have been correlated with psychophysiologic measures of orgasm (90).

As with surgically oophorectomized women, evidence supports an increase in sexual problems in postmenopausal women (91). Diminished vaginal lubrication, atrophic vaginitis, and decreased pelvic vasocongestion are effectively reversed by estrogen replacement therapy. The addition of testosterone has been shown to help increase sexual desire, although no consistent evidence supports the effect of androgen supplementation on the vasocongestive responses in sexual arousal.

Cognitive and attentional factors and relationship difficulties are often more important in female sexual disorders than is organic dysfunction. The empiric treatment of female sexual disorders has focused primarily on orgasmic dysfunction, dyspareunia, and vaginismus using combinations of educational, cognitive-behavioral, and physical interventions (92). An overall paucity of well-designed outcome studies on the treatment of female sexual disorders remains, however.

Of particular relevance in the psychiatric patient is the effect of psychopharmacologic drugs on all three phases of sexual function. Antidepressant and antipsychotic medications are the two major drug classes associated with sexual side effects. Anorgasmia is particularly common with the widely used SSRIs. 5-HT2, 5-HT1A, and 5-HT3 receptors have all been implicated in female sexual function (93). Despite clinical reports of successful treatment for SSRI-associated anorgasmia with the addition of cyproheptadine or weekend "drug holidays," switching to another antidepressant class that is associated with a lower incidence of sexual side effects is generally the most effective maneuver. Buproprion, mirtazapine, and nefazodone are common choices. Besides the sexual side effects of psychopharmacologic drugs, chronic psychiatric illness itself may result in decreased sexual interest or responsiveness, as can physical illness associated with chronic pain, lowered self-esteem, body image problems, or fatigue (94). Some evidence suggests that a history of depression may be a determinant of hypoactive sexual desire disorder. In such cases, sexual dysfunction has its onset when the affective disorder is first manifested, yet fails to remit with resolution of the affective episode (95).

ANXIETY DISORDERS

Anxiety is a normal adaptive emotion experienced in response to threat. It acts as a signal to alter behavior and minimize physical and psychological vulnerability. Decrease in anxiety is achieved through either mastery or avoidance of the anxiety-provoking situation. Pathologic anxiety states are differentiated from normal anxiety by the degree and chronicity of the emotion, the stimulus that provokes it, or the behavioral response adapted.

Anxiety disorders are very common psychiatric disorders, with a 1 month prevalence of 10% in women (96). The mean age of onset for anxiety disorders is during adolescence or young adulthood. Many patients never seek help for these conditions, and of those who do, most present to nonpsychiatric physicians complaining of the somatic symptoms associated with anxiety. They often do not report their emotional symptoms due to embarrassment or fear of the stigma of a mental illness. In evaluating a woman with anxiety, certain common medical conditions should be excluded, including cardiac conditions, hyperthyroidism, and systemic lupus erythematosus. Drug intoxication and withdrawal, caffeine use, and over-the-counter medications such as diet pills and pseudoephedrine may exacerbate anxiety disorders. Medical evaluation should include a careful history and physical examination, routine laboratory tests, TSH, ECG, and urine toxicology screen. Neurologic conditions associated with anxiety include movement disorders, cerebral neoplasms, cerebrovascular disease, migraine, and epilepsy.

Anxiety disorders fall into five general groups: phobias, panic disorder, generalized anxiety disorder (GAD), obsessive-compulsive disorder (OCD), and post-traumatic stress disorder (PTSD). With the exception of OCD, which has the same incidence in men as in women, anxiety disorders are much more common in women. Women are three times as likely to have specific phobia or agoraphobia, 1.5 times as likely to develop panic with agoraphobia, twice as likely to suffer from GAD, and have twice the risk for PTSD. The reason for this preponderance of anxiety disorders in the female population is unknown (97). Both hormonal and sociologic learning theories have been proposed to explain the discrepancy.

Sociologic theories focus on conventional female sex role stereotypes that reinforce helplessness, dependence, the avoidance of assertive behavior, and the lack of mastery experiences necessary to overcome anxiety. New mothers often develop worries about their competence or their child's safety, and unwanted pregnancies or infertility can exacerbate anxiety disorders. The increasing expectations and conflict over female roles as wife, mother, homemaker, and career woman may also contribute to the elevated incidence of anxiety disorders in women.

Hormonal fluctuations have been implicated in anxiety disorders premenstrually, during pregnancy, and postpartum. OCD and GAD symptoms have been reported to worsen premenstrually; menopause, oral contraceptives, and HRT have all been associated with the onset of or changes in panic disorder and OCD. Pregnancy and the postpartum period are associated with exacerbation of preexisting panic disorder and OCD in 30% or more cases (5).

Progesterone metabolites have been postulated to act as partial GABA agonists and possible modulators of serotonergic neurotransmission linked to dysphoric and anxiolytic mood states. In contrast, estrogen has neuroprotective effects and appears to enhance serotonergic neurotransmission. Estrogen also enhances norepinephrine and dopamine activity by interfering with monoamine oxidase and tyrosine hydroxylase activity (5).

Comorbidity with other psychiatric diagnoses in the anxiety disorders is high. The most common are affective disorders, substance abuse, other anxiety disorders, and personality disorders. In panic disorder, for example, comorbidity with depression is higher than 50% and comorbidity with alcohol abuse is 20 to 40%. In the case of social phobia, comorbidity with panic disorder is as high as 50% in some studies.

The general management principles for anxiety disorders include evidence that combined pharmacotherapy and cognitive-behavioral techniques tend to be more effective than either alone. Animal studies and pharmacologic treatment response have implicated three major neurotransmitter systems: the noradrenergic, serotonergic, and GABAergic systems. Effective classes of drugs include the antidepressants, benzodiazepines, and beta-blockers.

All medications should be initiated at low doses and titrated upward every 2 to 3 days, or more slowly when poorly tolerated, to minimize side effects. Patients with anxiety disorders are often very sensitive to side effects, so gradual increases in dosage will maximize compliance by minimizing side effects. Patients should be educated about the 8- to 12-week onset of action for most antidepressants, warned about common side effects, encouraged to continue taking the medication long enough to complete a therapeutic trial, and told that some of the initial side effects are likely to abate. The choice of antidepressant drug should rely on side effect profile and patient symptoms. For example, a patient with insomnia may benefit from a more sedating antidepressant such as imipramine. When effective, treatment should be continued for 6 months to a year before attempting a medication taper.

Benzodiazepines may be a useful adjunct and provide rapid symptomatic relief early in the course of treatment, before the onset of action of the antidepressant. Long-term benzodiazepine use should be avoided because of abuse potential, risk of dependence, interdose withdrawal symptoms, and development of tolerance. When benzodiazepines are prescribed, the physician should educate the patient about these risks and the importance of viewing these drugs as temporary symptomatic treatment. Clonazepam 0.5 mg bid or lorazepam 0.5 mg qid for a limited period of 4 to 6 weeks may improve initial compliance with antidepressant treatment. If prescribed for longer than 4 to 6 weeks, the discontinuation of benzodiazepine treatment should be achieved with a gradual dose taper to minimize the anxiety associated with possible withdrawal symptoms.

Anxiolytic medications should be administered with caution in the pregnant woman. Tricyclic antidepressant drugs are the antianxiety agents with the safest and longest established record in the pregnant patient and fetus. There are few reports of the effect of benzodiazepines during the third trimester; however, several case reports have associated their use with neonatal withdrawal symptoms, transient agitation, hypotonia, respiratory distress, and low Apgar scores. Of the benzodiazepines, clonazepam is thought to have the least teratogenic potential and may be used with caution during pregnancy for severe anxiety. Management with nonpharmacologic techniques should always be the initial course of action in breast-feeding and pregnant women (98). When the use of benzodiazepines cannot be avoided postpartum, daily dosing with a shorter acting compound coupled with bottlefeeding timed to match high plasma levels is preferable. Diazepam, with its long half-life, accumulates in breast milk and should be avoided. See also Chapter 4.

Cognitive and behavioral techniques are the primary psychotherapeutic interventions used in the treatment of anxiety disorders. Cognitive therapy relies on education regarding symptoms and challenging false beliefs that contribute to avoidant behaviors. Relaxation techniques and respiratory training are also effective, as are systematic desensitization exercises in which patients work through a hierarchy of progressively more anxiety-provoking tasks. Referral to a psychologist or behavioral medicine clinic is often indicated.

Phobic Disorders

Three types of phobic disorders exist: specific phobias, social phobia, and agoraphobia. In all three, exposure to the feared situation provokes anxiety and may result in a panic attack.

Specific phobias are irrational circumscribed fears of specific situations or objects, resulting in their avoidance. Examples are fear of heights, fear of flying, and fear of spiders. Age of onset is generally before age 25, and in women, animal phobias occur earliest (97). Affected women rarely seek treatment because most phobias do not cause significant functional impairment and the stimulus (for example, snakes) is easily avoided. In some cases, however, a phobia such as fear of flying may impair a woman's career, in which case treatment is indicated. Simple phobias are relatively easy to manage using cognitive-behavioral techniques and systematic desensitization. Additionally, a single dose of 0.5 to 1 mg of lorazepam before an airplane trip may help in decreasing fear of flying.

Social phobia is the most common anxiety disorder and consists of a fear of situations in which the individual is open to scrutiny by others (99). This may take the form of incapacitating performance anxiety before a presentation or more generalized anxiety in social gatherings. It causes greater morbidity than simple phobias because the avoidance of anxiety-provoking situations rapidly limits work performance and social function. Although social phobia is more common in women, men predominate in clinical samples, perhaps because women with social phobia can more easily avoid anxiety-provoking situations by not working outside the home and because gender roles and social expectations for men include greater assertiveness. Movement disorders and epilepsy may contribute to social phobia, and in one study of Parkinson's disease patients, the prevalence of social phobia was 17%. The pharmacologic treatment of social phobia relies on the use of beta-blockers: propranolol 20 to 40 mg 1 hour before an anticipated performance, or atenolol 50 to 100 mg daily. These drugs block the autonomic arousal associated with anxiety. Antidepressant drugs, including tricyclics, SSRIs, or MAOIs in doses used to treat depression, can also be helpful. The preferred management is a combination of pharmacotherapy and psychotherapeutic techniques. These may include the short-term use of benzodiazepines or low-dose clonazepam or lorazepam in conjunction with cognitive-behavioral therapy and systematic desensitization exercises.

Agoraphobia is the fear and avoidance of crowded spaces from which escape may be difficult or embarrassing. It is often associated with panic disorder. In extreme cases, women with agoraphobia are unable to leave the home alone without experiencing tremendous anxiety and panic. They often rely on a spouse to accompany them everywhere. As with social phobia, agoraphobia is more common in women, but men are more likely to seek treatment, perhaps because their symptoms are less socially acceptable to themselves and to their families. The management of agoraphobia is primarily by systematic desensitization and cognitive-behavioral techniques. Because of the high comorbidity with panic disorder and major depression, antidepressant treatment is also effective.

Panic Disorder

A panic attack is the sudden onset of a period of intense fear and discomfort lasting several minutes, dissipating gradually, and associated with at least four of the following symptoms: palpitations, chest discomfort, diaphoresis, chills or hot flashes, shortness of breath or choking, trembling, paresthesias, dizziness or lightheadedness, nausea or abdominal distress, fear of death, or impending loss of control or "going crazy." Panic attacks can occur in all anxiety disorders. In panic disorder, they are unexpected, at least initially, and become associated with persistent anticipatory anxiety of future attacks, thus

leading to changes in behavior aimed at minimizing recurrent attacks. DSM-IV distinguishes panic disorder as occurring with or without agoraphobia, and 50% of cases develop agoraphobia over time. Agoraphobia is more common in women with panic disorder than in men. Panic attacks are also common in many intoxication states and in medical conditions such as emphysema. Women with panic disorder are at elevated risk for alcohol dependence, possibly as a complication of attempts to self-medicate their anxiety with alcohol (5).

Although the course of untreated panic disorder tends to be chronic, treatment is effective and most patients show dramatic improvement with a combination of cognitive-behavioral therapy and medication. Antidepressant drugs, specifically tricyclic antidepressants, SSRIs, and MAOIs at dosages similar to those used in the treatment of depression, are the initial drugs of choice (see Table 31.2). Imipramine or nortriptyline should be started at low doses of 10 to 25 mg per day and titrated upward by 25 mg every 3 days as tolerated to minimize side effects and maximize compliance. In the case of nortriptyline, therapeutic levels should be checked, with a goal of a blood level between 50 and 150 ng/mL. Imipramine should be titrated upward to doses of 100 to 300 mg qd. Fluoxetine, fluvoxamine, paroxetine, tranylcypromine, or phenelzine are other appropriate choices.

Generalized Anxiety Disorder

DSM-IV defines GAD as persistent, excessive, and poorly controlled worry about everyday activities such as work or school, which impairs function and is not limited to anxiety better characterized by one of the other anxiety disorders (for example, fear of having a panic attack in panic disorder). The anxiety is associated with three or more of the following six symptoms: restlessness, fatigue, poor concentration, irritability, muscle tension, and sleep disturbance. Risk is low in adolescents and young adults but increases with age. GAD often runs a chronic course and is characterized by the increased utilization of medical and mental health services and psychotropic medication. Comorbidity between GAD and other psychiatric disorders is very high, especially with panic disorder or major depression (100).

Management should be multimodal and should include psychotherapy and medication. Buspirone is a first-line agent for the treatment of GAD. The initial dose is 5 mg tid, titrated gradually over a few weeks to 10 to 15 mg tid. Alternatives are imipramine or an SSRI such as sertraline (see Table 31.2). Short-term treatment with a long-acting benzodiazepine, such as clonazepam, may help relieve symptoms during the 4- to 8-week period needed before the onset of action of buspirone or an antidepressant medication. Psychotherapeutic techniques used in the treatment of GAD include cognitive-behavioral therapy, supportive therapy, and insight-oriented approaches. Insight-oriented therapy is aimed at increasing the patient's tolerance for anxiety. Cognitive-behavioral techniques include relaxation, biofeedback, and identifying irrational beliefs. Supportive psychotherapy relies on education regarding symptoms and a chance for the patient to discuss her anxiety with an empathic physician, which often results in a marked lessening of the anxiety.

Obsessive-Compulsive Disorder

An obsession is an anxiety-provoking, recurrent, intrusive thought, impulse, or image. Examples are fears of contamination or of committing a shameful or aggressive act. An obsession is distinguished from a preoccupation or rumination in that the individual perceives it as excessive or irrational and tries to resist it.

Compulsions are repetitive behaviors such as handwashing, ordering, counting, or checking. They can also be mental acts such as counting, repeating words silently, or praying. The patient feels driven to perform these rituals to temporarily decrease the anxiety produced by an obsession or according to some idiosyncratic rule that must be rigidly followed to avert danger. In clinical cases, obsessions and compulsions interfere with function by taking up much of an affected individual's time.

Although the lifetime prevalence of OCD is nearly equal in men and women, OCD in women tends to have a later age of onset, between ages 26 and 35. The incidence of OCD markedly increases in females with puberty, surpassing that in males, although OCD is much more common in prepubescent boys than in girls. This flip in the gender ratio suggests a role for hormonal factors in the development of the disorder, as does the premenstrual worsening of symptoms reported by 41% of a clinical sample of subjects with OCD. A history of an eating disorder, depression, panic attacks, or obsessive cleaning behavior is associated with the development of OCD in women (5). Women often develop OCD symptoms in the setting of an episode of major depression, although symptoms usually persist beyond the resolution of the depressive episode. Some evidence suggests that OCD occurring with depression has a better prognosis. Obsessions about food and weight and washing and cleaning compulsions tend to be more common in women, whereas checking rituals tend to be more common in men. These differences probably reflect cultural forces associated with gender roles. One study found a 12% rate of past anorexia nervosa in women who develop OCD (101). Neurologic conditions associated with OCD include Tourette's syndrome, temporal lobe epilepsy, and postencephalitic conditions. Comorbidity is especially high in Tourette's syndrome, with 60% of patients meeting criteria for OCD. Patients with

Tourette's and OCD are also more likely to be female than male.

The management of OCD is effective and should rely on a combination of cognitive-behavioral therapy and pharmacologic treatment. Serotonergic antidepressant drugs are the first-line pharmacologic agents and include clomipramine, fluoxetine, sertraline, and fluvoxamine. Effective dosages are often higher than those used in the treatment of depression; for example, fluoxetine at 80 to 100 mg daily. All agents should be initiated at minimum doses and gradually titrated upward every 7 to 10 days to clinical response. An 8- to 16-week trial is often needed to assess maximal therapeutic benefit. Useful behavioral therapy techniques include exposure and response prevention, desensitization, thought stopping, and flooding techniques. These are often as effective as and longer lasting than pharmacologic responses to treatment. The natural course of OCD is associated with at least partial symptom remission over time in about 50% of patients (5).

Post-Traumatic Stress Disorder

PTSD remains a relatively ill-defined disorder, that sometimes follows exposure to an event of a magnitude that would be traumatic to any individual. Examples of such events include combat, rape, assault, life-threatening accidents, or sudden bereavement. Diagnosis requires reexperiencing of the event through dreams or thoughts, accompanied by avoidance of reminders of the trauma, emotional numbing, and persistent sympathetic hyperarousal. Of individuals exposed to trauma, 1 in 4 develop this symptom cluster, and rape is associated with twice the risk of PTSD in women as are nonsexual crimes (101). Personality traits, life stressors, genetic or familial vulnerability to psychiatric illness, and perceptions of helplessness over the control of one's environment may explain why some people develop PTSD and others do not after exposure to identical traumatic events. One study found that women are more susceptible than are men to developing chronic symptoms of PTSD extending over a year (102). A biologic mechanism may help explain the preponderance of PTSD in women and its differential course.

Biologic theories of PTSD include limbic system dysfunction and a dysregulation of the catecholamine and endogenous opiate systems. Recent neuroimaging studies confirm structural, functional, and neurophysiologic brain abnormalities in individuals with PTSD, principally in the amygdala and hippocampus. Persistent alterations have been observed in physiologic reactivity and cortisol release, suggesting the involvement of neural circuits relevant to fear conditioning, extinction, and sensitization (103). Symptoms in women have been reported to worsen in the luteal phase of the menstrual cycle (104). Given the known variations in levels of endogenous opiates across the menstrual cycle, a link between endogenous opiate levels and PTSD symptoms has been postulated, and monthly estrogen fluctuations could play a role in the increasing neurotoxic processes precipitated by elevated stress hormone levels (14).

As many as 80% of individuals with PTSD also meet criteria for another psychiatric disorder. The most common comorbid conditions are depression, anxiety disorders, and substance abuse. Somatization symptoms are also common. Treatment for PTSD should include medication and psychotherapy. Few published placebo-controlled randomized trials have been undertaken, and most focus on men with combat-related PTSD. Imipramine or an SSRI are initial drugs of choice. Fluoxetine and sertraline have both been shown to be superior to placebo in randomized controlled trials, but medication is rarely a panacea and psychotherapy may be more effective. Psychotherapeutic interventions include stress management, cognitive-behavioral interventions, supportive therapy, education about the disorder, and graded exposure to those avoided stimuli that remind the patient of the trauma, with a goal of mastery.

In summary, anxiety disorders are more common in women than in men. Affected women often do not present for treatment because of feelings of embarrassment or fears associated with the stigma of mental illness. Differences in social role expectations that make anxiety disorders more understandable in women may also contribute to lower rates of seeking care. When women do present for treatment, they often report only the associated somatic symptoms, thus leading to elaborate, unproductive medical evaluations and inadequate psychiatric care. Although treatable, undiagnosed anxiety disorders often run a chronic course and may seriously impair function. The discrepancies observed in the prevalence and course of anxiety disorders across gender are largely unexplained. Future research aimed at elucidating these differences should focus on vulnerability factors, sociocultural factors, and biochemical differences, including menstrual cycle–linked fluctuations in symptoms.

SOMATOFORM DISORDERS AND FACTITIOUS DISORDERS

Somatization as a psychiatric phenomenon is the expression and experience of psychologic distress as somatic symptoms. It is common in many psychiatric conditions, including anxiety disorders and depressive disorders, and is of particular relevance to somatoform disorders, factitious disorders, and malingering. These psychiatric diagnoses have in common complaints of unexplained symptoms that are inconsistent with, or not wholly explained by, medical or neurologic disease. The motivation of indi-

viduals with such disease-simulating or abnormal illness behavior is to attain the *sick role* (105). This intention may vary from being entirely unconscious, as in conversion disorder, to being entirely conscious, as in malingering. The attainment of the sick role leads to secondary gain or reinforcement of the abnormal illness behavior in the form of increased attention from family and medical professionals and decreased social responsibilities and obligations.

Although epidemiologic evidence is inconclusive, most sources find higher community rates of somatic complaints and disability in women than in men (106). Biologic differences in the experience or tolerance of physical discomfort between the sexes may be one contributing factor. Women appear to have a lower threshold and tolerance for pain in experimental studies and nociception appears to vary over the course of the menstrual cycle, being most heightened during the luteal phase. The modulation of both gamma amino butyric acid and opioid neurotransmission by estrogen has been implicated in these phenomena (107). Cultural and social norms often shape somatized symptoms and may also play a role in the gender differences observed in the epidemiology and psychopathology of these conditions. Men are socialized to tolerate discomfort and suppress expressions of weakness and distress. Women are often more willing to seek help and admit to physical discomfort. As the most frequently designated "family health monitor," women tend to be attuned to the physical symptoms of both themselves and family members. Although hysteria is now recognized not to be an exclusively female affliction, abnormal illness behavior and adoption of the sick role has traditionally remained more socially acceptable for women (106). Finally, women are more likely than men to be victims of physical and sexual abuse, both of which can lead to an increased risk of both acute and chronic pain complaints (107). As such, questions regarding a history of physical or sexual abuse are appropriate when evaluating patients with somatic complaints that appear disproportionate with respect to medical signs of pathology.

Factitious Disorder and Malingering

Factitious disorders involve the deliberate and conscious production of signs of physical or mental disorders in order to assume the sick role. An illustrative example is the self-administration of insulin to induce a hypoglycemic coma resulting in hospital admission. By contrast, malingerers do not achieve gratification from the patient role per se and volitionally feign or induce signs and symptoms of illness to achieve some other practical goal. They may seek hospitalization to evade criminal arrest or in the hope of qualifying for disability income.

Somatoform Disorders

Four common somatoform disorders exist: somatization disorder, conversion disorder, hypochondriasis, and pain disorder. All these disorders present with physical symptoms that are inadequately explained by medical disease. Symptoms often fall into the neurologic realm and are not under conscious voluntary control, unlike in factitious disorder or malingering. By definition, symptoms must be severe enough to impair the individual's emotional, social, occupational, or physical function and to be associated with excessive medical help–seeking behavior. Because these patients present with a disease interpretation of their symptoms, one of the primary management challenges is to provide them with the psychiatric diagnosis in a form that will not be perceived as critical, condescending, or stigmatizing (108). Delivering the diagnosis involves building an alliance with the patient, psychoeducation, and reformulation of the patient's symptoms. Once the physician has established a diagnosis of somatoform disorder, the initial goal is to acquire the patient's trust and to validate her symptoms and suffering. The physician should convey to the patient that she is not being accused of volitionally inducing her symptoms. The next step is to elucidate the links between symptom exacerbations and life stressors, depression, or anxiety states. The goal is to explain that life stressors or comorbid psychiatric illness can exacerbate physical symptoms. Avoiding authoritative assertions of symptom cause is recommended, and suggesting a link (e.g., "one thought I have is that perhaps…") is often better accepted by the patient. An illustrative example, such as the effect of stress on ulcer healing, often helps patients start to address their symptoms in relationship to their current psychosocial environment. The importance of treating any comorbid depression or anxiety is stressed, together with the suggestion, when indicated, that the patient be evaluated by a psychiatrist to obtain a comprehensive assessment of the problem. Such an approach minimizes the risk of a patient leaving treatment because she feels misunderstood or labeled as "crazy" or "faking" her symptoms.

Somatization Disorder

Somatization disorder characteristically involves a multiplicity of somatic symptoms that affect several organ systems and has a chronic course beginning before age 30. DSM-IV diagnostic criteria require a history of at least four pain symptoms, two gastrointestinal symptoms, one sexual symptom, and one pseudoneurologic symptom, none of which are wholly explained by physical or laboratory examination. Patients are often vague and inconsistent historians. Affected women outnumber men by approximately 5:1. Lifetime prevalence in women is over 1%, and the disorder is inversely related to educational level and social class. Comorbidity with other psychiatric conditions, especially affective disorders and anxiety disorders, approximates 50% and is of particular importance with respect to management considerations (109). The etiology of somatization disorder is probably multifactorial and may include the use of somatic symptoms as a means of communicating mental distress, learned behavior following genuine physical illness, or imitative behavior in children copying an ill parent.

Treatment should start with a thorough history and medical evaluation to assess the extent of organic disease and any comorbid psychiatric conditions. Patients with somatization disorder often seek help from multiple care providers. Identifying a primary provider to coordinate care can be crucial for successful treatment. Frequent, short, regularly scheduled visits at monthly intervals often help reassure the patient that she is being heard and minimize overuse of health services. Psychotherapy, both individual or group, is often effective in helping a patient reformulate her illness.

Conversion Disorder

Conversion disorder is characterized by one or more neurologic symptoms that cannot be explained by a known medical or neurologic disorder, are not intentionally produced, and are believed to be initiated or exacerbated by psychologic distress or conflict. Symptoms may be sensory (as in conversion blindness or stocking–glove anesthesia), may be motor (as in astasia–abasia gait or paralysis and paresis), or may mimic complex neurologic disorders (as in pseudoseizures). Histrionic personality traits and inappropriate lack of concern over symptoms "la belle indifference" have been incorrectly labeled typical of conversion patients. Most patients do not have these characteristics.

As with somatization disorder, conversion disorder is up to five times as prevalent in women as in men, and the gender difference is even higher in childhood. Onset is most common in children and young adults, and prevalence is higher in rural areas, among the less educated, and in lower socioeconomic classes (109). High rates of neurologic and psychiatric comorbidity are associated with conversion disorders. Comorbidity with depression, anxiety disorders, and schizophrenia is elevated, but conversion symptoms can be seen in any psychiatric conditions and are also common in somatization disorder.

Frequently associated neurologic conditions include seizure disorders, movement disorders, and multiple sclerosis (110). These may occur with or be mistaken for conversion disorder. In the case of pseudoseizures, 25% of patients have coexisting epilepsy, but the nonepileptic seizures usually differ in presentation and symptomatology from the patient's epileptic seizures (111) (see also Chapter 32). It is difficult to definitively exclude an organic cause for symptoms, and 25% of patients initially diagnosed with conversion disorder eventually receive a neurologic or medical diagnosis (112). The resolution of symptoms with suggestion, hypnosis, or amytal interview increases the likelihood that symptoms constitute a pure conversion phenomenon.

The course of conversion disorder is usually brief and most cases resolve spontaneously over days or weeks. A single counseling session, including a sensitive presentation of the diagnosis and suggestion that the symptoms can be expected to gradually resolve, is often sufficient treatment (113). Supportive psychotherapy, education about the influence of stress on bodily function, coping and relaxation skills, and family counseling are also helpful. Family interventions should focus on explaining the patient's symptoms as a maladaptive mode of communication, encouraging more open communication of needs within the family, and avoiding attentional reinforcement of the conversion symptoms. In patients with comorbid personality disorders, long-term therapy is often needed (114). Occasionally, when diagnosis is followed by symptom resolution, the patient may later develop further conversion symptoms.

Hypochondriasis

Hypochondriasis is the result of a misinterpretation of normal bodily sensations as being caused by serious disease pathology. This fear persists even in the face of medical evaluation and reassurance that the patient is healthy. Typically, patients do not present with the plethora of symptoms seen in somatization disorder. They seek care because of a fear of having a specific disease rather than for the alleviation of symptoms. Unlike somatization disorder, conversion disorder, or pain disorder, hypochondriasis is not more common in women, and gender distribution is equal in men and women. Comorbidity with depression and anxiety disorders is estimated at 80% (109). The course is generally episodic and, when hypochondriasis occurs with other psychiatric conditions, it tends to manifest during exacerbations of the depression or anxiety disorder. Follow-up studies indicate recovery rates of up to 50% (115). Patients are often resistant to treatment, however, and may "doctor shop," believing that the "right physician" can correctly diagnose them. Frequent, scheduled visits may help reassure the patient that she is being taken seriously. Diagnostic tests should be administered only when they are clearly indicated. When comorbid depression or anxiety is present, treatment is essential. Psychotherapeutic techniques that are useful in treating hypochondriasis include group therapy, cognitive-behavioral therapy, and educational strategies.

Pain Disorders

Pain disorder is characterized by pain at one or more sites that cannot be fully accounted for by a medical or neurologic condition. Neurologic conditions commonly associated with pain disorder include low back pain and headaches. Pain disorder is twice as frequent in women as in men, and peak onset is in the forties and fifties. A familial pattern is common, suggesting either genetic predisposition or learned behavior. Secondary gain from the sick role can be a reinforcing factor. The disorder tends to be chronic; patients have long medical histories, seek medical and surgical services, and visit multiple providers. Pain disorder may be complicated by substance abuse or prescription drug abuse in attempts to self-medicate. Comorbid major depression is present in 25 to 50% of pain disorder patients (109). Management includes a combination of psychopharmacology and psychotherapeutic techniques. Tricyclic antidepressant drugs often help to control pain and may be effective at doses lower than those needed to treat depression. Patients should be started on 25 mg of amitriptyline or nortriptyline and increased gradually over several weeks to therapeutic doses for depression (see Table 31.2) or until symptomatic improvement is observed. Additionally, biofeedback, relaxation techniques, transcutaneous nerve stimulation, and nerve blocks may be helpful. Cognitive-behavioral techniques and group therapy with other pain patients are also effective. When a patient does not respond to these measures, or is dependent on high doses of narcotic drugs without pain relief, admission to a psychiatric specialty pain unit that employs a multidisciplinary approach can be extremely helpful in tapering the patient off narcotics, completing an antidepressant drug trial, and assessing the patient in a controlled environment.

Most somatoform disorders are much more common in women. The reasons for this gender discrepancy are unclear. Further research is needed to clarify differences in predisposing factors, psychopathology, and treatment response between genders for all of these disorders.

SCHIZOPHRENIA

Schizophrenia is a clinical syndrome of markedly abnormal mental experiences, including hallucinations, delusions, and disorganized thoughts and behavior. DSM-IV diagnostic criteria require at least two of the following: delusions, hallucinations, disorganized speech, disorganized or catatonic behavior, or negative symptoms including affective flattening or avolition. Bizarre delusions or auditory hallucinations of a voice that provides a running commentary on the patient's actions are sufficient to meet the criteria. Symptoms usually persist for at least 6 months. Impairment in work, interpersonal relationships, or self-care is also a necessary criterion for diagnosis. The diagnosis of schizophrenia requires that mood symptoms or cognitive impairment are not prominent features of the clinical presentation. Women and men have different symptom patterns: Women experience more affective symptoms, paranoia, and auditory hallucinations, whereas men have more of the "negative" symptoms such as flat affect, social withdrawal, and lack of motivation.

Women have a later age of onset and are more likely to marry and have children than are men with the illness (116). Adolescent boys are twice as likely to develop the illness as are girls, whereas women over the age of 50 are at high risk for late-onset schizophrenia, previously termed paraphrenia, which is seven times more common in women. Although the mechanisms for this pattern are not known, one theory proposes that female hormones such as estrogen may have a protective effect in premenopausal women. Animal studies have shown estrogen to be antidopaminergic (117), and symptoms of schizophrenia have been observed to worsen during the low estrogen premenstrual and follicular phases of the menstrual cycle in premenopausal female patients (13).

Although the prevalence of delusions and hallucinations is the same as in earlier-onset schizophrenia, late-onset schizophrenics have a distinctive clinical presentation with more complex hallucinations and delusions of a paranoid nature (118). Nonauditory hallucinations such as smelling gas are relatively common. Patients with late-onset schizophrenia also have less thought disorder and less flattening of affect (119). Women who are socially isolated and have hearing impairment are at particular risk for this disorder (120).

Schizophrenia does not have a known etiology and involves a complex relationship of genetic predisposition and environmental factors. Genetics has a central role in the disorder; numerous studies have demonstrated that first-degree relatives of schizophrenics have an increased prevalence of schizophrenia (121).

The management approach is the same for early- and late-onset schizophrenia: antipsychotic medications to treat positive symptoms (such as hallucinations and delusions) combined with individual, supportive, and psychosocial therapies. Antipsychotic medications are of two major classes: dopamine-receptor antagonists and "novel" antipsychotics with combined serotonin and dopamine receptor effects. The selection of a specific medication is based on its side effect profile. Low-potency antipsychotic medications such as chlorpromazine and thioridazine are more sedating and cause orthostatic hypotension. In contrast, high-potency neuroleptic medications such as haloperidol and fluphenazine are more likely to cause akathisia, acute dystonia, and parkinsonian symptoms of rigidity and tremor. Clozapine, risperidone, olanzapine, quetiapine, and ziprasidone, the newer antipsychotic medications, reportedly have a greater impact on negative symptoms (such as flat affect, lack of motivation, and decreased social interaction) than the classic antipsychotic drugs. With all antipsychotic medications, the lowest dose should be used to control the target symptoms. Tardive dyskinesia and neuroleptic malignant syndrome are the most serious side effects associated with antipsychotic medications. Long-term treatment with traditional antipsychotic medication, increasing age, and female gender are all risk factors for tardive dyskinesia.

Overall, women have better outcomes than do men when they are treated for schizophrenia. Women benefit more than men from both antipsychotic medication and psychosocial treatment (122). Issues of compliance and use of available services may also contribute to the positive results in women. In the Hillside Hospital First Episode Study, a higher percentage of women (87% versus 55% of men) had a complete remission of symptoms when they were treated with a standardized medication protocol (123). The later age of onset in women may contribute to a superior treatment outcome, as they have a longer symptom-free period.

DELIRIUM

The diagnosis of delirium should be considered in the differential diagnosis of any patient with psychiatric symptoms. The hallmark of the diagnosis is global cognitive impairment with a change in level of consciousness. This typically is of abrupt onset and relatively brief duration. Cognitive impairment usually involves disturbance in attention, sleep-wake cycle, and behavior, but it may include a wide variety of symptoms. Although the syndrome has an organic etiology, diagnosis is clinical and does not require that the etiology be known. The pathophysiology is multifactorial, with disturbances in acetylcholine modulation and impairment of function in the reticular formation hypothesized to be key elements.

Patients with comorbid medical or neurologic conditions are at a higher risk for delirium, as are those taking multiple medications. Pre-existing brain damage, sensory impairment, and age greater than 60 years are predisposing factors (124,125). Because any medical condition may cause delirium, a complete evaluation is critical. Clinically, a prodrome of restlessness, anxiety, and irritability usually is followed by a waxing and waning course with a varying level of consciousness. Disorientation for time is more common than for place. The syndrome may also include altered perception or hallucinations and delusions. Visual and auditory hallucinations are most common. The sleep-wake cycle often reverses, with worsening of confusion and disorientation in the evenings, referred to as "sundowning."

Patients with a history of psychiatric illness are often at increased risk for delirium, particularly if they have a history of substance abuse or are taking medications with anticholinergic side effects (126,127). Increased serum lithium levels also increase the risk of delirium characterized by lethargy, dysarthria, muscle fasciculations, and ataxia. Patients taking benzodiazepines are at risk for withdrawal delirium, as are patients with alcohol dependence. Alcohol withdrawal delirium can be complicated by Wernicke encephalopathy resulting from thiamine deficiency. The differentiation of symptoms arising from delirium rather than from a pre-existing psychiatric condition can be challenging but is critical. For example, swift diagnosis and treatment of Wernicke encephalopathy may prevent Korsakoff dementia. The differential diagnosis of delirium and dementia is important because patients with dementia are at increased risk for a superimposed delirium. Because these patients have impaired cognitive functioning at baseline, the diagnosis is based on monitoring their ability to attend to tasks and changes in their level of orientation (128). Additionally, collateral history from family and fluctuations in symptoms throughout the day are also important.

In addition to a careful history, physical examination, and mental status examination, information from an outside informant may be critical, particularly in establishing baseline functioning and whether a recent change has occurred. Serial examinations with a tool such as the Mini-Mental Status Examination (MMSE) (129) help document changes in cognitive functioning. The MMSE assesses orientation, memory, attention, recall, and language with a series of 30 questions. Laboratory studies may be necessary to establish the causes of delirium and should be tailored to the individual patient. Because delirium arises from numerous causes, including infection, metabolic abnormality, or brain infarction, the evaluation may include CSF studies, blood chemistry panel, or brain imaging. An electroencephalogram may be helpful in evaluation because most patients will have either generalized slowing or the low-voltage fast activity associated with withdrawal states. Nonconvulsive epileptic states can also be excluded by EEG.

The basic treatment principle for delirium is the identification and treatment of the underlying causes. General supportive care should include close monitoring of vital signs and behavior, frequent reassurance and reorientation, and appropriate sensory stimulation. Anticholinergic medications should be minimized, and the medication regimen should be simplified as much as possible. Neuroleptic medications or benzodiazepines should be used sparingly to treat psychotic symptoms or agitated behavior because they may contribute to the level of confusion. Benzodiazepines are important, however, in the treatment of alcohol and benzodiazepine withdrawal states.

The careful evaluation of delirious patients is a medical emergency because delirium carries a 20 to 30% mortality rate (128). The waxing and waning nature of the symptoms and the multitude of possible etiologies make diagnosis difficult. A patient with delirium may present with any psychiatric symptom. The patient's level of consciousness and cognitive examination are the critical elements in the diagnosis.

CONCLUSION

Psychiatric illnesses are common, underdiagnosed, and undertreated. Most cases present in nonpsychiatric settings, and all physicians should be attuned to the symptoms and signs of the common diagnostic syndromes. Simple first-line interventions and referral options for specialized treatment or consultation should be familiar to all clinicians. For two of the most common psychiatric disorders—depression and anxiety disorders—prevalence rates for women are at least twice as high as those for men. Medically and neurologically ill individuals have elevated rates of comorbid mental illness, which may worsen their prognosis and compliance with treatment. Patients who are frequent users of medical service are especially likely to present with somatic symptoms if they have a comorbid depressive illness. Given the availability of effective treatment, early diagnosis and psychiatric care should decrease medical morbidity and mortality as well as overall health care expenditure.

Gender-specific data are limited on the differential epidemiology, psychopathology, and management of psychiatric illness. Given the increasing body of evidence on gender differences in neurobiology, psychology, and social conditioning, research addressing treatment response and outcome in women is urgently needed. Psychotropic medications are prescribed with increasing frequency, and research addressing their use in women at different stages of the lifecycle—childhood, during pregnancy and breasfeeding, and among the rapidly increasing elderly population—are of particular salience.

References

1. Narrow WE, Rae DS, Robins LN, Regier DA. Revised Prevalence estimates of mental disorders in the United States. *Arch Gen Psychiatry* 2002;59:115–123.
2. Blumenthal SJ. Women's mental health: the new national focus. *Ann NY Acad Sci* 1996;789:1–16.
3. Rodin J, Ikovics J. Women's health: review and research agenda as we approach the 21st century. *Am Psychol* 1990;45:1018–1034.
4. Hamilton JA, Parry B. Sex-related differences in clinical drug response: Implications for women's health. *J Am Med Wom Assoc* 1983;38:126–132.
5. Pigott T. Gender differences in the epidemiology and treatment of anxiety disorders. *J Clin Psychiatry* 1999; 60:4–15.
6. Eisenberg L. Sounding board: treating depression and anxiety in primary care. *N Engl J Med* 1991;16:1080–1083.

7. Bridges KW, Goldberg DP. Somatic presentation of DSM-III psychiatric disorders in primary care. *J Psychosom Res* 1985;29:563–569.

8. Henk HJ, Katzelnick DJ, et al. Medical costs attributed to depression among patients with a history of high medical expenses in a health maintenance organization. *Arch Gen Psychiatry* 1996;53:899–904.

9. Okiishi CG, Paradiso S, Robinson RG. Gender differences in depression associated with neurologic illness: clinical correlates and pharmacologic response. *J Gend Specif Med* 2001;4:65–72.

10. Von Korff M, Ormel J, Katon W, Lin EHB. Disability and depression among high utilizers of health care. *Arch Gen Psychiatry* 1992;49:91–100.

11. Greenberg PE, Stiglin LE, Finkelstein SN, Berndt, ER. The economic burden of depression in 1990. *J Clin Psychiatry* 1993;54:405–418.

12. Rupp A. The economic burden of not treating depression. *Br J Psychiatry* 1995;166(suppl 27):29–33.

13. Hendrick V, Altshuler LL, Burt V. Course of psychiatric disorders across the menstrual cycle. *Harv Rev Psychiatry* 1996;4:200–207.

14. Seeman MV. Psychopathology in women and men: focus on female hormones. *Am J Psychiatry* 1997;154:1641–1647.

15. Robison J, Moen P, Dempster-McClain D. Women's caregiving: changing profiles and pathways. *J Gerontol Psychol Sci Soc Sci* 1995;50(6):S362–S373.

16. Zee RF, Trivedi MA. Effects of hormone replacement therapy on cognitive aging and dementia risk in postmenopausal women: a review of ongoing large-scale, long-term clinical trials. *Climacteric* 2002;5:122–134.

17. McHugh PR, Slavney PR. *The perspectives of psychiatry, 2nd ed.* Baltimore: Johns Hopkins University Press, 1986.

18. Frank, JD, Frank JB. *Persuasion and healing: a comparative study of psychotherapy, 3rd ed.* Baltimore: Johns Hopkins University Press, 1991.

19. Practice guideline for eating disorders. American Psychiatric Association. *Am J Psychiatry* 1993;150(2):212–228.

20. Szmukler GI, Tantam D. Anorexia nervosa: starvation dependence. *Br J Med Psychol* 1984;57:303–310.

21. McHugh, PR. Eating disorder and the behavioral perspective: grand rounds minutes. Baltimore: Johns Hopkins Department of Psychiatry, 1996.

22. American Psychiatric Association. *Diagnostic and statistical manual of mental disorders, 4th ed.* Washington, D.C.: American Psychiatric Association, 1994.

23. Holland AJ, Murray R, Russell GFM, Crisp AH. Anorexia nervosa: a study of 34 pairs of twins and one set of triplets. *Br J Psychiatry* 1984;145:414–419.

24. Treasure JL, Holland AJ. Genetic factors in eating disorders. In: Szmukler G, Dare C, Treasure J, (eds.) *Handbook of eating disorders: theory, treatment and research.* New York: Wiley, 1995;65–81.

25. Strober M, Lampert C, Morrell W, Burroughs J, Jacobs C. A controlled family study of anorexia nervosa: evidence of familial aggregation and lack of shared transmission with affective disorders. *Int J Eat Disord* 1990;9:239–253.

26. Theander S. Long term prognosis in anorexia nervosa: a preliminary report. Conference on Anorexia Nervosa, Toronto, Canada, Sept. 10–11, 1981.

27. Keys A, Brozek J, Henshel A, Mickelsen O, Taylor HL. *The biology of human starvation.* Minneapolis: University of Minnesota Press, 1950.

28. Mitchell J, Specker SM, de Zwaan M. Comorbidity and medical complications of bulimia nervosa. *J Clin Psychiatry* 1991;52(10):13–20.

29. Halmi KA, Eckert E, Marchi P, et al. Comorbidity of psychiatric diagnoses in anorexia nervosa. *Arch Gen Psychiatry* 1991;48:712–718.

30. Crisp AH, Callender JS, Halek C, Hsu LKG. Long term mortality in anorexia nervosa. *Br J Psychiatry* 1992;161:104–107.

31. Fluoxetine bulimia nervosa collaborative study group: Fluoxetine in the treatment of bulimia nervosa. A multicenter, placebo controlled, double blind trial. *Arch Gen Psychiatry* 1992;49:139–147.

32. Kaye WH, Nagata T, Weltzin, et al. Double-blind placebo-controlled administration of fluoxetine in restricting- and restricting-purging-type anorexia nervosa. *Biol Psychiatry* 2001;49(7):644–652.

33. Halmi KA. Eating disorder research in the past decade. *Ann N Y Acad Sci* 1996;789:67–77.

34. Fairburn CG, Norman PA, et al. A prospective study of outcome in bulimia nervosa and the long term effects of three psychological treatments. *Arch Gen Psychiatry* 1995;52:304–312.

35. Agras WA, Rossiter EM, et al. Pharmacologic and cognitive-behavioral treatment for bulimia nervosa: a controlled comparison. *Am J Psychiatry* 1990;149(1):82–87.

36. Weissman MM, Merikangas KR, Boyd JH. Epidemiology of affective disorders. In: Michels R, Cooper AM, Guze SB, et al., (eds.) *Psychiatry.* Vol. 1, Section 60. Philadelphia: Lippincott, 1991;1–14.

37. Weissman MM, Bland RC, Canino GJ, et al. Cross-national epidemiology of major depression and bipolar disorder. *JAMA* 1996;276:293–299.

38. Wilhelm K, Parker G. Sex differences in lifetime depression rates: fact or artefact? *Psychol Med* 1994;24:97–111.

39. Gallo JJ. Epidemiology of mental disorders in middle age and late life: conceptual issues. In: Anthony JC, Eaton WW, Henderson AS, (eds.) *Epidemiologic reviews.* Vol. 17, Number 1. Baltimore: Johns Hopkins University School of Hygiene and Public Health, 1995;83–94.

40. Angola A, Worthman CW. Puberty onset of gender differences in rates of depression: developmental, epidemiologic and neuroendocrine perspective. *J Affect Disord* 1993;29:145–158.

41. DSM-IV Research Criteria. American Psychiatric Association. *Diagnostic and statistical manual of mental disorders,* 4th ed. Washington: American Psychiatric Association, 1994;715–718.

42. Rubinow DR, Roy-Burne P. Premenstrual syndrome: overview from a methodological perspective. *Am J Psychiatry* 1984;141:163–172.

43. Yonkers KA, Halbreich U. Freeman EW, et al. Symptomatic improvement of premenstrual dysphoric disorder with sertraline treatment. *JAMA* 1997;278:983–988.

44. Steiner M, Steinberg S, Stewart D, et al. Fluoxetine in the treatment of premenstrual dysphoria. *N Engl J Med* 1995;332:1529–1534.

45. Dimmock PW, Wyatt KM, Jones PW, O'Brien PMS. Efficacy of selective serotonin-reuptake inhibitors in premenstrual syndrome: a systematic review. *Lancet* 2000;356:1131–1136.

46. Wikander I, Sundblad C, Andersch B, et al. Citalopram in premenstrual dysphoria: is intermittent treatment during luteal phases more effective than continuous medication throughout the menstrual cycle. *J Clin Psychopharmacol* 1998;18:390–398.

47. Sundblad C, Wikander I, Andersch B, Eriksson E. A naturalistic study of paroxetine in premenstrual syndrome: efficacy and side-effects during ten cycles of treatment. *Eur Neuropsychopharmacol* 1997;7:201–206.

48. Freeman EW, Rickels K, Sondheimer SJ, Polansky M. Differential response ro antidepressants in women with premenstrual syndrome/premenstrual dysphoric disorder. *Arch Gen Psychiatry* 1999;56:932–939.

49. Endicott J. The menstrual cycle and mood disorders. *J Affect Disord* 1993;29:193–200.

50. Gotlib IH, Whiffen VE, Mount JH, Milne K, Cordy Nl. Prevalence rates and demographic characteristics associated with depression in pregnancy and the postpartum. *J Consult Clin Psychol* 1989;57:269–274.

51. O'Hara MW. Social support, life events, and depression during pregnancy and the puerperium. *Arch Gen Psychiatry* 1986;43:569–573.

52. Kupfer DJ, Frank E, Perel JM, et al. Five-year outcome for maintenance therapies in recurrent depression. *Arch Gen Psychiatry* 1992;49:769–773.

53. Suppes T, Baldessarini RJ, Faedda GL, Tohen M. Risk of recurrence following discontinuation of lithium treatment in bipolar disorder. *Arch Gen Psychiatry* 1991;48:1082–1088.

54. Viguera AC, Nonacs R, Cohen LS, Tondo L, Murray A, Baldessarini RJ. Risk of Recurrence of bipolar disorder in pregnant and nonpregnant women after discontinuing lithium maintenance. *Am J Psychiatry* 2000;157:179–184.

55. Altshuler LL, Cohen L, Szuba MP, et al. Pharmacologic management of psychiatric illness during pregnancy: dilemmas and guidelines. *Am J Psychiatry* 1996;153:592–606.

56. Wisner KL, Gelenberg AJ, Leonard H, Zarin D, Frank E. Pharmacologic treatment of depression during pregnancy. *JAMA* 1999;282:1264–1269.

57. Kumar R, Robson KM. A prospective study of emotional disorders in childbearing women. *Br J Psychiatry* 1984;144:35–47.

58. Craig M, Abel K. Drugs in pregnancy. Prescribing for psychiatric disorders in pregnancy and lactation. *Best Pract Res Clin Obstet Gynaecol* 2001;15:1013–1030.

59. Schmidt PJ, Rubinow DR. Menopause-related affective disorders: a justification for further study. *Am J Psychiatry* 1991;148:844–852.

60. Writing group for the Women's Health Initiative Investigators. Risks and benefits of estrogen plus progestin in healthy postmenopausal women. Principal results from the Women's Health Initiative randomized controlled trial. *JAMA* 2002;288:321–333.

61. Anthony JC, Petronis KR. Suspected risk factors for depression among adults 18–44 years old. *Epidemiology* 1991;2:123–132.

62. Cadoret RJ. Evidence for genetic inheritance of primary affective disorder in adoptees. *Am J Psychiatry* 1978;135:463–466.

63. Merikangas KR, Kupfer DJ. Mood disorders: Genetic aspects. In: Kaplan HI, Sadock BJ, (eds.) *Comprehensive textbook of psychiatry, 6th ed.* Baltimore: Williams & Wilkins, 1995;1102–1116.

64. MacKinnon DF, Jamison KR, DePaulo JR. Genetics of manic depressive illness. *Ann Rev Neurosci* 1997;20:355–373.

65. Maas J. Biogenic amines and depression. *Arch Gen Psychiatry* 1975;32:1357–1361.

66. Maes M, Meltzer HY. The serotonin hypothesis of major depression. In: Bloom FE, Kupfer DJ, (eds.) *Psychopharmacology: the fourth generation of progress.* New York: Raven Press, 1994;933–944.

67. Schatzberg AF, Schildkraut JJ. Recent studies on neuroepinephrine systems in mood disorders. In: Bloom FE, Kupfer DJ, (eds.) *Psychopharmacology: the fourth generation of progress.* New York: Raven Press, 1994;911–920.

68. Cohen LS, Friedman JM, Jefferson JW, Johnson EM, Weiner ML. A reevaluation of risk of the in utero exposure to lithium. *JAMA* 1994;271:146–150.

69. Cohen LS, Heller VL, Rosenbaum JF. Treatment guidelines for psychotropic drug use in pregnancy. *Psychosomatics* 1989;30:25–33.

70. Renst CL, Goldberg JF. The reproductive safety profile of mood stabilizers, atypical antipsychotics, and broad-spectrum psychotropics. *J Clin Psychiatry* 2002;63(suppl 4):42–55.

71. Horwath E, Weissman MM. Epidemiology of depression and anxiety disorders. In: Tsuang MT, Tohen M, Zahner GE, (eds.) *Textbook in psychiatric epidemiology.* New York: Wiley, 1995;317–344.

72. Kessler RC, McGonagle KA, Swartz M, Blazer DG, Nelson CB. Sex and depression in the National Comorbidity survey. I: Lifetime prevalence, chronicity and recurrence. *J Affect Disord* 1993;29:85–96.

73. Cummings, JL. Depression and Parkinson's disease: a review. *Am J Psychiatry* 1992;149:443–454.

74. Sadovnick AD, Remick RA, Allen J, et al. Depression and multiple sclerosis. *Neurology* 1996;46:628–632.

75. Minden SL, Schiffer RB. Affective disorders in multiple sclerosis: review and recommendations for clinical research. *Arch Neurol* 1990;47:98–104.

76. Lipsey JR, Parikh RM. Depression and stroke. In: Robinson RG, Rabins PV, (eds.) *Depression and coexisting disease.* New York: Igaku-Shoin, 1989;186–201.

77. Moore R, Bone LR, Geller G, et al. Prevalence, detection and treatment of alcoholism in hospitalized patients. *JAMA* 1989;261:403–407.

78. Brienza RS, Stein MD. Alcohol use disorders in primary care: do gender-specific differences exist? *J Gen Intern Med* 2002;17(5):387–397.

79. Cyr MG, Moulton AW. The physician's role in prevention, detection, and treatment of alcohol abuse in women. *Psychiatr Ann* 1993;23:454–462.

80. Blume SB. Women and alcohol. A review. *JAMA* 1986;256:1467–1470.

81. Lex BW. Alcohol and other psychoactive substance dependence in women and in men. In: Seeman MV, (ed.) *Gender and psychopathology.* Washington: American Psychiatric Press, 1995;311–358.

82. Smith-Warner SA, Spiegelman D, Yaun S, et al. Alcohol and breast cancer in women: a pooled analysis of cohort studies. *JAMA* 1998;279:535.

83. Heizer JE, Pryzbeck TR. The co-occurrence of alcoholism and other psychiatric disorders in the general population and its impact on treatment. *J Stud Alcohol* 1988;49:219–224.

84. McLeod DR, Foster GV, Hoehn-Saric R, Svikis DS, Hipsley PA. Family history of alcoholism in women with generalized anxiety disorder who have premenstrual syndrome: patient reports of premenstrual alcohol consumption and symptoms of anxiety. *Alcohol Clin Exp Res* 1994;18:(3)664–670.

85. Blum LN, Nielsen NH, Riggs JA. Alcoholism and alcohol abuse among women: report of the Council on Scientific Affairs. American Medical Association. *J Womens Health* 1998;7(7):861-871.

86. Ewing JA. Detecting alcoholism: the CAGE questionnaire. *JAMA* 1984;252:1905–1907.

87. Fleming MF, Barry KL, Manwell LB, Johnson K, London R. Brief physician advice for problem drinkers: a randomized controlled trial in community-based primary care practices. *JAMA* 1997;277:1079.

88. Sherwin B, Gelfand M, Brender W. Androgen enhances sexual motivation in females: a prospective, crossover study of sex steroid administration in the surgical menopause. *Psychosom Med* 1985;47:339–351.

89. Schievi RC, Segraves RT. The biology of sexual function. *Psychiatr Clin North Am* 1985;18(1):7–23.

90. Carmichael MS, Warburton VL, Dixen J, et al. Relationships among cardiovascular, muscular and oxytocin responses during human sexual activity. *Arch Sex Behav* 1994;23:59.

91. Rosen RC, Taylor JF, Leiblum SR, Bachmann GA. Prevalence of sexual dysfunction in women: results of a survey of 329 women in an outpatient gynecological clinic. *J Sex Marital Ther* 1993;19(3):171–188.

92. Rosen RC, Leiblum SR. Treatment of sexual disorders in the 1990s: an integrated approach. *J Consult Clin Psychol* 1995;63:877–890.

93. Meston CM, Frolich PF. Update on female sexual function. *Curr Opin Urol* 2001;11:603-609.

94. Rosen RC, Leiblum SR. Hypoactive sexual desire. *Psychiatr Clin North Am* 1995;18(1):107–121.

95. Schreiner-Engel P, Schiavi RC. Lifetime psychopathology in individuals with low sexual desire. *J Nerv Ment Dis* 1986;174:646–651.

96. Regier DA, Boyd JH, Burke JD, et al. One month prevalence of mental disorders in the United States. *Arch Gen Psychiatry* 1988;45:977–986.

97. Yonkers KA, Gurguis G. Gender differences in the prevalence and expression of anxiety disorders. In: Seeman MV, (ed.) *Gender and psychopathology*. Washington: American Psychiatric Press, 1995;113–130.

98. Zerbe KJ. Anxiety disorders in women. *Bull Meninger Clin* 1995;59(suppl A):A38–A52.

99. Weinstock L. Gender differences in the presentation and management of social anxiety disorder. *J Clin Psychiatry* 1999;60:9–13.

100. Howell HB, Brawman-Mintzer O, Monnier J, Yonkers KA. Generalized anxiety disorder in women. *Psychiatr Clin North Am* 2001;24:165–178.

101. Foa EB. Trauma and women: course, predictors and treatment. *J Clin Psychiatry* 1997;58:25–28.

102. Breslau N, Davis G. Posttraumatic stress disorder in an urban population of young adults: risk factors for chronicity. *Am J Psychiatry* 1992;149:671–675.

103. Seedat S, Stein DJ. Trauma and post-traumatic stress disorder in women: a review. *International Clinical Psychopharmacology* 2000;15:S25–S33.

104. Hamilton JA. Clinical pharmacology panel report: In: Blumenthal SJ, Parry B, Sherwin B, (eds.) Forging a women's health research agenda (conference proceedings). Washington: National Women's Health Resource Center, 1991;1–27.

105. Slavney P. *Perspectives on hysteria*. Baltimore: Johns Hopkins University Press, 1990;137–160.

106. Wool AC, Barsky AJ. Do women somatize more than men? *Psychosomatics* 1994;35:445–452.

107. Barsky AJ, Peekna HM, Borus JF. Somatic symptom reporting in women and men. *J Gen Intern Med* 2001;16:266–275.

108. Goldberg D, Gask L, O'Dowd T. The treatment of somatization teaching techniques of reattribution. *J Psychosom Res* 1989;33:(6):689–695.

109. Kaplan HI, Sadock BJ. Kaplan and Sadock's synopsis of psychiatry: behavioral sciences. *Clinical Psychiatry*, 7th ed. Baltimore: Williams & Wilkins, 1994;617–631.

110. Boffeli TJ, Guze SB. The simulation of neurologic disease. *Psychiatric Clin North Am* 1992;15(2):301–310.

111. Devinsky O, Thacker K. Nonepileptic seizures. *Neurol Clin* 1995;13(2):298–319.

112. Watson CG, Buranen C. The frequency and identification of false positive conversion reactions. *J Nerv Ment Dis* 1979;167:243–247.

113. Lesser RP. Psychogenic seizures. *Neurology* 1996;46:1499–1507.

114. Blomhoff S, Malt UF. Psychiatric perspectives on psychogenic seizures and their treatment. In: Gram L, Johannessen SI, Osterman PO, Sillanpaa M, (eds.) *Pseudo-epileptic seizures*. Briston, Penn: Wrightson Biomed, 1993;99–108.

115. Kellner R. Diagnosis and treatment of hypochondriacal syndromes. *Psychosomatics* 1992;33(3):278–289.

116. Goldstein JM. The impact of gender on understanding the epidemiology of schizophrenia. In: Seeman MV, (ed.) *Gender and psychopathology*. Washington: American Psychiatric Press, 1995;159–199.

117. Lewine RRJ, Seeman MV. Gender, brain, and schizophrenia. Anatomy differences/differences of anatomy. In: Seeman MV, (ed.) *Gender and psychopathology*. Washington: American Psychiatric Press, 1995;131–157.

118. Pearlson GD, Kreger L, Rabins PV, et al. A chart review study of late-onset and early-onset schizophrenia. *Am J Psychiatry* 1989;146:1568–1574.

119. Rabins PV. Schizophrenia and psychotic states. In: Birren JE, Sloane RB, Cohen GD, (eds.) *Handbook of mental health and aging*. San Diego: Academic Press, 1992;463–475.

120. Almeida OP, Howard RJ, Levy R, David AS. Psychotic states arising in late life (late paraphrenia). The role of risk factors. *Br J Psychiatry* 1995;166:215–228.

121. Kendler KS, Diehl SR. The genetics of schizophrenia: a current genetic-epidemiologic perspective. *Schizophr Bull* 1993;19:261–284.

122. Seeman MV. Gender differences in treatment response in schizophrenia. In: Seeman MV, (ed.) *Gender and psychopathology*. Washington: American Psychiatric Press, 1995;227–51.

123. Syzmanski S, Lieberman JA, Alvir JM, et al. Gender differences in onset of illness, treatment response, course, and biologic indices in first-episode schizophrenic patients. *Am J Psychiatry* 1995;152:699–703.

124. Lishman WA. *Organic psychiatry, 2nd ed.* Oxford: Blackwell Scientific Publications, 1987.

125. Lipowski ZJ. *Delirium—acute brain failure in man, 2nd ed.* New York: Oxford University Press, 1990.

126. Tune LE, Bylsma FW. Benzodiazopine-induced and anticholinergic-delirium in the elderly. *Int Psychogeriatr* 1991;3:397–408.

127. Tune L, Carr S, Hoag E, Cooper T. Anticholinergic effects of drugs commonly prescribed for the elderly: potential means for assessing risk of delirium. *Am J Psychiatry* 1992;149:1393–1394.

128. Rabins PV, Folstein MF. Delirium and dementia. Diagnostic criteria and fatality rates. *Br J Psychiatry* 1992;140:1393–1394.

129. Folstein M, Folstein S, McHugh P. "Mini mental state": a practical method for grading the cognitive state of patients for the clinician. *Psychiatr Res* 1975;12:189–198.

32 Nonepileptic, Psychogenic, and Hysterical Seizures

Allan Krumholz, MD and Tricia Ting, MD

N onepileptic seizures, or what have also been termed psychogenic, pseudo-, or hysterical seizures, are a serious problem, particularly in women. Nonepileptic seizures occur in men but are approximately three times as frequent among women (1–3). Nonepileptic seizures pose major problems for physicians who care for patients with seizures. Such seizures account for approximately 20% of all intractable epilepsy referred to comprehensive epilepsy centers in the United States (1–3), and present with an annual incidence of about 4% that of true epileptic seizures (4).

Advances in video-EEG monitoring and a greater awareness of nonepileptic seizures have improved our ability to correctly diagnose patients with this disorder. Despite these advances and our better understanding of nonepileptic seizures, optimal management remains a problem.

HISTORY

Historically, what today are called nonepileptic or psychogenic seizures originated with the concept of *hysteria*. First described by the ancient Egyptians, hysteria was classically regarded as a disorder of women and related to a dysfunction of female organs, such as the uterus or womb. Hysteria was conceptualized as a disorder caused by a barren uterus wandering about the body in search of nourishment (5,6).

The specific symptoms were thought to depend on the portion of the body to which the uterus migrated. For example, if a wandering uterus were to come to rest in an extremity, it might cause paralysis, and if it pressed on the diaphragm, it could cause seizures (5,6).

The ancient Greeks adopted this Egyptian idea of hysteria; indeed the word *hysteria* derives from the Greek word for *uterus*. The Romans, strongly influenced by Greek medicine, modified this belief. They proposed that hysteria could affect both men and women, although it was more common in women. Moreover, based on human dissections that showed little variability in the position of the uterus, they related hysteria not to a wandering uterus but to the adverse effects of humors arising from the disturbed uterus or its related structures (5,6).

These original rational efforts to explain hysteria were replaced during the Dark or Middle Ages by mystical beliefs of a supernatural cause such as possession by demons. With the Renaissance, however, was a rediscovery of ancient Greek and Roman medicine and an attempt to again rationally or scientifically account for disorders like hysteria. Disorders of the reproductive system were again held responsible for hysteria, and women were principally implicated (5,6).

In the late 1800s, Jean Charcot, a founder of neurology, firmly established hysterical seizures as a clinical entity with his elegant and detailed descriptions of the patients that he observed at the Salpêtrière Hospital. He termed this disorder *hysteroepilepsy* or *epileptiform hysteria* (7). Charcot proposed that hysterical seizures were organic disorders of the brain, but still emphasized their relation to disturbance of the female reproductive system. He demonstrated that these hysterical seizures could be influenced by the manipulation of regions of the body that he termed *hysterogenic* zones (Figure 32.1), and specifically described how compression of the ovaries could abort these attacks in some women. In fact, he demonstrated a device that was used specifically for that purpose, an ovarian compressor belt (Figure 32.2). Charcot used such techniques as well as suggestion to both treat and provoke hysteria. Although he considered hysteria and hysterical seizures a disease that principally affected women, he also noted its occurrence in men, but his depictions of what he termed the *stages of hysteroepilepsy* are based on his observations in women (Figures 32.3 and 32.4) (6-8).

One of Charcot's most famous students was the neurologist Sigmund Freud. Freud observed Charcot's demonstrations (Figure 32.5), but drew different conclusions. He proposed that hysteria and hysterical seizures were not organic disorders of the brain, as Charcot assumed, but were rather emotional disorders of the unconscious mind caused by repressed energies or drives. Still, portions of the older concept of hysteria as a disorder of women persisted in Freud's theories. He proposed that hysteria was principally a disorder that affects women because it represented a conversion of repressed sexuality or sexual drive into an emotional disorder (5–6,9).

Today, we still consider hysteria within the broad framework of psychologic disorders known as *conversion disorders* or *reactions*, but we recognize that its causes are multifactorial and involve psychologic, environmental, and biologic influences (9–12). Recent evidence suggests that dissociation mechanisms may also be important in patients with conversion reactions (1). The exact reasons for this female preponderance are not entirely clear but may in part be sociologic or cultural. A more "feminine" psychological profile seems to promote conversion-related coping mechanisms (9–12).

DEFINITIONS

The term *epilepsy* should be restricted to well-defined disorders of the brain caused by electrical disturbances of normal brain function. The word *seizure* can be used in a more general sense. Consequently, disorders that are mistaken for epilepsy but are not due to abnormal electrical discharges in the brain are best termed *nonepileptic seizures*.

Historically, many other terms have been used to describe such events, including *hysterical seizures, hysteroepilepsy* (8), *pseudoseizures* (13), and *psychogenic seizure* (1,2). These disorders are not necessarily equivalent (1).

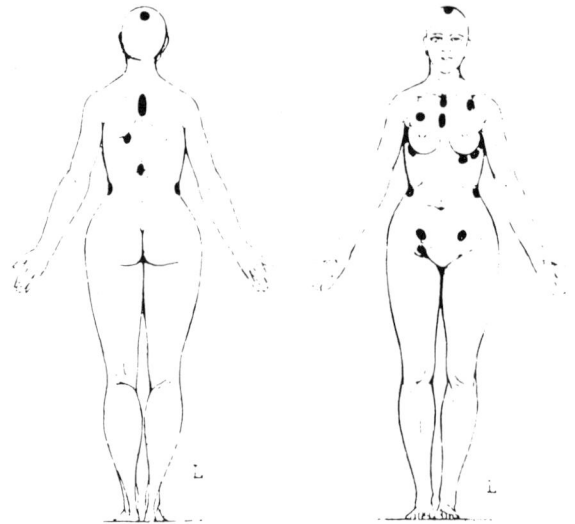

FIGURE 32.1

Charcot's map of a patient's hysterogenic zones, including the ovarian regions, but also other sensitive areas. (Reproduced with permission from: Iconographie Photographique de la Salpêtrière, 2:182,1878.)

Nonepileptic Seizures

Nonepileptic seizure describes all conditions, both physiologic and psychologic, that are mistaken for epilepsy (Table 32.1). Indeed, the clinical manifestations of epilepsy are so varied that many disorders can be mis-

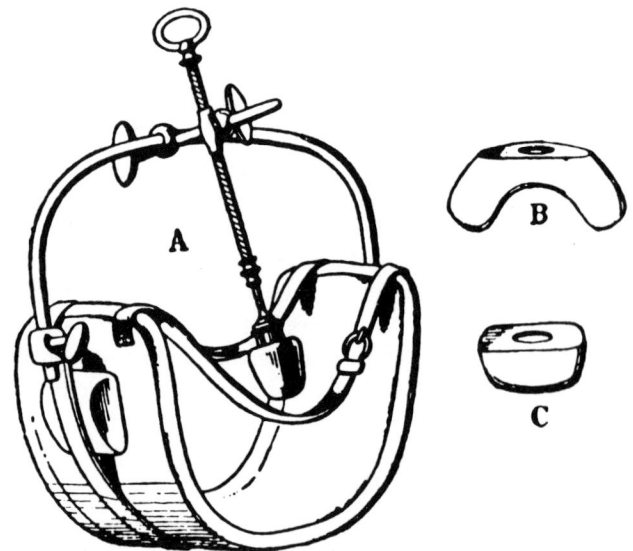

FIGURE 32.2

An ovarian compressor belt described by Charcot to prevent hysterical attacks in some patients with "ovarian" forms of hysteria. (Reproduced with permission from: Iconographie Photographique de la Salpetriere, 2:165,1878.)

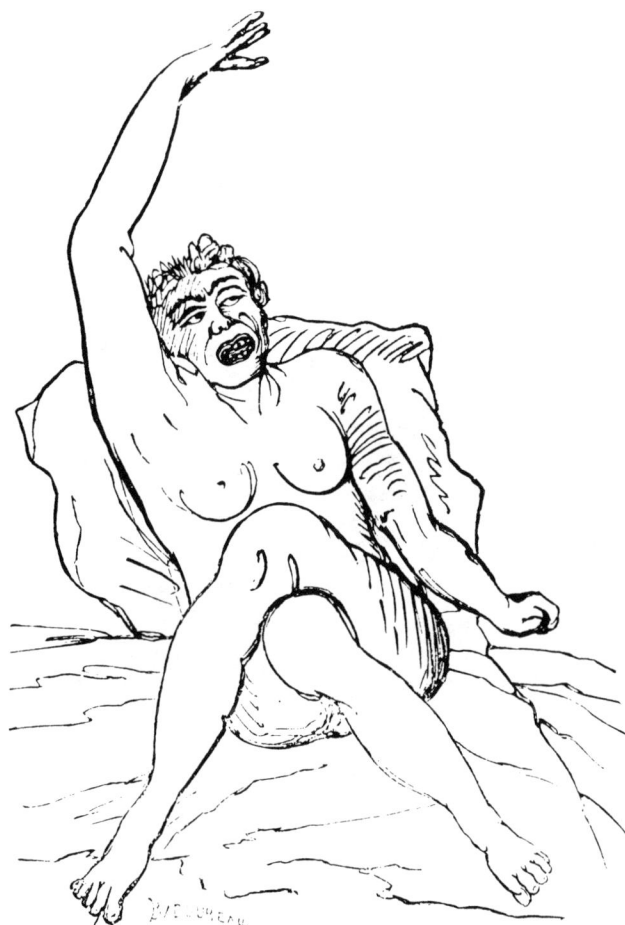

FIGURE 32.3

A drawing of one of Charcot's more famous hysterical seizure patients, Ler, during an attack. (Reproduced with permission from: Lectures on the diseases of the nervous system by JM Charcot [translated by G Sigerson] 1879;279.)

taken for epileptic seizures. In particular, some physiologic disorders that may imitate epilepsy include syncope, migraine, and transient ischemic attacks (TIAs). Such physiologic disorders may also have a psychologic component when symptoms are exaggerated or embellished by anxious or emotional patients who may be misinterpreting their symptoms. Still, nonepileptic physiologic events are responsible for only a small proportion of patients with nonepileptic seizures.

Psychogenic Seizures

The majority of patients with nonepileptic seizures have psychogenic seizures (Table 32.1). In general, any patient with a psychologic disorder that mimics epilepsy can be considered to have psychogenic seizures. In contemporary thought, the notion that all psychogenic seizures are a result of "hysteria" has been abandoned in favor of a

---

TABLE 32.1
Classification of Nonepileptic Seizures

I. Physiologic nonepileptic seizures (e.g., syncope, complicated migraine, night terror, breath-holding spells)

II. Psychogenic seizures
- Somatoform disorder
- Dissociative disorder
- Factitious disorder (e.g., Munchausen's syndrome)
- Malingering

---

growing appreciation for the heterogeneity and diversity of these patients (12).

Rather than treating psychogenic seizure patients uniformly as one group, it is useful to classify psychogenic seizure patients into four major categories (Table 32.1): (i) somatoform disorders, (ii) dissociation disorders, (iii) factitious disorders and, (iv) malingering (1,11). These subgroups are not mutually exclusive, and the causes of psychogenic seizures may be multifactorial (1,12,14).

Somatoform Disorders

The principal somatoform disorders that apply to individuals with psychogenic seizures are somatization disorders, conversion disorders, and undifferentiated somatoform disorders, as classified by the *Diagnostic and Statistical Manual of Mental Disorders* (15). The essential feature for a diagnosis of somatization disorder is a history of recurrent and multiple somatic complaints of long duration and early onset. In contrast, conversion disorder implies a more restricted range of somatic complaints, the expression of which is based on unconscious psychodynamic processes and is classically symbolic of a repressed psychologic conflict or need. Other categories of somatoform disorders include patients who do not meet these specific criteria.

Some patients with dramatic and disabling proven somatoform disorders such as nonepileptic seizures fail to demonstrate other major psychopathology on evaluation and testing and instead have relatively mild stress and coping disorders causing these severe symptoms. This may cause confusion and raises doubts about the diagnosis of nonepileptic seizures, but it does occur. In this group of nonepileptic psychogenic seizure patients, the balance between the stresses in their lives and their capacity to cope with them is disturbed (1). They may have predisposing vulnerabilities that lower their threshold for coping with stress and anxiety (e.g., mental retardation, learning disability, or cognitive changes associated with head injury), or their lives may have been burdened by

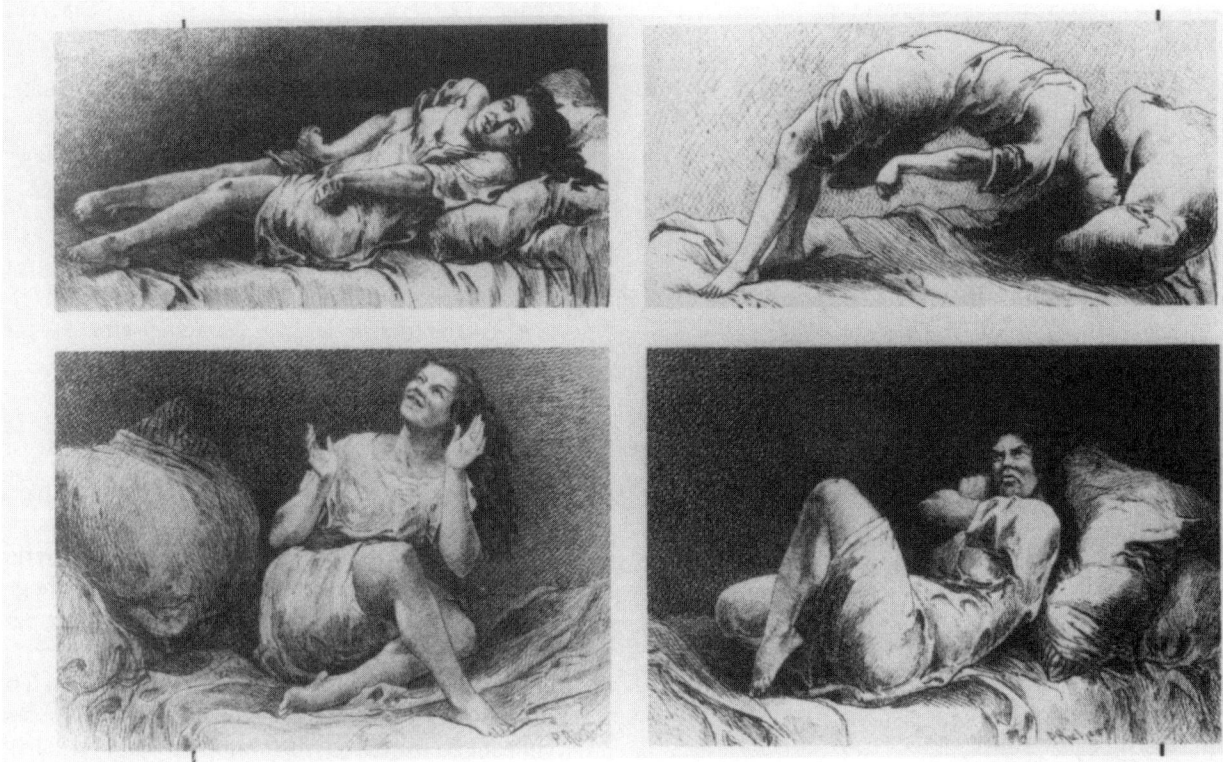

FIGURE 32.4

Drawing of the typical phases of a "hysteroepileptic" attack as defined by Charcot. The phases included from top left and clockwise: A. Epileptoid phase (predominantly tonic spasms), B. Acrobatic phase (exotic postures such as arching [arc en cercle] or rhythmic body rocking), C. (bottom left and right) Delirium with emotionally expressive postures such as happiness, ecstasy, or fright. (Reproduced with permission from: Études Cliniques sur la Grande Hystérie ou l' Hysteroépilepsie. P Richer, 1885.)

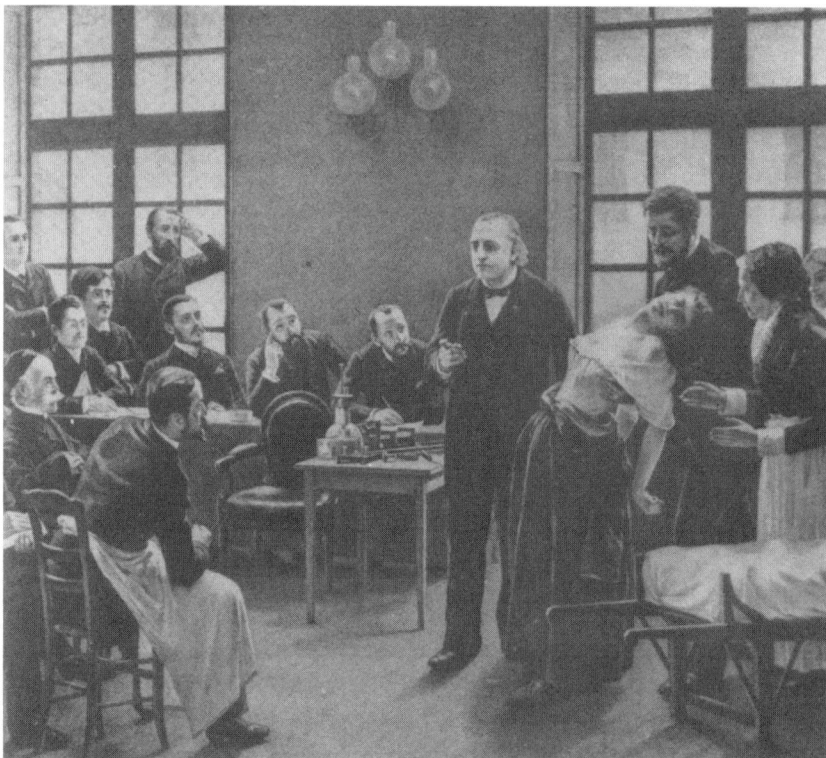

FIGURE 32.5

Lithograph of the Brouillet painting: A Clinical Lesson at the Salpêtrière (1887). This shows Charcot using suggestion to induce hysterical collapse in a woman. This is the type of presentation that Freud undoubtedly observed.

extraordinary stresses (e.g., post-traumatic stress disorder, multiple losses, or true epilepsy) (1,14). Apart from their psychogenic seizures, such patients do not have major or severe, definable psychopathology (1). Their psychogenic events are not volitional, but are usually temporally related to certain stressful life events (1).

Dissociative Disorders

In some patient with nonepileptic psychogenic seizures, the symptoms may be better related to dissociative mechanisms than to conversion (1,16). The essential feature of the dissociative disorders is a disruption of consciousness, memory, identity, or perception of the environment. These disruptions vary in nature and may be sudden or gradual, transient, or more chronic (15). Although psychogenic nonepileptic seizures have been traditionally considered conversion disorders, they have been more recently proposed to be related to psychodynamic mechanisms associated with dissociation and to have a high association with childhood sexual and physical abuse (1,16). The degree of demonstrable psychopathology may vary considerably, as it does in somatoform disorders, and underlying or causal psychopathology can be difficult to find (1,16).

Factitious Disorders and Malingering

The shared feature of these two groups of psychogenic seizure patients is the conscious fabrication of seizure-like symptoms. An important difference between factitious disorders and malingering patients is the purpose of the intentionally produced or simulated seizure symptoms. The goal of the psychogenic seizure patient with a factitious disorder (e.g., Munchausen's syndrome) is to maintain the role of a patient. Hence, they fake symptoms, exaggerate existing physical symptoms, or self-induce their symptoms through, for example, drug ingestion. In contrast, the intent of the malingerer is to obtain a recognizable external benefit (e.g., financial gain or release from prison) (15).

EPIDEMIOLOGY

Nonepileptic seizures and psychogenic seizures occur with greater frequency in women. The exact incidence varies, but women generally account for about 70 to 80% of all individuals with nonepileptic seizures (1–3). The reason for this is not clear. Most patients with nonepileptic seizures have psychogenic seizures, a type of somatoform disorder or conversion symptom, and a female preponderance is well noted for conversion reactions (10–13,16).

Sociologic and cultural factors influence the occurrence and nature of somatoform disorders such as conversion reactions. Patients with somatoform disorders are highly suggestible; they tend to meet the expectations for their illness (9–12). Changes in society and in the perception of various illnesses have influenced the manifestations of hysteria (9–12).

Economic and social restraints on women in society may be one factor that account for the high incidence of conversion in women. Western social structure traditionally has expected the female role to be more passive and accommodating. Limiting the potential to express anger, violence, competitiveness, or sexuality may lead to conversion of such repressed energies into physical symptoms or conversion reactions (9–12,16).

The male dominated nature and sexist attitudes of society have been blamed for the higher incidence of hysteria in women and the disparaging manner in which hysteria has been viewed by the medical profession. As women assume a more active and assertive role in society, they are also becoming more economically, socially, and sexually independent. In contrast, some men are feeling more threatened and dependent in their roles. Some experts believe that this accounts for the rising incidence of hysterical types of disorders in men and a change in the characteristics of conversion reaction in general (9–12).

Nonepileptic seizures occur in all age groups from childhood (17,18) to the elderly, but most patients present between the ages of 15 to 35 years (1,4). Very young children and infants are more likely to have physiologic nonepileptic events that may be mistaken for seizures rather than psychogenic seizures. These types of events include gastroesophageal reflux, night terrors, breath-holding spells, and pallid infantile syncope (1,17,18). The annual incidence of nonepileptic seizures is reported in one population-based study to be about 4% that of the incidence of true epileptic seizures (4).

PROVOKING FACTORS

Environmental factors may contribute to the risk for developing nonepileptic seizures, particularly psychogenic seizures. Sexual abuse is one such important factor. Historically, this issue is important because hysteria since Freud's early observations has been related to repressed sexual drives and associated with sexual abuse in women (5,6). Recent studies emphasize that a history of sexual or physical abuse may be quite common in patients with psychogenic seizures. One such series reports a history of sexual abuse in almost 25% of patients with nonepileptic seizures; and history of either sexual abuse, physical abuse, or both in 32% of patients (19). Unfortunately, sexual and physical abuse are relatively common problems in our society, so such a history does not exclude the possibility of true epilepsy. In fact, in this series, a control population of patients with epileptic seizures reported an almost 9% rate of sexual or physical abuse (19). Thus, this issue should be explored and integrated into treatment as necessary.

Head trauma has recently been recognized as another provoking factor for nonepileptic seizures. For example, one recent study reported that approximately 20% of psychogenic seizure patients attributed their seizures to head trauma, often rather mild head trauma (20). It may be that various types of environmental trauma or stress are potential provoking factors for conversion reactions like psychogenic seizures in susceptible individuals (1).

DIAGNOSIS

Clinical observation has long been the basis for distinguishing nonepileptic from epileptic seizures. In recent years, clinical observation has been greatly aided by the use of video-EEG monitoring, serum prolactin levels, and neuropsychologic assessments.

A complicating factor in diagnosis is that both nonepileptic and epileptic seizures may occur in a given patient. Indeed, approximately 10 to 40% of patients identified to have nonepileptic or psychogenic seizures also have been reported to have true epileptic seizures (1–3). There are several possible explanations for this. Some patients with epilepsy may learn that seizures result in attention and fill certain psychologic needs. Alternatively, they may have concomitant neurologic problems, personality disorders, cognitive deficits, or impaired coping mechanisms that predispose them to psychogenic symptoms. Fortunately, in such patients with combined seizure disorders, the epileptic seizures are usually well controlled or of only historical relevance at the time a patient develops psychogenic seizures (1,2).

Clinical Observations

No pathognomonic clinical signs allow one to distinguish nonepileptic or psychogenic seizures from epileptic seizures. Nonepileptic seizures are varied and may present with generalized convulsive manifestations, signs of altered consciousness or loss of consciousness, and focal motor or sensory symptoms (21–23).

Some clinical observations can be useful (Table 32.2). In particular, psychogenic seizures often last considerably longer than epileptic seizures, which typically persist for less than 3 minutes, excluding the postictal state. The nature of the convulsive activity in patients with psychogenic seizures differs from that seen in generalized convulsive epilepsy. With psychogenic seizures, the movements are more often purposeful or semipurposeful, asymmetric, or asynchronous, such as thrashing or writhing motions, rather than the tonic-clonic activity of epileptic seizures (21–23). It is more difficult to distinguish the movements of psychogenic seizures from the automatisms of complex partial epileptic seizures, however, particularly frontal lobe seizures (1,22).

Other clinical differences are present between psychogenic and epileptic seizures. For example, conscious-

TABLE 32.2		
Clinical Characteristics of Epileptic versus Nonepileptic Seizures		
	Epileptic	**Nonepileptic**
Age at onset	All ages: children and adolescents more common	All ages: 15 to 35 most common
Sex	Male and female about equal	Female more common: 3 to 1 ratio
Psychologic history	Occasionally present	Commonly noted
Motor	In generalized convulsions: bilateral movements are usually synchronous	Flailing, thrashing, and asynchronous movements more common, side-to-side head movements, pelvic thrusting
Vocalization	Vocaliziation or cry at onset	Weeping, or screaming; screaming more common
Incontinence	Frequent	Occasional
Duration of seizure	Usually less than 2 to 3 minutes	Often prolonged, more than 2 to 3 minutes
Injury	Frequent tongue biting	Uncommon
Amnesia	Common, unconscious during seizure	Variable, sometimes conscious during seizure
Suggestion provokes seizure	No	Often

ness and responsiveness may be surprisingly retained during psychogenic seizures. Crying and weeping are more common for psychogenic seizures (24). Although incontinence and self-injury are frequently reported by patients with nonepileptic seizures (25), they are rarely actually witnessed (23). Additionally, unlike epileptic seizures, psychogenic seizures characteristically do not respond well to antiepileptic drug treatment (1,2,20,23).

Psychogenic seizures also are more likely to be provoked by emotional stimuli and suggestion (26). In fact, provocative procedures may be useful for reproducing events during EEG recording. Provoking or suggesting seizures can be done in several ways, such as injecting saline or placing a tuning fork on the body or head (26–29). Hypnosis has also been used (30). These are all accompanied by a strong suggestion by the physician that this procedure is likely to bring on a typical seizure (1,26–29). EEG recording and sometimes video recording is undertaken simultaneously to enable the confirmation of the nonepileptic nature of the induced event.

Provoking psychogenic seizures raises some ethical controversies, however. Misleading a patient when provoking a seizure can be harmful to the patient–physician relationship and should be avoided. Nonetheless, provocative testing can be done with honesty, and benefits the patient (31).

Video-EEG Monitoring

A diagnosis of nonepileptic or psychogenic seizures is most secure during simultaneous video-EEG monitoring and demonstrates no evidence of epileptic activity. Patients with generalized convulsive epileptic seizures invariably demonstrate significant EEG changes during ictal EEG recordings. Individuals with complex partial seizures, who may have small or deep seizure foci, still show significant ictal EEG abnormalities in perhaps 85 to 95% of such seizures. Even patients with simple partial seizures—seizures that do not impair consciousness—have EEG abnormalities noted in about 60% of those seizures and, if one records multiple seizures, nearly 80% will demonstrate some EEG abnormality (32). The ictal EEG record-

ing is particularly important because interictal or routine EEGs occasionally may be misleading. For example, between seizures, some patients with epilepsy may have normal EEGs, and some patients with psychogenic seizures may have minor EEG abnormalities (Table 32.3) (1,2,23).

A clinical seizure may be captured in several ways during EEG monitoring. Outpatient monitoring is particularly useful for patients who have daily events or seizures that can be provoked by suggestion. Patients with less frequent events may require extended inpatient video-EEG monitoring. Simultaneous video-EEG recording offers the advantage of permitting the careful observation and review of the clinical manifestations of seizures. This can be especially useful when assessing patients with psychogenic seizures because video-EEG recordings are particularly helpful in distinguishing epileptic discharges from movement and muscle artifact.

Epileptic seizures commonly arise during sleep. Patients with psychogenic seizures, however, are usually awake at the time a seizure starts. This can be difficult to evaluate by history or behavior, because patients with psychogenic seizures may report seizures arising from sleep, or may appear to be sleeping when seizures begin. Video-EEG monitoring can be useful in showing that the patient with psychogenic seizures is not actually asleep when an event begins (33,34).

Prolactin Levels

The serum prolactin level is useful in patients with suspected psychogenic seizures (35,36). Prolactin levels rise approximately five- to tenfold after tonic-clonic seizures, and somewhat less so but still significantly (typically at least two- to threefold) after complex partial seizures (37). This increase in serum prolactin is maximum in the initial 20 minutes to 1 hour after a seizure (35–37). Although measurements of serum prolactin may be useful in distinguishing nonepileptic from epileptic seizures, some false positives and false negatives occur (1,37,38). In particular, simple partial seizures or mild complex partial seizures, particularly those with little motor activity, may not significantly raise prolactin levels. Serum

---

TABLE 32.3
EEG Characteristics of Epileptic versus Nonepileptic Seizures

	Epileptic	Nonepileptic
Interictal EEG	Spikes and sharp waves common	Normal or nonspecific abnormalities, such as mild slow activity
Pre-ictal EEG	Spikes, sharp waves	Movement artifact or rhythmic ictal activity
Ictal EEG	Spikes, sharp waves	Movement artifact or rhythmic ictal activity
Post-ictal EEG	Slow activity	Normal EEG, preserved alpha

prolactin elevations have also been reported after syncope (39).

Neuropsychologic Testing

Another important consideration in evaluating patients with suspected psychogenic seizures is their psychological status. Such an assessment requires a referral to mental health professionals who are experienced in psychologic and psychiatric assessment, psychometric assessment, and psychotherapeutic intervention in patients with neurologic disorders (1).

Mental health professionals should not be expected to determine whether an individual is having psychogenic rather than epileptic seizures, however, because these professionals generally lack the necessary neurologic training or experience. Moreover, neuropsychologic testing cannot in itself either diagnose or exclude the possibility that a seizure disorder is nonepileptic because of the considerable overlap between epileptic and nonepileptic test results (1,40,41). The distinction between psychogenic and epileptic seizures is best made by a neurologist, particularly one who has expertise in epilepsy, and should be based on a consideration of both clinical data and neuropsychologic assessments. Neuropsychologic evaluations aid this assessment by (i) determining the potential or likelihood of significant contributing psychopathology or cognitive difficulties, (ii) defining the nature of the associated psychological or psychosocial issues, and (iii) assessing how a patient might benefit from various psychologically based interventions (1,42).

TREATMENT

A correct diagnosis is essential for patients with nonepileptic seizures because early diagnosis is associated with better outcome (43). Yet, even after a diagnosis of nonepileptic seizures is established, physicians should follow up with such patients. Many psychogenic seizure patients benefit from education and support that can readily be provided by the neurologist or primary care physician (Table 32.4) (1,44,45). If the neuropsychologic assessment suggests a clinical profile that requires a professional mental health intervention, then an appropriate referral should be made.

The management of patients with psychogenic seizures is similar to that of patients with other types of so-called "abnormal illness behavior" (Table 32.4). The first consideration should be the manner in which the diagnosis of psychogenic seizures is presented to the patient and family. It is important to be honest with the patient and demonstrate a positive approach to the diagnosis (45). The physician should emphasize as favorable

---

TABLE 32.4
Management of Nonepileptic Seizure Patients

- Present the diagnosis of nonepileptic seizures positively, emphasizing the potential for better seizure control.
- After patients are referred to mental health professionals, the diagnosing neurologist should provide some follow-up and support.
- Regular follow-up visits should be scheduled that are not contingent on persistent, new, or worsening symptoms.
- Give patients attention when they do well.
- Avoid prescribing unnecessary medications, unwarranted tests, and excessive referrals to specialists.
- Permit the continuation of some symptoms. A patient's optimal well-being and function, rather than eradication of seizures, is the goal.

---

or good news the fact that the patient does not have epilepsy, and should also stress that the disorder, although serious and "real," does not require treatment with antiepileptic medications and that once stress or emotional issues are resolved, the patient has the potential to gain better control of these events (1).

Nevertheless, not all patients readily accept the diagnosis or this type of approach. Some patients may seek other opinions, and this should not be discouraged. An adversarial relationship with the patient should be avoided. The patient should be encouraged to return if desired, and records should be made available to avoid a duplication of services.

After the diagnosis of psychogenic seizures is presented, supportive measures should be initiated. Regular follow-up visits for the patient are useful, even if a mental health professional is involved. This allows the patient to get medical attention without demonstrating illness behavior. It also offers support to the involved mental health professional. Patient education and support are stressed at these visits. Because family issues are often important contributing factors, physicians should consider involving family members (1).

PROGNOSIS

The outcomes of patients with psychogenic seizures vary. Long-term follow-up studies show that about half of all patients with psychogenic seizures function reasonably well following their diagnosis. Only approximately one-third of patients will completely stop having psychogenic seizures or related problems, however, and approximately 50% percent have poor functional outcomes (1,2). When the diagnosis of psychogenic seizures is based on reliable criteria such a video-EEG monitoring, misdiagnosis is unlikely. Instead, the usual cause for a poor outcome is related to a patient's chronic psychologic and social problems (1,2,42,46).

It is noteworthy that children with psychogenic seizures appear to have a much better prognosis than adults (17,18). In fact, children may have psychogenic seizures related to transient stress and coping disorders, whereas adults are more likely to have psychogenic seizures within the context of more chronic psychologic maladjustment, such as personality disorders (17,18). Another factor that accounts for the better outcomes in children is that they are usually properly diagnosed earlier (17,18).

Patients with milder psychopathology respond better to supportive educational or behavioral therapeutic approaches (Table 32.4) (1). In contrast, patients with more severe psychopathology and factitious disorders more often have associated chronic personality problems and correspondingly, a poorer prognosis (1,42).

As knowledge about the nature of psychogenic seizures and their associated psychopathology is gained, better treatment strategies can be developed that will improve the care and prognosis of these difficult and challenging patients.

References

1. Krumholz A. Nonepileptic seizures: diagnosis and management. *Neurology* 1999;S76-83.
2. Krumholz A, Niedermeyer E. Psychogenic seizures: a clinical study with follow-up data. *Neurology* 1983;33: 498–502.
3. Meierkord H, Will B, Fish D, Shorvon S. The clinical features and prognosis of pseudoseizures diagnosed using video-EEG telemetry. *Neurology* 1991;41:1643–1646.
4. Sigurdardottir KR, Olafsson E. Incidence of psychogenic seizures in adults: a population-based study in Iceland. *Epilepsia* 1998;39:857–862.
5. Slavney PR. *Perspectives on hysteria.* Baltimore: Johns Hopkins University Press, 1990.
6. Veith I. *Hysteria: the history of a disease.* Chicago: University of Chicago Press, 1965.
7. Goetz CG. *Charcot the clinician. The Tuesday lessons.* New York: Raven Press, 1987.
8. Massey EW, McHenry LC. Hysteroepilepsy in the nineteenth century: Charcot and Gowers. *Neurology* 1986;36:65–67.
9. Lazare A. Current concepts in psychiatry: conversion symptoms. *N Engl J Med* 1981;305:745–748.
10. Stepfanis C. Markidis M, Christodoulou G. Observations on the evolution of hysterical symptomatology. *Brit J Psychiat* 1976;128:269–275.
11. Zeigler FJ, Imboden JB, Meyer E. Contemporary conversion reactions: a clinical study. *Am J Psychiatry* 1960; 116:901–910.
12. Pilowsky I. From conversion hysteria to somatization to abnormal illness behavior? *J of Psychosomatic Res* 1996; 40:345–350.
13. Liske E, Forster FM. Pseudoseizures: a problem in the diagnosis and management of epileptic patients. *Neurology* 1964;14:41–49.
14. Vanderzant CW, Giordani B, Berent S, Dreifuss FE, Sackellares JC. Personality of patients with pseudoseizures. *Neurology* 1986;36:664–668.
15. *Diagnostic and Statistical Manual of Mental Disorders. DSM-IV™ Fourth Edition.* Washington DC: American Psychiatric Association, 1995.
16. Bowman ES. Etiology and clinical course of pseudoseizures: relationship to trauma, depression, and dissociation. *Psychosomatics* 1993;34:333–342.
17. Metrick ME, Ritter FJ, Gates JR, Jacobs MP, Skare SS, Loewenson RB. Nonepileptic events in childhood. *Epilepsia* 1991;32:322–328.
18. Wyllie E, Friedman D, Luders H, Morris H, Rothner D, Turnbull J. Outcome of psychogenic seizures in children and adolescents compared to adults. *Neurology* 1991;41: 742–744.
19. Alper K, Devinsky O, Perrine K, Vazquez B, Luciano D. Nonepileptic seizures and childhood sexual and physical abuse. *Neurology* 1993;43:1950–1953.
20. Barry E, Krumholz A, Bergey C, Alemayehu S, Grattan L. Nonepileptic posttraumatic seizures. *Epilepsia* 1998; 39:427–431.
21. Gates JR, Ramani V, Whalen S, Loewenson R. Ictal characteristics of pseudoseizures. *Arch Neurol* 1985;42: 1183–1187.
22. Leis AA, Ross MA, Summers AK. Psychogenic seizures: ictal characteristics and diagnostic pitfalls. *Neurology* 1992;42:95–99.
23. Gulick TA, Spinks IP, King DW. Pseudoseizures: ictal phenomena. *Neurology* 1982;32:24–30.
24. Walczak TS, Bogolioubov. Weeping during psychogenic nonepileptic seizures. *Epilepsia* 1996;37:207–210.
25. Peguero E, Abou-Khalil B, Fakhoury, Mathews G. Self-injury and incontinence in psychogenic seizures. *Epilepsia* 1995;36:586–591.
26. Cohen RJ and Suter C. Hysterical seizures: suggestion as a provocative EEG test. *Ann Neurol* 1982;11: 391–395.
27. Walczak TS, Williams DT, Berton W. Utility and reliability of placebo infusion in the evaluation of patients with seizures. *Neurology* 1994;44:394–399.
28. Slater JD, Marland CB, Jacobs W, Ramsey RE. Induction of pseudoseizures with intravenous saline placebo. *Epilepsia* 1995;36:580–585.
29. Bazil CW, Kothari M, Luciano D, et al. Provocation of nonepileptic seizures by suggestion in a general seizure population. *Epilepsia* 1994;35:768–770.
30. Barry JJ, Atzman O, Morrell MJ. Discriminating between epileptic and nonepileptic events: the utility of hypnotic seizures induction. *Epilepsia* 2000;41:81–84.
31. Devinsky O, Fisher RS. Ethical use of placebos and provocative testing in diagnosing nonepileptic seizures. *Neurology* 1996;47:866–870.
32. Barre MA, Burnstine TH, Fisher RS, Lesser RP. Electroencephalographic changes during simple partial seizures. *Epilepsia* 1999;35:715–720.
33. Thacker K, Devinsky O, Perrine K, Alper K, Luciano D. Nonepileptic seizures during apparent sleep. *Ann Neurol* 1993;33:414–418.
34. Orbach D, Ritaccio A, Devinsky O. Psychogenic, nonepileptic seizures associated with video-EEG-verified sleep. *Epilepsia* 2003;44:64–68.

35. Trimble MR. Serum prolactin levels in epilepsy and hysteria. *BMJ* 1978;2:1682.

36. Laxer KD, Mullooly JP, Howell B. Prolactin changes after seizures classified by EEG monitoring. *Neurology* 1985;35:31–35.

37. Pritchard PB, Wannamaker BB, Sagel J, Nair R, DeVillier C. Endocrine function following complex partial seizures. *Ann Neurol* 1983;14:27–32.

38. Tomson T, Lindbom U, Nilsson BY, Svanborg E, Andersson DE. Serum Prolactin during status epilepticus. *J Neurol Neurosurgery Psychiatry* 1989;52:1435–1437.

39. Oribe E, Rohullah A, Nissenbaum E, Boal B. Serum prolactin concentrations are elevated after syncope. *Neurology* 1996;47:60–62.

40. Henrichs TF, Tucker DM, Farha J, Novelly RA. MMPI indices in the identification of patients evidencing pseudoseizures. *Epilepsia* 1988;29:184–188.

41. Wilkus RJ, Dodrill CB. Factors affecting the outcome of MMPI and neuropsychological assessments of psychogenic and epileptic seizure patients. *Epilepsia* 1989;30:339–347.

42. Rueber M, Pukrop T, Bauer J, Helmstaedter C, Tessendorf N, Elger CE. Outcome in psychogenic nonepileptic seizures: 1 to 10-year follow-up in 164 patients. *Ann Neurol* 2003;53:305–311.

43. Lempert L, Schmidt D. Natural history and outcome of psychogenic seizures: a clinical study in 50 patients. *J Neurol* 1990;237:35–38.

44. Aboukasm A, Mahr G, Gahry BR, Thomas A, Barkley GL. Retrospective analysis of the effects of psychotherapeutic interventions on outcomes of psychogenic nonepileptic seizures. *Epilepsia* 1998;39:470–473.

45. Shen W, Bowman ES, Markand ON. Presenting the diagnosis of pseudoseizure. *Neurology* 1990;40:756–759.

46. Walzack TS, Papacostas S, Williams DT, Scheuer ML, Lebowitz N, Notarfrancesco A. Outcome after the diagnosis of psychogenic nonepileptic seizures. *Epilepsia* 1995;36:1131–1137.

Index

Note: Boldface numbers indicate illustrations; *t* indicates a table.